CARDIOVASCULAR CANCER

Collected Reprints
(1962-2019)

By

William C. Roberts, MD

and

Colleagues

ISBN: 979-8-88862-154-7
Printed in the United States of America on acid-free paper.

Table of Contents

*Articles are numbered based on WCR's CV.

A Functional Carotid-Body-Like Tumor

Secreting Levarterenol

G. G. GLENNER, M.D.

J. R. CROUT, M.D.

AND

W. C. ROBERTS, M.D.

BETHESDA, MD.

Since the initial suggestion of de Castro[1,2] that the carotid body served a chemoreceptor function, the work of Heymans[3] and of Schmidt and Comroe[4] has established the role of the carotid and aortic bodies in response to changes in pH and CO_2 and O_2 tension of the circulating blood. However, evidence has been presented that the carotid body may also subserve a secretory function.[5,6] Although tumors of the so-called "nonchromaffin" paraganglionic or chemoreceptor system have been described arising from the carotid body,[7-10] the glomus jugulare,[11-13] the aortic arch bodies,[10,14] the ganglion nodosum,[10,15,16] and tissues of the thigh and retroperitoneum,[17] to the best of our knowledge no functioning tumor having the morphologic and histochemical characteristics of a carotid-body-like tumor has been previously described. The purpose of the present paper is to report a tumor of this type that secreted levarterenol.

Report of a Case

The patient was a 12-year-old white male admitted to the National Heart Institute on Nov. ., 1959, because of a painless mass present for 2 years in the left side of the neck at the angle of the jaw. During this time the mass had slowly enlarged and had been associated with progressive drooping of the left eyelid, a generalized increase in sweating, but decreased perspiration on the left side of the face relative to the right. There had been frequent episodes of nasal congestion and sneezing during the past 2 years, especially during autumn, attributed to "hay fever." There was no past history of hypertension. Growth and development were normal. The family history revealed that a paternal great-grandfather had died following surgical removal of a mass in the neck, said to have been present for many years; death followed "an injury to the artery in the neck during the operation." There was no history of hypertension in the family. On physical examination

Submitted for publication July 14, 1961.

National Institutes of Health.

Chief, Section of Histochemistry, Laboratory of Experimental Pathology, National Institute of Arthritis and Metabolic Diseases (Dr. Glenner); Experimental Therapeutics Branch, National Heart Institute, present address: 3d Medical Division, Bellevue Medical Center, New York (Dr. Crout); Department of Pathology, National Institutes of Health, Clinical Center (Dr. Roberts).

Urinary Excretion of Pressor Amines and Their Metabolites in Case of Levarterenol-Producing Carotid-Body-Like Tumor

	Patient	Normal (Refs. 18, 23)
evarterenol	1030μg/24 hr	10-70μg/24 hr
pinephrine	Not detected	0-20μg/24 hr
ormetanephrine	5.5 mg/24 hr	0.2-1.3 mg/24 hr
methoxy-4-hydroxy-mandelic acid	19 mg/24 hr	2-6 mg/24 hr
hydroxyindole acetic acid (serotonin metabolite)	Not detected	2-11 mg/day
evarterenol (2-hour period *before* massage of neck)	25μg/hr	0.5-4μg/hr
evarterenol (2-hour period *after* massage of neck)	39μg/hr	0.5-4μg/hr

ie patient was a normally developed prepubertal 2-year-old boy appearing in good general health. he blood pressure in the sitting position was 8/92 in the right arm and 128/92 in the left m. A left-sided Horner's syndrome was noted. here was a 7×5×4 cm. firm, nontender mass low the angle of the jaw on the left; the left mmon carotid artery and its branches could be lt overlying the superficial aspect of the mass. o cervical adenopathy was detected. The re-ainder of the physical examination was within ormal limits. Laboratory studies revealed the moglobin to be 13.2 gm/ml, the hematocrit 43%, e white blood cell count 8,300 cells per cubic llimeter, and the urinalysis to be normal. The sting blood sugar was 96 mg/100 ml, the blood ea nitrogen 18 mg/100 ml, the total serum olesterol 191 mg/ml, and the alkaline phosphatase King-Armstrong units. A chest roentgen survey, ctrocardiogram, and intravenous pyelogram were within normal limits. A skeletal roentgen survey iled to reveal any abnormalities.

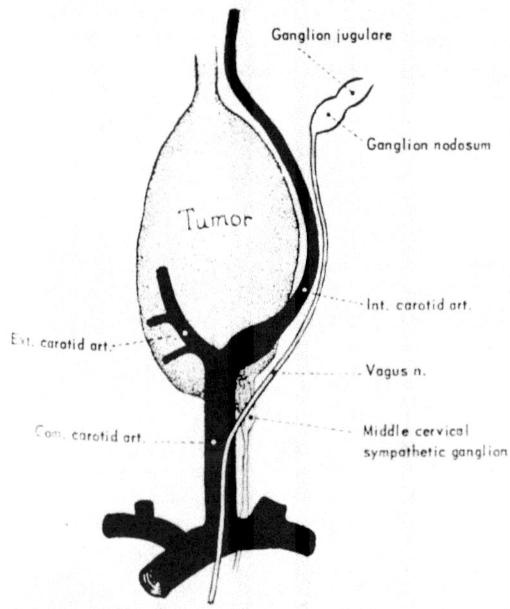

Fig. 1.—Relation of tumor to surrounding structures.

It had been noted prior to admission by the referring physician that massage of the tumor produced a rise in blood pressure from 94/64 to 132/100, which was accompanied by profuse sweating, moderate pallor, and a sense of anxiety. In the hospital the blood pressure varied spontaneously from 110/60 to 170/110; the pulse ranged from 78 to 116 beats per minute. The patient was consequently studied for the possible presence of a catecholamine-secreting tumor. Chemical analyses (Table) revealed the presence of increased amounts of levarterenol and its major metabolites in the urine.[18] Furthermore, massage of the tumor caused an increase in both the blood pressure and the urinary excretion of levarterenol. No evidence of increased serotonin production was found. On the basis of these findings a preoperative diagnosis of pheochromocytoma or ganglioneuroma[19] of the neck was made. On Dec. 1, 1959, the tumor was removed under general anesthesia—nitrous oxide, meperidine hydrochloride (Demerol), and succinylcholine chloride (Anectine) by Dr. Robert R. Smith of the National Cancer Institute. The fusiform tumor (Fig. 1) lay deep to the left carotid artery and displaced the common carotid and its branches laterally. The tumor completely surrounded the left sympathetic chain and at its lower pole received a number of small filaments from the sympathetic plexus. At the superior margin the tumor tapered off to a diameter of 3 to 4 mm. and extended as a firm white band over a distance of 3 cm., finally entering the foramen

Fig. 2.—Gross surgical specimen of levarterenol-secreting tumor.

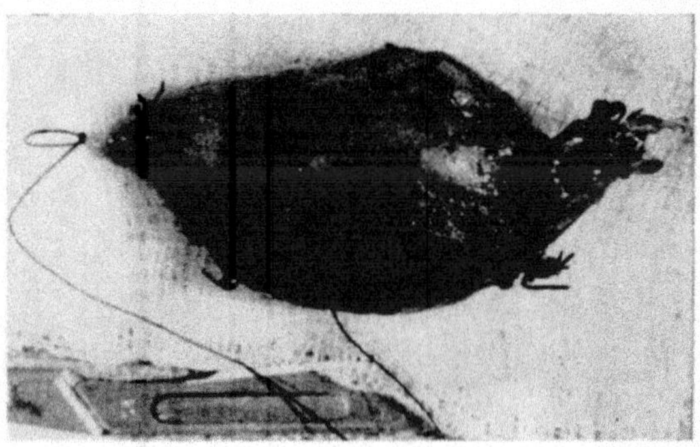

lacerum at the base of the skull. The tumor appeared to receive no blood supply from the carotids and was easily dissected from the carotid artery and its branches. The vagus nerve was well away from the mass and not involved in the tumor. The hypoglossal nerve was identified and was normal in position. During the operation the blood pressure ranged between 104/85 and 150/120; the heart rate increased midway during the procedure from 120 to 180 beats per minute and remained elevated in the region of 180-200 beats per minute for the remainder of the surgical procedure. Blood loss was minimal. Phentolamine hydrochloride (Regitine) was not administered. Immediately following removal of the tumor, the blood pressure fell to 60/40, and an infusion of levarterenol at a rate of 40μg/min was required to maintain the blood pressure at 90/60. As the patient was waking up, he suddenly developed a cardiac arrest. Resuscitative measures, including immediate cardiac massage, were unsuccessful, and the patient was pronounced dead.

Pathologic Study

Tumor

Gross.—The tumor (Fig. 2) was a well-circumscribed, relatively soft mass measuring 6×3.5×2 cm. The surface of the tumor was smooth and red-gray with 2 fibrous tags on the largest diameter which protruded about 0.3 cm. from the main portion of the mass. On section, this mass varied from red-purple to tan and was without cysts.

Microscopic.—The tumor was surrounded by a relatively thin fibrous capsule which was free of tumor cell infiltration except at the superior surgical margin. Here neoplastic cells infiltrated the thin fibrous capsule to within less than 1 mm. of its surface. The tumor was composed of alveolar cell groups separated by delicate connective tissue stroma. The cells were quite variable, and the majority were large, polygonal to pyriform, with abundant faintly eosinophilic cytoplasm and ill-defined cell borders. The nuclei were quite variable in size and shape with many bizarre forms and mitotic figures evident. Occasional binucleate and multinucleate varieties were present. The cell groups had a monotonous organoid arrangement (Fig. 3) and in areas appeared alveolar. The tumor was highly vascular, the cell groups being separated by delicate sinusoids and large, dilated, thin-walled vascular channels (Fig. 4). Reticulum stains revealed a fine stromal component separating nests of cells in a manner typical of the normal carotid body (*Zellballen* arrangement) (Fig. 5). Marginated within the cell nests proper around each group of the pyriform, pale eosinophilic cells, and occasionally within their midst, were fusiform to ovoid, finely granular cells with large centrally located nuclei and pale eosinophilic cytoplasm. With the Masson silver nitrate and Gomori methenamine silver nitrate methods on formalin-fixed tissue, these cells gave an argentaffin reducing reaction [10] in the numerous granules (Fig. 6). The aforementioned reactions frequently revealed these cells to have elongated cytoplasmic processes (Fig. 7). The granules of these cells were also stained by the ferric ferricyanide reaction (20) (Fig. 8). With the Giemsa stain the argentaffin cells were identified by their light-green-staining granules. An alkaline azo coupling reaction with the stabilized diazonium salt of *o*-aminoazotoluene (Fast Garnet GBC*) [20] revealed prominent reactivity by the presence of an orange-yellow to brown-yellow color. The chromaffin reaction in the argentaffin-positive cells, using Orth fixed tissue, was weak but definitely positive (Fig. 9). Oil red O and Sudan black B stains [21] on lipids in the argentaffin cells. The paraffin sections revealed the absence of

* Obtained through the courtesy of Verona Dyestuffs Corp., Union, N.J.

Fig. 3.—Hematoxylin and eosin stained section of tumor. × 30.

Fig. 4.—Relationship of tumor cells to capillaries. × 995.

Fig. 5.—Wilder's reticulum stain showing fine stromal component surrounding organoid groups of cells. × 155.

Fig. 6.—Argentaffin cells localized predominantly to periphery of cell nests of tumor. Masson silver nitrate reaction; × 205.

Fig. 7.—Argentaffin cells in tumor showing elongated cell processes. Masson silver nitrate reaction; × 735.

Fig. 8.—Ferric ferricyanide reduction reaction in argentaffin cells of tumor. × 315.

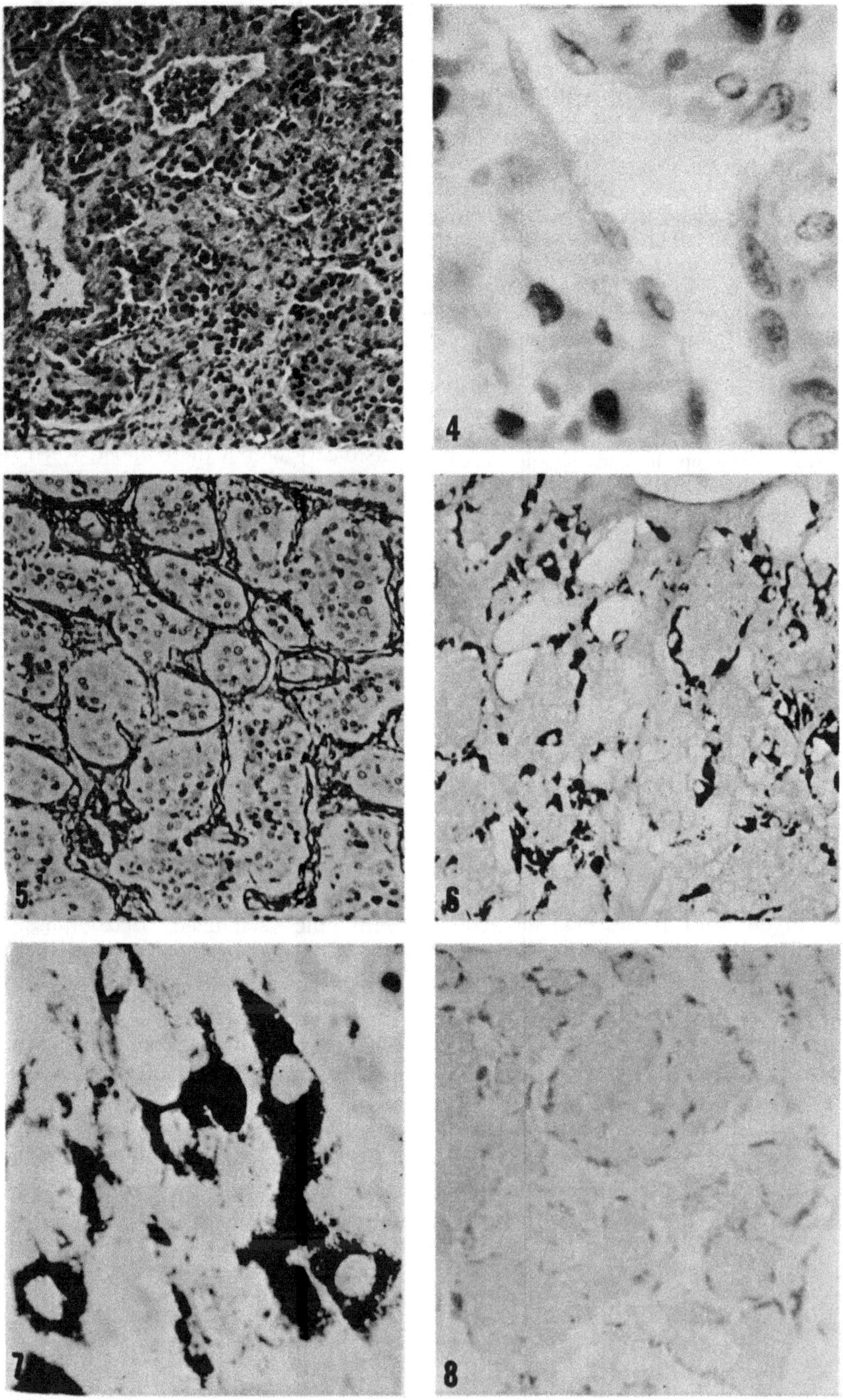

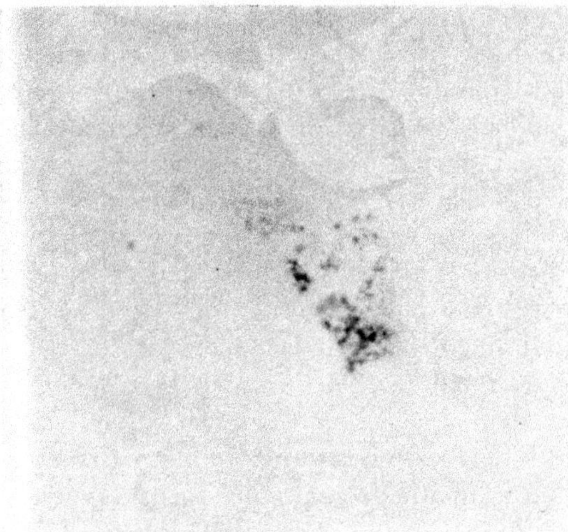

Fig. 9.—Chromaffin reaction in tumor in argentaffin cell. Orth's fixation; × 1,150.

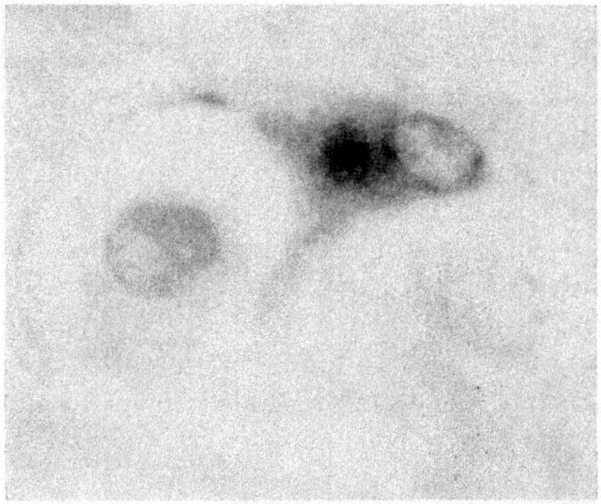

Fig. 10. Ferric ferricyanide reaction in normal carotid-body argentaffin cell. Note cytoplasmic processes extending between 2 nonargentaffin cells. Reduced 11% from mag. × 505.

ninhydrin [22] reaction for tryptamine derivatives and Clara's dilute hematoxylin [20] stain were also negative. Perls's iron reaction [21] revealed hemosiderin deposits focally in the stroma but not in the argentaffin cells.

Ancillary Studies.—Formalin-fixed, gelatin embedded models of crystalline levarterenol gave histochemical reactions identical to those of the argentaffin cell granules.

Eight carotid bodies were removed at necropsy, fixed immediately in formalin, and after routine processing were examined by the Masson silver nitrate reduction reaction, the ferric ferricyanide reaction, the azo coupling reaction, and the ninhydrin reaction. Argentaffin cells identical in appearance to those in the tumor were noted in one carotid body and were located predominantly at the periphery of the cell nests (Fig. 10). These cells also gave positive ferric ferricyanide and azo coupling reactions, but were unreactive to ninhydrin.

Through the courtesy of Dr. A. J. French, Department of Pathology, University of Michigan, 2 typical carotid body tumors No. 7192 AZ and No. 1093 BA were obtained and studied histochemically. In both cases typical argentaffin cells arranged at the periphery of the cell nests were demonstrated throughout the tumors.

Significant Autopsy Findings

Gross.—The heart weighed 220 gm., and the left ventricle was 1.4 cm. thick. Hemorrhage in the epicardium, myocardium, and on the endocardial surface of the right ventricle, hemorrhage into the pleura and parenchyma of the left lung and pulmonary atelectasis were noted and were thought to be sequelae of the cardiac massage. No attempt was made by the prosector to identify the carotid bodies or all cervical ganglia.

Microscopic.—There was present moderate hypertrophy of the myofibrils of the left ventricle with irregular intimal thickening and medial hypertrophy of the coronary arteries, most prominent at the ostia of the vessels. Examination of the vascular system and viscera, in particular the kidneys, adrenal glands, and brain, revealed no abnormalities. Small nests of neoplastic cells identical to those found in the surgically removed tumor mass were noted in the tissue surrounding the internal carotid artery where it entered the temporal bone. Tumor tissue was not identified elsewhere in the body.

Chemical and Chromatographic Analysis of Tumor.—A portion of the tumor was frozen immediately upon removal, and 1.5 gm. of a central section of this piece was later ground in 5 ml. of 5% trichloracetic acid. The clear supernatant from this mixture was assayed fluorimetrically for catecholamines and chromatographed on paper for catecholamines and phenols.[23] The tumor was found to contain 1.5 mg per gram of levarterenol but no detectable epinephrine. The chromatographic studies confirmed the presence of levarterenol and the absence of other catecholamines, including epinephrine and dopamine. In addition, a small normetanephrine spot was detected, but no other phenolic compounds were found.

Comment

Clinical findings of hypertension coupled with an increased excretion of levarterenol and its metabolites in the urine demonstrate that the patient was being subjected to a levarterenol effusion. The high levarterenol content of the tumor, the increased blood pressure with massage of the tumor, and the rapid drop in blood pressure following final ligation of the tumor implicate the tumor as the site of this levarterenol production. The objectives of the pathologic and histochemical study were to determine (1) the site or tissue of origin of the tumor and (2) the cellular site of levarterenol production in the tumor.

Morphology and Anatomic Location.—The histologic pattern in this tumor of a delicate highly vascularized reticular stroma surrounding well-circumscribed cell groups (cf. Ref. 17, Figs. 10 and 11) and having unique peripheral, ovoid to fusiform, argentaffin cells with centrally located nuclei and branching pseudodenditric cytoplasmic processes is characteristic of carotid-body-like tumors.[6,24] This tumor, therefore, appears to be morphologically and/or histochemically distinct from the reported neuroblastoma and ganglioneuroma catecholamine-secreting tumors[19] and from functional tumors of the adrenal medulla.[25] However, this statement in no way rules out the possibility that a levarterenol-secreting adrenal medullary tumor may be found which will have similar histologic and histochemical characteristics. We have to the present been unable to find such a case in the literature or in the functional adrenal tumors we have examined. Functional levarterenol-secreting tumors purported to have arisen from the organs of Zuckerkandl and reported to be of nonchromaffin nature have been described.[26,27] The argentaffin cells of the present tumor are morphologically distinct from the argentaffin cells of the intestine and carcinoid tumors. The latter cells have no cytoplasmic processes but are pyramidal to globular with basally situated nuclei.

The location of this tumor, surrounding the sympathetic chain and easily removed by blunt dissection from the carotid fork, militates somewhat against but does not completely exclude origin of the tumor from the carotid body. A tumor in many respects similar in location and histologic appearance to the one herein described was reported by Stout[15] as arising from the paraganglion of the ganglion nodosum of the vagus nerve. Argentaffin cells, demonstrated by the Fontana silver nitrate method, were also noted by him in the tumor. Lattes[10] has described 2 further cases of tumors believed to have arisen from the paraganglionic cells of the ganglion nodosum, one with an independent tumor of the carotid body on the opposite side of the neck and the other case with independent tumors at the carotid bifurcation and the arch of the aorta. A functioning tumor of the neck has been reported[28] in a child who had an adrenal pheochromocytoma removed 2½ years previously. The tumor in the neck was found to contain levarterenol but no significant amounts of epinephrine. Its anatomical location, surrounding the cervical sympathetic chain, was similar to that of the tumor we have described, but evidence as to its tissue of origin was not established.

Site of Norepinephrine Production.—At the time of the histochemical study of the present tumor, it was known that the tumor contained large quantities of levarterenol. Unfortunately, however, fresh tissue was no longer available at this time to perform the specific histochemical iodate and fluorescence tests for levarterenol.[29] On the basis of experiments with formalin-fixed models of levarterenol, it was found that this compound could be identified in tissues by its positive chromaffin, argentaffin, ferric ferricyanide, and azo coupling reactions. When applied to the tumor sections, all these reactions were given by the cells located predominantly at the periphery of the cell nests, cells to which we will henceforth refer, for the sake of identification only, as *carotid-body-type argentaffin cells.*

The significance of the histochemical reactions can be briefly summarized. The chromaffin reaction is evidence that a phenolic substance has formed a colored polymer as the result of chromate-effected oxidative dehydrogenation.[30,31] The chromaffin reaction itself does not identify the compound, since epinephrine, levarterenol, and serotonin (and perhaps other phenolic substances) will all give an insoluble colored polymer on exposure to chromate fixatives. The argentaffin reactions indicate again the presence of a reducing substance; however, the specificity of this reaction is less than that of the chromaffin reaction, since formalin-treated serotonin, levarterenol, melanin, and lipofuscin are among the compounds known to reduce basic silver nitrate. Relative to this Eränkö reported a positive argentaffin reaction in the adrenal medulla only in the specific levarterenol secretory cells.[32] Eränkö [33] has observed that in the specific levarterenol-secreting cells of the adrenal medulla a selective bathochromatic effect (shift in color to lower frequencies) occurs following alkaline azo coupling, indicating the presence of a compound with a reactive phenolic or quininoid substituent. The color produced with the stable diazonium salt Fast Garnet GBC was orange-yellow to brown-yellow in both levarterenol models and the carotid-body-type argentaffin cells of the tumor. The ferric ferricyanide reaction again indicates a reducing site and has approximately the same specificity as the ammonical silver reactions. However, it is important to note that adequate reduction of the ferric to ferrous ion to form Prussian blue or green with ferricyanide was delayed with formalin-fixed levarterenol as compared to comparably treated serotonin (5-hydroxytryptamine). In the present case the carotid-body-type argentaffin cells were adequately stained only after 10 minutes, while cells of formalin-fixed serotonin-secreting carcinoid tumors reduced the ferric salt in 5 minutes.[20]

Costero [6,24] has related the carotid-body-type argentaffin cells to the argentaffin cells of the intestine (enterochromaffin system) and serotonin production. We, therefore, felt it necessary to investigate whether a chemical relationship between these morphologically dissimilar cell types existed, i.e. whether both contained serotonin. The absence of a red to red-brown bathochromic shift in the granules of the carotid-body-type argentaffin cells following alkaline azo coupling with Fast Garnet GBC,[20] the delayed ferric ferricyanide reaction,[20] the absence of positive ninhydrin [22] and Clara's hematoxylin [20] reactions indicated the substance in the carotid-body-type argentaffin cells differed from serotonin. The absence of staining with Oil red O and Sudan black B appeared to eliminate the possibility that a lipofuscin pigment had caused the positive argentaffin and ferric ferricyanide reactions. The histochemical and biochemical findings, therefore, are both consistent with a levarterenol-secreting function for the carotid-body-type argentaffin cells.

As Costero [6] and Costero and Barroso-Moguel [24] have noted in human carotid body tumors, as Villasana has found in the normal human carotid body,[34] and as we have confirmed in this study, 2 histochemically distinct cell types can be identified. One is the peripherally located argentaffin cell and the other a nonargentaffin cell comprising the central group of the cell nests. Stout also described similar argentaffin cells in a tumor arising from the ganglion nodosum of the vagus.[15] Biochemical and histochemical proof of the presence of levarterenol in the normal carotid body has been demonstrated only in the calf.[35] On the basis of histochemical evidence this compound is also present in specific cell groups in the pig carotid body.[36] Electron microscopy examination of the rabbit[37] and cat[38] carotid bodies has revealed numerous osmophilic bodies in cells described in the respective species as "dark," and sustentacular." In the cat[39,40] and rabbit[39] chromaffin-positive cells have been described. Reserpine, a compound which is known to release catecholamines, has been shown to degranulate these cells[5] and to produce a burst of chemoreceptor impulses in Hering's nerve.[41] However, proof that the argentaffin, chromaffin, "sustentacular," and "dark" cells of the carotid body of the various species are functionally identical is, at present, lacking.

Since one of the main histologic distinctions between chromaffin bodies and paraganglia rests on the presence or absence of chromaffin cells,[42] the use of the term "nonchromaffin" paraganglia to describe the carotid body, aortic arch bodies, cell groups of the ganglion nodosum and glomus jugulare may in one sense be too limiting if evidence from the study of the carotid body as cited below is an indication. Since experimental evidence has indicated that anoxia produces degranulation of specific carotid body cells[5,43] which have been described as containing chromaffin granules,[39] it would be unlikely that chromaffin granules in these cells could be readily demonstrated histologically unless the carotid body was removed prior to the onset of tissue anoxia. In this regard it is of interest to note that in 8 normal carotid bodies removed and examined by us at *necropsy* only 1 could be demonstrated to give in the characteristic cells the histochemical reactions for levarterenol reported here. Yet, the presence of chromaffin cells has been reported in several *surgically* removed carotid body tumors.[7,8] It is possible, therefore, that certain cells in the human carotid body and other members of the so-called chemoreceptor system may in vivo contain levarterenol, but at death this substance would be depleted or lost as the result of anoxic discharge. In addition to the depletion of these granules in anoxia, several other factors may act to decrease the ability to identify a chromaffin reaction in levarterenol-containing cells. First, Hillarp and Hökfelt[44] have reported that it is epinephrine that is responsible for the dark-brown color of the chromaffin reaction in the adrenal medulla, while oxidized levarterenol gives a yellow or yellow-brown color. Tissue from an adrenal medullary tumor containing only levarterenol has been reported to give a color on chromate fixation that could be distinguished only with difficulty from the yellow color imparted to normal tissues by the chromate fixative.[25] Second, the absence of a histochemically demonstrable reaction for catecholamines or hydroxyindole ethylamines in various tissue sites, in various species in the same tissue site, and in some functional tumors[20,25] having a high biochemical assay for these substances may be due to absent or defective synthesis of a protein or proteolipid to which these amines are thought to be bound.[33,45] In such cases, therefore, consequent solubilization and loss of the free amine from in situ localization might occur during the fixation, dehydrating, and embedding procedures. Third, the chromaffin reaction is an extremely insensitive and capricious histochemical method upon which to base an absolute classification of a tumor type.[25,46]

Since the chemoreceptor function of the organs comprising the so-called paraganglia[42] (other than the carotid and aortic arch bodies) has not been established, it would seem convenient to use the term *carotid-body-like* in classifying these organs and their tumors in order to distinguish them from tumors of purely neuroblastic,[19] ganglionic,[19] and adrenal medullary origin. From the evidence at present available these tumor types appear to be morphologically[47] and/or histochemically distinct.

Conclusions

The morphological and histochemical evidence presented suggests that the tumor in the present case originated in carotid-body-like tissue and indicates that it contained levarterenol in specific argentaffin cells. A logical possibility is that the similar cells in the normal human carotid body may also be involved in levarterenol production. Although definitive evidence of partial innervation of the carotid body by the sympathetic system as well as origin of any one of its cellular components from neural crest tissue is lacking, the presence of levarterenol in carotid-body-type argentaffin cells would imply a neural crest origin for these cells. The presence of levarterenol also suggests a functional participation of these cells in the sympathoadrenal system,[48] perhaps as a local modulator of baroreceptor response [49] or as a levarterenol store responsive to local or generalized tissue anoxia (viz. Lever and Lewis, Ref. 5).[50,51] It may be significant in the latter regard that anoxia is known both to degranulate carotid body argentaffin cells [5,43] and to produce a vasopressor response.[4,52]

Summary

A case of a functioning tumor in the neck producing symptoms of hypertension and having morphological and histochemical characteristics suggestive of origin from carotid-body-like tissue is described. Biochemical analysis revealed the tumor to contain levarterenol, and histochemical examination localized this catecholamine to unique and characteristic argentaffin cells. Possible implications of this case with regard to the total function of carotid-body-like tissues, their relationship to the autonomic nervous system, and their embryonic origin are suggested.

We wish to acknowledge the technical assistance of Mr. Sherman Mason and the photography of Mr. John McGuire, and express our appreciation to Dr. I. Costero, Mexico City, for permission to review his sections of normal carotid bodies and carotid body tumors.

G. G. Glenner, Chief, Section of Histochemistry, National Institute of Arthritis and Metabolic Diseases, Bethesda 14, Md.

REFERENCES

1. de Castro, F.: Sur la Structure et l'innervation de la glande intercarotidienne (glomus carotocium) de l'homme et des mammifères, et sur un nouveau système d'innervation autonome du nerf glossopharyngien, Trav. Lab. Recherches Biol. Univ. Madrid 24:365-432, 1926.

2. de Castro, F.: Sur la Structure et l'innervation du sinus carotidien de l'homme et des mammifères: Nouveaux faits sur l'innervation et la fonction du glomus caroticum, Trav. Lab. Recherches Biol. Univ. Madrid 25:331-380, 1927-28.

3. Heymans, C., and Bouckaert, J. J.: Les Chémorécepteurs du sinus carotidien, Erg. Physiol. 41:28-55, 1939.

4. Schmidt, C. F., and Comoroe, J. H., Jr.: Functions of the Carotid and Aortic Bodies, Physiol. Rev. 20:115-157, 1940.

5. Lever, J. D., and Lewis, P. R.: A Possible Mechanism for the Initiation of Chemoreceptive Impulses, J. Physiol. (Proc.) 149:26, 1959.

6. Costero, I.: Symposium sobre tumor del cuerpo carotideo: IV. Histopatologia, Gac. Med. Mex. 90:679-690, 1960.

7. Mönckeberg, I. G.: Die Tumoren der Glandula carotica, Beitr. Path. Anat. 38:1-66, 1905.

8. Keen, W. W., and Funke, J.: Tumors of the Carotid Gland, J.A.M.A. 47:469-479, 1906.

9. Keen, W. W., and Funke, J.: Tumors of the Carotid Gland, J.A.M.A. 47:566-570, 1906.

10. Lattes, R.: Nonchromaffin Paraganglion of Ganglion Nodosum, Carotid Body and Aortic Arch Bodies, Cancer 3:667-694, 1950.

11. Ladenheim, J. C., and Sachs, E., Jr.: Familial Tumors of the "Glomus Jugulare": Report of 2 Cases, with a Note on the Vascular Origin of the Glomera, Neurology 11:303-309, 1961.

12. Lattes, R., and Waltner, J. G.: Nonchromaffin Paraganglion of the Middle Ear (Carotid Body-like Tumor, Glomus-Jugulare Tumor), Cancer 2:447-468, 1949.

13. Kipkie, G. F.: Simultaneous Chromaffin Tumors of the Carotid Body and Glomus Jugularis, Arch. Path. 44:113-118, 1947.

14. MacDonald, R. A.: A Carotid-Body-like Tumor on the Left Subclavian Artery, A.M.A. Arch. Path. 62:107-111, 1956.

15. Stout, A. P.: The Malignant Tumors of the Peripheral Nerves, Amer. J. Cancer 25:1-36, 1935.

16. Proctor, B.: Tumor of the Ganglion Nodosum of the Vagus Nerve, Laryngoscope 66:1577-1581, 1956.

17. Smetana, H. F., and Scott, W. F., Jr.: Malignant Tumors of Nonchromaffin Paraganglia, Milit. Surg. 109:330-341, 1951.

18. Crout, J. R.; Pisano, J. J., and Sjoerdsma, A.: Urinary Excretion of Catecholamines and Their Metabolites in Pheochromocytoma, Amer. Heart J. 61:375-381, 1961.

19. Vorhees, M. L., and Gardner, L. I.: Urinary Excretion of Norepinephrine, Epinephrine and 3-Methoxy-4-Hydroxy Mandelic Acid by Children with Neuroblastoma, J. Clin. Endocr. 21:321-335, 1961.

20. Lillie, R. D., and Glenner, G. G.: Histochemical Reactions in Carcinoid Tumors of the Human Gastrointestinal Tract, Amer. J. Path. 36: 623-651, 1960.

21. Lillie, R. D.: Histopathologic Technic and Practical Histochemistry, New York, The Blakiston Company, Division of McGraw-Hill Book Company, Inc., 1954, 501 pp.

22. Holcenberg, J., and Benditt, E. P.: A New Color Reaction for Tryptamine Derivatives: Histochemical Application to Enterochromaffin Cells, Lab. Invest. 10:144-158, 1961.

23. Sjoerdsma, A.; Leeper, L. C.; Terry, L., and Udenfriend, S.: Studies on the Biogenesis and Metabolism of Norepinephrine in Patients with Pheochromocytoma, J. Clin. Invest. 38:31-38, 1959.

24. Costero, I., and Barroso-Moguel, R.: Structure of the Carotid Body Tumor, Amer. J. Path. 38:127-135, 1961.

25. Sherwin, R. P.: Histopathology of Pheochromocytoma, Cancer 12:861-877, 1959.

26. Attia, A.; Golden, R. L., and Ziffer, H.: Nonchromaffin-Staining Functional Tumor of the Organs of Zuckerandl, N. Engl. J. Med. 264: 1130-1133, 1961.

27. Malinatti, G. M.; Camanni, F., and Pizzini, A.: Malignant Hypertension in a Case of Nonchromaffin Paraganglioma with a High Concentration of Catecholamine, Cancer 12:878-883, 1959.

28. Cone, T. E., Jr.: Recurrent Pheochromocytoma: Report of a Case in a Previously Treated Child, Pediatrics 21:994-999, 1958.

29. Eränkö, O.: Histochemistry of Noradrenaline in the Adrenal Medulla of Rats and Mice, Endocrinology 57:363-368, 1955.

30. Eriksen, N.; Martin, G. M., and Benditt, E. P.: Oxidation of the Indole Nucleus of 5-Hydroxytryptamine and the Formation of Pigments: Isolation and Partial Characterization of a Dimer of 5-Hydroxytryptamine, J. Biol. Chem. 235:1662-1667, 1960.

31. Gérard, P.; Cordier, R., and Lison, L.: Sur la Nature de la réaction chromaffine, Bull. Histol. Appliq. Physiol. 7:133-139, 1930.

32. Eränkö, O.: On the Histochemistry of the Adrenal Medulla of the Rat, with Special Reference to Acid Phosphatase, Acta Anat. (Supp. 17) 16:1-60, 1952.

33. Eränkö, O.: Personal communication to the authors, 1961.

34. Villasana, A.: Symposium sobre tumor del cuerpo carotideo: II. Morfologia del cuerpo carotideo del hombre, Gac. Med. Mex. 90:661-670, 1960.

35. Muscholl, E.; Rahn, K. H., and Watzka, M.: Nachweis von Noradrenalin im Glomus caroticum, Naturwissenschaften 47:325, 1960.

36. Muratori, G., and Battaglia, G.: Osservazioni sulla reazione iodaffine nel paraganglio carotico, Boll. Soc. Ital. Biol. Sper. 36:401-405, 1960.

37. Lever, J. D., and Boyd, J. D.: Osmophile Granules in the Glomus Cells of the Rabbit Carotid Body, Nature (Lond.) 179:1082-1083, 1957.

38. Ross, L. L.: Electron Microscopic Observations of the Carotid Body of the Cat, J. Biophys. Biochem. Cytol. 6:253-262, 1959.

39. Lever, J. D.; Lewis, P. R., and Boyd, J. D.: Observations on the Fine Structure and Histochemistry of the Carotid Body in the Cat and Rabbit, J. Anat. 93:478-490, 1959.

40. Goormaghtigh, N., and Pannier, R.: Les Paraganglias du coeur et des zones vaso-sensible carotidienne et cardio-aortique chez le chat adulte, Arch. Biol. (Liege) 50:455-533, 1939.

41. Dontas, A. S.: Effects of Reserpine and Hydralazine on Carotid and Splanchnic Nerve Activity and Blood Pressure, J. Pharmacol. Exp. Ther. 121:1-7, 1957.

42. Hollinshead, W. H.: Chromaffin Tissue and Paraganglia, Quart. Rev. Biol. 15:156-171, 1940.

43. Hollinshead, W. H.: Effects of Anoxia upon Carotid Body Morphology, Anat. Rec. 92:255-26[illegible], 1945.

44. Hillarp, N-Å., and Hökfelt, B.: Histochemical Demonstration of Noradrenaline and Adrenaline in the Adrenal Medulla, J. Histochem. Cytochem. 3:1-5, 1955.

45. Glenner, G. G., and Lillie, R. D.: Pepsin Release of Guinea Pig Enterochromaffin Substance, J. Histochem. Cytochem. 7:204, 1959.

46. Kennedy, J. S.; Symington, T., and Woodger, B. A.: Chemical and Histochemical Observations in Benign and Malignant Phaeochromocytoma, J. Path. Bact. 81:409-418, 1961.

47. Le Compte, P. M.: Tumors of the Carotid Body and Related Structures (Chemoreceptor System), in Atlas of Tumor Pathology, Section IV, Fascicle 16, 40 pp., Subcommittee on Oncology of the Committee on Pathology of the National Research Council, Armed Forces Institute of Pathology, Washington, D.C., 1951.

48. Goodall, McC., and Kirshner, J.: Biosynthesis of Epinephrine and Norepinephrine by Sympathetic Nerves and Ganglia, Circulation 17:366-371, 1958.

49. Peterson, L. H.; Feigl, E. O., and Gouras, P.: On the Mechanism of Carotid Sinus Function, Abstract, J. Clin. Invest. 39:1017, 1960.

50. Comline, R. S., and Silver, M.: Response of the Adrenal Medulla of the Sheep Foetus to Asphyxia, Nature (Lond.) 81:283-284, 1958.

51. Comline, R. S., and Silver, M.: The Release of Adrenaline and Noradrenaline from the Adrenal Glands of the Foetal Sheep, J. Physiol. 156:424-444, 1961.

52. Dripps, R. D., and Comroe, J. H., Jr.: The Clinical Significance of the Carotid and Aortic Bodies, Amer. J. Med. Sci. 208:681-694, 1944.

The Cardiac Disease Associated with the Carcinoid Syndrome (Carcinoid Heart Disease)*

WILLIAM C. ROBERTS, M.D. *and* ALBERT SJOERDSMA, M.D., PH.D.
Bethesda, Maryland

IN THE EARLY 1930's three patients were described who had metastasizing carcinoid tumors and, in addition, fibrous thickening of the valves on the right side of the heart and reddish discoloration of the skin [*1–4*]. Similar reports followed [*5–8*], and by 1954 three groups independently had recognized what is now referred to as the malignant carcinoid syndrome [*9–11*]. Recently, the clinical and biochemical aspects of this disorder have been emphasized; however, little attention has been given to the morphology of the associated cardiac disease.

The chief purpose of this communication is to describe the pathologic condition of the heart in carcinoid syndrome based on clinical and pathologic studies of seventeen patients with metastatic carcinoid tumors. The present experience and that previously recorded will be discussed in terms of morphology and pathogenesis of the cardiac lesions and clinical features of the patients studied.

PATIENTS STUDIED

Clinical and pathologic features in the seventeen patients are summarized in Table I (nine patients with carcinoid heart disease) and Table II (eight patients without carcinoid heart disease). The nine patients with carcinoid heart disease are described in detail in the appendix. Of the various features listed in the tables, only the presence of a cardiac murmur suggestive of pulmonic stenosis or tricuspid regurgitation served to separate the two groups during life. The cardiac silhouette as seen on chest roentgenogram was of no diagnostic importance. Pathologically, there was no distinguishing feature between the two groups other than the presence of cardiac lesions *per se*. The types of cardiovascular lesions seen in the nine patients with carcinoid heart disease are illustrated in Figures 1 through 11.

SUMMARY OF PATHOLOGIC FINDINGS IN PATIENTS WITH CARCINOID HEART DISEASE

The Carcinoid Tumor. In all nine patients the site of the primary tumor was the small intestine, the ileum in seven and the jejunum in two. Hepatic metastases occurred in all nine patients, and in six the liver weighed more than 1,800 gm. In some patients the hepatic parenchyma was largely replaced by carcinoid implants. The hepatic tissue not involved by tumor showed centrolobular congestion in all but one patient, three to a severe degree, and in seven there was an increase in periportal fibrous tissue which usually contained some chronic inflammatory cells. In five of the nine patients there was fatty change in the liver. Metastases to organs other than the liver occurred in eight of the nine patients. In the one patient without extrahepatic metastases there was recurrence of tumor at the site of intestinal anastomosis (ileum) and at the site of appendectomy. Thus, in all nine patients there was extraportal as well as portal venous drainage of tumor tissue. The regional lymph nodes were involved in all eight patients with extrahepatic metastases. Bone metastases, which occurred in five, were the next most frequent. Metastases to the heart, pancreas and spleen occurred in each of three patients, and metastases to the ovary

Table I

CLINICAL AND PATHOLOGIC DATA IN NINE PATIENTS WITH MALIGNANT CARCINOID TUMORS AND CARCINOID HEART DISEASE

Case No.	Age (yr.) Sex and Race	Length of Illness from Onset of Symptoms (yr.)	Initial Sign and/or Symptom	Diarrhea	Flushing	Bronchoconstriction "Asthma"	Heart Murmur(s)*	Electrocardiogram	Urinary 5-HIAA Excretion† (mg./24 hr.)	Immediate Cause of Death	Site of Primary Tumor	Liver Size (gm.)	Liver Metastases	Other Metastases	Heart Size (gm.)	Location of Carcinoid Fibrous Plaques	Foramen Ovale	Spleen Size (gm.)
I	41,M,W	3	Weight loss, diarrhea	+	+	0	+	Normal	500–700	Hepatic failure	Ileum	7,400	+	Lymph node (regional), lung, pancreas, thyroid gland, bone, heart, pericardium	220	Right atrium, tricuspid valve, pulmonic valve	Closed	120
II	50,F,W	12	Flushing	+	+	+	+	"Metabolic derangement"	1,209–1,270	Hepatic failure	Ileum	4,500	+	Lymph node (regional, supraclavicular, mediastinal), lung, bone, heart, spleen, kidney, ovary, pituitary, adrenal glands	250	Right atrium, coronary sinus, tricuspid valve, right ventricle, pulmonic valve	Closed	100
III	67,M,W	7	Diarrhea, abdominal pain	+	+	+	+	Normal	...	Arrhythmia (?)	Ileum	2,500	+	Lymph node (regional, retroperitoneal), appendix	280	Right atrium, tricuspid valve, right ventricle, pulmonic valve	Closed	110
IV	59,M,W	6	Diarrhea	+	+	+	+	Low voltage, right axis deviation	380–580	Congestive heart failure, arrhythmia	Ileum	1,800	+	Recurrence at ileoileal anastomosis and at appendiceal scar	350	Superior vena cava, inferior vena cava, right atrium, tricuspid valve, right ventricle, pulmonic valve	Patent	200
V	57,F,W	4	Diarrhea	+	+	+	+	First degree heart block	161–283	Gastrointestinal hemorrhage	Ileum	2,300	+	Lymph node (regional), bone, thyroid, adrenal glands, kidney, gallbladder	270	Superior vena cava, right atrium, tricuspid valve, right ventricle, pulmonic valve	Closed	400
VI	64,M,W	1.5	Diarrhea, flushing, abdominal pain	+	+	0	+	Low voltage	300–400	Hepatic failure, acute renal shutdown, arrhythmia	Jejunum	1,600	+	Lymph node (regional), bone, pancreas	400	Right atrium, tricuspid valve, right ventricle, pulmonic valve, pulmonary trunk, mitral valve, left ventricle	Closed	160
VII	57,F,W	4	Acute intestinal obstruction	+	+	0	+	Low voltage, vertical axis, prominent P waves	187–274	Electrolyte disturbances	Ileum	1,800	+	Lymph node (regional), pancreas, ovary, spleen, heart	210	Superior vena cava, inferior vena cava, innominate vein, coronary sinus, right atrium, tricuspid valve, right ventricle, pulmonic valve, pulmonary trunk, mitral valve, left ventricle, aorta	Closed	120

TABLE I (*Continued*)

CLINICAL AND PATHOLOGIC DATA IN NINE PATIENTS WITH MALIGNANT CARCINOID TUMORS AND CARCINOID HEART DISEASE

Case No.	Age (yr.) Sex and Race	Length of Illness from Onset of Symptoms (yr.)	Initial Sign and/or Symptom	Diarrhea	Flushing	Broncho-constriction "Asthma"	Heart Murmur(s)*	Electro-cardiogram	Urinary 5-HIAA Excretion† (mg./24 hr.)	Immediate Cause of Death	Site of Primary Tumor	Liver: Size (gm.)	Liver: Metastases	Other Metastases	Heart Size (gm.)	Location of Carcinoid Fibrous Plaques	Foramen Ovale	Spleen Size (gm.)
VIII	52,F,W	1.5	Diarrhea, flushing, wheezing, abdominal pain	+	+	+	+	Low voltage	180–220	Hepatic failure	Jejunum	2,800	+	Lymph node (regional), ovary, bone (vertebrae), spleen	200	Inferior vena cava, coronary sinus, right atrium, tricuspid valve, right ventricle, pulmonic valve, pulmonary trunk, mitral valve	Closed	130
IX	69,M,W	1	Abdominal pain, weight loss	+	+	+	+	Left axis deviation, left ventricular ischemia, old anterior myocardial infarct	80–120	Arrhythmia (?)	Ileum	2,600	+	Lymph node (regional)	475	Tricuspid valve, pulmonic valve pulmonary trunk	Closed	475

NOTE: + = present; 0 = absent.
* Murmur of tricuspid and/or pulmonic valvular disease. † Normal urinary 5-hydroxyindoleacetic acid excretion, 2 to 9 mg. per twenty-four hours.

occurred in three of the four women. Metastases to the kidney, lung, adrenal glands and thyroid glands occurred in each of two patients. There was no apparent correlation between the urinary excretion of 5-hydroxyindoleacetic acid and the number of carcinoid metastases or the size of the liver. (Table I.) The spleen weighed 200 gm. or less in seven patients and was enlarged in only two.

Distribution of Fibrous Lesions in the Heart and Great Vessels. Fibrous plaques of the carcinoid type were present on both tricuspid and pulmonic valves in all nine patients studied. Generally the involvement of each valve was diffuse and uniform. Occasionally, however, involvement of one valve was more extensive than that of the other. For example, in Case I there was severe diffuse fibrosis of the pulmonic valve and only two or three focal minute fibrous plaques on the tricuspid valve. In Case VIII the reverse was true. The tricuspid valve was diffusely involved whereas the pulmonic valve cusps were delicate and contained only small fibrous plaques. In eight patients the right atrium contained carcinoid plaques and the right ventricle in seven of nine patients. The process was always more extensive in the right atrium. Usually the right ventricular involvement was limited to "white capping" of the papillary muscles or only a rare mural plaque. In only one patient (Case V) was the right ventricular plaquing diffuse. Carcinoid plaques were present in the pulmonary trunk in four patients, and in each instance the involvement was limited to that portion lining the sinus of the pulmonic valve or immediately above it. In no case were the pulmonary arteries or veins involved by carcinoid fibrosis.

The systemic veins in several patients contained fibrous plaques. In each of three patients these plaques were seen on the intima of the superior and inferior vena cavae and coronary sinus and in one on the intima of the innominate vein. In Cases I, II and III the great veins were not available for re-examination.

Involvement of the left side of the heart occurred in three of the nine patients, and in none was there an intracardiac communication. The one patient (Case IV) who did have an intracardiac communication (patent foramen ovale) had no cardiac lesions on the left side. The mitral valve was involved by the fibrous process in three, the left ventricle in two and the aorta in one.

Table II

CLINICAL AND PATHOLOGIC DATA IN EIGHT PATIENTS WITH MALIGNANT CARCINOID TUMORS WITHOUT CARCINOID HEART DISEASE

Case No.	Age (yr.) Sex, and Race	Length of Illness from Onset of Symptoms (yr.)	Initial Sign and/or Symptom	Diarrhea	Flushing	Bronchoconstriction "Asthma"	Cardiac Murmur	Electrocardiogram	Urinary 5-HIAA Excretion (mg./24 hr.)	Immediate Cause of Death	Site of Primary Tumor	Liver		Other Metastases	Heart Size (gm.)	Cardiac Valves and Chambers	Foramen Ovale	Spleen Size (gm.)
												Size (gm.)	Metastases					
X	47,M,W	3	Flushing	+	+	0	0	Normal	90–124	Hepatic failure	Caecum	2,100	+	. . .	300	Normal	Closed	550
XI	69,M,W	9	Diarrhea	+	+	0	0	Normal	717–854	Hepatic failure	Meckel's diverticulum	3,800	+	Lymph node (regional), lungs, bone, spleen, pituitary gland	270	Normal	Patent	150
XII	75,M,W	1	Diarrhea	+	+	0	+*	Suggestion of old anterior myocardial infarct, left axis deviation	40–60	Gastrointestinal hemorrhage	Ileum	1,700	0	Lymph node (regional), lung, bone, heart	320	Arteriosclerotic heart disease	Closed	300
XIII	74,M,W	1.5	Abdominal swelling	+	+	0	+*	Normal	200–400	Hepatic failure	Uncertain, probably small intestine	2,500	+	Lymph node (abdominal and hilar), lung, bone, kidney, spleen, small and large intestine, heart, pancreas, prostate, parathyroid gland	290	Severe arteriosclerotic heart disease, calcification, focal, mitral and aortic valves	Closed	65
XIV	45,M,W	5	Flushing	+	+	+	0	Normal	487–588	Bronchial obstruction by tumor, bronchopneumonia	Uncertain, probably bronchus	6,100	+	Lymph node (abdominal and thoracic), lungs, bone, kidneys, pancreas, gallbladder, heart, adrenal, thyroid, pituitary gland	450†	Hypertensive cardiovascular disease (left ventricular hypertrophy)	Closed	400
XV	67,M,W	8	Abdominal mass	+	+	0	0	Normal	17–43	Hepatic failure	Ileum	2,100	+	Lymph node (regional), spleen, gallbladder, adrenal, stomach, small and large intestine	300	Arteriosclerotic heart disease	Closed	130
XVI	67,M,W	1	Abdominal pain, weakness	0	+	0	+*	Normal	Markedly positive‡	Renal failure (acute pyelonephritis)	Bronchus	1,650	+	Lung	270	Normal	Closed	270
XVII	40,F,W	4	Flushing, intestinal obstruction	+	+	0	0	Low voltage, left ventricular ischemia(?)	30–60	Atelectasis, miliary tuberculosis	Ileum	3,500	+	Lymph node (adnexal), ovary, jejunum, pancreas, pituitary gland	230	Normal	Closed	200

Note: + = present; 0 = absent.
* Murmur not characteristic of tricuspid insufficiency or pulmonic stenosis.
† Intermittent systemic hypertension.
‡ Screening test for urinary 5-HIAA.

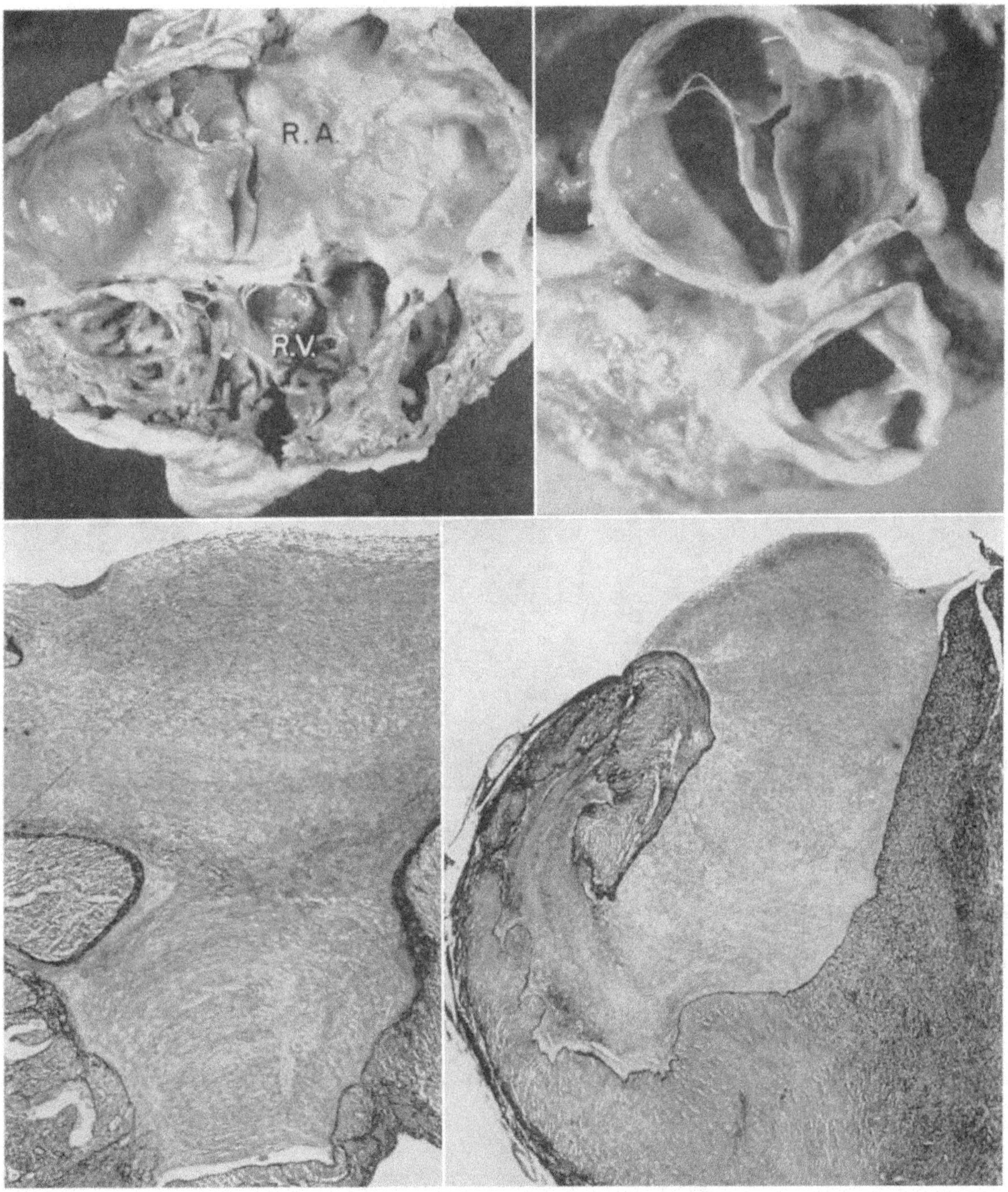

FIG. 1. Case v. *Upper left,* the right atrium (R.A.), tricuspid valve and right ventricle (R.V.) are opened. Each chamber is dilated, but neither is hypertrophied. Diffuse fibrous plaquing covers the endocardium of each chamber. The tricuspid valvular leaflets and chordae are shortened and thickened. *Upper right,* the pulmonic (smaller) and aortic valves (larger) from above. The pulmonic valve cusps are thickened, its commissures mildly interadherent and its opening fixed. The aortic valve cusps, in contrast, are delicate. Normally, in the adult, the aortic valve "ring" is larger than the pulmonic one. The reverse is frequently the case in carcinoid heart disease. *Lower left,* photomicrograph of a section of right atrium showing marked deposition of carcinoid fibrous tissue on the endocardium. The superimposed fibrous plaque is much thicker than is the true right atrial wall. Verhoeff-Van Gieson elastic tissue stain, original magnification × 43. *Lower right,* photomicrograph of a section of pulmonic valve. The valvular cusp is clearly demarcated from the superimposed fibrous tissue by the elastic membrane (black). The distal portion of the cusp is folded inward, and the fibrous deposition takes place almost entirely within the sinus of the valve. The fibrous deposit in this instance completely fills the sinus and contacts the pulmonary trunk. Verhoeff-Van Gieson elastic tissue stain, original magnification × 25.

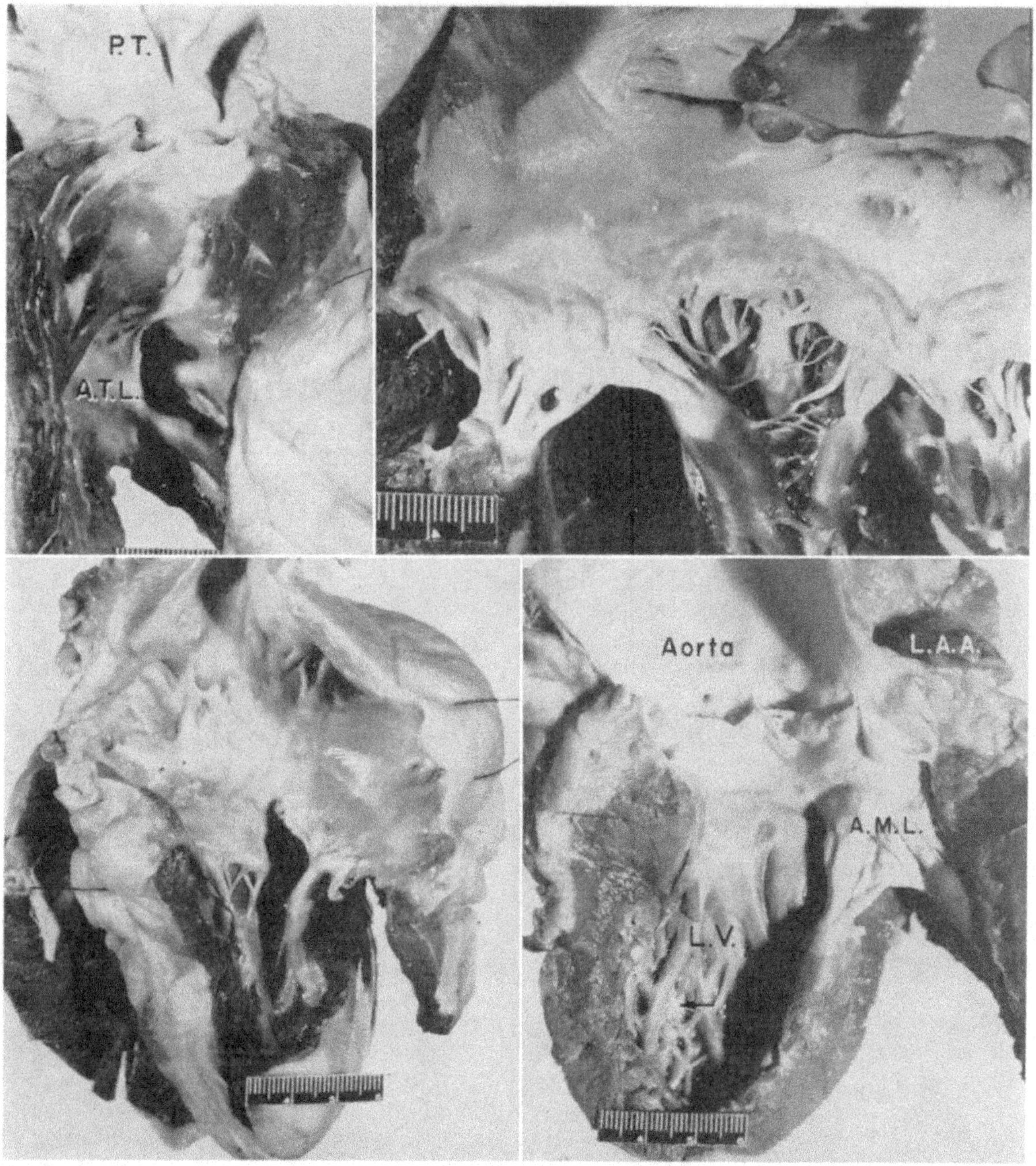

FIG. 2. Case VI. *Upper left*, the pulmonary trunk (P.T.), pulmonic valve and right ventricle are opened. Note the marked contraction of the pulmonic valve. Its cusps are thickened, but the commissures are not fused. The fibrous plaquing of the right ventricle and of the anterior leaflet of the tricuspid valve (A.T.L.) is apparent. *Lower left*, the superior vena cava, right atrium, tricuspid valve and right ventricle are opened. The right atrium is dilated and hypertrophied. Carcinoid plaquing is apparent on the right atrial endocardium, particularly that portion covering the atrial septum. The tricuspid valvular leaflets are shortened, thickened and insert at times directly into the papillary muscles, which also are covered by fibrous plaques ("white capping"). The chordae tendineae are thick and fused. The right ventricle is hypertrophied. *Upper right*, the left atrium, mitral valve and left ventricle are opened. The leaflets and chordae of the mitral valve are thick and white, and there is "white capping" of the papillary muscles. The left atrial endocardium is thicker than normal but free of fibrous plaques. *Lower right*, the ascending aorta, aortic valve and left ventricle (L.V.) are opened. Again note the marked thickening of the anterior mitral leaflet (A.M.L.). The arrow points to a small carcinoid plaque in the left ventricle. A small fibrotic nodule, noncarcinoid in type, is present on the aortic valve. L.A.A. = left atrial appendage.

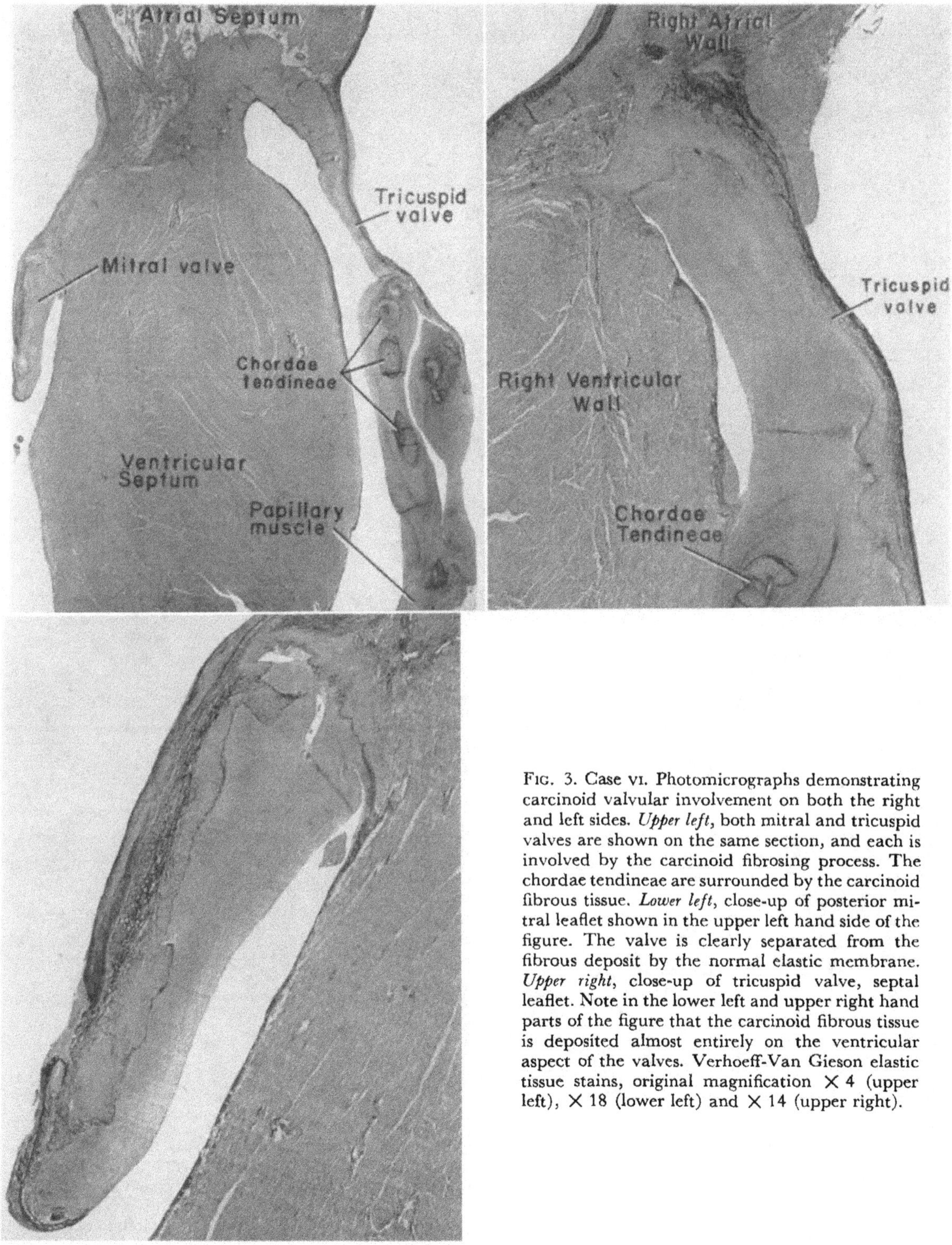

FIG. 3. Case VI. Photomicrographs demonstrating carcinoid valvular involvement on both the right and left sides. *Upper left,* both mitral and tricuspid valves are shown on the same section, and each is involved by the carcinoid fibrosing process. The chordae tendineae are surrounded by the carcinoid fibrous tissue. *Lower left,* close-up of posterior mitral leaflet shown in the upper left hand side of the figure. The valve is clearly separated from the fibrous deposit by the normal elastic membrane. *Upper right,* close-up of tricuspid valve, septal leaflet. Note in the lower left and upper right hand parts of the figure that the carcinoid fibrous tissue is deposited almost entirely on the ventricular aspect of the valves. Verhoeff-Van Gieson elastic tissue stains, original magnification × 4 (upper left), × 18 (lower left) and × 14 (upper right).

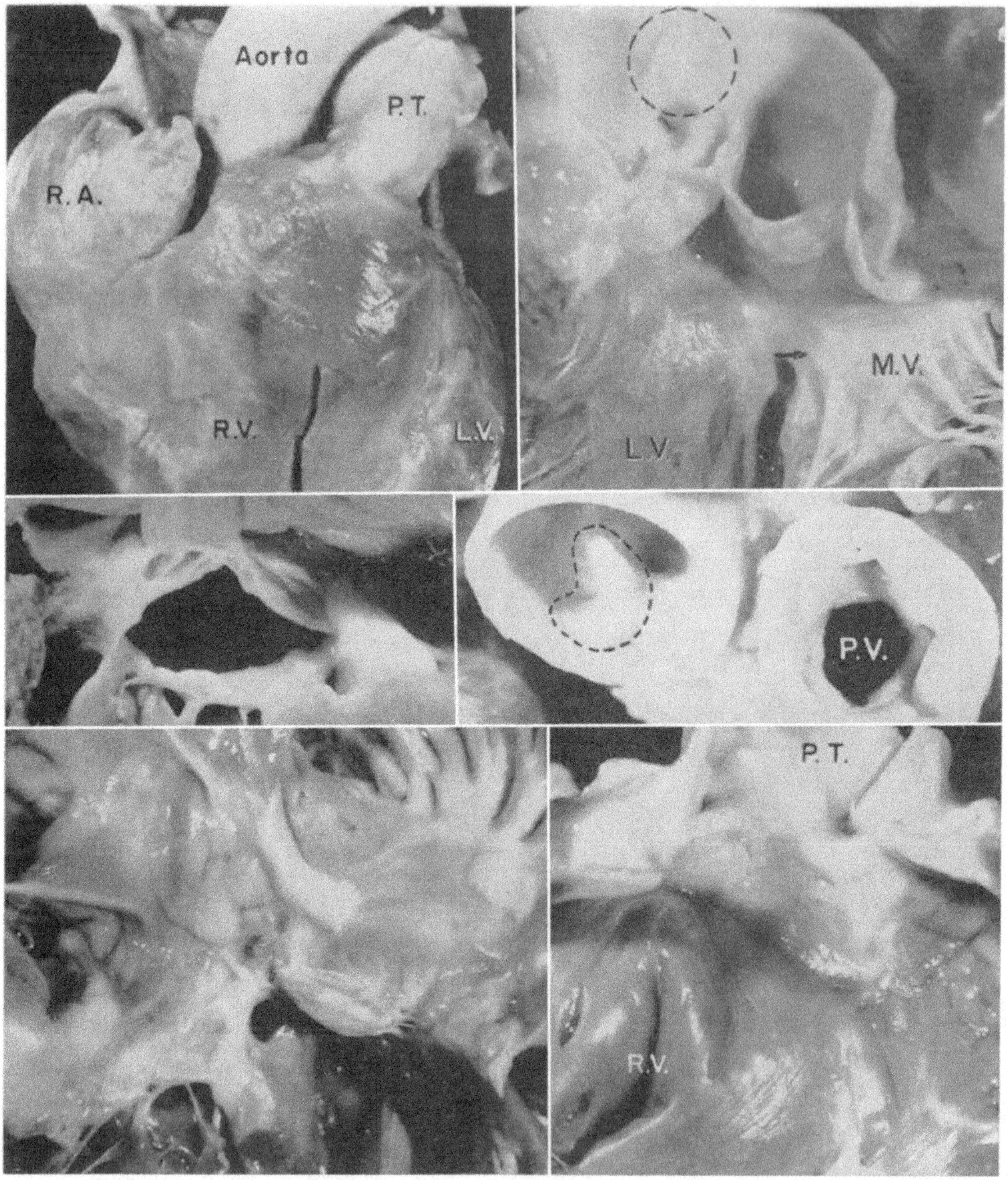

FIG. 4. Case VII. *Upper left*, external view of heart showing dilatation of the right atrium (R.A.) and right ventricle (R.V.) and serous atrophy of the subepicardial adipose tissue. Only a small portion of the left ventricle (L.V.) is visible anteriorly, and the left atrial appendage is almost completely obscured by the pulmonary trunk (P.T.). *Upper right*, the left ventricle (L.V.), aortic valve and ascending aorta are opened. The arrow designates a small carcinoid plaque on the anterior leaflet of the mitral valve (M.V.). The dashed circle encloses another carcinoid plaque in the ascending aorta. *Middle left*, the tricuspid valvular orifice as seen from the right ventricle. The valve orifice is open and consequently regurgitant. *Middle right*, the pulmonic valvular orifice (P.V.) and aorta are seen from above. The pulmonic valvular orifice is fixed and is both stenotic and regurgitant. The carcinoid fibrous plaque in the ascending aorta is again enclosed by the dashed lines. *Lower left*, the right atrium, tricuspid valve and right ventricle. Note the multiple smooth, pearly white fibrous plaques in the right atrium. The tricuspid valvular leaflets and chordae are shortened and thickened. *Lower right*, the pulmonary trunk (P.T.), pulmonic valve and right ventricle (R.V.). The pulmonic valve is diffusely involved by the pearly white fibrosing process.

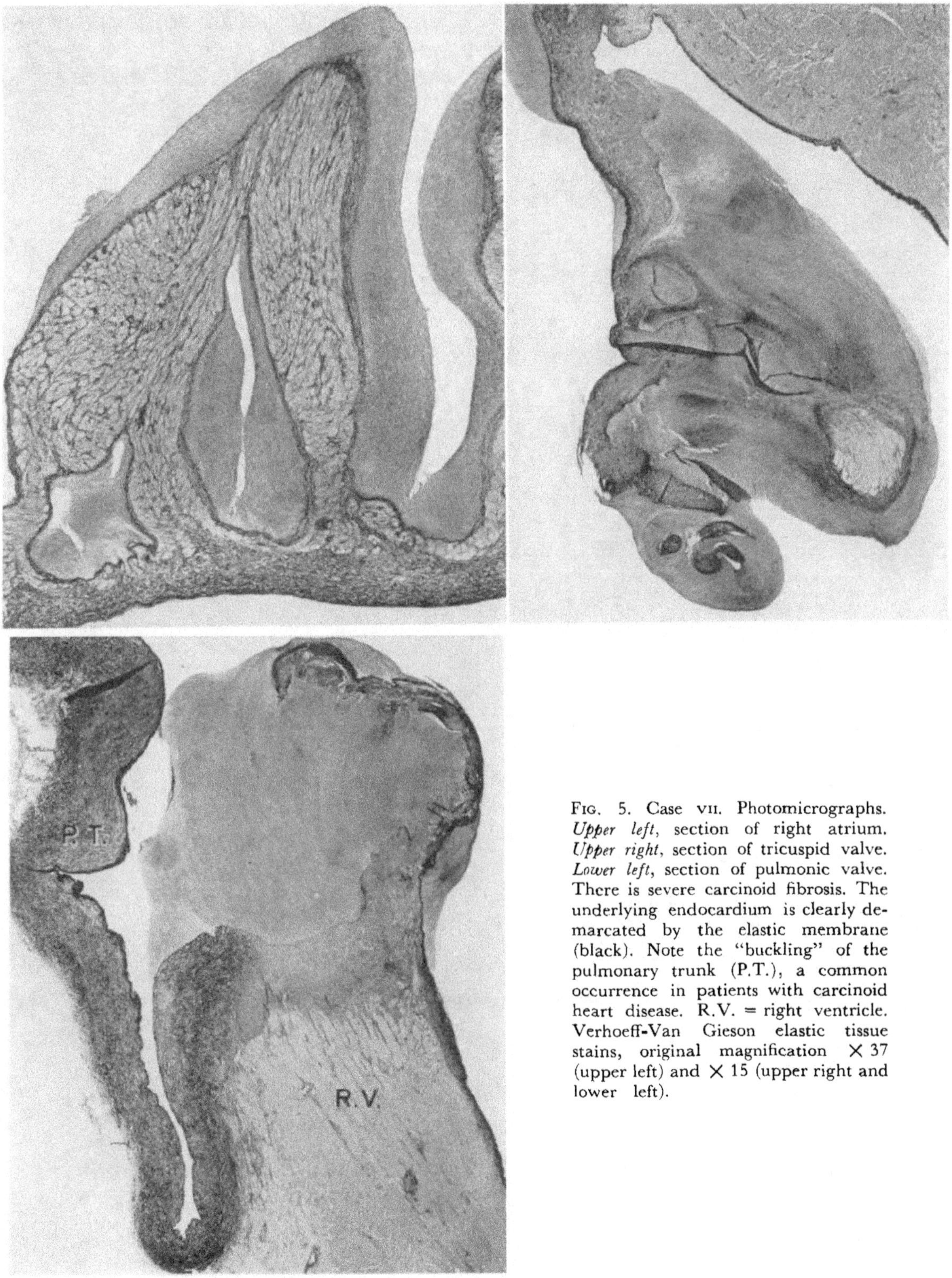

FIG. 5. Case VII. Photomicrographs. *Upper left*, section of right atrium. *Upper right*, section of tricuspid valve. *Lower left*, section of pulmonic valve. There is severe carcinoid fibrosis. The underlying endocardium is clearly demarcated by the elastic membrane (black). Note the "buckling" of the pulmonary trunk (P.T.), a common occurrence in patients with carcinoid heart disease. R.V. = right ventricle. Verhoeff-Van Gieson elastic tissue stains, original magnification × 37 (upper left) and × 15 (upper right and lower left).

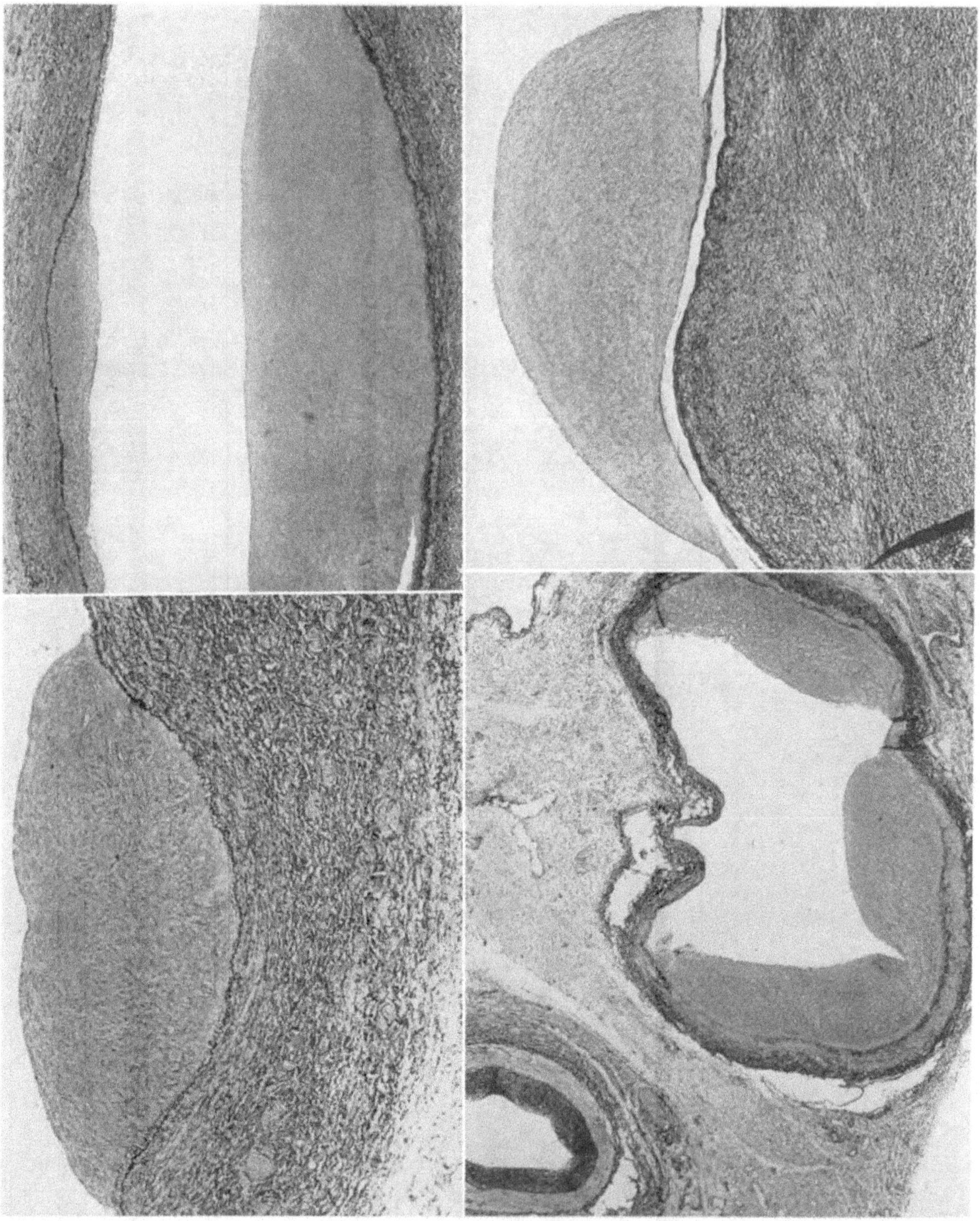

Fig. 6. Case vii. Systemic vessels involved by the carcinoid fibrosing process. *Upper left*, innominate vein. *Lower left*, inferior vena cava. *Upper right*, ascending aorta with a superimposed carcinoid fibrous plaque. The latter became disassociated from the underlying aorta during sectioning. *Lower right*, coronary sinus (large vessel) and coronary artery (small vessel, left lower corner). There is marked carcinoid fibrous plaquing involving the intima of the coronary sinus. The elastic intimal proliferation in the coronary artery, in contrast, is the result of "early" atherosclerosis and bears no resemblance to the process in the coronary sinus which is free of elastic fibrils. Verhoeff-Van Gieson elastic tissue stains; original magnification × 52 (lower left), × 37 (upper left), × 140 (lower right) and × 43 (upper right).

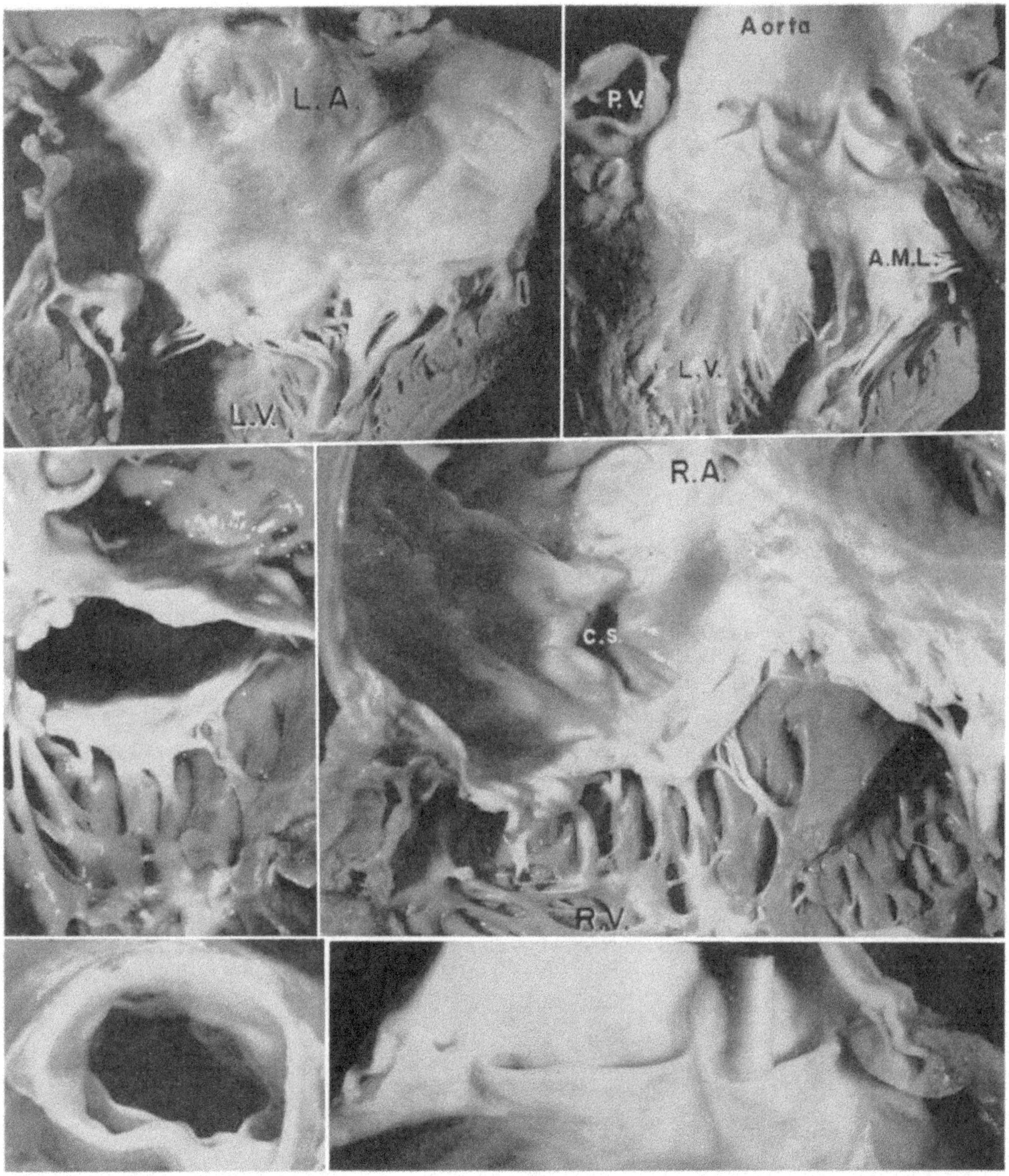

FIG. 7. Case VIII. *Upper left,* the left atrium (L.A.), mitral valve and left ventricle (L.V.). The mitral valvular leaflets and chordae are pearly white and thick. The left atrium is slightly dilated but free of carcinoid fibrous plaques. *Upper right,* the ascending aorta, aortic valve and left ventricle (L.V.) are opened showing the involved anterior leaflet of the mitral valve (A.M.L.) from this view. P.V. = pulmonic valve. *Middle left,* the tricuspid valve as seen from the right ventricle. The orifice is open; the consequence is regurgitation. *Middle right,* right atrium (R.A.) tricuspid valve and right ventricle (R.V.). The right atrium and tricuspid valve are extensively involved by the carcinoid fibrosing process. A single carcinoid plaque is present in the right ventricle. C.S. = ostium of coronary sinus. *Lower left,* the pulmonic valve from above. The appearance of this valve would suggest that it functioned normally. *Lower right,* the pulmonic valve opened. Its cusps are delicate. The lack of gross carcinoid fibrosis of this valve contrasts sharply with the marked involvement of the tricuspid valve.

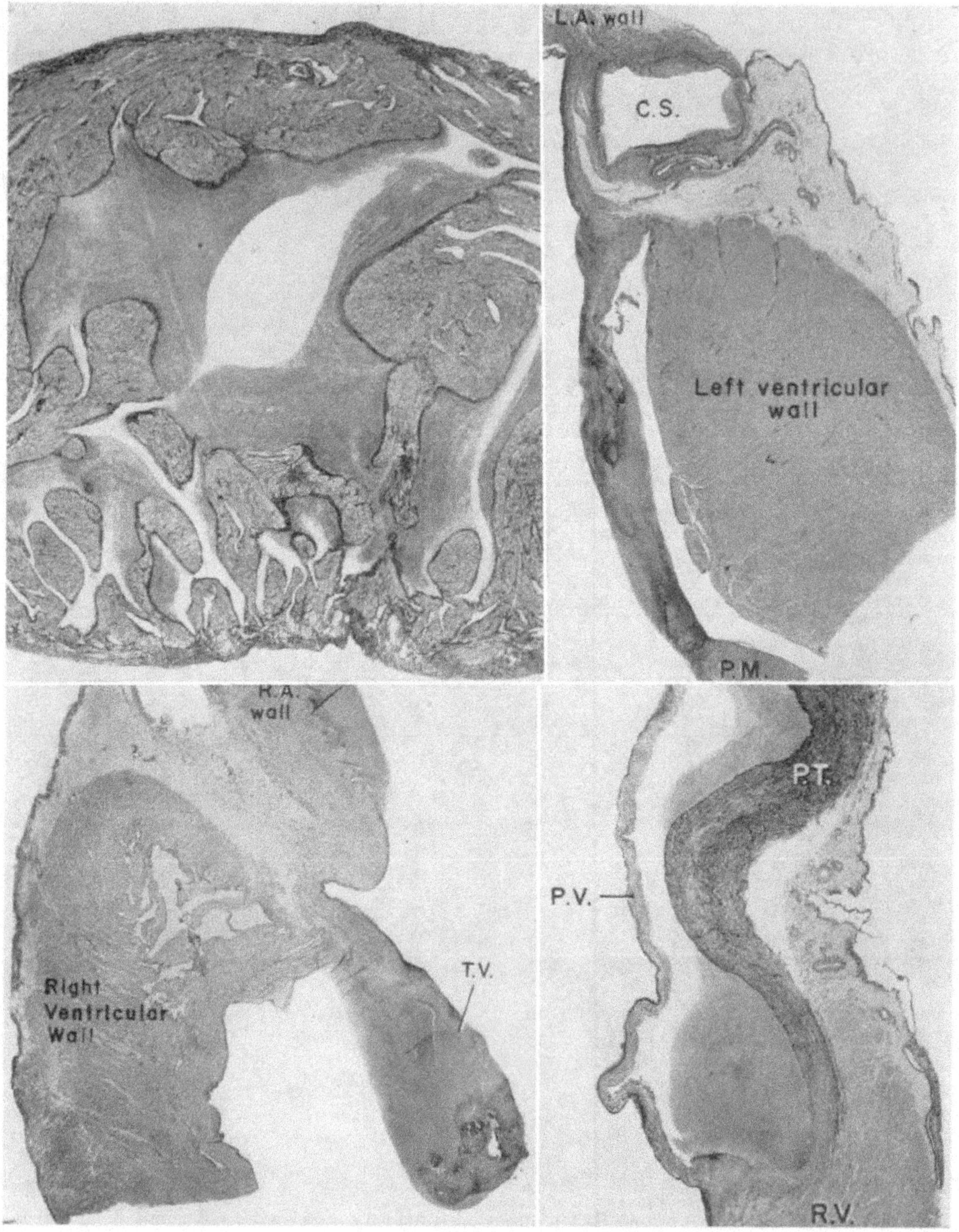

FIG. 8. Case VIII. Photomicrographs of sections demonstrating carcinoid fibrosis of the heart. *Upper left*, cross-section of right atrial appendage. Its lumen is considerably reduced by the widespread carcinoid fibrosis between the pectinate muscles. Note the "blood spaces" in the fibrous tissue. The underlying endocardium is well-demarcated by the black staining elastic membrane. *Upper right*, mitral valve, posterior leaflet. The fibrous process extends down and surrounds the chordae tendineae. Note also the carcinoid plaquing on the intima of the coronary sinus (C.S.). L.A. = left atrium; P.M. = papillary muscle. *Lower left*, tricuspid valve. The deposition of the fibrous stroma occurs on the ventricular aspect of the leaflet. Note also the fibrous plaquing on the right atrial (R.A.) endocardium. T.V. = tricuspid valve. *Lower right*, pulmonic valve. The carcinoid fibrous deposition in this instance occurs only on the intima of the pulmonary trunk (P.T.) causing it to "buckle." The pulmonic-valve (P.V.) cusp is free of fibrous material. R.V. = right ventricle. Verhoeff-Van Gieson elastic tissue stains; original magnification × 18 (upper left), × 7 (lower left), × 10 (lower right) and × 4 (upper right).

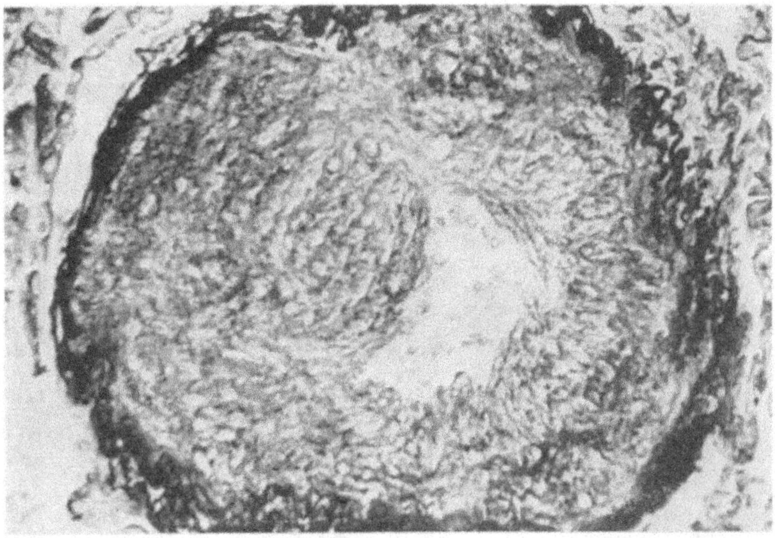

FIG. 9. Case VIII. Small pulmonary vein showing marked intimal fibrous proliferation. Since the fibrous tissue contains elastic fibrils (stained black) the fibrous proliferation is not of the carcinoid type but probably is secondary to increased pulmonary venous pressure, a result of mitral valvular disease. The pulmonary veins in this patient were diffusely and severely involved by this process, but, in addition, there was medial hypertrophy and intimal proliferation, although of only mild degree, of the muscular pulmonary arteries and arterioles. Verhoeff-Van Gieson elastic tissue stain, original magnification × 290.

COMMENTS

Cardiac Pathology. Histology of the fibrous deposits: The cardiovascular disease associated with the metastasizing "clinically functional" carcinoid is pathognomonic. The involvement consists of focal or diffuse collections of a peculiar type of fibrous tissue, which is free of elastic fibers and is deposited on the endocardium of the valvular cusps, on the endocardium of the cardiac chambers and on the intima of the great veins, coronary sinus and occasionally great arteries. The valvular cusps *per se* remain normal as does the mural endocardium, and each is clearly separated from the fibrosing process by the internal elastic membrane. Within the superimposed atypical fibrous tissue there is also a metachromatic ground substance, a few spindle-shaped cells (fibroblasts), blood vessels, oval or round spaces, which frequently contain small hyperchromatic nuclei, usually some lymphocytes, plasmacytes and mast cells, but no fat or fibrin. The oval or round spaces tend to give the fibrous tissue a "cartilage-like" appearance. The borders of these spaces are nicely delineated by the silver stain. The blood vessels, which frequently have thick walls, are located almost exclusively immediately adjacent to the valvular leaflets, usually on the side of the cusp which has initial contact with the stream of blood. The lymphocytes and plasma cells are located almost entirely in the perivascular regions, also immediately adjacent to the cusps. The mast cells, which are considerably increased in number in comparison to hearts of control subjects [*12*], are usually found in the subepicardial adipose tissue, interstitial myocardium, superimposed valvular fibrous tissue and rarely in the mural endocardial fibrous plaques. The ground substance, which is positive for Rinehart stain, lies between the open spaces and the spindle-shaped fibroblasts. These latter cells have elongated densely eosinophilic anisotropic cytoplasm which takes the periodic acid-Schiff and diastase-periodic acid-Schiff stains. Cosh et al. [*13*] described three patients in whom electron microscopic examination of the endocardial fibrous plaques was performed. Their findings indicate that the carcinoid plaques are composed of a material which is consistent in its features with young collagen. To our knowledge the carcinoid fibrous plaques have not been analyzed chemically.

Distribution of the Fibrous Deposits. Right-sided cardiac lesions: The curious atypical fibrous tissue is limited in the majority of instances to the right side of the heart. When the pulmonic valve is involved, the fibrous tissue is deposited almost entirely on the arterial aspect of the pulmonic valve cusps, sometimes contacting the

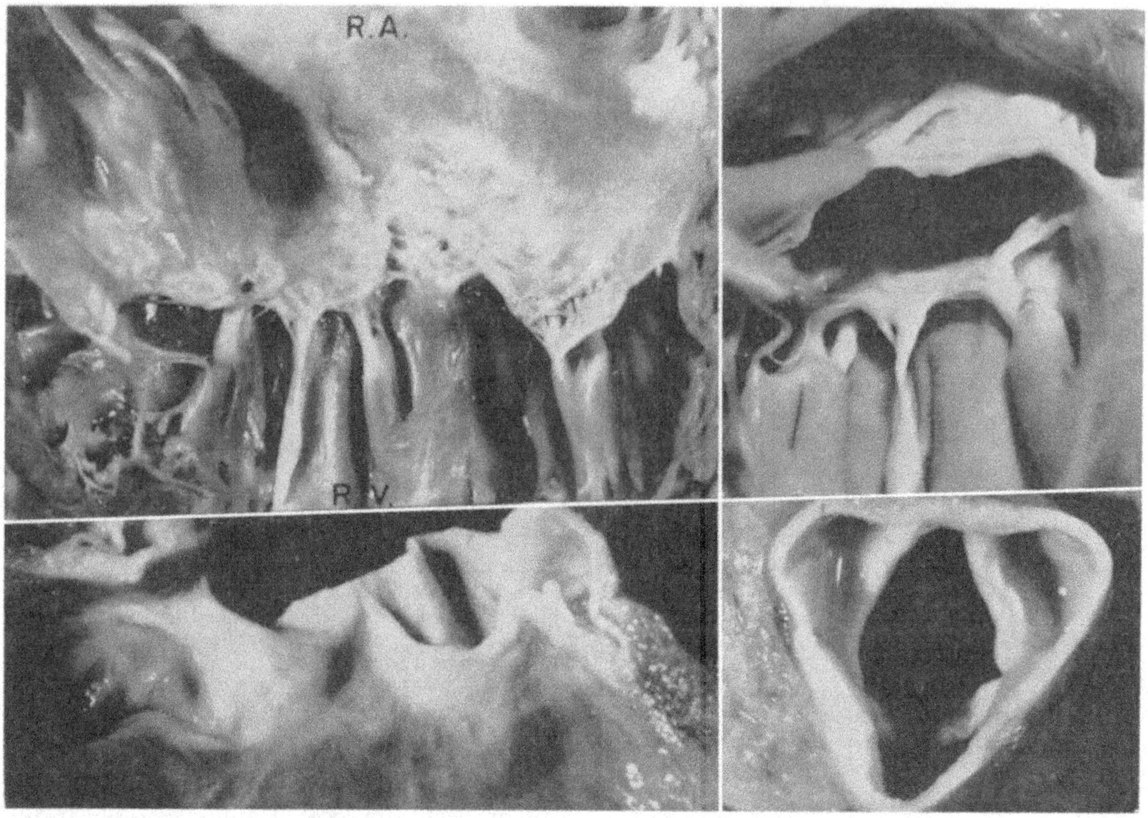

FIG. 10. Case IX. Interior of the heart showing severe carcinoid fibrosis of the tricuspid and pulmonic valves. *Upper left,* the right atrium (R.A.), tricuspid valve, involved by carcinoid fibrosis, and right ventricle (R.V.). The cardiac chambers on the right side are dilated but free of carcinoid plaques. *Upper right,* tricuspid valve as viewed from the right ventricle. The orifice is regurgitant. *Lower left,* pulmonic valve opened. The cusps are thick but the commissures are not fused. *Lower right,* pulmonic valve from above prior to opening. The orifice is rigid. The predominant functional derangement is probably regurgitation although some degree of stenosis is present as well.

intima of the pulmonary trunk. The fibrotic process causes infolding of the distal portion of the valvular cusp toward the sinus of the valve. When the posterior and septal leaflets of the tricuspid valve are involved, the fibrous tissue is located predominately on the ventricular aspect of the leaflets, frequently rigidly adhering the leaflets to the underlying ventricular wall. When the anterior tricuspid leaflet is involved, the fibrous tissue is deposited on the atrial as well as on the ventricular aspects of the leaflet and approximately in equal amounts. The fibrous tissue constricts the pulmonic and tricuspid valves, eventually producing fixed valvular orifices. The pulmonic valve becomes predominantly stenotic, although some regurgitation usually also occurs since the orifice is more or less the same size throughout both phases of the cardiac cycle. Despite the narrowing of its annulus, the tricuspid valve is usually fixed in a wide open position, and thus the predominant functional derangement produced is regurgitation although an element of stenosis generally is present as well. It is apparent that the basic process involving both valves is similar but that the size of the natural orifice of each determines the eventual predominant functional alteration. Thus, since the pulmonic valve orifice is small initially, the contracting process leads to stenosis. The tricuspid valve ring initially is large and, although it becomes contracted, stenosis is usually not the predominant lesion produced. An effective means of producing chronic right-sided cardiac failure in the experimental animal is by making the pulmonic valve stenotic and the tricuspid valve regurgitant [*14*]. It is, therefore, apparent why right-sided congestive failure may be a prominent problem in patients with carcinoid heart diseases.

The atypical fibrous deposits, which we prefer to call "carcinoid fibrous plaques," are commonly seen on the endocardial surface of the right atrium and ventricle as well as on the

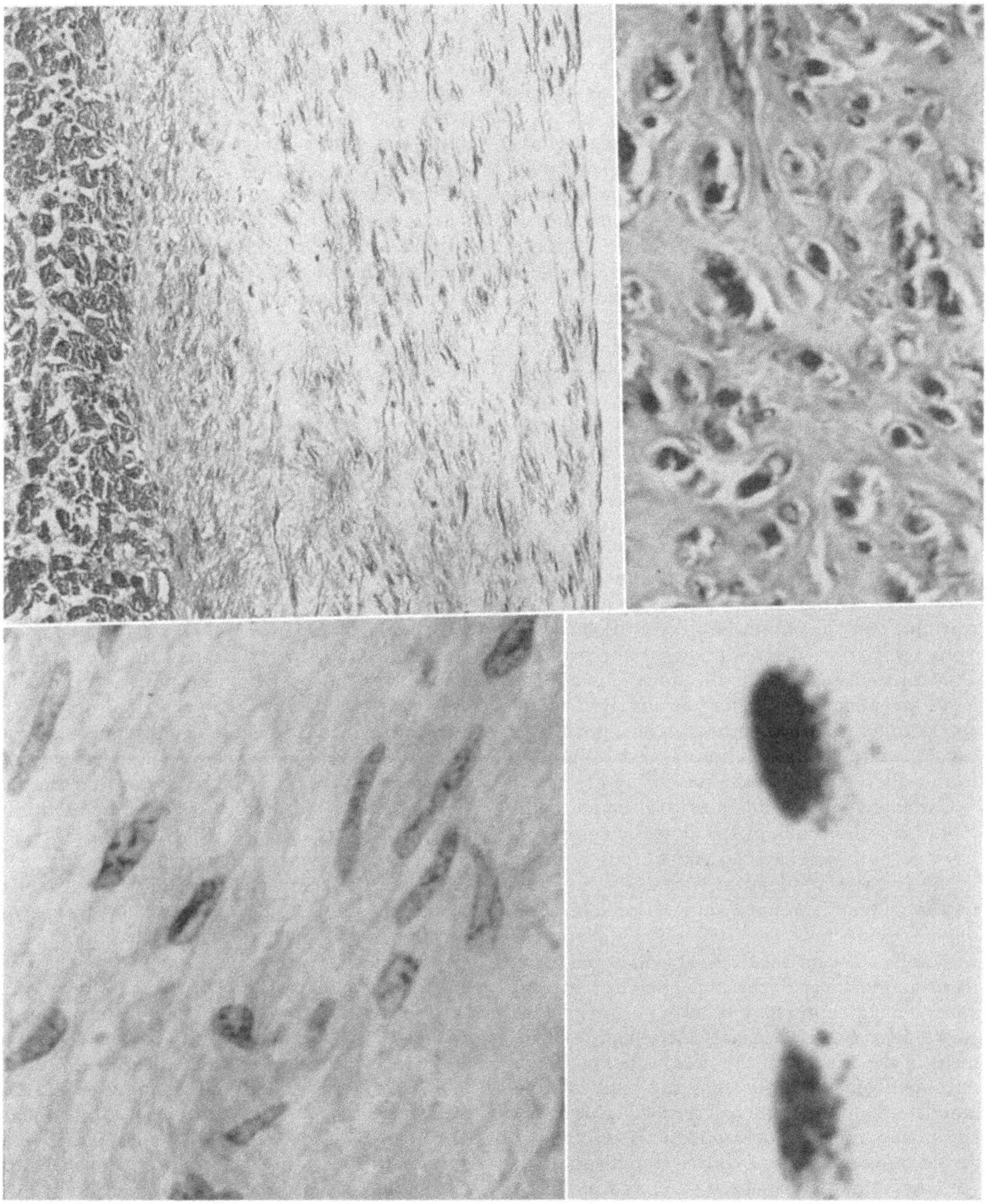

FIG. 11. The carcinoid fibrous plaque. *Upper left,* a mural plaque. The cells are arranged parallel to the surface (on the right), which is covered by cells similar to those in the interior of the plaque. The ground substance between the cells is evident. The underlying myocardium (to the left) is apparent. Hematoxylin and eosin stain, original magnification × 140. *Lower left,* close-up view of the spindle-shaped cells (fibroblasts) within the plaque. Hematoxylin and eosin stain, original magnification × 830. *Upper right,* toluidine blue stain of a plaque showing the "open spaces" which contain hyperchromatic nuclei. Original magnification × 830. *Lower right,* mast cells which are readily seen in the plaques adjacent to the endocardium of the chamber or valve or adjacent to the intima of the vessels. These cells also are present in the underlying myocardium and in the overlying subepicardial adipose tissue. Toluidine blue stain, original magnification × 2,080.

pulmonic and tricuspid valvular leaflets. The plaques are smooth, glistening and whitish gray elevations, which are usually focally distributed, although sometimes diffuse. The plaques appear to be preferentially located in areas of excessive turbulence of blood or in the paths of regurgitant streams. These lesions, therefore, are seen most commonly on the atrial septum immediately above the junction of the septal and anterior tricuspid valvular leaflets and in the right atrial appendage. When the tricuspid valve is involved by carcinoid fibrosis, plaques almost always are present in the right atrium as well.

Fibrous plaques in the right ventricle are less extensive than in the right atrium. Here they frequently are located on the papillary muscles, having extended down the chordae tendineae from the tricuspid valve. In one patient (Case v) the plaquing in the right ventricle was diffuse. Carcinoid fibrous lesions have not been reported in the right atrium or right ventricle unless the tricuspid or pulmonic valves also were involved. In the formalin-fixed hearts the fibrous carcinoid plaques overlying atrial or ventricular endocardium can sometimes be neatly displaced or "plucked" from the underlying endocardium. This procedure is difficult, however, on the fresh specimen. Also, since the involvement of the cardiac valves by this fibrous process is usually diffuse, this technic is not advisable from a therapeutic standpoint during life.

Carcinoid fibrous plaques are found commonly on the intima of the systemic veins. We have seen these characteristic fibrous deposits in the superior and inferior vena cavae, innominate vein and coronary sinus. The lesions in these regions may be attributable to contact with inferior vena caval blood which has been regurgitated through the incompetent tricuspid valve during ventricular systole.

Left-Sided Cardiac Lesions. Carcinoid involvement of the left side of the heart is less common than involvement of the right side but probably more common than generally realized. Many reports have appeared describing various changes in the mitral and aortic valves in patients with the carcinoid syndrome and carcinoid plaquing in the right side of the heart. In probably the first patient described with metastasizing carcinoid syndrome, flushes, diarrhea and endocardial fibrosis, Scholte [*2*] described "irregular, sharply limited, greyish-white, elevated areas" on the endocardium of the anterior mitral leaflet and left ventricle as well as on the endocardium of the pulmonic and tricuspid valves, right atrium and ventricle, and on the intima of the superior vena cava. In one of the patients (Case III) with the malignant carcinoid syndrome described by Isler and Hedinger [*9*] there was "severe fibrosing endocarditis" of the mitral as well as of the tricuspid and pulmonic valves. Of the two patients with the carcinoid syndrome described by Bean and co-workers [*15*], one had "thickening and sclerosis" of all four cardiac valves with "contraction" of the pulmonic and aortic valves, and the other had "valvulitis involving all cardiac valves, most marked in the pulmonic and tricuspid valves." Hand et al. [*16*] mentioned "thickening of the free edge and chordae tendineae of the mitral valve" in addition to typical carcinoid plaques on the pulmonic and tricuspid valves in still another patient with the carcinoid syndrome. These investigators also found changes, similar to those on the endocardium, on the intima of the pulmonary and renal vessels, and in the vessels in the vicinity of the carcinoid tumor. Bean and Funk [*17*] described yet another patient with malignant carcinoid and "lesions on the mitral and, to less degree, the aortic valve similar to" those in the tricuspid and pulmonic valves. Other patients with the syndrome have been described in whom focal thickening or fibrosis occurred on valves on the left side of the heart [*10,18–25*]. In no patient referred to by the authors was a defect in the cardiac septum described. It is probable that in some of these patients the valvular abnormalities on the left side were the result of carcinoid fibrosis, but it is not possible to rule out some other type of cardiac disease, particularly rheumatic, as being responsible.

There remain, to our knowledge, only three described patients in whom there is unequivocal evidence of carcinoid fibrosis on the left side of the heart, and in two others there was probably left-sided carcinoid plaquing. One of the three patients, a sixty-eight year old woman described by McKusick [*21*], had typical focal fibrous deposits on the endocardium of the mitral valve, aortic valve, left ventricle and possibly on the intima of the renal arteries in addition to the more severe ones involving the pulmonic and tricuspid valves, right atrium and ventricle. This patient, whose primary carcinoid tumor was located in the ileum, had a foramen ovale-type atrial septal defect (1.5 cm. in diameter). A similar patient, a seventy year old man, described by Fischer and Lindeneg [26], also had carcinoid plaquing involving the mitral and aortic valves in addition to more extensive deposits on the pulmonic valve, tricuspid valve, right atrium and inferior vena cava. This patient, whose primary carcinoid was situated in the ileum, also had an intracardiac communication, a "slit-like foramen ovale measuring 1 cm. in length." Von Bernheimer and associates [25] described a patient with a nonmetastasizing "clinically active" bronchial carcinoid, in whom there was carcinoid fibrous plaquing of the local pulmonary veins which drained the carcinoid tumor, and of the mitral and aortic valves and coronary arteries, without involvement of the cardiac valves or chambers on the right side. This latter patient thus had isolated left-sided cardiac lesions and appears to be the only one described with this unique distribution. Of all other described patients with clinically active primary bronchial carcinoid tumors proved at autopsy [27–37], none had carcinoid fibrous lesions on the left side, and only three [32,34,37] had endocardial abnormalities on the right side, none of which were unequivocally carcinoid in type. Davies [23] illustrated a mildly thickened mitral valve in a patient with the carcinoid syndrome who also had "capping of the papillary muscle" in the left ventricle, but no information regarding histologic studies was given. A patient with malignant carcinoid recently described by Wolfe et al. [24] had "early thickening of the edges of the mitral valve, and white capping of the papillary muscle" of the left ventricle. This patient had a defect in the atrial septum, a "small" patent foramen ovale.

Three of the nine patients with carcinoid heart disease in the present series had unequivocal carcinoid fibrous plaquing in the left side of the heart in addition to that occurring in the right side. In two patients (Cases VI and VIII) the mitral valve was diffusely involved by the carcinoid fibrous process, and in the third (Case VII) a focal carcinoid plaque was present on the ventricular aspect of the anterior mitral leaflet. The leaflets and chordae tendineae of the valve in the two former patients were shortened, thickened and grossly resembled rheumatic mitral disease. On histologic study of sections through this valve in these two patients, however, the characteristic fibrous tissue devoid of elastic fibers was present, being superimposed on the valvular cusps. The deposition was limited to the ventricular aspect of the posterior leaflet but was present in approximately equal amounts on the two surfaces of the anterior mitral leaflet. The primary tumor in each of these three patients was located in the small intestine, and in none was there an intracardiac communication, a pulmonary arteriovenous fistula or a carcinoid tumor in the lung. Thus, these three patients represent the first proved examples of carcinoid heart disease involving the left side of the heart, as well as the right side, in patients with primary intestinal carcinoid tumors without right to left shunts. In one patient (Case VII) there were typical carcinoid plaques in the aorta as well as on the mitral valve. We are not aware of any previous report describing carcinoid plaquing in the aorta. The aortic plaques in this patient were usually superimposed on atheromas, which appeared whitish grey rather than yellow. In no patient in the present series was there carcinoid plaquing of the aortic valve or of the pulmonary arteries or veins. There was minimal carcinoid plaquing of the left atrium in Case VI. These lesions, however, were limited to that portion of the left atrial endocardium immediately above the mitral valvular annulus. We are not aware of any previous report describing carcinoid fibrous lesions in the left atrium, and in only one [21] is aortic valve involvement well described or illustrated, and in this instance it consisted only of "mild change in one aortic cusp." In Case VI the patient had a 0.6 cm. sized nodule on one cusp of the aortic valve, but it bore no resemblance to endocardial fibrosis of the carcinoid type. Nodules of calcium were present on the aortic valvular cusps in Case III. In two patients (Cases VI and VII) there were focal carcinoid plaques on the endocardium of the left ventricle. In one (Case VII) there was only "white capping" of the left ventricular papillary muscles, and in the other (Case VI) only a rare plaque on the mural endocardium.

Differentiation from other cardiac diseases: Cardiac involvement in malignant carcinoid is specific and bears little resemblance to other types of cardiac disease. MacDonald and Robbins [12] compared the cardiac lesions of carcinoid syndrome to those of rheumatic heart disease, congenital pulmonic stenosis, congenital fibroelastosis, bacterial and nonbacterial thrombotic endocarditis and various collagen diseases. These investigators, and we have confirmed their findings, found the cardiac lesions in the carcinoid syndrome unlike those in any of these other conditions. In rheumatic heart disease the involvement is principally on the left side of the heart, and when the tricuspid and pulmonic valves are involved the mitral or the mitral and aortic valves are almost invariably involved as well. In rheumatic valvular disease the scarring involves the valvular cusp itself, with deposition of densely eosinophilic masses of fibrous tissue within the cusp. There are also strands of elastic fibers within this fibrous stroma. Likewise, in congenital pulmonic stenosis a few elastic fibrils are present within the valvular cusp. Congenital fibroelastosis presents no problem in differentiation since the thickened endocardium in this instance contains a great number of elastic fibers. The African heart disease, namely endomyocardial fibrosis, is readily distinguished from the carcinoid fibrous plaques, in that the structure and location of the lesions are different [*38*]. In this disease the endocardial fibrosis generally begins at the apex of the ventricles, spreads to the atrioventricular valves and spares the semilunar valves. The lesions in the right side of the heart are usually less extensive than those in the left, and isolated right ventricular involvement is unusual. Superimposed thrombi and vegetations are common, and strands of fibrous tissue penetrate the underlying myocardium to varying depths. So called "jet lesions" are distinguished readily from the carcinoid plaques in that these lesions contain a number of elastic fibers and are more frequently present in the left side of the heart except in ventricular septal defect with a left to right shunt. The cardiac lesions of the collagen diseases are generally vascular and myocardial in location and bear no resemblance to the carcinoid plaques. Atypical verrucal endocarditis presents no problem in differentiation from the carcinoid plaque.

Clinical Correlation. Physical findings: The diagnosis of carcinoid heart disease is usually readily established by physical examination. The most characteristic sign of cardiac disease in a patient with the carcinoid syndrome is the presence of a precordial murmur. This was found in all nine patients with endocardial carcinoid fibrosis in the present study. The most frequent murmur in this disease is fairly harsh in quality, grade 1 to 4/6 in intensity, systolic in time and located along the upper left sternal border. This murmur is generally interpreted to represent valvular pulmonic stenosis. The diagnosis of tricuspid valvular disease by clinical examination has proved to be more difficult. A systolic blowing murmur, which became accentuated during inspiration, was audible along the lower left sternal border in only two of the nine patients with carcinoid heart disease described herein. The other patients in this series who were found to have tricuspid insufficiency at autopsy, clinically did not have a precordial murmur which increased in intensity with inspiration. In neither of the two patients with carcinoid mitral involvement was the diagnosis of left-sided valvular disease established prior to autopsy. The cardiac murmurs in the three patients with malignant carcinoid but no heart disease (Table II) were of a nonspecific nature, and none suggested organic valvular involvement. The murmurs in each of these three patients may have been on the basis of anemia (hemoglobin 10 gm. per cent or less in each). It has been noted previously [*39*] that the cardiac murmurs and sounds tend to increase in intensity during the flushing episodes. A rare patient with carcinoid heart disease may have an audible murmur only during cutaneous flushes. The intensity of the cardiac murmur also appears to increase as the disease progresses (Case II). A precordial lift, right ventricular in type, and a systolic thrill often are palpable in these patients.

Supportive evidence for the presence of carcinoid heart disease is obtained by examination of the neck veins and the liver. The superficial jugular veins in the upright position are distended in the majority of these patients, and frequently V waves and occasionally A waves are clearly discernible. A pulsatile liver, confirmative evidence for the presence of tricuspid regurgitation, is present in some patients. However, as pointed out by Thorson [*18*], "cyanosis," hepatomegaly, peripheral edema, ascites, dyspnea and distended systemic veins are not diagnostic of valvular heart disease in patients with the carcinoid syndrome. These signs may result simply from hepatic enlargement secondary to metastatic carcinoid. The intrahepatic metastases may produce portal hypertension which in turn may lead to ascites and peripheral edema, and the large liver may displace the diaphragms, leading to dyspnea. Hypoproteinemia is commonly present in patients with the carcinoid syndrome, and this also may contribute to development of peripheral manifestations of cardiac failure.

Roentgenographic findings: Routine roentgenologic examination of the chest appears to be of little value in determining the presence or absence of carcinoid heart disease. Carcinoid involvement of the heart in itself rarely produces significant thickening of the wall of a cardiac chamber, although histological sections from the right atrium and ventricle usually show hypertrophy of many of the myocardial fibers. If the size of the heart is increased in a patient with the carcinoid syndrome, an associated cardiac disease unrelated to carcinoid should be suspected. The right side of the heart in these patients, however, is frequently dilated to a mild or moderate degree. Poststenotic dilatation of the pulmonary trunk appears not to be a feature of the roentgenogram in patients with carcinoid heart disease.

Electrocardiographic findings: The electrocardiogram is rarely of benefit in determining the presence or absence of carcinoid cardiac disease. The most frequent electrocardiographic abnormality is probably low voltage [*18*], and this was observed in four of our nine patients. Its mechanism is unclear. Pericardial effusion (150 ml.) occurred in only one of four patients with low voltage in the present series, and none had frank pericarditis, although small foci of round cells (primarily lymphocytes) were seen in the subepicardial adipose tissue immediately beneath the visceral pericardium in several patients studied. Prominent P waves suggesting right atrial enlargement occur occasionally. Electrocardiographic evidence of right ventricular hypertrophy was absent in all nine patients with involvement of the heart in this series, and only one had right axis deviation. Right bundle branch block, right ventricular strain, S-T segment depression and flattening of the T waves have been recorded in patients with carcinoid heart disease by others [*18*]. In summary, the electrocardiographic changes in carcinoid heart disease generally are nonspecific.

Hemodynamic findings: Relatively few patients with the carcinoid syndrome have undergone cardiac catheterization [*8,22,40–45*], and studies reported thus far have been limited to the right side of the heart. Tricuspid insufficiency has been the most common hemodynamic alteration reported in patients with carcinoid valvular disease [*8,40,42–44*], followed by pulmonic stenosis [*22,43,44*]. The least common lesion described has been tricuspid stenosis [*22,44*]. V waves up to 34 mm. Hg have been recorded in the right atrium (Case IV). The highest end-diastolic gradient reported across the tricuspid valve was 9 mm. Hg [*22*]. Minimal pulmonary arterial hypertension was found in one patient, described by Charms et al. [*42*], who also had significant valvular disease (tricuspid regurgitation). Arterial oxygen saturation is usually slightly below normal.

An intriguing hemodynamic aspect of the carcinoid syndrome concerns the state of the cardiac output. Recently, Schwaber and Lukas [*45*] reported elevated cardiac outputs in two patients with "metastatic carcinoid and the typical flush syndrome." Neither of these patients had hemodynamic evidence or, in one, necropsy evidence of right-sided valvular cardiac disease. The cardiac outputs were elevated even more during a flush or during exercise than at rest. These authors, in addition, briefly described two further patients with metastatic carcinoid and elevated urinary excretion of 5-hydroxyindoleacetic acid who did "not manifest chronic cutaneous erythema or repeated episodes of flushing." Cardiac outputs in each of these patients, neither of whom had hemodynamic evidence of right-sided valvular heart disease, were low normal. These authors attributed the hyperkinemia in the two patients with chronic cutaneous erythema to the cardiovascular effects of serotonin and concluded that hyperkinemia of itself may contribute to the high incidence of cardiac failure in the carcinoid syndrome. A patient examined earlier with malignant carcinoid, described by Schneckloth et al. [*41*], also was found to have an elevated resting cardiac output. There was no apparent evidence of valvular cardiac disease in this patient. In other reports of patients with carcinoid valvular disease the resting cardiac outputs have not been elevated but, indeed, low [*8,22,42*] or, occasionally, normal [*43*]. In a patient described by Goble et al. [*22*], however, the cardiac output, although low at rest, increased to a normal level during a cutaneous flush, returning to the resting level during an attack of wheezing. Thörson [*39*] noted an increase in the amplitude of the ballistographic waves, as well as an increase in the intensity of the cardiac sounds and murmurs, and in the cardiac rate during episodes of cutaneous flushing in four patients with metastasizing carcinoid.

A word of caution seems advisable in regard to cardiac diagnostic procedures in this disease. A patient with the carcinoid syndrome described by Biörck et al. [*8*] died immediately following angiocardiography, and one patient described by Schwaber and Lukas [*45*] died following routine right heart catheterization.

Pathogenesis of the Cardiac Lesions. The pathogenesis of the endocardial carcinoid plaques remains the subject of controversy. The morphologic appearance of the endocardial lesion would suggest that it was the result of the deposition of a material from the blood. That the underlying endocardium, with its internal elastic membrane, remains intact is evidence that the deposition may come from the blood and not from the underlying endocardium or myocardium. The substance which produces the endocardial fibrosis is unknown, but serotonin (5-hydroxytryptamine) has been implicated to play a major role in the pathogenesis of these lesions. This material is presumed to be liberated in greatest quantity from liver metastases. Unless carcinoid metastases to the liver are present or unless there is drainage of carcinoid tumor by routes other than the portal vein, the endocardial carcinoid lesions do not occur [*18*]. The relative scarcity of left-sided cardiac lesions has been explained by the inactivation of serotonin by monoamine oxidase during its passage through the lungs [*22,46*]. If serotonin does indeed play a role in the production of these endocardial plaques, the occurrence of left-sided cardiac lesions in a third of the patients with carcinoid heart disease in the present series would suggest that plasma serotonin is by no means totally inactivated during its passage through the lungs. This conclusion is in support of the earlier observations of Sjoerdsma and associates [*40*] who were unable to detect significant differences between arterial and venous blood levels of serotonin in patients with the carcinoid syndrome.

Efforts to produce the endocardial carcinoid lesions in experimental animals have been unsuccessful with the possible exception of the work of Spatz [*47*] who made guinea pigs tryptophan-deficient or niacin-deficient and then injected serotonin intraperitoneally for six to eight weeks. The endocardial lesions, mainly on the right side, were described as "early" and bore little resemblance to the typical carcinoid plaques seen in man. Spatz suggested, however, that longer-term experiments might be productive of lesions more similar to those found in man. One of the curious features of the endocardial plaques in man, however, is their uniformity of structure. The histologic appearance of the plaques in the same patient is similar, and there is virtually no variation in this structure from one patient to the next. The concept of an "early" endocardial carcinoid plaque does not appear to apply in man.

Although the inability to produce the carcinoid type of cardiac lesion in animals with serotonin is perhaps not surprising, sufficient work has now been carried out to raise considerable doubt about the role of this substance in the pathogenesis of these lesions. The observations in the present series of patients raise further questions in this regard. The present study, for example, showed no significant difference in the urinary levels of 5-hydroxyindoleacetic acid in those patients with carcinoid heart disease and in those without carcinoid cardiac involvement. (Tables I and II.) It appears that the total serotonin production, by the carcinoid tumor and by its metastases, is similar both in patients with carcinoid heart disease and in those without endocardial lesions. The quantity of hepatic metastases and the distribution of metastases in these two groups also were similar. (Tables I and II.) Why one patient with the carcinoid syndrome has endocardial plaquing and why another one does not is difficult to explain.

Thus, in conclusion, the pathogenesis of the endocardial carcinoid lesions remains obscure. Since no definitive evidence has been obtained that serotonin is responsible for the lesions, investigation should also be directed at mechanisms independent of this substance.

SUMMARY

The clinical and pathologic features of seventeen patients with the carcinoid syndrome are reviewed. Nine had carcinoid heart disease. The only clinical feature which distinguished those patients with carcinoid heart disease from those without was the presence of a precordial systolic murmur suggestive of tricuspid regurgitation or pulmonic stenosis. Urinary excretion of 5-hydroxyindoleacetic acid was similar in the two groups. The chest roentgenogram and the electrocardiogram was of no help in determining presence or absence of carcinoid heart disease. Cardiac catheterization in patients with carcinoid heart disease has shown that tricuspid regurgitation and pulmonic stenosis are the most frequent valvular alterations. Cardiac output appears to be increased in some patients who do not have carcinoid cardiac involvement.

The cardiac lesions associated with the carcinoid syndrome were pathognomonic and bore little resemblance to lesions found in other cardiac diseases. Cardiac involvement in the carcinoid syndrome consisted of focal or diffuse collections of a peculiar type of fibrous tissue, which was free of elastic fibers and which was deposited on the endocardium of the valvular cusps, on the endocardium of the cardiac chambers and on the intima of the great veins, coronary sinus and occasionally great arteries. The valvular cusps *per se* remained normal as did the mural endocardium, and each was clearly separated from the fibrosing process by the elastic membrane which covered its surface. Left-sided cardiac lesions were commoner in the carcinoid syndrome than previously thought and were found in the absence of a right to left shunt or a pulmonary carcinoid tumor.

The pathogenesis of the carcinoid cardiac lesions (carcinoid fibrous plaques) remains unknown. The morphologic appearance of the endocardial lesion suggests that it might be the result of the deposition of a material, possibly collagen, from the blood, but the identity of the substance which either directly or indirectly produced the endocardial fibrosis is unknown. The inability to produce these cardiac lesions in animals with serotonin and the present observation that the urinary excretion of 5-hydroxyindoleacetic acid was similar in the patient with carcinoid heart disease irrespective of the presence or absence of cardiac involvement suggest that mechanisms other than that involving serotonin should be considered.

Acknowledgment: We wish to thank the following: Miss Mary Catherine Bowling for the staining of the histologic sections; Mr. Gebhard Gsell for the photomicrographic work; Mr. Kenzie Edwards for the gross photographic work; and Mrs. Katharine Nichols for the labelling of the photographs.

REFERENCES

1. CASSIDY, M. A. Abdominal carcinomatosis with probable adrenal involvement. *Proc. Roy. Soc. Med.*, 24: 139, 1930.
2. SCHOLTE, A. J. Ein Fall von Angioma teleangiectaticum Cutis mit chronischer Endokarditis und malignem Dünndarmcarcinoid. *Beitr. path. Anat.*, 86: 440, 1931.
3. CASSIDY, M. A. Postmortem findings in case shown on October 10, 1930, as one of abdominal carcinomatosis with probable adrenal involvement. *Proc. Roy. Soc. Med.*, 24: 920, 1931.
4. CASSIDY, M. A. Abdominal carcinomatosis associated with vasomotor disturbances. *Proc. Roy. Soc. Med.*, 27: 220, 1934.
5. MILLMAN, S. Tricuspid stenosis and pulmonary stenosis complicating carcinoid of the intestine with metastases to the liver. *Am. Heart J.*, 25: 391, 1943.
6. GOLD, I. R. and GRAYZEL, D. M. Multiple argentaffinomas in ileum with metastases in lymph nodes and in the liver. *Am. J. Surg.*, 60: 144, 1943.
7. CURRENS, J. H., KINNEY, T. D. and WHITE, P. D. Pulmonary stenosis with intact interventricular septum, report of eleven cases. *Am. Heart J.*, 30: 491, 1945.
8. BIÖRCK, G., AXÉN, O. and THÖRSON, Å. Unusual cyanosis in a boy with congenital pulmonary stenosis and tricuspid insufficiency. Fatal outcome after angiocardiography. *Am. Heart J.*, 44: 143, 1952.
9. ISLER, P. and HEDINGER, C. Metastasierendes Dünndarmcarcinoid mit schweren, vorwiegend das rechte Herz betreffenden Klappenfehlern und Pulmonalstenose—ein eigenartiger Symptomenkomplex? *Schweiz. med. Wchnschr.*, 83: 4, 1953.
10. ROSENBAUM, F. F., SANTER, D. G. and CLAUDON, D. B. Essential telangiectasia, pulmonic and tricuspid stenosis, and neoplastic liver disease. A possible new clinical syndrome. (Abstract.) *J. Lab. & Clin. Med.*, 42: 941, 1953.
11. THÖRSON, Å., BIÖRCK, G., BJÖRKMAN, G. and WALDENSTRÖM, J. Malignant carcinoid of the small intestine with metastases to the liver, valvular disease of the heart (pulmonary stenosis and tricuspid regurgitation without septal defects), peripheral vasomotor symptoms, bronchoconstriction, and an unusual type of cyanosis. A clinical and pathologic syndrome. *Am. Heart J.*, 47: 795, 1954.
12. MACDONALD, R. A. and ROBBINS, S. L. Pathology of the heart in the carcinoid syndrome. A comparative study. *Arch. Path.*, 63: 103, 1957.
13. COSH, J., CATES, J. E. and PUGH, D. W. Carcinoid heart disease. *Brit. Heart J.*, 21: 369, 1959.
14. BARGER, A. C., ROE, B. B. and RICHARDSON, G. S. Relation of valvular lesions and of exercise to auricular pressure, work tolerance, and to development of chronic, congestive failure in dogs. *Am. J. Physiol.*, 169: 384, 1952.
15. BEAN, W. B., OLCH, D. and WEINBERG, H. B. The syndrome of carcinoid and acquired valve lesions of the right side of the heart. *Circulation*, 12: 1, 1955.
16. HAND, A. M., MCCORMICK, W. F. and LUMB, G. Malignant carcinoid tumor. A case report with discussion of systemic manifestations. *Am. J. Clin. Path.*, 30: 47, 1958.
17. BEAN, W. B. and FUNK, D. The vasculocardiac syndrome of metastatic carcinoid. *Arch. Int. Med.*, 103: 189, 1959.
18. THÖRSON, Å. H. Studies on carcinoid disease. *Acta med. scandinav.*, supp.: 334, 1958.

19. ALTMAN, V. and MANN, N. Metastasizing carcinoid tumor of the appendix and caecum. *Am. J. Surg.*, 76: 434, 1948.
20. RATZENHOFER, M. and LEMBECK, F. Über den Gehalt an 5-Oxytryptamin in Carcinoiden des Darmtraktes. *Ztschr. Krebsforsch.*, 60: 169, 1954.
21. MCKUSICK, V. A. Carcinoid cardiovascular disease. *Bull. Johns Hopkins Hosp.*, 98: 13, 1956.
22. GOBLE, A. J., HAY, D. R., HUDSON, R. and SANDLER, M. Acquired heart disease with argentaffin carcinoma. *Brit. Heart J.*, 18: 544, 1956.
23. DAVIES, A. J. Carcinoid tumors (Argentaffinomata). *Ann. Roy. Coll. Surgeons England*, 25: 277, 1959.
24. WOLFE, H. R. I., DAVIES, A., MATHIAS, A. P. and SCHACHTER, M. Metastatic argentaffinoma secreting 5-hydroxytryptamine in a patient with a patent foramen ovale. *Brit. M. J.*, 5177: 929, 1960.
25. VON BERNHEIMER, H., EHRINGER, H., HEISTRACHER, P., KRAUPP, O., LACHNIT, V., OBIDITSCH-MAYER, I. and WENZL, M. Biologisch aktives, nicht metastasierendes Bronchuscarcinoid mit Linksherzsyndrom. *Wien. klin. Wchnschr.*, 72: 867, 1960.
26. FISCHER, S. and LINDENEG, O. Cardiac changes in argentaffinomatosis. *Acta path. et microbiol. scandinav.*, 44: 128, 1958.
27. WARNER, R. R. P. and SOUTHREN, A. L. Carcinoid syndrome produced by metastasizing bronchial adenoma. *Am. J. Med.*, 24: 903, 1958.
28. SAUER, W. G., DEARING, W. H. and FLOCK, E. V. Diagnosis and clinical management of functioning carcinoids. *J. A. M. A.*, 168: 139, 1958.
29. SCHNECKLOTH, R. E., MCISAAC, W. M. and PAGE, I. H. Serotonin metabolism in carcinoid syndrome with metastatic bronchial adenoma. *J. A. M. A.*, 170: 1143, 1959.
30. JOSEPH, M. and TAYLOR, R. R. Argentaffinoma of the lung with carcinoid syndrome. *Brit. M. J.*, 2: 568, 1960.
31. WILLIAMS, E. D. and AZZOPARDI, J. G. Tumors of the lung and the carcinoid syndrome. *Thorax*, 15: 30, 1960.
32. GRAMLICH, V. F. and WIETHOFF, E. O. Das Carcinoidsyndrom unter Mitteilung eines metastasierenden Bronchialcarcinoids. *Deutsche. med. Wchnschr.*, 85: 1750, 1960.
33. ANLYAN, W. G., HARGROVE, M. D., RUFFIN, J. M., WALLACE, D. K., WEAVER, W. T. and KIRSHNER, N. Metastasizing bronchial adenoma. *J. A. M. A.*, 174: 415, 1960.
34. VON HÜSSELMANN, H. and WENDT, K. H. Metastasierendes Bronchusadenom vom Karzinoidtyp mit atypischem Carcinoid-syndrom. *München. med. Wchnschr.*, 103: 663, 1961.
35. ESCOVITZ, W. E. and REINGOLD, I. M. Functioning malignant bronchial carcinoid with Cushing's syndrome and recurrent sinus arrest. *Ann. Int. Med.*, 54: 1248, 1961.
36. SANDLER, M., SCHEUER, P. J. and WATT, P. J. 5-hydroxytryptophan-secreting bronchial carcinoid tumor. *Lancet*, 2: 1067, 1961.
37. MCCONAGHIE, R. J. The malignant carcinoid syndrome associated with a metastasizing bronchial adenoma. *J. Thoracic & Cardiovasc. Surg.*, 43: 303, 1962.
38. DAVIES, J. N. P. and BALL, J. D. The pathology of endomyocardial fibrosis in Uganda. *Brit. Heart J.*, 17: 337, 1955.
39. THÖRSON, Å. H. Hemodynamic changes during "flush" in carcinoidosis. (The carcinoid syndrome.) *Am. Heart J.*, 52: 444, 1956.
40. SJOERDSMA, A., WEISSBACH, H., TERRY, L. L. and UDENFRIEND, S. Further observations on patients with malignant carcinoid. *Am. J. Med.*, 23: 5, 1957.
41. SCHNECKLOTH, R., PAGE, I. H., DEL GRECO, F. and CORCORAN, A. C. Effects of serotonin antagonists in normal subjects and patients with carcinoid tumors. *Circulation*, 16: 523, 1957.
42. CHARMS, B. L., KOHN, P., APPLEBAUM, H. I. and GELLER, J. Hemodynamic studies in a case of carcinoid cardiovascular syndrome. *Circulation*, 20: 208, 1959.
43. THORSON, Å. and NORDENFELT, O. Development of valvular lesions in metastatic carcinoid disease. *Brit. Heart J.*, 21: 243, 1959.
44. LEVINE, R. J. and FOLSE, R. Hemodynamic observations in a case of carcinoid heart disease associated with an atrial right-to-left shunt. *Am. Heart J.*, 62: 830, 1961.
45. SCHWABER, J. R. and LUKAS, D. S. Hyperkinemia and cardiac failure in the carcinoid syndrome. *Am. J. Med.*, 32: 846, 1962.
46. BRADLEY, T. R., BUTTERWORTH, R. F., REID, G. and TRAUTNER, E. M. Nature of the lung enzyme which inactivates serum vasoconstrictor. *Nature, London*, 166: 911, 1950.
47. SPATZ, M. Carcinoid syndrome in tryptophan- and niacin-deficient guinea pigs. *Univ. Michigan M. Bull.*, 27: 289, 1961.

APPENDIX

Case Reports

CASE I. A forty-one year old white man (D. W., 01-19-90*) died on March 5, 1957. He had been well until June 1954 when he noted the onset of weight loss, easy fatiguability and diarrhea. In October 1955 acute pain in the right upper quadrant associated with fever and leukocytosis led to an exploratory laparotomy. Both the liver and mesenteric lymph nodes were enlarged and contained metastatic carcinoid. A carcinoid tumor 2 cm. in size was resected from the terminal ileum.

He was first seen at the Clinical Center in January 1956 and since operation had gained weight and strength and was asymptomatic. He weighed 68 kg. and measured 154 cm. in height. His blood pressure was 110/70 mm. Hg. There was no skin erythema. The heart was not enlarged. A short, early, grade 2/6 systolic murmur was heard along the upper left sternal border. The liver was greatly enlarged; the spleen was not felt. There was no ascites or peripheral edema. The chest roentgenogram disclosed an elevated right diaphragm. The electrocardiogram was interpreted to be normal. The urinary excretion of

* The clinical aspects of this case were previously reported by Sjoerdsma et al. [*40*], Case VIII.

5-hydroxyindoleacetic acid ranged from 157 to 192 mg. per 24 hours.

During this three week period of hospitalization facial flushing appeared. Following discharge the flushes increased in length and frequency. Diarrhea, easy fatiguability and abdominal fullness recurred, and in August 1956 he was hospitalized again. Physical findings were unchanged except for loss of weight and a more enlarged liver. The urinary excretion of 5-hydroxyindoleacetic acid now averaged 600 mg. per 24 hours. The electrocardiogram and chest roentgenogram were unchanged. His course was progressively downhill and was not significantly altered by therapy with 6-azouracil or 6-mercaptopurine. Terminally, hypotension and hypoglycemia appeared.

At autopsy (A57-49) he was emaciated, weighing 46 kg. The abdomen was greatly distended by a massively enlarged liver (weight, 7,400 gm.) which was largely replaced by a metastatic carcinoid tumor. Many fibrous adhesions bound loops of bowel to one another, to the undersurface of the liver and to the peritoneal surfaces. No residual tumor was seen in the intestinal tract; however, the mesenteric lymph nodes were large and matted together. The peritoneum was thick and gray, and the abdominal cavity contained 200 ml. of serous fluid.

The heart weighed 220 gm. A firm, white carcinoid tumor 1 cm. in size was present in the parietal pericardium. The carcinoid fibrosing process grossly was limited to the pulmonic valve. Its cusps were thickened, contracted and rigid, and the pulmonic valvular orifice was fixed in a more or less open position. A rare fibrous plaque was seen in the right atrium but not in the right ventricle. Grossly, the tricuspid valvular leaflets and chordae appeared normal, but histologically a few focal fibrous plaques were seen on the leaflets. The right ventricle was mildly dilated but not hypertrophied. The cardiac chambers on the left side and valves were normal. Histologically, metastatic tumor was widespread. (Table I.)

Case II. A fifty year old housewife (E. W., 01-14-46) died on November 18, 1957. She had been well until 1945 (age thirty-eight) when she noted the onset of transient episodes of flushing of the face and neck. These "blushing" attacks were not especially bothersome to her, however, until age forty-seven when they became more frequent and lasted longer. Each of three more severe attacks continued for several hours and was associated with wheezing, dyspnea and facial puffiness. In addition, at this time, diarrhea became apparent, and intermittent abdominal pain led to the discovery of an abdominal mass. Exploratory laparotomy was undertaken two and a half years before death, and multiple ileal tumors which histologically proved to be carcinoid were found along with metastatic deposits in the liver.

When first seen at the Clinical Center six months later (November 1955) she appeared healthy. Her blood pressure was 120/80 mm. Hg. There was marked erythema of the face. The heart was not enlarged, and the sounds were of good quality. A grade 1/6 soft blowing systolic murmur was heard in the second left intercostal space. The lungs were clear. The liver was greatly enlarged, nodular and nontender. The spleen was not palpable. There was no ascites or peripheral edema. Heberden's nodes and spindle-shaped deformities of the first interphalangeal joints were noted, but there was no limitation of motion. The electrocardiogram and chest roentgenogram appeared normal. The urinary excretion of 5-hydroxyindoleacetic acid ranged from 294 to 380 mg. per 24 hours.

Following one week in the hospital she returned home and continued to perform her usual household chores without difficulty until a year later (one year before death) when the diarrhea worsened, abdominal pain intermittently recurred and fatiguability, weight loss, low grade fever, pedal edema and anorexia appeared. An increase in the dosages of paregoric and thorazine, and the initiation of salt restriction and periodic injections of mercurial diuretics allowed her to remain comfortable and fairly active until two months before death when these remedies no longer controlled the signs and symptoms. She was rehospitalized and now showed evidence of marked weight loss. The neck veins were distended with the patient sitting up, and a deep systolic jugular pulsation was noted. A massive right pleural effusion was present. The heart was not enlarged, but the previously described murmur had become much louder and harsher, now of grade 4/6 intensity. In addition, a grade 3/6 early and mid-diastolic murmur also was heard along the lower left sternal border. The liver had enlarged, but no ascitic fluid was apparent. There was severe wasting of the extremities and 2 plus pitting edema of the lower part of the legs. The electrocardiogram showed a slight increase in the magnitude of the T waves as compared to the previous tracings. The chest roentgenogram confirmed the presence of a right pleural effusion. The urinary excretion of 5-hydroxyindoleacetic acid averaged approximately 1,250 mg. per 24 hours during her last two months. Treatment with 6-mercaptopurine failed to be of benefit. She became progressively weaker and died in hepatic failure with a "metabolic flap," jaundice and finally coma.

At autopsy (A57-238) she weighed 38 kg. and measured 158 cm. in length. Three discrete carcinoid tumors were found in the ileum with metastases to the regional, mediastinal and supraclavicular lymph nodes, liver (4,500 gm.), spleen (100 gm.), kidneys, ovary, adrenal and pituitary glands, bone marrow and heart. The abdominal cavity contained 200 ml., the right pleural space 1,000 ml., the left pleural space 1,500 ml. and the pericardial sac 100 ml. of serous fluid. Esophageal varices were present, and the stomach contained material the color of coffee grounds.

The heart weighed 250 gm. A metastatic carcinoid tumor was present in the ventricular septum. All chambers were dilated. The endocardium of the right atrium and the leaflets and chordae of the tricuspid valve were irregularly thickened by the deposition of smooth, white, fibrous tissue. This fibrosis extended irregularly over the papillary muscles of the right ventricle. The pulmonic valvular cusps were contracted and thickened by the deposition of similar fibrous material which produced a small, fixed pulmonic orifice. The sinuses of the pulmonic valve were much smaller than normal. The chambers and valves of the left side of the heart were normal. The right ventricle measured 0.3 cm. and the left, 1.2 cm. in thickness. The valve circumference measurements (in centimeters) were: tricuspid, 10.5; mitral, 10.0; pulmonic, 5.5; and aortic, 6.5.

Histologically, sections from the ileal tumors and from the metastatic implants disclosed carcinoid tumor. There was severe fatty change of the liver. In sections from the heart microscopic-sized carcinoid metastases were seen in the right and left atria, in the subepicardial adipose tissue overlying the right ventricle and in the ventricular septum. Sections from the coronary sinus, right atrium, tricuspid and pulmonic valves, and papillary muscles of the right ventricle confirmed typical carcinoid fibrosis in these regions.

Case iii. A sixty-seven year old white man (G. M., 03-51-98) died on September 30, 1959. He had been well until 1952 (age sixty) when he noted the onset of periodic severe abdominal pain and diarrhea. An exploratory laparotomy in December 1953 revealed metastatic carcinoid in the mesenteric lymph nodes and in the liver. No search was made for the primary tumor. Following recovery from the operation, he returned to work and did well until January 1957 when he began to feel weak. In July 1958 facial flushing appeared. His liver now was greatly enlarged. He was believed to be in mild congestive cardiac failure and was treated thereafter with digitalis and a low salt diet. His weakness progressively worsened, and in January 1959 he had to discontinue working.

On admission to the Clinical Center June 1959, he was thin and appeared chronically ill. His blood pressure was 110/70 mm. Hg. The skin over the face and neck was thickened, erythematous, "cyanotic" and telangiectatic. The skin over the rest of the body and especially over the legs had a faint purple hue which blanched on pressure. Moderate sized A waves were present in the superficial jugular veins, and a systolic pulse was noted in the deep jugular veins. The anteroposterior diameter of the chest was increased, and occasional wheezes were heard. The heart sounds were distant. A short, high-pitched presystolic murmur, which strikingly increased in intensity with inspiration, was heard along the lower left sternal border. This murmur was discrete and terminated prior to the first sound. In addition, there was a loud systolic murmur in the same area, which began early after the first sound and did not increase with inspiration. After mild exercise a protodiastolic gallop was heard along the left sternal border. The liver was greatly enlarged, nodular and nontender. The spleen was not felt, and there was no ascites or peripheral edema. The electrocardiogram was normal. Chest roentgenogram disclosed a normal-sized heart and normal appearing lungs. His course, unaltered by dichloromethotrexate therapy, was progressively downhill; he became confused, comatose and died.

At autopsy (A59-192) he weighed 66 kg. and measured 183 cm. in length. The skin, particularly over the upper half of the body, was purple. The peritoneal cavity contained 700 ml., the left pleural space, 1000 ml., and the pericardial sac 50 ml. of serous fluid. The ileum, particularly in its distal portion, was matted together and bound to a large retroperitoneal mass which represented matted lymph nodes. Metastatic carcinoid tumor was seen in the mesenteric lymph nodes, as well, and also in the appendix and liver (2,500 gm.). Multiple carcinoid tumors, the largest of which measured 2.0 cm. in diameter, were present in the ileum. The largest ileal tumor burrowed through the bowel wall and was adherent to the omentum, mesentery and to other loops of small intestine and produced a partial intestinal obstruction.

The heart weighed 280 gm. and there was typical carcinoid fibrosis involving the tricuspid and pulmonic valves, right atrium and ventricle. The right atrium was dilated and its endocardium was smooth, thickened and whitish grey in appearance. The tricuspid valve leaflets and its chordae were shortened and thickened. The wall of the right ventricle measured up to 0.3 cm. in thickness, and the chamber was dilated. The three pulmonic valvular cusps were markedly thickened, rigid and contracted and the valve orifice stenotic. The valves and chambers of the left side of the heart were normal. There was moderate atherosclerosis of the coronary arteries.

Case iv. A fifty-nine year old white man (K. W., 01-04-45*) died on November 7, 1959. He had been well except for pulmonary tuberculosis, treated by pneumothorax from 1923 to 1926, until 1953 when he noted the onset of intermittent, explosive diarrhea, increasing fatiguability and weight loss. Erythematous flushes of the face and neck appeared in July 1954 and were noted daily thereafter. Needle biopsy of the liver in November 1954 was thought to show

* The clinical aspects of this case were previously reported by Sjoerdsma et al. [*40*], Case iii.

"hepatoma." On exploration the following month, a segment of distal ileum containing two small carcinoid tumors was resected. Extensive metastatic carcinoid was seen in the liver. The flushes and diarrhea continued unabated. During 1955 dependent ankle edema and paroxysmal respiratory distress, characterized by a slightly productive cough, dyspnea and substernal oppression, appeared.

On admission to the Clinical Center April 1955, he weighed 77.1 kg.; his blood pressure was 115/80 mm. Hg. He appeared well but had frequent transient crimson flushes of the face and neck and blotchy erythema of the trunk and extremities. A and V waves were noted in the superficial jugular veins, and systolic pulsations were seen in the deep jugular veins. Wheezes were audible over both lung fields during paroxysms of cough and dyspnea. The heart was not enlarged, and the heart sounds were normal. A soft systolic blowing murmur, which increased in intensity with inspiration, was heard along the lower left sternal border. The upper part of the abdomen was protuberant, the liver extremely large and nodular. Vasomotor episodes were induced repeatedly by manual massage over the liver. The spleen was not felt. There was 2 plus pedal and pretibial pitting edema.

The chest roentgenogram showed extensive pleural and parenchymal changes in the right hemithorax and a slightly enlarged heart. On cardiac fluoroscopy the right atrium was believed to be enlarged. The electrocardiograms were interpreted as normal. Right cardiac catheterization revealed elevated pressures in the right atrium with V waves up to 34 mm. Hg, and a pressure curve typical of tricuspid insufficiency. The A waves were also elevated and tricuspid stenosis was suspected as well, but the catheter could not be passed through the tricuspid valvular orifice. Peripheral arterial oxygen saturation was 95 per cent. The urinary 5-hydroxyindoleacetic acid assays during his seventy-four days in the hospital ranged from 380 to 580 mg. per 24 hours.

In August 1955 the flushes increased in severity, his abdomen increased in size, his ankles and lower legs swelled, and his strength lessened. These signs were improved greatly by diuretic therapy and a single abdominal paracentesis. Thereafter, until his final hospitalization in October 1959, his peripheral edema and abdominal swelling were well controlled by a low salt diet and periodic treatment with diuretics. The diarrhea was well controlled by the administration of paregoric. Physical examination on readmission was unchanged except for a slightly large liver. Electrocardiogram now showed low voltage and right axis deviation. Chest roentgenogram disclosed a left pleural effusion and probably an increase in cardiac size in addition to the changes noted previously. On November 6, 1959, eighteen days following admission, early one morning while sitting on the bedpan, he suddenly collapsed, became hypotensive and comatose. Repeat electrocardiograms showed only bigeminal rhythm and frequent premature ventricular contractions. The following day he died.

At autopsy (A59-223), he weighed 56 kg. and measured 183 cm. in length. The skin over the face, neck and upper anterior chest had a purplish discoloration. The abdomen was protuberant, and there was 2 plus pitting edema of the lower part of the legs. The peritoneal cavity contained excessive fluid. The peritoneum and serosal surface of the bowel were thickened. At the ileoileal anastomosis, two feet proximal to the ileocecal valve, there was a small carcinoid tumor. No other tumor was seen in the intestine except for a small nodule on the serosal surface of the appendix. The liver (1,800 gm.) contained numerous carcinoid implants. No other metastases were seen.

The heart weighed 350 gm. Focal fibrous plaques, carcinoid type, were present on the intima of both the superior and inferior vena cavae. Both the right atrium and ventricle were dilated. The foramen ovale was probe-patent but valvular-competent. The endocardium of the right atrium was thickened, smooth and whitish grey. The tricuspid valvular cusps and chordae were thickened, shortened and fibrotic. This valve measured 15 cm. in circumference and easily admitted three fingers. Only one small endocardial plaque was seen in the right ventricle. Its wall measured 0.4 cm. in thickness. The pulmonary valvular cusps were contracted, shortened and fibrotic, and the orifice, although contracted, was fixed in an open position. The chambers and valves of the left side of the heart were normal. There was severe coronary arterial atherosclerosis.

Case v. A fifty-seven year old white woman (S. W., 09-97-07) died on February 22, 1961. She had been well until 1957 when intermittent diarrhea (eight to ten watery movements daily) and pedal edema appeared. On examination she was found to have cardiomegaly and hepatomegaly. In 1959, one to one and a half years later, she noted periodic wheezing and dyspnea. Nine months thereafter facial flushing and abdominal pain of the right upper quadrant appeared. From 1957 to 1960 her weight decreased from 118 to 82 kg.

On admission to the Clinical Center in May 1960, she was still obese. Her blood pressure was 170/100 mm. Hg. Her face and neck were plethoric and contained telangiectases. No abnormal pulsations were seen in the superficial or deep jugular veins. The anteroposterior diameter of the chest was increased. Breath sounds were distant, but no wheezes were heard. A faint right ventricular lift was felt. The first heart sound at the apex was diminished, but an atrial sound was heard at the lower left sternal border during deep inspiration. A grade 2/6 systolic blowing murmur, which did not increase with inspiration, and an early diastolic rumble without presystolic accentuation, were heard along the lower left sternal border. The liver was markedly enlarged; the spleen was not felt. There was 2 plus pitting edema of the lower part of the legs.

The chest roentgenogram showed the heart to be slightly enlarged and the aorta, tortuous. Electrocardiograms demonstrated normal sinus rhythm, digitalis effect and prolongation of the P-R interval. A gastrointestinal series of the upper part of the gastrointestinal tract disclosed a "markedly irritable" small intestine. The urinary determinations of 5-hydroxyindoleacetic acid varied from 161 to 283 mg. per day during her 117 days in the hospital. She was treated with methyl-dopa, isoniazid and cyproheptidine without detectable benefit.

Following discharge in September 1960 and until her final admission four months later, she noted increasing dyspnea, edema and weight gain despite diuretic and digitalis therapy. The flushes and intermittent abdominal pains persisted. She was readmitted on January 25, 1961, and the physical findings, other than evidence of increased edema and hepatomegaly, were unchanged. On February 21, bronchopneumonia developed, and she died the following day.

At autopsy (A61-68) she was obese (weight 60.6 kg., height 141 cm.). The body cavities contained no excessive fluid. A carcinoid tumor 0.8 cm. in size was present immediately proximal to the ileocecal valve. Other carcinoid nodules were present in the periappendiceal, omental and mesenteric tissues, liver (2300 gm.), kidney and thyroid gland. Carcinoid nodules, microscopically, also were seen in the gallbladder. The lungs were congested and contained foci of bronchopneumonia.

The heart (Fig. 1) weighed 270 gm. The right atrium and ventricle were dilated and their walls "brittle-like" in consistency. The endocardium of the right atrium and right ventricle, tricuspid and pulmonic valves was diffusely involved by the carcinoid fibrosing process. The valves and chambers of the left side of the heart appeared normal.

Case vi. A sixty-four year old white man (B. E., 03-61-20) died on August 12, 1961. He had been well until approximately 1956 when angina pectoris developed which thereafter was present intermittently. In 1958 he noted the onset of weight loss, and during the next three years his weight decreased from 70 to 50 kg. On May 9, 1960, he had an attack of prolonged substernal chest pain not relieved by nitroglycerin treatment and associated with severe weakness and dyspnea, and was hospitalized for two weeks. The following month pedal and sacral edema and occasional paroxysmal nocturnal dyspnea appeared, but these were ameliorated by diuretic therapy. Also, in June 1960, he noted the onset of diarrhea (four to eight bowel movements daily), periodic flushes of the face and upper trunk, intermittent severe abdominal cramps and weakness. In January 1961, on examination at another hospital, he was found to have hepatomegaly and elevated urinary excretion of 5-hydroxyindoleacetic acid.

On admission to the Clinical Center June 13, 1961, he appeared weak and undernourished. The blood pressure was 130/80 mm. Hg. There was a marked reddish blue discoloration of the nose and malar areas of the face, hands, arms, feet and lower part of the legs. V waves were seen in the superficial jugular veins. The lungs were clear. The heart was enlarged, the point of maximal impulse being in the fifth left intercostal space in the left anterior axillary line. Right and left ventricular precordial lifts were palpated. The first heart sound at the apex was normal. The second heart sound over the aortic area was louder than the second heart sound over the pulmonary area and paradoxically split. A protodiastolic gallop was heard at the apex and along the lower left sternal border, and a loud ejection sound was heard at the lower left sternal border. A grade 2/6 short, soft systolic murmur was audible at the base and a grade 3/6 ejection-type systolic murmur, at the apex and along the left sternal border. Also, a grade 2/6 low-pitched diastolic murmur was present at the apex, and a similar but higher pitched diastolic rumble, which increased in intensity with inspiration, along the lower left sternal border. The abdomen was distended. The liver was large, nontender and nodular. There was 3 plus pitting edema of the lower part of the legs. The urinary excretion of 5-hydroxyindoleacetic acid averaged approximately 350 mg. per 24 hours. The electrocardiogram showed only low voltage. Chest roentgenogram revealed slight left ventricular hypertrophy. The gastrointestinal series of the upper part of the gastrointestinal tract and the small bowel series as well as a barium enema were interpreted to be normal.

During his two months in the hospital, the abdominal cramps, diarrhea and flushing episodes continued. He was treated by a salt restricted diet, intermittent diuretics, opiates and two experimental chemotherapeutic agents (methyl-dopa and MK-485) without significant benefit. During the final five weeks his condition rapidly deteriorated. The abdominal pains became severe, and right-sided congestive cardiac failure became evident. He died in hepatic coma.

At autopsy (A61-193) he weighed 50 kg. and measured 138 cm. in length. There was no excessive fluid in the body cavities. The small intestine from the ligament of Treitz to the ileocecal valve, following formalin-fixation, measured 3.1 M. in length. Twelve distinct, firm, white carcinoid tumors were found in the small intestine beginning 147 cm. distal to the ligament of Treitz and ending 75 cm. proximal to the ileocecal valve; the largest measured 2 cm. in diameter, the smallest 0.4 cm. in diameter. Some of the tumors were centrally ulcerated. The serosal surface beneath the tumors was smooth. There was no evidence of bowel obstruction. The liver (1,600 gm.), mesenteric lymph nodes and pancreas contained metastatic carcinoid. The spleen weighed 160 gm., and its surface had a "frost-like" appearance.

The heart weighed 400 gm. All chambers were dilated and hypertrophied. There was severe fibrous involvement, carcinoid type, of the mitral valve as well as of the pulmonic and tricuspid valves and right atrium (Fig. 2 and 3). There was no intracardiac communication. The tricuspid valve appeared incompetent, the pulmonic and mitral valves stenotic. The pulmonic valvular cusps were contracted and thickened. Distinct white fibrous plaques were seen at the base of the pulmonary trunk. The mitral valvular cusps and chordae were thickened and shortened. A fibrous plaque was present on the endocardial surface of the left ventricle. There was severe coronary arterial atherosclerosis.

Histologically, sections from the lungs disclosed proliferation of the intima of the pulmonary veins and, to a lesser extent, of the small muscular pulmonary arteries and arterioles. The media of the muscular pulmonary arteries was thickened. In addition, there was mild fibrous thickening of the alveolar septa, and some of the alveolar spaces contained numerous hemosiderin-laden macrophages. (These changes in the lung are seen commonly in patients with mitral valvular disease.) Also, there was mild focal acute pneumonia. Sections from the pancreas disclosed the presence of acute pancreatitis. Foci of inflammatory cells also were present in the hypothalamus and midbrain. An acute infarct was noted in the spleen. Carcinoid metastases were seen in sections of vertebral bone marrow.

Case vii. A fifty-seven year-old white woman (R. W., 03-85-05) died on November 19, 1961. In 1951 (age forty-seven) she had had a left radical mastectomy for carcinoma of the breast. There had been no evidence of recurrence thereafter, and she had been well until February 1958 when a sudden attack of fecal vomiting prompted the diagnosis of acute intestinal obstruction and a laparotomy was performed. A carcinoid tumor was found in the terminal ileum and was resected along with the ascending colon. Carcinoid metastases were seen in three of twenty-seven mesenteric lymph nodes. Immediately after the operation, the urinary excretion of 5-hydroxyindoleacetic acid was found to be elevated. Shortly thereafter, however, the urinary excretion of 5-hydroxyindoleacetic acid was reported to have dropped to normal levels and remained so until February 1959 when it again became elevated. In June 1960 hepatomegaly was noted. From November 1960 until her death one year later, she was in bed, getting up only to go to the bathroom. During this last year of life, anorexia, watery diarrhea, weight loss and marked weakness appeared. There was no history of asthma or facial blushing.

On admission to the Clinical Center October 4, 1961, she appeared thin and chronically ill. Her blood pressure was 110/65 mm. Hg. There was an atypical symmetric "cyanosis" from the forehead to the umbilicus. Prominent V waves were noted in the superficial jugular veins. A right ventricular precordial lift was felt. A soft, right ventricular diastolic gallop was heard. A grade 2/6 ejection-type systolic murmur was present at the cardiac base, most prominent in the pulmonic area, and a grade 3/6 holosystolic blowing murmur, which increased with inspiration, was heard at the apex. The predominant cardiac lesion was believed to be tricuspid insufficiency. The liver was massively enlarged and pulsatile. The spleen was not felt. There was evidence of a right pleural effusion, otherwise the lungs were clear. There was 1 plus pitting pedal and pretibial edema and 3 plus pitting sacral edema.

Chest roentgenogram disclosed a left pleural effusion but no cardiomegaly. The electrocardiogram showed low voltage, prominent P waves suggestive of right atrial enlargement and a vertical axis. The values for urinary 5-hydroxyindoleacetic acid on two occasions were 187 and 274 mg. per 24 hours. Her final month of life was characterized by multiple electrolyte derangements, azotemia and oliguria. Death came quietly.

At autopsy (A61-266) she was emaciated (weight 50 kg., height 134 cm.). The skin of the face, neck and anterior trunk was "cyanotic" and telangiectatic. There was no evidence of recurrence of tumor in the healed left radical mastectomy incision. Both axillary and supraclavicular regions were free of lymphadenopathy, and no nodules were present in the right breast. The abdomen was protuberant. There was 2 plus pitting pedal, pretibial and sacral edema. Excessive fluid was present in the abdominal cavity (525 ml.), left pleural (300 ml.) and right pleural (450 ml.) spaces. The pericardial cavity contained 15 ml. of watery fluid. The small intestine was matted together by tumorous adhesions but there was no evidence of intestinal obstruction. The ileocolonic anastomosis was intact. No tumor was found in the bowel. The peritoneum was thick, leathery and studded with carcinoid implants. Numerous carcinoid tumors also were seen on the surfaces of the pelvic organs and in the pancreas and liver.

The heart (Fig. 4 and 5) weighed 200 gm. There was serous atrophy of the subepicardial adipose tissue and brown atrophy of the myocardium. The wall of the inferior vena cava was markedly thickened and its intima, white, and a few focal whitish grey elevations were present on the intima of the superior vena cava. (Fig. 6.) The right atrium and ventricle were dilated. The endocardium of the right atrium contained numerous focal greyish white fibrous plaques, most pronounced on the septum.

The foramen ovale was closed. The tricuspid and pulmonic valvular leaflets and the tricuspid chordae were fibrotic, thickened and contracted. Only one fibrous plaque was seen in the right ventricle, and it was located just below the papillary muscle of the conus. The orifice of both the tricuspid and pulmonic valves were fixed. The base of the pulmonary trunk folded double over the pulmonic valve, a result of the fibrous proliferative process within the sinuses of the pulmonic valve. A single fibrous plaque was present on the ventricular aspect of the anterior mitral leaflet and in the ascending aorta. Multiple carcinoid-type plaques also were present throughout the aorta, usually superimposed on atherosclerotic lesions.

Case viii. A fifty-two year old white woman (H. M., 03-41-30) died on January 12, 1962. She had been well until May 1960, when she noted the onset of diarrhea (eight to ten loose bowel movements daily), periodic flushing of the face, neck and upper part of the arm, wheezing, intermittent pain of the right upper part of the abdomen and low grade fever. Because of the persistence of these symptoms she underwent exploratory laparotomy in September 1960, and peritoneal carcinoid implants were found. No search for the site of the primary was undertaken. Following the operation, weight loss and weakness continued unabated.

On admission to the Clinical Center February 14, 1961, she appeared chronically ill (weight 56 kg.). The blood pressure was 120/80 mm. Hg. Numerous telangiectases were noted in the skin over the entire body. No abnormal venous pulsations were seen in the neck. The lungs were clear to auscultation. The heart was not enlarged. The second heart sound was louder at the left than at the right second intercostal space. A grade 2/6 ejection-type systolic murmur was heard along the left sternal border. Also, a grade 2/6 blowing systolic murmur and a grade 1/6 low-pitched diastolic rumble were heard at the apex. The liver was large but nontender. The spleen was not felt. There was no peripheral edema. Urinary excretion of 5-hydroxyindoleacetic acid on numerous occasions averaged approximately 200 mg. per 24 hours. Chest roentgenogram disclosed a normal-sized heart. The electrocardiogram showed generalized diminution in QRS and T wave amplitudes.

During her almost one year period of hospitalization, she was treated with several cancer chemotherapeutic agents without detectable benefit. During the final four months she became extremely cachectic and noted the development persistent peripheral edema and ascites. Her last week of life was characterized by vomiting, extreme weakness and finally coma.

At autopsy (A62-9) she weighed 43 kg. and measured 161 cm. in length. The skin over the anterior chest and neck was plethoric. The abdomen was protuberant. The abdominal cavity contained 4,600 ml. of serous fluid. Portions of the bowel were matted together by multiple adhesions. There also were adhesions of the intestine to the liver, peritoneum and omentum. The liver weighed 2,800 gm. and contained multiple carcinoid metastases, many of which were necrotic. The spleen weighed 130 gm. An annular carcinoid tumor 1 cm. in size was found in the jejunum. No other intestinal tumors were seen. The lungs, pulmonary arteries and veins appeared normal.

The heart weighed 250 gm. There was marked serous atrophy of the subepicardial adipose tissue and brown atrophy of the myocardium. The right atrium and ventricle were dilated. Focal fibrous plaques were present on the intima of the inferior and superior venae cavae, coronary sinus and on the endocardium of the right atrium, tricuspid valve and its chordae, right ventricle, pulmonic valve and mitral valve and its chordae. (Fig. 7 and 8.) Although fibrous plaques were present within the sinuses of the pulmonic valve, its cusps were freely movable, and the appearance of this valve suggested that it had functioned normally. The left atrium was slightly dilated and its endocardium, although uniformly thickened, was free of fibrous plaques. The foramen ovale was closed. The mitral valvular leaflets and chordae were thickened, but the commissures were not fused. The appearance of this valve suggests that it probably was neither significantly stenotic nor regurgitant. No fibrous lesions were seen in the left ventricle. The aortic valve was normal. Histologic study of sections of the lung disclosed marked intimal proliferation in the pulmonary veins. (Fig. 9.)

Case ix. A sixty-nine year old white man (T. M., 04-00-87) died on February 11, 1962. He had been well until March 1961 when he noted anorexia, weight loss and intermittent pain of the lower abdomen. In June 1961 intermittent diarrhea developed (twelve watery bowel movements daily) as well as periodic flushes of the face and neck and, rarely, wheezing respirations. In September 1961 he experienced acute intestinal obstruction and underwent laparotomy. Two carcinoid tumors were found in the ileum. These tumors compressed the mesenteric arteries, producing gangrene of a portion of the small intestine, which was resected. Carcinoid metastases were found in the liver and in the mesenteric lymph nodes. During the six months before operation he had lost 30 kg. During the first four months following operation, he regained 8 kg. Diarrhea did not recur following operation. He had had orthopnea, paroxysmal nocturnal dyspnea and systemic hypertension intermittently for a number of years, but there was no history of angina pectoris.

On admission to the Clinical Center January 8, 1962, he weighed 57.9 kg. and was slightly dyspneic.

His initial blood pressure was 180/110 but thereafter remained in the vicinity of 120/80 mm. Hg. The superficial jugular veins were distended with the patient sitting upright. The anteroposterior diameter of the chest was increased, and inspiratory rales and occasional expiratory wheezes were heard throughout the lung fields. The point of maximum cardiac impulse was in the fifth left intercostal space, just to the right of the left anterior axillary line. The second cardiac sound was louder in the aortic than in the pulmonic area. A grade 2/6 blowing systolic murmur was heard at the apex, and a grade 1/6 low-pitched, ejection-type systolic murmur was heard along the lower left sternal border. No abnormal jugular venous waves and no hepatic pulsations were noted. The liver was enlarged, the spleen not palpable. There was slight pretibial pitting edema.

The chest roentgenogram showed enlargement of the left ventricle and tortuosity of the ascending aorta. The electrocardiogram disclosed normal sinus rhythm, left axis deviation, left ventricular ischemia and absent R waves in leads V_2 and V_3, suggesting an old anterior myocardial infarct. The urinary excretion of 5-hydroxyindoleacetic averaged approximately 100 mg. per 24 hours.

While in the hospital, he had many transient flushes, and occasionally these were associated with hypotension. The number of flushes was decreased considerably during treatment with phenoxybenzamine. On the day of death the patient collapsed while defecating, became cyanotic, complained of left precordial chest pain, had convulsions and died.

At autopsy (A62-34) he was cachectic (weight 51.6 kg., height 177 cm.). The skin of the chest was plethoric and telangiectatic. No excessive fluid was present in the abdominal, pleural or pericardial cavities. Carcinoid metastases were found in the regional lymph nodes and in the liver (2,600 gm.). An intact ileoileostomy was present approximately 60 cm. proximal to the ileocecal valve. No nodules were found in the intestinal tract.

The heart weighed 475 gm. The right atrium, right ventricle and left atrium were dilated. No fibrous plaques were noted on the intima of the vena cavae or on the endocardium of the right atrium. The tricuspid valvular orifice was smaller than normal but fixed in an open position. (Fig. 10.) Its leaflets and chordae were considerably shortened and thickened. The right ventricular wall measured up to 4.5 cm. in thickness. The pulmonic valvular cusps were thickened and pearly white, and the orifice was fixed in an open position. The left atrium and mitral valve were normal. The foramen ovale was closed. The left ventricular wall measured up to 1.0 cm. in thickness. In the apex of the left ventricle and involving the most caudal portion of the ventricular septum there was an old healed myocardial infarct which measured 2 by 4 cm. in size. Foci of calcium were present within each of the aortic sinuses of Valsalva, but there was no fusion of the commissures of the aortic valve. The coronary arteries were markedly tortuous and atherosclerotic.

ADDENDUM

Since this manuscript was submitted for publication, we have studied both clinically and at autopsy two additional patients with the carcinoid syndrome. One, a forty year old Negro man (L. P., 03-10-65), died in April 1963 with widespread carcinoid tumor from a primary tumor in the small intestine. The total length of his illness was three years, during which time he had severe weight loss, diarrhea, flushes, wheezing, exertional dyspnea, hepatomegaly, ascites, peripheral edema and terminally, severe hepatic and renal failure (total serum bilirubin 22 mg. per 100 ml., serum urea nitrogen 199 mg. per 100 ml.). On examination the heart was not enlarged. A blowing pansystolic murmur which increased in intensity with inspiration was audible over the entire precordium, and a rumbling diastolic murmur along the left sternal border. The urinary excretion of 5-hydroxyindoleacetic acid ranged from 296 to 432 mg. per twenty-four hours. Electrocardiogram disclosed low voltage and peaked P waves characteristic of right atrial hypertrophy. At autopsy (A63-96) there was typical carcinoid fibrosis involving the tricuspid, pulmonic and mitral valves and right atrium. There was no intracardiac communication and no carcinoid tumor in the lungs. The mitral valvular fibrosis was less extensive than that of the tricuspid and pulmonic valves. The involvement of the mitral valve, which also included a few of its chordae tendineae, was probably not hemodynamically significant. Carcinoid metastases were present in the peritoneum, appendix, liver (2,900 gm.), pancreas, biliary tree, spleen (200 gm.), prostate gland, testes, bone, abdominal and thoracic lymph nodes, and heart (myocardium of left ventricle and visceral pericardium).

The second patient, a sixty-five year old white woman (L. C., 03-38-59), also died in April 1963 following a three year illness characterized by diarrhea, flushes, partial intestinal obstruction and progressive emaciation. Widespread peritoneal metastases and a primary tumor of the ileum were found at ileotransverse colon anastomosis two years before death. There were no precordial murmurs. Electrocardiogram showed low voltage. The urinary excretion of 5-hydroxyindoleacetic acid before operation ranged from 14 to 23 mg. per twenty-four hours and during the two years after operation was normal (2 to 6 mg. per twenty-four hours). (These are the lowest levels of urinary 5-hydroxyindoleacetic acid recorded at the Clinical Center in a patient with the carcinoid syndrome.) At autopsy (A63-67) the patient weighed only 28 kg. The heart weighed 150 gm., and its valves and chambers were normal. Carcinoid implants were extensive throughout the peritoneal surfaces and abdominal and retroperitoneal lymph nodes. The liver weighed 500 gm. and contained only a few small carcinoid implants, the largest of which measured 1 cm. in diameter. The spleen weighed 30 gm.

Cyanotic Malformations of the Heart with Pheochromocytoma

A Report of Five Cases

By Gordon M. Folger, Jr., M.D., William C. Roberts, M.D., Ali Mehrizi, M.D., K. D. Shah, M.D., D. L. Glancy, M.D., Charles C. J. Carpenter, M.D., and John R. Esterly, M.D.

ALTHOUGH the occurrence of pheochromocytoma in patients with neurocutaneous defects has been reported,[1-3] the occurrence of this rare tumor in patients with congenital cardiac malformations, to the best of our knowledge, has not previously been recorded. During the past 13 years, five patients with pheochromocytoma and cyanotic congenital malformations of the heart have come to our attention at The Johns Hopkins Hospital. A description of the clinical and pathologic features of these five patients forms the subject of this report.

Case Reports

Case 1

R.D. (JHH no. A 511024), a 26-year-old white man, who, although cyanotic at birth, was acyanotic during early childhood, grew and developed well and only suffered mild to moderate exertional dyspnea. At 7 years of age, cyanosis reappeared, squatting became apparent, and the dyspnea and fatigability increased. In spite of these symptoms the patient finished high school and was able to perform light farm chores. By age 18 the cyanosis had become persistent. In 1949, at the age of 26, he was referred to the Harriet Lane Home because of severe incapacity.

On examination, the blood pressure was 140/80 mm. Hg, pulse 80, respiratory rate 20, and temperature 39 C. The patient was small in stature, undernourished, and deeply cyanotic, and the digits were severely clubbed. A systolic thrill and murmur, most prominent in the third left intercostal space along the sternal border, were present.

The electrocardiogram showed right axis deviation and right ventricular hypertrophy. Chest radiogram showed a normal-sized heart and reduced pulmonary vascularity. Cardiac catheterization and venous angiocardiography confirmed the diagnosis of tetralogy of Fallot. Oximetry revealed a resting oxygen saturation of 89 per cent, which fell to 54 per cent with exercise. The hematocrit value was 74 per cent.

A Blalock-Taussig operation was performed on September 10, 1949. Prior to operation the patient had no symptoms other than exertional dyspnea and easy fatigability. His blood pressure had ranged from 110/80 to 142/90 mm. Hg. During the operation, the blood pressure dropped abruptly when the left pulmonary artery was clamped and he became deeply cyanosed. The blood pressure gradually rose to preoperative levels after removal of the pulmonary arterial clamp and the operation was continued; the blood pressure remained satisfactory throughout the remainder of the procedure. The patient, however, did not regain consciousness and died 3 hours following completion of the procedure.

At autopsy (no. 22006), the heart weighed 480 Gm. The foramen ovale was patent but guarded by a competent valve. There was biventricular hypertrophy. The aorta was dextroposed and overriding a 3 by 2 cm.-sized defect in the basal portion of the ventricular septum. Infundibular pulmonary stenosis was present; the pulmonic valve was bicuspid but of normal size. The left pulmonary artery was larger than the right. The surgical anastomosis between the left subclavian artery and the left pulmonary artery was patent. The bronchial arteries were dilated and tortuous.

A firm, encapsulated tumor, measuring 4.5 by 3.5 by 3.5 cm. was found immediately inferior to the left renal vein and just anterior to the abdominal aorta. On section, the tumor was reddish-brown, slightly friable, and contained flecks of calcium and two distinct nodules. On histologic

From the Cardiac Clinic of the Harriet Lane Home, The Johns Hopkins Hospital, and the Departments of Pediatrics, Medicine, and Pathology, The Johns Hopkins University School of Medicine, Baltimore, Maryland.

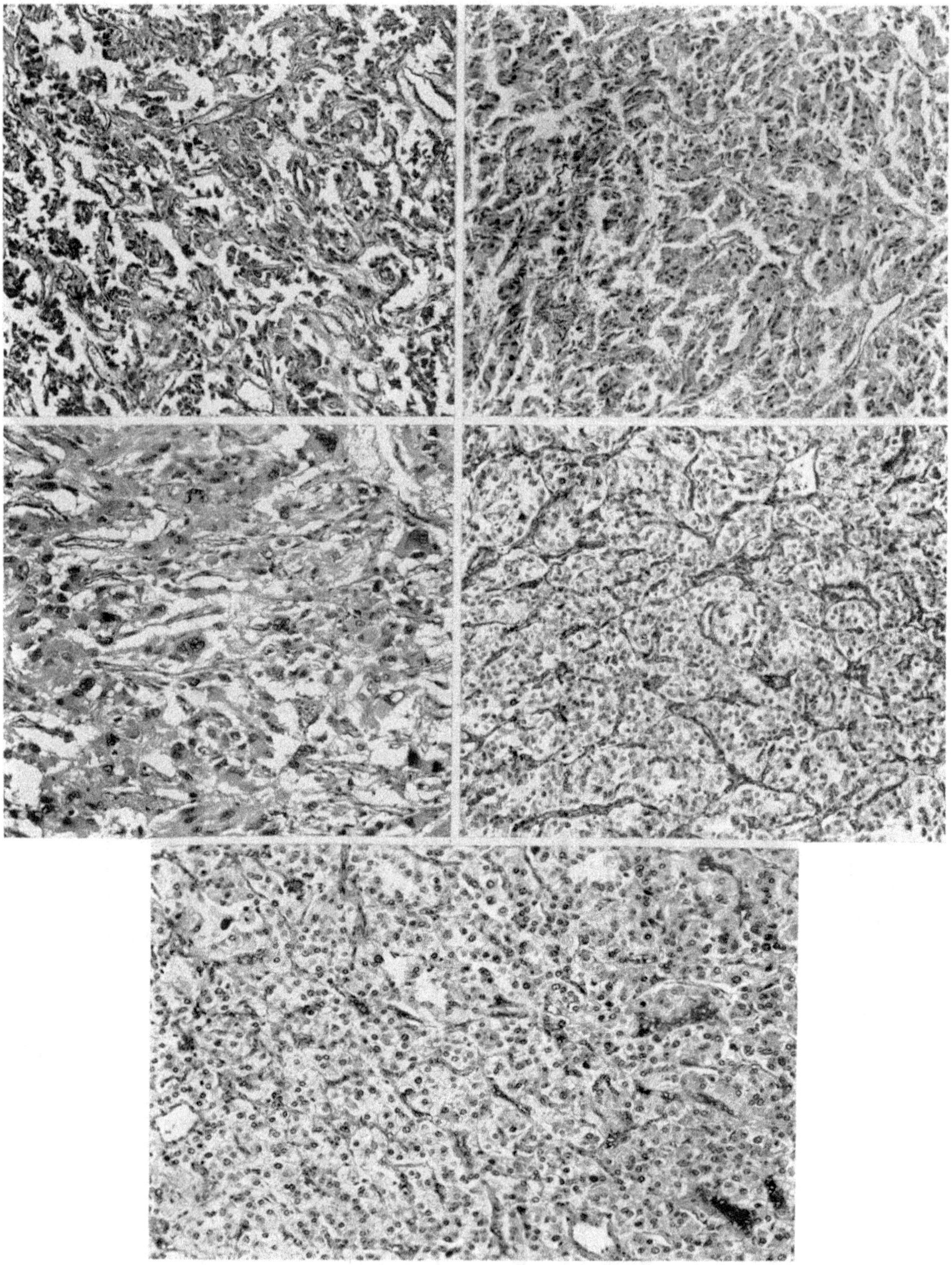

Figure 1

Photomicrographs of sections of the pheochromocytomas in cases 1 to 5. Upper left, *case 1.* Upper right, *case 2.* Middle left, *case 3.* Middle right, *case 4.* Lower, *case 5. Hematoxylin and eosin stains. Original magnification × 100 in cases 1, 2, and 4; × 150 in cases 3 and 5.*

section (fig. 1), the tumor consisted of irregular groups of cells, varying in size and shape, resembling those characteristic of adrenal medulla. Fibrous tissue was present surrounding the chromaffin cells. The adrenal glands were intact and were in no way remarkable. The final anatomic diagnosis was tetralogy of Fallot and pheochromocytoma.

Case 2

E.H.* (JHH no. 855746), a 14-year-old girl was followed in the Cardiac Clinic of the Harriet Lane Home from 1946 until her death in 1959. Throughout this period she was markedly cyanotic and presented clinical findings compatible with transposition of the great vessels. Two years before death she began having attacks of extreme nervousness, recurrent frontal headaches, profuse sweating, insomnia, periodic vomiting, and tachycardia. The blood pressure varied from 98/70 to 150/110 mm. Hg. The arterial oxygen saturation was 77 per cent. Shortly before death a phentolamine (Regitine) test was positive. She died during surgical exploration for a suspected brain abscess.

Autopsy (no. 29292), confirmed the diagnosis of transposition of the great vessels. A pheochromocytoma weighing 47 Gm. was present in the left adrenal gland with metastases in a regional lymph node and in the liver. Histologically (fig. 1), the tumor consisted of cells similar to those seen in case 1. They were arranged in an irregular cord-like pattern. The cells had hyperchromatic, pyknotic nuclei and eosinophilic cytoplasm. There were considerable vascularity and hemorrhage. Fetal fat was present at the periphery. The final anatomic diagnosis was transposition of the great vessels and pheochromocytoma.

Case 3

R.J. (JHH no. 423829), a 16-year-old white boy, had cyanosis and a cardiac murmur from birth. Growth and development were slow. When 18 months of age, following a convulsion, the child developed left hemiplegia. At 3 years of age he was sent from his home in Oregon to the Cardiac Clinic of the Harriet Lane Home.

Physical examination revealed a small child with clubbing of the extremities and intense cyanosis. The heart was located in the right hemithorax and was not enlarged. A grade IV/VI systolic murmur was present over the entire precordium, loudest in the fourth intercostal space to the right of the sternum. The hematocrit value was 61 per cent. The arterial oxygen saturation was 43 per cent. Chest roentgenograms showed the heart to lie in the right hemithorax. The lung fields were hypovascular. Although the patient did not appear to have a tetralogy of Fallot, he was suffering from a decrease in pulmonary blood flow. A right subclavian-to-right pulmonary artery anastomosis was performed with immediate and striking improvement.

When 13 years old (1957), during re-examination by his physician in Oregon, he was found to have hematuria, pyuria, proteinuria, and cylindruria; these findings persisted throughout the remainder of his life. Serum urea nitrogen remained normal until his terminal illness. During his last 3 years, his heart enlarged, dyspnea reappeared, and terminally he developed anasarca. The blood pressure, which had been checked on many occasions throughout his life, had always been normal (approximately 110/70 mm. Hg). He died on April 14, 1960, at age 16, in severe congestive heart failure.

At autopsy* (no. 30329) the heart was markedly enlarged (600 Gm.) and located predominantly in the right hemithorax. The right subclavian-to-right pulmonary artery anastomosis was occluded by an organized thrombus. A large oval defect was present in the lowermost portion of the atrial septum. The foramen ovale was closed. The tricuspid and mitral valves were continuous across the midline through a common atrioventricular defect. The aorta and the pulmonary artery arose from the anterior chamber, which anatomically was the right ventricle. The ascending aorta lay anterior to the pulmonary trunk. The pulmonary trunk was hypoplastic and the pulmonic valve was bicuspid and stenotic.

Both adrenal glands were partially replaced by a solid, brown-colored tumor measuring 6 by 4 by 3 cm., which connected one gland with the other by a wide bar and extended across the aorta to form a dumbbell-shaped tumor. Histologic sections (fig. 1) of the tumor disclosed that it consisted of cells of varying size and shape with uniform cytoplasm, and frequently large, pyknotic, irregular, and bizarre nuclei. Many of the cells were multinucleated. Occasional oncocytic and ganglion-like cells were present.

The kidneys were enlarged; the glomeruli were much larger than normal, slightly hypercellular, and a few were hyalinized. A number of large juxtaglomerular bodies were seen. The renal arterioles were normal. The final anatomic diagnosis was origin of both great vessels from the right ventricle with pulmonary stenosis and pheochromocytoma.

* This patient is being reported in detail by Drs. Arthur Grollman and John R. Esterly.[4]

* The authors are indebted to the Department of Pathology, Sacred Heart General Hospital, Eugene, Oregon, for sending the organs and histologic sections from this patient.

Case 4 *

A.O. (JHH no. 644014), a 44-year-old man, was cyanotic from birth. He was admitted on several occasions to The Johns Hopkins Hospital with complaints of palpitation, breathlessness, weakness, and right parasternal chest pain. The diagnosis of atrial fibrillation was made, and he was successfully treated with quinidine. Later cardiac catheterization was performed and this procedure combined with intracardiac electrocardiogram was compatible with the diagnosis of Ebstein's anomaly of the tricuspid valve.

He was subsequently seen at the Baltimore City Hospital and was diagnosed as having a pheochromocytoma. The tumor was successfully removed surgically. Histologic examination of the tumor (fig. 1) demonstrated pigment-containing cells arranged in cord-like groups resembling the pattern characteristic of the adrenal medulla. The final clinical diagnosis was Ebstein's anomaly of the tricuspid valve and pheochromocytoma.

Case 5

J.E. (JHH no. 528646), a 20-year-old white college student, who was cyanotic at birth, squatted frequently, and fatigued easily was first seen in the Cardiac Clinic of the Harriet Lane Home at age 7 years. The hematocrit level was 77 per cent. The patient was found to have a tetralogy of Fallot, and an end-to-side right subclavian-to-right pulmonary artery anastomosis was performed with considerable improvement. During the following 3 years the hematocrit level ranged between 52 and 56 per cent and the blood pressure between 95/45 and 120/80 mm. Hg.

In 1955, at the age of 12 years the cyanosis began to increase and the exercise tolerance to diminish. The hematocrit level was 60 per cent and the blood pressure 150/90 mm. Hg. In 1958, in addition to a gradual increase in exertional dyspnea the patient developed nosebleeds, headaches, polyphagia with weight gain, polydipsia, profuse sweating, insomnia, several episodes of diplopia, and extreme nervousness. The blood pressure recorded at his clinic visit was 130/80 mm. Hg and the hematocrit was 75 per cent.

At 17 years of age, prior to consideration for corrective surgery, an angiocardiogram was performed, which confirmed the diagnosis of tetralogy of Fallot. During this admission in 1960 he was noted to complain bitterly of intolerance to the heat on the ward and to have unexplained episodes of sweating and irritability. His blood pressure was 170/110 mm. Hg. The possibility of a pheochromocytoma was considered. A 24-hour urine sample was positive for catecholamines (greater than 180 micrograms/24 hours). The patient, however, returned to his home in New York before the results of the test were known, and he was subsequently not seen for a period of 18 months. During this interval he had frequent episodes of headache, nervousness, epistaxis, sweating, insomnia, and diplopia. The patient was finally readmitted for study of a possible pheochromocytoma in 1962.

Physical examination revealed a temperature of 37.8 C, a pulse of 90, a respiratory rate of 20, and a blood pressure of 190/130 mm. Hg. The nailbeds were cyanotic, and clubbing was prominent. The heart was enlarged. A loud continuous murmur was present over the right hemithorax, and a grade-III/VI systolic murmur was present over the precordium, maximal along the lower left sternal border. The hematocrit value was 72 per cent.

While on the ward, the patient sweated frequently and his blood pressure was noted to vary from 140/100 to 200/150 mm. Hg. Twenty-four-hour urinary excretion of norepinephrine was 876 micrograms (normal 10 to 90 micrograms) and of epinephrine 25 micrograms (normal 5 to 40 micrograms). The diagnosis of a pheochromocytoma was thus established.

On March 15, 1962, the patient underwent laparotomy. A 2 by 4 by 1.5 cm. mass was found at the junction of the aorta and the left renal artery. The tumor was removed and histologic examination (fig. 1) revealed it to be similar to that seen in case 4. The pattern and individual cells were similar to those seen in the normal adrenal gland. Fetal fat was adherent to the fibrous tissue.

During the postoperative period, the patient's blood pressure ranged from 120/75 to 150/100 mm. Hg. Histamine and phentolamine tests performed postoperatively were negative. Repeat 24-hour urinary excretions of norepinephrine and epinephrine were 167 and 23 micrograms, respectively.

On March 20, 1963, 1 year following removal of the pheochromocytoma, the patient returned to The Johns Hopkins Hospital for corrective cardiac surgery. Although he complained of dyspnea and fatigue on exertion, he no longer had headaches, nosebleeds, or sweats and his voracious appetite and excessive thirst had disappeared. The blood pressure now varied from 135/95 to 150/110 mm. Hg. The hematocrit value was 83 per cent. The phentolamine, histamine, and cold pressor tests were negative, and the urinary catecholamines were normal (less than 180 micrograms per 24 hours). On March 26, 1963, he underwent closure of the ventricular septal defect and removal of the hypertrophied musculature of the right ventricular infundibulum

* This case is being reported in detail elsewhere by Dr. A. R. Christlieb et al.

by Dr. David Sabiston. In spite of difficulty during surgery and the early postoperative period, he did well. Since operation his blood pressures have varied between 110/60 and 120/80 mm. Hg. The cyanosis disappeared rapidly and the hematocrit fell to 50 per cent.

Discussion

The association of endocrine tumors with heart disease has recently been noted by Roberts et al.[5] These authors described five patients, ages 21 to 57 years, three with congenital cardiac malformations (total anomalous pulmonary venous connection in two and complete transposition of the great vessels in one) leading to cyanosis, and two with isolated calcific aortic stenosis of uncertain etiology. The associated endocrine tumor in three of these five patients was of adrenocortical origin (in each of the two patients with calcific aortic stenosis and in the one patient with complete transposition of the great vessels). A pituitary adenoma associated with the clinical picture of Cushing's syndrome was present in one of the patients with anomalous pulmonary venous connection, and an islet-cell carcinoma of the pancreas was present in the other patient with this malformation. Those authors believed that the association of endocrine tumors with congenital cardiac malformations was more than coincidental.

Our observation of pheochromocytoma in five patients with cyanotic congenital cardiac malformations is indeed unusual. This tumor is rare; its reported incidence among autopsies varies from 1:400 to 1:3,000.[6–8] Barbeau[9] found 626 cases of pheochromocytoma reported up to 1957. Insley and Smallwood[10] were able to collect 62 cases in patients under 14 years of age up to 1961. Only 21 cases of histologically proved pheochromocytoma were found among 31,227 autopsies performed at The Johns Hopkins Hospital from 1901 to 1962, and three of these (cases 1–3) are included in this report. Two of these (cases 2 and 3) represent the youngest instances of pheochromocytoma found at autopsy at this hospital.

The cause of the association between this rare endocrine tumor and cyanotic congenital malformations of the heart is obviously only speculative. Because clinical manifestations of the tumor did not appear until 12 to 41 years after birth, the pheochromocytoma in these instances does not appear to be congenital in origin. Chronic arterial hypoxemia may possibly be a factor in the production of the pheochromocytoma. Asphyxia and anoxia in the experimental animal are known to cause a striking increase in secretion of epinephrine and norepinephrine from the adrenal medulla.[11], [12] This is especially true of norepinephrine production. Cheek et al.[13] recently found considerably elevated plasma levels of epinephrine and norepinephrine in premature infants with placental insufficiency and postmaturity. These authors related their findings to hypoxia. Propst[14] has suggested a compensatory hyperplastic mechanism as an etiologic factor in the production of a pheochromocytoma, and recently Sherwin[2] noted a histologic relation between adrenal medullary hyperplasia and neoplasia. Bialestock[15] reported hyperplasia of the adrenal medulla in each of two patients who died with severe hypertension and related its occurrence to an increase in function of the adrenal medulla. Medullary adrenal hyperplasia has also been noted by Bongiovanni et al.[16] to occur in patients with long-standing cystic fibrosis of the pancreas. It is conceivable that persistent hypoxemia could produce adrenal medullary hyperplasia and finally an autonomously functioning medullary tumor (pheochromocytoma). Such a sequence of events would be analogous to that suggested by Albright and Reifenstein[17] in which hypocalcemia was thought to lead to hyperplasia of the parathyroid gland and eventually to parathyroid adenoma.

Three of the five patients in this study had clinically functional pheochromocytomas (cases 2, 4, and 5). In each of these patients the tumor was diagnosed during life; in two of the three patients the tumor was successfully removed. The sign that initially led to the consideration of a pheochromocytoma was systemic hypertension. Although systemic hypertension occurs not infrequently in severely

Table 1

Summary of Five Cases with Pheochromocytoma

Patient age, race, and sex	Cardiac malformation	Signs and symptoms of pheochromocytoma	Highest blood pressure mm Hg	Highest hematocrit value, %	O_2 Sat., %	Diagnostic studies for pheochromocytoma	Diagnosis of pheochromocytoma confirmed by
1. R. D. 26 years WM	Tetralogy of Fallot	Hypotensive episode at time of Blalock-Taussig operation	142/90	74	85* 54	None	Autopsy
2. E. H. 14 years CF	Transposition of great vessels	Sweating, nervousness, anorexia, headaches, tachycardia, insomnia	150/110	70	77	Positive Regitine and benzodioxane	Autopsy
3. R. J. 16 years WM	Transposition of great vessels; both vessels from RV; dextrocardia; AV communis	None	110/70	61	43	None	Autopsy
4. A. O. 44 years WM	Ebstein's anomaly	Arrhythmias, palpitation, sweating, dizziness, paresthesias	240/150	66	90	Positive Regitine, norepinephrine (urine)—1390 μg., 3900 μg.	Surgery
5. J. E. 19 years WM	Tetralogy of Fallot	Nervousness, headaches, heat intolerance, sweating, insomnia, epistaxis, polydipsia	200/150	83	80	Positive Regitine and benzodioxane, norepinephrine (urine)—876 μg., epinephrine (urine)—25 μg.	Surgery

* Highest saturation at rest; lower saturation following activity.

cyanotic patients, excessive sweating and nervousness are uncommon. These findings in addition to periodic headaches, paroxysmal arrhythmias, hyperglycemia, and glucosuria offer helpful clues to the clinical recognition of a pheochromocytoma. Indeed some of these symptoms or signs were present in each of the three patients in whom the diagnosis was made clinically (table 1).

The recognition of the presence of a pheochromocytoma in these patients prior to cardiac catheterization or other operation is important in view of the occasional occurrence of sudden death in patients with pheochromocytoma during surgical procedures or during the induction of anesthesia.[18-20] Although none of the five present patients manifested any difficulty attributable to the pheochromocytoma at the time of cardiac catheterization or angiocardiography, the severe hypotensive episode during operation and the early postoperative death in one patient (case 1) may have been directly related to the associated pheochromocytoma.

Summary

The clinical and pathologic features of five patients with pheochromocytoma associated with congenital cyanotic cardiac malformations have been described. This association appears to be more than mere coincidence. Chronic hypoxemia may be a significant factor in the development of this rare endocrine tumor in such patients. The finding of systemic hypertension combined with episodes of nervousness and sweating or repeated severe headaches initially aroused suspicion of a pheochromocytoma in the three patients in which this tumor was diagnosed clinically.

Acknowledgment

The authors gratefully acknowledge the help and advice of Dr. Helen B. Taussig and Dr. Richard S. Ross in the preparation of this manuscript. We are also indebted to Dr. J. G. Wiswell for the determination of the urinary epinephrine and norepinephrine levels in case 5.

References

1. Glushien, A. S., Mansuy, M. M., and Littman, D. S.: Pheochromocytoma. Its relationship to neurocutaneous syndromes. Am. J. Med. **14:** 318, 1953.
2. Sherwin, R. P.: Histopathology of pheochromocytoma. Cancer **12:** 861, 1959.
3. Koonce, D. H., Pollock, B. E., and Glassy, F. J.: Bilateral pheochromocytoma associated with neurofibromatosis (death following aortography). Am. Heart J. **44:** 901, 1952.
4. Grollman, A. P., Jr., and Esterly, J. R. In press.
5. Roberts, W. C., Mason, D. T., and Braunwald, E.: Survival to adulthood in a patient with complete transposition of the great vessels. Including a note on the association of endocrine tumors with heart disease. Ann. Int. Med. **57:** 834, 1962.
6. Berkheiser, S. W., and Rappoport, A. E.: Unsuspected pheochromocytoma of the adrenal: Report of 5 cases. Am. J. Clin. Path. **21:** 657, 1951.
7. Blacklock, J. W. S., Ferguson, J. W., Mack, W. S., Shafar, J., and Symington, T.: Pheochromocytoma. Brit. J. Surg. **35:** 179, 1947.
8. Minno, A. M., Bennett, W. A., and Kvale, W. F.: Pheochromocytoma: A study of 15 cases diagnosed at necropsy. Proc. Staff Meet., Mayo Clin. **30:** 394, 1955.
9. Barbeau, A.: Le phéochromocytoma: Une revue générale du sujet. Union méd. Canada **86:** 1045, 1957.
10. Insley, J., and Smallwood, W. C.: Pheochromocytoma in children. Arch. Dis. Childhood **37:** 606, 1962.
11. Vogt, M.: Epinephrine and norepinephrine. *In* Hormones in Human Plasma. Edited by H. N. Antonaides. Boston, Little, Brown and Company, 1960, p. 581.
12. Goldfien, A., Ganong, W. F., and Wise, B.: Specific neural stimulation of norepinephrine secretion by the adrenal medulla during anoxia. J. Clin. Invest. **40:** 1043, 1961.
13. Cheek, D. B., Malinek, M., and Fraillon, J. M.: Plasma adrenaline and noradrenaline in the neonatal period, and infants with respiratory distress syndrome and placental insufficiency. Pediatrics **31:** 374, 1963.
14. Propst, A.: Über Regulationen bei Geschwulsten endokriner Drüsen. Krebsarzt **11:** 275, 1956.
15. Bialestock, D.: Hyperplasia of the adrenal medulla in hypertension of children. Arch. Dis. Childhood **36:** 465, 1961.
16. Bongiovanni, A. M., Yakovac, W. C., and Steiker, D. D.: Study of adrenal glands in childhood: Hormonal content correlated with morphologic characteristics. Lab. Invest. **10:** 956, 1961.
17. Albright, F., and Reifenstein, E. C.: The Parathyroid Glands and Metabolic Bone Dis-

ease. Baltimore, Williams & Wilkins Co., 1948.
18. Crockett, K. A., Snow, E., and Rees, V. L.: Pheochromocytomas as cause of unexpected operating room deaths. Am. Surgeon **27**: 395, 1961.
19. Seward, E. H.: Death from pheochromocytoma. Lancet **2**: 903, 1961.
20. Neill, C. A., and Smith, G.: Bilateral pheochromocytoma in a six year old boy. Arch. Dis. Childhood **27**: 286, 1952.

THE NONDISTENSIBLE RIGHT ATRIUM OF CARCINOID DISEASE OF THE HEART

WILLIAM C. ROBERTS, M.D., DEAN T. MASON, M.D., AND LOUIS D. WRIGHT, JR., M.D.

Laboratory of Pathology, Clinic of Surgery, the Cardiology Branch, National Heart Institute, and the Pathologic Anatomy Department, Clinical Center, National Institutes of Health, Bethesda, Maryland

Approximately half of the patients with the carcinoid syndrome have carcinoid heart disease.[1] The endocardial fibrous lesions, which are pathognomonic of this disease, almost always involve the tricuspid and pulmonic valves, and whenever the deposits on the tricuspid valve are extensive, similar lesions are generally also present on the endocardium of the right atrium. The chief hemodynamic consequence of diffuse fibrosis of the tricuspid valve in patients with the carcinoid syndrome is tricuspid regurgitation, although some degree of stenosis is almost always present as well. The endocardial fibrous plaques in the right atrium, when diffuse, may prevent this chamber from expanding during ventricular systole as would be expected with tricuspid regurgitation, and thus the right atrial pressure during ventricular contraction may be excessively elevated. This was the case in 2 patients with carcinoid heart disease who underwent cardiac catheterization and finally came to autopsy. Few reports have appeared describing the cardiac morphology in patients with carcinoid heart disease who have undergone catheterization. This paper describes the clinical, hemodynamic, and pathologic features of these 2 patients and calls particular attention to their right atrial pressure pulses.

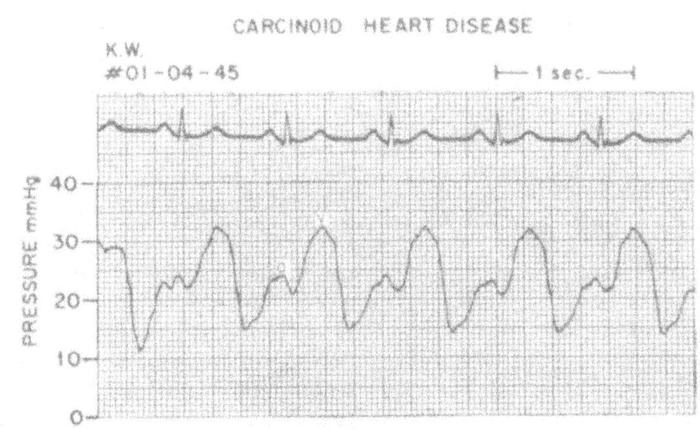

FIG. 1. Right atrial pressure tracing in patient K. W. showing marked elevation of peaks of the v- and a-waves.

REPORT OF CASES

Each of the 2 patients had elevated values of urinary 5-hydroxyindoleacetic acid (range 265 to 580 mg. per 24 hr.), and at autopsy the carcinoid primary in each was in the ileum and the only metastases in each were to the liver and regional lymph nodes. One patient (K. W., 01-04-45) was a 59-year-old man who died 6 years after the onset of diarrhea and facial flushing. He had cardiac catheterization 4 years before he died, and the right atrial a-wave pressure was elevated to 24 and the v-wave to 34 mm. Hg (Fig. 1). The second patient (C. G., 05-49-35) was a 32-year-old woman who died 9 years after the onset of diarrhea and facial flushing. At catheterization (Figs. 2 and 3), performed 8 months before death, the right atrial a-wave pressure was 18, v-wave 23, and mean pressure 15 mm. Hg. The right ven-

Received, June 1, 1965.

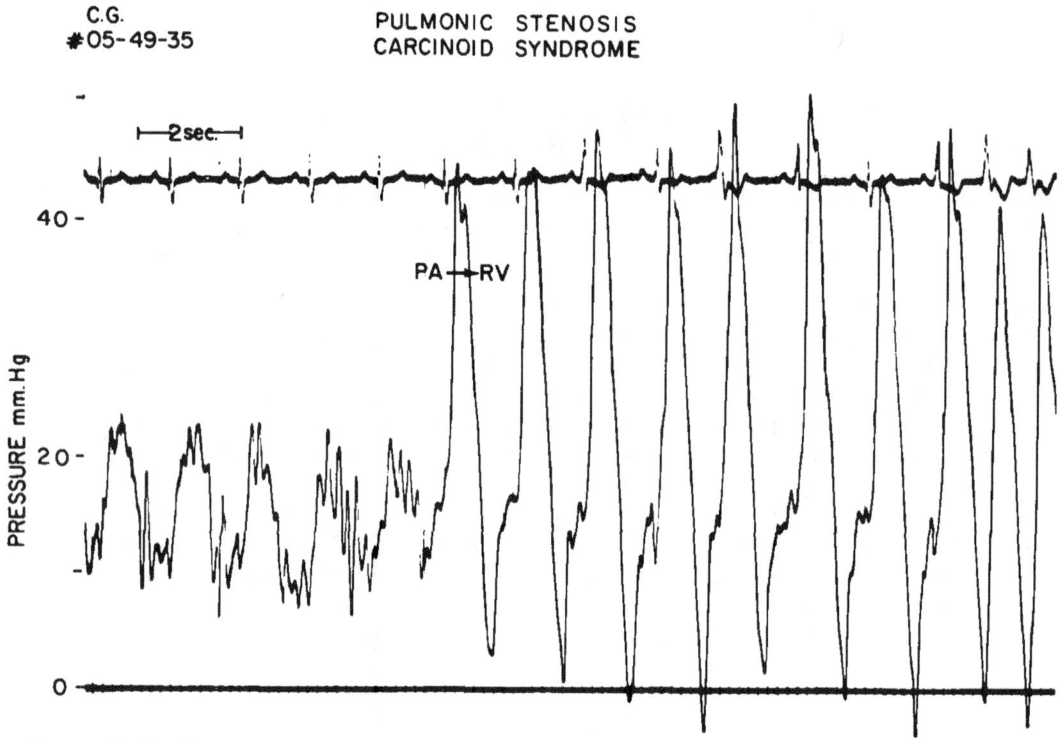

FIG. 2. Pullback pressure tracing from the pulmonary artery (*PA*) into the right ventricle (*RV*), demonstrating the systolic pressure gradient.

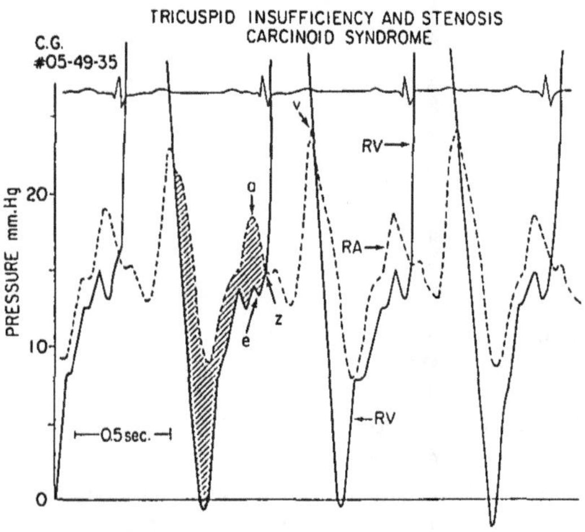

FIG. 3. Simultaneously recorded right atrial (*RA*) and right ventricular (*RV*) pressures showing the tall right atrial v-waves with rapid descent, elevated right atrial mean pressure, increased right ventricular end-diastolic pressure (*e*), and small diastolic pressure gradient (*dashed area*). *Z* = z-point, *a* = a-point.

tricular pressure was 45/13, and the pulmonary arterial pressure, 20/8 mm. Hg. Cardiac output (dye dilution method) was 4.95 liters per min., and the cardiac index was 3.25 liters per min. per M² B.S.A. The arterial hemoglobin oxygen saturation was 92.5 per cent.

On examination, each of the patients was emaciated and demonstrated hepatomegaly, ascites, leg edema, and greatly distended neck veins. A blowing systolic murmur, which increased in intensity during inspiration, was present over the lower left sternal border, and a harsh systolic murmur was present over the upper left sternal border in each patient. Electrocardiograms (Fig. 4) in both patients revealed low voltage and right axis deviation. In addition, right ventricular hypertrophy was present in one (C. G.)

At autopsy, both patients had extensive endocardial fibrosis involving the tricuspid and pulmonic valves and right atrium (Figs. 5 to 7). The heart of K. W. weighed 350 Gm., and that of C. G., 250 Gm.

COMMENT AND CONCLUSIONS

The valvular and mural lesions in carcinoid heart disease are specific and characterized by the deposition of an unusual

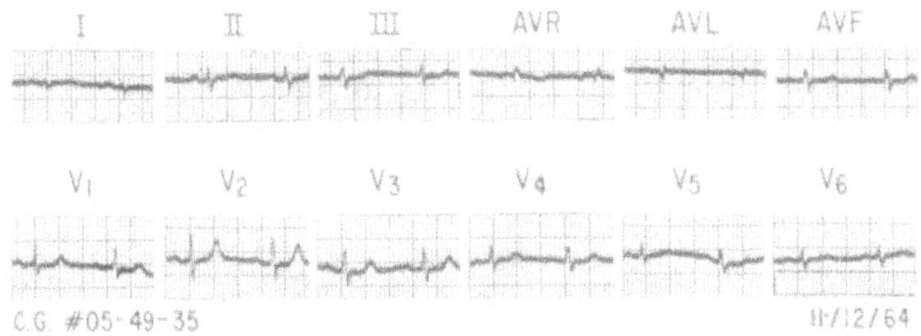

FIG. 4. Electrocardiogram in Patient C. G. Low voltage was present in each of the 2 patients described herein and is the most frequent electrocardiographic abnormality found in patients with carcinoid heart disease.[1]

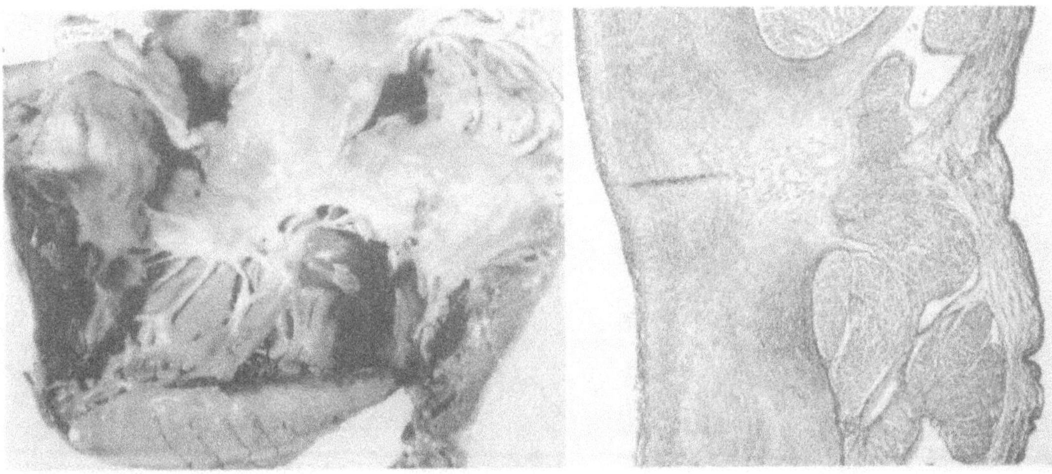

FIG. 5. The heart of Patient K. W. *Left,* the right atrium, tricuspid valve, and right ventricle are opened. There is marked carcinoid-type endocardial fibrosis involving the tricuspid valve leaflets and the right atrial wall. The tricuspid valve is incompetent. *Right,* photomicrograph of section of right atrium showing severe thickening of its wall by the deposition of fibrous tissue on the endocardium. The endocardial surface is toward the left, the epicardial surface is on the right. The thickness of the superimposed fibrous tissue at times is greater than that of the right atrial wall. Elastic tissue stain. Reduced 30 per cent from × 40.

type of fibrous tissue on the endocardial surface. The deposits, which are devoid of elastic fibrils, are located almost entirely on the under or ventricular surface of the tricuspid valve leaflets and on the arterial surface of the pulmonic valve cusps. The underlying valve leaflets and ventricular walls are not involved by this fibrous process and are clearly separated from it by the normal endocardial elastic membrane. The fibrous plaques frequently bind the posterior and septal leaflets of the tricuspid valve to the underlying right ventricular wall, and the result is a fixed regurgitant and slightly stenotic orifice. Tricuspid regurgitation is the most frequent clinical cardiac lesion resulting from this type of fibrosis. When the tricuspid valve is involved, this fibrosing process almost always involves the right atrial endocardium, as well. From study of the extensive right atrial deposits at autopsy in the 2 patients presented, it would seem that the wall of this chamber in these instances is relatively inelastic and consequently not able to distend or to contract normally. This reduction in right atrial elasticity or distensibility as a result of the thick endocardial fibrous deposits probably significantly altered the hemodynamic findings in the right atrial pulse. Thus, there was in each of these 2 patients a greater

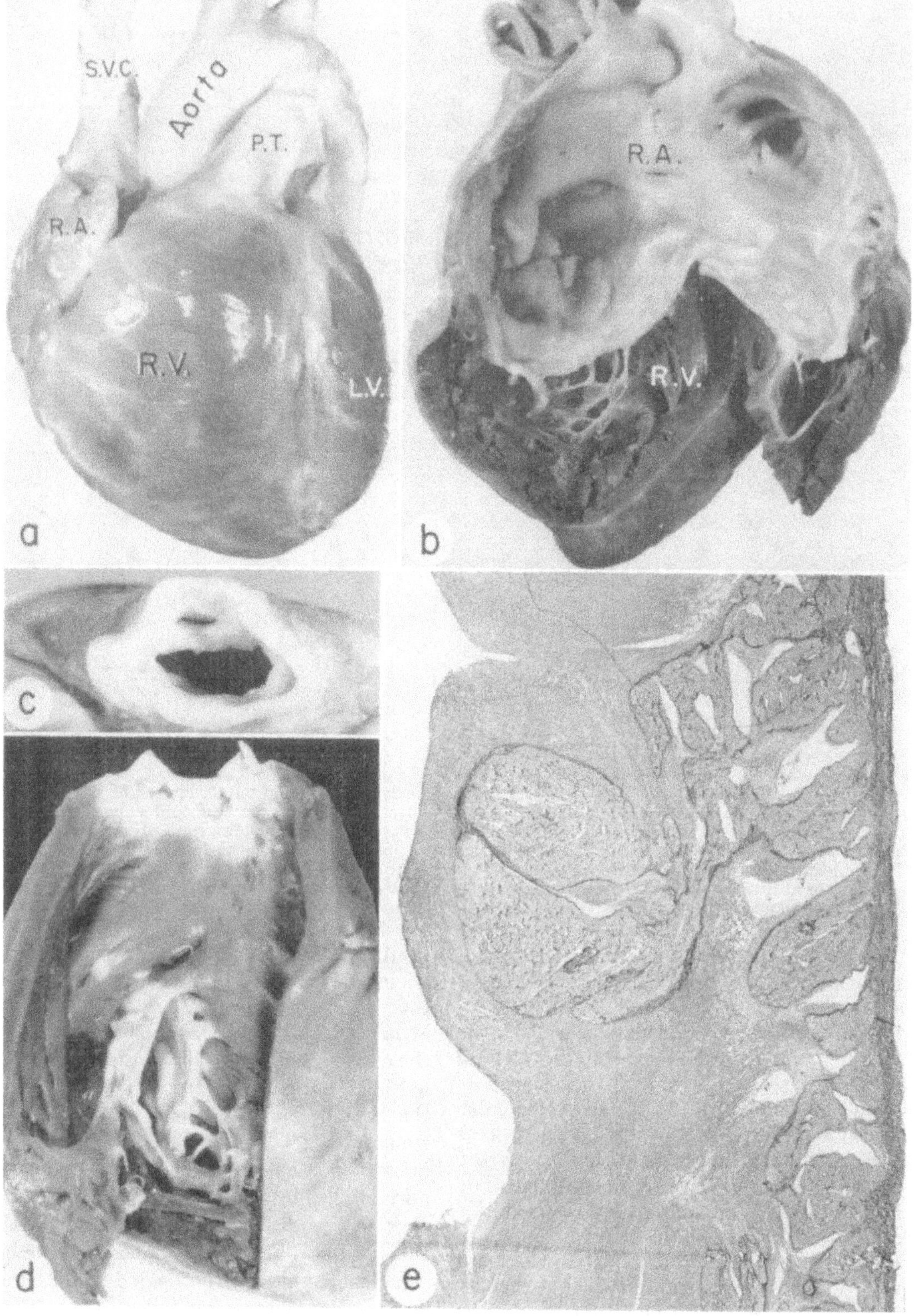

FIG. 6. The heart of Patient C. G. *a*. Exterior view showing a dilated right ventricle (*R.V.*) and right atrium (*R.A.*). The apex of the heart is formed by the right ventricle. *S.V.C.* = superior vena cava. *P.T.* = pulmonary trunk. *b*. Opened right atrium, tricuspid valve, and right ventricle. There is marked fibrous thickening of the tricuspid-valve leaflets with fusion of their commissures, and diffuse carcinoid-type fibrosis of the dilated right atrium and superior vena cava. *c*. Unopened, immobile pulmonic valve. *d*. Opened right ventricle and pulmonic valve disclosing marked carcinoid-type fibrosis of both tricuspid and pulmonic valve leaflets producing stenotic and regurgitant orifices. *e*. Photomicrograph of section of right atrial wall which is severely thickened by the deposition of the fibrous tissue which is devoid of elastic fibrils. Elastic tissue stain. × 19.

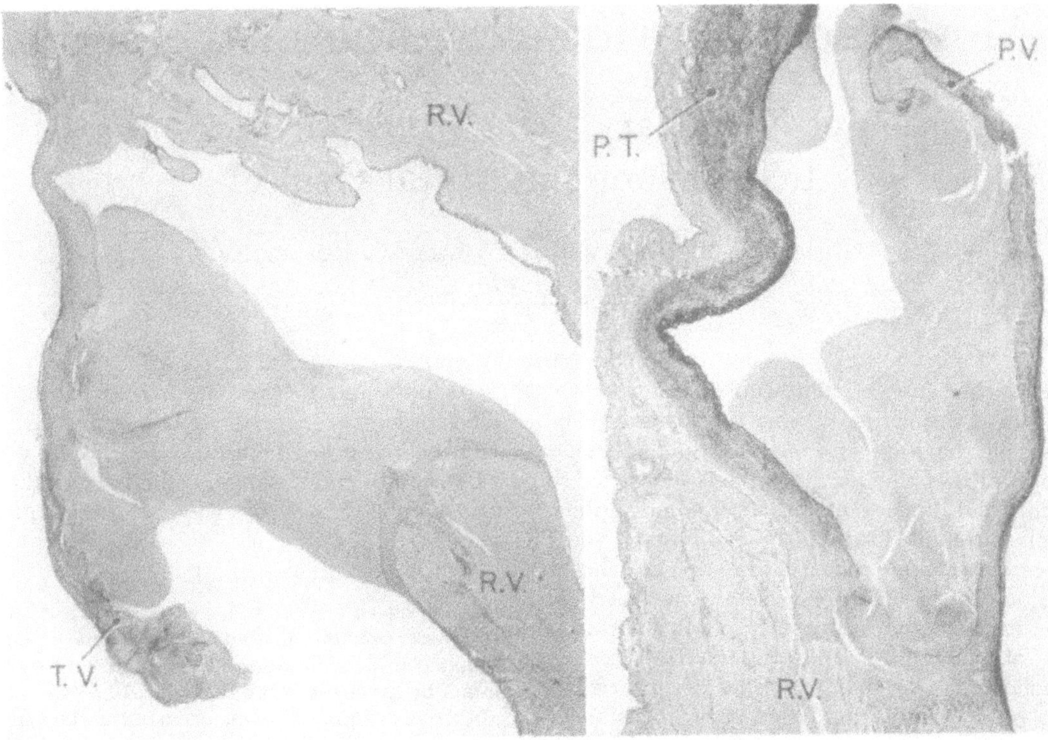

FIG. 7. Photomicrographs of right-sided cardiac valves in patient C. G. *Left*, tricuspid valve (*T.V.*). The superimposed atypical fibrous tissue is deposited only on the undersurface of the leaflet, binding it to the underlying right ventricular (*R.V.*) wall. *Right*, pulmonic valve (*P.V.*). The cusp itself is normal and sharply outlined by its black-staining elastic membrane, but the superimposed fibrous tissue is adherent to its entire arterial surface and fills much of the sinus. A small deposit also is present on the pulmonic trunk (*P.T.*). The surface of the pulmonic valve cusp which has the initial contact with blood ejected from the right ventricle is free of fibrous deposits. Elastic tissue stains. Reduced 20 per cent from × 15.

elevation of the right atrial pressures than would have been expected from the sizes of the tricuspid valve orifices observed at autopsy. It is suggested that even mild tricuspid carcinoid disease may produce significant elevation of right atrial pressures, whereas an equal degree of rheumatic tricuspid disease would not cause right atrial hypertension.

Acknowledgment. Dr. Albert Sjoerdsma, Chief, Experimental Therapeutics Branch, National Heart Institute, gave permission to report these 2 patients and reviewed the manuscript.

REFERENCE

1. Roberts, W. C., and Sjoerdsma, A.: The cardiac disease associated with the carcinoid syndrome (carcinoid heart disease). Am. J. Med., *36:* 5–34, 1964.

Metastatic Choriocarcinoma of the Lung

Invasion of Pulmonary Veins with Extension into the Left Atrium and Mitral Orifice*

JAMES D. MACLOWRY, M.D. *and* WILLIAM C. ROBERTS, M. D.

Bethesda, Maryland

AMONG the causes of stenosis of the pulmonary veins are primary and metastatic neoplasms of the lung and mediastinum, chronic mediastinitis, phlebitis, thrombosis, constrictive pericarditis and congenital malformations. Neoplasms may obstruct the pulmonary veins by extravascular compression or by direct invasion of the wall of the vessel by intravascular growth. The tumor most commonly associated with obstruction of the pulmonary veins is bronchogenic carcinoma. Studies in recent years have demonstrated that gross invasion of the pulmonary veins occurs in approximately 40 per cent of patients with this tumor,[1–3] and in an equal number of patients the pulmonary arteries also are invaded.[3] The peripheral pulmonary vessels are the ones usually involved and the extraparenchymal pulmonary veins, far less frequently.[2] Review of the reports describing neoplastic invasion of the major pulmonary veins with extension of tumor into the left atrium discloses this occurrence in bronchogenic[1,4–10] and metastatic thyroid carcinoma.[11] The present report describes a patient with choriocarcinoma metastatic to the lung with extension of the tumor into the left atrial cavity and mitral orifice by way of the pulmonary veins.

REPORT OF PATIENT

A 28 year old woman, gravida IV, para II, abortus II, whose previous pregnancy five years earlier terminated in a hydatidiform mole, delivered a normal infant by caesarean section on Mar. 10, 1965. Thereafter, daily vaginal bleeding occurred, and two months following delivery unilateral headaches, facial weakness and blurred vision suddenly appeared, and bilateral papilledema was observed. Carotid arteriograms disclosed a space-occupying lesion in the right parietal area; at craniotomy on June 7, this mass was removed and diagnosed histologically as choriocarcinoma.

One week later she was admitted to the Clinical Center of the National Institutes of Health. The uterus was twice normal size and the 24-hour urinary chorionic gonadotrophin titer was between 2 and 5

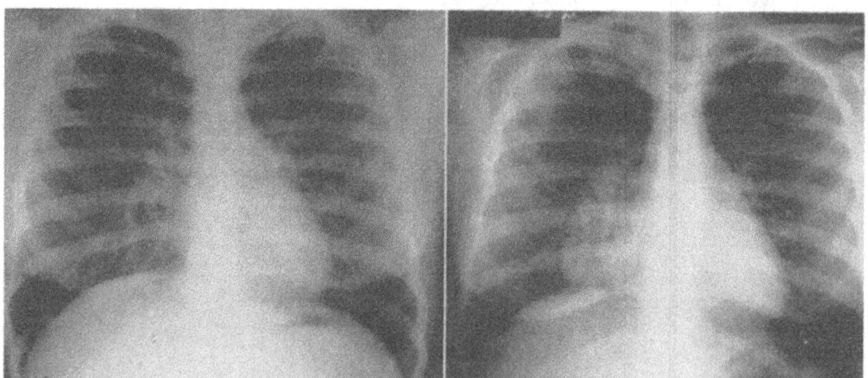

FIG. 1. *Chest roentgenograms.* A, taken four years before death when the patient was well. B, taken two weeks before death. There is a mass in the right lung but no cardiomegaly.

* From the Pathologic Anatomy Branch, National Cancer Institute, National Institutes of Health, Bethesda, Md.

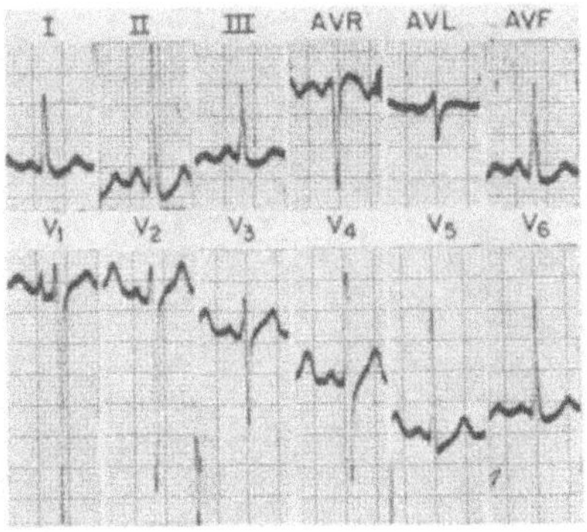

FIG. 2. *Electrocardiogram*, recorded one day before death, shows peaked P waves and prominent QRS complexes.

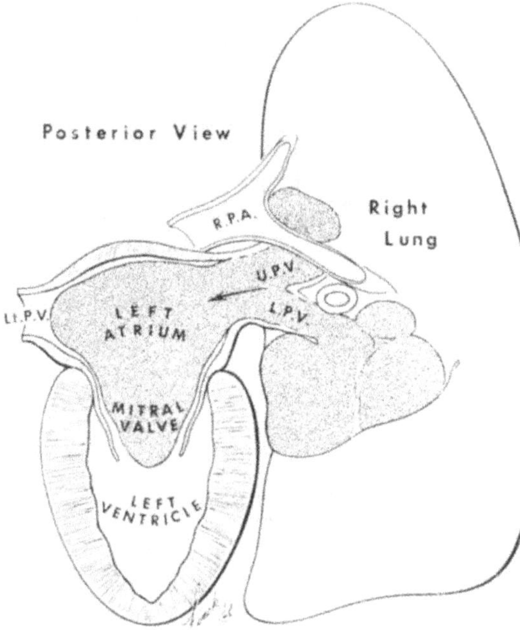

FIG. 3. *Diagram depicts the tumor in the right lung*, growing into the upper (U.P.V.) and lower (L.P.V.) pulmonary veins, and extending into the left atrium and mitral valvular endocardium, but firmly attached to the walls of the pulmonary veins. R.P.A. = right pulmonary artery; Lt. P.V. = left pulmonary veins.

FIG. 4. *Posterior view of the tumor in the right lung* extending into the right lower (R.L.) and right upper (R.U.) pulmonary veins and into the left atrium (L.A.) completely filling its cavity. The pulmonary artery (P.A.) to the right lung is free of tumor. L.U. and L.L. = left upper and lower pulmonary veins, respectively; L.A.A. = left atrial appendage; L.V. = left ventricle; B. = bronchus.

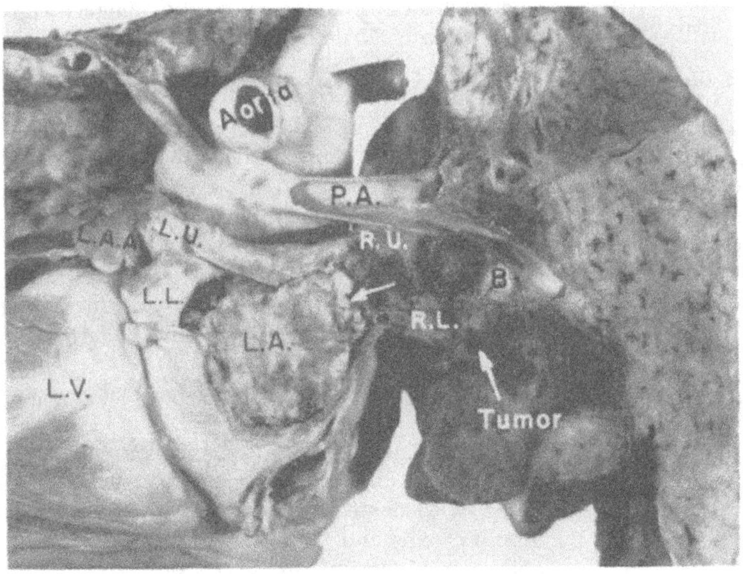

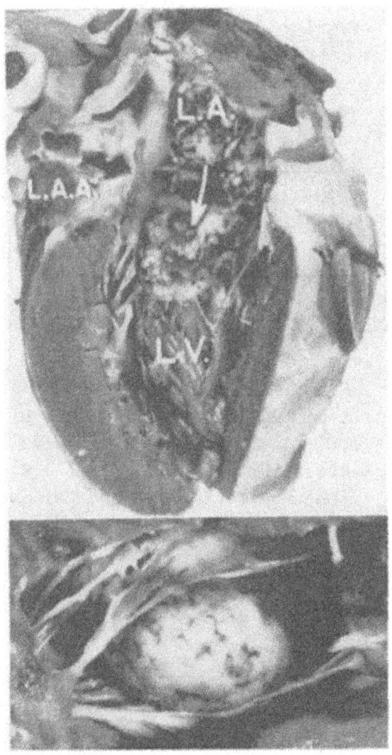

FIG. 5. *The left atrium (L.A.), mitral valve and left ventricle (L.V.)* are opened (upper photograph) showing the tumor filling the atrium and extending through the mitral orifice. The tumor in the mitral orifice, as seen from the left ventricular aspect, is shown in the lower photograph.

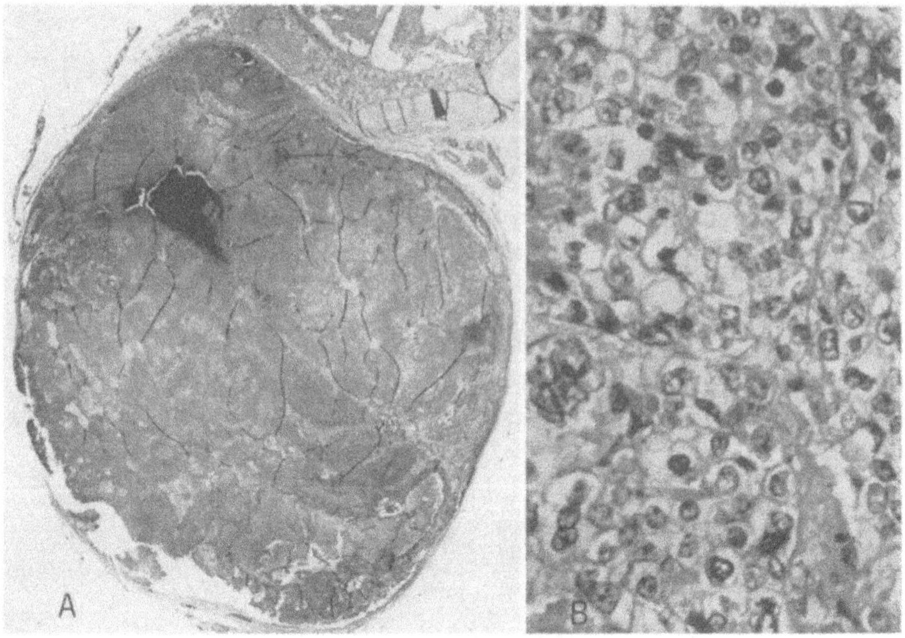

FIG. 6. *Photomicrograph of the choriocarcinoma* filling the right lower pulmonary vein (A), and a high power photomicrograph of the neoplastic cells (B). Viable tumor cells are located only at the periphery, and the main mass of tumor is necrotic. Hematoxylin and eosin stains; original magnification × 10 reduced by 30% (A), and × 380 reduced by 30% (B).

million mouse units. The heart was not enlarged by roentgenogram, but a mass was present in the mid and lower lung fields (Fig. 1). The electrocardiogram disclosed prominent P waves and large QRS complexes (Fig. 2). Methotrexate and prednisolone were administered, but she died on June 30 from increased intracranial pressure. At no time was a precordial murmur detected, nor could any of her symptoms be attributed to cardiopulmonary disease.

Autopsy (*A65-123*) revealed choriocarcinoma in the uterus, lungs, spleen, liver, kidneys, small intestine, brain and perineum. The middle and lower lobes of the right lung contained tumor which totally obstructed the right superior and inferior pulmonary veins, extended into and almost filled the left atrial cavity, and projected through the mitral valvular orifice (Fig. 3–5). The choriocarcinoma was totally adherent to the major pulmonary veins from the right lung (Fig. 6) but was not adherent to the endocardium of the normal-sized left atrium or mitral valve.

The heart was of normal size and weighed 270 gm. The right ventricular cavity was moderately dilated, and the right ventricular wall measured 0.2 cm. in maximal thickness. The left ventricular cavity was of normal size and its wall measured 1.1 cm. in maximal thickness.

COMMENTS

Despite the extension of this tumor through the mitral valvular orifice and the total obstruction of the right major pulmonary veins, there were no symptoms of cardiac disease, no precordial murmur and no cardiomegaly. The electrocardiogram, however, did suggest right heart strain. Histologically, the left atrial tumor was necrotic except for a thin rim of viable tumor at the periphery. Whether or not the tumor would have fragmented or become dislodged from its attachment to the wall of the pulmonary veins when these remaining tumor cells degenerated, possibly as a result of chemotherapy, is a matter of speculation. It is possible that the tumor deposits in the brain, spleen, liver, kidney and small intestine were the result of dislodged fragments of left atrial tumor.

SUMMARY

The clinical and pathologic features of a patient with choriocarcinoma, metastatic to the lungs, with obstruction of the right major pulmonary veins and extension into the left atrium and mitral valvular orifice are described.

ADDENDUM

Since this paper was submitted, Sterns and associates[12] reported on a 33 year old man who died of a metastatic rhabdomyosarcoma to the lung with invasion of the right upper lobe pulmonary vein and extension into the left atrial cavity and into the mitral valvular orifice. Most of this chamber and mitral orifice were filled with tumor. The patient had had systolic and diastolic apical murmurs and atrial fibrillation.

References

1. Aylwin, J. A. Avoidable vascular spread in resection for bronchial carcinoma. *Thorax*, 6: 250, 1951.
2. Hinson, K. F. W. and Nohl, H. C. Involvement of the pulmonary veins by bronchogenic carcinoma. *Brit. J. Dis. Chest*, 54: 54, 1960.
3. Pryce, D. M. and Walter, J. B. The frequency of gross vascular invasion in lung cancer with special reference to arterial invasion. *J. Path. & Bact.*, 79: 141, 1960.
4. Andrew. Primary cancer of the left lung and of the mediastinal glands. *Tr. Path. Soc. London*, 16: 51, 1865.
5. West, S. Cases of mediastinal tumor. *Tr. Path. Soc. London*, 37: 141, 1886.
6. Wolf, K. Der primäre Lungenkrebs. *Fortschr. Med.*, 13: 725, 1895.
7. Geipel, P. Geschwultsbildung im Herzen. *Zentrabl. allg. Path.*, 10: 846, 1899
8. Jeannée, H. Zur Frage der Metastasenbildung bei Einbrüchen von Carcinomen in den grossen Kreislauf. *Virchows Arch. path. Anat.*, 256: 684, 1925.
9. Müller, R. F. Über multiple, nichtsystematisierte Primärcarcinome und ihre Häufigkeit. *Ztschr. Krebsforsch.*, 31: 339, 1930.
10. Spencer, H. Pathology of the Lung, pp. 668–669. New York, 1962. The MacMillan Co.
11. Kaufmann, E. Pathology for Students and Practitioners, pp. 85–86. Translated by Reimann, S. P. Philadelphia, 1929. P. Blakiston's Sons and Co.
12. Sterns, L. P., Eliot, R. S., Varco, R. L. and Edwards, J. E. Intracavitary cardiac neoplasms. A review of fifteen cases. *Brit. Heart J.*, 28: 75, 1966.

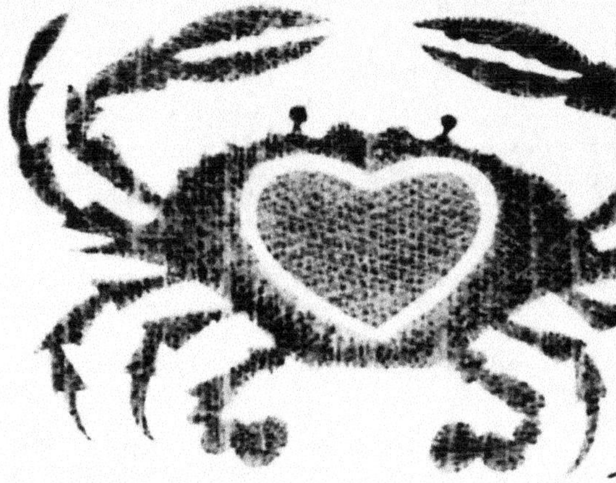

THE HEART IN THE CARCINOID SYNDROME

WILLIAM C. ROBERTS, M.D.

Laboratory of Pathology, Clinic of Surgery, National Heart Institute, National Institutes of Health, Bethesda, Maryland

The carcinoid syndrome, recognized as a distinct entity only twelve years ago, is caused by a metastasizing carcinoid tumor usually located in the small intestine, and occasionally in the bronchus, or stomach, and rarely in the pancreas, ovary, or biliary tract. The tumor produces several biologically active substances including serotonin (5-hydroxytryptamine), histamine, and kinin peptides (bradykinin) (Oates *et al.*). The diagnosis of the syndrome is established by increased excretion in the urine of 5-hydroxyindole acetic acid, a breakdown product of serotonin. Dermal flushing and diarrhea occur in almost all patients with the carcinoid syndrome, wheezing occurs in approximately a third, and a peculiar but specific cardiac disease is present in over half. This report describes the clinical and pathologic features of carcinoid heart disease, and is based on the clinical and autopsy study of 24 patients with the carcinoid syndrome seen at the National Heart Institute. Fourteen of these 24 patients had carcinoid heart disease.

pathology

The cardiovascular disease associated with the carcinoid syndrome is pathognomonic, and bears little resemblance to lesions found in other cardiac diseases (Roberts and Sjoerdsma). The involvement consists of focal or diffuse collections of a peculiar type of fibrous tissue which is deposited on the endocardium of the valvular cusps and cardiac chambers, and on the intima of the great veins, coronary sinus, and occasionally great arteries (Figures 1 through 7). The distinctive feature of this fibrous tissue is the complete absence of elastic fibers. The valvular cusps *per se* and mural endocardium are normal, and are clearly separated from the fibrosing process by the endocardial elastic membrane. The deposits, often referred to as fibrous, white, or carcinoid plaques, are more frequent in the right side of the heart. Of the 14 patients with carcinoid heart disease, these plaques were present on the tricuspid and pulmonic valves in every patient, on the right atrium also in 13, right ventricle in nine, vena cava in seven, coronary sinus in six, and pulmonary trunk in four. In every patient, the tricuspid and pulmonic valves were contracted, relatively rigid, and both stenotic and incompetent. The predominant finding of the tricuspid valve, however, was regurgitation, and that of the pulmonic valve, stenosis. When the tricuspid valve was diffusely involved, a similar diffuse deposit of fibrous tissue usually was also present on the endocardium of the right atrium, causing its wall to be more or less rigid (Roberts *et al.*).

Left-sided cardiac lesions in the carcinoid syndrome are far more common than initially believed. Of the 14 patients with cardiac involvement, six had carcinoid plaques in the left side of the heart: the mitral valve was involved in all six, left ventricle in three, aortic valve in one, and ascending aorta in one. Although two of these patients had diffuse mitral valvular deposits, the valvular orifices did not appear stenotic or incompetent. None of the six patients with left-sided lesions had circulatory shunts or carcinoid tumor in the lung. The right-sided lesions in these six patients

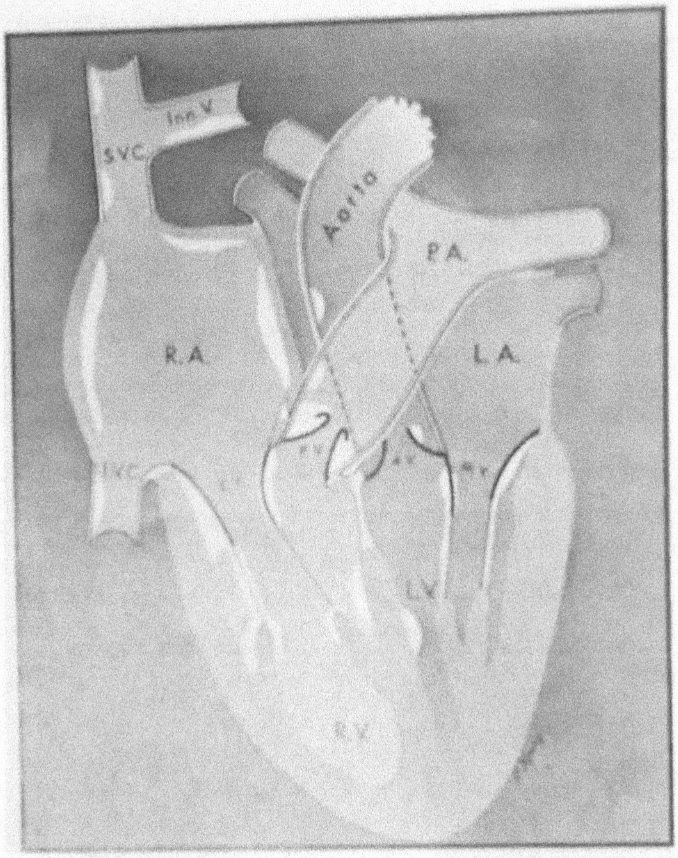

Figure 1. Summary diagram demonstrating (in white) the sites where fibrous plaques occur in patients with the carcinoid syndrome. In patients with abdominal carcinoid tumors the lesions are always more numerous and more extensive on the right side of the heart. The white plaques are usually diffuse over the endocardial surface of the right atrium (R.A.), and tricuspid (T.V.) and pulmonic valves (P.V.). The lesions have never been observed in the pulmonary arteries (P.A.), except in the immediate vicinity of the pulmonic valve, or in the left atrium (L.A.). Inn. V. = innominate vein; S.V.C. = superior vena cava; I.V.C. = inferior vena cava; R.V. = right ventricle; M.V. = mitral valve; L.V. = left ventricle, and A.V. = aortic valve.

Figure 2. The carcinoid heart. This 32-year-old woman, whose electrocardiogram and intracardiac pressure tracings are shown in Figures 9 and 10 respectively, had severe tricuspid regurgitation and pulmonic stenosis. The heart is typical of that seen in carcinoid heart disease. There is atrophy of the subepicardial adipose tissue. The right-sided chambers are dilated, and the cardiac apex is formed by the right ventricle (R.V.)

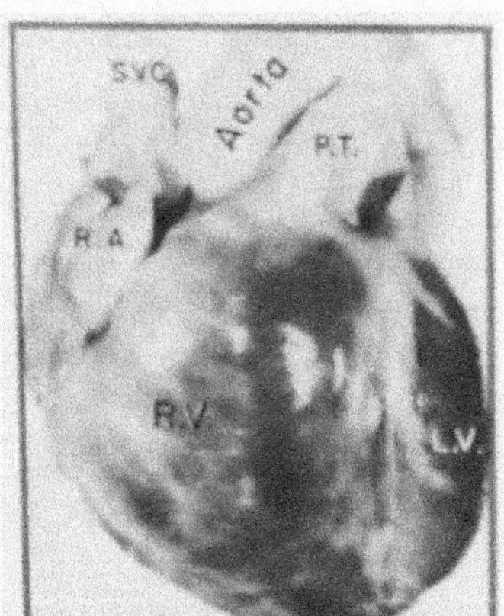

were in every instance more extensive than the left-sided ones. Carcinoid plaquing limited entirely to the left side of the heart, however, has been reported by Melmon and co-workers in patients with bronchial carcinoid.

The right ventricle and right atrium were mildly hypertrophied and dilated in each of the 14 patients with carcinoid heart disease. The hearts weighed more

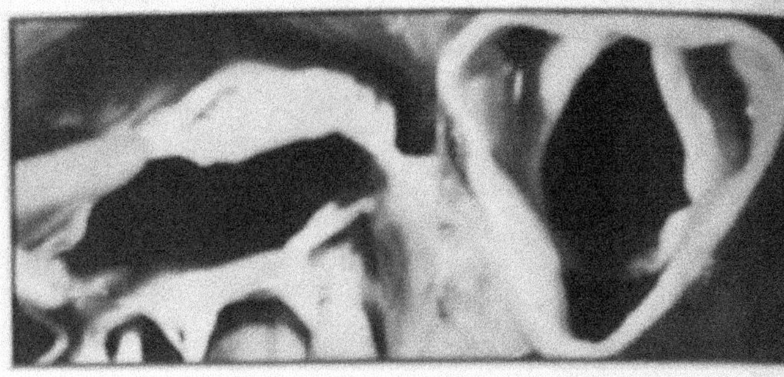

Figure 3. The tricuspid orifice from below (left) and the pulmonic orifice from above (right) in a 69-year-old man with carcinoid heart disease. Both orifices are incompetent and stenotic.

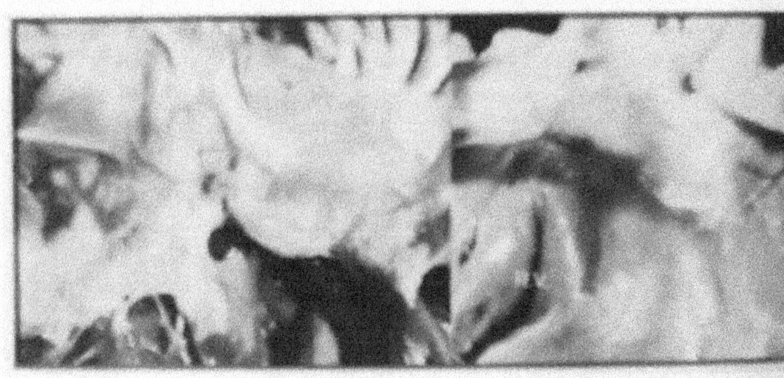

Figure 4. The opened tricuspid valve (left) and pulmonic valve (right) in a 57-year-old woman with carcinoid heart disease. Both valves are severely thickened and immobile. White fibrous plaques also are present in the right atrium (left). R.V. = right ventricle; P.T. = pulmonary trunk.

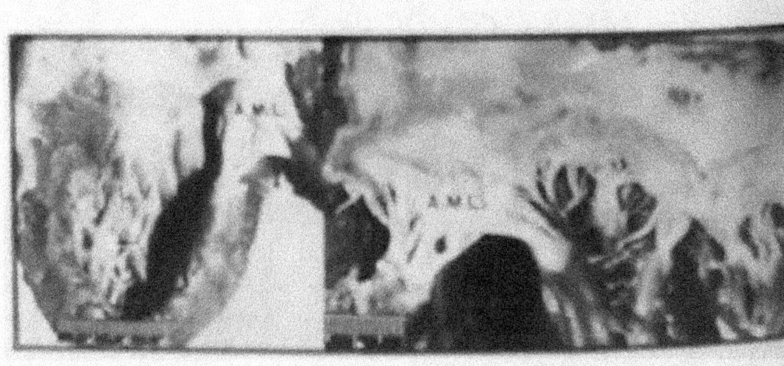

Figure 5. Carcinoid mitral disease. This 57-year-old man had carcinoid fibrosis on the right side of his heart causing tricuspid regurgitation and pulmonic stenosis, and he also had extensive mitral disease. Grossly, the mitral involvement cannot readily be differentiated from rheumatic disease, but sections of this valve, illustrated in Figure 6, are pathognomonic of carcinoid heart disease. One carcinoid plaque (arrow) also is located in the left ventricle (L.V.), but none are present in the left atrium or aortic valve. A.M.L. = anterior mitral leaflet.

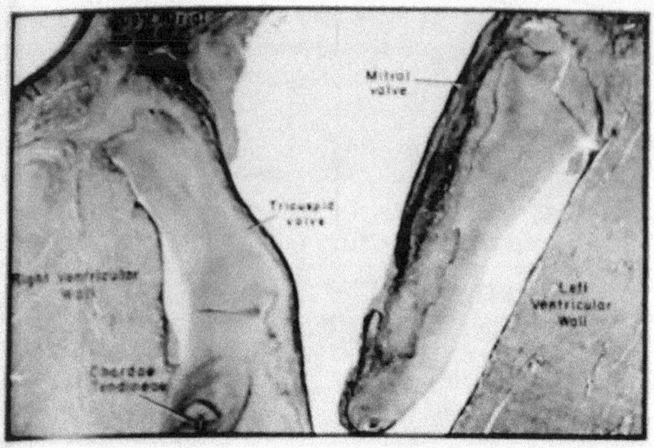

Figure 6. The atrioventricular valves in carcinoid heart disease. The diagnostic feature of this disease histologically is the absence of elastic fibers in the superimposed fibrous tissue. The elastic tissue in these two photographed sections stains black. Each of the valve leaflets is clearly separated from the superimposed fibrous tissue by the black stained endocardial membrane. The deposits occur entirely on the undersurfaces of the posterior and septal tricuspid leaflets, and posterior mitral leaflets, but on both surfaces of the anterior tricuspid and anterior mitral leaflets. Left: Posterior leaflet of tricuspid valve which is adherent to the right ventricular endocardium by the fibrous tissue. Reduced from x14. Right: Posterior mitral leaflet demonstrating similar though less extensive deposition. Elastic tissue stains. Reduced from [illegible]

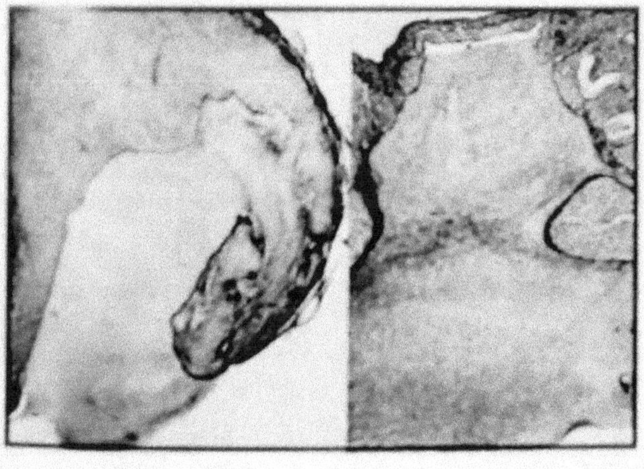

Figure 7. Photomicrographs of right atrial wall (left), and pulmonic valve cusp (right) in a patient with carcinoid heart disease. Left: The superimposed fibrous deposits are far thicker than is the original right atrial wall. Reduced from x43. Right: The fibrous tissue is deposited entirely within the sinus, filling it completely. The distal segment of the cusp is retracted into the sinus and totally surrounded by the fibrous deposits. Elastic tissue stains. Reduced from x25.

than 300 gms in only four patients, however, and each of these patients had a history of systemic hypertension, or associated coronary arterial or chronic pulmonary disease.

clinical features

The clinical finding which distinguishes patients with carcinoid heart disease from those without is the presence of a murmur suggestive of tricuspid regurgitation or pulmonic stenosis. The most frequent murmur in the 14 patients was fairly harsh in quality, Grade 1 to 4/6 in intensity, systolic in time, and located along the upper left sternal border. A systolic blowing murmur, which became louder with inspiration was located along the lower left sternal border, and was heard less frequently. In none of the six patients with mitral carcinoid disease was the diagnosis established

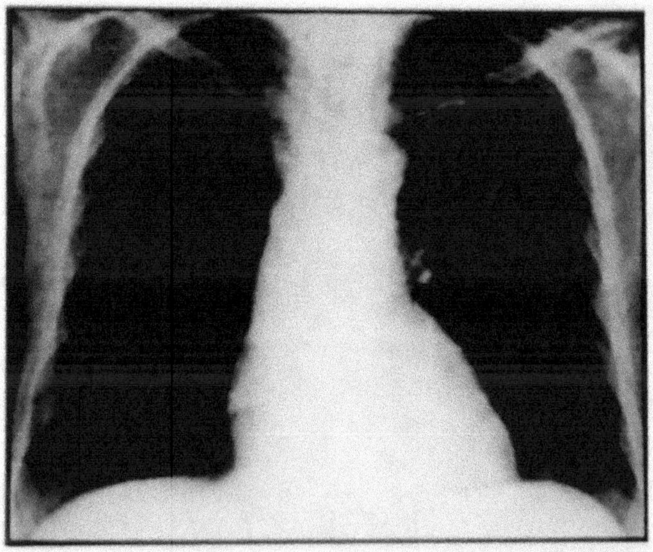

Figure 8. A typical chest roentgenogram in a patient with carcinoid heart disease. The transverse diameter is usually normal. This patient's tricuspid and pulmonic valves are illustrated in Figure 4.

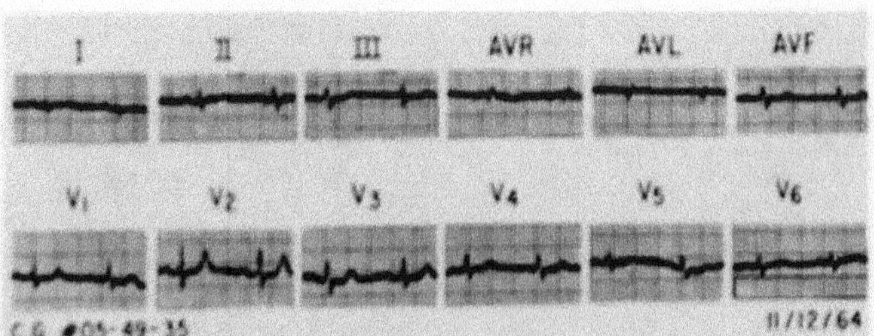

Figure 9. The most frequent electrocardiographic change in carcinoid heart disease is low voltage, but this finding is occasionally seen in patients with the carcinoid syndrome without cardiac involvement.

before autopsy. Prominent V and occasionally prominent A waves often were detectable in the superficial jugular veins, and the liver was sometimes pulsatile.

The chest roentgenogram (Figure 8) and electrocardiogram (Figure 9) are of little value in determining the presence or absence of carcinoid heart disease.

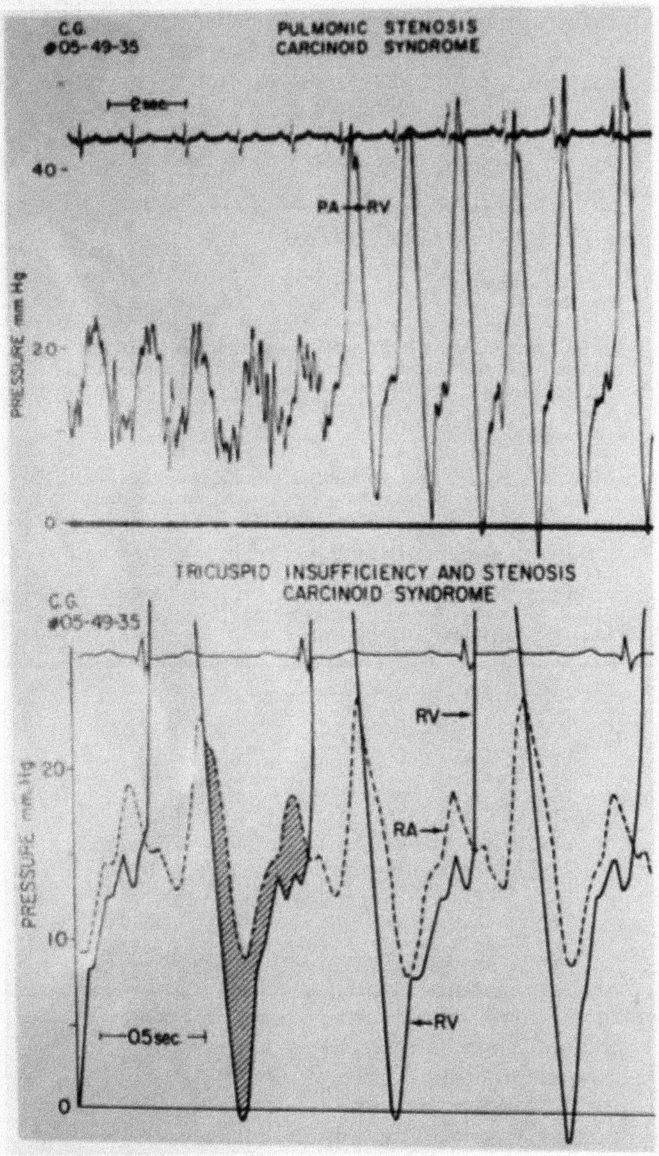

Figure 10. A typical right-sided cardiac pressure tracing in a patient with carcinoid heart disease. A. Pullback from pulmonary trunk (PA) to right ventricle (RV) disclosing a 20 mm. Hg peak systolic pressure gradient. B. The right atrial tracing is superimposed on the high-sensitivity right ventricular pressure tracing. The right atrial pressures are markedly elevated, particularly the V wave. A small mean diastolic pressure gradient (hatched area) is present. The right ventricular end-diastolic pressure also is elevated.

Although the lateral x-ray film sometimes discloses enlargement of the right ventricle, the over-all size of the heart on posteroanterior projection is usually normal. Low voltage seems to be the most frequent electrocardiographic abnormality observed in patients with the carcinoid syndrome. This finding was present in six of the 14 patients with carcinoid heart disease and in two of the ten patients without it. Electrocardiographic evidence of right ventricular hypertrophy occurred in two patients, and evidence of right atrial enlargement (peaked P waves) occurred in three patients with carcinoid heart disease.

Cardiac catheterization in patients with carcinoid heart disease has disclosed tricuspid regurgitation and pulmonic stenosis to be the most frequent valvular findings (Figure 10). The right atrial pressures are commonly elevated, and probably are higher than would be expected with rheumatic tricuspid regurgitation of similar severity (Roberts and co-workers). Although the cardiac output has been reported to be elevated in patients with the carcinoid syndrome without carcinoid heart disease, it is generally normal or low in patients who have carcinoid heart disease.

prognosis

One of the best means of producing severe right-sided cardiac failure in animals is by making the pulmonary trunk stenotic and the tricuspid valve incompetent. These are the two principal valvular lesions which occur in patients with carcinoid heart disease. Interestingly, the presence of this cardiac disease in patients with the carcinoid syndrome does not seem to alter the prognosis. The length of illness from the onset of symptoms to death in the 14 patients with carcinoid heart disease averaged 4.4 years (range ten months to twelve years), whereas the length of illness in the ten patients without carcinoid cardiac disease averaged 3.9 years (range one to nine years). Peripheral edema and ascites appear to be worse, however, in these patients with cardiac disease.

pathogenesis of the cardiac lesions

The pathogenesis of the carcinoid plaque is uncertain. The morphologic appearance of the endocardial lesion suggests that it is the result of the deposit of a material from the blood. That the internal elastic membrane of the underlying endocardium remains intact is evidence that the deposit does not come from the endocardium or myocardium. Initially, serotonin

(Continued on page 40)

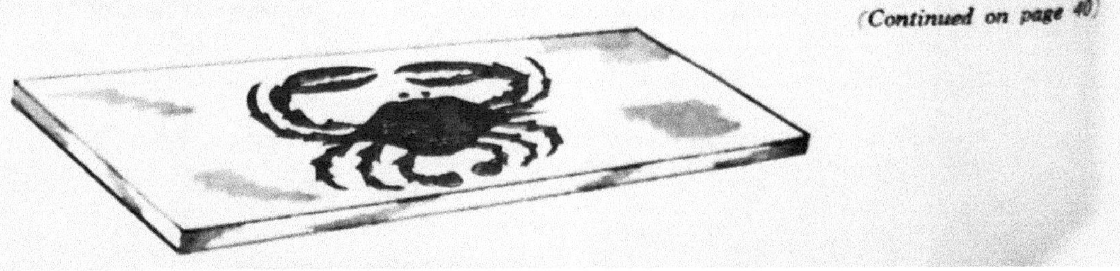

CARCINOID SYNDROME

(Continued from page 24)

was believed to cause the endocardial fibrosis, but there is no evidence to substantiate this belief. It has not been possible to produce the cardiac lesions in animals by giving serotonin or other substances. The breakdown product of serotonin in the urine (5-hydroindoleacetic acid) and the blood serotonin levels have been similar in carcinoid patients with heart disease and in those without cardiac involvement (Roberts and Sjoerdsma). Serotonin initially also was believed responsible for the dermal flush in this syndrome, but recently this hypothesis has been discounted (Levine and Sjoerdsma). A kinin peptide such as bradykinin now seems to be the more likely cause of the flush, and possibly may be involved in the pathogenesis of the carcinoid endocardial lesions (Oates *et al.*).

summary

Among 24 patients with the carcinoid syndrome, studied both clinically and at autopsy, 14 were found to have carcinoid heart disease. The cardiac involvement in this syndrome is characterized by the presence of a peculiar type of fibrous tissue, which is deposited on the endocardium of the cardiac valves and chambers, and on the intima of the veins and arteries attached to the heart. The lesions are most extensive on the right side of the heart and produce tricuspid and pulmonic stenosis and regurgitation. Less extensive lesions occurred in six of the 14 patients on the left side of the heart, and none had a left-to-right shunt or a pulmonary carcinoid. The presence of a precordial murmur suggestive of tricuspid regurgitation or pulmonic stenosis is the only clinical feature which separates those patients with carcinoid heart disease from those without cardiac involvement. The presence of carcinoid heart disease does not seem to alter the prognosis. The carcinoid heart lesions seem to result from the deposition of a material from the blood. Present evidence suggests that serotonin is not responsible for these lesions, and that kinin peptides may play a part in pathogenesis.

acknowledgment

The patients were studied clinically by Dr. Albert Sjoerdsma, Chief, Experimental Therapeutics Branch, National Heart Institute, and the author is indebted to him for free access to the clinical data.

references

MELMON, K. L., *et al.*: Distinctive Clinical and Therapeutic Aspects of the Syndrome Associated with Bronchial Carcinoid Tumors, Am. J. Med. 39:568 (Oct.) 1965.

OATES, J. A., *et al.*: Release of a Kinin Peptide in the Carcinoid Syndrome, Lancet 1:514 (March) 1964.

ROBERTS, W. C., and SJOERDSMA, A.: The Cardiac Disease Associated with the Carcinoid Syndrome (Carcinoid Heart Disease), Am. J. Med. 36:5 (Jan.) 1964.

ROBERTS, W. C., *et al.*: The Nondistensible Right Atrium in Carcinoid Heart Disease, Am. J. Clin. Path. 44:627 (Dec.) 196

ARTERIAL SURGERY

(Continued from page 31)

"subclavian steal" syndrome. In this condition the occlusive lesion is in the subclavian artery directly proximal to the origin of the vertebral artery. Because of the lowered intraluminal pressure in the subclavian as compared to the vertebral arterial trunk, the direction of flow in the vertebral artery is reversed and the vessel becomes a collateral branch of the subclavian artery, drawing blood from the brain to the arm. Cure is readily accomplished by correction of the subclavian lesions.

Other visceral arteries. The celiac, superior mesenteric and inferior mesenteric arteries participate in the occlusive process of systemic arteriosclerosis probably to the same degree as most peripheral arteries but rarely cause clinically detectable physiologic disturbances. The reason for this semeiotic silence is undoubtedly the existence of rich collateral circulation in all the splanchnic regions. When clinical manifestations d appear, they are either high-grade stenoses, or a com plete obliteration in more than one main arterial ster or some anatomical anomaly has reduced the potenti collateral bed.

Only one such arterial lesion has given rise to a syn drome of some frequency: the occlusive involveme of the superior mesenteric artery. When symptomati this lesion is almost always associated with an a vanced stenosis of the celiac artery and it manifes itself in postprandial midabdominal pain and in the ev dences of small bowel malabsorption. The diagnosis often suspected but seldom proven; its proof is th demonstration of the arterial stenosis in an arteriogra taken in a lateral view. The lesion is well suited f surgical correction (by endarterectomy, as a rule).

Part I of this article appeared in the November-Decemb 1966 issue of THE HEART BULLETIN. Part II appeared in t January-February 1967 issue of THE HEART BULLETIN.

The Heart in Acute Leukemia

A Study of 420 Autopsy Cases*

WILLIAM C. ROBERTS, M.D., F.A.C.C., GERALD P. BODEY, M.D. and PAUL T. WERTLA~

Bethesda, Maryland

> There is no organ or tissue in the body which has not been involved by leukemic infiltration, with or without the production of clinical signs and symptoms.
>
> *M. M. Wintrobe and D. M. Mitchell*[1]

THE HEART of a patient with acute leukemia may function abnormally because of several factors: leukemic cell infiltrates or hemorrhages in its wall, hypoxia resulting from associated severe anemia, a cardiac or systemic infection, an underlying cardiac disease or a combination of these factors. Most previous studies of the heart in patients with acute :eukemia have centered mainly on the incidence and extent of the cardiac leukemic cell infiltrates and on the clinical and electrocardiographic alterations resulting from them. Few reports have mentioned cardiac hemorrhages or the types and incidence of cardiac infections that are prevalent in patients with acute leukemia. The present study describes the cardiac findings in 420 patients with acute leukemia and attempts to correlate the pathologic observations with the clinical features.

PATIENTS STUDIED AND METHODS

The clinical records of patients with acute leukemia who underwent autopsy at the Clinical Center from 1954 through 1964 were reviewed. Excluding those patients in whom the autopsy permit did not allow examination of the heart, a total of 420 patients with acute leukemia, either myelogenous or lymphocytic, were studied (Fig. 1). Sixty per cent of the 420 patients had acute lymphocytic leukemia, and 40 per cent had acute myelogenous leukemia. The majority of patients with acute lymphocytic leukemia were between 2 and 10 years of age (54 per cent), and 80 per cent of the patients with acute myelogenous leukemia were over 20 years of age. The diagnosis of leukemia in each was made by bone marrow examination during life. Each patient received some form of antileukemic therapy (6-mercaptopurine, methotrexate, cyclophosphamide, vincristine, adrer steroids, or experimental drugs).

The hearts of 402 patients were re-examined grossly; the hearts of the other 18 were unavailable for re-examination, but histologic sections of them

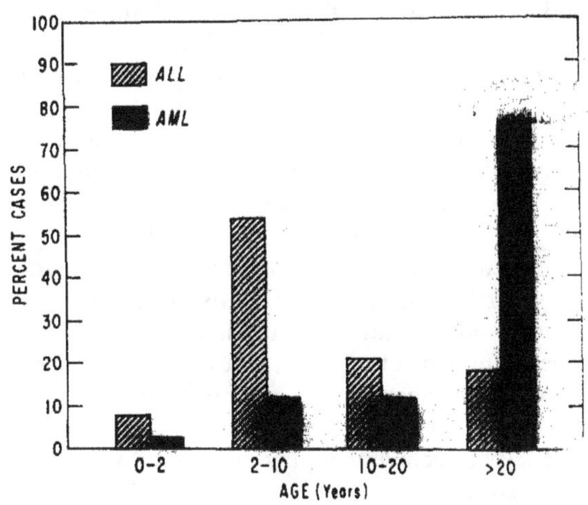

FIG. 1. *Age distribution* of the 420 patients with acute lymphocytic (ALL) and acute myelogenous (AML) leukemia.

* From the Laboratory of Pathology, Clinic of Surgery, National Heart Institute, and Branches of Medicine and Pathologic Anatomy, National Cancer Institute, National Institutes of Health, Bethesda, Md. 20014.

Address for reprints: William C. Roberts, M.D., Laboratory of Pathology, Clinic of Surgery, National Heart Institute, Department of Health, Education, and Welfare, Bethesda, Md. 20014.

were reviewed. In all patients, however, the cardiac descriptions and diagnoses were reviewed in the autopsy protocols. In each of the 420 patients usually four microscopic sections of the heart had been taken at the time of the necropsy, and in most patients these sections were re-examined. Addi- were cut in approximately 250 of the .02 hearts re-examined grossly, and each of these sections was studied histologically. In a number of patients re-examination of the gross heart and of the additional carefully selected histologic sections dis-closed the presence of pathologic alterations that had ot been recorded in the autopsy protocols.

The chest roentgenograms and electrocardiograms, the reports in the charts, were reviewed patients w... unusual or severe cardiac alterations observed at necropsy.

Clinical Observations

Symptoms: Twenty patients had symptoms that clearly could be related to abnormalities of the heart. Thirteen of the 20 had *chest pain*, always substernal or precordial, and 9 of them had pericarditis at necropsy. The chest pain in all 9 subjects was aggravated by inspiration, and each had a pericardial friction rub. The pericarditis was the result of leukemic cell infiltrates into the pericardia in only 2 of the 9 subjects; in 4 patients it was hemorrhagic; in 2 pyogenic; and in 1 of uncertain etiology, being fibrinous and unassociated with pericardial leukemic infiltrates, hemorrhages, or organisms. In each of the other 4 patients with anteriorly located chest pain, a focus of myocardial necrosis was observed at necropsy. In none of them was the myocardial necrosis associated with leukemic in- but 1 had focal myocardial hemor- massive mucor infection of the myocardial wall, and 1 focal bacterial myocarditis; the fourth had myocardial toxoplasmosis. At least 2 additional patients had transient but severe anterior chest pain, but at necropsy there were no abnormalities of the heart or pericardia; each was a 6 year old child with transient subendocardial injury revealed by electrocardiogram.

Seven additional patients had severe *dyspnea* resulting from acute cardiac failure, and 6 of the had leukemic infiltrates and hemorrhages in myocardium. In 2 of the 6 subjects the myocardial hemorrhages and leukemic cell infiltrates were massive. One of the 6, a 51 year old woman, had severely narrowed coronary arteries in addition to the myocardial infiltrates, and another patient, a 7 year old boy, had staphylococcal septicemia with high fever in addition to the myocardial infiltrates. The seventh patient had cytomegalic inclusion disease involving the myocardium and lungs.

Dyspnea occurred occasionally in patients other than these 7, but in them it was attributed to an associated pleural or peritoneal effusion, associated anemia, infection (usually pneumonia), fever related to the leukemic process itself, or an enlarged liver or spleen pushing the diaphragm cephalad.

Precordial Murmurs: These were described in 127 patients. In all but 4 the murmurs were believed to be functional or hemic in nature, and often occurred transiently when the patients were febrile or severely anemic. The ventricles and atrioventricular rings were dilated at necropsy in some patients, and functional mitral or tricuspid regurgitation, or both, may have occurred. The murmurs in all patients were systolic; none had diastolic murmurs. Pericardial friction rubs were described in 20 patients.

Cardiac Enlargement: Cardiac size was often difficult to evaluate. By precordial examination cardiac enlargement rarely was noted. By *chest roentgenogram*, however, the cardiac silhouette was enlarged in 45 patients, but cardiac hypertrophy was found at autopsy in only 10 of these patients. Furthermore, 68 additional subjects at necropsy were considered to have enlarged hearts, and in none of them was cardiomegaly described in the chest roentgenogram. Not infrequently, however, a considerable period of time had elapsed between the last chest roentgenogram and death. Almost certainly in some patients the impression of cardiac enlargement on chest roentgenogram was the result of an enlarged spleen or liver that had pushed the heart upward and to the left, or was the result of mediastinal lymphadenopathy causing enlargement of the "cardiac silhouette." Left ventricular dilatation without hypertrophy was the most frequent cause of the enlargement, and right ventricular dilatation was next. It appears clear that cardiomegaly occurs in a significant percentage of patients with acute leukemia and that ventricular dilatation without hypertrophy is its most frequent cause. Most patients received large volumes of fluid intravenously, including frequent transfusions of blood and blood products, and hypervolemia may have been a factor causing cardiac enlargement.

Electrocardiographic Findings: Electrocardiograms were recorded in the majority of the adult patients, but many of the children never had an electrocardiogram. In some cases tracings were made only during the early part of the patients's illness, and often electrocardiograms were not recorded during the last week of life. Multiple tracings were available for only a few patients. Sinus tachycardia, the result of anemia, fever, infection, and the like, was the most frequent electrocardiographic alteration recorded. Various nonspecific abnormalities of the P or T waves, QRS complexes, or S-T segments were observed in 83 patients; in 24 the alterations were attributed to so-called metabolic disturbances.

Various arrhythmias were recorded in 20 patients: atrial premature contractions (8 patients); ventricular premature contractions (4); atrial fibrillation (5); paroxysmal atrial tachycardia (4); wandering atrial pacemaker (3); sinus pauses, or arrest, or nodal escape (3); sinus bradycardia (2), and ventricular tachycardia (1). Two of the 5 patients with atrial fibrillation had underlying cardiac disease (coronary heart disease in 1, and rheumatic heart disease in the other). In 1 patient, a 42 year old man, with ventricular tachycardia the arrhythmia developed terminally, and at necropsy he was found to have widespread Clostridium perfringens infection, including numerous gas bubbles and organisms in the myocardium. The P-R interval was prolonged (>0.20 sec.) in 5 patients, atrioventricular dissociation was recorded in 1 patient, and intraventricular conduction defects were seen in 2 patients, aged 4 and 9 years. The 48 year old woman with atrioventricular dissociation had an anatomically normal heart at necropsy.

Right bundle branch block of unknown cause was recorded in 2 patients, and left bundle branch block in 1. The latter patient had cytomegalic inclusion disease of the heart and lungs with acute pulmonary edema, and the tracing was made terminally during this episode. Left axis deviation was recorded in 2 elderly patients (aged 70 and 82 years, respectively), and each had coronary heart disease. Right axis deviation was recorded in the 1 patient with a ventricular septal defect.

Observations at Necropsy

CARDIAC HEMORRHAGES AND LEUKEMIC CELL INFILTRATIONS (FIG. 2 TO 18)

Of the 420 hearts examined, 288 (69 per cent) had hemorrhages, or leukemic cell infitrates, or both, and 132 hearts (31 per cent) were free of leukemic cells or extravasated erythrocytes. Of 171 hearts (41 per cent) that were normal grossly, 39 had hemorrhages, or leukemic infiltrates, or both, on histologic examination. Of the 288 hearts containing hemorrhages and/or leukemic cell infiltrates, 132 had hemorrhages only, 96 had both hemorrhages and leukemic cell infiltrates, and 60 had leukemic cell infiltrates only (Table I). Leukemic cell infiltrates with or without hemorrhages, therefore, were observed in 156 of the 420 hearts (37 per cent), and hemorrhages with or without leukemic infiltrates were seen in 228 hearts (54 per cent). The incidence of cardiac leukemic infiltrates and hemorrhages was relatively constant during each of the 11 years included in this study.

The cardiac hemorrhages and leukemic cell infiltrates occurred in the walls of all cardiac chambers as well as in the visceral and parietal pericardia and subepicardial adipose tissue. In addition, these lesions often were seen grossly in the adventitia of the great vessels attached to the heart. The hemorrhages and leukemic cell infiltrates were almost always focal and were most frequently located in, or immediately beneath, the endocardium. Involvement of the myocardium, however, was by no means unusual. The endocardial and pericardial hemorrhages were detected on gross examination of the heart in almost every patient, since their color was distinctly different from that of the surrounding structures. In contrast, pure leukemic cell infiltrates, which had not been noted grossly, occasionally were found in the histologic sections of heart. Leukemic cell infiltrates usually were found in the endocardium, in the interstitial and perivascular regions of the myocardium and in various portions of the pericardium but had not altered the basic architecture or color of these regions of the heart. Consequently, unless the leukemic cell infiltrates were associated with hemorrhages or were distinct tumorous nodules, their presence on gross examination of the hearts was usually not appreciated. Localized, white, firm leukemic cell nodules were found grossly in the hearts of only 3 patients and in only 1 (Fig. 18) were the nodules multiple. On histologic study of sections of hearts, however, foci of leukemic cells were seen fairly frequently. In at least 14 patients the hemorrhages and/or leukemic cell infiltrates extended through the entire wall of a cardiac chamber. In 1 patient the entire free walls of both atria and the atrial septum

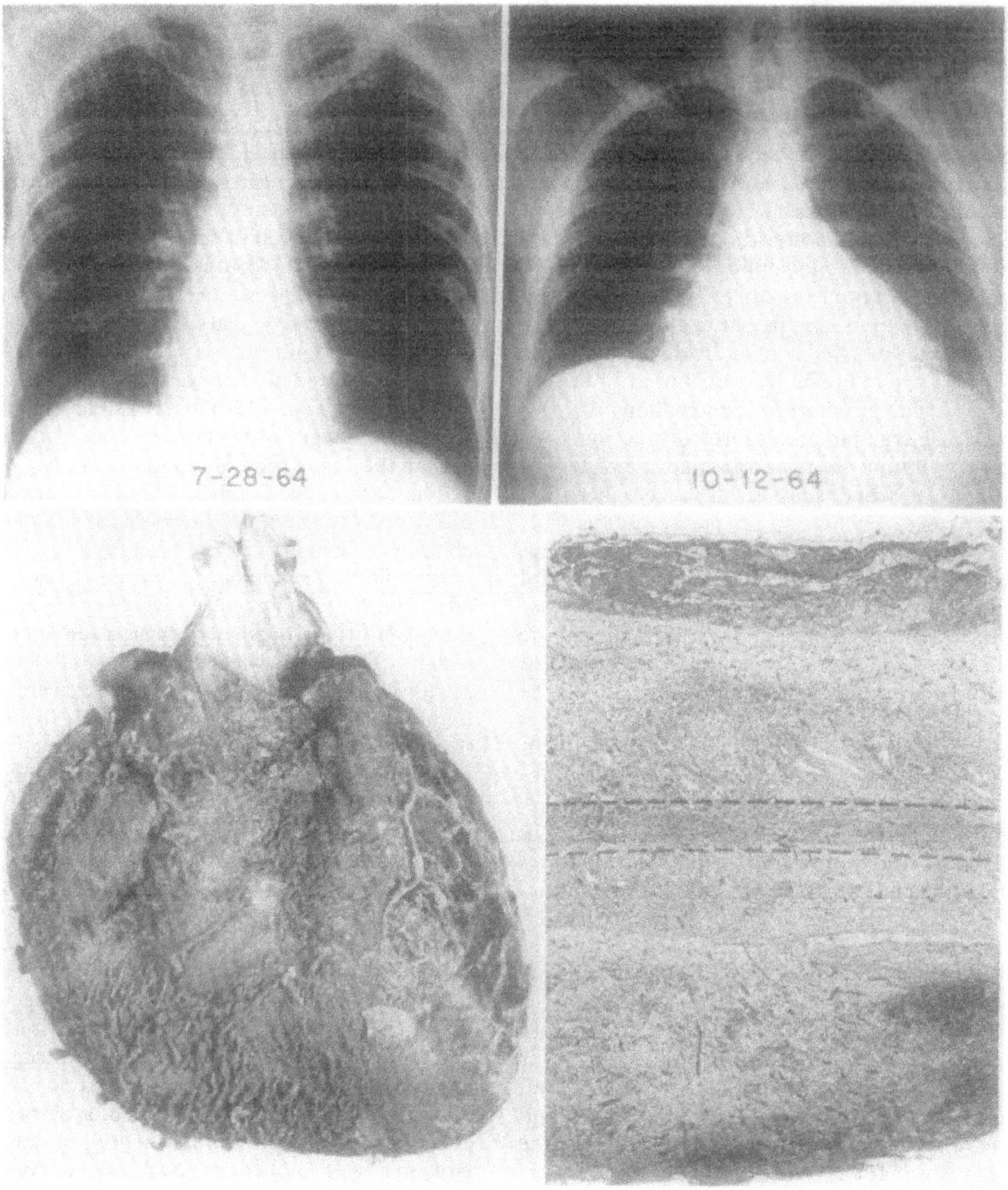

FIG. 2. *Acute Pericarditis. Chest roentgenograms, anterior surface of heart (lower left), and section of parietal pericardium (lower right) in a 32 year old man with acute myelogenous leukemia.* This patient's presenting symptom was chest pain typical of acute pericarditis, and this symptom predominated throughout his entire seven month illness. At the first appearance of chest pain the white blood cell count was 7,700 per cu. mm. with 56 per cent polymorphonuclear leukocytes and 44 per cent lymphocytes; a diagnosis of leukemia was not considered. Fifteen days later the white cell count was 73,000 per cu. mm., the blood smear showed 90 per cent myeloblasts, and a diagnosis of acute myelogenous leukemia was made. A precordial friction rub was audible intermittently. The precordial pain became so severe during the patient's final two weeks that he received mediastinal irradiation for it. He died on October 27, 1964. Shaggy adhesions obliterated most of the pericardial space, which contained 30 ml. of serosanguinous fluid. The heart weighed 450 gm. *Lower right*, the dashed lines indicate what is believed to be the thickness of the parietal pericardium before the pericarditis appeared. Organizing connective tissue containing extravasated erythrocytes and a few leukemic cells produced the marked thickening of the pericardium. (Hematoxylin and eosin, × 26 reduced by 16%.)

Table I

TYPE OF CARDIAC INVOLVEMENT IN ACUTE LEUKEMIA

	No.	% of Total	Region of Heart Involved					
			RA	RV	LA	LV	Pericardium	TV
No hemorrhages or leukemic cells grossly or microscopically	132	31.4						
Leukemic cells + hemorrhage	96	22.9	54	37	32	55	61	1
Leukemic cells only	60	14.3	14	11	5	19	34	0
Hemorrhages only	132	31.4	58	34	21	76	68	2
TOTAL	420	100.0	126	82	58	150	163	3

ABBREVIATIONS: RA = right atrium; RV = right ventricle; LA = left atrium; LV = left ventricle; TV = tricuspid valve leaflets.

were hemorrhagic; the ventricular walls, in contrast, were nearly entirely free of hemorrhages and leukemic cells (Fig. 10). In 4 patients hemorrhages and/or leukemic cell infiltrates were located in the atrioventricular bundle (Fig. 12), and in a fifth patient a focal hemorrhage involved the proximal portion of the left bundle branch (Fig. 13). Electrocardiograms were not recorded for any of these 5 patients, but in none was the pulse rate slow terminally. When a cardiac wall was massively hemorrhagic, the myocardial fibers often were necrotic. Occasionally, complete lysis of myocardial fibers was observed in areas of hemorrhage or leukemic cell infiltration (Fig. 15 and 16).

Sites of the leukemic cell infiltrates and/or hemorrhages: These are listed in Table I, and in Table II the number of cardiac sites involved in each patient is tabulated. The most frequent site of involvement was the pericardium, followed by the left ventricle, right ventricle and left atrium in that order. The infiltrates listed as occurring in the left ventricle most frequently were limited to the left side of the ventricular septum, usually the outflow portion in, or immediately below, the endocardium. Extensive infiltrates occasionally occurred in the atria and left ventricle but were rare in the right ventricle. Three patients had petechiae or leukemic cell infiltrates in a cardiac valve: in 2 minute hemorrhages only were present and in 1, leukemic cells as well as erythrocytes were observed. Only the basal portion of one leaflet of the tricuspid valve was involved in each of the 3 patients. Hemorrhages and leukemic cell infiltrates occurred in all areas of the pericardium, but a particularly prominent site was the atrioventricular sulcus, which frequently contained large collections of erythrocytes, and less commonly, leukemic cells. The infiltrates were most often limited to the wall of one cardiac chamber, and next, to one chamber plus the pericardium (Table II). Only 20 patients had leukemic infiltrates and/or hemorrhages in the walls of all four chambers, and in 16 of them the pericardium also was involved.

PERICARDIAL DISEASES (FIG. 2 TO 8)

Disease of the pericardium other than, or in addition to, petechiae or infiltrations of leukemic cells occurred in 56 of the 420 patients (13 per cent). In 39 patients the pericardial space contained quantities of fluid ranging from 25 to 1,100 ml. (>25 ml. in children; >50 ml. in

Table II

SITE OF CARDIAC HEMORRHAGE OR LEUKEMIC CELL INFILTRATE IN ACUTE LEUKEMIA

	NUMBER	% OF TOTAL
No hemorrhage or leukemic cells grossly or microscopically*	132	31.4
One cardiac chamber only	62	14.8
Two cardiac chamber	17	4.1
Three cardiac chamber	10	2.4
Four cardiac chamber	4	0.9
Pericardium only	31	7.3
Pericardium plus one chamber	52	12.4
Pericardium plus two chamber	33	7.9
Pericardium plus three chamber	29	6.9
Pericardium plus four chamber	16	3.8
Site not specified (grossly normal)	33	7.9
Tricuspid valve only	1	.2
TOTAL	420	100.0

*39 additional hearts normal grossly but contained hemorrhages or leukemic infiltrates microscopically. Thus, hearts normal grossly = 40.7% of total.

adults); over 300 ml. of fluid was recorded in 4 patients. In 28 of the 39 patients there was no associated fibrinous, fibrous, purulent, or hemorrhagic pericarditis; grossly these effusions were serous in 22 and blood-tinted in 6. The effusions in the remaining 11 were associated with gross lesions, other than petechiae or leukemic nodules, of the pericardium. Four of the 9 patients with fibrinous pericarditis had effusions, and each of the 7 patients with hemorrhagic pericardial linings had effusions. Significant effusions were absent in each of the 6 patients with fibrous pericarditis, in the 1 patient with fibrinofibrous pericarditis, and in the 5 patients with purulent pericarditis.

The etiology of the pericardial disease in the 56 patients was variable. Nearly all of the 28 patients with effusions unassociated with pericarditis also had effusions in the pleural and abdominal spaces as well as peripheral edema. Therefore, it would appear that these pericardial effusions were more likely a part of a generalized process, probably related to leukemic infiltrations, severe anemia, or hypoproteinemia. One of the 7 patients with hemorrhagic pericarditis died of cardiac tamponade, and at autopsy the parietal pericardium was 4 cm. thick (Fig. 5). Of the 5 patients with grossly purulent pericarditis, 4 were associated with Gram-negative organisms: in 2 the infections resulted from esophageal rupture and mediastinitis; a pulmonary Escherichia coli abscess was the probable source in another; and Gram-negative septicemia appeared to be the underlying cause in the fourth. Aspergillus organisms were the cause of the pericarditis in the other patient with grossly purulent pericarditis. This patient also had myocardial abscesses associated with aspergillus organisms. An additional patient—not included in the 56 with gross pericardial disease—was found on histologic sections to have aspergillus organisms focally in the subepicardial adipose tissue. In the patients with fibrinous and fibrinofibrous pericarditis, leukemic cell infiltrates frequently were observed in the pericardium. The precise cause of the pericarditis, however, was not apparent from histologic study of the pericardium in most of the patients. One patient with fibrous pericarditis had had acute rheumatic fever many years earlier.

Endocardial Diseases

Twenty-four patients had chronic cardiac

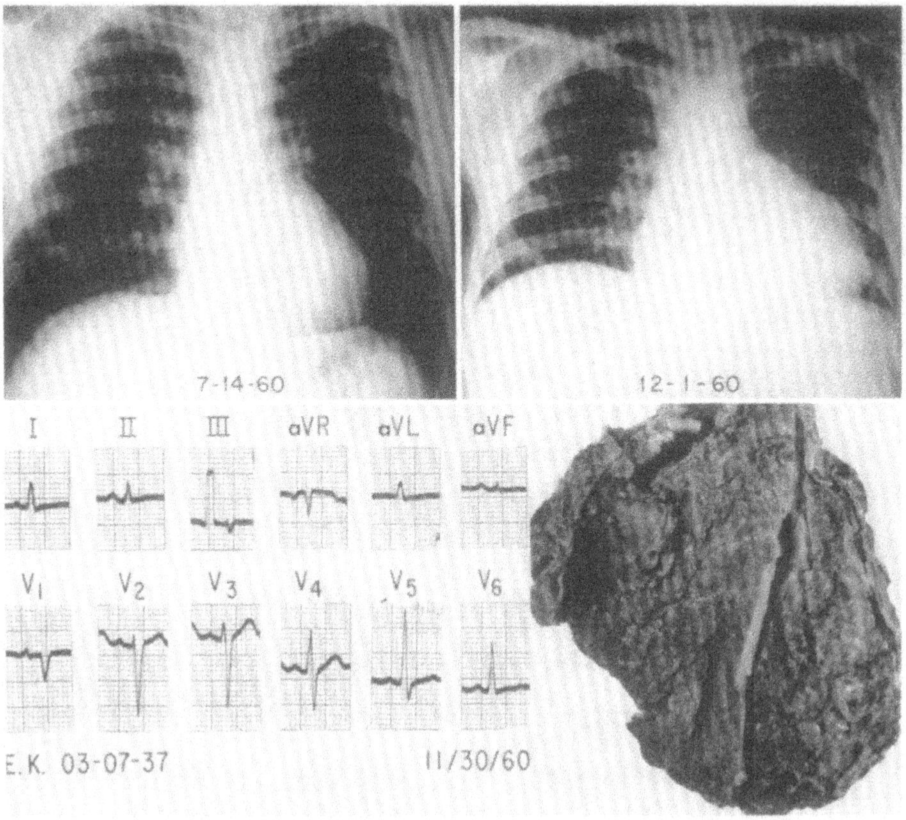

FIG. 3. *Hemorrhagic Pericarditis. Chest roentgenograms, electrocardiogram, and anterior surface of heart in a 29 year old man with acute myelogenous leukemia.* He died on December 21, 1960, and at necropsy 1,100 ml. of blood was found in the pericardial sac. Clinically, he had no signs of symptoms of cardiac tamponade. The electrocardiogram shows low voltage. The heart is covered by hemorrhagic organizing connective tissue (*lower right*).

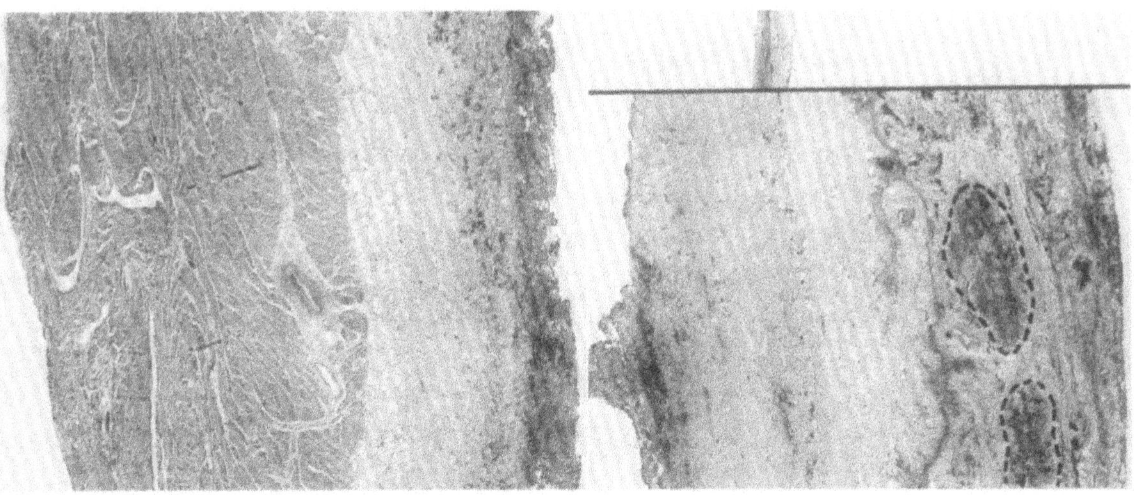

FIG. 4. *Same Case. Photomicrographs of visceral* (*left*) *and parietal* (*right*) *pericardia.* Both pericardia are markedly thickened, and the parietal pericardium, in addition to fibrous tissue, contains clumps of leukemic cells (dashed areas) within which are located calcium deposits (stained black). A section of normal parietal pericardium taken at the same magnification is shown at the upper right for comparison. (Hematoxylin and eosin, × 14 reduced by 28%.)

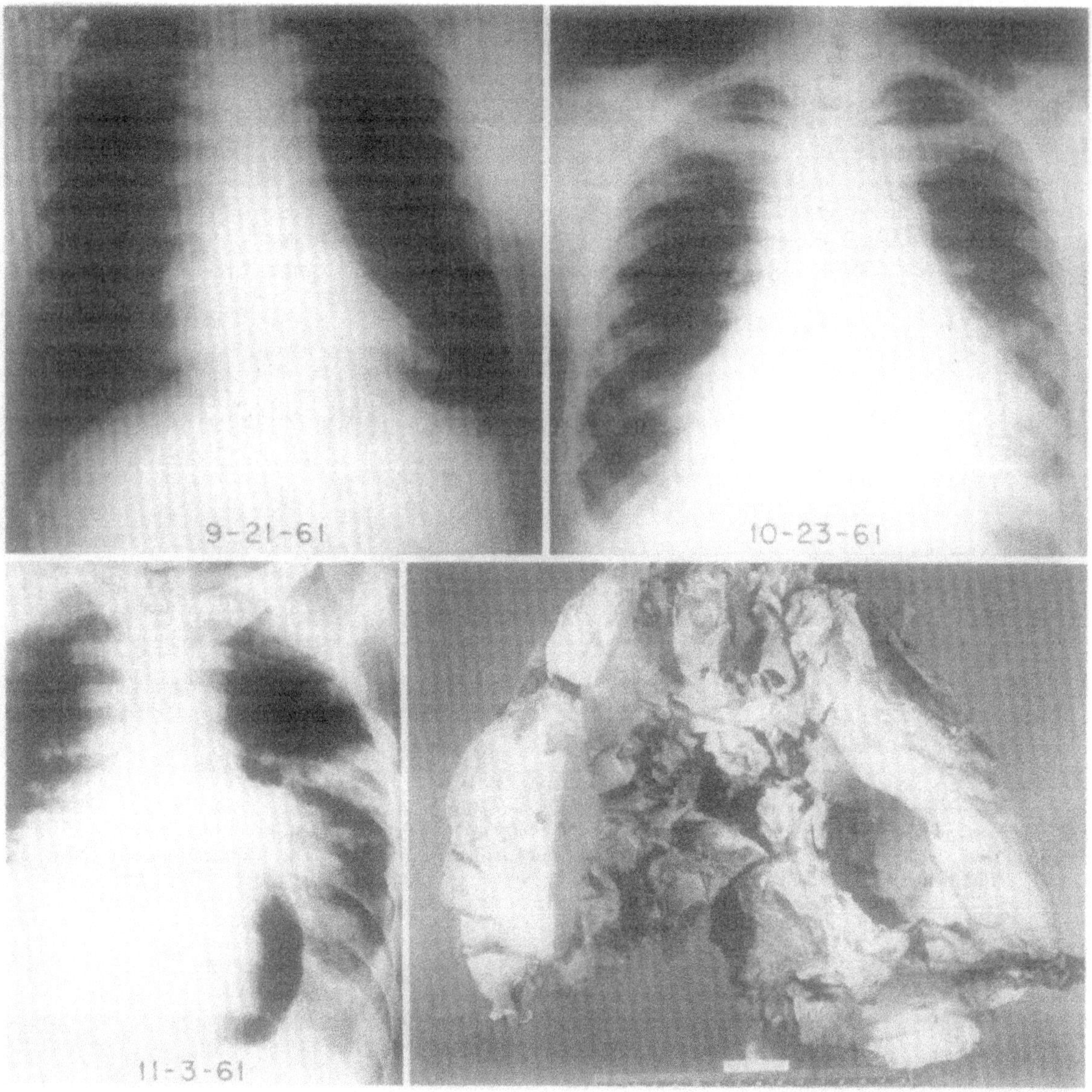

FIG. 5. *Hemorrhagic Pericarditis and Cardiac Tamponade. Chest roentgenograms and massively thickened parietal pericardium in a 22 year old man with acute lymphocytic leukemia.* During the last week of life (he died on November 4, 1961) severe dyspnea developed and signs of increased central venous pressure, hepatic tenderness and marked paradoxic pulsation. The electrocardiogram showed low voltage and sinus tachycardia. Pericardiocentesis, performed two days before death, yielded 100 ml. of serous fluid, which contained 102,000 lymphocytes per cu. mm. and virtually no erythrocytes; the total protein was 6.6 gm. with albumin 3.6 gm. per 100 ml. After removal of this fluid, 100 ml. of air was injected into the pericardial space (*lower left*). At necropsy, the heart weighed 350 gm., and 200 ml. of bloody fluid was present in the pericardial space. The parietal pericardium (*lower right*) measured 4 cm. in thickness and was massively infiltrated by leukemic cells. No leukemic cells were seen in the epicardium, which was covered by fibrin.

valvular lesions: in 20 the mitral valve only was involved; in 2 the aortic valve only; and in 2 both mitral and aortic valves were involved. In only 1 patient did the valvular lesion appear to cause any hemodynamic abnormality as judged from gross examination of the hearts. Rheumatic heart disease was believed to be the basis of the valvular deformities in 7 patients. In the remainder, the changes were generally in the older patients, nonspecific in appearance, and usually focal, i.e., only one cusp or a portion of it was involved.

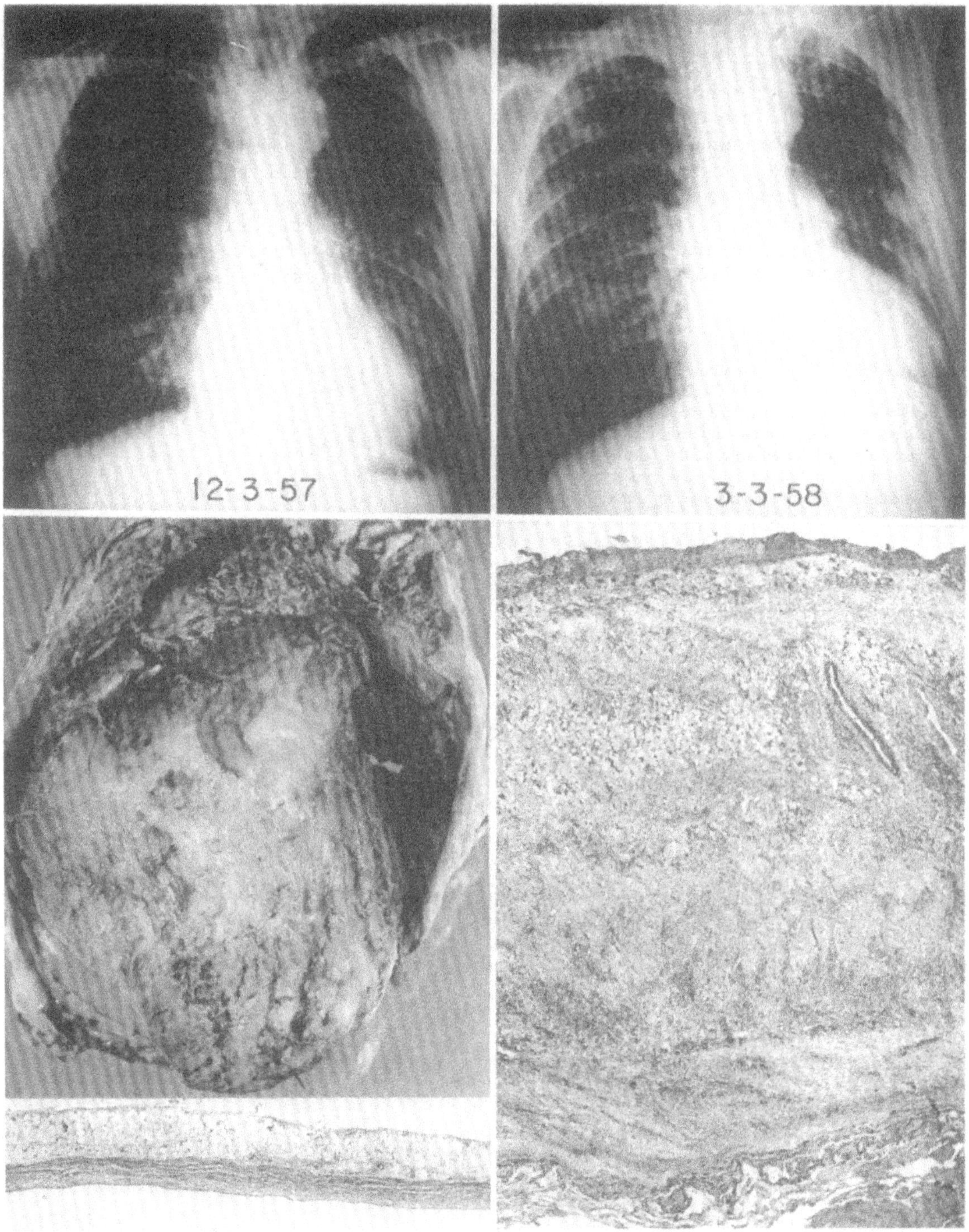

Fig. 6. *Hemorrhagic Pericarditis and Gram-Negative Infection. Chest roentgenograms, gross heart (middle left) and photomicrograph of parietal pericardium (lower right) in a 55 year old man with acute myelogenous leukemia.* The visceral and partial pericardia are thick and contain numerous leukemic cells and clumps of Gram-negative bacilli (culture grew E. coli, proteus sp. and pseudomonas sp.). He died on March 14, 1958, of Gram-negative pneumonia. He had episodes of supraventricular tachycardia (rate 200/min.) during his last two months. At necropsy, the pericardial space contained 300 ml. of bloody fluid, and the lungs contained huge quantities of iron (pulmonary hemosiderosis). A cross-section of normal parietal pericardium is shown (*lower left*) for comparison with the thickness of the parietal pericardium in this patient (*lower right*). [Hematoxylin and eosin (lower left and lower right), × 22.]

MYOCARDIAL AND ENDOCARDIAL INFECTIONS (FIG. 19 TO 24)

Myocardial abscesses or foci of inflammation containing stainable organisms were found in 31 of the 420 patients (7 per cent). Of the 18 caused by bacteria, Pseudomonas was the etiologic agent in 7 (Fig. 20), Staphylococcus aureus in 6, Clostridium perfringens in 2 (Fig. 20), Cl. sphenoides in 1,[2] and E. coli in 1. Fungi were responsible for myocardial abscesses in 10 patients (Fig. 19 and 24); in 5 Candida albicans was present; in 2 each mucor and aspergillus organisms, respectively, were identified; and in 1 patient both aspergillus and candida species were found. In 2 patients large cytoplasmic and smaller nuclear inclusions, consistent with cytomegalic inclusion disease, were found in the myocardium, and in 1 patient were associated with a focal inflammatory response (Fig. 21).[3] This latter patient died of acute pulmonary edema probably resulting from salivary gland virus infection of the heart and lungs. Or-

FIG. 7. Right, *Focal Epicardial Hemorrhages with Hypothrombocytopenia. Anterior surface of heart showing focal hemorrhages in a 56 year old man with acute myelogenous leukemia.* The epicardial hemorrhages seen here are typical of those observed in many patients studied, and are believed to be the result of severe hypothrombocytopenia. This man's platelet count two days before death was 500 per cu. mm.

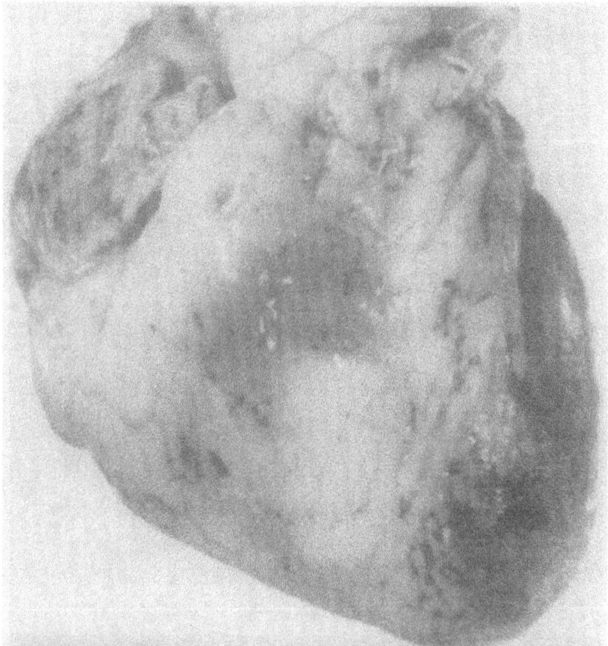

FIG. 8. Below, *Pericardial Leukemic Infiltration. Photomicrographs of visceral pericardium in 2 additional patients showing heavy leukemic infiltrations in each. Left,* a band of leukemic cells (enclosed by dashed lines) is covered by fibrous tissue in this 39 year old woman with acute myelogenous leukemia. *Right,* the subepicardial adipose tissue is diffusely infiltrated by leukemic cells in this 57 year old woman with acute lymphocytic leukemia. Cardiac symptoms and signs were absent in each of these patients. [Hematoxylin and eosin, × 37 (left) and × 60 (right) both reduced by 15%.]

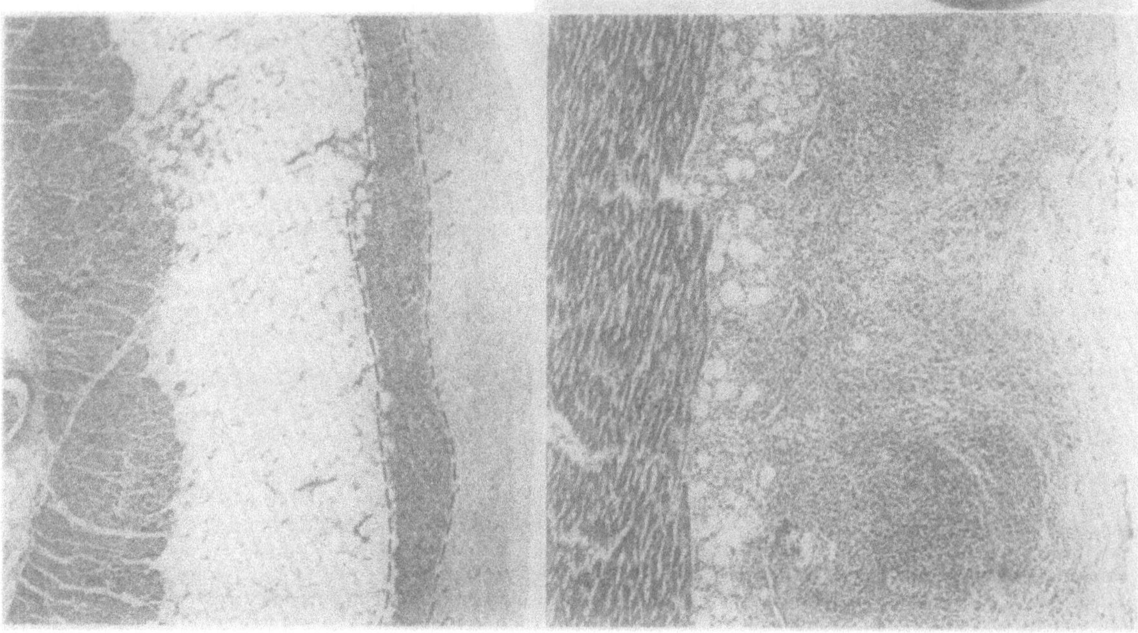

ganisms morphologically consistent with Toxoplasma gondii were found in the myocardium of 2 patients. Each had focal myocarditis, in 1 it was associated with the protozoal organisms, in the other at some distance from the organisms. One patient with toxoplasmosis of the heart (Fig. 22) had various electrocardiographic abnormalities including atrial fibrillation, atrial tachycardia, severe T wave changes, and finally ventricular fibrillation[4]; in the second patient electrocardiographic findings were normal, but he had substernal chest pain and persistent tachycardia.

The myocardial infections in 26 of the 28 patients appeared to be secondary to widespread systemic infection. With the exception of the 2 patients with cardiac toxoplasmosis, similar bacterial, fungal and cytoplasmic inclusion disease lesions were present in other body organs; usually the organisms had been cultured from the peripheral blood during the last several days of life, or from the heart blood at autopsy. Systemic bacterial infections, with the exception of clostridium, usually were diagnosed during life, but fungal infections more commonly were not diagnosed until necropsy. Cytomegalic inclusion disease (2 patients) and toxoplasmosis (2 patients) were unsuspected findings at autopsy.

Endocardial vegetations were found at autopsy in 3 patients, but in none were stainable organisms identifiable. Thus, each had noninfective thrombotic endocarditis. Their ages were 11, 23 and 26 years; 2 were men. The period of time from the onset of signs or symptoms of acute leukemia to death in these 3 patients ranged from three to nine months, and each had the myelogenous type of acute leukemia. The vegetations were located on the mitral valve in 2 patients, and on the left ventricular aspect of the membranous ventricular septum in the third (Fig. 23).

CONGENITAL MALFORMATIONS OF HEART OR GREAT VESSELS

Eight (2 per cent) of the 420 patients had congenital malformations of the heart or great vessels, but in only 3 were these of hemodynamic significance as judged from anatomic study. One of the 3 had an atrial septal defect of the secundum type, 1 both atrial and ventricular septal defects and 1 coarctation of the aorta. The defects of no functional significance included a barely valvular-incompetent atrial septal defect (1 patient), bicuspid aortic valve (1), bicuspid pulmonic valve (1), malformed but tricuspid pulmonic and aortic valves (4), and origin of right subclavian artery as the fourth branch of the aortic arch (1). Five of the 420 patients had mongolism, and 1 of them had a congenital cardiovascular malformation. Valvular-competent patent foramens ovale were found in 82 patients (20 per cent). In 2 patients isolated indentations in the ventricular septum were considered evidence of spontaneous closure of ventricular septal defect.[5]

COMMENTS

Cardiac leukemic cell infiltrates and hemorrhages were observed in 69 per cent of the 420 patients with acute leukemia, cardiac hemorrhages alone in 54 per cent and leukemic cell infiltrates alone in 37 per cent. Comparison of these figures with those of others is difficult since most previous studies have not separated patients with chronic leukemia from those with the acute form. When both types of leukemia are considered together leukemic cell cardiac infiltrates have been found in 34 to 53 per cent of necropsy cases.[6–25] Krasovskiĭ[24] in 1965 found leukemic cell infiltrates in the hearts of 100 of 643 patients (16 per cent) with acute leukemia. The most frequently quoted study regarding the cardiac involvement in leukemia is that of Kirshbaum and Preuss[8] in 1943. These authors found leukemic infiltrations in the hearts of 43 of 123 subects (75 had acute leukemia), and stated that next to the kidney the heart was the organ most frequently involved by these infiltrations. Of the 420 patients described in the present study, the bone marrow, lymph nodes, liver, spleen and kidneys were infiltrated by leukemic cells in virtually every patient; in this study the heart at best ranks sixth in a list of organs most frequently infiltrated by leukemic cells.

Cardiac hemorrhages in leukemia have been mentioned infrequently in previous reports. Kirshbaum and Preuss[8] in 1943 stated that cardiac hemorrhages occurred "mainly" in the acute form of leukemia, and were "most frequently" located in the epicardium and endocardium. No mention of cardiac hemorrhages in leukemia was made by Forkner[7] or by Dameshek and Gunz[23] in their books on leukemia, although cardiac leukemic cell infiltrates were discussed. Cardiac hemorrhages apparently were present in most of the 260 necropsy patients with acute leukemia studied by Ponomareva[22] in 1964. Krasovskiĭ[24] described endocardial and

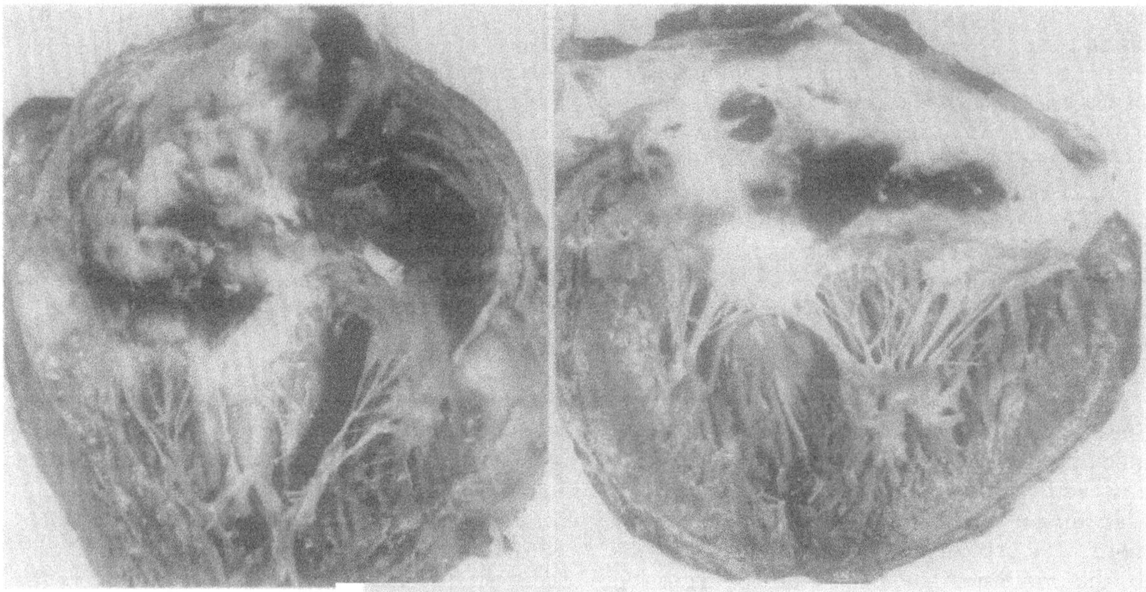

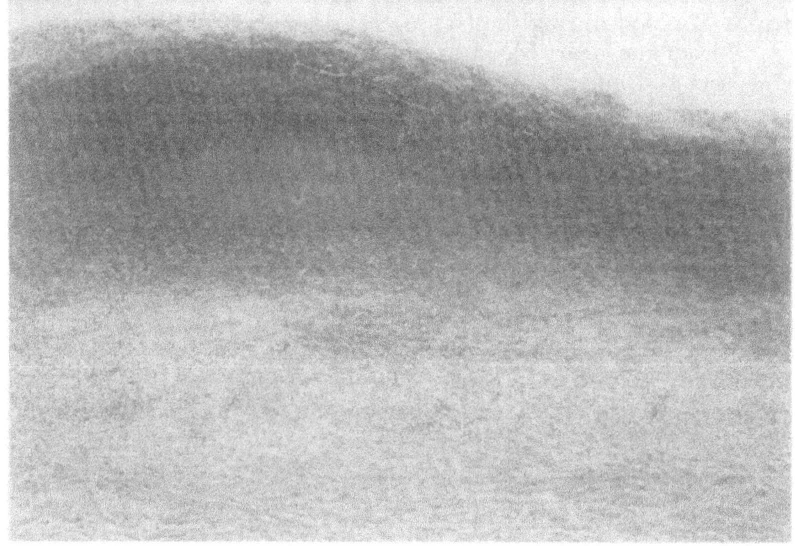

FIG. 9. *Extensive atrial hemorrhages in patient described in Figure 2. Upper left,* opened right atrium, tricuspid valve and right ventricle. *Upper right,* opened left atrium, mitral valve, and left ventricle. Focal but extensive hemorrhages are present in the atrial septum and in the free walls of each atrium. The cardiomegaly (450 gm.) is attributed to severe anemia of seven months' duration. *Below,* photomicrograph of the hemorrhage in the left atrium. The blood is located predominantly in the endocardium. Some leukemic cells are present in the connective tissue between the endocardium and myocardium. (Hematoxylin and eosin, × 50 reduced by 7%.)

pericardial hemorrhages in 31 per cent and myocardial hemorrhages in 11 per cent of 643 autopsy cases of with acute leukemia.

The explanation for the difference in location of the hemorrhages and/or leukemic cell infiltrates in the various areas of the heart is not known. The differences in the amount of surface area, or the degree of vascularity between the walls of the four chambers and the pericardium, or both, may be significant factors. The infiltrates were found most frequently in the pericardium (39 per cent), and its surface area almost certainly is greater than that of any of the cardiac chambers, and the epicardium contains many vascular channels. The cardiac wall most frequently involved was the left ventricle (36 per cent). Again, its surface area is probably greater than that of any other chamber, and its myocardium is highly vascularized since its work load is the heaviest. The left atrial wall was involved least frequently of the four chambers. The infiltrates in all chambers were most pronounced, as a rule, in the endocardium, and the endocardium of the left atrium, although thickest, is the least vascularized. The least common site of hemorrhage and/or leukemic cell infiltration was the cardiac valves,[26] and these structures normally are relatively avascular.

10A 10B

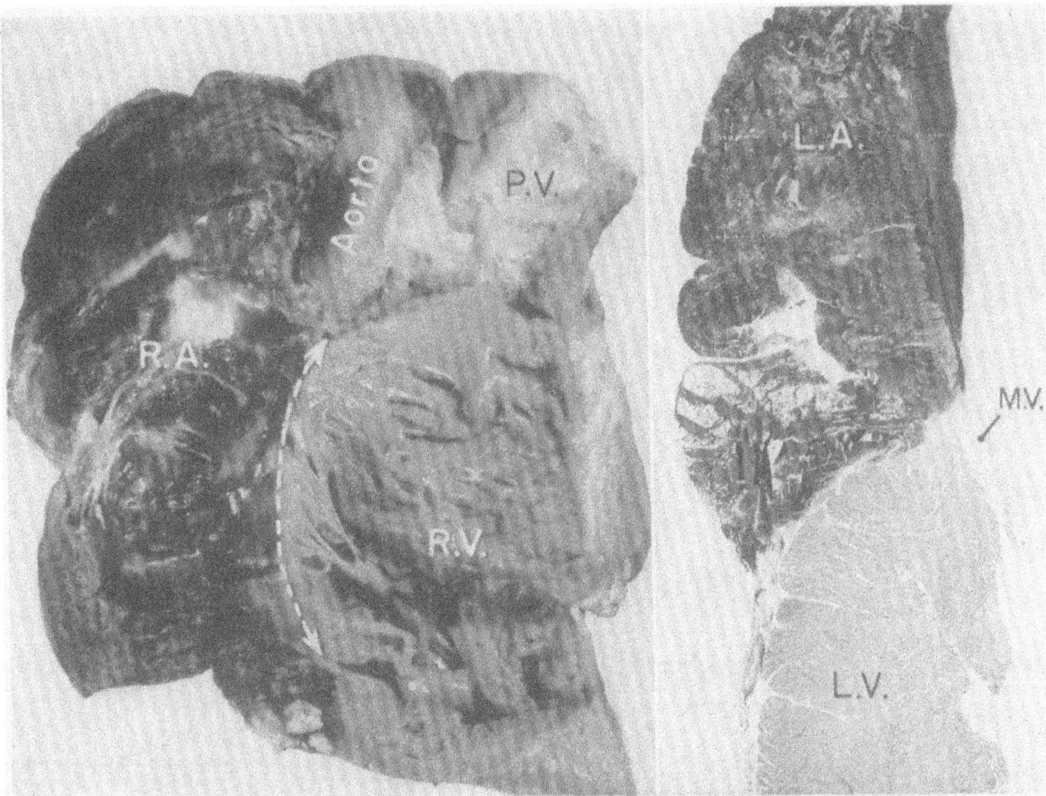

11

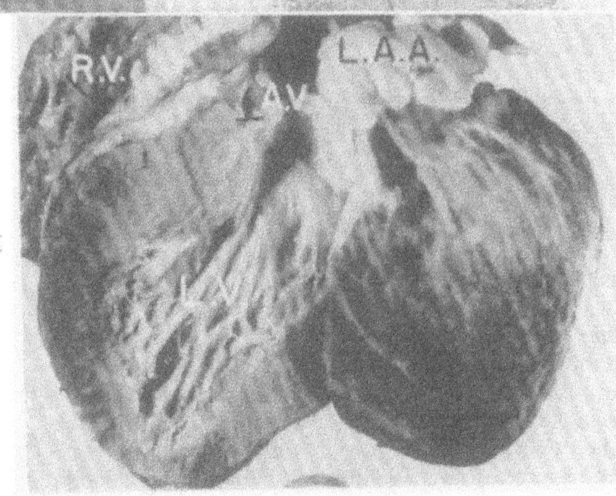

FIG. 10. *Massive Atrial Hemorrhages. Heart of a 15 month old girl with acute lymphocytic leukemia of two months' duration.* She died of generalized bleeding (platelet count 600 per cu. mm.). None of her clinical features could be attributed to cardiac involvement; an electrocardiogram was not recorded. Necropsy disclosed massive diffuse hemorrhage in the walls of both atria and atrial septum, but only rare minute hemorrhages in the ventricles. A, opened right atrium (R.A.), tricuspid valve ring (dashed line), right ventricle (R.V.), and pulmonic valve (P.V.). The atrial walls are hemorrhagic (black) and the ventricular walls appear normal. B, section of left atrial wall (L.A.), posterior leaflet of the mitral valve (M.V.), and left ventricle (L.V.). There is massive hemorrhage in the adipose tissue of the atrioventricular sulcus, and the atrial wall shows hemorrhagic necrosis. The ventricular wall, in contrast, is free of hemorrhages. (Hematoxylin and eosin, × 5.)

FIG. 11. *Massive Myocardial Hemorrhage in a 5½ Month Old Boy with Acute Myelogenous Leukemia.* This child appeared well until three weeks before death when a hemorrhagic swelling of the scrotum developed; he was hospitalized and found to have a white blood cell count of 158,000 per cu. mm. with 90 per cent abnormal cells, platelet count 11,000 per cu. mm. and hemoglobin 6.3 gm./100 ml. He died of massive subarachnoid and gastrointestinal hemorrhage, and at autopsy had widespread focal hemorrhages in nearly every organ and tissue. Interestingly, however, dermal hemorrhages were absent, except at sites of venopunctures. Twenty-five ml. of blood was present in the pericardial sac, and several transmural hemorrhages were present in the wall of the left ventricle. Many myocardial fibers in the areas of hemorrhage were degenerated. None of his symptoms could be attributed to the cardiac hemorrhages.

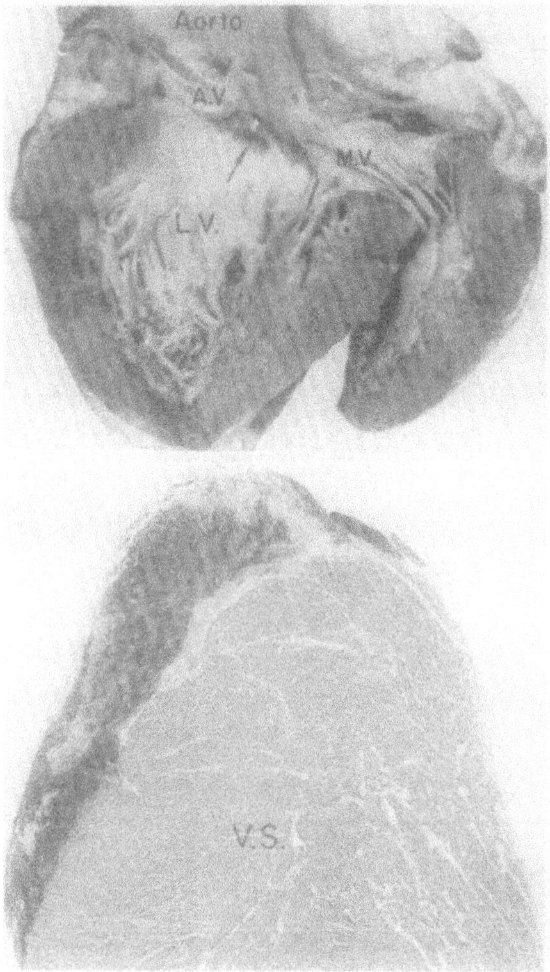

FIG. 12. *Hemorrhage in A-V Bundle. Heart (upper) and section of ventricular septum (V.S.) (lower) in an 8 year old boy with acute lymphocytic leukemia.* This child died of subarachnoid hemorrhage (platelet count = 1,600 per cu. mm.), and at necropsy a large hemorrhage was found in the atrioventricular bundle (arrow). Despite the large hemorrhage in the A-V bundle, the pulse terminally ranged from 100 to 160/min. No electrocardiogram was recorded. *Upper*, opened aorta, aortic valve (A.V.) and left ventricle (L.V.) disclosing several hemorrhages, one of which involved the A-V bundle (arrow). M.V. = anterior leaflet of mitral valve. *Lower*, section of ventricular septum (V.S.) showing the large hemorrhage in the A-V bundle and in the proximal portion of the left bundle branch. (Hematoxylin and eosin, × 15 reduced by 7%.)

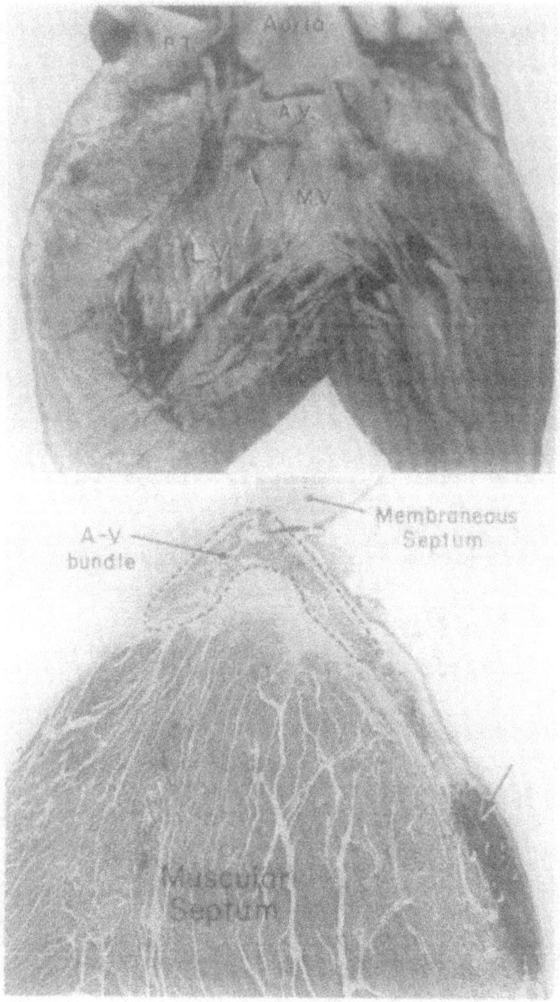

FIG. 13. *Focal Hemorrhage in A-V Bundle and Left Branch. Heart (upper) and section of ventricular septum in a 23 year old man with acute lymphocytic leukemia.* He died of massive gastrointestinal hemorrhage (platelet count = 3,800 per cu. mm.). At necropsy several focal hemorrhages were observed in the myocardium and pericardium. One of the hemorrhages grossly appeared to be in the area of the A-V bundle (*upper*, at arrow). A.V. = aortic valve; P.T. = pulmonary trunk; M.V. = anterior leaflet of mitral valve; L.V. = left ventricle. *Lower*, section through membraneous and muscular ventricular septa disclosing the A-V bundle, and a focal hemorrhage (arrow) in the left bundle branch. Terminally, the pulse rate was 140/min. No electrocardiogram was recorded. (Hematoxylin and eosin, × 14 reduced by 28%.)

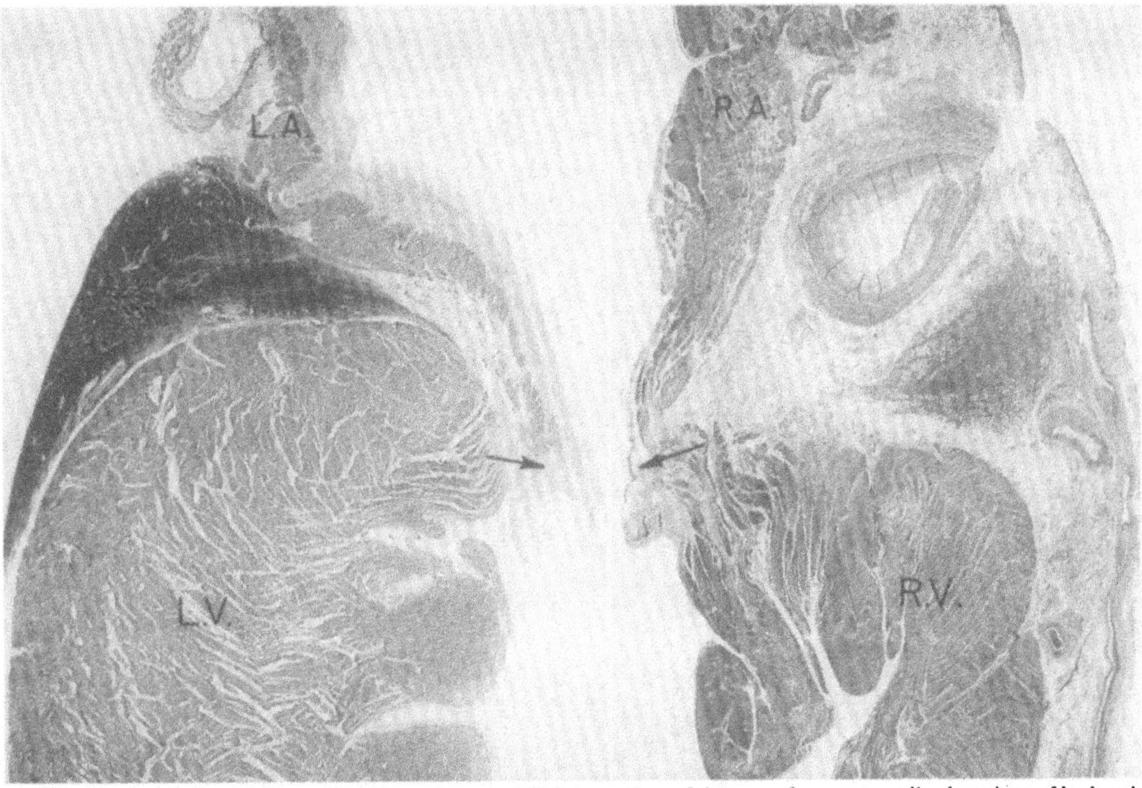

FIG. 14. Above, *Leukemic Infiltrates and Hemorrhages in A-V Sulcus.* One of the more frequent cardiac locations of leukemic cell infiltrates and hemorrhages was the subepicardial adipose tissue of the atrioventricular sulcus. Shown here are photomicrographs of this region in each of 2 patients with acute leukemia. *Left,* the left A-V sulcus is massively infiltrated by erythrocytes. *Right,* the right A-V sulcus in this 71 year old woman with acute myelogenous leukemia contains large focal collections of leukemic cells and no significant numbers of extravasated erythrocytes. L.V. = left ventricular wall; L.A. = left atrial wall; R.V. = right ventricular wall; R.A. = right atrial wall. The arrows point to the atrioventricular valve annuli. [Hematoxylin and eosin, × 12 (left), × 5 (right) reduced by 13%.]

FIG. 15. Below, *Myocardial Necrosis and Calcification. Photomicrographs of left ventricular wall in a 25 year old man with acute lymphatic leukemia.* In this patient acute pulmonary edema and cardiomegaly developed terminally (confirmed by roentgenogram; weight of heart at autopsy was 440 gm.). Sections of the left ventricle at autopsy showed foci of myocardial necrosis (*left*) and calcification (*right*). The calcium deposits are surrounded by leukemic infiltrates. The right photograph is a close-up of the area in brackets. The electrocardiogram terminally showed only sinus tachycardia. [Hematoxylin and eosin, × 50 (left), × 205 (right) reduced by 7%.]

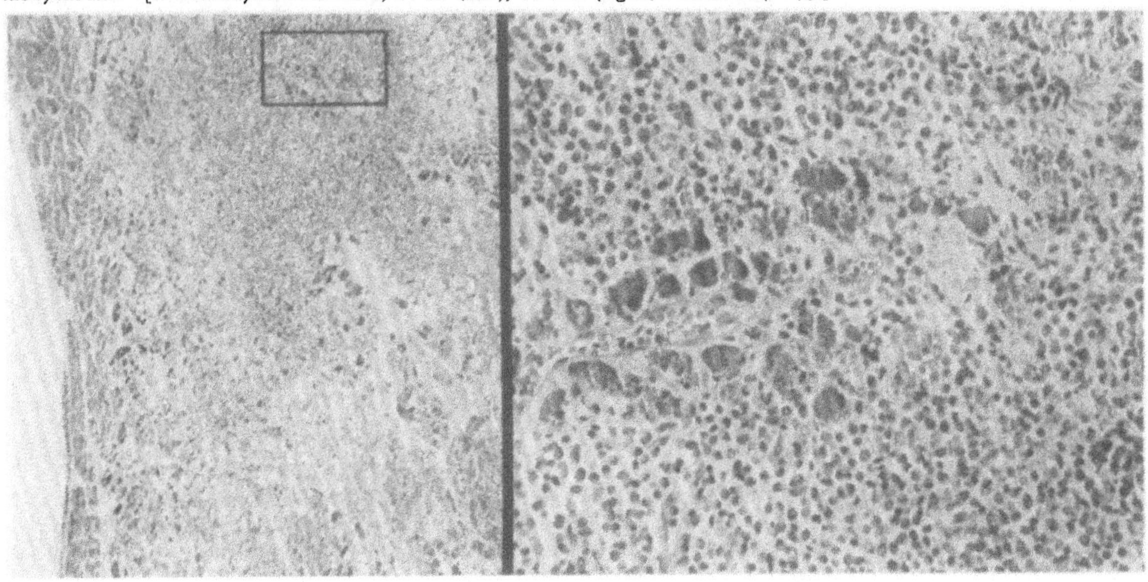

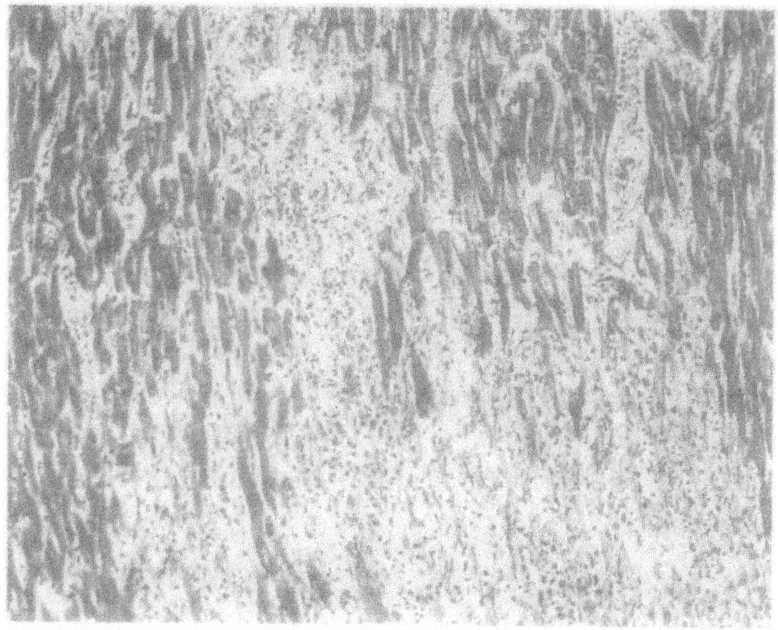

FIG. 16. Above, *Focal Myocardial Necroses. Photomicrograph of a section of left ventricle in a 26 year old man with acute myelogenous leukemia.* These foci of myocardial fiber lysis associated with leukemic cell infiltrates were present in many areas of the left ventricle. Their cause is uncertain. The patient did have a small vegetation which contained no organisms on the mitral valve (noninfective thrombotic endocarditis), but embolic material was not observed in any of the coronary arteries. No electrocardiogram was recorded. (Hematoxylin and eosin, × 120 reduced by 6%.)

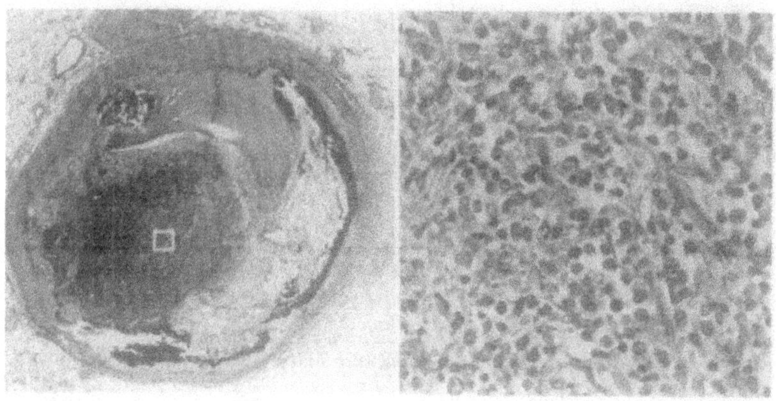

FIG. 17. Center, *Leukemic Cell Coronary Occlusion. Cross-section of right coronary artery (left) and close-up of the intraluminal material (right) in a 41 year old man with acute myelogenous leukemia.* In this patient hypotension, tachypnea and diaphoresis developed terminally, but at no time did he have chest pain. He was normotensive and the total serum cholesterol was 71 mg./100 ml. No electrocardiogram was recorded. Necropsy disclosed severe diffuse coronary arterial atherosclerosis, complete occlusion of the right coronary artery and focal fibrous scars in the left ventricle. The final occlusion of this vessel (*left*) was produced by leukemic cells (*right*). The right photograph represents a close-up of the area in brackets shown in the left one. [Hematoxylin and eosin stains, × 4 (left), × 315 (right) reduced by 20%.]

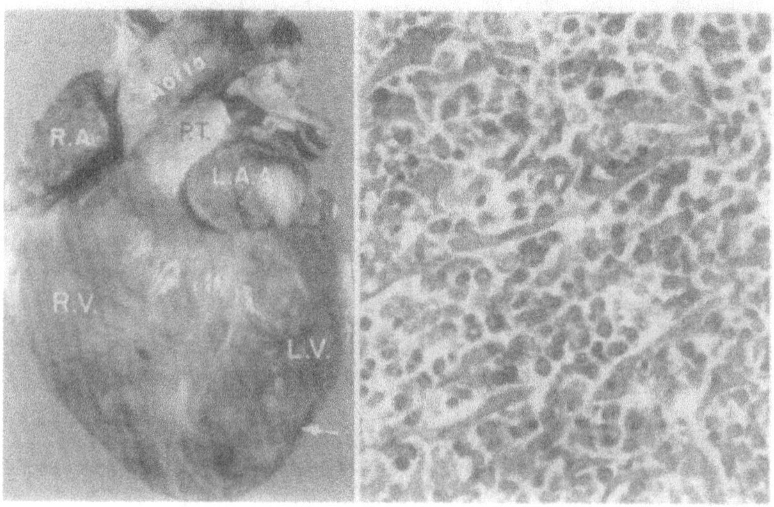

FIG. 18. Below, *Leukemic Nodules in Myocardium. Heart (left) and close-up of leukemic nodule (right) in an 18 month old girl with acute lymphocytic leukemia whose total illness lasted only three weeks.* The white blood cell count one day before death was 69,000 per cu. mm. with 82 lymphocytes and 18 per cent unclassified forms. She died of massive intracerebral hemorrhage (the platelet count during the final week ranged from 5,000 to 36,000 per cu. mm.), and at necropsy nodular leukemic infiltrations were present in many organs. White nodules of leukemic cells were present in the walls of each cardiac chamber. R.A. = right atrium; R.V. = right ventricle; P.T. = pulmonary trunk; L.V. = left ventricle; and L.A.A. = left atrial appendage. A section of the nodule designated by the arrow is shown at right. The degenerating myocardial fibers are widely separated by the leukemic cells. (Hematoxylin and eosin, × 360 reduced by 26%.)

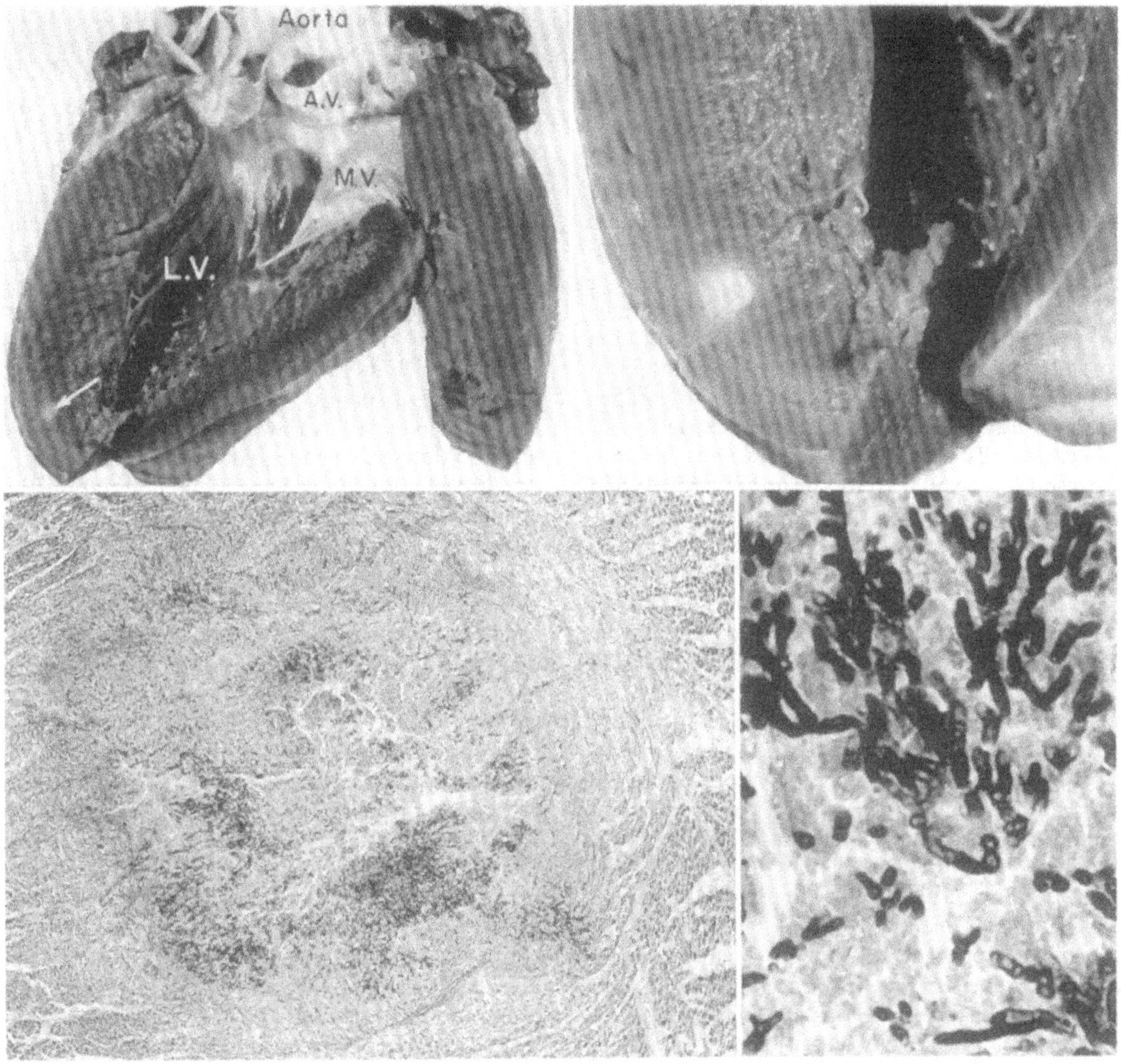

FIG. 19. *Myocardial Abscess in a 25 Year Old Man with Acute Lymphocytic Leukemia who Died of Generalized Fungal Infection.* Electrocardiogram 20 days before death showed sinus tachycardia and nonspecific T wave changes. Aspergillus fumigatus was cultured at necropsy from a pulmonary abscess, and similar abscesses were present in many organs. *Upper left*, opened aorta, aortic valve (A.V.) and left ventricle (L.V.) showing an abscess (arrow) near the apex. M.V. = anterior leaflet of mitral valve. *Upper right*, close-up of the myocardial abscess. *Lower left*, section of the abscess. All of the dark-staining structures represent fungal organisms. (Hematoxylin and eosin, × 31.) *Lower right*, close-up view of the fungal organisms which morphologically are consistent with aspergillas species. (Methenamine silver, × 610 reduced by 16%.)

The myocardial infiltrates were usually focal, and did not alter the basic architecture of the heart. In some patients there was lysis or hydropic, fatty or eosinophilic degeneration of myocardial fibers adjacent to the infiltrates. Krasovskiĭ[24] described "dystrophic changes" in the myocardial fibers, usually fatty or parenchymatous degeneration, in 222 of 643 patients with acute leukemia. When the myocardial fibers were altered, the hemorrhages and/or leukemic cell infiltrates usually were quite large. The extravasated cells, composed usually of massive numbers of erythrocytes and only a few leukemic cells, which extended through an entire cardiac wall, almost always caused severe degeneration or frank necrosis of the myocardial fibers at the site of the infiltration. Costa[27] reported on a 28 year old woman with acute myelogenous leukemia whose left atrial wall was nearly perforated by a heavy infiltrate of leukemic cells.

This same author[28] described rupture of the aorta in a 30 year old man with lymphatic leukemia, probably acute. It is not certain, however, whether the aortic wall was weakened by leukemic cell infiltration or by associated infection. Tumor-like leukemic nodules in the wall of the heart were observed in 3 patients in this study, and similar nodular infiltrates, although unusual, have been recorded by others in patients with acute leukemia.[29–31]

All of the patients studied with cardiac hemorrhages at necropsy had thrombocytopenia (platelet count <50,000 per cu. mm.), and usually the platelet counts were less than 10,000 per cu. mm. The presence or absence of extravasated leukemic cells in the hearts, however, did not correspond as well with the terminal white blood cell counts. Many patients with severe leukopenia terminally had extensive leukemic cell infiltrates in their hearts, but 40 of the 98 patients with peripheral white blood cell counts over 50,000 per cu. mm. during their last week of life had no leukemic cell infiltrates in their hearts at autopsy.

Cardiac Infection: In addition to leukemic infiltrates and hemorrhages, the hearts of patients with acute leukemia occasionally contain foci of acute inflammation (mature polymorphonuclear leukocytes) in response to specific infectious agents. Focal myocarditis or frank myocardial abscesses associated with stainable organisms in the sections of heart were found in 31 of the 420 patients (7 per cent). The myocardial infections, in general, were produced by organisms that were rarely reported as causing infection in man before the advent of antibiotics or cancer chemotherapeutic agents. Except for the 2 patients with cardiac toxoplasmosis, the myocardial inflammations in each patient were associated with widespread systemic infection. Obviously, cardiac muscle was destroyed in those patients with frank myocardial abscesses, but it also showed signs of degeneration in several patients with infective myocarditis. The cardiac pseudomonas infections caused acute necrotizing vasculitis of the intramural coronary arteries with at times virtual replacement of the vessel wall with colonies of organisms.[32] Microscopic-sized myocardial infarcts often were seen distal to these involved coronary arteries. The mucor and aspergillus cardiac infections also caused acute coronary arteritis, usually with focal occlusions of the vessels by thromboembolic material containing numerous fungal organisms. In 2 of the 5 patients with mucor or aspergillus infections of the heart focal hemorrhagic necrosis extending through an entire cardiac wall was observed. In 1 of these patients, a 43 year old man, severe precordial pain occurred during his last seven days of life, and necropsy showed extensive hemorrhagic necrosis of the myocardium associated with mucor organisms. Cardiac infections have rarely been discussed in previous reports of the heart in leukemia. None of the 123 necropsy patients with acute leukemia described in the prechemotherapeutic era by Kirshbaum and Preuss[8] apparently had cardiac infections, although pneumonia, tuberculosis and hyperthyroidism were mentioned. These authors stated that these associated diseases were "no doubt coincidental and have no relationship to leukemia." Myocardial abscess was described in only 1 of the 643 necropsy patients with acute leukemia reported in 1965 by Krasovskiĭ,[24] and Ponomareva[22] made no mention of cardiac infection in a study of the cardiac findings in 260 patients dying of acute leukemia.

CLINICAL CARDIAC MANIFESTATIONS

Despite their frequent occurrence at autopsy, the cardiac leukemic infiltrates and hemorrhages rarely produced clinically detectable signs or symptoms. Although a number of patients in this study and others[8,22,24,33,34] had dyspnea, pleural and pericardial effusions, ascites, peripheral edema and tachycardia, these features could usually be attributed to the associated anemia, hypoproteinemia, blockage of vascular or lymphatic channels by leukemic cells, or infection, particularly pneumonia, without implicating the cardiac leukemic cell infiltrates or hemorrhages. It is doubtful, however, that the extensive myocardial infiltrates—those that extended through an entire wall of a cardiac chamber or involved portions of the conduction system—were truly clinically "silent." It appears more probable that the signs and symptoms produced by these cardiac infiltrations were simply masked or overshadowed by those resulting from associated infiltrations into other organs and tissues, particularly the central nervous system and gastrointestinal tract, or by those resulting from infection, particularly pneumonia and septicemia, or by both. All of the patients included herein with cardiac leukemic infiltrates and/or hemorrhages always had similar infiltrates in other organs, although apparently this is not always the case. Kravoskiĭ[24] described hemorrhages limited entirely to the heart in 18 of 643 patients with acute leukemia. Forkner[7] in 1938 in his monograph stated that the leukemic cell "infiltrations in the myocardium are not uncommon, but rarely do they lead to alteration in the mechanism of heart action. . . Later in the course of leukemia when anemia is severe patients may exhibit signs of progressive heart failure, but this is due, in all probability, to myocardial degeneration and failure associated with anemia and anoxemia." Dameshek and Gunz[23] in their 1964 monograph stated that "heart failure is, of course, quite common in leukemia as a result, not of specific lesions, but of myocardial degeneration from long-continued anemia."

The reported incidence of clinical cardiac manifestations has ranged from 0 to 30 per cent of patients with leukemia, including the chronic as well as the acute variety.[8,17,22,24,33–36] Of 322 patients with acute leukemia observed by Boggs and associates,[33] none had significant cardiac manifestations. Of 143 patients with leukemia studied clinically by Bregani and Perrotta,[34] 4 had congestive cardiac failure, 3 peripheral edema, 1 angina pectoris and 3 evidence of pericarditis. Of 260 patients with acute leukemia reported by Ponomareva,[22] 10 had "acute disturbance of the coronary circulation," 13 had pulmonary edema, and 12 fibrinous and hemorrhagic pericarditis. All of these patients at necropsy had "marked degenerative changes in the myocardium" and foci of leukemic infiltration and hemorrhages in the myocardium or epicardium. Ponomareva did not mention associated systemic or cardiac infection but did state that the cardiac manifestations correlated relatively well with the level of the blood hemoglobin. Interestingly, no cardiac symptoms occurred in a 20 year old woman with acute leukemia and a blood hemoglobin of 1 gm./100 ml.

Pericardial Involvement: Although clinical manifestations resulting from leukemic cell infiltrates or hemorrhages into the myocardium are usually not detected because they are absent or overshadowed by signs and symptoms resulting from involvement of other systems, a number of patients have been described in whom the clinical picture was characterized by pericardial involvement. Nine patients in the present study had chest pain typical of pericarditis, although 28 patients at necropsy had pericarditis and a number of others had pericardial effusions. Even though pericardial involvement in acute leukemia is often not apparent clinically, evidence of pericardial disease may be the initial manifestation, or the predominent clinical feature of acute leukemia, or both, or it may be a part of the terminal illness. In this series one of the patients with symptomatic pericardial involvement presented initially with precordial pain typical of pericardial disease. When he was first seen, the peripheral white blood cell count and smear were in no way suggestive of leukemia (Fig. 2). Several weeks later, however, the leukemic nature of the involvement became apparent, and his entire illness was predominated by cardiac signs and symptoms. Similar patients have been reported by others.[37–41] Wendkos[41] described a 15 year old girl with acute lymphocytic leukemia in whom massive pericardial effusion was "the earliest and most outstanding manifestation" of her illness. Raynolds and associates[38] and others[37,39] have described polyserositis including pericardial effusion as a complication of acute leukemia and, rarely, as the initial manifestation of the blood dyscrasia.

Some clinical features of acute leukemia, namely, pallor, anemia, precordial murmur, fever and joint pains, may cause this disease to be mistaken initially for acute rheumatic fever or infective endocarditis.[1,17] In older patients acute leukemia has presented a clinical picture of acute myocardial infarction.[1] Wintrobe and Mitchell[1] described a 50 year old woman (their Case 9) who was treated for several months for paroxysmal tachycardia and precordial discomfort before it became apparent that she had acute myelogenous leukemia. Of the 125 patients with leukemia (75 acute, 48 chronic) reported by Kirchbaum and Preuss,[8] the initial diagnosis in 7 was "rheumatic heart disease with sepsis" or "coronary occlusion."

Electrocardiographic Alterations: These have been described in 12 to 35 per cent of patients with acute leukemia.[13–15,20,22,24,35,36,42] With rare exception these percentages are based on random rather than serial electrocardiograms. Unquestionably, the more frequently electrocardiograms were recorded, the more often abnormalities were found. The most frequent changes are sinus tachycardia, nonspecific S-T segment and T wave changes, premature atrial and ventricular contractions, prolonged P-R and Q-T intervals and low voltage. Rare abnormalities in acute leukemia include right and left bundle branch block, complete atrioventricular block or dissociation, atrial and ventricular tachycardia, atrial fibrillation, left and right axis deviation and the Wolff-Parkinson-White syndrome. To our knowledge, right or left ventricular hypertrophy has not been recorded in patients with acute leukemia unless there was some underlying cardiac disease.

Aronson and Leroy[35] in 1947 attempted to determine if the electrocardiogram could be of value in demonstrating leukemic involvement of the heart. From a clinical electrocardiographic-necropsy correlative study of 8 patients with leukemia they concluded that changes in the electrocardiogram depended upon the extent and location of the myocardial leukemic infiltrates. Popescu and Grozea[16] in 1959 from a similar study of 42 patients with acute leukemia and 102 patients with chronic leukemia found no parallelism between myopericardial leukemic lesions and electrocardiographic alterations. It does appear from the present study and from the reports of others that the more extensive the infiltrates in the heart, the more likely are electrocardiographic alterations. There remains, however, a large number of patients with acute leukemia who have electrocardiographic abnormalities and no leukemic cell infiltrates, hemorrhages, or infective foci in their hearts. The electrocardiographic changes in this group of patients consist mainly of T wave, S-T segment and P-R interval abnormalities, and these may disappear after elevation of the blood hemoglobin level. Similar observations have been made by Faivre and associates.[13,40] Abnormalities of the T wave and S-T segment, occasionally suggesting myocardial hypoxia, as well as low voltage

FIG. 20. *Myocardial Bacterial Infections. Left, section of myocardium in a 47 year old man with acute myelogenous leukemia who died of Pseudomonas septicemia with shock.* Infarcts associated with Pseudomonas species organisms were found at autopsy in the heart, lung and brain. Colonies of Gram-negative organisms (dark structures) consistent with pseudomonas species infiltrate the entire wall of this intramural coronary artery and spread into adjacent connective tissue and myocardium. (Giemsa, × 108.) *Right, section of myocardium in a 43 year old woman with acute myelogenous leukemia who died of Clostridium perfringens septicemia* and had gas gangrene of many organs including the heart. The endocardium of the cardiac valves and the intima of the arteries were pink-stained, the result of intravascular hemolysis secondary to the gas gangrene infection. The source of the Cl. perfringens infection probably was an ulceration in the gastrointestinal tract. Colonies of large Gram-positive bacilli were present in every section of myocardium. The postmortem culture of heart blood grew Cl. perfringens. (Hematoxylin and eosin, × 14 reduced by 16%.)

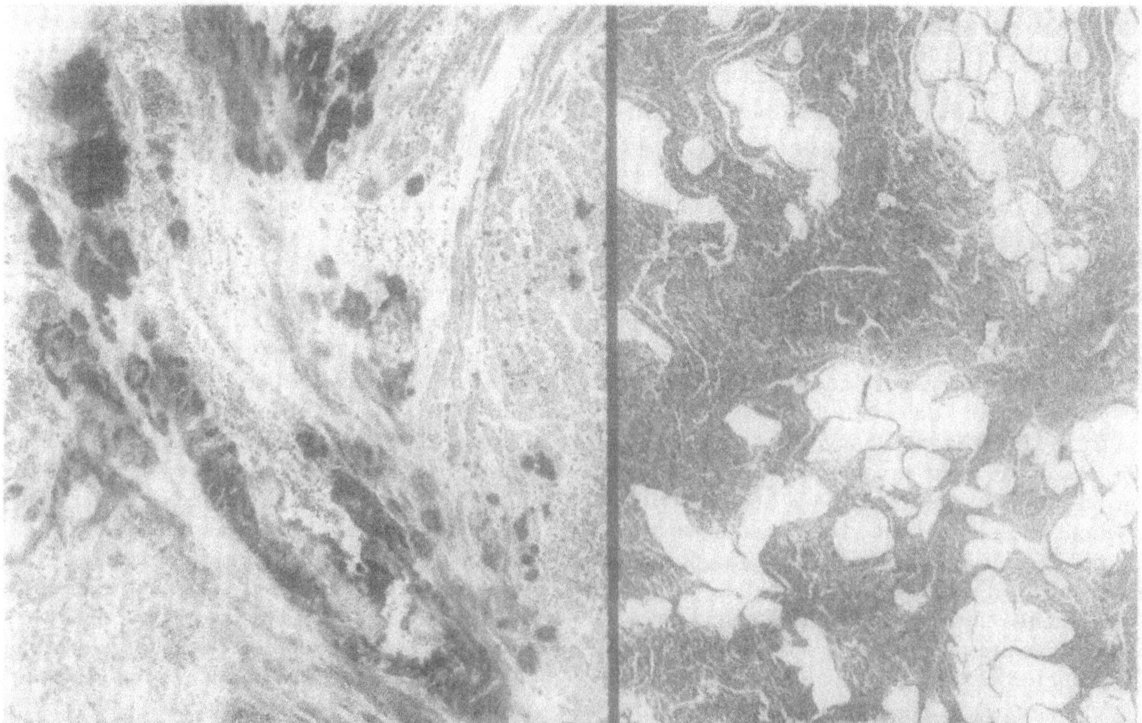

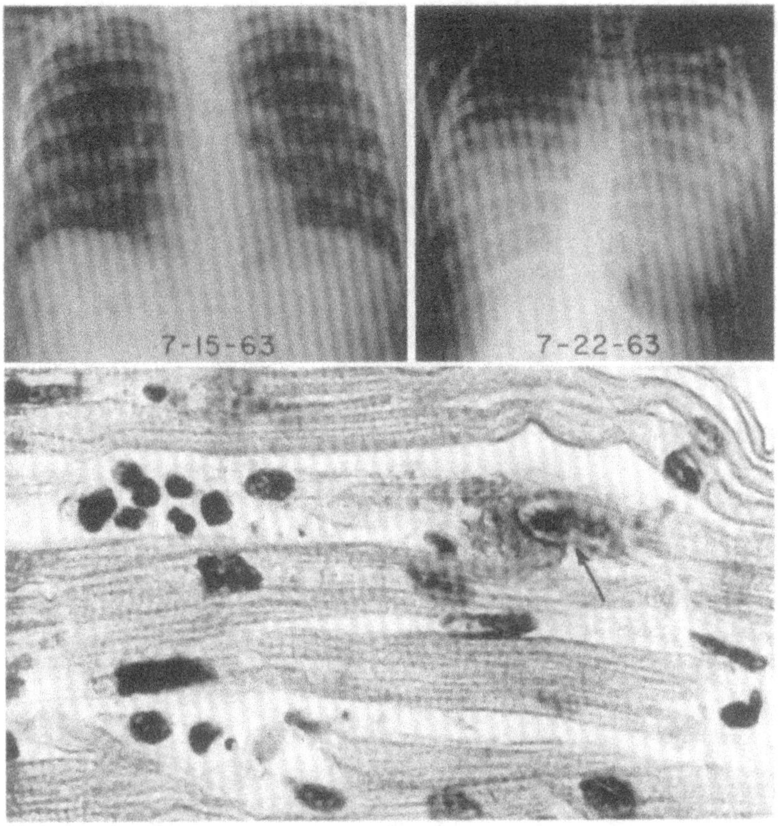

FIG. 21. *Cytomegalic Inclusion Disease of the Heart.* This 8 year old girl with acute lymphocytic leukemia of eight months' duration had clear lung fields by chest roentgenogram (*upper left*) seven days before death. During her last four days she gained 3 kg. in weight, and fever (to 41° C.), tachypnea (to 80/min.), pulmonary rales and, finally, hypotension developed. Electrocardiogram 24 hours before death showed left bundle branch block, and chest roentgenogram 30 minutes before death (*upper right*) showed changes consistent with acute pulmonary edema. At necropsy, cytomegalic inclusion bodies were found in numerous organs including the heart. *Lower,* section of myocardium showing cytomegalic inclusion body (arrow) and surrounding acute inflammatory cells. (Hematoxylin and eosin, × 900 reduced by 14%.)

and prolongation of the P-R interval, are recognized electrocardiographic changes in severe anemia (hemoglobin <8 gm./100 ml.).[43] Also, correction of electrolyte disturbances in several patients included herein was followed by return of the electrocardiogram to normal. The more serious abnormalities, such as arrhythmias, heart block including bundle branch block, and altered axis and conduction disturbances may reasonably be attributed to infiltration of the myocardium by leukemic cells, hemorrhages or infectious foci if underlying cardiac disease can be excluded. At least 3 patients with acute leukemia have been described in whom complete heart block or atrioventricular dissociation was the result of leukemic cell infiltrates in the atrioventricular bundle.[44–46] Leukemic cell infiltrates or hemorrhages were observed in 5 patients in the present study, but none had had electrocardiograms to determine if cardiac conduction was altered. Dresdale and associates[45] emphasized that heart block may be overlooked in a patient with acute leukemia because the associated anemia or fever may prevent the pulse from slowing markedly. Heart block secondary to leukemic infiltration of the conduction tissue may disappear after irradiation.[44]

The significance of the cardiac lesions in causing or contributing to the death of the patient with acute leukemia is difficult to determine. In the 14 patients in this study in whom the leukemic cell infiltrates and/or hemorrhages extended through the entire myocardial wall, it appears reasonable to believe that death was related to these lesions. However, probably many of the intramyocardial hemorrhages or leukemic infiltrates that were not transmural at least contributed significantly to death. In at least 10 patients pericardial involvement was considered a major cause of death, and cardiac infection was the chief factor in 2

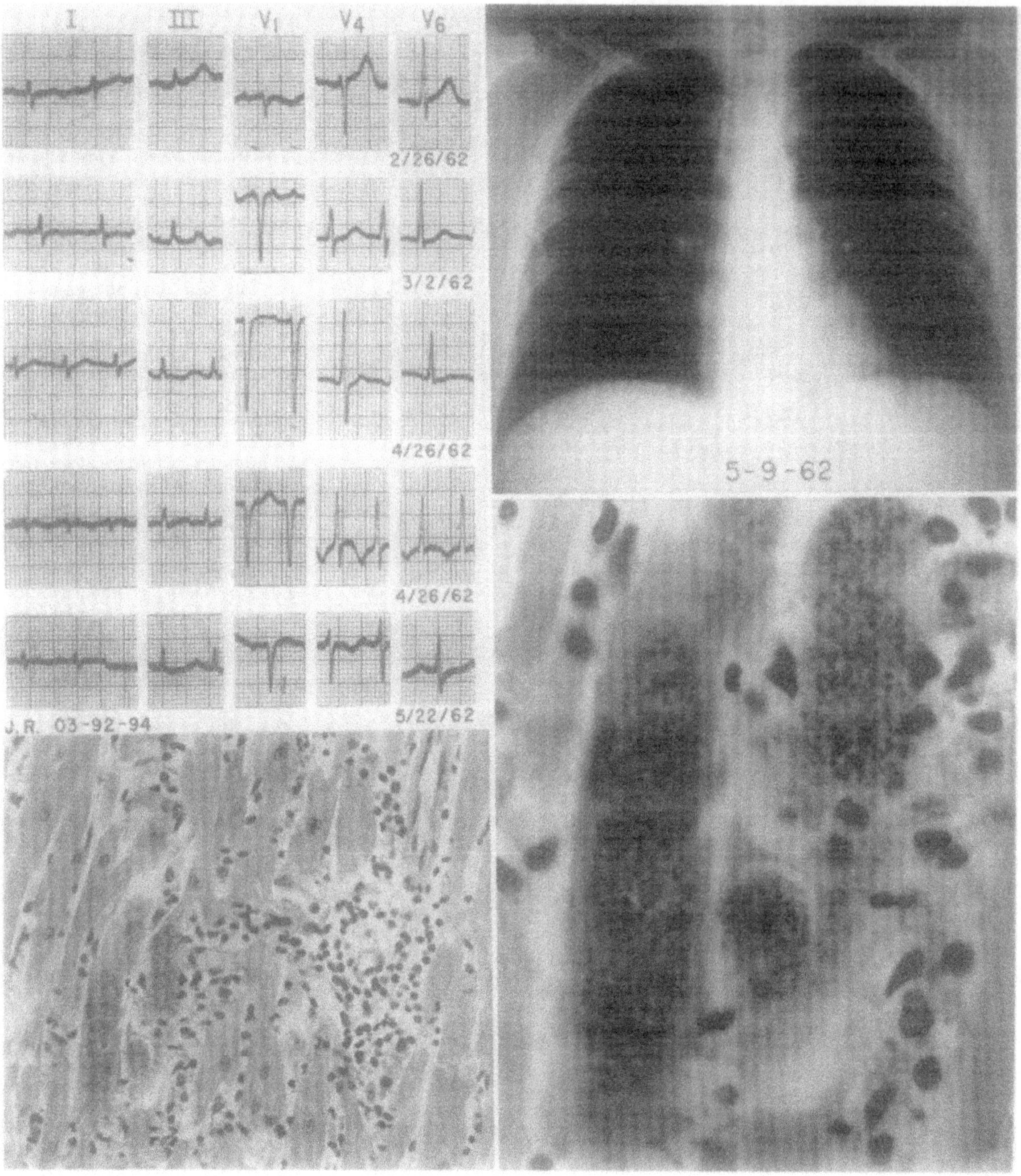

FIG. 22. *Toxoplasmosis of the Heart of a 27 Year Old Man with Acute Lymphocytic Leukemia.* His illness was characterized by recurrent Aerobacteria cloaca septicemia and paroxysmal arrhythmias (atrial fibrillation, atrial tachycardia). He died with ventricular fibrillation on May 24, 1962, and organisms consistent with Toxoplasma gondii were found in sections of myocardium. The cardiac arrhythmias probably were the result of the protozoan cardiac infection. *Lower left*, area of focal myocarditis associated with T. gondii organisms. *Lower right*, close-up view of the encysted organisms. [Hematoxylin and eosin, × 275 (lower left), × 915 (lower right) reduced by 6%.]

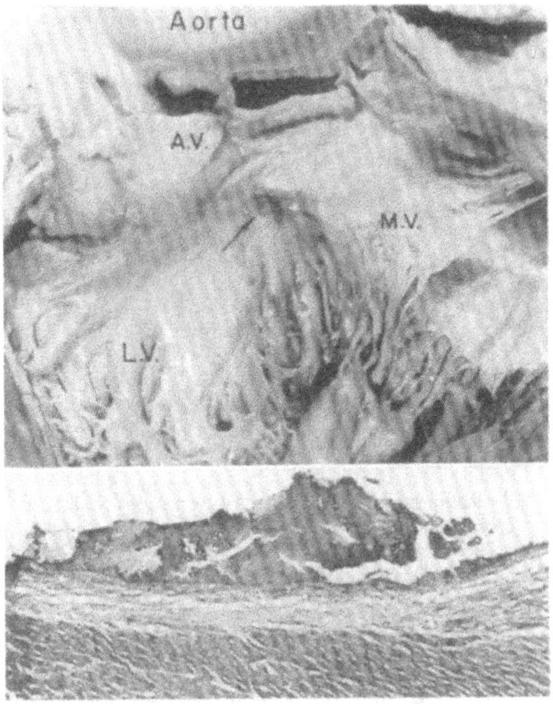

FIG. 23. *Noninfective Thrombotic Endocarditis in a 23 Year Old Man with Acute Myelogenous Leukemia. Upper*, the arrow points to a vegetation at the junction of the membraneous and muscular ventricular septa, and the photomicrograph (*lower*) reveals that it consists entirely of fibrin and platelets. No organisms were present in the vegetation, and culture of the heart blood at autopsy was sterile. The total length of this man's illness was only three months. A.V. = aortic valve; L.V. = left ventricle; M.V. = anterior leaflet of mitral valve. (Hematoxylin and eosin, × 60 reduced by 26%.)

others. A huge "leukemic thrombus" in the left ventricle apparently was the cause of death in a reported patient with acute leukemia.[47] Acute pulmonary edema is often a terminal event in these patients, and it is probably often of cardiac origin. Hemorrhage and infection in sites other than the heart appear to be the major causes of death in patients with acute leukemia,[48,49] but cardiac alterations are probably of more significance than previously appreciated.

SUMMARY

The clinical and necropsy features of 420 patients with acute leukemia, either lymphogenous or myelogenous, are reviewed. Leukemic infiltrates were present at necropsy in

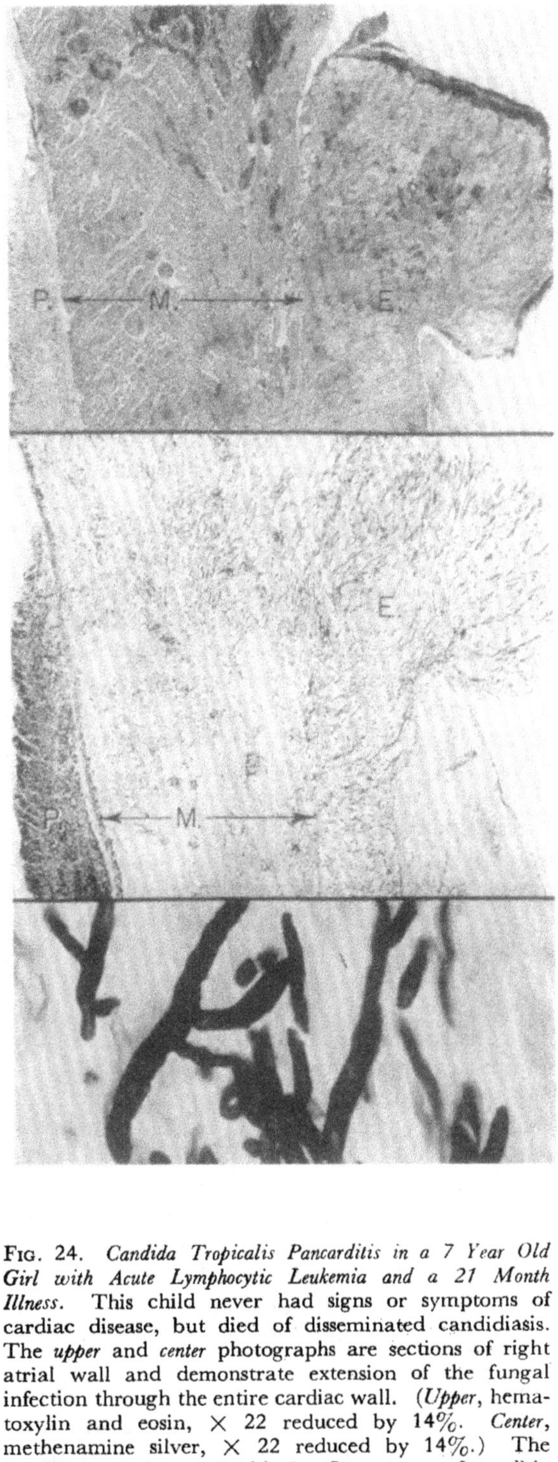

FIG. 24. *Candida Tropicalis Pancarditis in a 7 Year Old Girl with Acute Lymphocytic Leukemia and a 21 Month Illness.* This child never had signs or symptoms of cardiac disease, but died of disseminated candidiasis. The *upper* and *center* photographs are sections of right atrial wall and demonstrate extension of the fungal infection through the entire cardiac wall. (*Upper*, hematoxylin and eosin, × 22 reduced by 14%. *Center*, methenamine silver, × 22 reduced by 14%.) The candida organisms stain black. P. = mass of candida organisms on pericardial surface; M. = myocardial wall; E. = endocardial vegetation. *Lower*, close-up of organisms. (Methenamine silver, × 690 reduced by 14%.)

the hearts of 156 subjects (37 per cent), and cardiac hemorrhages were observed in 228 (54 per cent). In 96 of the 288 patients with cardiac involvement both hemorrhages and leukemic cell infiltrates were present in the heart. The hearts of only 132 patients (31 per cent) were free of hemorrhages or leukemic cell infiltrates. The leukemic cell infiltrates and hemorrhages were focal, usually few in number, located most frequently in the pericardium and walls of the left ventricle and right atrium, and only occasionally extended through the entire cardiac wall.

The cardiac leukemic cell infiltrates and hemorrhages, a frequent finding at autopsy, rarely produced clinically detectable signs or symptoms. This discrepancy between the, at times, striking cardiac findings at necropsy and the lack of detectable symptoms resulting from them may be due in part to the cardiac symptoms being masked or overshadowed by clinical manifestations resulting from leukemic cell infiltrates or hemorrhages in other body organs or tissues. Although they occurred in a number of the patients, dyspnea, tachycardia, pleural, pericardial and peritoneal effusions and edema often disappeared after transfusions for anemia, antibiotics for infection, particularly pneumonia, or antineoplastic agents for decreasing the size of the liver or spleen. In 20 subjects chest pain or dyspnea clearly resulted from leukemic cell infiltrates or hemorrhages or inflammatory foci in the heart; 9 of the 13 patients with chest pain had pericarditis with thickening of the visceral and parietal pericardia.

Various abnormalities were observed on random electrocardiograms in a number of patients. The most frequent findings were nonspecific T wave and S-T segment changes, suggesting myocardial ischemia, and these occasionally disappeared after transfusions. So-called metabolic disturbances also were common. Arrhythmias, heart block and abnormal axis deviation were unusual electrocardiographic findings.

Myocardial infections occurred in 31 of the 420 patients and were associated with systemic infection in all but 2. The focal myocarditis or myocardial abscesses were produced by organisms which rarely caused infection in man before the advent of potent antibiotics or cancer chemotherapeutic agents. Five patients, including 1 with myocarditis, had grossly purulent pericarditis, but infective endocarditis occurred in none of the subjects.

Acknowledgments

The photomicrographs were taken by Mr. Gebhard Gsell, and the gross pathology photographs by Mr. Kensie Edwards.

References

1. Wintrobe, M. M. and Mitchell, D. M. Atypical manifestations of leukaemia. *Quart. J. Med.*, 9: 67, 1940.
2. Roberts, W. C. and Berard, C. W. Gas gangrene of the heart in clostridial septicemia. *Am. Heart J.*, (In press).
3. Bodey, G. P., Wertlake, P. Y., Douglas, G. and Levin, R. H. Cytomegalic inclusion disease in patients with acute leukemia. *Ann. Int. Med.*, 62: 899, 1965.
4. Wertlake, P. T. and Winter, T. S. Fatal toxoplasma myocarditis in an adult patient with acute lymphocytic leukemia. *New England J. Med.*, 273: 438, 1965.
5. Glancy, D. L. and Roberts, W. C. Complete spontaneous closure of ventricular septal defect. Necropsy study of five subjects. *Am. J. Med.*, 43: 846, 1967.
6. Tedeschi, C.: Appunti per la istologia patologica delle leucemie. *Bull. Soc. Med. Chir. Modena*, 35: 373, 1935.
7. Forkner, C. E. Leukemia and Allied Disorders, p. 97. New York, 1938. Macmillan.
8. Kirshbaum, J. D. and Preuss, F. S. Leukemia. A clinical and pathologic study of 123 fatal cases in a series of 14,400 necropsies. *Arch. Int. Med.*, 71: 777, 1943.
9. Bellini, E. Sulle miocardiopatie leucemiche. *Gior. sc. med.*, 4: 161, 1949.
10. Lucia, S. P., Mills, H., Lowenhaupt, E. and Hunt, M. L. Visceral involvement in primary neoplastic diseases of the reticuloendothelial system. *Cancer*, 5: 1193, 1952.
11. Bisel, H. F. Wróblewski, F. and LaDue, J. S. Incidence and clinical manifestations of cardiac metastases. *J.A.M.A.*, 153: 712, 1953.
12. Burnett, R. C. and Shimkin, M. B. Secondary neoplasms of the heart. *Arch. Int. Med.*, 93: 205, 1954.
13. Faivre, G., Lamy, P. and Larcan, A. Le coeur des leucémiques. *Arch. mal. coeur*, 48: 1156, 1955.
14. Visioli, O. Aspetti clinici ed anatomo-pathologici del cuore nelle leucemie. *Ateneo parmense*, 27: 91, 1956.
15. Giraud, G., Latour, H., Puech, P., Roujon, J. and Pages, A. Infiltration lymphoblastique du myocarde; troubles rythmiques dissociatifs intéressant les trois étages du coeur. *Arch. mal. coeur*, 50: 720, 1957.
16. Popescu, J., Enescu, V. and Grozea, P. Leukemic heart changes. *Helvet. med. acta*, 26: 860, 1959.
17. Hayhoe, F. G. J. Leukemia. Research and Clinical Practice, p. 235. Boston, 1960. Little, Brown.
18. Saphir, O. Neoplasms of the pericardium and heart. In: Pathology of the Heart, ed. 2, p. 886. Edited by Gould, S. E. Springfield, Ill., 1960. Charles C Thomas.

19. Hanfling, S. M. Metastatic cancer to the heart. Review of the literature and report of 127 cases. *Circulation*, 22: 474, 1960.
20. Horeau, J. and Robin, C. Cardiac manifestations of leukemia. *Actualites Cardiol. Angeiol. Int.*, 10: 193, 1961.
21. Thurber, D. L. Edwards, J. E. and Achor, R. W. P. Secondary malignant tumors of the pericardium. *Circulation*, 26: 228, 1962.
22. Ponomareva, E. D. On cardiovascular disorders in acute leukemia. *Sovet. med.*, 28: 3, 1964.
23. Dameshek, W. and Gunz, F. Leukemia, ed. 2, p. 187. New York, 1964. Grune & Stratton.
24. Krasovskiĭ, I. I. Izmeneniia serdechno-sosudistoĭ sistemy pri ostrykh leĭ Kozakh. *Klin. med.*, 43: 102, 1965.
25. Javier, B., Yount, W., Crosby, D. and Hall, T. Cardiac metastasis in lymphoma and leukemia. Unpublished data.
26. Köberle, F. Über leukämische Infiltrate in den Herzklappen. *Ztschr. Kreislaufforsch.*, 29: 785, 1937.
27. Costa, A. Rara forma di rottura dell'atrio sinistro del cuore per infiltrati leucemici nel miocardio. *Sperimentale*, 85: 117, 1931.
28. Costa, A. Una lesione non nota dell'aorta: infiltratio laeucemica aortae. *Sperimentale*, 87: 7, 1933.
29. Mönckeberg, J. G. In: Henke, F. and Lubarsch, O. Handbuch der Speziellen Pathologischen Anatomie und Histologie. Vol. 2. Herz and Gefasse, p. 498. Berlin, 1924. J. Springer.
30. Willius, F. A. and Amberg, S. Two cases of secondary tumor of the heart in children, in one of which the diagnosis was made during life. *M. Clin. North America*, 13: 1307, 1930.
31. Reim, A. Ein seltener Herzbefund bei akuter lymphatischer Leukämie. *Klin. Wchnschr.*, 53: 475, 1916.
32. Forkner, C. E., Jr., Frei, E., Edgcomb, J. H. and Utz, J. P. Pseudomonas septicemia. Observations on twenty-three cases. *Am. J Med.*, 25: 877, 1958.
33. Boggs, D. A., Wintrobe, M. M. and Cartwright, G. E. The acute leukemias. Analysis of 322 cases and review of the literature. *Medicine*, 41: 163, 1962.
34. Bregani, P. and Perrotta, P. Il cuore nelle leucemie: Aspetti clinici ed elettrocardiografici. *Folia cardiol.*, 19: 193, 1960.
35. Aronson, S. F. and Leroy, E. Electrocardiographic fingings in leukemia. *Blood*, 2: 356, 1947.
36. Correa-Suárez, R., Loaeza, M. C., Bravo, J. L. and Villaseñor, J. B. Manifestaciones electrocardiográficas en las leucemias. *Arch. Inst. cardiol. México*, 26: 193, 1956.
37. Bouvrain, Y., Piguet, B. and Potter, M. Leucose aiguë révélée par un tableau de péricardite aigüë. *Arch. mal. coeur*, 54: 460, 1961.
38. Raynolds, A. H., Olivetti, R. G. and Ekstrand, R. W. Aleukemic stem cell leukemia with polyserositis. Report of case. *Blood*, 10: 81, 1955.
39. Bierman, H. R., Perkins, E. K. and Ortega, P. Pericarditis in patients with leukemia. *Am. Heart J.*, 43: 413, 1952.
40. Faivre, G., Rauber, G., Lamy, P., Larcan, A. and Gilgenkrantz, J.-M. Leucose aigüë avec atteinte myocardo-péricardique: Péricardite leucémique. *Presse méd.*, 65: 1943, 1957.
41. Wendkos, M. H. Leucemic pericarditis. Report of a case of lymphatic leucemia in whch massive pericardial effusion was the earliest and most outstanding manifestation. *Am. Heart J.*, 22: 417, 1941.
42. Gigante, D. and Serra, N. Sul comportamento dell'elettrocardiogramma in 56 casi di leucemia, *Folia cardiol.*, 13: 131, 1954.
43. González-de-Cossío, A., Sánchez-Medal, L. and Smith, J. F. Electrocardiographic modifications in anemia. *Am. Heart J.*, 67: 166, 1964.
44. Blotner, H. and Sosman, M. C. X-ray therapy of the heart in a patient with leukemia, heart block and hypertension. *New England J. Med.*, 230: 793, 1944.
45. Dresdale, D. T., Spain, D. and Perez-Pina, F. Heart block and leukemic cell infiltration of interventricular septum of heart. *Am. J. Med.*, 6: 530, 1949.
46. Mahaim, I. and Rossier, P. H. Leucémic myéloïde aiguë, deathèse hémorragique, bloc auriculo-ventriculaire. Lésions du tissu spécifique. *Cardiologica*, 15: 196, 1950.
47. Puech, A., Vidal, J. and Dufoix, M. Thrombose totale intra-cardiaque au cours d'une leucémie aigue. Présentation de pièces. *Arch. Soc. Sc. Mèd. et Biol. de Montpellier*, 13: 23, 1932.
48. Leach, W. B. Acute leukemia: A pathologic study of the causes of death in 157 proved cases. *Canad. M. A. J.*, 85: 345, 1961.
49. Hersh, E. M., Bodey, G. P., Nies, B. A. and Freireich, E. J. Causes of death in acute leukemia. A ten-year study of 414 patients from 1954–1963. *J.A.M.A.*, 193: 99, 1965.

Angiosarcoma of the Heart*

D. LUKE GLANCY, M.D., JORGE B. MORALES, JR., M.D. and WILLIAM C. ROBERTS, M.D., F.A.C.C.

Bethesda, Maryland and Washington, D. C.

ANGIOSARCOMA is a rare, malignant tumor that most often occurs in the skin and subcutaneous tissue, including breast, but that may arise from any blood vessel. When it originates in the heart, obstruction to filling of the right-sided cardiac chambers by a large right atrial tumor, or extensive pericardial invasion, or both, almost uniformly occurs. This report describes a patient with primary cardiac angiosarcoma and summarizes the clinicopathologic features in previously reported patients with angiosarcoma of the heart.

REPORT OF PATIENT

A 35 year old Negro woman who died on Feb. 9, 1967, had been well until two months earlier when occipital headaches appeared. These recurred daily and became progressively more severe. Cough, chills and fever appeared one week before death, and vomiting and mental obtundity were present on the day of death, when she was admitted to Providence Hospital.

Examination disclosed stupor, slurred speech, nuchal rigidity, early papilledema and vertical and horizontal nystagmus. There were no precordial murmurs or abnormal sounds, and there was no evidence of cardiomegaly or peripheral edema. Dullness to percussion and diminished breath sounds were noted over the right hemithorax. The temperature was 99.8° F., pulse 112/min. and blood pressure 140/80 mm. Hg. An electrocardiogram showed sinus tachycardia and nondiagnostic ST-T wave changes. Chest roentgenogram (Fig. 1) revealed a prominent right cardiac border, diffuse, finely nodular infiltration of both lungs and a right pleural effusion.

On lumbar puncture the opening pressure was 36 cm. cerebrospinal fluid, which was xanthochromic and contained 1,200 erythrocytes and 70 leukocytes (90 per cent polymorphonuclear cells) per cu. mm., 140 mg. protein and 70 mg. glucose per 100 ml. The patient had a generalized seizure 45 minutes later, followed by coma and slow (10/min.) Cheyne-Stokes type respirations, and she died.

AUTOPSY

Numerous tumor nodules were present in the subepicardial adipose tissue (Fig. 1). The larger ones invaded the underlying myocardium of all four cardiac chambers and the overlying parietal pericardium, thus producing obliterative tumor pericarditis. A 6 by 6 by 5 cm. mass of tumor in the anterolateral right atrial wall had caused the bulging right cardiac border on roentgenogram. It involved epicardium, myocardium and endocardium and projected as a 2 by 2 by 2 cm. mass into the right atrial cavity (Fig. 1). Large subepicardial tumor deposits surrounded the pulmonary trunk, the ascending aorta enclosed by pericardium and both atria; they also infiltrated the atrial septum.

A 1.5 cm. tumor nodule was present in each cerebellar hemisphere, and smaller ones were present in the midbrain. In both lungs there were diffuse, miliary metastases, most of which were less than 0.5 cm. in diameter. Tumor also was found in the ovaries, uterus, spleen, liver, thyroid gland, kidney and lymph nodes (paratracheal, periaortic and retroperitoneal). The skin was normal.

Histologically, the tumor in some areas consisted of large, thin-walled, vascular spaces filled with blood, and in other areas it consisted mainly of sheets of spindle-shaped cells (Fig. 2). Both histologic patterns often were present in the same tumor nodule, as well as intermediate patterns containing small vascular spaces.

COMMENTS

The clinical and pathoanatomic features in 40 previously reported patients[1–40] with angiosarcoma of the heart are summarized in Table I. In each the heart was considered the site of the primary tumor, but in 26 this was not unequivocally established since extracardiac tumor also was present. As in the present patient, however, the largest mass of tumor in each was in the heart, and the cardiac findings were similar, both clinically and pathologically, in those with

* From the Laboratory of Pathology, Clinic of Surgery, National Heart Institute, National Institutes of Health, Bethesda, Md., and the Department of Pathology, Providence Hospital, Washington, D. C.

Address for reprints: William C. Roberts, M.D., Laboratory of Pathology, Clinic of Surgery, National Heart Institute, National Institutes of Health, Department of Health, Education and Welfare, Bethesda, Md. 20014.

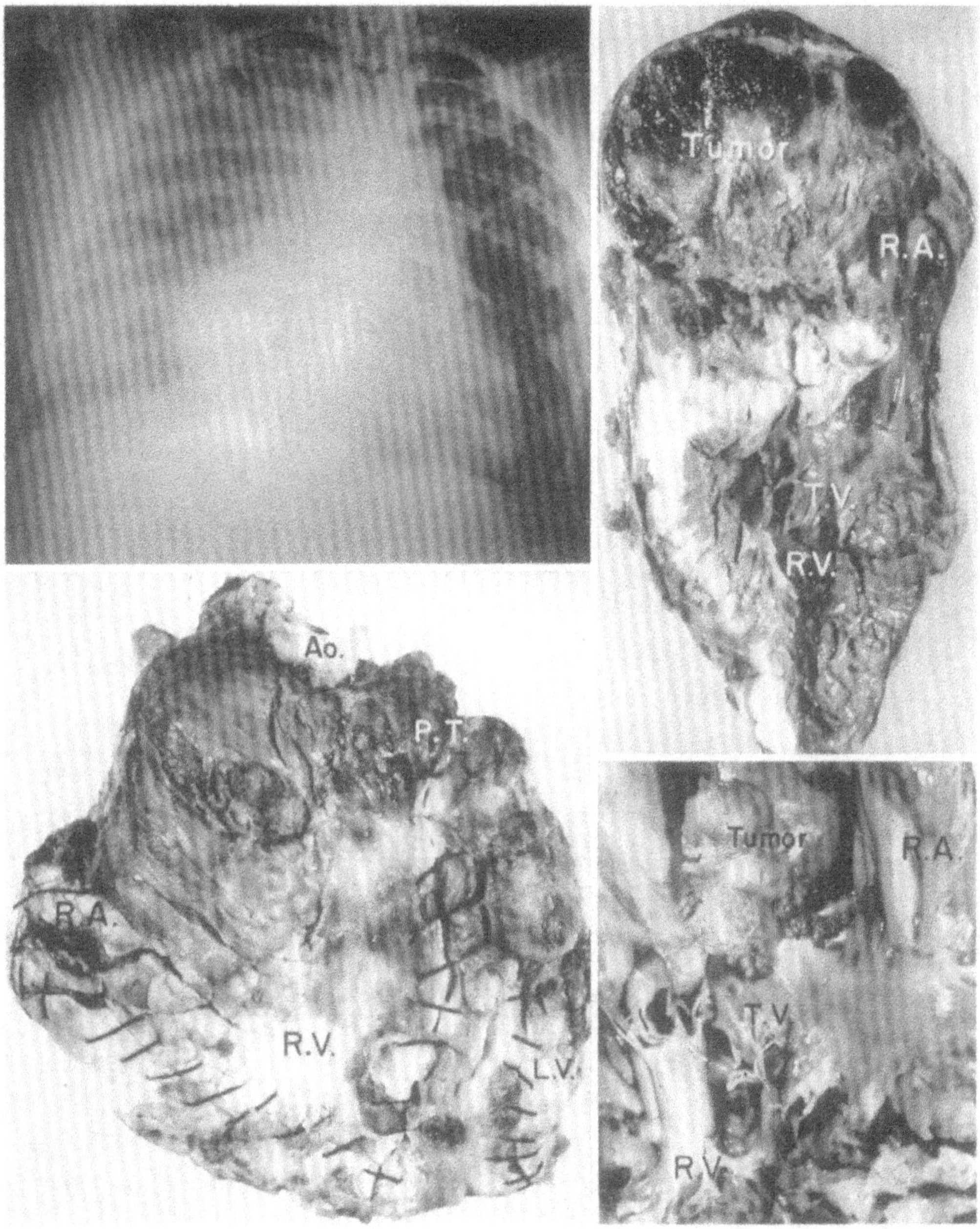

FIG. 1. Above, *chest roentgenogram and heart*. Upper left, *anteroposterior projection*, taken with the patient supine, shows generalized cardiac enlargement, prominence of the right cardiac border and right ventricular outflow tract, finely nodular infiltrates in both lungs, and a right pleural effusion. Lower left, *anterior surface of the heart* after removal of the adherent parietal pericardium. A large right atrial tumor (R.A.) caused the prominent right cardiac border on roentgenogram. Large masses of epicardial tumor surround the aorta (Ao.) and pulmonary trunk (P.T.), and smaller nodules are in the right (R.V.) and left (L.V.) ventricular epicardium. Upper right, *the free walls of the right atrium and right ventricle*. A partially hemorrhagic tumor, 6 cm. in diameter, involves the right atrial epicardium, myocardium and endocardium and projects into the right atrial cavity just above the tricuspid valve (T.V.). Lower right, *the intracavitary projection of the tumor* shown at upper right measures 2 cm. in diameter.

FIG. 2. Opposite page, *photomicrographs of the cardiac angiosarcoma*. Upper left, *epicardial tumor nodule* with both cellular areas and large vascular spaces (× 25). Upper right, *large vascular spaces* separated by cords of endothelial cells (× 160). Lower left, *spindle-shaped cells* with inconspicuous vascular spaces between them. This histologic pattern is indistinguishable from that of Kaposi's sarcoma (× 251). Lower right, *high power photomicrograph* of the tumor cells (× 628). All sections stained with hematoxylin and eosin.

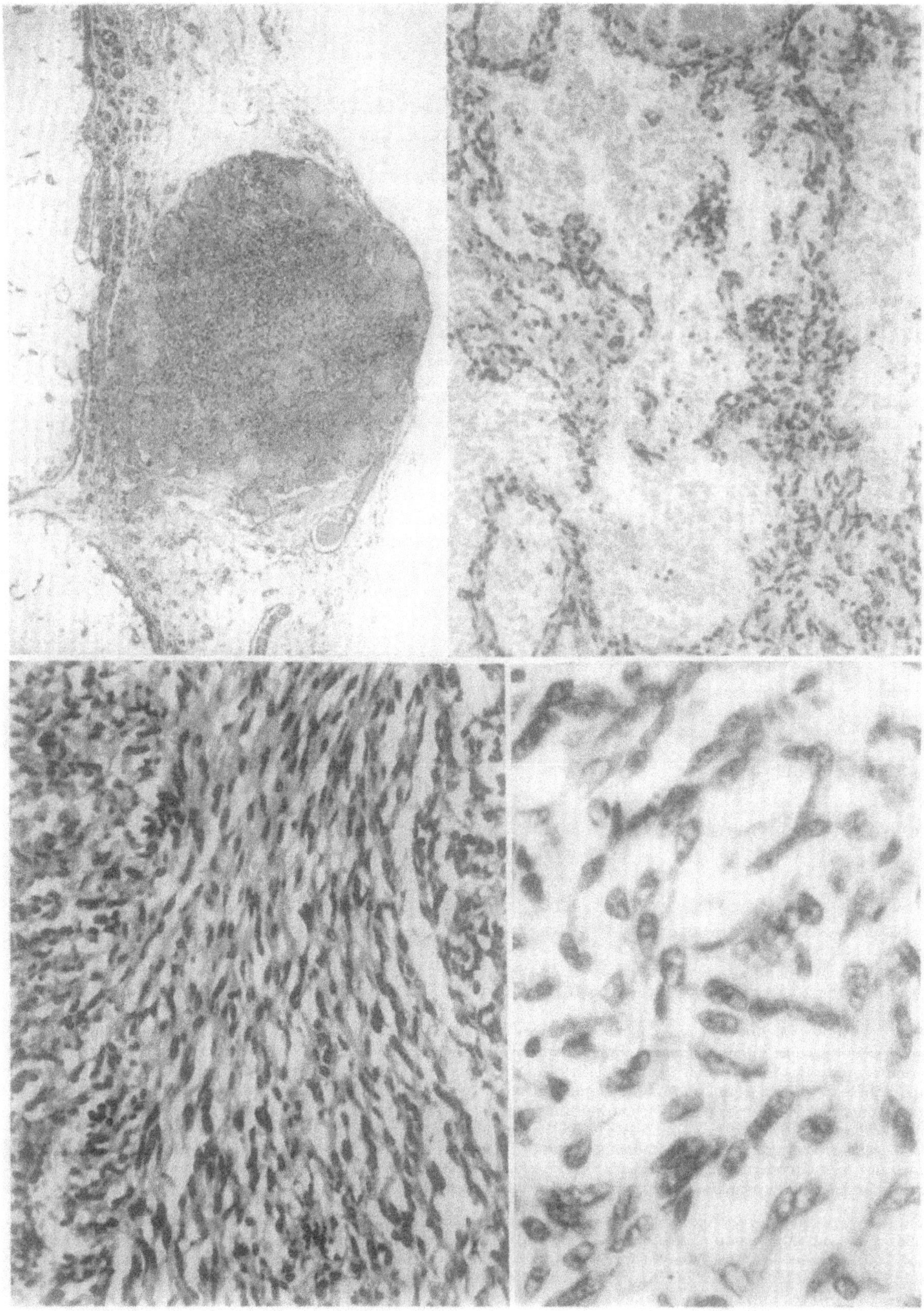

and those without extracardiac tumor. The angiosarcomas were described under a variety of names: angiosarcoma,[1,10,12,13,16,18,19,21,25,27–29,31,35–37,40] angioendothelial sarcoma,[24] hemangiosarcoma,[23] endothelioma,[11] hemangioendothelioma,[4,34,39] malignant hemangioendothelioma,[3,20,38] hemangioendotheliosarcoma,[8,15,17,22,26] hemangioendothelioblastoma,[14] malignant hemangioblastoma,[5] hemangioreticuloendothelioma,[9] telangiectatic and cavernous spindle-cell sarcoma[2] and primary Kaposi's sarcoma of the heart.[6,7,30,32,33] Judged by the histologic features in published photomicrographs, "primary Kaposi's sarcoma of the heart" (Table I, Cases 6, 7, 31 and 33) is identical to primary cardiac angiosarcoma (Fig. 2) and in the absence of cutaneous manifestations of Kaposi's sarcoma should be classified as angiosarcoma.

CLINICAL FEATURES

The clinical features in the 41 patients with cardiac angiosarcoma were remarkably uniform (Table I). All were adults, and 35 were under age 50 years (range 22 to 68, average 40 years); 29 were men. Of the 37 patients for whom adequate clinical information was available, 32 had evidence of obstruction to filling of the right-sided cardiac chambers. All 32 had cardiomegaly. Dyspnea was described in 23, systemic venous distention in 19, hepatomegaly in 17, edema in 16, cyanosis in 11, diminished cardiac sounds in 11, systemic arterial pulse pressures of 25 mm. Hg or less in 6, pulsus paradoxus in 5 and syncope in 4 of the 32 patients. Venous distention, edema and cyanosis were at times limited to the head and upper trunk. A few reports simply stated that the patient had superior vena caval obstruction or cardiac tamponade without listing each sign and symptom. Orthopnea, paroxysmal nocturnal dyspnea, pulmonary alveolar edema, pulsus alternans and other manifestations of left-sided cardiac failure rarely occurred.

Precordial pain, often typically pericarditic in type, was present in 23 of 34 patients, and pericardial friction rubs were heard in 8 of 32 subjects (Table I). Temperatures over 100° F. were recorded in 16 of 22 patients whose temperature was stated. Of 30 patients, 13 had cough and 8, including 2 without pulmonary metastases, had hemoptysis. The combination of fever, hemoptysis and evidence of a pericardial effusion led to a diagnosis of tuberculosis in at least 5 patients.

X-ray and Electrocardiographic Findings: All 28 patients with chest roentgenograms had cardiomegaly. In 20 the enlargement was generalized, and often the cardiac silhouette was globular and massive; in 7 generalized enlargement was present, but the most striking finding was a prominent right cardiac border (Fig. 1); in 1 the right ventricular outflow tract was prominent. In addition, chest roentgenograms demonstrated pulmonary metastases in 4 patients and rib metastases in 3. All but 1 of 24 patients had electrocardiographic abnormalities: ST-T wave changes, which were usually nonspecific but were occasionally typical of pericarditis, in 15 patients; low QRS voltage in 13; right axis deviation in 5; supraventricular arrhythmias in 4; right bundle branch block in 2; QRS changes suggesting an old myocardial infarct in 2; and in 2 patients changes suggesting a recent myocardial infarct, which was found at necropsy in 1 of them.

Clinical Diagnosis and Prognosis: A malignant, primary cardiac tumor was suspected clinically in 12 patients, and this diagnosis was supported by a positive biopsy of bone, lung or the primary tumor in 4 patients, by finding tumor cells in pericardial fluid in 1, by visualizing the tumor by pneumopericardium in 1 and by venous angiocardiogram in 1. The duration of symptoms from their onset until death was nine months or less in 29 of the 33 patients in whom this interval could be determined. Each of the 4 patients (Table I, Cases 15, 22, 25, 28) who lived longer than nine months after the onset of symptoms had a biphasic illness, and it is possible that the initial phase in them was unrelated to angiosarcoma.

PATHOANATOMIC FEATURES

Site of Primary Tumor: The pathoanatomic features in the 41 patients were even more uniform than the clinical features. The site of the primary tumor was the right side of the heart (almost always the right atrium) or the pericardium (usually the epicardium) in all but 1 patient (Table I, Case 4), and her left atrial tumor was an incidental autopsy finding. In each of the other patients, tumor involved the right atrium (Fig. 1); this chamber almost invariably was the one most extensively involved. Right atrial intracavitary projections of tumor were usually present, and measured up to 12 cm. in diameter In 17 patients tumor obstructed one or both venae cavae, or the tricuspid valvular orifice, or both. The epicardium was involved by tumor in all but

1 patient (Table I, Case 14). At times only the epicardium over a right atrial tumor was invaded, but usually there was extensive invasion of the epicardium and subepicardial adipose tissue, and in at least 11 patients, the heart was encased by a layer of tumor over 1 cm. thick. The pericardial cavity was obliterated by tumor, or organized hemorrhage, or both, in 13 patients; it contained hemorrhagic fluid in 24, serous fluid in 1 and was normal in 2. Pericardial tumor most often limited right ventricular filling by producing hemopericardium with tamponade, but ventricular constriction by a thick layer of epicardial tumor was probably another mechanism, and each of these mechanisms at times coexisted with vena caval obstruction.

TABLE I
Cardiac Angiosarcoma: Clinical and Pathologic Data in 41 Cases

		Clinical Features							Pathoanatomic Features			
Case No. (Ref.)	Age/Sex	RV Inflow Obstruction	Pericardial Rub	Chest Pain	Fever (>100° F.)	Hemoptysis	Heart on X-ray	Duration of Symptoms (mo.)	Primary Site	Pericardial Cavity	Venous or Valvular Obstruction by Tumor	Extracardiac Metastases
1[1]	22/M	+	+	+	+	0	...	4	P	Hemo.	VC	L
2[2]	44/M	+	0	+	...	+	...	1.5	RA	Oblit.	SVC	L, CNS
3[3]	62/F	0	0	0	...	+	...	6	RA	Hemo.	0	L, B, LN, Om.
4[4]	45/F	0†	...	...	...	...	...	†	LA	Normal	0	0
5[5]	44/M	+	0	0	...	0	GE	6	P	Hemo.	SVC	L, Liv.
6[6,7]	26/M	+	0	0	+	0	GE	2	RA	Oblit.	TV	L, Liv., LN, Om
7[6,7]	30/M	+	0	0	+	+	GE	1.5	RA	Hemo.	SVC, IVC, TV	0
8[8]	40/M	0	0	+	+	0	GE	9	P	Oblit.	SVC	L, Liv., S, B, K, Pan., T, A
9[9]	46/M	...	...	...	...	...	...	...	P or RA	Oblit.	0	L, Liv., LN, B
10[10]	60/M	+	...	...	...	...	...	‡	RA	Hemo.	0	LN
11[11]	45/M	+	0	...	...	...	GE	1.2	RA	Hemo.	IVC	0
12[12]	47/M	+	0	0	0	0	GE	2	P, RA, or RV	Hemo.	0	L, LN, SM
13[13]	27/M	+	0	0	+	0	GE	5	P	Oblit.	SVC, IVC, PV	0
14[14]	54/M	+	0	0	0	0	GE	8	RA, RV, or TV	Normal	SVC, IVC, TV, RVI	0
15[15]	23/F	+	0	+	+	0	GE	?21, ?7	RA	Hemo.	SVC, IVC, TV	0
16[16]	46/M	...	...	...	...	...	...	...	RA or RV	Oblit.	0	L, Liv., K, A, B
17[17]	26/M	+	0	+	+	0	RVO	2.5	RA or RV	Oblit.	0	L, Pr.
18[18]	45/F	+	0	+	0	0	R	2	RA	Hemo.	SVC, IVC, TV, CS	L
19[19]	27/M	0	0	0	+	0	R	...	RA	Hemo.	0	0
20[20]	25/M	+	+	+	+	0	GE	4	RA	Hemo.	SVC	L, Liv., LN, A
21[20]	33/M	+	0	+	0	0	GE	4	RA	Oblit.	0	L, Liv., B, LN
22[21]	37/M	+	+	+	+	+	GE	?23, ?3	RA	Hemo.	0	L, S
23[22]	46/M	+	+	+	+	0	R	8	RA	Oblit.	SVC	CNS, Liv., A, B
24[23]	32/F	+	0	0	+	0	GE	2	RA	Hemo.	0	0
25[24]	35/M	+	+	+	+	+	GE	?24, ?5	RA	Hemo.	0	0
26[25]	47/M	...	...	+	...	...	...	5	P	Oblit.	0	L, Liv., LN
27[26]	45/M	+	0	+	...	+	GE	1.2	RA	Hemo.	SVC, ?TV	L
28[27]	29/F	+	0	+	+	0	R	?15, ?8	P	Hemo.	IVC, ?SVC	0
29[28]	38/M	+	0	+	...	0	R	8	RA or RV	...	0	L, Liv., B, A
30[29]	59/F	+	...	+	...	...	...	...	RA	Hemo.	0	L
31[30]	43/M	+	0	+	...	+	GE	...	P or RA	Hemo.	0	L
32[31]	39/F	+	...	...	...	...	...	...	RA	Oblit.	TV, IVC	L
33[32,33]	38/M	+	0	0	...	0	GE	5	P	Serous	0	0
34[34]	38/F	0	0	+	...	0	R	6	RA	Oblit.	SVC	L, Liv.
35[35]	52/F	+	...	+	...	...	...	0.3	RA	Hemo.	0	0
36[36]	43/M	+	+	+	+	+	GE	3	RA	Hemo.	LSV	L, LN
37[37]	25/M	+	...	...	...	...	...	0.3	RA	Hemo.	0	0
38[38]	33/M	+	0	+	...	0	...	5	P	Hemo.	0	0
39[39]	68/M	+	+	+	0	...	GE	1	RA	Hemo.	0	L, LN
40[40]	26/F	+	+	+	+	0	GE	5	RA	Hemo.	0	L, Ov.
41*	35/F	0	0	0	0	0	R	2	RA	Oblit.	0	L, CNS, Ov., U, S, Liv., T, K, LN

(Ref.) = reference describing the patient; + = present; 0 = absent; ... = insufficient information; A = adrenal gland; B = bone; CNS = brain; CS = coronary sinus; GE = generalized enlargement; Hemo. = hemopericardium; IVC = inferior vena cava; K = kidney; L = lung and/or pleura; Liv. = liver; LA = left atrium; LN = lymph nodes; LSV. = left subclavian vein; Oblit. = obliterated; Om. = omentum; Ov. = ovary; P = pericardium; Pan. = pancreas; Pr. = prostate; PV = pulmonary veins; R = prominent right cardiac border; RA = right atrium; RV = right ventricle; RVI = right ventricular infundibulum; RVO = prominent right ventricular outflow tract; S = spleen; Serous = serous effusion; SM = skeletal muscle; SVC = superior vena cava; T = thyroid; TV = tricuspid valve; U = uterus; VC = vena cava.

* Present patient.

† Died of rheumatic mitral stenosis. Angiosarcoma an incidental necropsy finding.

‡ Died suddenly of hemopericardium with tamponade. Dyspnea for one year and cardiac murmur probably due to cardiac disease other than angiosarcoma.

Metastatic Tumors: Metastases were present in 27 patients and occurred in the lung in 25 of them. Pleural effusions were present in at least 24 patients, and were bilateral in 14 and hemorrhagic in 16. Benign hepatic hemangiomas were described in 5 patients. Widely metastasizing angiosarcomas, however, not uncommonly have a "benign" histologic appearance in some or all portions of the tumor,[41–43] and it is likely that many of the hepatic hemangiomas were in fact angiosarcomatous metastases. Brain metastases were found in only 2 of the 40 previously reported patients with cardiac angiosarcoma (Table I). We have found reports of brain metastases in only 2 patients with angiosarcomas originating in extracardiac sites,[44,45] and brain metastases have not been reported in patients with cutaneous Kaposi's sarcoma. Cerebellar and midbrain metastases caused the present patient's death before significant cardiac dysfunction developed.

Incidence: Although it is a rare tumor, angiosarcoma may be the most common primary malignant tumor of the heart. It originates in the heart about as frequently as does rhabdomyosarcoma, and probably more frequently than does fibrosarcoma, reticulum-cell sarcoma, or lymphosarcoma. Angiosarcomas accounted for 23 of the 177 malignant primary cardiac tumors summarized in reviews through 1959.[46–48] In addition, there have been at least 6 patients with metastases to the heart from angiosarcomas originating elsewhere,[41,43,45,49–51] and 1 of them[49] both clinically and pathologically closely resembled the patients listed in Table I. Cardiac metastases also have been reported in patients with Kaposi's sarcoma and typical cutaneous involvement.[33]

Summary

The clinical and pathoanatomic features in a 35 year old woman with angiosarcoma of the heart are described, and the findings in previously reported patients with cardiac angiosarcoma are summarized. Obstruction to filling of the right-sided cardiac chambers by hemopericardium with tamponade, constriction of the ventricles by a thick layer of epicardial tumor, vena caval or tricuspid valvular obstruction, or a combination of these mechanisms was almost uniformly present in the previously reported patients. The present patient's right atrium and epicardium were massively invaded by tumor, but she died of metastases to the brain, an unusual finding in patients with angiosarcoma, before significant cardiac dysfunction developed.

References

1. Redtenbacher, L. Ein Fall von Angiosarcoma pericardii. *Wien klin. Wschnschr.*, 2: 214, 1889.
2. Gödel, A. Zur Kenntnis der primären Herzgeschwülste. *Zentralbl. Herz. u. Gefässkr.*, 14: 99, 1922.
3. Hewer, T. F. and Kemp, R. P. Malignant hemangio-endothelioma of the heart: Report of a case. *J. Path. & Bact.*, 43: 511, 1936.
4. Gross, P. and Englehart, C. E. Primary hemangio-endothelioma of the heart: Report of a case. *Am. J. Cancer*, 30: 102, 1937.
5. Scheidegger, S. Malignes Hämangioblastom des Perikards. (Beitrag zur Frage der Deckzellengeschwülste.) *Frankfurt. Ztschr. Path.*, 51: 286, 1937–8.
6. Choisser, R. M. and Ramsey, E. M. Angioreticuloendothelioma (Kaposi's disease) of the heart. *Am. J. Path.*, 15: 155, 1939.
7. Weller, G. L., Jr. The clinical aspects of cardiac involvement (right auricular tumor) in idiopathic hemorrhagic sarcoma (Kaposi's disease). *Ann. Int. Med.*, 14: 314, 1940.
8. Jucker, P. Die Diagnose der primären Bösartigen Geschwülste des Perikards und der das Perikard infiltrierenden Herzwandtumoren. Bericht uber zwei an der Basler Medizinischen Klinik beobachteten primäre Perikardsarkome. *Ztschr. klin. Med.*, 139: 208, 1941.
9. Da Cunha Motta, L. Hemangio reticulo-endothelioma. *Ann. Fac. med. São Paulo*, 17: 627, 1941.
10. Aegerter, E. E. and Peale, A. R. Kaposi's sarcoma. A critical survey. *Arch. Path.*, 34: 413, 1942.
11. Reisinger, J. A., Pekin, T. J. and Blumenthal, B. Primary tumor of the inferior vena cava and heart with hemopericardium and alternation of the ventricular complexes in the electrocardiogram *Ann. Int. Med.*, 17: 995 1942.
12. Lange, H. F. and Christiansen, T. Hemopericardium-angiosarcoma cordis. A case of primary heart tumor, diagnosed intra vitam. *Acta med. scandinav.*, 127: 107, 1947.
13. Greenberg, M. and Angrist, A. Primary vascular tumors of the pericardium: A report of two cases. *Am. Heart J.*, 35: 623, 1948.
14. Amsterdam, H. J., Grayzel, D. M. and Louria, A. L. Hemangio-endothelioblastoma of the heart. *Am. Heart J.*, 37: 291, 1949.
15. Lübschitz, K., Lundsteen, E. and Forchhammer, E. Primary malignant heart tumor diagnosed in vivo with the aid of artificial pneumopericardium. *Radiology*, 52: 79, 1949.
16. Tatsumi, T., Nagatomo, T. and Kashiwai, K. An autopsy case of primary heart tumor. *Gann*, 40: 174, 1949.
17. Glassy, F. J. and Massey, F. C. Primary hemangio-endothelial sarcoma of the heart. *Am. J. Med.*, 8: 544, 1950.
18. Tacket, H. S., Jones, R. S. and Kyle, J. W. Primary angiosarcoma of the heart. *Am. Heart J.*, 39: 912, 1950.
19. Bruzzone, P. L. and Guglielmini, G. Immagini anatomo-radiologiche cistosimili del diaframma

di destra e dell'angolo cardio-frenico (pseudoernia del diaframma e angiosarcoma del cuore). *Minerva med.*, 1: 968, 1951.

20. Blanchard, A. J. and Hetherington, H. Malignant hemangioendothelioma of the heart. *Canad. M. A. J.*, 66: 147, 1952.
21. Schwartz, N. H. and Loder, M. Primary tumor of the heart. *New York J. Med.*, 52: 2658, 1952.
22. Deloach, J. F. and Haynes, J. W. Secondary tumors of the heart and pericardium. Review of the subject and report of one hundred and thirty-seven cases. *A.M.A. Arch. Int. Med.*, 91: 224, 1953.
23. Schwarzkopf, H. and Gais, H. Primäres Hämangiosarkom im Gebiet der rechten Kranzarterie. *Frankfurt. Ztschr. Path.*, 64: 483, 1953.
24. Brandenburg, R. O. and Edwards, J. E. Cardiac sarcoma: Report of a case and comparison with a case of metastatic carcinoma of the pericardium. *Proc. Staff. Meet. Mayo Clin.*, 29: 437, 1954.
25. Florange, W. Über die Beobachtung eines angioplastischen Sarkoms des Perikards; zugleich ein Beitrag zur Frage des ausgangsortes der Sarkome des Herzbeutels. *Zentralbl. allg. Path.*, 91: 413, 1954.
26. Cheng, T. O. and Sutton, D. C. Primary hemangioendotheliosarcoma of heart, diagnosed by angiocardiography: Review of the literature and report of a case. *Circulation*, 11: 456, 1955.
27. Grosse-Brockhoff, F. and Schreiber, H. W. Angiosarkom des Herzbeutels. *Ztschr. Kreislaufforsch.*, 44: 866, 1955.
28. Groom, D. Electrocardiogram of the month. *J. South Carolina M. A.*, 52: 10, 1956.
29. Kurashova, M. V. and Kogan, R. P. [Angiosarcoma of the Heart.] *Klin. med.*, 34(11): 77, 1956. Abstr. in *Abstr. Soviet Med.*, 2-B: 352, 1958.
30. Contrearas, R. Angiosarcoma de Kaposi primario del corazón; revisión de la literatura y descripción del sexto caso. *Arch. Inst. cardiol. México*, 27: 463, 1957.
31. Kogan, R. P. [Tumors of Heart.] *Arkh. Pat.*, 19 (1): 66, 1957. Abstr. in *Excerpta med. sect. 16*, 5: 703, 1957.
32. Gelfand, M. Kaposi's hemangiosarcoma of the heart. *Brit. Heart J.*, 19: 290, 1957.
33. Lothe, F. and Murray, J. F. Kaposi's sarcoma: Autopsy findings in the African. *Acta Unio internat. cancum.*, 19: 429, 1962.
34. Crenshaw, J. F., Dowling, E. A. and Cresswell, W. F., Jr. Primary hemangio-endothelioma of the heart. *Ann. Int. Med.*, 50: 1289, 1959.
35. Harris, H. R. Angiosarcoma of the heart. *J. Clin. Path.*, 13: 205, 1960.
36. McNalley, M. C., Kelble, D., Pryor, R. and Blount, S. G., Jr. Angiosarcoma of the heart: Report of a case and review of the literature. *Am. Heart J.*, 65: 244, 1963.
37. Wright, R. P., Jr., McCall, M. M. and Wenger, N. K. Primary atrial tumor. Evaluation of clinical findings in ten cases and review of the literature. *Am. J. Cardiol.*, 11: 790, 1963.
38. Berlov, G. A. and Pigarev, Yu. G. [A peculiar form of systemic tumour-like angiomatosis (malignant hemangioendothelioma of the pericardium, angiomatous polyp of the endocardium and progressive hemangiomatosis of the liver).] *Arkh. Pat.*, 26(8): 74, 1964.
39. Robinson, D. S. and Machanic, P. B. Hemangioendothelioma of the heart. *J.A.M.A.*, 189: 1026, 1964.
40. Lukash, W. M., Schneider, P. J. and Sennett, C. O. Angiosarcoma presenting as acute rheumatic pancarditis. *J.A.M.A.*, 193: 975, 1965.
41. Shennan, T. Histologically non-malignant angioma with numerous metastases. *J. Path. & Bact.*, 19: 139, 1914.
42. Robinson, J. M. and Castleman, B. Benign metastasizing hemangioma. *Ann. Surg.*, 104: 453, 1936.
43. Stout, A. P. Hemangio-endothelioma: A tumor of blood vessels featuring vascular endothelial cells. *Ann. Surg.*, 118: 445, 1943.
44. Nesbitt, S., Mark, P. F. and Zimmerman, H. M. Disseminated visceral idiopathic hemorrhagic sarcoma (Kaposi's disease): Report of a case with necropsy findings. *Ann. Int. Med.*, 22: 601, 1945.
45. Tibbs, D. Metastasizing hemangiomata: A case of malignant haemangio-endothelioma. *Brit. J. Surg.*, 40: 465, 1952–3.
46. Whorton, C. M. Primary malignant tumors of the heart: Report of a case. *Cancer*, 2: 245, 1949.
47. Brucker, E. A., Jr. and Glassy, F. J. Primary reticulum-cell sarcoma of the heart with review of the literature. *Cancer*, 8: 921, 1955.
48. Somers, K. and Lothe, F. Primary lymphosarcoma of the heart: Review of the literature and report of 3 cases. *Cancer*, 13: 449, 1960.
49. Grayson, R. R. Hemangioendotheliosarcoma of the ileum with metastases to the right auricle, rupture of the heart, and hemopericardium at least 10 days before death: A case report. *Ann. Int. Med.*, 41: 151, 1954.
50. Bourne, M. S., Cook, T. A. and Williams, G. Hemangiosarcomatosis: Two cases presenting as haematological problems. *Brit. M. J.*, 2: 275, 1965.
51. Crymes, T. and Taylor, R. G. Angiosarcoma metastatic to the tongue: Report of a case. *J. Oral Surg.*, 24: 63, 1966.

The Heart in Malignant Melanoma

A Study of 70 Autopsy Cases*

D. Luke Glancy, M.D. *and* William C. Roberts, M.D., F.A.C.C.

Bethesda, Maryland

Cardiac metastases have been found at necropsy in 1.5[1] to 21 per cent[2] of patients with malignant tumors. In absolute numbers, carcinoma of the lung and breast metastasize to the heart most often,[3-8] but the highest percentage of cardiac involvement occurs in malignant melanoma, leukemia[9] and malignant lymphoma,[10] in that order. The present study reviews the cases of 70 patients with metastatic malignant melanoma who underwent autopsy at the Clinical Center and summarizes the clinical cardiac findings and the frequency and extent of the metastases to the heart.

Patients Studied

From 1954 through 1966, 74 patients with a histologic diagnosis of malignant melanoma underwent autopsy at the Clinical Center. Four of the 74 are excluded from this review: 2 because the material available for review was inadequate and 2 because they had no metastases at necropsy. One of the latter subjects died 10 days after resection of a malignant melanoma of the vulva; the second died of a cerebellar hemorrhage 7 months after resection of melanoma of the ear. In each of the remaining 70 patients metastatic malignant melanoma was present at necropsy: in 69 the metastases were widespread, and in the seventieth metastases were present in only one organ (the brain).

The clinical records, chest roentgenograms, electrocardiograms and necropsy protocols of each of the 70 patients were reviewed. The heart of each was re-examined by us, and the histologic sections taken at the time of autopsy were reviewed. Additional histologic sections of the heart were taken for many patients. On the average, we examined microscopically five sections per heart. Since the parietal pericardium was rarely available for re-examination, the data on the pericardium concern the visceral layer.

Observations At Necropsy

Of the 70 patients with metastatic melanoma, there were 38 men and 32 women. Their ages ranged from 15 to 89 years; the average age at death was 44 years for the men, and 45 years for the women. Only 1 patient was less than 21 years of age. All were white. The site of the primary tumor in the 70 patients is listed in Table I. The time of removal of the primary

Table I
Site of Primary Tumor in 70 Patients with Metastatic Melanoma

	Men	Women
Eye	1	1
Head and neck	6	6
Shoulder	2	4
Arm	0	1
Anterior trunk	7	2
Posterior trunk	13	7
Anus	0	1
Leg	4	4
Foot	2	2
Unknown	3	4
Total	38	32

* From the Laboratory of Pathology, Clinic of Surgery, National Heart Institute, and the Pathologic Anatomy Department, National Cancer Institute, National Institutes of Health, Bethesda, Md.

Address for reprints: D. Luke Glancy, M.D., Laboratory of Pathology, Clinic of Surgery, National Heart Institute, National Institutes of Health, Bethesda, Md. 20014.

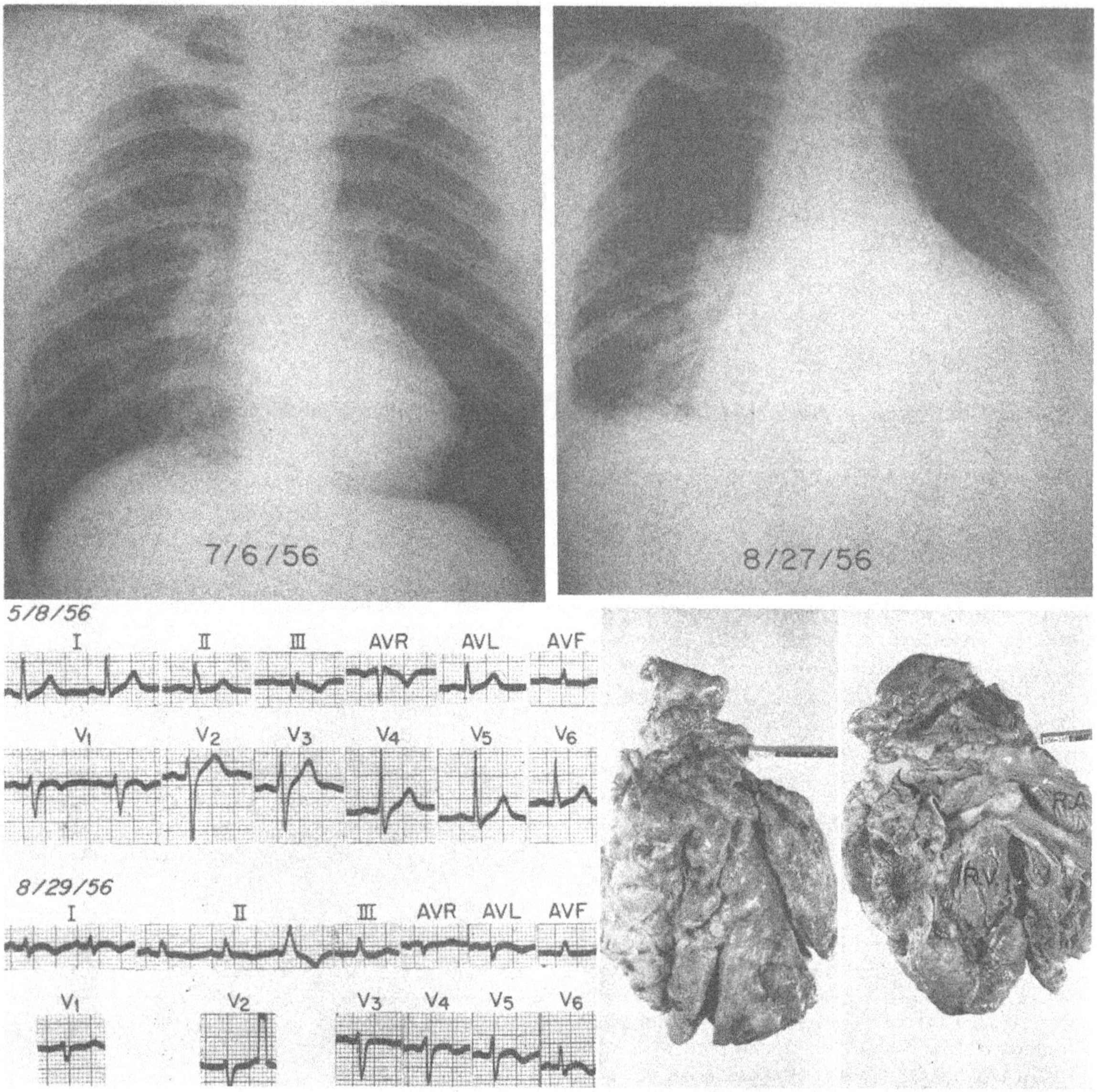

FIG. 1. *Pericarditis with Effusion and Tamponade. Chest roentgenograms, electrocardiograms and the heart in a 33 year old man who died on Oct. 23, 1956, four years after removal of a melanoma of the back.* Two months before death dyspnea, cough and chest pain typical of pericarditis developed. He also had tachypnea, pulsus paradoxus (20 mm. Hg), an enlarged area of precordial percussion dullness without palpable pulsations, faint heart sounds, elevated venous pressure (23 cm. water) and a prolonged circulation time (17 sec.).

Chest roentgenogram (8/27/56) revealed a huge cardiac silhouette. The electrocardiogram (8/29/56) showed sinus tachycardia, low voltage, and ST-T wave changes consistent with pericarditis. Pericardiocentesis yielded 700 ml. of bloody fluid containing malignant cells. Other pericardiocenteses were necessary for relief of cardiac tamponade during the patient's last two months. At necropsy, the heart with its metastases weighed 880 gm., and there was a generalized fibrofibrinous pericarditis (**lower middle**). Tumor extended from the epicardium into the right ventricular (**R.V.**) myocardium (**lower right**). R.A. = opened right atrium.

FIG. 2. *Pericarditis with Atrial Flutter. Anteroposterior chest roentgenogram, electrocardiograms and the heart in a 43 year old woman who died on Oct. 19, 1957, 11 years after removal of a melanoma of the eye.* Numerous pulmonary metastases were noted on x-ray examination. One week before death a pericardial friction rub was noted. The day before death, October 18, 1957, atrial flutter with 2:1 block developed, and the QRS voltage had decreased strikingly since the previous electrocardiogram (2/20/57). At necropsy, there was 200 ml. of pericardial fluid, and the heart with its metastases weighed 520 gm. On its external surface (**lower left**), there were numerous tumor nodules and diffuse fibrinous pericarditis. (The arrows indicate subendocardial tumor nodules in the opened right atrium.) There were massive, pigmented metastases in the region of the atrioventricular sulcus (**lower right**). L.A. = opened left atrium; L.V. = opened left ventricle.

tumor was known for 61 patients. The average survival time after this operative procedure was 3.1 years in the 33 men and 4.2 years in the 28 women. The longest survival period after initial excision of the primary tumor was 15 years, and the shortest, 5 weeks. The primary tumor in the latter patient first appeared four months before death. Of the 61 patients, 14 (10 women and 4 men) survived five or more years.

Site and Extent of Cardiac Metastases: Of the 70 patients 45 (64 per cent) had cardiac metastases, and each also had metastases to many other organs. The portions of the heart involved by these metastases are listed in Table II. Diffuse fibrinous pericarditis secondary to epicardial melanoma occurred in 2 patients (Fig. 1 and 2). By gross examination, the extent of cardiac involvement by tumor was classified as extensive in 13 patients, moderate in 14 and slight in 15.* In addition, minute foci of metastatic tumor were demonstrated histologically in three hearts that on gross examination appeared normal. In another patient no cardiac metastases were ob-

* The classification was based on both the number of cardiac sites invaded by tumor (Table II) and the number and size of metastases in those sites. For example, in each patient whose cardiac involvement by tumor was classified as extensive there were endocardial, epicardial and myocardial metastases. In all but 1 of these patients, all four cardiac chambers were invaded by tumor, and metastases were numerous and usually large. In contrast, in patients whose cardiac involvement by tumor was classified as slight, on the average, only one or two cardiac chambers were involved; when more sites were involved, the metastases in each site were few in number and small in size. When the involvement was classified as moderate, the extent of cardiac invasion by tumor was intermediate between these two.

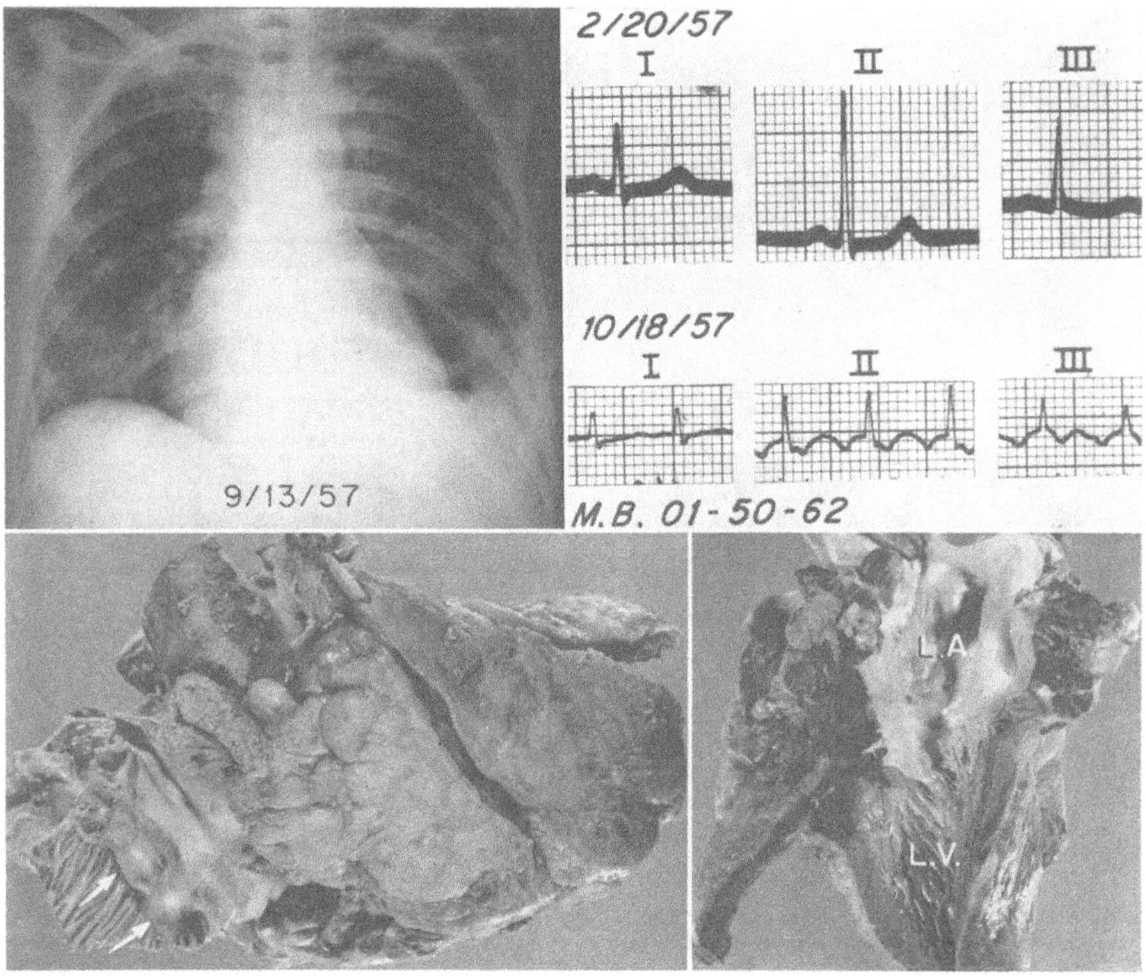

FIG. 2. **See opposite page**

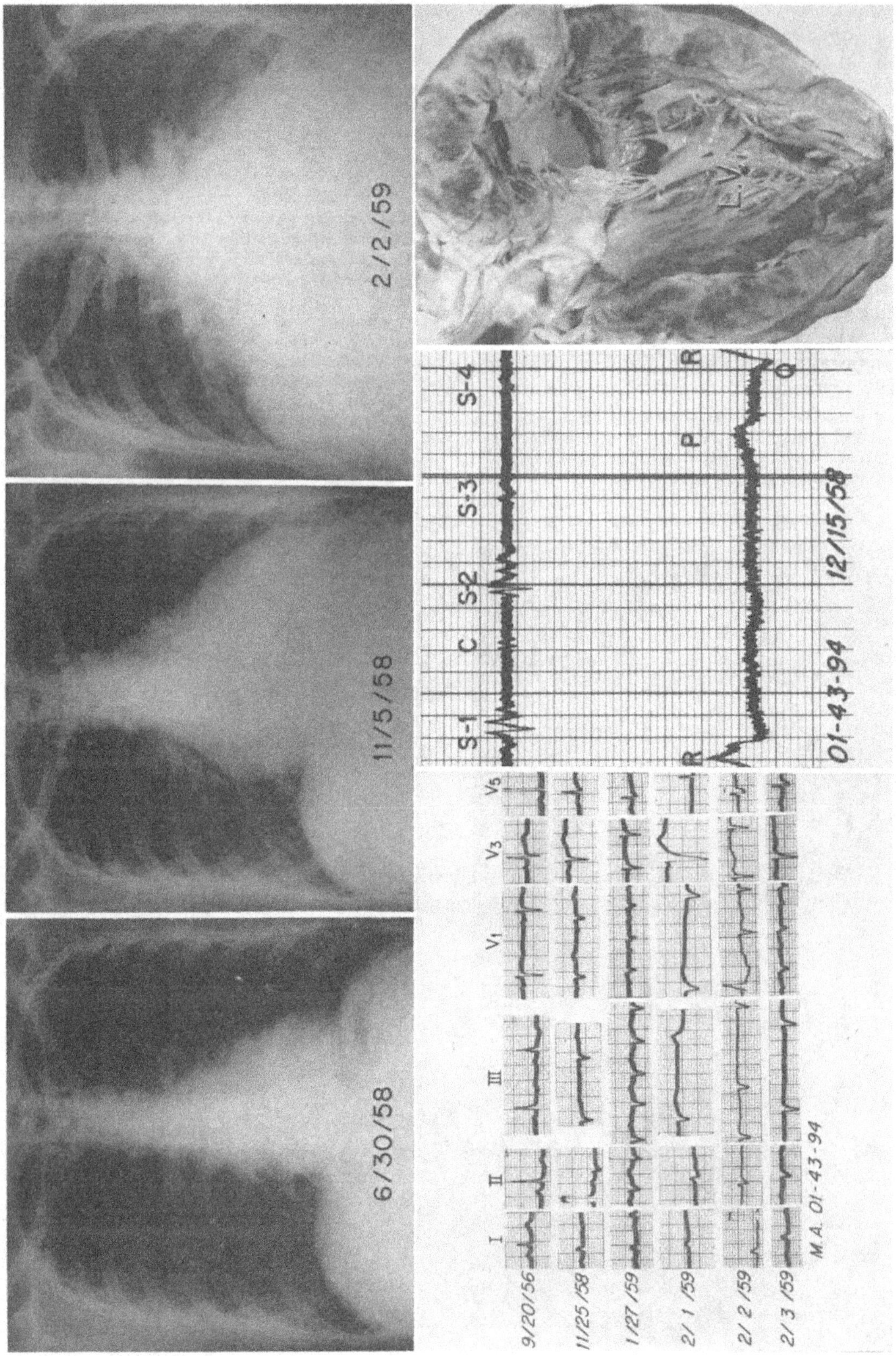

FIG. 3. **See opposite page**

Fig. 3. **Opposite page.** *Massive Myocardial Metastases with Congestive Failure. Chest roentgenograms, electrocardiograms, phonocardiogram* (**lower middle**), *and the opened left ventricle and aortic valve* (**lower right**) *in a 43 year old woman who died on February 6, 1959, eight years after removal of a melanoma of the leg.* Dyspnea began three months before death, and the chest roentgenogram (11/5/58) revealed an enlarged cardiac silhouette. Low QRS voltage and left axis deviation were observed on electrocardiogram (11/25/58). A phonocardiogram (12/15/58) revealed a widely and persistently split second heart sound (S-2); atrial (S-4) and ventricular (S-3) gallops, and a mid-systolic click (c). On January 27, 1959, dyspnea increased; pulmonary rales and sacral edema were noted; venous pressure was 15 cm. water; circulation time was 27 sec.; and sinus tachycardia (135 beats/min.) with premature atrial contractions was present. Digitalis and diuretics slowed the sinus rate to 60/min. and effected an eight pound diuresis. The blood pressure, however, fell from 110/70 to 80/60 mm. Hg, suggesting that in addition to myocardial failure pericardial tamponade was responsible for the cardiac failure. Atrial fibrillation with frequent aberrant conduction developed on Feb. 1, 1959. The next day an intermittent right bundle branch block pattern also was present, and chest roentgenogram revealed pulmonary congestion and bilateral pleural effusions. On February 3 there was sinus rhythm with alternating first and second (2:1) degree A-V block; digitalis was discontinued. The patient died suddenly on February 6. *At necropsy*, 500 ml. of fluid was present in each pleural space, 200 in the pericardial sac. The heart weighed 600 gm.; tumor was present in the walls of all chambers. The left ventricular (L.V.) myocardium (**lower right**) was massively infiltrated by tumor.

Table II
Sites of Cardiac Metastases in 45 Patients with Malignant Melanoma of the Heart

Site	No. of Patients	Per Cent
Endocardium	33	73
Mural endocardium	33	73
Tricuspid valve	2	4
Myocardium	44	98
Right atrium	34	76
Left atrium	23	51
Atrial septum	22	49
Right ventricle	30	67
Left ventricle	33	73
Ventricular septum	26	58
Epicardium	35	78

served, but a minute tumor embolus was found within a small intramural coronary artery. Patients with extensive cardiac metastases had larger hearts on the average than other patients (Table III). Clinical and pathologic findings of 10 who had extensive cardiac tumor are illustrated in Figures 1 to 10.

Tumor extended through the entire wall of one or more cardiac chambers in at least 15 patients. It extended through the wall of the right atrium in 11 patients, the left atrium in 5, atrial septum in 3, right ventricle in 2, left ventricle in 2 and ventricular septum in 1 (Fig. 3 and 4). Marked invasion by tumor was encountered more frequently in the right than in the left cardiac chambers. The atrioventricular sulcus was the most common site of epicardial invasion, and often it contained huge tumor deposits (Fig. 2). Invasion of intramyocardial veins, lymphatics and sinusoids was seen commonly, but, except in 2 patients, the walls of both large and small coronary arteries were not invaded by tumor.

The cardiac tumors in 33 of the 45 patients contained melanin pigment; in 4 the pigment

Table III
Weight of Heart

Extent of Metastases	No. of Patients	Heart Weight (gm.) Range	Heart Weight (gm.) Average
None	25	220–460	313
Microscopic only	2	300 & 310	305
Slight	15	160–420	300
Moderate	14	180–410	300
Extensive	13	240–880	409
Total	69	160–880	326

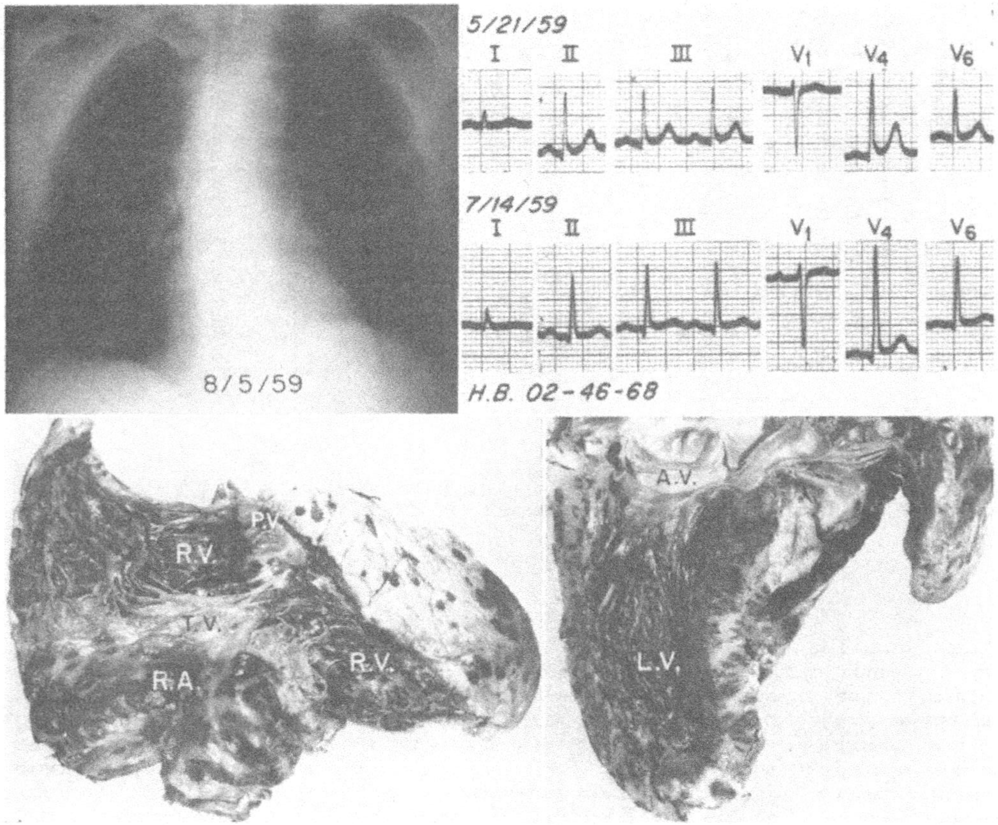

FIG. 4. *Extensive Pericardial and Myocardial Metastases. Anteroposterior chest roentgenogram, electrocardiograms and the heart in a 56 year old man who died on August 5, 1959, four months after removal of a melanoma of the back.* During his last month of life, atrial and ventricular gallops and a pleuropericardial friction rub developed. Electrocardiograms were normal except for slight S-T segment elevation in leads II, III, V_1 and V_3. These changes suggested early repolarization rather than pericarditis since T wave inversion never occurred. At necropsy, the heart weighed 430 gm. On the **lower left** are the opened right atrium (R.A.), tricuspid valve (T.V.), right ventricle (R.V.) and pulmonic valve (P.V.). On the **lower right** are the opened left ventricle (L.V.) and aortic valve (A.V.). Black tumor metastases extended through the entire wall of each cardiac chamber, almost completely replaced the myocardium, and covered the endocardial surfaces. Pericardial metastases were present, but there was no epicarditis.

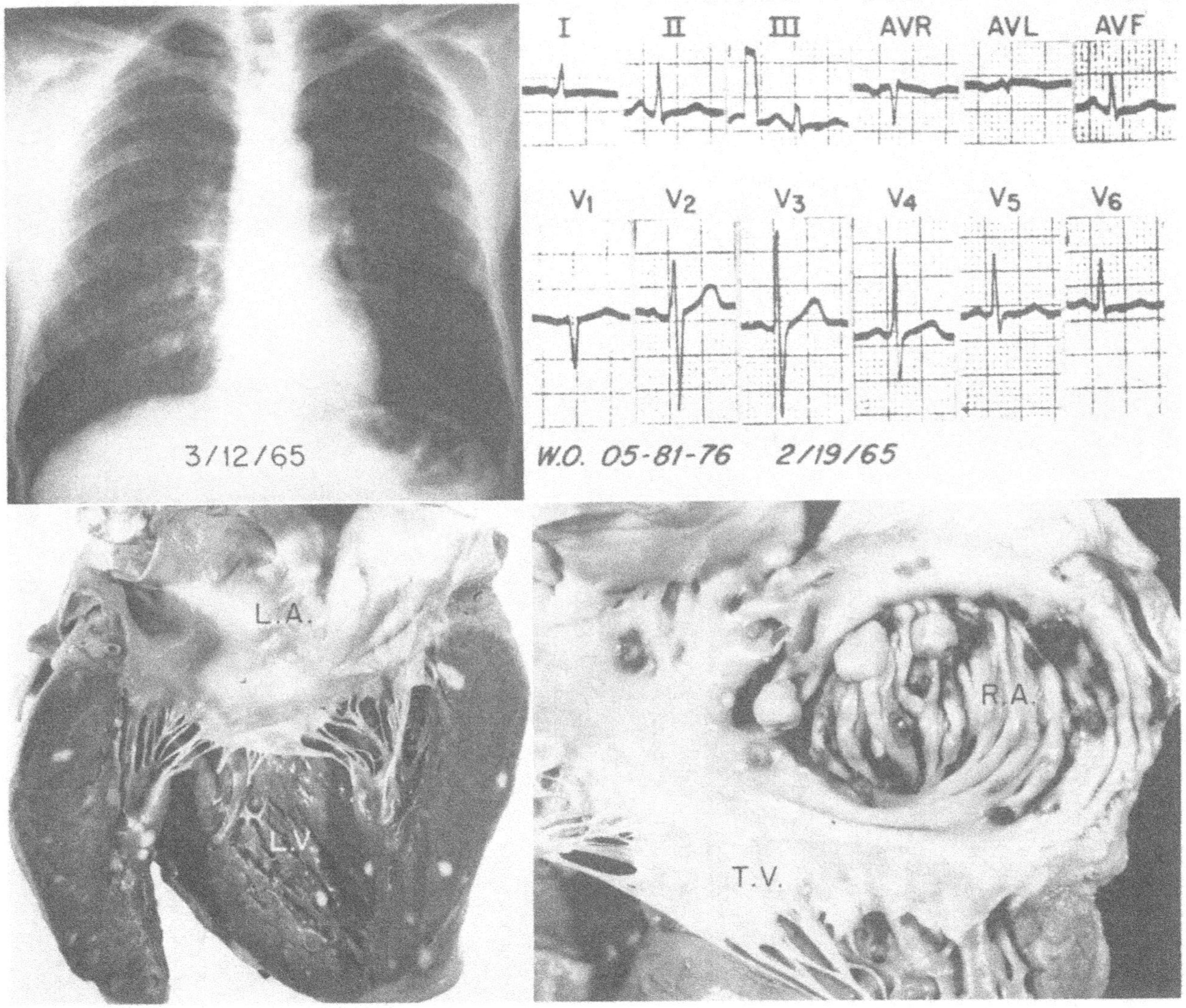

FIG. 5. *Tumor Nodules in Heart Without Dysfunction. The chest roentgenogram, electrocardiogram and heart in a 50 year old man who died of hemorrhage into a cerebral metastasis on March 28, 1965, six months after removal of a melanoma of the back.* (His 27 year old son also died of melanoma with widespread metastases, including to the heart.) There was never any evidence of cardiac dysfunction, and the electrocardiogram was normal. Chest roentgenogram revealed pulmonary metastases, but the cardiac silhouette was normal. At necropsy, the heart weighed 330 gm. There were numerous tumor nodules in the walls of all four cardiac chambers and in the atrial and ventricular septa. Those in the left ventricle (L.V.) (**lower left**) were white, whereas those in the right atrium (R.A.) were variably pigmented and pedunculated. L.A. = left atrium; T.V. = tricuspid valve.

was observed only histologically. Occasionally both pigmented and nonpigmented metastases were seen in the same heart (Fig. 5). Tumor invasion was usually nodular (Fig. 11) rather than interstitial; within most of the larger nodules few if any myocardial fibers remained. Areas of tumor necrosis, usually the central portions of large tumor nodules, were observed in cardiac metastases in 25 of the 45 subjects. The necrotic debris contained little pigment, but frequently large deposits of pigment were present in the zone between the necrotic and viable tumor. Rarely, fibrous tissue infiltrated the necrotic portions of tumor nodules. Polypoid intracavitary projections of endocardial metastases ("tumor thrombi") frequently had necrotic centers, but there was always an outer layer of viable tumor.

Noninfective thrombotic endocarditis was present in 4 patients: on the posterior mitral leaflet in 3 (Fig. 6) and on the left ventricular mural endocardium in the fourth. Cardiac infections were present in 2 patients: 1 had focal, microscopic Staphylococcus aureus myocardial abscesses, and the second clostridial myocardial gas cysts (Fig. 12). Each had septicemia. Endocardial, epicardial and myocardial hemorrhages were rare.

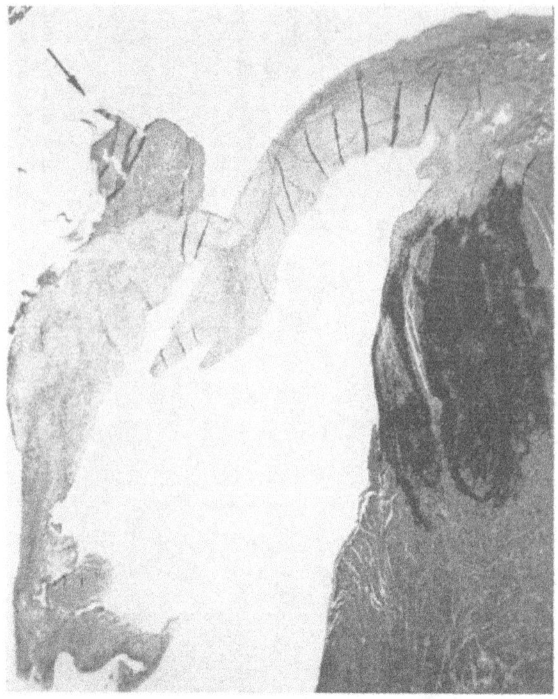

Fig. 6. *Noninfective Thrombotic Endocarditis of Mitral Valve. Photomicrograph of a section of posterior mitral leaflet and a portion of left ventricular wall in a 67 year old woman who had no evidence of cardiac dysfunction.* On the atrial aspect of the leaflet is a vegetation of noninfective thrombotic endocarditis (arrow). A dark-staining nodule of metastatic melanoma is present in the left ventricular myocardium just beneath the mitral annulus. Marantic endocarditis occurred in 3 other patients in this study. (Hematoxylin and eosin stain, × 10.)

Clinical Observations

Symptoms and Signs: Table IV records clinical features that might be associated with cardiac

Table IV
Clinical Features in 70 Patients

Extent of Cardiac Metastases	None	Microscopic Only	Slight	Moderate	Extensive	Total
No. of patients	25	3	15	14	13	70
Dyspnea	6	2	6	6	4	24
Peripheral edema	8	0	5	3	4	20
Precordial murmur*	5	1	3	5	3	17
Atrial gallop	0	0	1	2	3	6
Ventricular gallop	0	0	0	0	3	3
Pericardial or pleuropericardial rub	0	1	1	0	2	4
Pulsus alternans	0	0	0	0	1	1
Pulsus paradoxus	0	0	0	0	1	1
Venous pressure > 12 cm. water	1	0	1	1	2	5
Circulation time > 16 sec.	0	0	0	0	2	2
Pulmonary edema	0	0	0	0	2	2
Cardiomegaly by x-ray	2	0	0	0	5	7
Digitalis therapy	3	0	2	3	7	15
Effusions at necropsy†	13	2	13	5	9	42

* All 17 patients had systolic murmurs of grade 1 or 2/6 intensity. One patient, with mild rheumatic mitral stenosis, had a diastolic murmur as well.

† > 100 ml. fluid in the peritoneal or a pleural space, or > 30 ml. pericardial fluid.

FIG. 7. *Extensive Cardiac Metastases with Bundle Branch Block. Chest roentgenogram, electrocardiograms, the opened right atrium, tricuspid valve, and right ventricle* (**upper right**); *and the opened left ventricle and aortic valve* (**lower right**) *in a 33 year old man, who died on December 27, 1957, three years after removal of a melanoma of the scalp.* During the last month of life a ventricular gallop, pulsus alternans and orthostatic hypotension developed. Diabetes insipidus, the result of pituitary metastasis, and Addison's disease, the result of adrenal metastases, prevented the congestive phenomena of cardiac failure: the patient's blood volume was only one-half the predicted normal, and his venous pressure was 10 cm. water. There was an enlarged cardiac silhouette on chest roentgenogram (12/18/57). Electrocardiograms showed sinus tachycardia, low QRS voltage and inverted T waves in leads V_1 to V_4, and during the last week of life right bundle branch block was present (12/26/57). *At necropsy*, there was 350 ml. of pericardial fluid, and the heart weighed 320 gm. Extensive black metastases were present in the epicardium, myocardium and endocardium of all cardiac chambers, and numerous small tumor thrombi (arrows) projected from the right atrial, right ventricular, and left ventricular endocardium. T.V. = tricuspid valve; R.V. = right ventricle; A.V. = aortic valve.

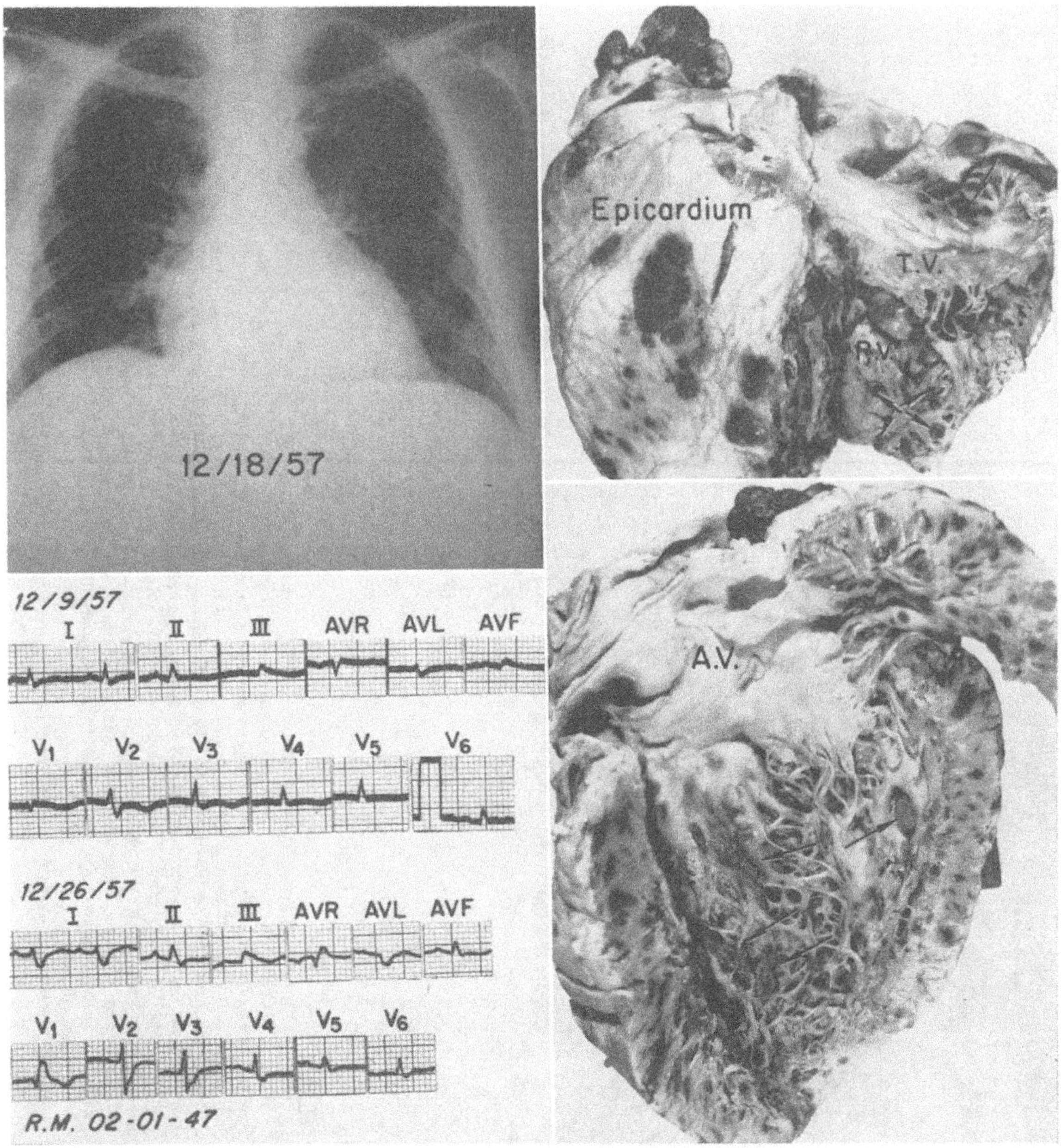

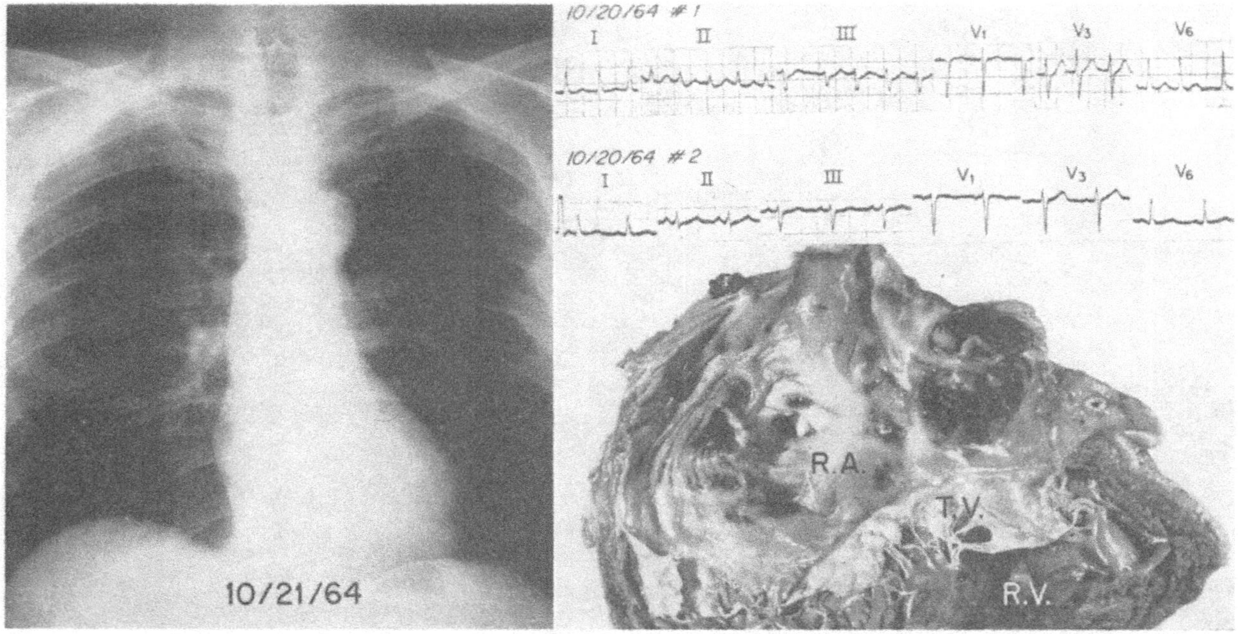

FIG. 8. *Cardiac Metastases with Atrial Fibrillation. Chest roentgenogram, electrocardiograms, and the heart at necropsy in a 58 year old man with systemic hypertension, who died on December 8, 1964, of widespread metastases 20 months after excision of a melanoma of the chest.* Atrial fibrillation developed seven weeks before death (electrocardiogram No. 1), but the patient reverted to sinus rhythm the same day after he was given digitalis (electrocardiogram No. 2). He had no further evidence of cardiac dysfunction. At necropsy, the heart weighed 440 gm., and all cardiac chambers were invaded by tumor. **Lower right,** the opened right atrium (R.A.), tricuspid valve (T.V.) and right ventricle (R.V.). There are numerous nodules of black tumor projecting from the right atrial endocardium (tumor thrombi).

FIG. 9. **Opposite page.** *Cardiac Metastases with Pleuropericarditis Due to Treatment. Chest roentgenograms, electrocardiograms and heart in a 25 year old woman who died on December 25, 1966, three years after removal of a melanoma of the back.* An intermittent atrial gallop and a systolic precordial murmur were present during the last six weeks of life. The electrocardiograms show sinus tachycardia, progressive decrease in QRS voltage in the limb leads and the development of nonspecific ST-T wave changes. (The patient was not on digitalis.) The earlier chest roentgenogram (8/8/66) is normal except for the presence of a right paratracheal mass. The later roentgenogram (12/13/66) shows bilateral pleural effusions and suggests the presence of a pericardial effusion as well. These effusions were probably the result of a reaction to bis-beta-chlorethyl nitrosourea (BCNU) given five days earlier (17 days before death) since at necropsy there were no pericardial nor pleural effusions, and the heart weighed only 240 gm. After an earlier dose of BCNU, the patient had had a similar transient adverse reaction consisting of severe respiratory distress associated with roentgenographic findings of diffuse pneumonitis and pleural effusions. Thus, at times, treatment itself may be the cause of clinical failure. **Upper right**, the right atrium (R.A.) is extensively involved by black tumor nodules. The arrow indicates the region of the sinus node. Ao. = ascending aorta; R.V. = right ventricle; S.V.C. = superior vena cava. **Lower middle**, the opened left atrium, mitral valve, and left ventricle (L.V.). Black metastases are seen in the myocardium of both chambers and project as polypoid masses from the endocardial surface. **Lower right,** the opened aortic valve (A.V.) and left ventricle (L.V.). A. = anterior mitral leaflet.

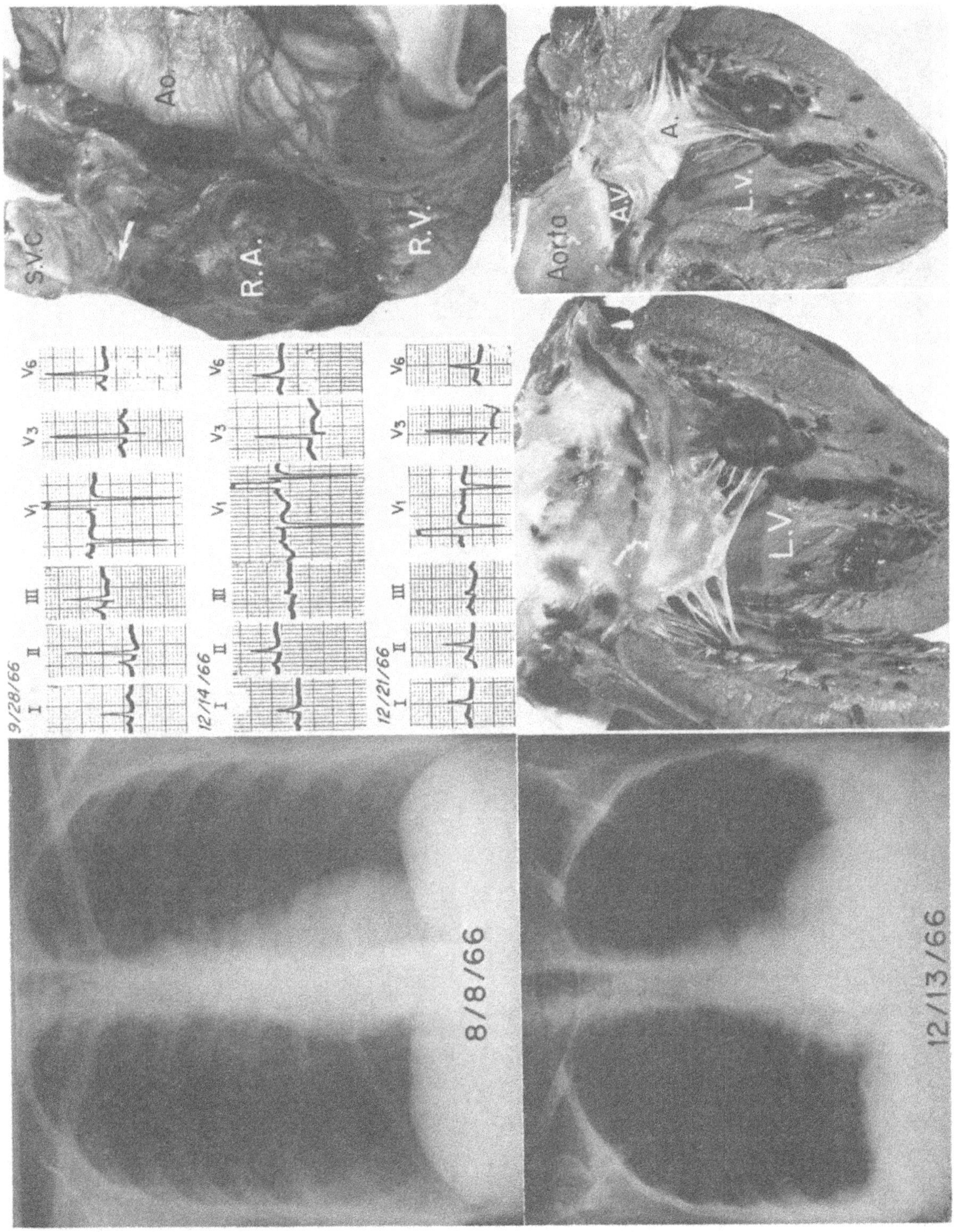

Fig. 9. See opposite page

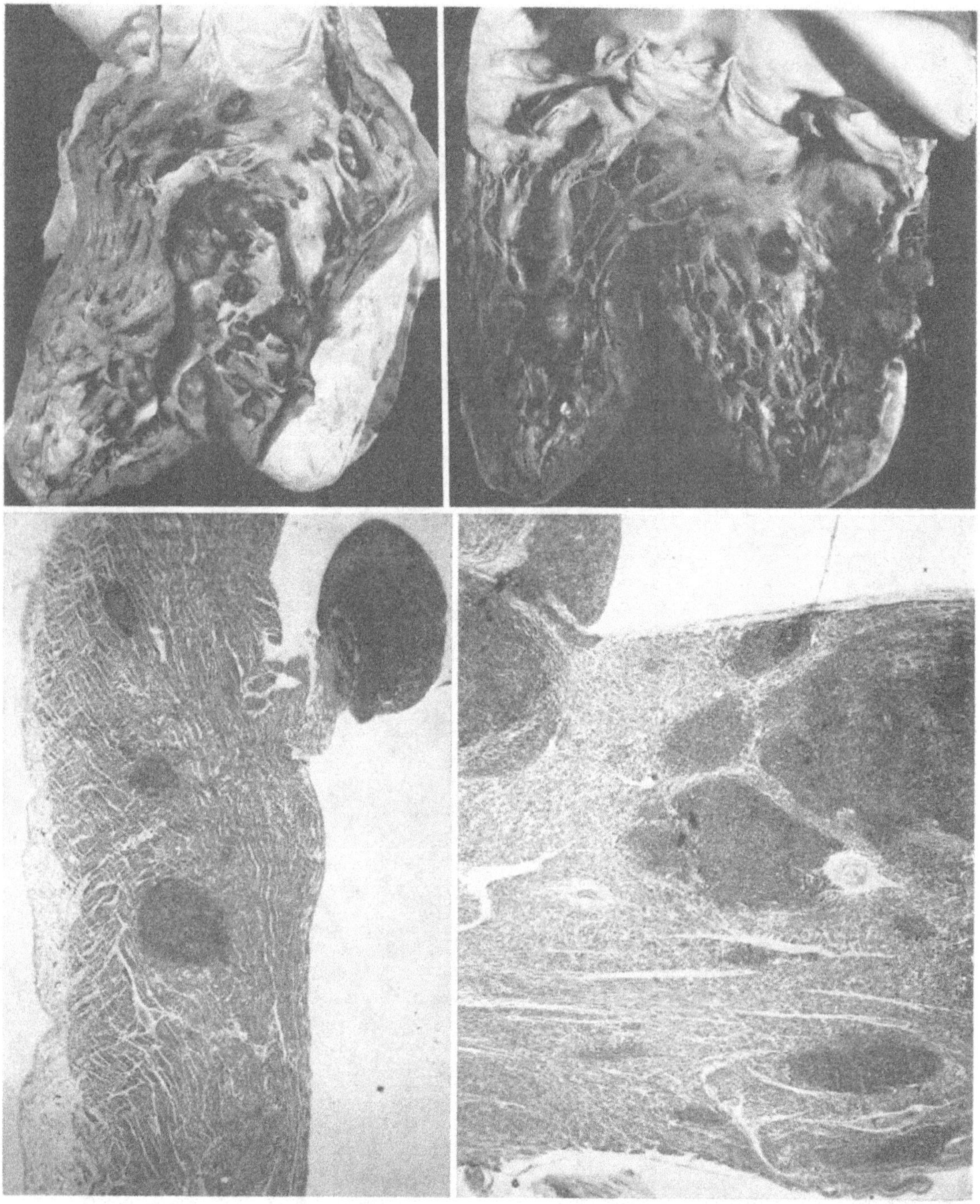

FIG. 10. *Polypoid Myocardial and Endocardial Metastases. The opened right ventricle and pulmonic valve* (**upper left**), *and the opened left ventricle and aortic valve* (**upper right**) *in a 44 year old woman who died of cerebral metastases.* There had been minimal pretibial edema, a soft systolic precordial murmur and nonspecific electrocardiographic changes, but no cardiomegaly, cardiac failure nor arrhythmias. The serum albumin had been 2.8 gm. and the hemoglobin 8.8 gm./100 ml. *At necropsy,* the heart weighed 310 gm. Numerous pigmented metastases projected from the endocardial surfaces of both ventricles. The photomicrograph of the right ventricular wall just below the pulmonic valve (**lower left**) shows three myocardial metastases and a polypoid endocardial metastasis. (Hematoxylin and eosin, × 10.) The photomicrograph of a left ventricular papillary muscle (**lower right**) shows numerous dark-staining myocardial metastases. (Hematoxylin and eosin, × 10.)

dysfunction and their frequency according to the extent of cardiac metastases. Most of these parameters did not differentiate patients with cardiac metastases from those without them. In fact, dyspnea, edema, effusions and precordial murmurs most often were not the result of cardiac disease. Extensive *pulmonary metastases* were the most frequent cause of dyspnea. *Hypoalbuminemia* was probably the most common cause of edema since the serum albumin, which was measured in 57 subjects, ranged from 1.1 to 3.9 gm. and averaged only 2.2 gm./100 ml. *Anemia*, which often appeared to be the result of chemotherapy, was present in 55 patients. The blood hemoglobin remained above 12 gm./100 ml. throughout the entire illness in only 15 subjects, and in 31 it fell below 8 gm./100 ml. Many systolic precordial murmurs were probably due to anemia. In several patients digitalis did not ameloriate tachycardia, dyspnea, or edema, presumably because these were the result of pulmonary metastases or hypoalbuminemia rather than cardiac disease. Pericardial, pleural and peritoneal effusions were usually the result of local tumor invasion.

Congestive cardiac failure was observed in 7 of the 70 patients. In 2 (Fig. 1 and 3), it was severe, and both had cardiac tamponade and extensive deposits of tumor in the heart. In the other 5 subjects the cardiac failure was mild: 2 had extensive cardiac metastases, and 1 moderate, 1 slight and 1 no cardiac tumor. Cardiac reserve was probably diminished in other patients, but the sedentary existence dictated by metastatic tumor in other organs prevented the development of overt congestive cardiac failure.

Cause of Death: Of the 70 patients, 26 died primarily of central nervous system metastases, hemorrhage within the tumor frequently being the terminal event. Most of the remainder died of the effects of widespread metastases, at times accompanied by terminal sepsis (Fig. 12). Pulmonary emboli were contributory causes of death in 3 patients. Five patients died suddenly, but in only 1 could cardiac disease be incriminated. This patient (Fig. 3) had marked cardiac involvement by tumor.

Electrocardiographic Changes: An electrocardiogram was recorded in 60 of the 70 patients, and 38 patients had more than 1 tracing. In only 13 of the 60 were all electrocardiograms normal (Table v). Sinus tachycardia, the most common abnormality, was present in at least 1 tracing in 37 patients, and low QRS voltage, in 20. Electrocardiographic abnormalities occurred as frequently in patients without cardiac metastases as in those with microscopic-sized, slight, or moderate involvement of the heart by tumor (Table v). The incidence of the various electro-

TABLE V
Electrocardiographic Abnormalities in 60 Patients

Extent of Cardiac Metastases	No. of Patients with ECG	All ECG's Normal	Low Voltage*	Sinus Tachycardia (>100/min.)	Ectopic Tachycardia	Atrioventricular Block	Other Abnormalities†
None	17	4	3	8	3‡	0	7
Microscopic only	3	1	1	2	0	1§	0
Slight	13	3	6	7	0	2‖	5
Moderate	14	4	3	9	0	0	7
Extensive	13	1	7	11	4¶	1#	7
Total	60	13	20	37	7	4	26

* Sum of QRS voltage in leads I, II and III less than 1.5 mv.

† Sinus bradycardia, premature atrial beats, premature ventricular beats, left and right axis deviation, right bundle branch block, intraventricular conduction disturbance, delayed precordial transition, ischemic, pericarditis, and nonspecific ST-T wave changes, hypokalemic and hyperkalemic changes, P wave abnormality, changes of acute cor pulmonale and combinations of these changes.

‡ 1 nodal tachycardia, 2 atrial fibrillation (1 chronic atrial fibrillation associated with chronic rheumatic mitral valvular disease).

§ First degree.

‖ Both first degree and both associated with hyperkalemia.

¶ 2 atrial flutter, 2 atrial fibrillation.

Second degree heart block in a patient on digitalis.

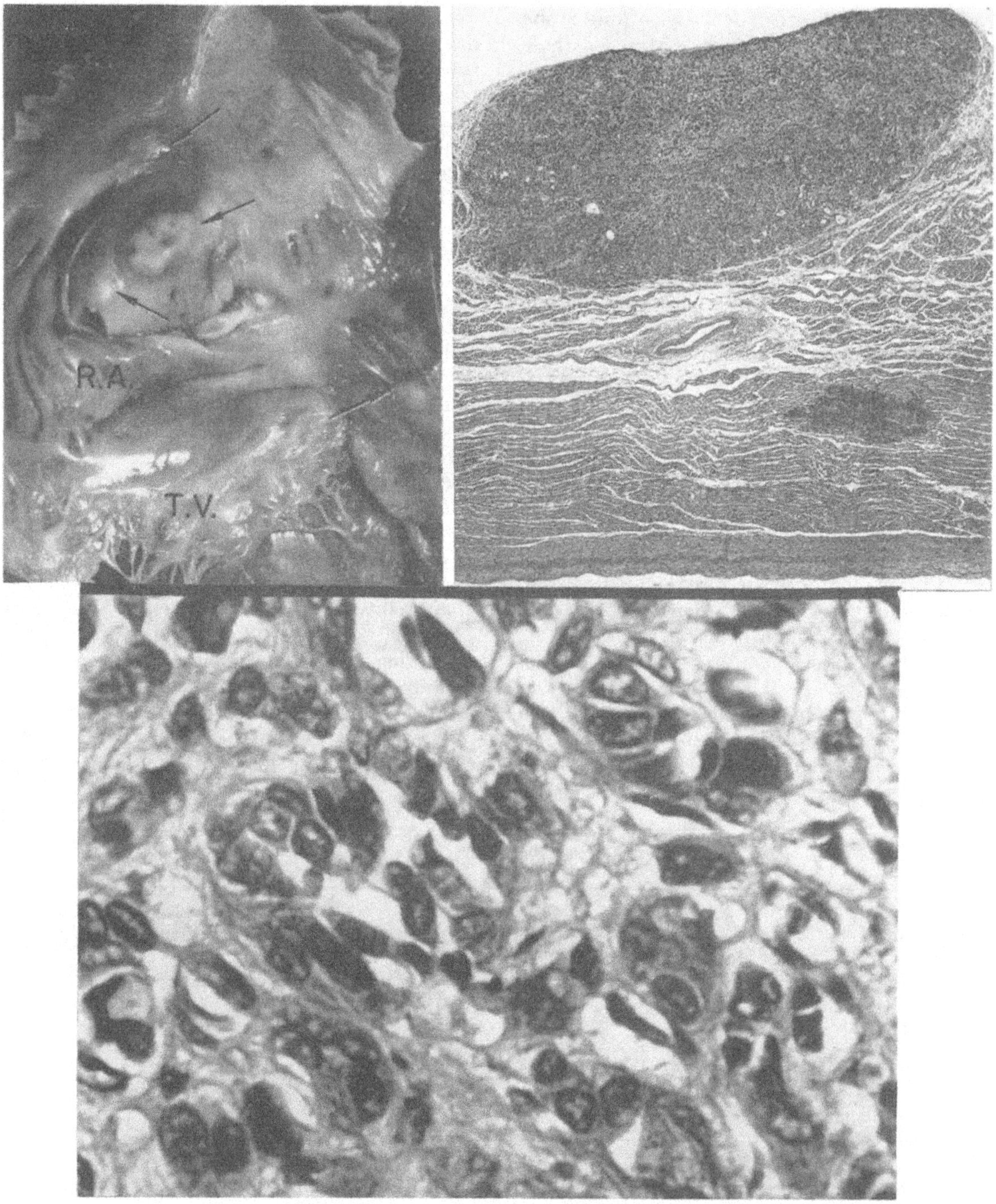

FIG. 11. *Cardiac metastases in a 21 year old man who had no evidence of cardiac dysfunction during life.* At necropsy, the extent of cardiac metastases was classified as moderate. **Upper left,** the opened right atrium (R.A.) and tricuspid valve (T.V.). Tumor nodules are indicated by arrows. **Upper right,** photomicrograph of the large tumor nodule on the right atrial surface of the atrial septum. A smaller metastasis is present deeper in the atrial septum. (Hematoxylin and eosin, × 19.) **Lower,** high power photomicrograph of the melanoma in the heart. (Hematoxylin and eosin, × 780.)

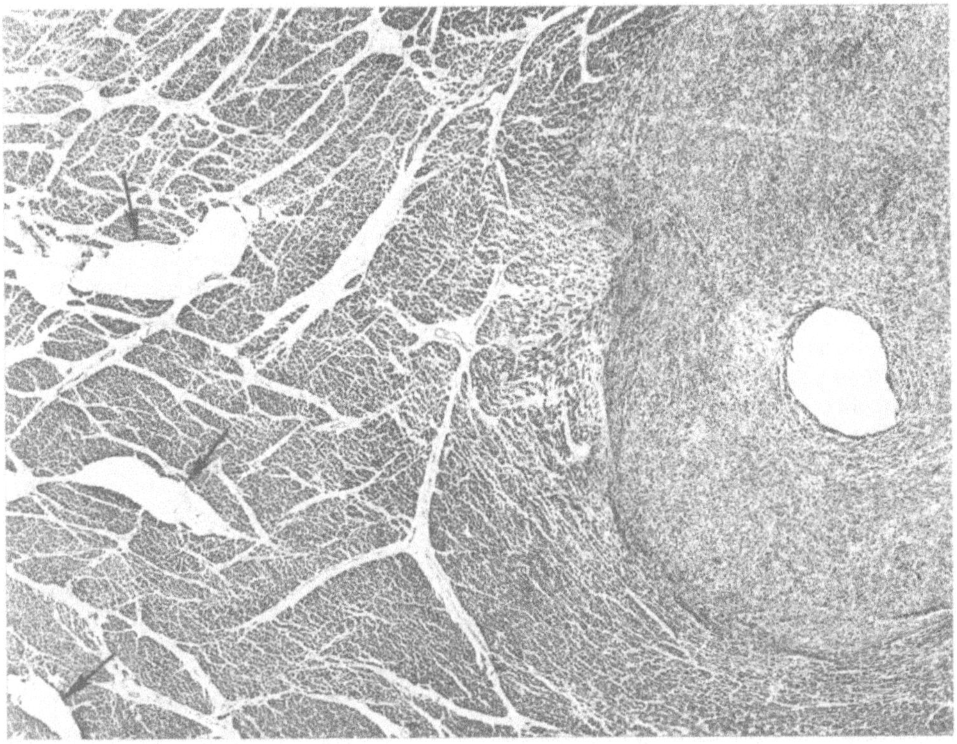

FIG. 12. *Cardiac Metastases with Clostridial Infection of Myocardium. Photomicrograph of a section of myocardium in a 23 year old man who died of clostridial peritonitis and septicemia following perforation of the small intestine through a necrotic mass of metastatic melanoma.* On the right is a nodule of metastatic melanoma containing a gas cyst. Other gas cysts are present among the myocardial fibers (arrows). Gram positive rods were present within the myocardium and tumor. (Hematoxylin and eosin, × 25.)

cardiographic abnormalities was slightly greater in the 13 patients with extensive cardiac involvement by tumor; in only 1 of them were all tracings normal. Excluding the patient with rheumatic mitral valvular disease and chronic atrial fibrillation, 4 of the 6 patients with ectopic tachycardias had extensive cardiac involvement by tumor. The incidence of abnormal electrocardiograms increased as death approached. All tracings were normal in only 2 of 37 patients for whom these were recorded during the last month of life. Sinus tachycardia was present in 26 of the 37 patients, and rates of 150 beats/min. were not uncommon. Low QRS voltage was present in 19 of the 37. In 5 of the 7 patients with ectopic tachycardia, the latter developed during the last three weeks of life.

Thus, in 11 of the 70 patients significant cardiac dysfunction developed: Cardiac failure in 7 (Fig. 1,3,4 and 7), atrial fibrillation in 3 (Fig. 3 and 8), atrial flutter in 2 (Fig. 2), nodal tachycardia in 1, second degree atrioventricular block in 1 (Fig. 3) and sudden death in 1. Of the 11 patients, 7 had extensive, 1 moderate, 1 slight and 2 no cardiac involvement by tumor. Tumor implants in the heart, therefore, did not appear to increase the likelihood of cardiac dysfunction unless the cardiac involvement by tumor was extensive.

COMMENTS

Numerous studies of cardiac involvement by metastatic tumor have been reported in the past.[1-8,11-27] Virtually all of these studies have had two major weaknesses: (1) the necropsy data were obtained from autopsy protocols rather than from examination of the hearts, both grossly and histologically, by only one or two observers; (2) the clinical data were derived solely from patients with cardiac metastases, without observations on patients with the same tumor but no cardiac metastases. In the present study, each heart was examined by us as well as by the prosector, and clinical data were tabulated for all patients with metastatic melanoma both with and without cardiac metastases. Thus, the data obtained should be more meaningful.

Cardiac metastases from malignant melanoma have previously been reported in at least 152 patients.[2–8,11–26,28,29] The percentage of cardiac metastases in the present series (64 per cent) is twice that of the only previous series of comparable size.[5] However, frequencies of over 50 per cent have been reported in smaller series.[4,16] Metastases to the heart by melanoma or any other tumor are almost always accompanied by metastases to other organs.[2,5,9,10,15,16,19] The high frequency of cardiac deposits of melanoma is largely a manifestation of the tumor's propensity to metastasize widely before causing death.

The multifocal distribution of the cardiac metastases in melanoma and their more frequent location in the myocardium than in the epicardium suggest that the tumor reaches the heart by the blood stream rather than by lymphatic channels or direct extension from adjacent intrathoracic structures.

Clinical Diagnosis of Cardiac Metastases: In the past a wide variety of clinical, electrocardiographic and roentgenographic findings have been used to diagnose cardiac dysfunction due to cardiac metastases. Some of these clinical features (listed in Tables IV and V) have little or or no correlation with the presence or extent of cardiac metastases. Sinus tachycardia, for example, which has frequently been suggested as a criterion for clinically determining the presence of cardiac metastases,[12,16,22,27] is found during the last weeks of life in at least one half of patients dying of malignant melanoma who have no cardiac metastases. Nevertheless, the presence of cardiac metastases can often be determined before death. Certainly, the development of cardiac dysfunction without other apparent cause in a patient known to have a malignant tumor suggests cardiac metastases. The problem, however, is being certain that the clinical findings really indicate cardiac dysfunction, rather than their being the result of associated anemia, hypoproteinemia, or pulmonary metastases. Dyspnea, tachypnea, tachycardia, systolic precordial murmurs, edema, effusions into body cavities, or any of several electrocardiographic abnormalities may occur in patients with malignant tumors but without cardiac metastases. On the other hand, one or more of the following clinical findings, in a patient with a malignant tumor and without previous heart disease, strongly suggests the presence of cardiac metastases: (1) acute pericarditis (Fig. 2); (2) cardiac tamponade (Fig. 1) or constriction; (3) rapid increase in the size of the heart as shown by roentgenogram (Fig. 1 and 3); (4) onset of an ectopic tachycardia (Fig. 2, 3 and 8); (5) development of second (Fig. 3) or third degree atrioventricular block; and (6) onset of unequivocal cardiac failure. Cytologic examination of pericardial fluid and angiocardiography obviously will increase the accuracy of diagnosing cardiac metastases. When the tumor is metastatic melanoma, the clinical diagnosis of cardiac metastases is aided by the knowledge that 2 of 3 patients will develop tumor of the heart before death.

Summary

Cardiac metastases were found in 45 of 70 patients (64 per cent) dying of metastatic melanoma. Of the 70 patients, 11 had significant cardiac dysfunction clinically. Tumor implants in the heart did not appear to cause dysfunction unless cardiac involvement by tumor was extensive. Many previously proposed criteria for clinically determining the presence of cardiac metastases were found to be unreliable.

References

1. Pic, A. and Bret, J. Contribution a l'etude du cancer secondaire du coeur. *Rev. méd.*, 11: 1022, 1891.
2. Bisel, H. F., Wróblewski, F. and La Due, J. S. Incidence and clinical manifestations of cardiac metastases. *J.A.M.A.*, 153: 712, 1953.
3. Scott, R. W. and Garvin, C. F. Tumors of the heart and pericardium. *Am. Heart J.*, 17: 431, 1939.
4. Young, J. M. and Goldman, I. R. Tumor metastasis to the heart. *Circulation*, 9: 220, 1954.
5. Gassman, H. S., Meadows, R., Jr. and Baker, L. A. Metastatic tumors of the heart. *Am. J. Med.*, 19: 357, 1955.
6. Goudie, R. B. Secondary tumors of heart and pericardium. *Brit. Heart J.*, 17: 183, 1955.
7. Cohen, G. U., Peery, T. M. and Evans, J. M. Neoplastic invasion of the heart and pericardium. *Ann. Int. Med.*, 42: 1238, 1955.
8. Raven, R. W. Secondary malignant disease of the heart. *Brit. J. Cancer*, 2: 1, 1948.
9. Roberts, W. C., Bodey, G. P. and Wertlake, P. T. The heart in acute leukemia. A study of 420 autopsy cases. *Am. J. Cardiol.*, 21: 388, 1968.
10. Roberts, W. C., Glancy, D. L. and DeVita, V. T., Jr. The heart in malignant lymphoma (Hodgkin's disease, lymphosarcoma, reticulum-cell sarcoma and mycosis fungoides). A study of 196 autopsy cases. *Am. J. Cardiol.*, in press.
11. Moragues, V. Cardiac metastases from malignant

melanoma: Report of four cases. *Am. Heart J.*, 18: 579, 1939.

12. Lefkovits, A. M. Neoplastic metastasis to the heart. *Am. Heart J.*, 36: 610, 1948.
13. Lymburner, R. M. Tumors of the heart: Histopathological and clinical study. *Canad. M. A. J.*, 30: 368, 1934.
14. Yater, W. M. Tumors of the heart and pericardium: Pathology, symptomatology and report of 9 cases. *Arch. Int. Med.*, 48: 627, 1931.
15. Prichard, R. W. Tumors of the heart: Review of the subject and report of one hundred and fifty cases. *A.M.A. Arch. Path.*, 51: 98, 1951.
16. DeLoach, J. F. and Haynes, J. W. Secondary tumors of the heart and pericardium: Review of the subject and report of one hundred thirty-seven cases. *A.M.A. Arch. Int. Med.*, 91: 224, 1953.
17. Burnett, R. S. and Shimkin, M. B. Secondary neoplasms of the heart. *A.M.A. Arch. Int. Med.*, 93: 205, 1954.
18. Piotti, A. Die Herztumoren; 30 Fälle von Tumor metastasen im Herzen. *Cardiologia*, 14: 129, 1949.
19. Herbut, P. A. and Maisel, A. L. Secondary tumors of the heart. *Arch. Path.*, 34: 358, 1942.
20. Ritchie, G. Metastatic tumors of the myocardium: A review of sixteen cases. *Am. J. Path.*, 17: 483, 1941.
21. Dimmette, R. M. The ante-mortem diagnosis of secondary tumors of the heart: Report of four cases. *U.S. Armed Forces M. J.*, 1: 750, 1950.
22. Hanfling, S. M. Metastatic cancer to the heart: Review of the literature and report of 127 cases. *Circulation*, 22: 474, 1960.
23. Ritz, N. D. Diffuse melanosis, pericardial effusion, and melanuria associated with malignant melanoma: Case report with autopsy findings. *Ann. Int. Med.*, 30: 184, 1949.
24. Lothe, F. and Somers, K. Secondary tumors of the heart and pericardium in Uganda Africans. *A.M.A. Arch. Path.*, 69: 158, 1960.
25. Krumbhaar, E. B. and Crowell, C. Spontaneous rupture of heart; clinicopathologic study based on 22 unpublished cases and 632 from literature. *Am. J. M. Sc.*, 170: 828, 1925.
26. Smith, D. S. Neoplastic involvement of the heart: Two cases diagnosed before death. *J.A.M.A.*, 109: 1192, 1937.
27. Levy, T. Metastatic malignancies involving the heart. *Postgrad. Med.*, 5: 407, 1949.
28. White, P. D. Other etiologic factors and relationships. In: Heart Disease, ed. 4, chap. 23, p. 593. New York, 1951. Macmillan.
29. Wenger, N. K. Rare causes of heart disease. In: The Heart, chap. 55, p. 950. Edited by Hurst, J. W. and Logue, R. B. New York, 1966. McGraw-Hill.

Heart in Malignant Lymphoma (Hodgkin's Disease, Lymphosarcoma, Reticulum Cell Sarcoma and Mycosis Fungoides)

A Study of 196 Autopsy Cases*

WILLIAM C. ROBERTS, M.D., F.A.C.C.,† D. LUKE GLANCY, M.D.† AND VINCENT T. DEVITA, JR., M.D.‡

Bethesda, Maryland

CARDIAC metastases are reported to occur in 1 to 21 per cent of patients with malignant tumors and to cause signs or symptoms of cardiac dysfunction in less than 10 per cent of those who have cardiac metastases. The tumors that most frequently metastasize to the heart are carcinomas of the lung and breast; both are relatively radioresistant, and there is no definitive treatment for them. In relative numbers malignant melanoma,[1] leukemia[2] and malignant lymphoma most frequently metastasize to the heart. Since leukemia and malignant lymphoma are relatively radiosensitive, diagnosis of cardiac involvement is important because radiotherapy can be beneficial.

The present report summarizes the clinical and necropsy observations of the hearts of 196 subjects with malignant lymphoma studied at the Clinical Center. The types, prevalence, extent, and clinical significance of cardiac abnormalities in these patients is described.

PATIENTS STUDIED AND METHODS

From 1954 through 1966, 196 patients who died of malignant lymphoma had complete autopsies recorded at the Clinical Center. Of these, 75 had Hodgkin's disease, 32 lymphosarcoma, 22 reticulum cell sarcoma, 51 mycosis fungoides and 16 undifferentiated or mixed cell lymphoma (Table I). Cases of both well and poorly differentiated (lymphoblastic) lymphoma of the lymphocytic type were included in the lymphosarcoma group, and these patients did not have associated leukemia. Eight of the 16 patients with undifferentiated lymphoma had Waldenstrom's macroglobulinemia. Of the 196 patients, 75 were female, and 121 were male; their ages ranged from 5 to 81 years (average 46).

The diagnosis of malignant lymphoma in each was made by biopsy, usually of a lymph node or skin, during life. The histopathologic diagnosis of cutaneous mycosis fungoides was based on the findings of a polymorphic intradermal infiltrate containing atypical reticulum cells and characteristic intraepidermal

TABLE I
Malignant Lymphoma of the Heart

Type of Lymphoma	No. of Necropsies	Patients with Cardiac Tumor No.	%
Hodgkin's disease	75	12 (4)	16
Lymphosarcoma	32	9 (5)	28
Reticulum cell sarcoma	22	6 (2)	27
Mycosis fungoides	51	17 (8)	33
Undifferentiated	16	4 (2)	25
Totals	196	48 (21)	24

Numbers in parentheses indicate those patients whose tumor was not observed grossly but only in histologic sections of the heart.

* From the Laboratory of Pathology, Clinic of Surgery, National Heart Institute,† and the Solid Tumor Service, Medicine Branch, National Cancer Institute,‡ National Institutes of Health, Bethesda, Md.

Address for reprints: William C. Roberts, M.D., Laboratory of Pathology, Clinic of Surgery, National Heart Institute, National Institutes of Health, Bethesda, Md. 20014.

Pautrier's abscesses. Cardiac mycosis fungoides was diagnosed when the cellular infiltrates were characteristic of a lymphoma: the infiltrate may have resembled a typical or atypical reticulum cell sarcoma, a lymphosarcoma, or Hodgkin's disease; or the cardiac cellular infiltrates may have closely resembled those in the skin. Each patient had received some form of antineoplastic therapy: local and, occasionally, whole body irradiation, nitrogen mustard, adrenal steroids, methotrexate, cyclophosphamide, vincristine, vinblastine, chlorambucil, methyl-GAG, thio-TEPA, methylhydrazine and its derivatives, daunomycin and bis-beta-chloronitroso urea.

The hearts of 161 patients were re-examined grossly; those of the other 35 subjects were not available for re-examination, but histologic sections of them were reviewed. In all patients the cardiac descriptions and diagnoses were reviewed in the autopsy protocols. Usually four histologic sections of heart had been taken at the time of necropsy, and in all subjects these sections were re-examined. In 75 of the 161 hearts re-examined, additional sections for histologic study were cut and examined.

The clinical records of all 196 patients were reviewed; in addition, the chest roentgenograms and electrocardiograms were reviewed in the cases in which unusual or severe cardiac alterations were observed at necropsy.

Necropsy Observations

Of the 196 patients, 48 (24 per cent) had lymphoma involving the heart. Twenty of the 75 female (25 per cent) and 28 of the 121 male patients (23 per cent) had cardiac implants. The average age of the 48 patients with cardiac lymphoma was identical to that of the 148 subjects without cardiac lymphoma (46 years). In 21 of the 48 hearts (44 per cent) containing lymphoma, the tumor was not observed grossly and was seen only on histologic examination. The percentages of cardiac metastases in the various lymphomas are shown in Table I. The cardiac metastases were focal, firm, usually uniformly whitish-tan nodules, only occasionally containing small hemorrhagic foci, and were located in the walls of all cardiac chambers and pericardium. ("Pericardium" in this study refers to visceral pericardium or epicardium since the parietal pericardium was rarely available for re-examination.) Some of the cardiac lymphomas are illustrated in Figures 1 to 14. The sites of the cardiac tumor nodules are listed in Table II and the number of such sites in each patient are tabulated in Table III. The type of lymphoma could not be determined from study of the size, appearance, or location of the cardiac implants observed grossly in 27 patients. A cardiac lymphosarcoma nodule grossly, for example, may have had an appearance, size and location virtually identical to a mycosis fungoides cardiac nodule but differentiated strikingly on histologic examination.

The most frequent site of involvement was the pericardium, which includes the subepicardial adipose tissue. The atrioventricular sulcus was the most common site of epicardial invasion and often very large tumor deposits occurred in it. The nodules listed as occurring in the left ventricle actually most frequently involved the left side of the ventricular septum. A cardiac valve (tricuspid) contained tumor in only 1 patient, and this was found only on histologic examination. In at least 9 subjects tumor nodules extended through the entire wall of a cardiac chamber or through the atrial septum. In no subject had cardiac tumor destroyed the atrioventricular node or bundle.

Effusions in Body Cavities and Subcutaneous Tissues: Pericardial effusions (>50 ml.) were recorded in 8 of 48 subjects (17 per cent) with cardiac lymphoma and in 21 of 148 (14 per cent) without cardiac lymphoma. Pleural effusions (>100 ml. on one side) occurred in 25 of 48 patients (52 per cent) with and in 77 of 148 (52 per cent) without cardiac lymphoma.

Table II
Specific Location of Cardiac Lymphoma

Region of Heart	No. with Cardiac Tumor
Pericardium	41 (15)
Right atrium	17 (2)
Right ventricle	18 (5)
Left atrium	11 (1)
Left ventricle	19 (5)
Valve (tricuspid)	1 (1)

Numbers in parentheses indicate those patients whose tumor was not observed grossly but only in histologic sections of the heart.

Table III
Number of Sites of Cardiac Metastases Involved n Each Patient with Malignant Lymphoma

Region of Heart	No. of Patients
Pericardium only	18
Pericardium plus 1 chamber	5
Pericardium plus 2 chambers	8
Pericardium plus 3 chambers	5
Pericardium plus 4 chambers	5
1 chamber only	5
2 chambers	2
Total	48

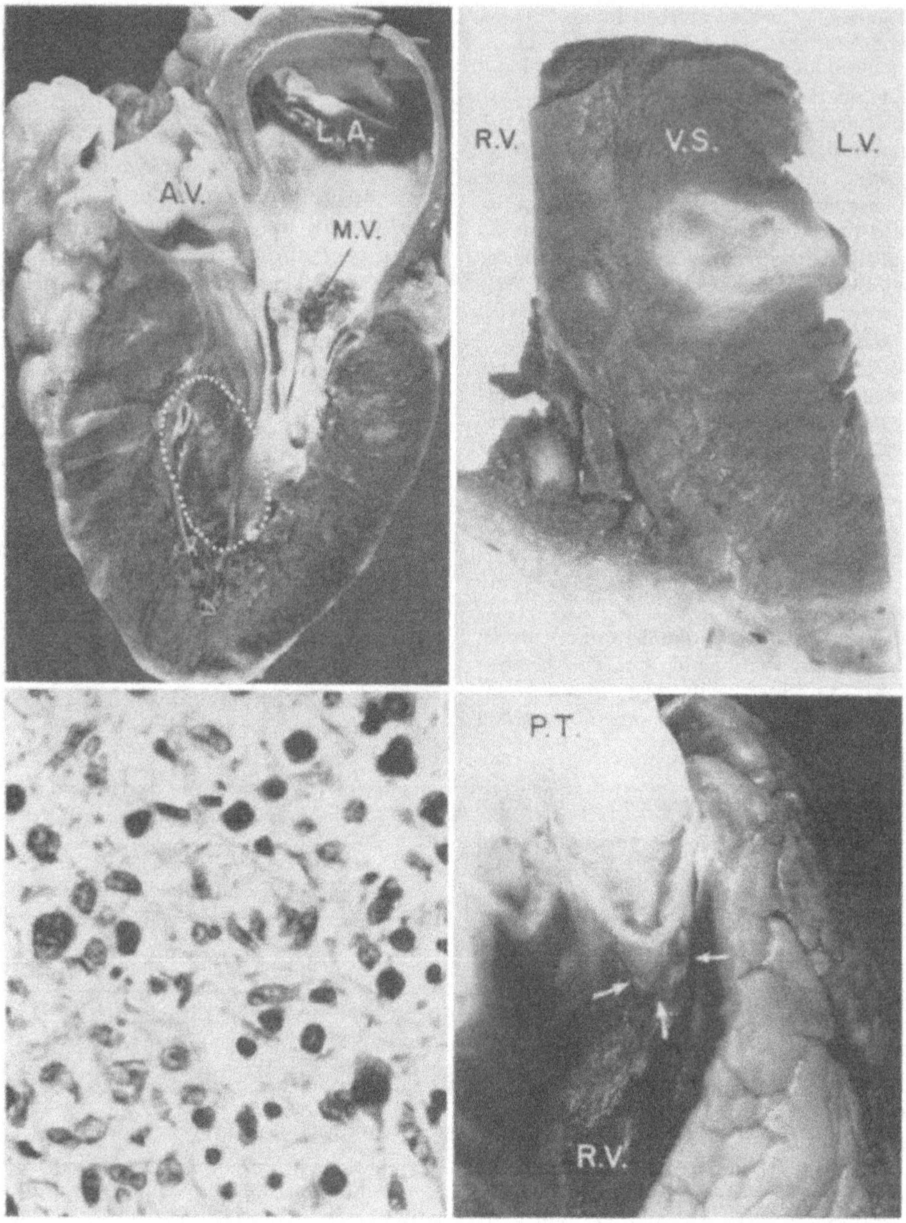

Figure 1. *Mycosis fungoides of the heart in a 51 year old man who also had rheumatic disease of the mitral and aortic valves.* **Upper left,** a portion of the free wall of the left ventricle has been excised. Within the dotted circle is a firm nodule located within the ventricular septum. The mitral (M.V.) and aortic (A.V.) valves are diffusely fibrotic and focally calcified. L.A. = left atrium. **Upper right,** section of ventricular septum (V.S.) demonstrating the extent of infiltration of tumor nodule into the septum. This is the nodule enclosed by dots in the upper left photograph. R.V. = right ventricular cavity; L.V. = left ventricular cavity. **Lower left,** photomicrograph showing the histology of this cardiac lymphoma. (Hematoxylin and eoxin × 628, reduced by 16%.) **Lower right,** another mycosis fungoides tumor nodule, designated by the arrows, in the right ventricular (R.V.) outflow tract just below the pulmonic valve. P.T. = pulmonary trunk.

This patient had typical mycosis fungoides of the skin, and tumor, like that shown in the lower left photograph, was found in many organs. He had no symptoms of cardiac dysfunction, although precordial murmurs were present. Terminally, the peripheral white blood cell count rose to 167,000 per cu. mm. with 68 per cent eosinophils.

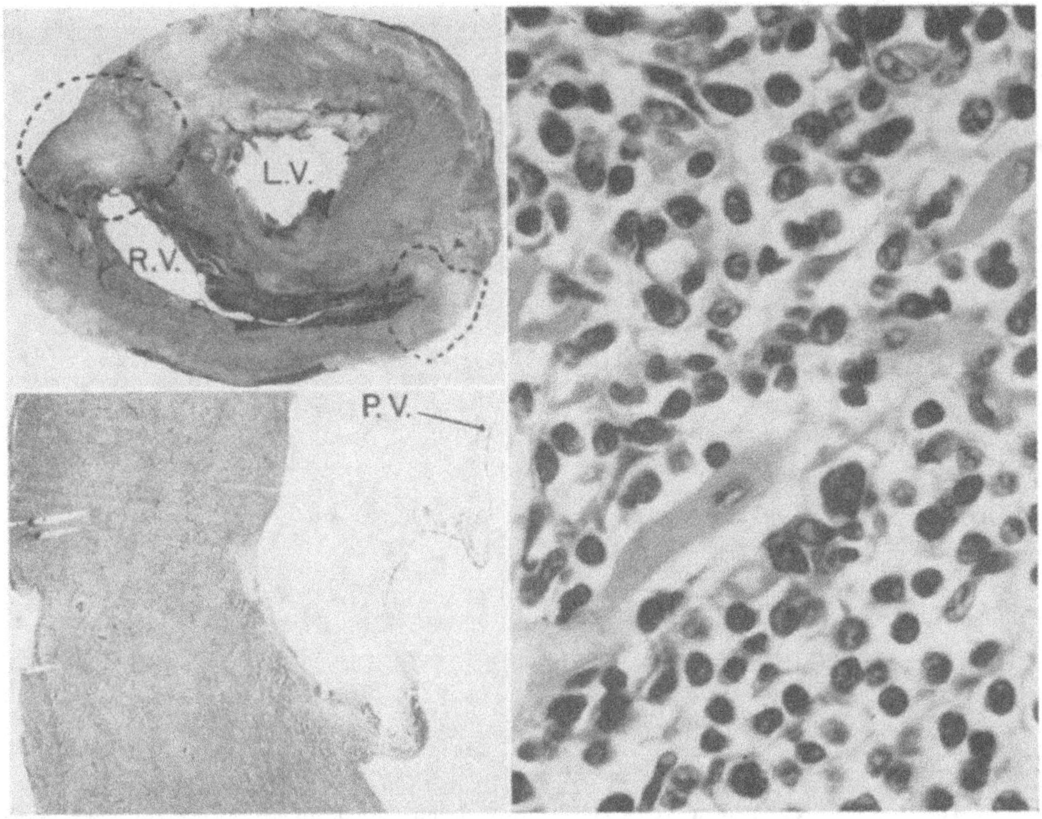

Figure 2. *Mycosis fungoides of the heart in a 58 year old man in whom dyspnea and pedal edema developed two weeks before death.* After digitalization the heart decreased in size, as shown by chest roentgenogram, and the dyspnea lessened. He died from a bleeding duodenal ulcer, probably secondary to corticosteroid medication. At necropsy, tumor nodules were observed in the wall of each cardiac chamber and in the pericardium.

Upper left, transverse section of right (R.V.) and left (L.V.) ventricles demonstrating firm white tumor nodules (enclosed by the dashes). **Lower left,** photomicrograph of pulmonic valve cusp (P.V.) and attached right ventricle and pulmonary trunk. Each of the latter structures is diffusely infiltrated by tumor cells. **Right,** closeup of tumor deposit in the right ventricle. Two myocardial fibers remain. (Hematoxylin and eosin × 5.5 [lower left] and × 628 [right].)

Peritoneal effusions (>100 ml.) were recorded in 22 of 48 patients (46 per cent) with lymphoma and in 58 of 148 (39 per cent) without it. Subcutaneous edema, usually of the legs or sacrum, or both, was recorded in 29 of 48 patients (59 per cent) with and in 67 of 148 (45 per cent) without cardiac lymphoma. With relatively few exceptions, these effusions were serous, and most of the patients had hypoalbuminemia. The serum albumin was less than 3.5 gm./100 ml. in 43 of 45 subjects (96 per cent) with and in 133 of 143 (93 per cent) without cardiac lymphoma; the low values averaged 2.1 (range 0.8 to 3.3) in the group with cardiac tumor and 2.1 gm./100 ml. (range 0.7 to 3.4) in the remaining subjects. Hypoalbuminemia even when severe, however, was not necessarily associated with effusions. Of the 35 patients without effusions or subcutaneous edema, the serum albumin was low in 31 of the 33 in whom this determination was recorded. A 64 year old man with Hodgkin's disease had a serum albumin of 0.9 gm./100 ml. and no body cavity effusions or subcutaneous edema. Two patients had chylous pleural and pericardial effusions, and several had hemorrhagic pleural or pericardial effusions.

Pericardial Diseases: Pericarditis was observed grossly and histologically in 10 of 48 patients (21 per cent) with and in 10 of 148 (7 per cent) without cardiac lymphoma. Infiltration of the pericardium by neoplastic cells appeared to cause the pericarditis in 8 patients, mediastinal irradiation in 2, infection (Aspergillus fumigatus) in 1; in 9 the cause was unknown. The pericarditis was diffuse in 10 patients and

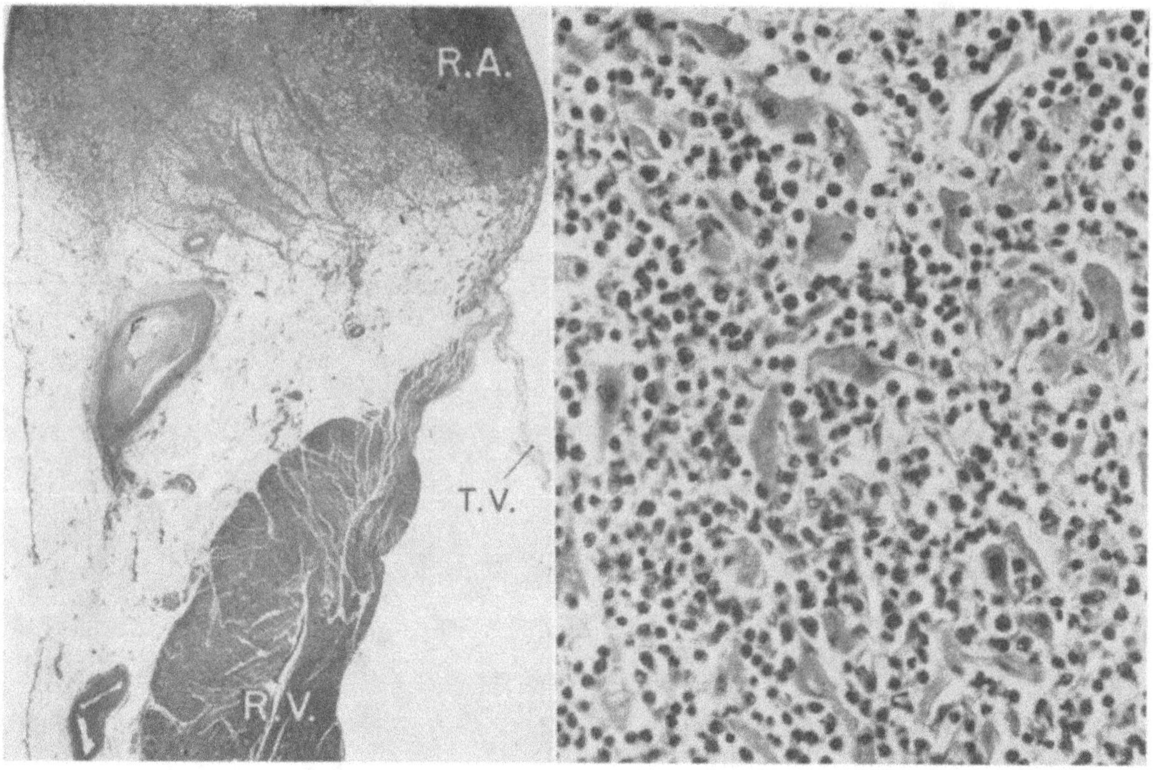

Figure 3. *Mycosis fungoides of the heart in a 68 year old woman who had extensive tumor deposits in the walls of all four cardiac chambers and in the pericardium.* This patient, who also had diffuse rheumatic-type fibrosis of the mitral valve, experienced atrial fibrillation, then atrial flutter, with a slow ventricular response (50 beats/min.) nine days before death. Two days later, complete atrioventricular dissociation with a nodal pacemaker appeared and persisted until her death. Right bundle branch block appeared three days before death as well as electrocardiographic evidence of left ventricular ischemia. These rhythm disturbances prompted the clinical diagnosis of cardiac mycosis fungoides, and at necropsy extensive cardiac deposits of tumor were found including involvement of the atrial septum and free wall of the right atrium.

Left, sections through right atrium (R.A.), tricuspid valve (T.V.) and right ventricle (R.V.) demonstrating virtual replacement of right atrial myocardium by tumor cells. **Right,** closeup of right atrial tumor. Similar tumor deposits occurred in the skin, lung, lymph nodes, tongue and thyroid gland. (Hematoxylin and eosin × 4.5 [left], × 220 [right], both reduced by 13%.)

focal in the other 10. It was fibrinous in 6, fibrinofibrous in 7 and fibrous in 7. Of the 20 patients with pericarditis, 11 had Hodgkin's disease, 3 mycosis fungoides, and 2 each lymphosarcoma, reticulum cell sarcoma and undifferentiated lymphoma. The focal pericarditis was clinically silent in the 10 patients in whom it occurred, but 5 of the 10 with diffuse pericarditis had clinical features that in part may have resulted from it. Of 2 patients with pericardial friction rubs 1 had in addition a ventricular gallop and 1 severe substernal chest pain of the pericardial type. The other 3 patients had evidence of pericardial constriction with distended neck veins, dyspnea and considerable peritoneal and subcutaneous effusions. Each of the 3 had Hodgkin's disease and thickened parietal as well as visceral pericardium. The pericardial disease in 2 was the result of tumor, and in the third, the result of widespread fibrosis secondary to irradiation for cardiac lymphoma present several years earlier. The clinical features of the latter patient, who died in 1966, were described in 1962 by Carney and associates,[8] and the pathologic features are illustrated in Figures 9 to 11. In another of these 3 patients the parietal pericardium was 5 cm. thick as a result of infiltrating Hodgkin's granuloma, but symptoms of cardiac involvement did not occur until several days before death.

In addition to the 20 patients with gross evidence of pericarditis, 7 others had evidence on histologic examination of focal epicarditis that was the result of tumor in 2, infection in 2, acute myocardial infarction in 1 and unknown causes

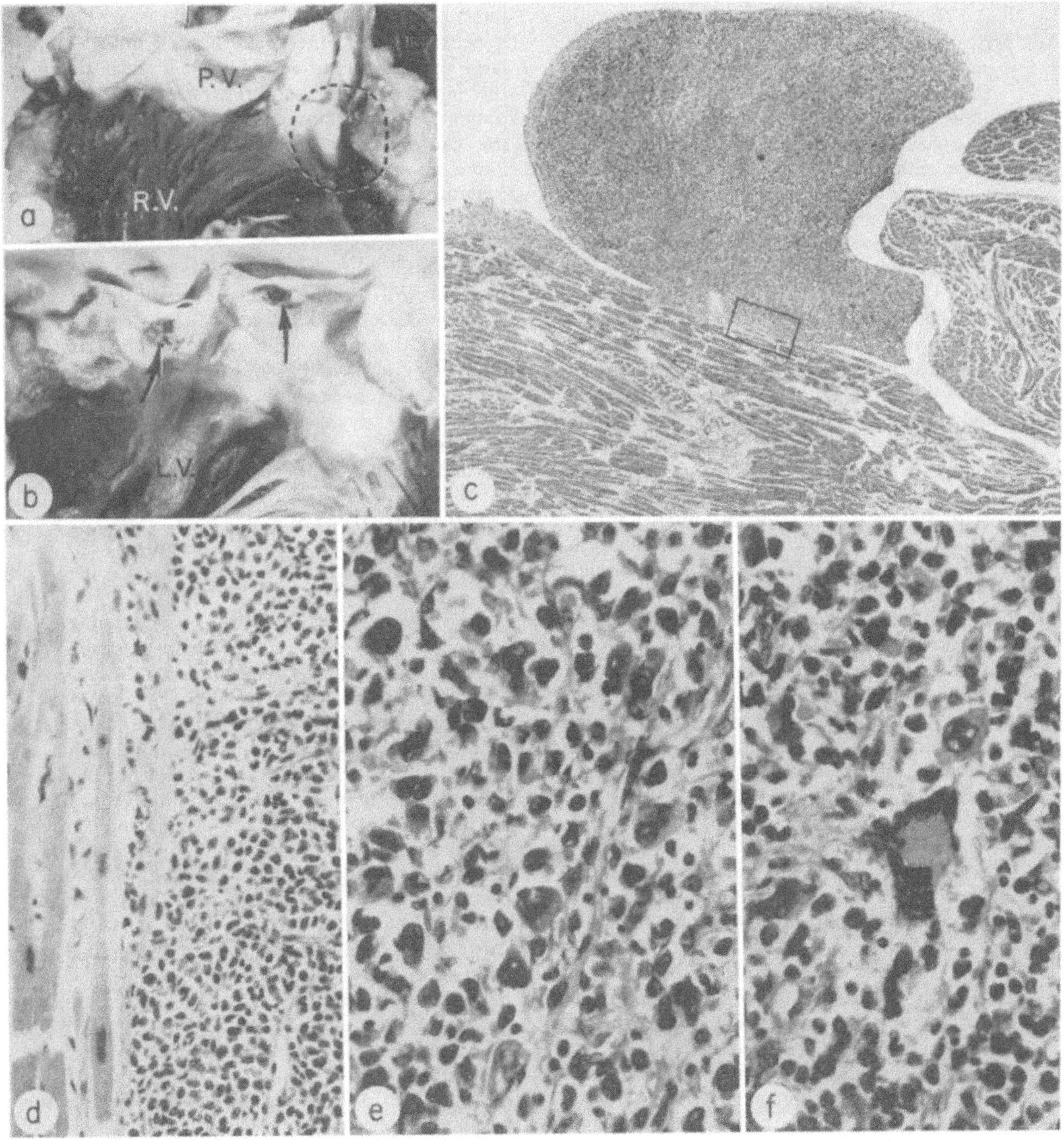

Figure 4. *Mycosis fungoides of the heart in a 79 year old man whose cardiac tumor histologically was similar to Hodgkin's disease.* This man had various skin lesions for 25 years, and a diagnosis of mycosis fungoides was made 11 years before death. Although at necropsy he had several tumor nodules in the walls of both ventricles, ventricular septum and in the subepicardial adipose tissue adjacent to the anterior descending coronary artery, he had no signs or symptoms of cardiac dysfunction. An electrocardiogram one day before death was normal. He also had tumor nodules in the lungs, lymph nodes, thyroid gland and skin. **a,** opened pulmonic valve (P.V.) and right ventricular outflow tract (R.V.) showing a tumor nodule (dashed circle) just below one of the pulmonic valve cusps. Another patient with mycosis fungoides had a similar lesion at the same site (Fig. 1). **b,** opened aortic valve and left ventricular outflow tract showing small thrombi (**arrows**) on two of the valvular cusps. No organisms were present in these lesions ("marantic" endocarditis). **c,** tumor thrombus on right ventricular endocardium. **d,** closeup of area in rectangle in c. **e,** high-power photomicrograph of area of tumor thrombus shown in c. Many tumor giant cells are present. **f,** another area of right ventricular tumor thrombus shows marked anaplasia of the tumor. (Hematoxylin and eosin × 22 [c], × 219 [d], × 400 [e and f], all reduced by 13%.)

in 2. None of these patients with "microscopic" pericarditis had signs or symptoms of cardiac dysfunction.

Cardiac Infections: Foci of inflammation containing stainable organisms were found in the hearts of 9 of the 196 patients (5 per cent). Of the 3 infections caused by bacteria, Staphylococcus aureus was the organism in 2 patients and mixed gram-negative organisms were stained and cultured in the third patient. Fungi were responsible for the cardiac infections in 4 subjects: Candida albicans in 1, mucor in 1, Cryptococcus neoformans in 1, and A. fumigatus in 1. Toxoplasma gondii was responsible for acute focal myocarditis in 2 patients. Two of the 9 subjects had staphylococcal endocarditis, which involved both mitral and aortic valves in 1 and the tricuspid valve alone in the other. Both patients also had focal acute myocarditis, and in neither was infective endocarditis suspected clinically. Four of the other 7 subjects had acute focal myocarditis, and the remaining 3 had acute pancarditis involving the epicardium and mural endocardium as well as the myocardium. The acute inflammatory process in each of the latter 3 patients extended through the wall of at least one cardiac chamber, and in each the necrotizing process was visible grossly. The infection in each of the 3 subjects with pancarditis was caused by fungi. Of the 9 with cardiac infections, 5 had Hodgkin's disease, 2 mycosis fungoides, 1 undifferentiated and 1 the lymphocytic type of lymphoma.

The cardiac infection in 8 of the 9 patients was associated with widespread systemic infection. With the exception of the patient with staphylococcal endocarditis of the left-sided cardiac valves, similar bacterial, fungal, or parasitic organisms were present in other organs of the body; usually the organisms had been cultured from the peripheral blood during the last few days of life or from the blood in the heart at necropsy. Despite extensive focal myocardial necrosis associated with acute inflammation in several subjects, none of the 9 patients had clinical signs or symptoms of cardiac dysfunction.

Heart Weight: The weight of the heart at the time of necropsy was recorded in 186 of the 196 patients: in 165 subjects it weighed less and in 21 it weighed more than 375 gm. (considered the upper limit of normal). The cardiomegaly in 11 of the 21 subjects was clearly the result of an underlying condition: systemic hypertension in 7 patients, rheumatic mitral and aortic valvular disease in 2, coronary heart disease with myocardial infarcts in 1 and nonrheumatic calcific aortic stenosis in 1. The large size of the cardiac tumor could account for the increased weight of the heart in another patient. In the remaining 9 patients, however, the cause of the cardiomegaly was unclear. None had underlying cardiac disease, and in the 5 with cardiac lymphoma the deposits were small. Although anemia was present in each of the 10 subjects (average blood hemoglobin 9.2 mg./100 ml.) it was similar to that in the 11 patients with cardiomegaly of definite cause (average 9.5 mg./100 ml.).

Of the 21 patients whose heart weighed more than 375 gm., 9 had evidence of cardiomegaly by chest roentgenogram, and 6 of ventricular hypertrophy by electrocardiogram. Each of the patients with roentgenographic or electrocardiographic evidence of cardiac enlargement had either systemic hypertension or underlying valvular heart disease.

Clinical Observations

Symptoms: Symptoms that are often attributed to cardiac involvement were frequent but usually were not the result of lymphoma of the heart. Dyspnea was recorded in 13 of 48 patients (27 per cent) with and in 35 of 148 patients (24 per cent) without cardiac lymphoma. Pleural effusions appeared to be the most common cause of this symptom, although acute pneumonitis, pulmonary and mediastinal lymphoma and anemia were also important factors. Precordial or substernal chest pain, or both, occurred in 3 of 48 patients (6 per cent) with and in 10 of 148 patients (7 per cent) without cardiac lymphoma. Mediastinal lymphadenopathy appeared to be an important cause of this pain although pericarditis, usually fibrinous and nonspecific, occasionally was present.

Physical Signs: Precordial murmurs were described in 18 of 48 patients (37 per cent) with and in 46 of 148 subjects (32 per cent) without cardiac lymphoma. In all but 4 patients, each of whom had underlying valvular heart disease, the murmurs were believed to be functional or hemic in nature. The blood hemoglobin was less than 10 gm./100 ml. at some time during the illness in 108 of the 196 (55 per cent) patients studied, and some degree of anemia was present in all but a few patients. The murmurs in all patients were systolic. Precordial friction rubs were recorded in 6 subjects, only 1 of whom had myocardial or epicardial lymphoma. A ventricular gallop was heard in 4 of 48 subjects (8

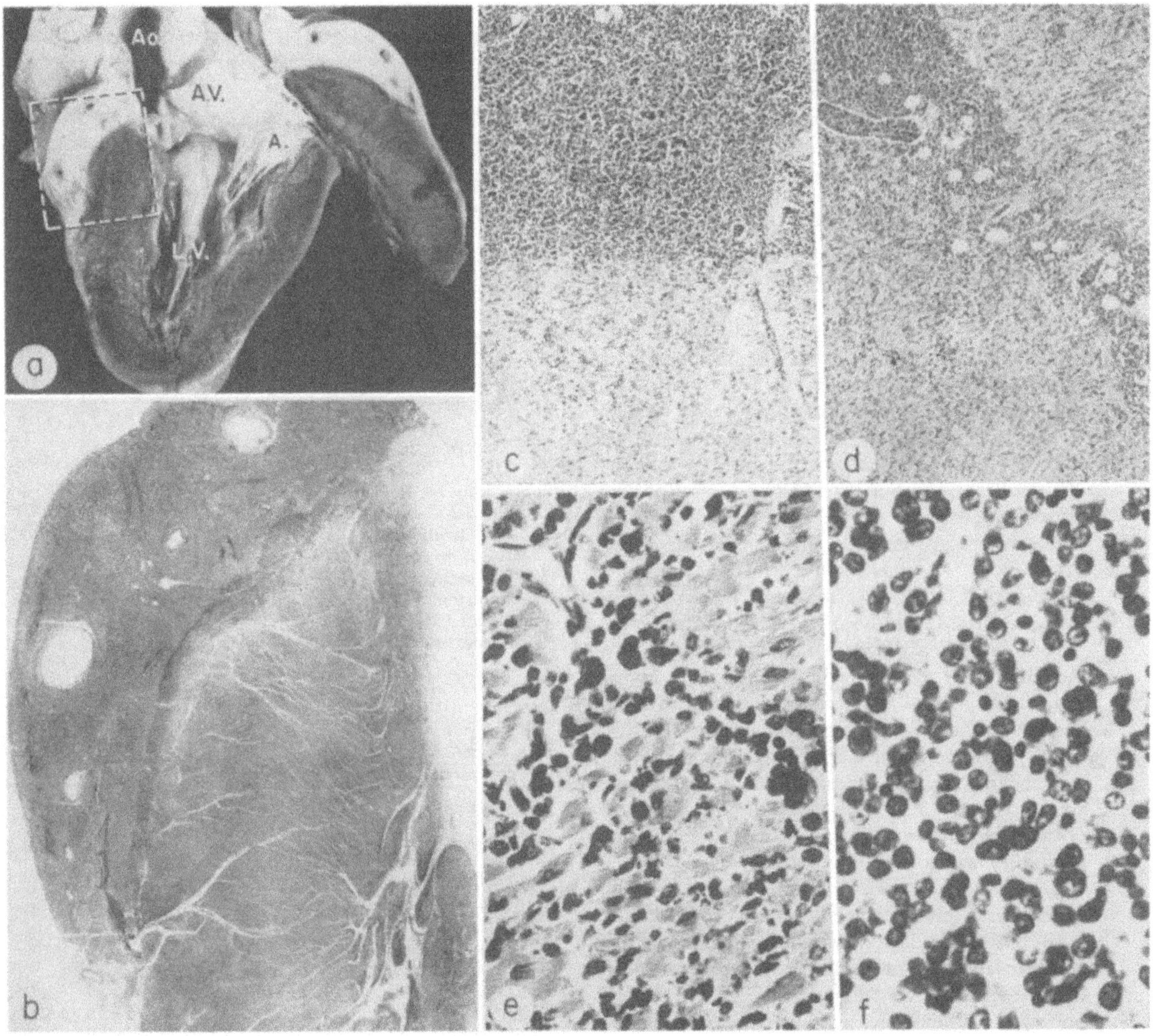

Figure 5. *Reticulum cell sarcoma of the heart in a 54 year old man who had no signs nor symptoms of cardiac dysfunction.* Large masses of tumor cells were present in the subepicardial adipose tissue and in the outer left ventricular wall. **a,** opened left ventricle (L.V.), aortic valve (A.V.), and aorta (Ao.) showing firm white tumor replacing the subepicardial tissue. A. = anterior mitral leaflet. **b,** photomicrograph of the area in the rectangle shown in a. The subepicardial adipose tissue is completely replaced by tumor cells. The lumen of the coronary artery, seen in cross-section, is not compromised by the tumor. **c,** section at junction of epicardium and myocardium, demonstrating replacement of the former by tumor cells, and focal infiltration into the outer myocardium by tumor cells. **d** and **e,** lymphoma cells in the interstitial myocardium. **f,** closeup of the subepicardial tumor. (Hematoxylin and eosin × 3.3 [b], × 63 [c and d], × 400 [e], × 628 [f], all reduced by 20%.)

per cent) with and in 7 of 148 patients (5 per cent) without cardiac lymphoma.

Chest Roentgenograms: These were interpreted as indicating cardiac enlargement in 8 of 48 patients (17 per cent) with and in 12 of 148 patients (8 per cent) without cardiac lymphoma.

Electrocardiograms: These were recorded, usually as part of a routine workup, in 156 of the 196 patients. Abnormal electrocardiograms were observed in 25 of 38 subjects (66 per cent) with and in 78 of 118 (66 per cent) without cardiac lymphoma. However, 5 of the 38 patients with and 14 of the 118 without lymphoma had underlying heart disease: hypertensive in 8 subjects, coronary in 6, valvular in 4 and pulmonary in 1. Excluding these 19 subjects with underlying heart disease, 20 of 33 patients (61 per cent) with and 64 of 104 (62 per cent) without cardiac lymphoma had an abnormal tracing. The electrocardiographic disturbances in these 137 subjects are tabulated in Table IV. Only 49 of the 137 patients (36 per cent) had more than one electrocardiogram recorded, and 63 of the 137 (46 per cent) had no electrocardiogram taken during the last month of life. Patients whose first tracings were judged abnormal tended to have additional records; those with normal initial tracings usually did not. The 84 patients with abnormal electrocardiograms averaged 50 years of age compared to 43 for the 53 patients who had normal electrocardiograms or whose only abnormality was sinus tachycardia.

The most frequent electrocardiographic disturbance recorded in the subjects without evidence of underlying cardiac disease was sinus tachycardia. Alterations in the S-T segment or T wave, or both, were the second most frequent findings. These changes usually were nonspecific and may often have been secondary to tachycardia or anemia. Alterations of the ischemic type also occasionally may have been the result of anemia. The abnormal electrocardiographic data in 2 patients returned to normal after blood transfusions for anemia. Low voltage, the third most common finding, appears to have been secondary most often to pleural or pericardial effusion, or both. Serum electrolytic disturbances in these patients were common, and many of the ST-T wave, Q-T interval abnormalities (6 patients) and U wave abnormalities (6 patients) appeared to be secondary to them. Only a few of the electrocardiographic disturbances could be attributed to lymphomatous deposits in the heart.

TABLE IV
Electrocardiographic Abnormalities

	Patients With Cardiac Lymphoma (no.)	Patients Without Cardiac Lymphoma (no.)	Totals
Electrocardiograms obtained	33	104	137
Abnormal tracing	20 (61%)	64 (62%)	84
Normal tracing*	13	40	53
More than 1 electrocardiogram	15	34	49
Recording obtained during last month of life	22	52	74
Sinus tachycardia (>100/min.)	15	46	61
Low voltage (sum of QRS in I, II, III < 1.5 mv.)	10	23	33
Ectopic tachycardia			
Atrial fibrillation	1	1	2
Atrial flutter	1	0	1
Atrial tachycardia	2	1	3
Atrioventricular block			
Prolonged P-R interval (>0.20 sec.)	1	3	4
Second degree	2	0	2
Complete A-V dissociation	1	1†	2
Premature contractions			
Nodal	0	2	2
Atrial	1	6	7
Ventricular	7	7	14
Left axis deviation	2	7	9
Right axis deviation	0	3	3
Right bundle branch block	1	0	1
ST-T wave changes			
Nonspecific	8	17	25
Ischemic	2	7	9
Digitalis effect	1	7	8
Potassium disturbance	0	8	8
Pericarditis type	2	1	3
P wave abnormality	1	5	6

* Normal except for sinus tachycardia.

† Lasted only 1 day on each of 2 occasions. Last tracing was entirely normal.

Correlation of Clinical Findings of Cardiac Dysfunction and Lymphomatous Infiltration of Heart: Although dyspnea, effusions, edema, precordial murmurs and electrocardiographic disturbances were common, these manifestations of cardiac dysfunction could be attributed to lymphomatous infiltration of the heart in only a few patients. Mycosis fungoides of the heart caused cardiac dysfunction in at least 3 patients. One (described in Fig. 3) had multiple, large (2 to 3 cm. in diameter) tumor nodules in the walls of all four cardiac chambers and clinical signs and symptoms of right- and left-sided congestive cardiac failure. Both of the other 2 subjects had large mycosis fungoides tumor nodules in the wall of the right atrium and atrial septum as well as multiple electrocardiographic disturbances. The latter included atrial fibrillation and flutter, nodal rhythm, first and second degree heart block, complete atrioventricular dissociation, right bundle branch block and aberrant ventricular conduction patterns. *One*

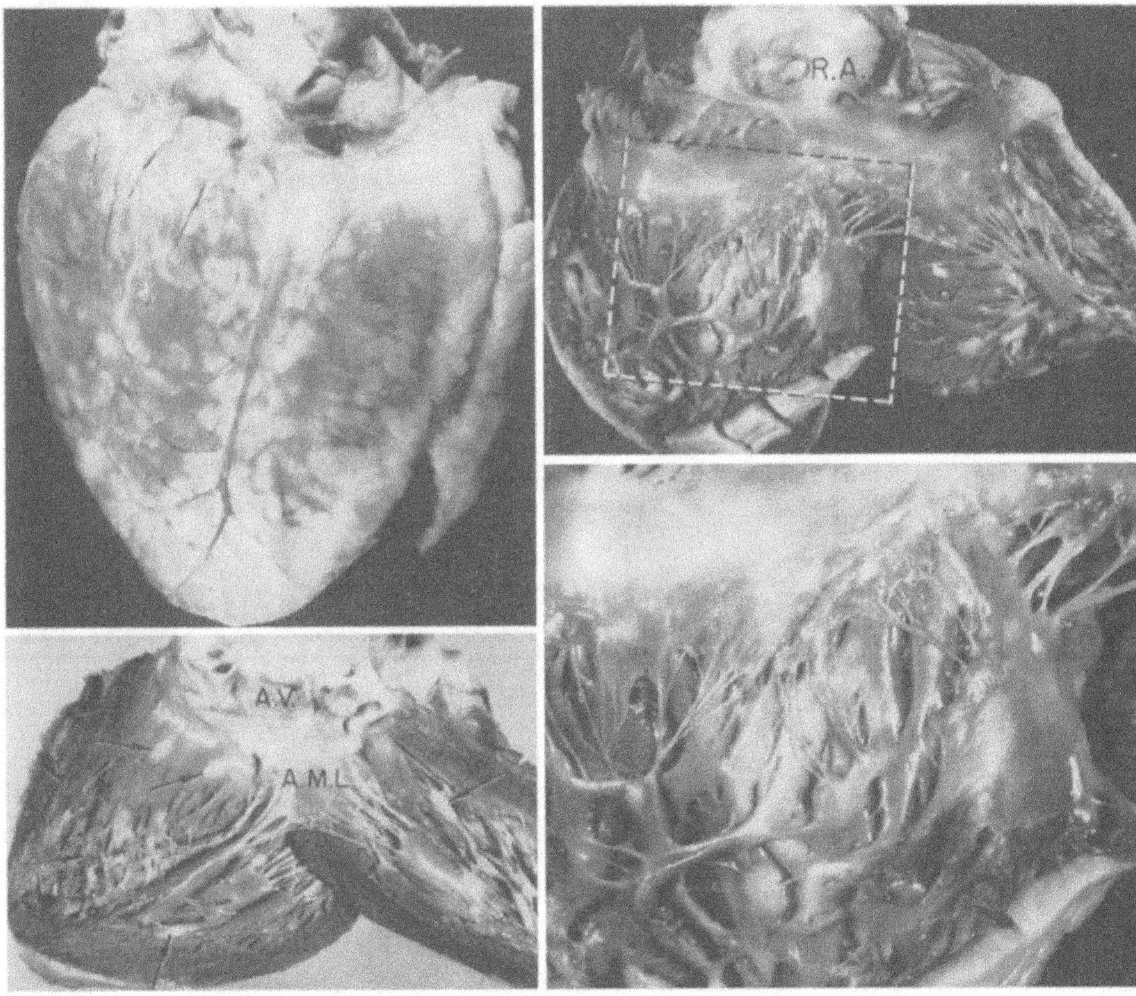

Figure 6. *Lymphosarcoma of the heart in a 21 year old man who never had signs or symptoms of cardiac dysfunction.* An electrocardiogram two days before death was normal, and the cardiac size was normal as shown by chest roentgenogram. The patient died suddenly and unexpectedly. At necropsy, the heart weighed 390 gm., and numerous deposits of tumor were present on the epicardial and endocardial surfaces.

Upper left, the posterior surface of the ventricles demonstrating numerous tumor nodules. There was no increased amount of fluid in the pericardial sac. **Lower left,** opened left ventricle and aortic valve (A.V.) showing several endocardial tumor implants (arrows). A.M.L. = anterior mitral leaflet. **Upper right,** opened right atrium (R.A.), tricuspid valve, and right ventricle, again demonstrating endocardial tumor implants. A closeup of the area in brackets is shown in the **lower right** photograph.

Figure 7, opposite page. *Photomicrographs of endocardial and myocardial lymphosarcoma* in the patient whose gross heart is shown in Figure 6. **Upper left,** the epicardium (upper portion of photograph) is nearly replaced by tumor cells and only a few fat cells remain. Neoplastic cells infiltrate the outer right ventricular myocardium. **Upper right,** the endocardium (lower portion of photograph) and inner right ventricular myocardium are extensively infiltrated by tumor cells. **Lower left,** closeup of right ventricular endocardial implant. **Lower right,** intramyocardial left ventricular tumor deposit. (Hematoxylin and eosin stains; original magnification × 25 [upper left and right, lower right] and × 400 [lower left], all increased by 12%.)

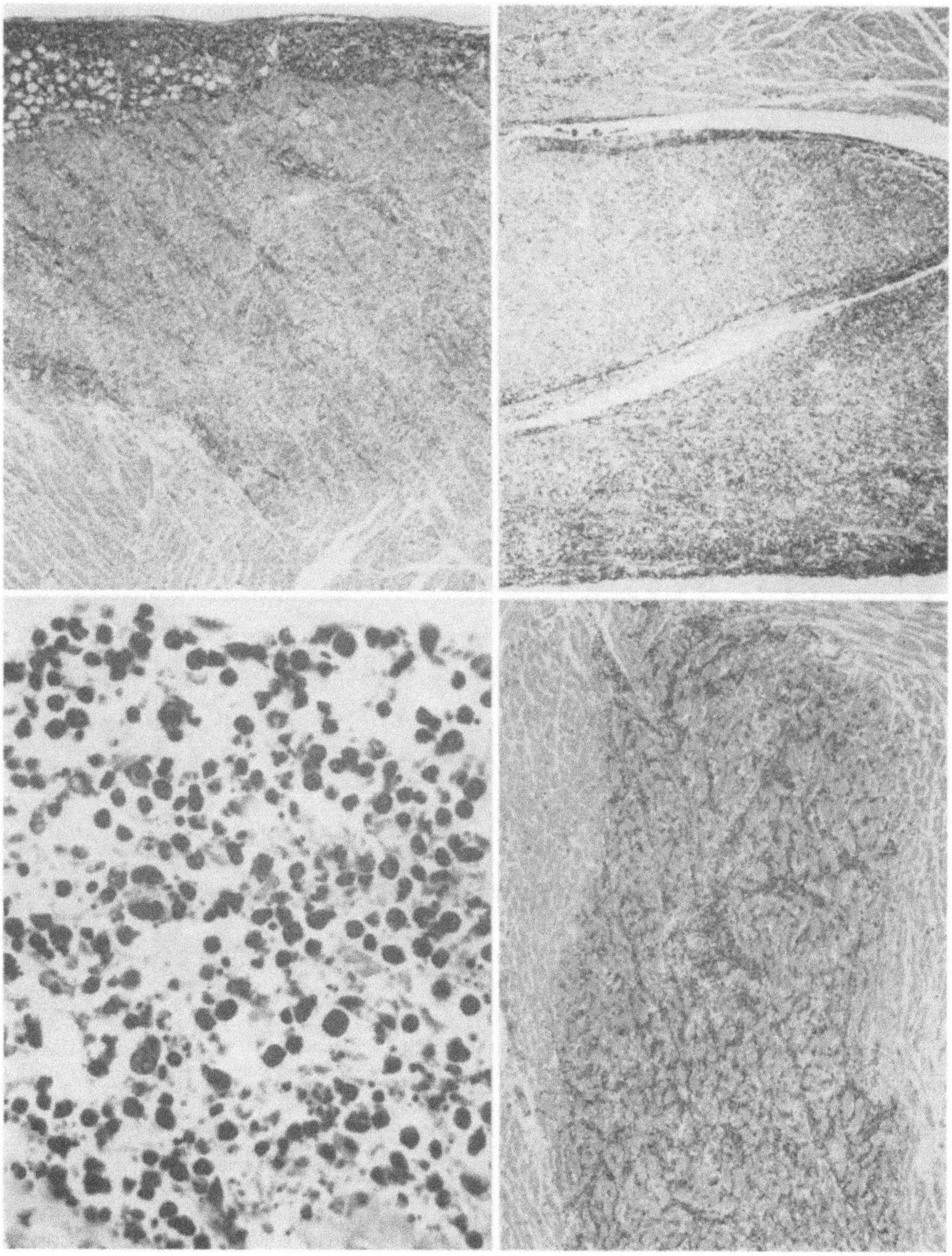

Figure 7, see opposite page.

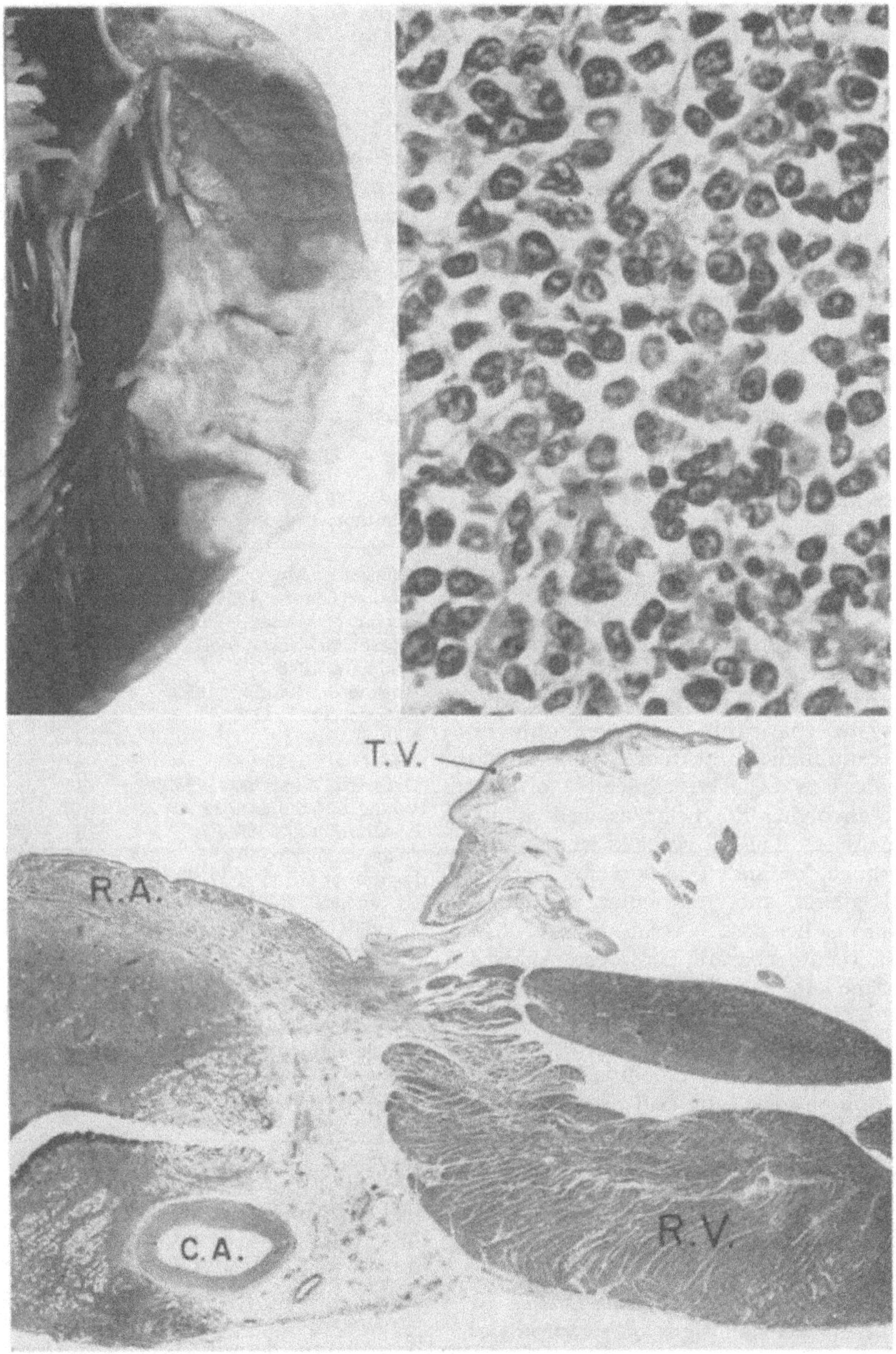

Figure 8. *Undifferentiated or mixed (histiocytic and lymphocytic) lymphoma of the heart in a 59 year old woman who had extensive deposits of tumor in the right atrium, left ventricle and pericardium but no signs nor symptoms of cardiac dysfunction.* Tumor was present at necropsy in 16 organs and tissues. **Upper left,** cut section of left ventricular free wall showing a tumor deposit extending through the wall. **Upper right,** photomicrograph (× 628) of an area of this tumor nodule. **Lower,** photomicrograph (× 5) of a section of right atrium (R.A.), tricuspid valve (T.V.) leaflet, and right ventricle (R.V.) showing extensive infiltration by tumor in the adipose tissue in the right atrioventricular sulcus. C.A. = coronary artery. (Hematoxylin and eosin stains on each of the histologic sections.)

patient with Hodgkin's disease had signs and symptoms of severe cardiac dysfunction probably secondary to tumor involving the pericardium. This man (described in detail in Fig. 9 to 11) had right ventricular outflow obstruction and second degree atrioventricular block; both disorders disappeared after mediastinal irradiation, but subsequently signs of constrictive pericarditis secondary to the radiation therapy occurred intermittently. Another patient with Hodgkin's disease, studied after completion of this series, had evidence of recurrent constrictive pericarditis with tamponade secondary to radiation fibrosis after therapy for mediastinal and probably pericardial Hodgkin's disease (Fig. 12 and 13). A third patient with Hodgkin's disease, a 25 year old man, had severe precordial and substernal chest pain with a pericardial friction rub during his last seven days of life but never had evidence of congestive cardiac failure. At necropsy, the parietal pericardium was 1 cm. thick, secondary to infiltration by Hodgkin's disease; although fibrinous pericarditis was present there were only minute foci of neoplastic deposits in the heart, and these were limited to the epicardium and seen only on histologic examination. A fourth with Hodgkin's disease was believed clinically to have lymphoma involving the heart as well as adjacent structures. This 27 year old woman had severe dyspnea, distended neck veins, ascites, peripheral edema, and ventricular and atrial gallops during her last several days of life. The chest roentgenogram, however, showed the area of the left lung to be totally radiodense; at necropsy it was atelectatic, infected, its pleura severely thickened, and the right lung contained foci of acute pneumonitis. Purulent infection from the left lung had extended into the pericardial sac causing obliterative pericarditis, but there was no anatomic evidence of constriction. The heart weighed only 240 gm., and Hodgkin's disease was found in the parietal and visceral pericardia, but only on histologic examination.

None of the patients with lymphosarcoma or reticulum cell sarcoma had signs or symptoms of cardiac dysfunction that justifiably could be attributed to lymphoma involving the heart. However, a 7 year old girl with lymphosarcoma had distended neck veins, pulmonary rales, a ventricular gallop and pedal edema during her last several days, and no improvement followed therapy with digoxin and aminophylline. At necropsy, a single small nodule of lymphosarcoma was found in the wall of the right atrium, but it did not appear to be of a size adequate to account for the clinical signs and symptoms.

Comments

A number of studies have described involvement of the heart in lymphoma.[4-22] The incidence of cardiac metastases in these reported necropsy series of patients with Hodgkin's disease, lymphosarcoma and reticulum cell sarcoma are tabulated in Tables v, vi and vii,*

Table v
Hodgkin's Disease of the Heart: Survey of Reported Series

Author, Year (Reference)	Total Autopsy Cases (no.)	Patients with Cardiac Metastases (no.)	(%)
Krueger & Meyer, 1936[4]	16	3	19
Scott & Garvin, 1939[5]	22	0	0
Herbut & Maisell, 1942[6]	13	2	15
Jackson & Parker, 1947[7]	98	2	2
Symmers, 1948[8]	30	0‡	0
Rottino & Hoffman, 1952[9]	63	5	8
Lucia et al., 1952[10]	18	3	17
Nabarro, 1953[11]	24	4	17
Bisel et al., 1953[13]	27	8	30
DeLoach & Haynes, 1953[12]	49	3*	6
Young & Goldman, 1954[14]	39	2	5
Gassman et al., 1955[15]	189	7†	4
Jakob & Zirkin, 1960[17]	15	3	20
Levitan et al., 1961[18]	112	4	4
Richmond, 1962[19]	272	33	12
Totals	987	79	8
Present series, 1968	75	12	16

* Includes only patients in whom cardiac tumor was observed grossly.

† Patient with tumor in parietal pericardium only excluded.

‡ Author described involvement in detail of virtually every organ except the heart.

respectively. The anatomic data presented in these studies were obtained entirely from autopsy protocols, and there was no re-examination of the hearts or of histologic sections from them. Also, with the exception of electrocardiographic findings in one study,[20] clinical data were described only in patients with cardiac metastases, and no mention was made of clinical observations in those with lymphoma but without tumor in the heart. It is hoped that the clinical and necropsy data presented in this study are more meaningful since most of the hearts and histologic sections from them

* See page 103 for Tables vi and vii.

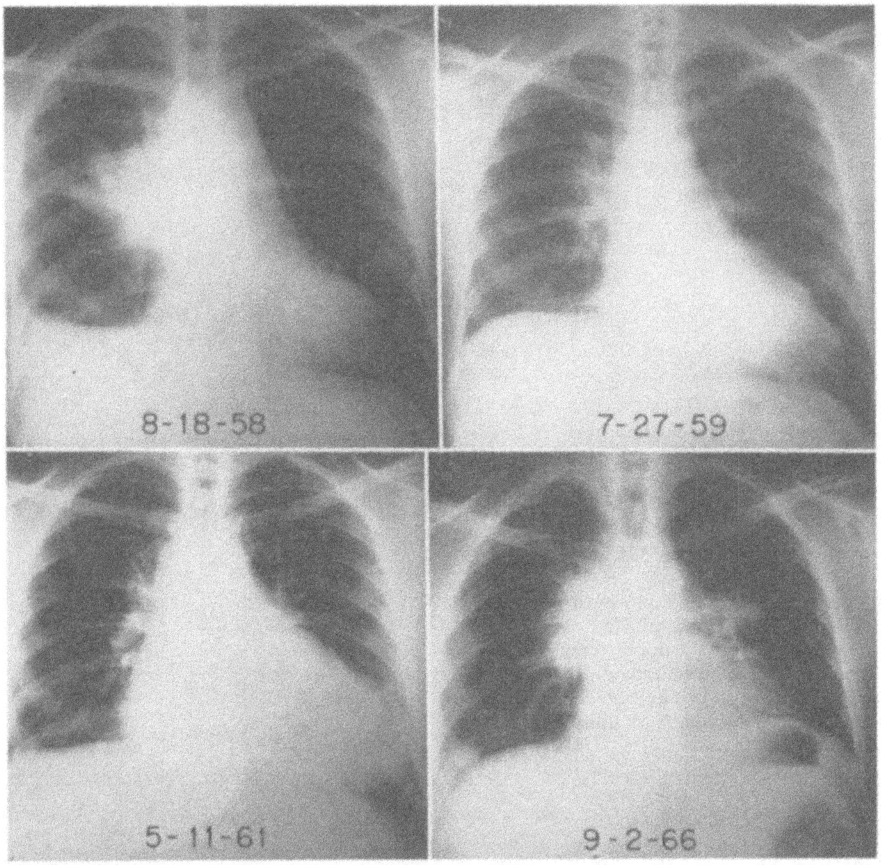

Figure 9. *Pericardial Hodgkin's disease causing right ventricular outflow obstruction.* This 36 year old man, who died on Sept. 24, 1966, was found to have a mediastinal mass on routine chest roentgenogram (**upper left**) in August 1958, and biopsy of the mass disclosed Hodgkin's disease. A pericardial effusion was present at the time of thoracotomy, but no tumor nodules were observed within the pericardium. A pericardiopleural window was created. Postoperatively, he received 3,000 rads to the mediastinum, and during the ensuing three months the mass disappeared. Four months after operation a supraclavicular mass appeared, and it was treated with 3,000 rads. He then was asymptomatic until March 1959 when cough, malaise and episodes of pressing substernal pain and dyspnea after exertion appeared. Large pulsations (*a* wave) developed in the jugular veins, and when examined in July 1959 the heart was enlarged (**upper right**), a grade 3/6 ejection-type systolic murmur was audible along the upper left sternal border, and the liver was enlarged and pulsated.

Cardiac catheterization in May 1961 disclosed significant systolic pressure gradients between the right ventricular body, infundibulum and pulmonary trunk (Fig. 10). There was also partial A-V block. Injection of contrast material into the right ventricle disclosed a large mass which compressed the pulmonary trunk and right ventricular outflow tract. No fluid was obtained by pericardiocentesis. Chest roentgenogram at this time revealed increased cardiac enlargement (**lower left**). During the 10 days after catheterization he received 1,480 rads to the mediastinum. Within a month the 2:1 A-V block had disappeared, the P-R interval had returned to normal, the *a* wave in the jugular venous pulse had diminished, the intensity of the precordial murmur had decreased, and he was asymptomatic with good tolerance to exercise. Repeat catheterization showed a normal right ventricular systolic pressure (Fig. 10).

The patient was well thereafter until December 1962 when exertional dyspnea and periodic precordial chest pain recurred, and he was digitalized. The precordial systolic ejection murmur was grade 3/6 intensity again, a ventricular gallop was present, but there was no right ventricular hypertrophy by electrocardiogram, which showed sinus rhythm, low voltage, abnormal P waves consistent with both right and left atrial enlargement, and periodic T wave inversion in the lateral precordial leads. In October 1965 he received 2,000 rads to the left hilar region of the lung because of radiodensities in this region. Also, at this time the dyspnea worsened but was lessened by treatment with vincristine and nitrogen mustard. In December 1965 the dyspnea worsened abruptly and he retained fluid. He was now cachetic and dyspneic while sitting. The chest roentgenogram was interpreted as showing radiation pneumonitis and fibrosis. With antidiuretic therapy the dyspnea lessened, the excess fluid disappeared, and thereafter he was able to walk up two flights of stairs with only mild dyspnea until May 1966 when acute pneumonitis, which responded to antibiotics, caused the return of severe dyspnea. From July until his death in September 1966 he was always mildly dyspneic and had mild subcutaneous edema The neck veins terminally were only mildly distended. Hepatic failure from serum hepatitis was the immediate cause of death. The **lower right** roentgenogram was taken 22 days before death.

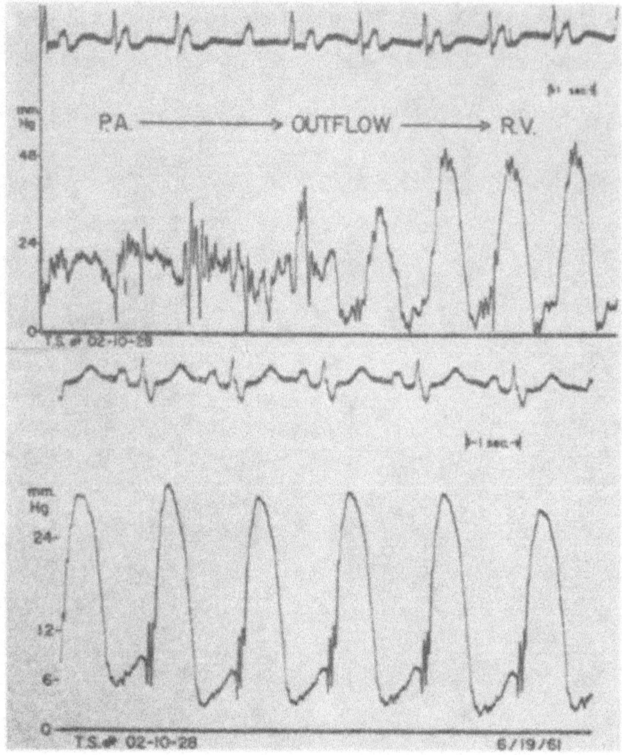

Figure 10. Same case. *Right-sided cardiac pressure tracings of the patient described in Figure 9.* The **upper panel** (May 1961) shows the pressure during withdrawal of the catheter from the pulmonary artery (P.A.) (24/10 mm. Hg) through the right ventricular outflow tract (34/6 mm. Hg) into the right ventricular body (R.V.) (52/6 mm. Hg). The **lower panel** shows the right ventricular pressure (30/8 mm. Hg) at catheterization one month after the upper tracing and after therapy. The electrocardiogram during the first catheterization (**upper**) showed second degree heart block, which had disappeared by the second study (**lower**).

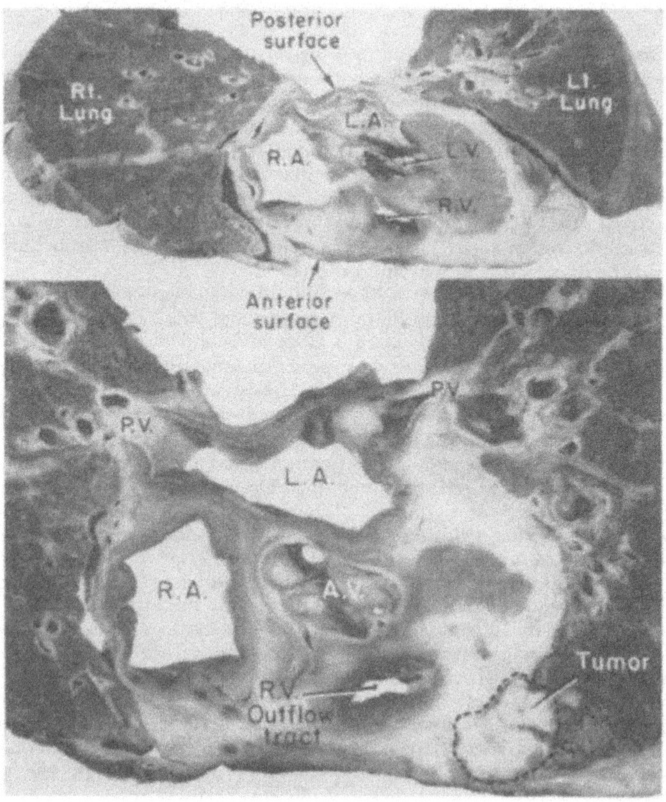

Figure 11. Same case. *Radiation fibrosis of the heart in the patient with Hodgkin's disease described in Figures 9 and 10.* **Upper,** transverse section of the heart and lung demonstrating severe fibrous thickening of the epicardium and fibrosis of the outer walls of the right (R.V.) and left (L.V.) ventricles. The body of the right ventricle is very small. **Lower,** closeup of transverse section of the heart at the level of the right ventricular outflow tract (infundibulum), which is severely narrowed. The only residual of Hodgkin's disease is at the junction of the right ventricle and left lung (enclosed by the dashed lines). R.A. = right atrium; L.A. = left atrium; A.V. = aortic valve; and P.V. = pulmonary vein.

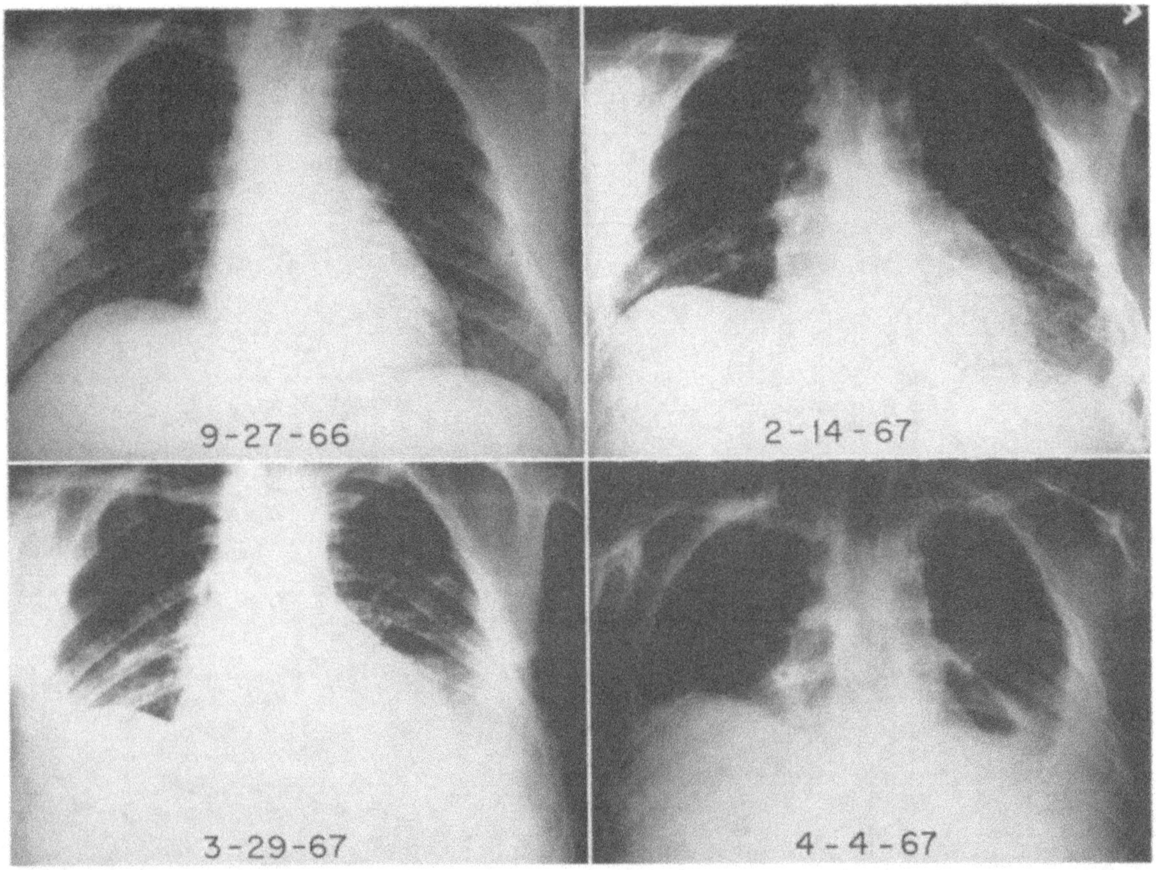

Figure 12. *Chest roentgenograms in a 26 year old man who died on April 5, 1967, of cardiac tamponade and Hodgkin's disease.* (This patient is not included as one of the 196 subjects tabulated in this study since he died after Dec. 31, 1966.) In September 1964 biopsy of a painless unilateral swelling in the neck disclosed Hodgkin's disease. The heart and lungs appeared normal on chest roentgenogram in December 1964. In January 1965 he received 6,000 rads to the upper chest and neck, 6,000 to the lower mediastinum, 6,000 to the abdominal periaortic regions, 2,000 to the splenic area, and 1,800 to the pelvis. Except for acute esophagitis in February 1965, presumably secondary to the irradiation, he was asymptomatic until Jan. 24, 1967, when exertional and nocturnal dyspnea, precordial pain, and swelling of the legs and abdomen suddenly appeared. Examination on Feb. 1, 1967 disclosed dyspnea on sitting up in bed, a 25 mm. Hg decrease in the brachial arterial systolic pressure during inspiration, rapid respirations (40/min.), distended neck veins, a pericardial friction rub, sinus tachycardia (150/min.) with atrial premature contractions, ascites, pitting lower leg edema and large pleural effusions. No murmurs or gallops were audible and a precordial impulse was not palpable. Left thoracentesis yielded 1,200 ml. serous fluid and pericardiocentesis yielded 200 ml. of bloody fluid. The patient then felt better and the heart sounds were louder on precordial auscultation.

His last two months were characterized by repeated reaccumulations of pleural fluid (a total of 9,200 ml. was removed from the pleural spaces during nine thoracenteses) and continued evidence of right- and left-sided cardiac failure. A second pericardiocentesis yielding 210 ml. of fluid was performed on Feb. 7, 1967, and he then was digitalized. Approximately eight days before death the dyspnea worsened, hypotension, oliguria and hyperkalemia appeared and he gained weight. Pericardiocentesis was repeated on April 4 and 330 ml. of fluid was obtained. Several hours later he died.

At necropsy, 350 ml. of fluid was present in the pericardial sac, 2,500 ml. in each pleural space, and 1,200 in the peritoneal cavity.

The date of each roentgenogram shown is indicated. Eighty ml. of air was injected into the pericardial sac (**lower right**) after the third and final pericardiocentesis, and this study demonstrates the thickened parietal pericardium.

were re-examined, and the clinical data were recorded in patients without as well as with cardiac lymphoma.

Mycosis Fungosides: From review of previous studies of cardiac involvement in lymphoma and from analyses of the patients studied by us, mycosis fungoides appears to involve the heart most frequently. Mention of the frequency of cardiac involvement by this lymphoma was initially made by Block and associates[23] and Edgcomb et al.[24] These authors described the necropsy findings in the first 17 patients with

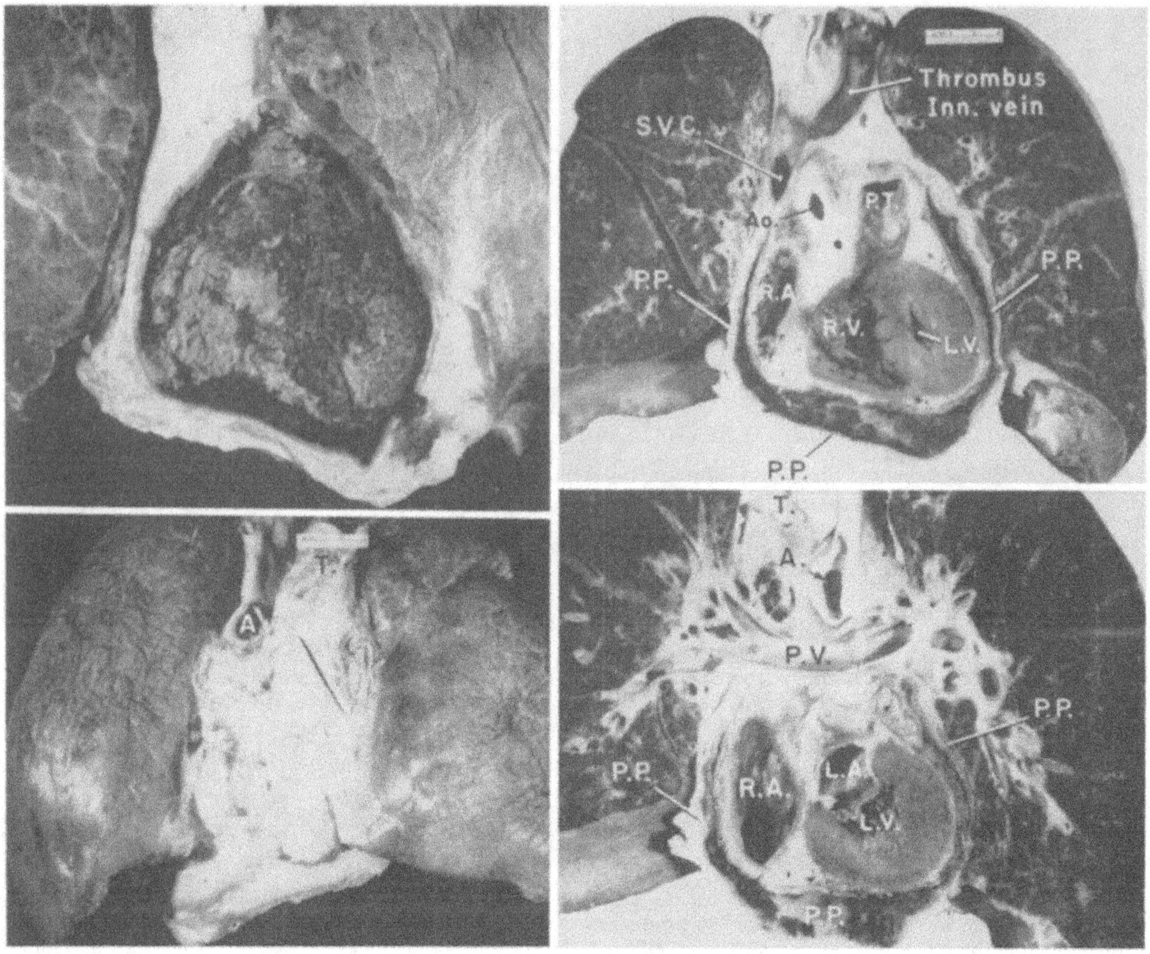

Figure 13. Same case. *Exterior and interior of the heart in the patient with Hodgkin's disease described in Figure 12.* **Upper left,** the anterior portion of the parietal pericardium has been excised, exposing the ragged hemorrhagic epicardial surface of the heart. The parietal pericardium is tightly adherent to the left lung. **Lower left,** posterior surface of the heart and lungs showing severe fibrosis of the mediastinal structures. Both lungs are adherent posteriorly to the parietal pericardium. A. = aorta at level of isthmus; T. = trachea. **Upper right,** frontal section of heart and lungs. The parietal pericardium (P.P.) and epicardium are thick. An antemortum thrombus occludes the innominate (Inn.) vein. Ao. = ascending aorta; S.V.C. = superior vena cava; R.A. = right atrium; R.V. = right ventricle; L.V. = left ventricle; and P.T. = pulmonic trunk. **Lower right,** another section of heart and lungs, but it is more posterior than the upper right view. There is marked fibrosis of the tissues adjacent to the pulmonary veins. The lymph nodes adjacent to the trachea (T.) are large. L.A. = left atrium.

mycosis fungoides who underwent necropsy at the Clinical Center of the National Institutes of Health, and 6 (35 per cent) had tumor in the heart. In the present report this number had increased to 51 subjects and 17 (33 per cent) had tumor in the heart. That the internal organs are frequently involved in patients with mycosis fungoides is now indisputable[23,24,25–27] but lymph nodes, spleen and liver appear to be involved more frequently than the heart.[23] Recently, Cyr and associates[28] summarized certain necropsy observations in 42 patients with mycosis fungoides, and at least 2 had lymphoma in the heart. At least 8 case reports of patients who died of mycosis fungoides have mentioned involvement of the heart.[29–36]

Lymphosarcoma and Hodgkin's Disease: The incidence of cardiac involvement (about 25 per cent) is similar in patients with lymphosarcoma and reticulum cell sarcoma (Tables I, VI, VII), and in Hodgkin's disease the incidence is lowest (about 10 per cent). In addition to being summarized in several reports of large series of patients with malignant lymphoma, cardiac involvement by tumor has been the subject of a number of detailed case reports of

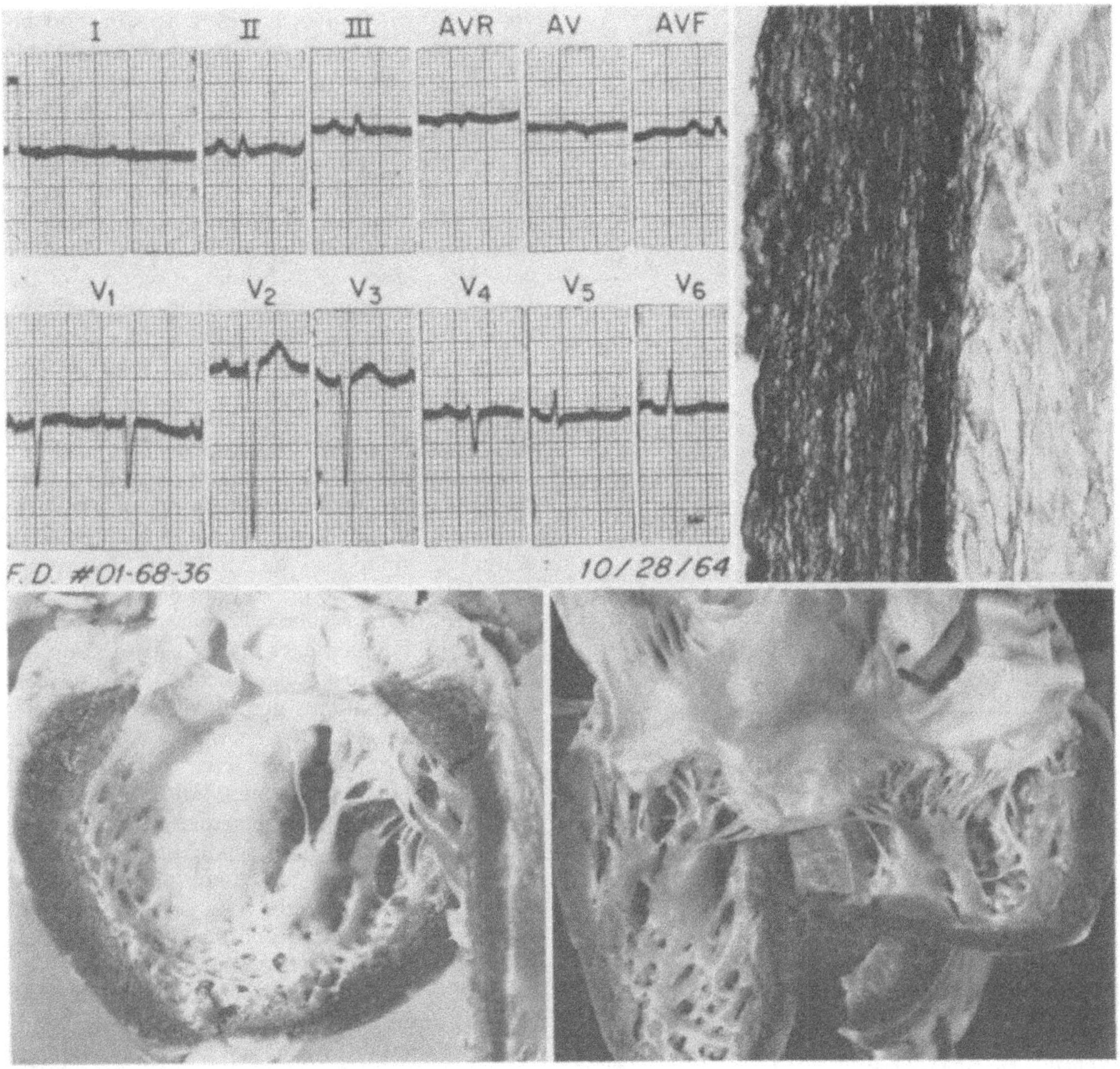

Figure 14. *Low voltage and endocardial fibroelastosis in a 27 year old woman who died in 1964 of Hodgkin's disease.* The diagnosis of lymphoma was established at age 17 by biopsy of an enlarged axillary lymph node. Her course was characterized by lesions in the lungs and bones, generalized lymphadenopathy and severe pleuritis of undetermined cause. She received antineoplastic agents plus local radiotherapy. In 1954 and 1956 she received a total of 21,800 rads to the chest and mediastinum. Although she was examined often during the 10 year illness, cardiomegaly was never revealed by roentgenogram, and there were no precordial murmurs, arrhythmias, nor symptoms suggesting cardiac disease. The electrocardiogram recorded in April 1958 (six and a half years before death) showed normal sinus rhythm and low voltage, and the repeat electrocardiogram (**upper left**) one month before death was unchanged.

At autopsy there was widespread Hodgkin's sarcoma involving bone marrow, spleen, liver, lymph nodes, lungs, stomach, dura mater and diaphragm. The heart weighed 200 gm. and showed diffuse endocardial thickening of the left ventricle (**lower and upper right**) and left atrium. The underlying ventricular myocardium was normal, as were the coronary arteries and cardiac valves. There was no endocardial thickening of the right atrium or ventricle.

Lower left, opened left ventricle and aortic valve. There is diffuse thickening of the mural endocardium. **Lower right,** opened left atrium, mitral valve and left ventricle. The mitral leaflets and chordae are probably normal. **Upper right,** histologic section demonstrating the thickened left ventricular endocardium, which consists primarily of elastic fibers (stained black). (Elastic van Gieson × 160, reduced by 8%.)

Table vi
Lymphosarcoma of the Heart: Survey of Reported Series

Author, Year (Reference)	Total Autopsy Cases (no.)	Patients with Cardiac Metastases (no.)	(%)
Scott & Garvin, 1939[5]	13	1	8
Herbut & Maisel, 1942[6]	16	3	19
Symmers, 1948[8]	17	6	35
Lucia et al., 1952[10]	24	9	37
DeLoach & Haynes, 1953[12]	33	14*	42
Bisel et al., 1953[13]	15	2	13
Young & Goldman, 1954[14]	12	5	42
Gassman et al., 1955[15]	142	16†	11
Goudie, 1955[16]	12	0	0
Richmond et al., 1962[19]	188	41	22
Madianos & Sokal, 1963[20]	170	25	15
Wright, 1964[21]	50‡	16	32
Totals	692	138	20
Present series, 1968	32	9	28

* Includes only patients whose cardiac tumor was observed grossly.

† Two patients with involvement of parietal pericardium only are excluded.

‡ Burkitt tumor.

Table vii
Reticulum Cell Sarcoma of the Heart: Survey of Reported Series

Author, Year (Reference)	Total Autopsy Cases (no.)	Patients with Cardiac Metastases (no.)	(%)
Scott & Garvin, 1939[5]	9	6	67
Jackson & Parker, 1947[7]	28	6	21
DeLoach & Haynes, 1953[12]	45	18*	40
Bisel et al., 1953[13]	23	7	30
Young & Goldman, 1954[14]	7	2	29
Goudie, 1955[16]	28	3	11
Richmond et al., 1962[19]	230	50	22
Madianos & Sokal, 1963[20]	41	11	27
Wilkinson et al., 1967[22]	20†	8	40
Totals	431	111	26
Present series, 1968	22	6	26

* Includes only patients in whom cardiac tumor was observed grossly.

† Of the 20 patients, 18 had reticulum cell sarcoma and 2 had lymphosarcoma. All were under 15 years of age.

patients with systemic lymphosarcoma,[37–40] reticulum cell sarcoma,[11,41–44] and Hodgkin's disease.[45–58]

Sites of Cardiac Involvement: Any portion of the heart may be infiltrated by lymphoma. Involvement of a valve, however, is rare, and involvement of the pericardium is common (Table ii). In the present study lymphoma in the left side of the heart was about as frequent as involvement of the right side. The tumor was always focal, sometimes appearing as discrete nodules on the pericardium or endocardium or in the intramural myocardium, and at times no tumor was apparent grossly but foci of tumor cells were observed in histologic sections of the heart. The infiltrates observed histologically were most commonly found in the subepicardial adipose tissue but also frequently in the interstitial areas between myocardial fibers. When the infiltrates were large, adjacent myocardial fibers often were destroyed. In 9 patients studied by us the tumor extended through the entire free wall or septal wall of a cardiac chamber. In contrast to their frequency in acute leukemia,[2] cardiac hemorrhages were observed rarely in the present patients, and no reports describing systemic lymphoma have commented on hemorrhages in the heart despite the frequency of thrombocytopenia. In at least 81 of the 196 patients described herein, platelet counts below 50,000 per cu. mm. were recorded, and in 34 the counts were below 10,000. Lymphoma in the subepicardial adipose tissue, particularly the atrioventricular sulci, was observed frequently in our patients. A similar preferential location for tumor also was found in the hearts of patients with acute leukemia.[2]

Clinical Manifestation of Cardiac Dysfunction: Although a frequent finding at autopsy, lymphoma of the heart rarely produced clinical signs or symptoms of cardiac dysfunction. This clinicoanatomic discrepancy has been noted by many observers. A recent study of malignant melanoma showed that only patients with extensive or huge tumor nodules in the hearts had signs or symptoms of cardiac dysfunction. None of the patients in the present study had tumor nodules in the heart approaching the size of some of the larger cardiac malignant melanoma metastases,[1] and in 21 of the 48 patients with cardiac lymphoma, tumor was found in the heart only on histologic examination.

Of the malignant lymphomas, Hodgkin's disease is the one most likely to be associated with signs of cardiac dysfunction. This appears to be caused by its tendency to involve the mediastinal lymph nodes in an extensive manner. With irradiation to the mediastinum the parietal pericardium tends to adhere to the epicardium. If the former thickens, because of lymphomatous infiltration or fibrosis secondary to irradiation, signs and symptoms of constrictive pericarditis may occur.[59] In each of 2 patients (Fig. 9 to 13) signs of pericardial constriction occurred, and right ventricular outflow obstruction occurred in one. In the latter patient the cause of the outflow obstruction initially was tumor since the stenosis disappeared after irradiation. Pericardiectomy was performed in 6 patients with Hodgkin's disease at the Clinical Center by Dr. Donald Morton, and each is still living and has received substantial benefit from this procedure. In 2 the constriction resulted from Hodgkin's disease infiltrating the parietal pericardium, and in the others, from fibrous thickening of the pericardium secondary to mediastinal irradiation. Pericardial constriction has been described previously in patients with Hodgkin's disease by several authors.[18,47–49,53,56,58]

Signs and symptoms of cardiac dysfunction may be the initial manifestation of a systemic lymphoma. Hagens[56] described 1 and Brun and associates[58] 2 patients with Hodgkin's disease who initially presented with signs of pericardial tamponade. Greiner[42] described a 40 year old man with reticulum cell sarcoma whose initial presenting symptoms were substernal pain and dyspnea. At necropsy, the heart was encased in tumor, the pericardial space was obliterated and the mediastinum contained a huge mass of tumor. Lisa et al[38] described a 17 year old girl whose initial manifestation of lymphosarcoma was intractable congestive cardiac failure and bloody pericardial and pleural effusions. At necropsy, she had extensive tumor implants in the endocardium, myocardium and pericardium. Steven[39] also described a patient, a 25 year old man, with lymphosarcoma whose initial manifestation was intractable cardiac failure. Nabarro[11] described a patient with reticulum cell sarcoma in whom congestive cardiac failure was the initial manifestation of his illness. At necropsy, however, no gross deposits of tumor were seen in the heart, although tumor was observed on histologic sections of this organ. The author attributed the cardiac failure in this patient to the microscopic-sized implants since the patient had no underlying cardiac disease and was young (aged 32 years). Goggio and associates[57] described a 58 year old man whose initial manifestation of Hodgkin's disease was complete heart block. The diagnosis of systemic lymphoma was not made until three months after the onset of heart block. During his entire five month illness congestive cardiac failure was present. At autopsy, large deposits of tumor were present in the epicardium and in the right atrium. A 5 cm. mass of tumor in this chamber protruded into the tricuspid valve orifice and also invaded the atrioventricular bundle.

Effusions and Edema: Effusions into body cavities or subcutaneous edema, or both, occurred in 82 per cent of the 196 patients with lymphoma studied by us. Wong and associates[60] at necropsy found effusions or edema, or both, in 80 per cent of 141 patients with Hodgkin's disease. Pleural or peritoneal effusions, or both, have even been the initial clinical manifestation of malignant lymphoma.[61]

The causes of fluid retention in patients with lymphoma appear to be: (1) lymphatic or venous obstruction by enlarged lymph nodes; (2) transudation or exudation from invaded organs; (3) complicating associated illness; and (4) hypoalbuminemia. Of the four, hypoalbuminemia occurs most frequently. The serum albumin was less than 3.5 gm./100 ml. in 94 per cent of our patients and in 80 per cent of those studied by Wong et al. in whom this determination was recorded. The serum albumin was less than 4 gm./100 ml. in 83 per cent of the 112 patients with Hodgkin's disease studied at necropsy by Levitan and associates.[18] The cause of the hypoalbuminemia is uncertain. Levitan and co-workers[19] and Wong and associates[60] found no correlation between the presence of hepatic Hodgkin's disease and hypoalbuminemia. Similarly, infiltration of the kidneys by lymphoma does not cause the hypoalbuminemia.[19] Also, excessive loss of protein by the intestinal tract has rarely been demonstrated in patients with lymphoma.[62] Although the effusions into body cavities in subjects with lymphoma are usually serious, heart failure uncommonly appears to be the cause.[60] Pleural, pulmonary and mediastinal lymphomatous deposits are common in the subjects with pleural effusions, and nearly all patients with pericardial effusions also have pleural effusions. Wong and associates found little correlation between the presence of ascites and the incidence of severely enlarged retroperitoneal lymph nodes or hepatic Hodgkin's disease. Likewise, these authors found little correlation between edema of the legs and the incidence of compression of the inferior vena cava by enlarged lymph nodes, tumor invasion, or thrombus, or the incidence of severely enlarged inguinal or iliac lymph nodes. Malnutrition, decreased protein production and increased protein catabolism probably play important roles in causing hypoalbuminemia in these patients.

Electrocardiographic Changes: Although various arrhythmias and heart block secondary to lymphomatous infiltration of the heart have been described,[17,41,57] the present study indicates that electrocardiographic disturbances occur as commonly in patients with lymphoma and no cardiac involvement as in those with lymphoma and cardiac involvement. Nevertheless, the sudden appearance of second or third degree heart block or of an ectopic tachycardia in a patient with lymphoma (or any other malignant tumor) and no underlying cardiac disease certainly suggests cardiac involvement. Premature contractions, ST-T wave changes, low voltage and bundle branch block are not useful in distinguishing patients with from those without cardiac lymphoma. Low voltage occurred commonly, and usually these patients had pleural effusions or, less often, pericardial effusions. Irradiation may cause disappearance of heart block, as illustrated by the patient described in Figures 9 to 11. Davies[63] described a patient with lymphosarcoma who had periodic syncope that he attributed to infiltration of the left vagus nerve by lymphoma since the heart was free of lymphoma. Heart block, however, was not documented by electrocardiogram in this case.

Primary Lymphoma of Heart: Although they occur rarely in patients with systemic lymphoma, signs and symptoms of cardiac dysfunction occur uniformly in patients with primary lymphoma of the heart. Hodgkin's disease and mycosis fungoides lymphoma originating in the heart have not been described, but at least 7 patients with primary cardiac lymphosarcoma[64–67] and 11 with primary cardiac reticulum cell sarcoma[68–77] have been reported. No patient in the present study had primary lymphoma of the heart. Systemic lymphosarcoma and reticulum cell sarcoma involving the heart, however, are identical histologically to primary cardiac lymphoma of corresponding types. Primary lymphosarcoma or reticulum cell sarcoma of the heart may occur at any age, reported from 1 to 84 years,[74,75] and signs and symptoms caused by cardiac involvement or obstruction of the venae cavae are nearly always the most impressive clinical feature. The primary cardiac lymphomatous tumors are large, may involve the pericardium and any chamber, most frequently the right atrium, and lead to death within months after the onset of symptoms.

Lymphomas in Animals: Lymphosarcoma and reticulum cell sarcoma occur spontaneously in a number of animals, probably most commonly the cow. Mycosis fungoides appears to be limited to human beings, and there is debate whether or not true Hodgkin's disease occurs in animals.[78–80] When malignant lymphoma occurs in animals, metastases to the heart are frequent. Smith[81] found cardiac tumor nodules in 586 of 1,113 cows with lymphoma. The heart, after the lymph nodes, was the organ most frequently involved. This author found the cardiac metastases most frequently in the atrial walls, but they also occurred in the ventricular free walls and septum. Clinical signs or symptoms of cardiac dysfunction were uncommon in the cows, although "a few" with tumor in the heart died suddenly. Other reports have described and illustrated systemic lymphosarcoma and reticulum cell sarcoma with involvement of the heart in cows, dogs and rabbits.[82–84]

Summary

Of 196 patients with malignant lymphoma studied at autopsy, 48 (24 per cent) had lymphoma involving the heart. In 27 subjects the cardiac lymphoma was observed on gross examination, and in the other 21 it was found only on study of histologic sections. Lymphoma in the heart occurred most frequently in mycosis fungoides (33 per cent) and least frequently in Hodgkin's disease (16 per cent). Cardiac lymphoma was found in approximately 25 per cent of patients with lymphosarcoma, reticulum cell sarcoma and undifferentiated or mixed cell malignant lymphoma. The cardiac metastases when observed grossly were usually firm white focal nodules located most frequently in the pericardium but also often in the walls of the chambers. In 9 patients the cardiac lymphoma extended through the wall of a cardiac chamber or septum.

The incidence of dyspnea, chest pain, effusions into body cavities, precordial murmurs, ventricular gallops, edema and electrocardiographic disturbances was similar in patients with and without cardiac lymphoma, and these clinical findings most often were the result of mediastinal, pleural or pulmonary lymphoma, anemia, hypoalbuminemia, or an underlying cardiac condition. Signs or symptoms of cardiac dysfunction could be attributed to lymphomatous involvement of the heart in only 5 of the 48 patients with cardiac lymphoma. Three of them had mycosis fungoides, and 2, Hodgkin's disease.

References

1. Glancy, D. L. and Roberts, W. C. The heart in malignant melanoma. A study of 70 autopsy cases. *Am. J. Cardiol.*, 21: 555, 1968.
2. Roberts, W. C., Bodey, G. P. and Wertlake, P. T. The heart in acute leukemia. A study of 420 autopsy cases. *Am. J. Cardiol.*, 21: 388, 1968.
3. Carney, E. K., Oppelt, W. W., Gleason, W. L. and Brindley, C. O. Cardiac Hodgkin's disease. A clinical, hemodynamic, and angiocardiographic evaluation of a case. *Am. Heart J.*, 64: 106, 1962.
4. Krueger, F. J. and Meyer, O. O. Lymphogranulomatosis (Hodgkin's disease). A review of sixty cases. *J. Lab. & Clin. Med.*, 21: 682, 1936.
5. Scott, R. W. and Garvin, C. F. Tumors of the heart and pericardium. *Am. Heart J.*, 17: 431, 1939.
6. Herbut, P. A. and Maisel, A. L. Secondary tumors of the heart. *Arch. Path.*, 34: 358, 1942.
7. Jackson, H., Jr. and Parker, F., Jr. Hodgkin's Disease and Allied Disorders, p. 177. New York, 1947. Oxford University Press.
8. Symmers, D. Lymphoid diseases. Hodgkin's granuloma, giant follicular lymphadenopathy, lymphoid leukemia, lymphosarcoma and gastrointestinal pseudoleukemia. *Arch. Path.*, 45: 73, 1948.
9. Rottino, A. and Hoffman, G. T. Cardiac involvement in Hodgkin's disease. *Am. Heart J.*, 43: 115, 1952.
10. Lucia, S. P., Mills, H., Lowenhaupt, E. and Hunt, M. L. Visceral involvement in primary neoplastic diseases of the reticulo-endothelial system. *Cancer*, 5: 1193, 1952.
11. Nabarro, J. D. N. Cardiac involvement in malignant lymphoma. *Arch. Int. Med.*, 92: 258, 1953.
12. DeLoach, J. F. and Haynes, J. W. Secondary tumors of the heart and pericardium: Review of the subject and report of one hundred thirty-seven cases. *Arch. Int. Med.*, 91: 224, 1953.
13. Bisel, H. F., Wróblewski, F. and LaDue, J. S. Incidence and clinical manifestations of cardiac metastases. *J.A.M.A.*, 153: 712, 1953.
14. Young, J. M. and Goldman, I. R. Tumor metastasis to the heart. *Circulation*, 9: 220, 1954.
15. Gassman, H. S., Meadows, R., Jr., and Baker, L. A. Metastatic tumors of the heart. *Am. J. Med.*, 19: 357, 1955.
16. Goudie, R. B. Secondary tumors of the heart and pericardium. *Brit. Heart J.*, 17: 183, 1955.
17. Jakob, H. G. and Zirkin, R. M. Hodgkin's disease with involvement of the heart and pericardium. *J.A.M.A.*, 173: 338, 1960.
18. Levitan, R., Diamond, H. D. and Craver, L. F. The liver in Hodgkin's disease. *Gut*, 2: 60, 1961.
19. Richmond, J., Sherman, R. S., Diamond, H. D. and Craver, L. F. Renal lesions associated with malignant lymphomas. *Am. J. Med.*, 32: 184, 1962.
20. Madianos, M. and Sokal, J. E. Cardiac involvement in lymphosarcoma and reticulum cell sarcoma. *Am. Heart J.*, 65: 322, 1963.
21. Wright, D. H. Burkitt's tumour. A post-mortem study of 50 cases. *Brit. J. Surg.*, 51: 245, 1964.
22. Wilkinson, H. A. iii, Hutchins, G. M. and Hartman, W. H. Occurrence of "African lymphoma syndrome" in Baltimore, Maryland. *Johns Hopkins M. J.*, 121: 21, 1967.
23. Block, J. B., Edgcomb, J., Eisen, A. and Van Scott, E. J. Mycosis fungoides. Natural history and aspects of its relationship to other malignant lymphomas. *Am. J. Med.*, 34: 228, 1963.
24. Edgcomb, J., Block, J., Eisen, A. and Van Scott, E. Mycosis fungoides. In: Conference on Biology of Cutaneous Cancer, National Cancer Institute Monograph No. 10, 1963, pp. 278–280.
25. Liechti, E. Über Tumoren innerer Organe bei Mycosis fungoides. *Arch. Dermat. u. Syph.*, 154: 246, 1928.
26. Berman, L. Pathologic nature of mycosis fungoides. *Arch. Path.*, 29: 530, 1940.
27. Gall, E. A. Enigmas in lymphoma. Reticulum cell sarcoma and mycosis fungoides. *Minnesota Med.*, 38: 674, 1955.
28. Cyr, D. P., Geokas, M. C. and Worsley, G. H. Mycosis fungoides. Hematologic findings and terminal course. *Arch. Dermat.*, 94: 558, 1966.
29. Paltauf, R. and Scherber, G. Ein fall von Mycosis fungoides mit Erkankung von Nerven und mit Lokalisation in den inneren Organen. *Virchows Arch. path. Anat.*, 222: 9, 1916.
30. Gödel, A. Zur pathologischen Anatomie der Mycosis fungoides. *Arch. Dermat. u. Syph.*, 130: 172, 1921.
31. Goldsmith, W. N. Specimens from a case of mycosis fungoides of internal organs. *Brit. J. Dermat.*, 43: 528, 1931.
32. Zinck, K. H. Die neubildung lymphoiden Gewebes bei der Mycosis fungoides. *Virchows Arch. path. Anat.*, 296: 319, 1935.
33. Pautrier, L. M., Hoerner, G. and Woringer, F. Résultats fournis par l'autopsie du cas de mycosis fongoide avec tumeurs, présente à la séance de mars dermier. *Bull. Soc. franc. dermat. et syph.*, 47: 8, 1940.
34. Hemmingson, H. Ein Fall von Mycosis fungoides mit Metastasierung als polymorphzelliges Sarkom. *Acta radiol.*, 22: 606, 1941.
35. Arzt, L. Mycosis fungoïdes (Alibert) et lymphogranulomatose (Palt-auf-Sternberg), leur pathogenese et leur diagnostic différentiel. *Bull. Soc. franc. dermat. et syph.*, 54: 204, 1947.
36. Curtis, A. C., Cawley, E. P. and Leach, J. E. K. Is mycosis fungoides a reticuloendothelial neoplastic entity? *A.M.A. Arch. Dermat.*, 64: 255, 1951.
37. Morris, L. M. Metastases to the heart from malignant tumors. *Am. Heart J.*, 3: 219, 1927.
38. Lisa, J. R., Hirschhorn, L. and Hart, C. A. Tumors of the heart. Report of four cases and review of literature. *Arch. Int. Med.*, 67: 91, 1941.
39. Steven, R. A. Heart tumor: Report of a case. *Am. Heart J.*, 30: 411, 1945.
40. Pilcher, R. B. Lymphosarcoma invading the heart: A report of three cases with autopsy findings. *M. J. Australia*, 2: 366, 1950.
41. Fishberg, A. M. Auricular fibrillation and flutter in metastatic growths of the right auricle. *Am. J. M. Sc.*, 180: 629, 1930.
42. Greiner, D. J. Reticulum cell sarcoma involving

the heart and pericardium. *Bull. School Med. Univ. Maryland*, 25: 44, 1940.

43. BRICK, J. B. and GREENFIELD, M. Reticulum cell sarcoma with cardiac metastasis. Report of two cases with ante-mortem diagnosis of one. *Am. Heart J.*, 34: 599, 1947.
44. HURST, J. W. and COOPER, H. R. Neoplastic disease of the heart. *Am. Heart J.*, 50: 782, 1955.
45. TERPLAN, K. and MITTELBACH, M. Beiträge zur Lymphogranulomatose und zu anderen Eigenartigen, verallgemeinerten Granulomen der Lymphknoten. *Virchows Arch. path. Anat.*, 271: 759, 1929.
46. BARONE, V. G. Sopra un caso di linfogranulomatosi maligna cervico-mediastinica, con infiltrazione secondaria del cuore e del polmone. *Riforma med.*, 46: 1949, 1930.
47. RIMBAUD, P. L'évolution de la lymphogranulomatose maligne. Développement insidieux d'une forme médiastinale avec localisations viscérales multiples. *Ann. d'anat. path.*, 11: 43, 1934.
48. DALOUS, J. F. and PONS, H. Un cas de pancardite Hodgkinienne. *Arch. mal coeur*, 29: 89, 1936.
49. HARRELL, G. T. Hodgkin's disease with invasion of pericardium and gallbladder. Review of the literature and report of a case with autopsy. *Arch. Path.*, 28: 58, 1939.
50. RITVO, M. Hodgkin's disease. Report of a case with unusual longevity and invasion of the heart and pericardium. *New England J. Med.*, 223: 891, 1940.
51. GARVIN, C. F. Hodgkin's disease of the heart and pericardium. *J.A.M.A.*, 117: 1876, 1941.
52. CATSARAS, J. and PATSOURI, E. Über eine Blastomatös wachsende Form von Herz- und Leberlymphogranulomatose. *Virchows Arch. path. Anat.*, 307: 297, 1941.
53. AYERZA, L. and CERNICH, R. Granuloma maligno primitivo del pericardio (caso princeps). *Rev. Asoc. méd. argent.*, 57: 981, 1943.
54. RAST, H., WEBER, F. P. and GREENFIELD, J. G. Hodgkin's disease of unusual distribution apparently primarily of mediastinum, with multiple involvement of heart (epicardium). *M. Press & Circular*, 214: 30, 1945.
55. MCCOY, J. J., JR. Hodgkin's disease involving the epicardium. Report of a case. *U.S. Nav. M. Bull.*, 48: 272, 1948.
56. HAGANS, J. A Hodgkin's granuloma with pericardial effusion. An unusual case of Hodgkin's disease presenting initially the signs and symptoms of pericarditis with effusion. *Am. Heart J.*, 40: 624, 1950.
57. GOGGIO, A. F., HARKNESS, J. T. and PALMER, W. S. Stokes-Adams syndrome in Hodgkin's granuloma. *J.A.M.A.*, 176: 687, 1961.
58. BRUN, F., FREYCON, F. and FROMENT, R. Deux observations de maladie d'Hodgkin a forme de péricardite liquidienne initiale. *Lyon med.*, 211: 811, 1964.
59. COHN, K. E., STEWART, J. R., FAJARDO, L. F. and HANCOCK, E. W. Heart disease following radiation. *Medicine*, 46: 281, 1967.
60. WONG, F. M., GRACE, W. J. and ROTTINO, A. Pleural effusions, ascites, pericardial effusions and edema in Hodgkin's disease. *Am. J. M. Sc.*, 246: 678, 1963.
61. YUEH-SHU, C., KUEI-JU, C., TA-EN, P., CHI-HSÜN, L. and SE-HSI, C. Malignant lymphomas with special manifestations. *Chinese M. J.*, 85: 229, 1966.
62. JEFFRIES, G. H., HOLMAN, H. R. and SLEISENGER, M. H. Plasma proteins and the gastrointestinal tract. *New England J. Med.*, 266: 652, 1962.
63. DAVIES, P. Sino-auricular block associated with intrathoracic new growths. *Brit. Heart J.*, 19: 431, 1957.
64. CERUTI, R. Un caso di neoplasia maligna del cuore. *Osservatore med.*, 3: 9, 1925.
65. MORRIS, J. J. Primary sarcoma of heart. *J. Lab. & Clin. Med.*, 18: 935, 1933.
66. KEAT, E. C. B. and TWYMAN, V. R. Cardiac involvement in lymphosarcoma with spontaneous rupture of the heart. *Brit. Heart J.*, 17: 563, 1955.
67. SOMERS, K. and LOTHE, F. Primary lymphosarcoma of the heart. Review of the literature and report of 3 cases. *Cancer*, 13: 449, 1960.
68. HARTMANN, G. Ungewöhnliche Metastasierung eines primären Rundzellensarkoms des Herzens. (Haemangiosis cutis et renum.) *Frankfurt Ztschr. Path.*, 53: 602, 1939.
69. TEDESCHI, C. Primary sarcoma of the heart. *Arch. Path.*, 37: 70, 1944.
70. WHORTON, C. M. Primary malignant tumors of the heart. Report of a case. *Cancer*, 2: 245, 1949.
71. DLUHOŠ, M. Primární retothelsarkom srdce. *Časop. lék česk.*, 87: 641, 1948.
72. DAGNINI, G. Reticolosarcoma primitivo del cuore. *Arch. ital. di anat. e istol. pat.*, 23: 470, 1950.
73. COURTOY, P. and POTVLIEGE, P. Cancer primitif du coeur. Considerations sur le bloc de branche. *Acta cardiol.*, 6: 1027, 1951.
74. GILLET, P. and PARMENTIER, R. Reticulosarcome à départ cardiaque chez un enfant de seize mois. *Acta paediat. belg.*, 7: 27, 1953.
75. BRUCKER, E. A., JR., and GLASSY, F. J. Primary reticulum-cell sarcoma of the heart with review of the literature. *Cancer*, 8: 921, 1955.
76. KAUFMAN, B. H. and COHEN, S. E. Primary tumor of the heart (reticulum cell sarcoma). *New York J. Med.*, 57: 2652, 1957.
77. SPIGOLON, G. and VANGELISTA, F. Su un raro tumore primitivo del duore: istiocitoblastoma ad evoluzione reticolosarcomatosa. *Arch. ital. anat. e istol. pat.*, 31: 50, 1957.
78. MACMAHON, H. E. A case of Hodgkin's disease in a dog. *Am. J. Path.*, 10: 309, 1934.
79. STALKER, L. K., SCHLOTTHAUER, C. F. and FELDMAN, W. H. Probable Hodgkin's disease in a dog: Report of a case. *Am. J. Cancer*, 28: 595, 1936.
80. MEDLAR, E. M. and SASANO, K. T. An interpretation of the nature of Hodgkin's disease. III. Report of a neoplasm in the rabbit which corresponds closely to Hodgkin's disease in man. *Am. J. Cancer*, 29: 102, 1937.
81. SMITH, H. A. The pathology of malignant lymphoma in cattle. A study of 1113 cases. *Path. vet.*, 2: 68, 1965.
82. SAVAGE, A. and ISA, J. M. Lymphocytoma in a cow's heart. *Cornell Vet.*, 36: 279, 1946.
83. SMITH, H. A. Malignant lymphomas in animals. A survey of present knowledge. *Am. J. Clin. Path.*, 38: 75, 1962.
84. JUBB, K. V. F. and KENNEDY, P. C. Pathology of Domestic Animals, Vol. I, pp. 305–313. New York, 1963. Academic Press.

Pericardiectomy for Radiation-induced Pericarditis with Effusion

Donald L. Morton, M.D., A. Robert Kagan, M.D., William C. Roberts, M.D., Kevin P. O'Brien, M.B., Ch.B., Elbert C. Holmes, M.D., and Paul C. Adkins, M.D.

The heart and pericardium were once assumed to be resistant to radiation damage [1], but recent reports [2–5, 7–10] have disproved this assumption. Chronic pericardial effusion appears to be the most frequent clinical manifestation of radiation injury. Sixteen patients who developed chronic pericardial effusions following mediastinal irradiation for Hodgkin's disease have been studied at the National Cancer Institute since 1966. This report describes observations in these 16 patients and the results of subtotal pericardiectomy in 11 of them.

CLINICAL MATERIAL

Each patient was referred to the Radiation or Medicine Branch of the National Cancer Institute for treatment of histologically proved Hodgkin's disease. Cardiac dysfunction first appeared in each only after mediastinal irradiation. The dose to the anterior mediastinum through anterior fields varied from

From the Branches of Surgery and Radiation, National Cancer Institute, and the Section of Cardiac Pathology and Cardiology Branch, National Heart Institute, National Institutes of Health, Bethesda, Md.; and George Washington University School of Medicine, Washington, D.C.

Presented at the Fifth Annual Meeting of The Society of Thoracic Surgeons, San Diego, Calif., Jan. 27–29, 1969.

Address reprint requests to Dr. Morton, Surgery Branch, National Cancer Institute, National Institutes of Health, Bethesda, Md. 20014.

3,000 rads in three weeks to 4,000 rads in four to six weeks. The dose to the anterior portions of the heart and pericardium varied from 4,500 rads in three weeks to 5,200 to 7,200 rads in four to six weeks and depended to some degree on the anterior-posterior diameter of the chest. Three patients were irradiated from several portals, often receiving repeated courses of irradiation for recurrent disease in the mediastinum. Fourteen patients who developed radiation pericarditis had mediastinal Hodgkin's disease when radiation therapy was initiated; however, 2 patients received mediastinal irradiation because lymph nodes involved with Hodgkin's disease were adjacent to the mediastinum.

Before August, 1967, most patients with radiation-induced pericarditis and effusion were treated only by pericardicentesis and supportive care. The results of nonoperative therapy were unsatisfactory, and 5 patients treated in this manner died. The usual response to conservative therapy is illustrated by G. S., a 26-year-old man admitted on February 1, 1967, with dyspnea, orthopnea, and swelling of the legs and abdomen. Two years previously he had received mediastinal irradiation with a maximum pericardial dose of 5,000 rads in five weeks for Hodgkin's disease. Examination revealed dyspnea with rapid respirations (40 per minute), tachycardia (150 beats per minute), distended neck veins, and pulsus paradoxus of 22 mm. Hg. Chest roentgenogram showed an enlarged cardiac silhouette and bilateral pleural effusions. The patient was much improved following pericardicentesis with removal of 200 ml. of bloody fluid. A week later, however, cardiac tamponade recurred requiring a second pericardicentesis of 210 ml. of fluid. Following digitalization he was again much improved, but seven weeks later signs of acute tamponade returned. Pericardicentesis was repeated and 330 ml. of fluid obtained. The patient died shortly thereafter with evidence of acute tamponade. Postmortem examination revealed thick, hemorrhagic visceral and parietal pericardia with 375 ml. of pericardial fluid (Fig. 1).

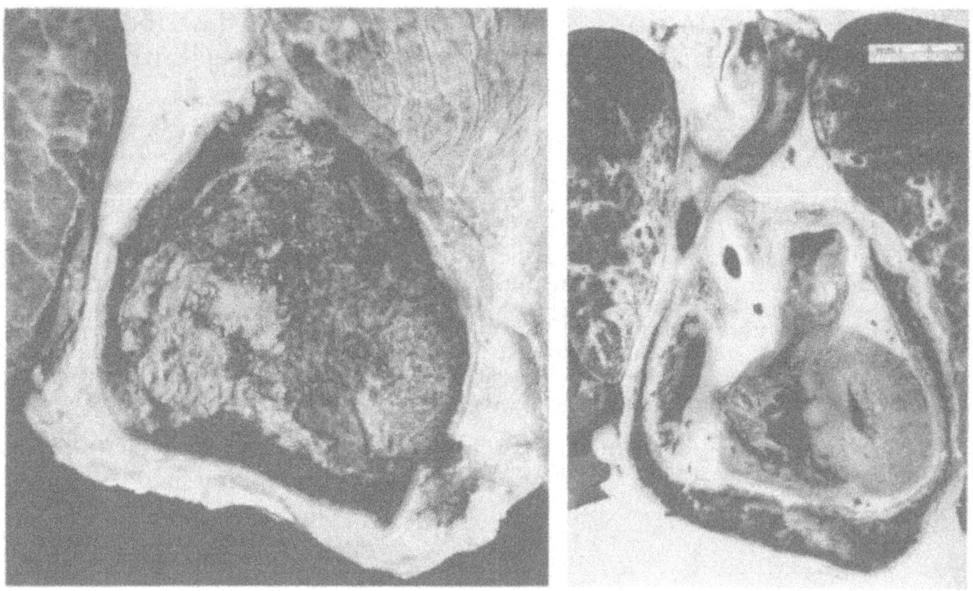

A B

FIG. 1. Heart of patient G. S. (A) The anterior parietal pericardium has been removed exposing the ragged hemorrhagic epicardium. (B) Longitudinal section through the lungs and heart. The parietal pericardium is thick and adherent to both lungs. A large pericardial effusion was present. A thrombus occludes the innominate vein.

Dissatisfaction with the results of conservative therapy for radiation-induced pericardial effusions, and the discovery that most of these effusions were not associated with recurrent Hodgkin's disease, prompted therapy by subtotal pericardiectomy. The clinical features of 11 patients who have undergone subtotal pericardiectomy are summarized in Table 1.

The interval between the initiation of radiation therapy and the appearance of pericardial effusion varied from 6 to 26 months (see Table 1). The course of these pericardial effusions was extremely variable. Most effusions produced no symptoms in the beginning; in fact, only patient No. 3 had evidence of acute pericarditis coincident with the appearance of the pericardial effusion. Some effusions persisted as long as 10 months (Fig. 2) while producing minimal signs of cardiac compression; others progressed to acute tamponade within four to six weeks. In patient No. 7 the effusion completely resolved and progressed to pericardial constriction with obliteration of the pericardial space in seven weeks (Fig. 3). In many patients an unexplained temporary decrease in the transverse cardiac diameter (Fig. 2) occurred shortly after the initiation of radiation therapy [9].

The duration of the effusion before signs of cardiac tamponade appeared in this group of patients is indicated in Table 1 as the time interval between the onset of the effusion and pericardiectomy. When pericardiectomy was performed, patients Nos. 1 through 7 had clinical features of cardiac tamponade including dyspnea, tachycardia, jugular venous distention, pleural effusion, and pulsus paradoxus. Four of these 7 patients (Nos. 1–4) had signs of acute tamponade necessitating emergency pericardicentesis. The other 4 patients (Nos. 8–11) were asymptomatic, although each had large pericardial effusions with elevated central venous pressures and pulsus paradoxus greater than 10 mm. Hg.

PREOPERATIVE EVALUATION

The diagnosis of pericardial effusion usually was suggested first by progressive enlargement of the cardiac silhouette on chest roentgenogram following mediastinal irradiation. Dyspnea, venous distension, pulsus paradoxus, and other signs of cardiac tamponade usually appeared only after enlargement of the cardiac silhouette had been present for some time. Cardiac scans with technetium-labeled albumin (Fig. 4) were obtained for 9 patients and helped to confirm the diagnosis of pericardial effusion. Conclusive diagnosis of pericardial effusion was made by pericardicentesis with injection of air (pneumopericardium). Pericardicentesis also helped in evaluating the extent to which the effusion contributed to cardiac compression. The elevated central venous pressure was usually returned toward normal after removing 200 to 300 ml. of pericardial fluid.

The electrocardiograms in all patients were abnormal. The most frequent changes were decreased voltages of the QRS complexes, but flattening and inversion of the T waves and ST segment changes were also seen.

Right-heart catheterization in 7 patients revealed abnormalities with mild to moderate elevations of the right atrial and right ventricular end-diastolic pressures in 5 patients (Table 2). The hemodynamic abnormalities were proportional to the severity of the clinical signs and symptoms of cardiac tamponade. Cardiac catheterization was performed in only 1 of the 4 patients with acute tamponade. In this patient (No. 4), removal of 1,500 ml. of pericardial fluid produced dramatic improvement in cardiac hemodynamics. Angiocardiography was performed at the time of cardiac catheterization in 7 patients and confirmed the presence of an effusion that previously had been demonstrated by cardiac scan.

The volume of pericardial fluid removed by pericardicentesis or at the time of pericardiectomy varied from 400 to 1,800 ml. (see Table 1). The effusions were serofibrinous exudates with total protein contents of 4 to 6 gm. per 100 ml. In 2 patients, the effusions were bloody, and in 8, "straw-colored." Cytological examination of the pericardial fluid was carried out in all cases, and in none were tumor cells observed.

TABLE 1. CLINICAL SUMMARY OF PATIENTS WITH PERICARDIAL EFFUSIONS TREATED BY PERICARDIECTOMY

Case No.	Patient's Age & Sex	Time Between Radiation and Effusion (mo.)	Time Between Effusion and Pericardiectomy (mo.)	Clinical Features: Elevated Venous Pressure	Pulsus Paradoxus	Dyspnea	Hypotension	Size of Effusion (ml.)	Postoperative Status: Length of Follow-up (mo.)	Recurrent Hodgkin's Disease
1	35,F	6	1	+	+	+	+	500	25	Yes; receiving radiation therapy
2	54,M	18	2	+	+	+	+	470	17	No
3	23,M	26	1	+	+	+	+	500	15	Yes; receiving chemotherapy
4	24,M	12	4	+	+	+	+	1,800	12	No
5	29,M	10	2	+	+	+	0	1,250	13	Yes; receiving chemotherapy
6	20,M	14	11	+	+	+	0	900	4	Yes; receiving chemotherapy
7	27,F	11	2	+	+	+	0	—[a]	1	No
8	29,M	15	6	+	+	0	0	400	11	No
9	18,M	16	6	+	+	0	0	700	8	No
10	21,M	11	6	+	+	0	0	800	3	No
11	20,F	6	9	+	+	0	0	600	2	Yes; receiving radiation therapy

[a]This patient developed pericardial constriction with obliteration of the pericardial space following complete resorption of a pericardial effusion.

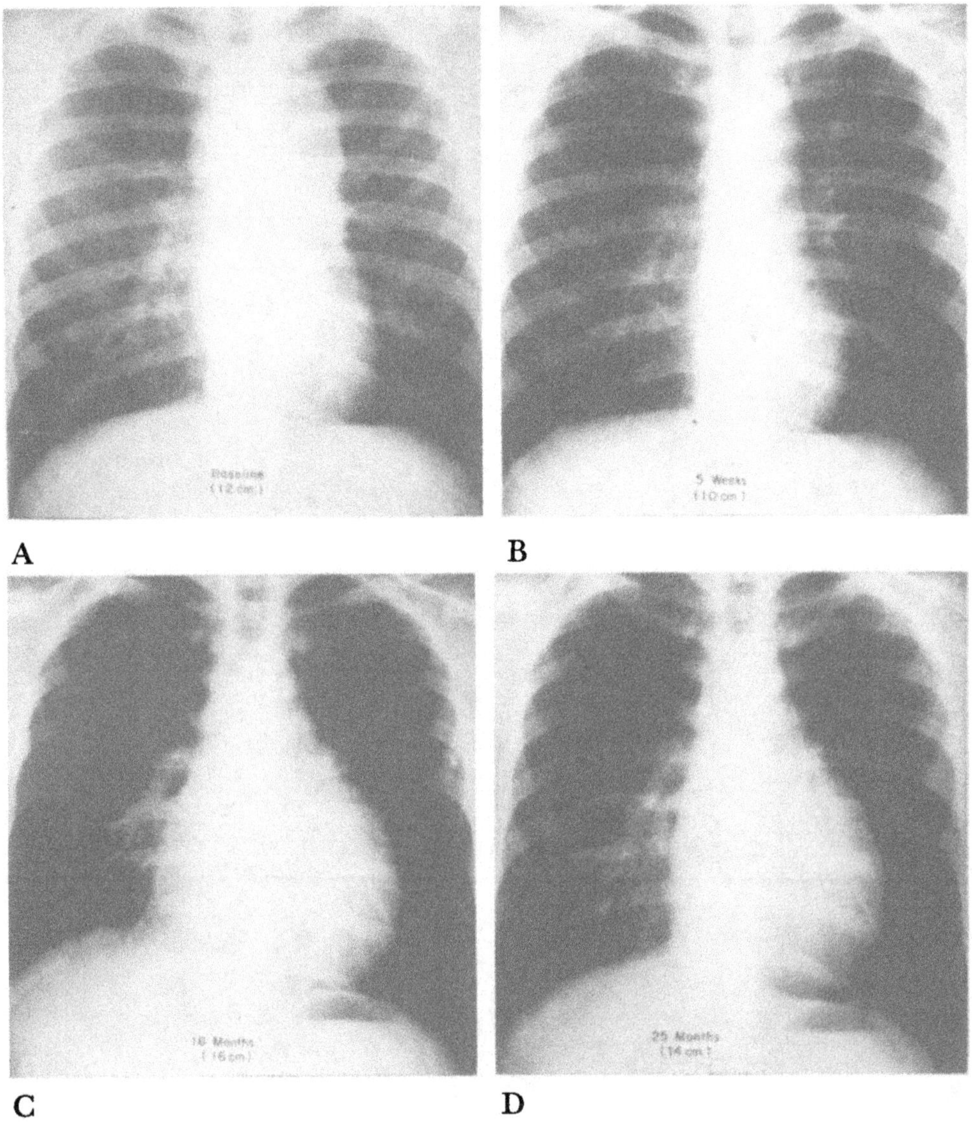

FIG. 2. (A) This 20-year-old man (No. 6, Table 1) received 5,400 rads of radiation in five weeks for mediastinal Hodgkin's disease. (B) Five weeks after radiation therapy was initiated his cardiac silhouette had decreased in size to 10 cm. transverse cardiac diameter. (C) An enlarging cardiac silhouette was first noted 14 months after irradiation and had increased to 16 cm. by 16 months after irradiation. (D) No symptoms of cardiac dysfunction occurred until 25 months after irradiation.

OPERATIVE MANAGEMENT

Pericardicentesis was performed preoperatively under local anesthesia in 6 patients with signs of cardiac tamponade to prevent acute cardiac decompensation at the induction of anesthesia. Pericardiectomy was accomplished through a left anterolateral thoracotomy incision. The parietal pericardium was usually thickened and stretched by the enclosed effusion. The thickening was most

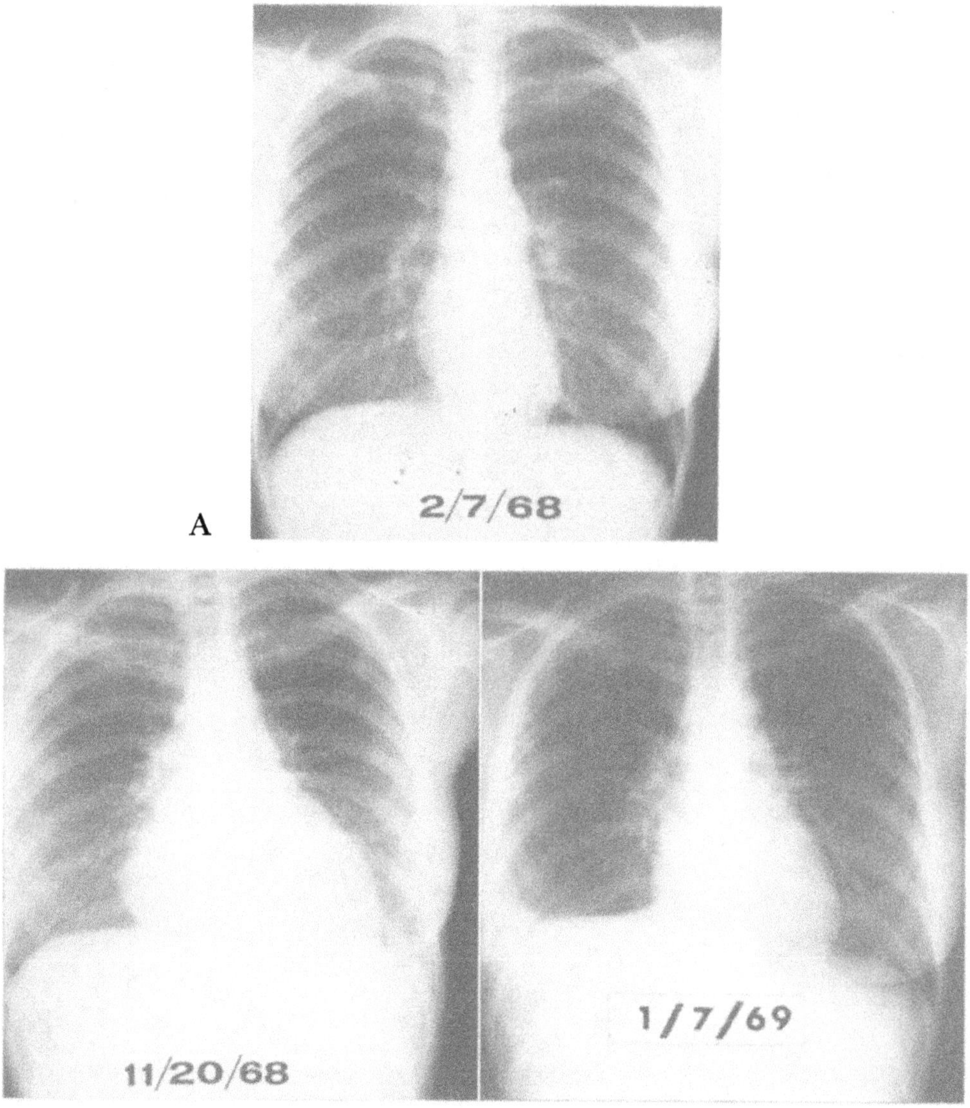

A

B C

FIG. 3. (A) This 27-year-old woman (No. 7, Table 1) received irradiation for mediastinal Hodgkin's disease in December, 1967. (B) She developed a pericardial effusion on November 20, 1968, associated with dyspnea, jugular venous distension, and pulsus paradoxus. (C) By January 7, 1969, her cardiac silhouette had returned to almost normal. Pericardial constriction with fusion of the visceral and parietal pericardia was found at the time of pericardiectomy.

marked anteriorly behind the sternum, the site that received the largest doses of irradiation. Similarly, the epicardium over the anterior surface of the right ventricle was always thickened, whereas the epicardium over the left ventricle was often normal. The epicardial fibrosis, however, was not sufficiently thick or confluent to cause cardiac constriction in any patient except patient No. 7. In 3 patients shaggy fibrinous exudates were present over the pericardial surfaces

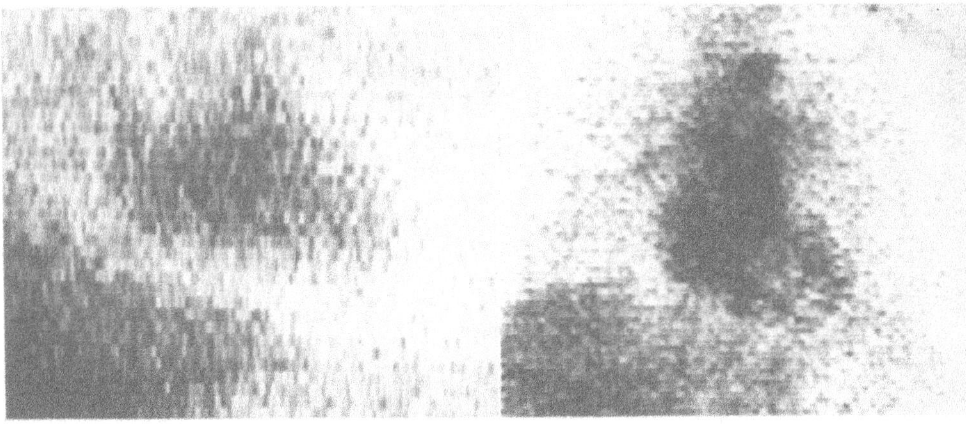

A B

FIG. 4. (A) Cardiac scan with technetium-labeled albumin (patient No. 4, Table 1), showing an abnormally wide space between the heart and liver produced by the pericardial effusion. (B) Scan showing the normal space between the heart and liver.

with adhesions between the visceral and parietal pericardia. These exudates had not yet organized and therefore could be separated easily from the underlying epicardium. Patient No. 7, however, had progressed to pericardial constriction with fusion of the visceral and parietal pericardia (Fig. 2). The thick fibrinous membrane that was closely adherent to the underlying epicardium in this patient was dissected free only with considerable difficulty. Tumor nodules were not observed on the cardiac surface of the parietal pericardium or on the epicardium in any of the 11 patients; however, 2 patients had tumor nodules on the pleural surface of the parietal pericardium.

A subtotal pericardiectomy was performed by removing as much of the damaged parietal pericardium as possible. The anterior parietal pericardium was dissected free from behind the sternum and removed from the diaphragm to the atrioventricular groove and to the base of the aorta and pulmonary trunk. Posteriorly, the excision extended to the junction of the inferior vena cava and right atrium, and posterolaterally, on the left to the most caudal pulmonary vein. The phrenic nerve and vessels were preserved with a 3-cm.-wide strip of underlying pericardium. A through-and-through biopsy of the right and left ventricular walls was carried out with a Vim Silverman needle in 3 patients to determine the extent of myocardial damage resulting from the irradiation. The entire operative procedure took one to two hours. Operative blood loss was less than 500 ml. in most patients, and only 3 patients received blood replacement.

Two operative complications occurred. The patient with constrictive pericarditis (No. 7) was reexplored for postoperative bleeding but afterward he made an uneventful recovery. A left phrenic nerve palsy occurred in patient No. 2 as a result of inadvertent division of the phrenic nerve, which was encased in an intensely fibrotic pericardium.

RESULTS OF PERICARDIECTOMY

All signs and symptoms of cardiac dysfunction that had been present preoperatively disappeared, and in all patients the central venous pressures returned to normal following pericardiectomy. The postoperative courses were uneventful in all patients, and all are now living and free of cardiac symptoms

TABLE 2. CARDIAC CATHETERIZATION DATA FROM PATIENTS TREATED BY PERICARDIECTOMY

Case No.	Right Atrial Pressure (mm. Hg) a/v	Right Atrial Pressure (mm. Hg) mean	Right Ventricular Pressure (mm. Hg) S/D	Pulmonary Arterial Pressure (mm. Hg) S/D	Pulmonary Arterial Pressure (mm. Hg) Mean	Cardiac Output (L/min.)	Cardiac Index (L/min./M^2)
4[a]	24/22	20	40/22	40/23	26	3.3	1.9
	8/5	5	24/7	26/10	—	6.4	3.6
5	17/15	13	28/16	33/17	23	7.0	2.9
6	12/10	8	23/10	23/11	13	5.6	3.0
8	9/7	6	24/7	24/10	14	5.6	2.9
9	8/6	6	20/8	20/14	16	5.3	3.1
10	10/8	8	24/10	24/12	16	7.2	3.7
11	8/7	7	20/7	20/10	12	5.0	2.9

[a]Measurements before and after removal of 1,500 ml. of pericardial fluid.

from 1 month to 2 years (average 9 months) after operation. Five patients have developed recurrent Hodgkin's disease, but none has had signs or symptoms of cardiac dysfunction. In each patient the tumor has been controlled by further irradiation or chemotherapy.

PATHOLOGY

Autopsies were performed in 4 of the 5 patients who died following non-operative management. In all 4 subjects the parietal pericardium was thickened, in 2 to severe degrees and in 2 to mild degrees. The latter 2 subjects, however, had large pericardial effusions of 800 and 900 ml. Of the 2 patients with severely thickened pericardia, 1 (Fig. 1) had an associated pericardial effusion of 375 ml. In the second patient the pericardial sac was totally obliterated by dense fibrous tissue. Recurrent Hodgkin's disease was not present within the pericardial sac or heart in any of the 4 autopsied subjects. All 4 had foci of interstitial myocardial fibrosis, most prominent in the right ventricular walls, and in addition, each had foci of mural and valvular endocardial thickening, all believed to be the result of irradiation.

The parietal pericardium was examined grossly and histologically in each of the 11 patients in whom pericardiectomy was carried out. In each the excised pericardium was thickened by fibrous tissue; the degree of thickness varied from two to nine times that of normal parietal pericardium. Several patients, in addi-

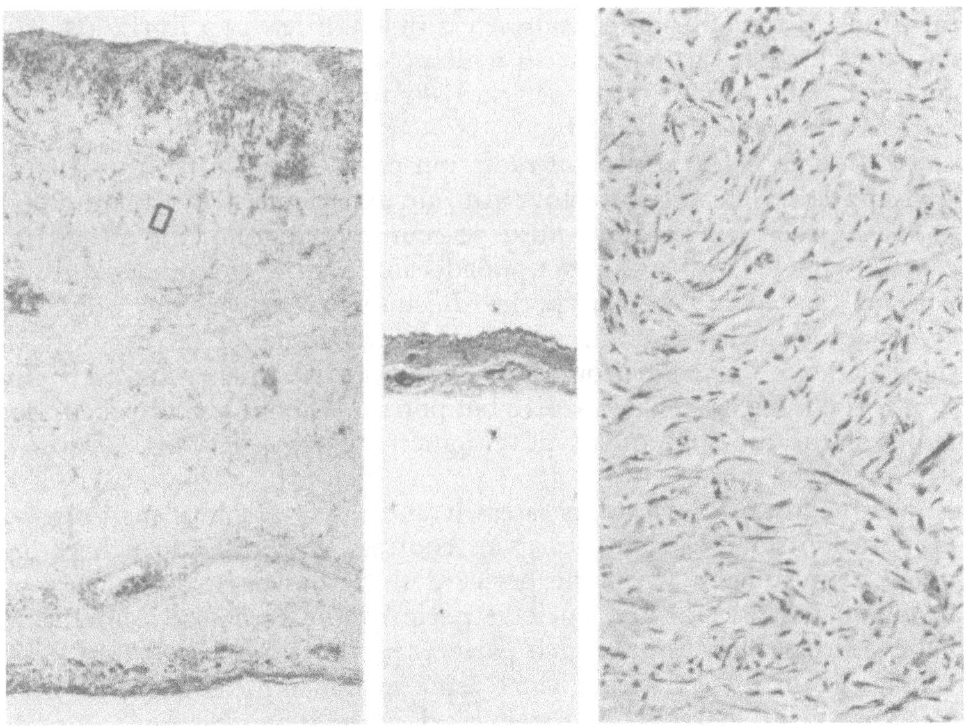

FIG. 5. Excised parietal pericardium (left) in patient No. 2. It is severely thickened (H&E; ×27). Normal parietal pericardium (center) in an adult patient without cardiac disease (H&E; ×27). Close-up view (right) of the thickened pericardium enclosed in the box in the photomicrograph at left. The fibroblasts show changes attributable to damage by irradiation (H&E; ×160).

tion, had focal deposits of fibrin on the cardiac surface of the parietal pericardium. Some degree of radiation damage was present in excised pericardia in 8 patients, as evidenced by atypical, hyperchromatic, and occasionally giant and bizarre-appearing fibroblasts and mesothelial cells and by increased numbers of vascular channels. Care should be taken to avoid confusing these radiation changes with Hodgkin's disease. Hodgkin's disease was found on the mediastinal surface of the parietal pericardia in 2 patients (Nos. 1, 10), but in none was tumor observed on the cardiac surface of, or within the substance of, the parietal pericardia. Myocardial biopsies carried out in 3 subjects disclosed mild interstitial fibrosis in the right ventricular walls in 2 of them. In the third patient the biopsied right ventricular myocardium appeared normal. The biopsied left ventricular myocardium in these 3 subjects appeared normal. Histological sections of the excised pericardia are illustrated in Figure 5.

COMMENT

Although large doses ($>$ 4,500 rads) of irradiation to the anterior mediastinum may injure myocardial fibers and cause patchy myocardial fibrosis, the mortality and morbidity from this irradiation usually results from pericardial injury. Radiation damage to the pericardium appears to cause an acute inflammation that often is followed first by a serofibrinous exudate and later by fibrosis and thickening of the pericardium. As the effusion is reabsorbed, it often leaves a fibrinous exudate over the pericardial surfaces which coagulates, becomes organized, and eventually may result in pericardial constriction with fusion of the visceral and parietal pericardia.

Conservative treatment of radiation pericarditis with chronic effusion appears to be unsatisfactory. In our experience with this method of management, pericardial fluid reaccumulated following pericardicentesis and led to cardiac tamponade and death. In contrast, all 11 patients treated by subtotal pericardiectomy are alive, and none has evidence of cardiac dysfunction. It is hoped that pericardiectomy in these patients with radiation-induced pericardial thickening and effusion will not only alleviate cardiac tamponade when it already exists but will prevent the subsequent development of constrictive pericarditis when it is not yet present.

Subtotal pericardiectomy is easily and safely accomplished during the effusion stage of the disease. In contrast, this procedure becomes much more difficult when the pericardial sac has been obliterated by fusion of the visceral and parietal pericardia. It seems reasonable to believe that removal of as much parietal pericardium as possible is advantageous in these patients, since some evidence of damage has been observed in all portions of the excised parietal pericardium. Simple pericardial drainage by creation of a pleuropericardial window only would not appear adequate, since it is probable that the damaged nonexcised pericardium will undergo further fibrosis which eventually may result in constriction.

Pericardiectomy is indicated in all patients with radiation pericarditis and chronic effusions who have symptoms of cardiac compression. In our experience, treatment by pericardicentesis alone often results in reaccumulation of the effusion and cardiac tamponade. Pericardiectomy is indicated even in patients with recurrent Hodgkin's disease, because improvements in the management of this disease with radiation therapy and chemotherapeutic agents permit significant long-term control and may be curative. Asymptomatic patients with chronic pericardial effusions persisting for more than six months also should undergo pericardiectomy to prevent the subsequent development of constrictive pericarditis. Moreover, a definitive diagnosis of the cause of the effusion will be established by pericardiectomy, and appropriate therapy can be carried out if recurrent Hodgkin's disease is present. Recurrent Hodgkin's disease was unexpectedly found in 2 of our 11 patients; further therapy was given, and now both patients are doing well.

Since intensive radiation therapy has greatly increased the cure rates in Hodgkin's disease [6], this method of therapy undoubtedly will be employed more widely in the future. Therefore, the incidence of radiation-induced pericarditis and effusion will probably increase as more patients with Hodgkin's disease survive sufficiently long to develop delayed heart disease from radiation damage. Hopefully, pericardiectomy will control the pericardial complications of this radiation injury; however, careful long-term follow-up is necessary to determine whether diffuse myocardial fibrosis or epicardial constriction will complicate the postpericardiectomy course of these patients.

SUMMARY

Although large doses of radiation to the anterior mediastinum may occasionally injure myocardial fibers and cause patchy myocardial fibrosis, the major morbidity and mortality from this irradiation usually results from pericardial injury. Radiation damage to the pericardium initially results in a serofibrinous effusion and pericardial thickening which frequently progresses to tamponade and constrictive pericarditis. Conservative therapy with pericardicentesis frequently results in reaccumulation of the effusion and reappearance of cardiac tamponade.

Removal of the radiation-damaged pericardium by subtotal pericardiectomy effectively relieves the cardiac tamponade and probably will prevent the subsequent development of constrictive pericarditis. Subtotal pericardiectomy can be accomplished easily and safely when an effusion is present. Eleven patients with radiation-induced pericardial effusions treated by subtotal pericardiectomy are living and well without evidence of cardiac dysfunction up to 2 years after operation.

Pericardiectomy appears indicated even in patients with effusions and recurrent Hodgkin's disease, since further irradiation or chemotherapy may be curative or provide long-term palliation.

REFERENCES

1. Ackerman, L. V., and Del Regato, J. A. *Cancer: Diagnosis, Treatment and Prognosis.* St. Louis: Mosby, 1954. P. 118.
2. Burch, G. E., Sohal, R. S., Sun, S. C., Miller, G. C., and Colgolough, H. L. Effects of radiation on the human heart: An electron microscopic study. *Arch. Intern. Med.* (Chicago) 121:230, 1968.
3. Cohn, K. E., Stewart, J. R., Fajardo, L. F., and Hancock, E. W. Heart disease following radiation therapy. *Medicine* 46:281, 1967.
4. Fajardo, L. F., Stewart, J. R., and Cohn, K. E. Morphology of radiation-induced heart disease. *Arch. Path.* (Chicago) 86:512, 1968.
5. Haas, J. M. Symptomatic constrictive pericarditis developing 45 years after radiation therapy to the mediastinum. A review of radiation pericarditis. *Amer. Heart J.* 77:89, 1969.
6. Kaplan, H. S. Clinical evaluation and radiotherapeutic management of Hodgkin's disease and the malignant lymphomas. *New Eng. J. Med.* 278:892, 1968.
7. Masland, D. S., Rotz, C. T., and Harris, J. H., Jr. Postradiation pericarditis with chronic pericardial effusion. *Ann. Intern. Med.* 69:97, 1968.
8. Muggia, F. M., and Cassileth, P. A. Constrictive pericarditis following radiation therapy. *Amer. J. Med.* 44:116, 1968.
9. Pierce, R. H., Haferman, M. D., and Kagan, A. R. Changes in the transverse cardiac diameter following mediastinal irradiation for Hodgkin's disease. *Radiology.* In press.
10. Stewart, J. R., Cohn, K. E., Fajardo, L. F., Hancock, W. E., and Kaplan, H. S. Radiation-induced heart disease. *Radiology* 89:302, 1967.
11. Vaeth, J. M., Fiegenbaum, L. Z., and Merrill, M. D. Effects of intensive radiation on the human heart. *Radiology* 76:755, 1961.

DISCUSSION

DR. CHARLES V. MECKSTROTH (Columbus, Ohio): I have quizzed our three radiologists and our hematologist at Ohio State University, and none of them has recognized such a case as these presented here today. I believe it is probably because of the fact that they give 20% less radiation.

We also have given up needle pericentesis of the pericardium because even though you use a fairly large needle catheter, 13-gauge, the fibrin usually plugs up these needles. In operating for pericardial effusions from other causes, we follow a procedure that we found in a British journal of thoracic surgery in 1967. We have used this procedure in 10 cases.

This operation can be done under local or under general anesthesia. It involves a 4-inch incision centered over the xiphoid. The xiphoid is then removed and we take advantage, of course, of the fact that the pericardium is lowered in these cases. After the xiphoid is removed, a stitch is placed at the connection between the diaphragmatic and the anterior surface of the pericardium. Retraction on this permits entry into the pericardial sac without getting into either pleural space.

I caution you to use a needle to make certain that there is pericardial effusion. All of you know that sometimes our medical men are wrong in diagnosing these cases. A patch of pericardium is taken out. It consists of a window the size of a commemorative stamp, perhaps. It is not as large, of course, as Dr. Morton's specimens, but we use this procedure for people in serious trouble from tamponade. As a matter of fact, the only time we use a needle is in cases of trauma from switchblade knives or cardiac catheters. When draining these, be sure to use a large-size catheter such as a 32 F-angled Argyle catheter.

The pericardia in our cases were not as thick as those in Dr. Morton's cases; perhaps this is why we have had no recurrence of fluid in our patients.

If the lesion is caused by malignancy, some chemotherapeutic agent is placed inside the catheter, such as nitrogen mustard. We usually use 30 mg. If the cause is unknown, as in many of our cases, no specific therapy is given and the catheter is removed two days later.

Dr. Juro Wada (Sapporo, Japan): What the author described as subtotal pericardiectomy is either a unilateral or bilateral procedure. If it is bilateral, what approach does the surgeon use when entering the chest from one side? Also, I would like to know, if the pericardium is normal, how much of the pericardium can be resected safely?

Radiation pericardial effusion is to me similar to pericardial effusion that develops after a human heart transplant, which I describe as "tissue- or immunoreactive pericarditis and effusion."

The first human heart transplant was performed in Japan on August 8, 1968. The recipient was an 18-year-old boy in a late stage of trivalvular disease with intractable cardiac failure. The donor was a 21-year-old who drowned at sea. The newly transplanted heart occupied only one-third of the recipient's pericardium. This difference in size was one of the causes of fluid collection.

The left side of the pericardium was cleared by a window, but not the right side. Retrospectively, I should have done extensive bilateral subtotal pericardiectomy at the time of the transplant operation. This patient died from tracheal obstruction caused by tracheobronchitis and general cachexia while recovering from infectious hepatitis on his eighty-third postoperative day.

This is a new type of pericarditis which we will be seeing more often and for which, as Dr. Morton has suggested, we must be prepared to perform subtotal pericardiectomy.

Dr. Donald B. Miller (Burlington, Vt.): I just want to mention a case that argues against attempting to prevent or treat this problem by pericardial drainage alone. In the course of a total left pneumonectomy for lung cancer, a portion of pericardium was resected and electively left open because of its size. The immediate postoperative course was smooth and uneventful, and the radiation therapy initiated preoperatively was completed to a total of 5,200 rads. During the seventh postoperative month, however, a downhill trend developed. The patient died 12 months after the pneumonectomy.

At autopsy, the area from which the pericardium had been removed at operation was easily identified, but the pericardium radiating from this area was markedly thickened and literally fused with the epicardium in a solid, leatherlike manner, just as Dr. Morton has so clearly described here today.

This patient was just 47 years old. No trace of residual carcinoma was found at autopsy. Obviously, ample drainage did no good, and unfortunately, the literature at the time contained very little mention of this type of problem and no mention of its management by pericardiectomy.

Dr. Morton: Dr. Meckstroth, I think the case reports presented by the other discussants illustrate that simple drainage of the effusion is not advisable. This procedure will frequently be followed by cardiac constriction from the radiation-damaged pericardium, and pericardiectomy at that time is much more difficult than in the effusion stage of the disease. However, pericardial fluid should be removed by pericardicentesis prior to pericardiectomy in patients with tamponade to prevent acute cardiac decompensation at the induction of general anesthesia.

Dr. Wada, an adequate pericardiectomy can be done through this left anterolateral thoracotomy incision by carefully dissecting the pericardium free from behind the sternum and pulling it toward the left. In this manner, part of the pericardium from the right side is removed. At the completion of the procedure, the only pericardium remaining is a 3 to 4 cm. strip along the right phrenic nerve and the pericardium surrounding the superior vena cava and parts of the right atrium.

In closing, I would like to emphasize again the importance of not giving up on these patients who have large hearts after undergoing radiation therapy for Hodgkin's disease. Our first patient had recurrent disease but would have died of acute tamponade if we had not operated on her. She is now living and well 25 months later after additional radiation therapy.

CLINICAL CASE RECORDS IN CHEMOTHERAPY

POSSIBLE RADIATION PERICARDITIS IN HODGKIN'S DISEASE [1,2]

Moderator: Arthur Serpick [3]

It is well known that radiotherapy for malignant disease of the thorax is capable of producing radiation pneumonitis and pulmonary fibrosis. It is now becoming better appreciated that there is a certain incidence of cardiac disease attributed to irradiation of the anterior mediastinum which we will call radiation heart disease. This radiation heart disease may be manifest as acute pericarditis, chronic pericardial effusion, pericardial thickening which may progress to tamponade and constrictive pericarditis, vascular phenomena, and by electrocardiographic abnormalities (most commonly T-wave changes), atrial arrhythmias, and conduction defects attributable to myocardial, endocardial, pericardial, and vascular changes.

The major morbidity and mortality from radiotherapy results from pericardial injury. Since many patients with Hodgkin's disease may be "cured" by radiotherapy, it is important to recognize the nature of the cardiac disease produced and to treat it appropriately.

Today's case presentation illustrates the dilemma posed in differential diagnosis and management of a patient with advanced Hodgkin's disease now showing cardiomegaly, and one who has had previous X irradiation to the anterior mediastinum.

Dr. Stanley Lowenbraun will present the case.

DR. LOWENBRAUN: The patient, a 32-year-old man, was well until spring 1967 when he developed right cervical adenopathy. A biopsy disclosed Hodgkin's disease. He was staged as 1-A after evaluation by history, physical, and laboratory findings at the National Cancer Institute, Bethesda, Maryland. The liver scan, lymphangiogram, and bone marrow biopsy at the time were normal. The patient was treated with radiotherapy to the neck, mediastinum, and right axilla, and was said to have received approximately 4000 rads to these areas. Radiotherapy was completed on June 30, 1967.

The patient did well until October 1968, when he developed fever, malaise, and night sweats. He was readmitted and was found to have an enlarged spleen and a positive lymphangiogram. Alkaline phosphatase on 3 occasions was 106, 107, and 162 King-Armstrong units. Liver scan showed a heterogeneous uptake of isotope, but liver biopsy was within normal limits. Between October and December of 1968 he was treated with 4000 rads to the node-bearing areas and the spleen. Shortly after he developed a palpable node in the left supraclavicular area which was biopsied with 4000 rads to the left supraclavicular area between February and March 1969. He then did well until readmission on April 18, 1969, after developing cough productive of purulent sputum, fever, and chest pain. Chest X ray showed bilateral hilar infiltrates and an increase in the cardiac size. Chest film on April 21, 1969, showed progression of the changes and development of a left pleural effusion. Cardiac scan on May 2, 1969, showed a probable pericardial effusion. Hematocrit was 37%, platelets 300,000/mm^3, and white blood count 12,200/mm^3 with a normal differential. Serum chemistries were normal, except for marked alkaline phosphatase elevations (215, 414, and 161). Sputum culture was positive for enterobacter and *Proteus*. The patient was treated initially intravenously with cephalothin with no improvement. He was believed to have Hodgkin's disease of lungs and pericardium, and was treated with cyclophosphamide, 10 mg/kg, and

[1] Received Mar 11, 1970.

[2] Management and diagnostic problems presented at joint conferences of the Oncology Department, The Johns Hopkins University Hospital, Baltimore, Md, and the National Cancer Institute's Baltimore Cancer Research Center.

[3] Medical Service, Baltimore Cancer Research Center, National Cancer Institute, Public Health Service (PHS), Baltimore, Md.

vinblastine, 0.1 mg/kg, intravenously. The patient's liver had become palpable 4–6 cm below the right costal margin in this hospitalization. He received these medications on April 21, April 28, May 12, and May 20, 1969. After the first 3 days of chemotherapy the patient became afebrile and there was improvement in his pulmonary symptomatology. Ten days after the onset of chemotherapy the liver size decreased and the alkaline phosphatase fell from a high of 414 to 161 on the day of discharge, May 21, 1969. Following chemotherapy the cardiac size also decreased. Neck veins, which had been mildly distended, improved. As his chest X ray also improved, it became apparent that he had a large mediastinal mass. At discharge, the chest X ray showed a residual left pleural effusion, but the pulmonary parenchyma was remarkably clear and the mediastinal widening had resolved. The heart remained enlarged. Clinically, there was a pleural-pericardial friction rub. He tolerated his chemotherapy well.

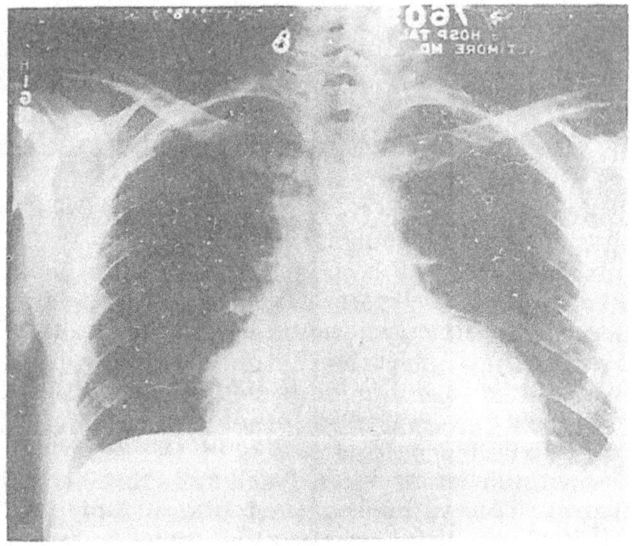

FIGURE 1

The patient was referred to the Baltimore Cancer Research Center Out-Patient Department on June 19, 1969, for further chemotherapy with probable stage IV-B Hodgkin's disease involving lung, liver, and pericardium. He was in complete remission clinically, but was leukopenic precluding reinstitution of therapy. By June 25, 1969, he developed fever, cough productive of mucoid sputum, dyspnea, and increased size of the cardiac silhouette on roentgenogram. Sputum culture grew no pathogens. He was believed to be in relapse and was treated with a combination of nitrogen mustard, vincristine, procarbazine, and prednisone. Within a week he was asymptomatic and afebrile and his cardiac size was smaller. However, by August 1, 1969, he developed substernal discomfort, aggravated by any change in position, and dyspnea and was admitted to the hospital. On examination the blood pressure was 120/75 mmHg, with a 5 mmHg pulsus paradoxus, pulse 100 per minute, temperature 99.4 F, and respiration 20. Neck veins were not distended. There was evidence of a left pleural effusion. Cardiac sounds were decreased and the liver was palpated 2 cm below the right costal margin. Neither the spleen nor lymph nodes were palpable. Chest X ray showed an enlarged globular cardiac silhouette and a left pleural effusion (fig 1). Electrocardiogram revealed borderline low voltage. Thoracentesis resulted in removal of 500 ml of straw-colored, slightly cloudy fluid with 1400 leukocytes, 80% lymphs, and the remainder polymononuclear cells. The fluid had 3.5 g/100 ml protein, 81 mg/100 ml glucose, and negative cultures for bacteria, fungi, and acid-fast organisms. Cytology was negative for malignant cells. The results of liver function tests were normal. Skin tests for mumps, histoplasmosis, and tuberculosis were negative.

The patient was treated again with 4-drug combination chemotherapy, but without response. By August 8, 1969, a right pleural effusion developed. Pleural biopsy revealed only mild acute and chronic pleuritis. On August 8 and August 9 he was given 100 mg/m^2 of BCNU intravenously. By August 20 his pulsus paradoxus increased to 20 mmHg. Pericardiocentesis was performed with marked difficulty thought to be due to fibrous tissue. A few milliliters of serosanguineous fluid was removed and sent for acid-fast and bacteriologic culture. A diagnostic and therapeutic thoracotomy was considered, but the pulsus paradoxus decreased with supportive measures, and the platelet count fell to 20,000 mm^3 secondary to the BCNU therapy.

On September 12, 1969, after a rise in platelet count, BCNU 100 mg/m^2 $\times$ 1 was administered again because the patient's pleural and pericardial disease had not progressed. By

September 24, the bilirubin rose to 3.2 mg, alkaline phosphatase to 41, and SGOT to 123 units. Prednisone, 150 mg daily, was begun on September 25. Since then the patient's fever has lysed. He now appears less icteric and has had some decrease in pleural fluid. His pulsus paradoxus is 5 mmHg and the heart size is slightly smaller.

DR. STUART SHEINBROT (Radiology Department, Baltimore PHS Hospital) : On June 24th, shortly after admission, generalized cardiomegaly with no specific chamber enlargement is present. The transverse cardiothoracic ratio is 0.53. There was some pulmonary fibrosis and a great deal of pleural thickening which is probably due to his previous radiation therapy to the mediastinum. He developed a right pleural effusion which isn't seen too well on the lateral film. A large number of films were taken between June and October and one that is pretty representative is shown (fig 1) where there is a large pleural effusion and the cardiac silhouette, which cannot be evaluated well, is enlarged. He now has a subpulmonic effusion rather than a pleural effusion, but it is a large amount. The cardiothoracic ratio is now 14 over 31 so it has decreased.

QUESTION: Did you attempt to outline the width of the pericardium or ventricular wall by other studies?

DR. SHEINBROT: If you mean angiography, no there were no such studies performed.

DR. KIRKLAND BRACE: The radiotherapy dosage on this patient is difficult to evaluate. I have just looked at the patient's old records prior to his admission here and there are several findings worth noting. The patient was treated initially through a single anterior field. When midplane dose to the mediastinum was carried to 4000 rads, the dose at the body surface may be very high. If we calculate the depth dose at 3 cm from the surface, which is approximately the anterior portion of the pericardium, a final tumor dose of approximately 6000 rads may have been reached. Also, when the radiotherapist treated the para-aortic

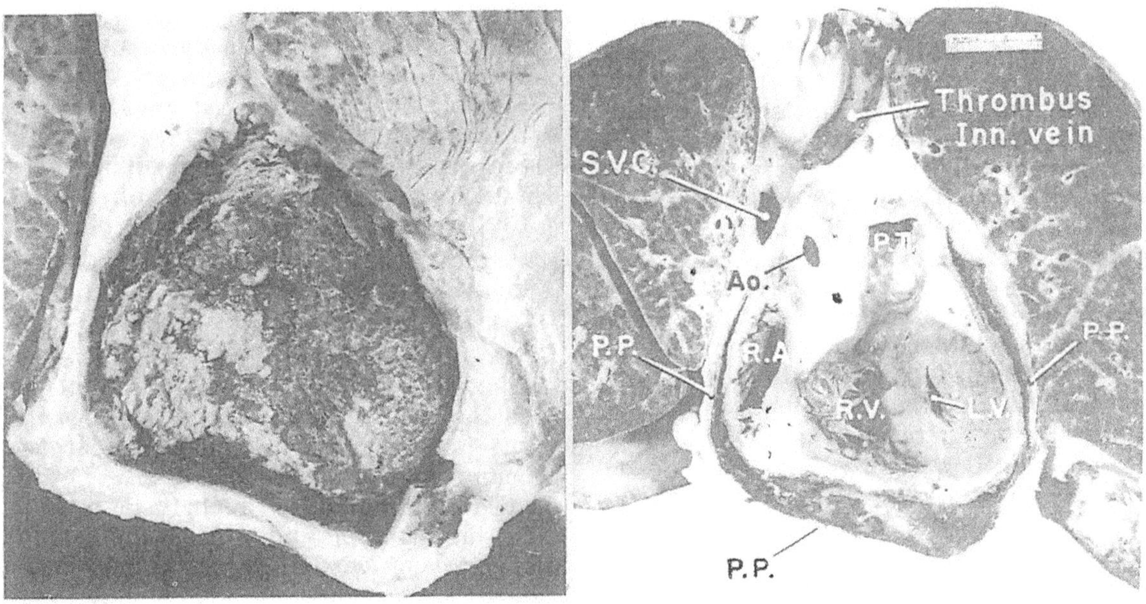

FIGURE 2.—Heart in a 26-year-old man (NIH A67-95) who died of Hodgkin's disease with cardiac tamponade. This man never underwent pericardiectomy. He received a total of 4000 rads to his mediastinum, neck, and upper chest. Three pericardiocenteses were performed during his last 5 weeks of life and 750 ml was removed. Pericardial fluid continued to accumulate and he died with typical clinical features of pericardial constriction. Another 350 ml of hemorrhagic pericardial fluid was aspirated at necropsy. *Left:* View of heart after anterior parietal pericardium had been excised at autopsy. *Right:* Longitudinal section of heart and lungs. The parietal pericardium (*P.P.*) is thick and the pericardial surfaces, saggy. Radiation changes also were present in the lungs but no tumor cells were present. The cause of the thrombus in the innominate (*Inn.*) vein is unknown. *S.V.C.* = superior vena cava; *R.A.* = right atrium; *R.V.* = right ventricle; *P.T.* = pulmonic trunk; and *L.V.* = left ventricle.

areas for his infradiaphragmatic disease it is difficult to evaluate how much, if any, overlap occurred between the splenic and para-aortic radiotherapy fields and the previously irradiated mediastial fields. These considerations make it probable that the patient could have received more than 4000 rads to various areas of the heart.

DR. SERPICK: Dr. Belcher, you saw this patient in surgical consultation when we were considering diagnostic and perhaps therapeutic pericardiectomy. Do you want to comment on your views at the time?

DR. V. BELCHER (Department of Surgery, Baltimore PHS Hospital): Perhaps it would be more appropriate if I waited to see what the experts are going to say about radiation pericarditis because my personal experience has been limited to surgical correction of pericardial disease due to tuberculosis and viral pericarditis.

QUESTION: Dr. Belcher, what are some of the clinical factors which would influence you to decide whether or not you would attempt a pericardiectomy in a patient like this?

ANSWER: Well, at the time, our major concern was the chemotherapy that the patient had recently received and with the expectation that he was going to develop leukopenia and thrombocytopenia. We were very reluctant to consider an operative procedure unless our hand was absolutely forced because we anticipated, at the time, that he would get his maximum hematopoietic depression at the day of surgery or the day after surgery. Our major concern was his 20 cm paradoxical pulse. Did this really indicate impending disaster in this man or could he be followed conservatively? If he did require an operative procedure, could it be prolonged until we saw what would be the effect of the BCNU? Under the circumstances, we decided that it would be more hazardous to do anything surgically at the time and I guess that the course of events proved that we were right.

QUESTION: In forcing your hand, is it the height of the paradoxical pulse that is critical or is the clinical condition more important?

DR. BELCHER: Well, I was not too concerned about the paradoxical pulse, particularly in the presence of a central venous pressure which wasn't significantly elevated. He had high normal venous pressure and was clinically doing well so I wasn't too alarmed about his 20 cm pulsus paradoxicus. I might mention that there was also another technical problem involved and it involved the radiation that the patient received. Ordinarily, we do a pericardiectomy through a sternal incision and Dr. Brace assured me if we had a sternal splitting incision, it would never heal and I'm sure he is right. At the NIH in Bethesda, there has been enough concern about previous irradiation and the fact that there would be delay in healing that in their patients they have employed a left thoracotomy incision and developed a dissection plane between the sternum and the heart to go over into the right chest and remove the major part of the pericardium, all through an incision in the left chest far enough removed from the radiation area.

DR. SERPICK: This patient is a bit unique from those in the literature in that the cases reported have had radiotherapy alone, whereas our patient had radiotherapy and, when we asked Dr. Belcher to see him, was in the midst of receiving chemotherapy as well. We were concerned with delayed leukopenia and thrombocytopenia from BCNU. Of course, in any patient with pericarditis and effusion, the cause must be determined. One must distinguish radiation heart disease from viral or idiopathic pericarditis and from actual neoplastic involvement of the heart or pericardium. Myxedema should not be a problem in the differential diagnosis if the thyroid is shielded from radiation.

Dr. Brace, do you know if the thyroid was shielded in this patient?

DR. BRACE: It was not shielded.

DR. SERPICK: Patients who have received radiotherapy to the mediastinum and heart by and large would include patients with Hodgkin's disease, carcinoma of the left breast, seminoma, lung and thymic cancer, esophageal cancer, and really any metastasis to this region that might need palliative radiotherapy. The incidence of cardiac or pericardial metastasis among solid tumors in autopsy studies in the literature varies from 5 to 20% (1). Involvement of the heart and pericardium by Hodgkin's disease in autopsy surveys varies from 2 to 25% with pericardial involvement much more frequent than myocardial involvement (2). However, antemortem diagnosis of this site of tumor involvement is quite difficult. At the NIH Clinical Center in Bethesda, 16% of patients with Hodgkin's disease had cardiac involvement. There are only a few adequate series in the literature which help gain experience in the recognition and management of the entity of radiation heart disease. One is the study reported from Stanford University in which 21 patients developed significant heart or pericardial disease following radiation of at least 4000 rads to the anterior portion of the heart (3). Among these patients, 5.8% had lymphoma, of which 6.7% had Hodgkin's disease and 3.4% had breast cancer. The most common manifestation was acute pericarditis usually transient, which developed either immediately following or during radiotherapy, or up to 4 years following completion of the radiotherapy. Four of the 13 patients who developed the acute pericarditis syndrome went on to develop chronic pericarditis with effusion or chronic constrictive pericarditis as the initial manifestation of their radiation heart disease. There is one patient in the literature who developed constrictive pericarditis some 20 years after receiving radiation to the heart (4). The causal relationship there may be a bit tenuous.

Since the installation of a new cobalt unit at the nearby Carlisle Hospital in Pennsylvania in 1962, among 30 patients who had received radiotherapy to the anterior mediastinum for various neoplasms, 3 developed chronic pericarditis with effusion (5). The cases in the literature suggest that at least 4000 rads to the anterior surface of the heart is necessary to produce these syndromes and it can be orthovoltage or supervoltage (6). The pericardial fluid transaminase levels may be high because of hemolyzed erythrocytes or the presence of tumor cells. The latter finding has only been occasionally reported even in demonstrated malignant effusions and in known malignant metastasis to the pericardium.

QUESTION: Dr. Brace, how much radiation does a heart get when the mediastinum is irradiated and what measures might radiotherapists take to deliver adequate tumoricidal radiotherapy and yet avoid prohibitive damaging effects to the heart?

DR. BRACE: Using a treatment scheme employing opposing fields which limit the dose to the pericardium to a fairly uniform 4000 rads should be useful in this regard. Since their initial paper was published the Radiation Branch of the NCI have changed to using parallel opposing fields. Their incidence of cardiomegaly from radiotherapy is said to have decreased remarkably. Kaplan reports rather low incidence of pericarditis in this series treated with 4400 rads using opposing fields. From this we may draw the conclusion that probably 4000 rads to the mediastinum in sufficiently symmetrical arrangement does not produce a significant incidence of pericarditis.

DR. SERPICK: Are you using opposing fields here now?

DR. BRACE: Yes.

DR. SERPICK: Do you count cardiomegaly as a complication of radiation?

DR. BRACE: No, we shouldn't really do that. Most cardiac enlargements are asymptomatic, and rarely result in a final pericarditis that is symptomatic. Most cases became apparent on a routine followup and disappeared without any further symptoms.

QUESTION: Does this resolve more quickly with diuretics?

DR. BRACE: I cannot answer that, but the cardiomegaly does disappear spontaneously in most cases.

I have a question for Dr. Serpick. The patient who had pericarditis in the Stanford series 4 years after radiation therapy—how was it documented that they had radiation pericarditis as opposed to some other type of pericarditis?

DR. SERPICK: In the Stanford paper, patients were included who had disease of the heart or pericardium which was evident clinically or at postmortem examination and who did not have direct tumor involvement of the heart or pericardium. All the patients had medical evaluation and chest X-rays before institution of radiotherapy, and in none was pre-existing heart disease detected. Pericardiocentesis and/or pericardiectomy was performed in most patients; therefore, tissue or pericardial fluid was examined.

DR. BLOCK: One of the problems faced by the clinicians was whether this patient had pericarditis due to Hodgkin's disease or to radiation heart disease, and finally the decision was made that it was related evidently to tumor because he was treated with BCNU and certainly he was not made any worse. I don't know of any diuretic effect of BCNU but it would suggest that there may have been tumor there. Now, if what you say is true, Dr. Brace, that he had in excess of 4000 rads to the heart, he had an excess of what is supposed to be a curative "sterilizing dose" of radiation therapy, at least as this concept is applied to lymph nodes. We don't know yet what happened in this patient, but are sterilizing doses of radiotherapy sterilizing per se or can this dose differ from tissue to tissue in terms of guaranteed eradication of Hodgkin's disease?

DR. BRACE: Well, I think the important thing here is that the mediastinum was treated some time before he had the recurrence in the abdomen. If he does have disease of the heart, and presumably he does, one could easily take the stand that this is an extension up, rather than a recurrence, from the untreated area immediately below the heart. The fact remains, however, that one can treat lymph nodes with Hodgkin's disease up to doses of 5000 rads and still on occasion have the tumor recur in that area without other evidence of recurrence. I do not think one can ever reach a final solution on this question.

QUESTION: Is there reason to think that many of these patients will have to be operated on? The effusion appears to be recurring in this patient despite BCNU therapy.

DR. SERPICK: I think we ought to defer to Dr. Roberts who has been involved with 11 patients who have been operated upon at the Clinical Center in Bethesda.

DR. WILLIAM C. ROBERTS (Section of Pathology, National Heart and Lung Institute, National Institutes of Health, Bethesda, Md): Before discussing the patients operated upon at the Clinical Center by Dr. Donald Morton (7), I thought I might summarize some studies (2) we have done on autopsy patients with Hodgkin's disease. We reviewed the hearts of 196 patients with malignant lymphoma in the heart (table 1). In 21 of the 48 patients, tumor was present only histologically, and in 27 on both gross and histologic examination. Of the 196 patients, 75 had Hodgkin's disease, and 12 of them had lymphoma in the heart at necropsy; in 4 the tumor was apparent only histologically.

TABLE 1.—Malignant lymphoma of the heart

Type of lymphoma	Number of necropsies	Number with cardiac tumor	Percentage with cardiac tumor
Hodgkin's disease	75	12 (4)*	16
Lymphocytic type	32	9 (5)	28
Reticulum cell sarcoma	22	6 (2)	27
Mycosis fungoides	51	17 (8)	33
Undifferentiated	16	4 (2)	25
Totals	196	48 (21)	24

*Numbers in parentheses indicate patients in whom tumor was not observed grossly but only in histologic sections of the heart.

TABLE 2.—Hodgkin's disease of the heart: survey of reported series

Author, year (reference)	Total No. autopsied patients	Number with cardiac metastases	Percentage with cardiac metastases
Krueger & Meyer, 1936 (4)	16	3	19
Scott & Garvin, 1939 (5)	22	0	0
Herbut & Maisell, 1942 (6)	13	2	15
Jackson & Parker, 1947 (7)	98	2	2
Symmers, 1948 (8)	30	0*	0
Rottino & Hoffman, 1952 (9)	63	5	8
Lucia et al, 1952 (10)	18	3	17
Nabarro, 1953 (11)	24	4	17
Bisel et al, 1953 (13)	27	8	30
DeLoach & Haynes, 1953 (12)	49	3†	6
Young & Goldman, 1954 (14)	39	2	5
Gassman et al, 1955 (15)	189	7‡	4
Jakob & Zirkin, 1960 (17)	15	3	20
Levitan et al, 1961 (18)	112	4	4
Richmond, 1962 (19)	272	33	12
Totals	987	79	8%
Present series, 1968	75	12	16%

* Author described involvement in detail of virtually every organ except the heart.
† Includes only patients in whom cardiac tumor was observed grossly.
‡ Patient with tumor in parietal pericardium only excluded.

TABLE 3.—Specific location of cardiac lymphoma

Region of heart	Number with cardiac tumor
Pericardium	41 (15)*
Right atrium	17 (2)
Right ventricle	18 (5)
Left atrium	11 (1)
Left ventricle	19 (5)
Valve (tricuspid)	1 (1)

* Numbers in parentheses indicate patients in whom tumor was not observed grossly but only in histologic sections of the heart.

This incidence is slightly higher than that reported by most observers (8–22) in the past (table 2). In 41 of the 48 patients with cardiac lymphoma the tumor was present in the epicardium (table 3). The incidence of involvement of parietal pericardium by lymphoma was probably greater but this tissue was not available for re-examination by us.

Electrocardiographic abnormalities have been common in patients with lymphoma. In our study of 196 patients, the percentage of patients with cardiac lymphoma with electrocardiographic abnormalities was 64%, but the percentage without cardiac lymphoma and electrocardiographic abnormalities also was 64%.

In addition to pericardial thickening (figs 2 and 3), excessive radiation to the area of the heart may also cause focal thickening of the valvular and mural endocardium. Focal myocardial fibrosis is another described complication of irradiation but we have not observed this complication in any patient we have studied at necropsy.

Dr. Donald L. Morton has operated on 11 patients with Hodgkin's disease and radiation-induced pericarditis. Cardiac dysfunction first appeared in each only after mediastinal irradiation. The dose to the anterior portions of the heart and pericardium varied from 4500 rads in 3 weeks to 5300–7200 rads in 4–6 weeks. The interval between initiation of radiation therapy and the appearance of pericardial effusion varied from 6 to 26 months (avg, 13). Initially the pericardial effusions

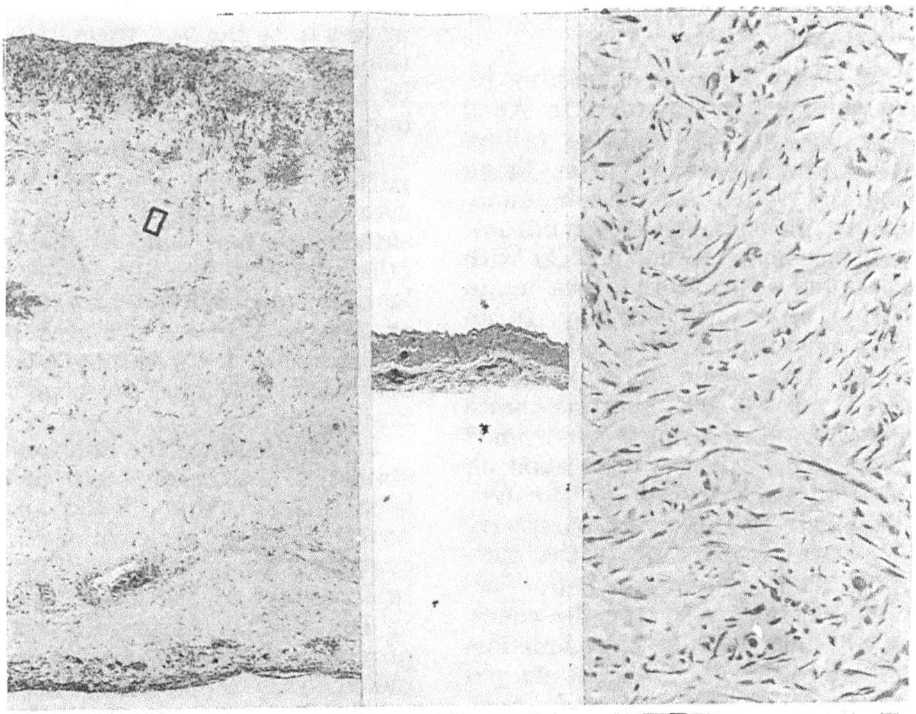

FIGURE 3.—Excised parietal pericardium in a 54-year-old man who underwent pericardiectomy because of cardiac tamponade secondary to mediastinal irradiation. The parietal pericardium (*left*) is severely thickened. Normal parietal pericardium in an adult without cardiac disease is shown in the center for comparison. *Right:* Close-up view of the thickened pericardium enclosed in the box in the photomicrograph at left. The fibroblasts show changes attributable to damage by irradiation. Hematoxylin and eosin stains; × 27 (*left* and *center*), × 160 (*right*).

usually did not produce signs of cardiac dysfunction. Pericardiocenteses preoperatively or at time of pericardiectomy in 10 patients yielded effusions ranging from 400 to 1800 ml (avg, 790). The fluid was serous in 8 and bloody in 2, and none contained tumor cells by cytologic examination. In the 11th patient the pericardial effusion resolved, and the pericardial space was obliterated by adhesions at the time of operation. Subtotal pericardiectomy was accomplished through left anterolateral thoracotomy incision. The parietal pericardium was 2–9 times thicker than normal and the thickening was the result of fibrous tissue proliferation. Some fibroblasts showed radiation damage in 8 patients and tumor cells were observed on the mediastinal surface of the parietal pericardia. At operation, the epicardium over the right ventricle was always thickened, but not over the left ventricle. Three patients had fibrinous pericardial adhesions.

All 11 patients were benefited by pericardiectomy. The signs and symptoms of cardiac dysfunction that had been present preoperatively disappeared in each of them after operation. All 11 patients are living and free of evidence of cardiac dysfunction 1–24 months (avg, 9) after pericardiectomy.

DR. MATTHEW CARR: There is something interesting about this patient's history. In April he had episodes of fever and cardiac failure and this disappeared apparently after being given chemotherapy which included immunosuppressive agents. The same type of syndrome recurred at least once more rather acutely with fever and pericardial effusion and once again seemed to improve after chemotherapy. In an adult who had a myocardial infarction a couple of months ago this would undoubtedly be called Dressler's syndrome. The question comes up, is this some type of Dressler's syndrome? Has anyone been able to demonstrate such an event following radiotherapy and can the syndrome be managed by immunosuppressive drugs? Is this patient responding to the steroids he was given each time? Or is it possible that the anti-inflammatory effect of the chemotherapeutic agent has actually been ameliorating an allergic carditis? Dr. Roberts, do you have any answer about whether such pericarditis or effusion may be similar to Dressler's syndrome?

DR. ROBERTS: I have never studied a patient with Dressler's syndrome at necropsy so I do not know. Have inflammatory changes occurred in patients with radiation pericarditis? One of our patients was operated on within a month after the onset of pericardial effusion. Two patients had a few polymorphonuclear cells in the excised parietal pericardia but the inflammation was minimal.

QUESTION: What is the morbidity of the pericardiectomy at the Clinical Center and how many patients, when they came to pericardiectomy, had advanced Hodgkin's disease with involvement of the liver and other viscera as our patient had?

DR. ROBERTS: All 11 patients, as mentioned earlier, were improved by pericardiectomy. The postoperative course, except in 2 patients, was uneventful. One was re-explored for postoperative bleeding but thereafter his course was smooth. The second had a left phrenic nerve palsy due to inadvertent division of this nerve which was encased in dense fibrous tissue. I do not know the extent of the Hodgkin's disease in our 11 patients.

QUESTION: Had any of these patients been given steroids alone and observed?

DR. ROBERTS: No. There are no controls for these 11 patients. Whether pericardiectomy proves to be the best form of therapy for radiation-induced pericardial constriction remains to be seen. This therapeutic approach is a new one.

DR. ALBERT OWENS: If you return to the patient at hand and weigh carefully what everyone has said, there are a number of considerations pertinent to his management and other patients like him. I already have a problem in fully appreciating a clinical situation even from the last protocol, but in reviewing the evidence I try to challenge myself with a series of questions to classify the patient's main problems.

In this instance the anatomic and functional states of the heart seem primary. We have been talking about "heart size," "cardiac silhouettes," and "pericardial effusion." I am not convinced how precisely we have delineated the basic nature of the lesion. Since the existence of constrictive pericarditis is likely, the appropriate diagnostic procedure should be completed. This is especially important since the studies have definite therapeutic implications.

The etiology of this disorder also relates to the selection of therapy. We have focused on the likely causative role of radiation therapy, but should not overlook the possibilities of tuberculosis or fungus infection. The changing pulmonary infiltrates could well be related to such infections. Bacteriologic studies and skin tests are not likely to be helpful and biopsy should be considered.

It is also possible that these problems stem from active Hodgkin's disease. It is not clear in my mind how active this patient's Hodgkin's disease is and how to manage it. Again biopsy material should help in making this decision.

It should also be noted that this patient is leukopenic and thrombocytopenic. Is this related to tumor infiltration in the marrow or is this marrow suppression due to cytotoxic treatment? Bone marrow biopsy would be helpful here.

A few larger questions arise that relate to the management of Hodgkin's disease. What do we know with certainty about the dose-levels and dose-schedules of cytotoxic agents in relation to preserving marrow function and maximizing antitumor effect? What can we expect from BCNU in a patient who apparently has progressed on a regimen containing nitrogen mustard, since BCNU may well function as an alkylating agent.

Similar questions could also be raised about the use of steroids. In addition, one might inquire as to whether modifications in steroid structure could be expected to lead to greater antitumor effect.

An obvious point relates to its prevention. It would be sound to alter the technical factors involved to avoid this situation.

I don't know whether these remarks have been helpful, but I did want to focus a bit more on this patient and his management. The problem at hand concerns how we procede with this patient.

Dr. Roberts, concerning studies of hemodynamic function in these patients, do you think they are useful?

DR. ROBERTS: I think they are useful. In addition to providing hemodynamic evidence for the presence or absence of pericardial constriction, this diagnostic procedure is excellent for judging objectively the effectiveness of the operation. All of these patients should have repeat cardiac catheterization postoperatively since pericardiectomy is a new therapeutic approach to this iatrogenic disease.

QUESTION: Is there anything about the clinical situation or related to the hemodynamic data you obtained on your patients which influenced the morbidity of the operation?

DR. ROBERTS: No. It should be remembered that all 11 patients had large effusions. To what degree the tamponade was due to thickening of the parietal pericardium or to what degree it was due to the effusion is not completely clear. In 2 patients right atrial and right ventricular pressures dropped virtually to normal in the cardiac catheterization laboratory by removing fluid from the pericardial sac. Since this occurred it might be worthwhile to use a pericardial window only in some of these patients.

DR. OWENS: I don't think that any of us feels the likelihood of an infectious pericarditis is very great. The major alternatives are those of Hodgkin's disease and radiation pericarditis.

We know that the patient has extensive Hodgkin's disease, but I am not confident that continued chemotherapy can be expected to improve his major impairment—that of cardiac function. Time considerations are pressing and there are no longer prime drugs available.

Might not a surgical procedure offer the most direct approach? It would provide the best material for diagnostic study and possible means of improving hemodynamic function.

QUESTION: Another point about trying not to get into this clinical situation: Dr. Brace you mentioned now that we are using at least 3800 rads to the mediastinum, is that correct, and not going up to 4000?

DR. BRACE: It depends a bit on the time duration of therapy.

QUESTION: I wonder if there are any telltale signs with lab tests or other enzyme tests that might tip us off that these patients might be more prone, even at a dosage of 3800 rads, to developing pericarditis?

DR. BRACE: You will recall Dr. Roberts' comments on the EKG being abnormal equally in patients with Hodgkin's disease whether they had cardiac tumor or not.

DR. SERPICK: This is a new entity and as Dr. Owens mentioned nobody has a lot of experience with this. I think it would behoove us to study our patients in a prospective manner.

With the increasing use of radical radiotherapy to cure malignant diseases and the longer survival of such patients, we may have the opportunity to observe more of the delayed cardiac and pericardial damage of such therapy.

SYNONYMS OF COMPOUNDS

BCNU: NSC-409962; urea, 1,3-bis(2-chloroethyl)-1-nitroso-

Cyclophosphamide: NSC-26271; 2*H*-1,3,2-oxazaphosphorine, 2-[bis-(2-chloroethyl)amino]tetrahydro-, 2-oxide, monohydrate; Cytoxan

Nitrogen mustard: NSC-762; diethylamine, 2,2′-dichloro-*N*-methyl-, hydrochloride

Prednisone: NSC-10023; pregna-1,4-diene-3,11,20-trione, 17,21-dihydroxy-

Procarbazine: NSC-77213; *p*-toluamide, *N*-isopropyl-α-(2-methylhydrazino)-, monohydrochloride

Vincristine: NSC-67574; leurocristine, sulfate (1:1)

REFERENCES

1. COHEN, G. V., PERRY, T. M., and EVANS, J. M. Neoplastic invasion of the heart and pericardium. Ann Intern Med 42:1238, 1955.
2. ROBERTS, W. C., GLANCY, D. L., and DEVITA, V. T., JR. Heart in malignant lymphoma (Hodgkin's disease, lymphosarcoma, reticulum cell sarcoma and mycosis fungoides). Amer J Cardiol 22:85–107, 1968.
3. COH, K. E., STEWART, J. R., FAJARDO, L. F., ET AL. Heart disease following radiation. Medicine 47:281–289, 1967.
4. STEINBERG, I. Effusive-constrictive radiation pericarditis. Amer J Cardiol 19:434–439, 1967.
5. MASLAND, D. S., ROTZ, C. T., JR., and HARRIS, J. H. Postradiation pericarditis with chronic pericardial effusion. Ann Intern Med 69:97–102, 1969.
6. MUGGIA, F. M., and CASSILETH, P. A. Constrictive pericarditis following radiation therapy. Amer J Med 44:116–123, 1968.
7. MORTON, D. L., KAGAN, A. R., ROBERTS, W. C., ET AL. Pericardiectomy for radiation-induced pericarditis with effusion. Ann Thorac Surg 8:195–298, 1969.
8. KRUEGER, F. J., and MEYER, O. Lymphogranulomatosis (Hodgkin's disease). A review of six cases. J Lab Clin Med 21:682, 1936.
9. SCOTT, R. W., and GARVIN, C. F. Tumors of the heart and pericardium. Amer Heart J 17:421, 1939.
10. HERBUT, P. A., and MAISEL, A. L. Secondary tumors of the heart. Arch Path 34:358, 1942.
11. JACKSON, H., JR., and PARKER, F., JR. Hodgkin's Disease and Allied Disorders. New York, Oxford University Press, 1947, p 177.
12. SYMMERS, D. Lymphoid diseases. Hodgkin's granuloma, giant follicular lymphadenopathy, lymphoid leukemia, lymphosarcoma and gastrointestinal pseudoleukemia. Arch Path 45:73, 1948.
13. ROTTINO, A., and HOFFMAN, G. T. Cardiac involvement in Hodgkin's disease. Amer Heart J 43:115, 1952.
14. LUCIA, S. P., MILLS, H., LOWENHAUPT, E., ET AL. Visceral involvement in primary neoplastic diseases of the reticuloendothelial system. Cancer 5:1193, 1952.
15. NABARRO, J. D. N. Cardiac involvement in malignant lymphoma. Arch Intern Med 92:258, 1953.
16. BISEL, H. F., WROBLEWSKI, F., and LADUE, J. S. Incidence and clinical manifestations of cardiac metastases. JAMA 153:712, 1953.
17. DELOACH, J. F., and HAYNES, J. W. Secondary tumors of the heart and pericardium: review of the subject and report of 137 cases. Arch Intern Med 91:224, 1953.
18. YOUNG, J. M., and GOLDMAN, I. R. Tumor metastasis to the heart. Circulation 9:220, 1954.
19. GASSMAN, H. S., MEADOWS, R., JR., and BAKER, L. A. Metastatic tumors of the heart. Amer J Med 19:357, 1955.
20. JAKOB, H. G., and ZIRKIN, R. M. Hodgkin's disease with involvement of the heart and pericardium. JAMA 173:338, 1960.
21. LEVITAN, R., DIAMOND, H. D., and CRAVER, L. F. The liver in Hodgkin's disease. Gut 2:60, 1961.
22. RICHMOND, J., SHERMAN, R. S., DIAMOND, H. D., ET AL. Renal lesions associated with malignant lymphomas. Amer J Med 32:184, 1962.

Endocardial Papillary Elastofibromas

Histologic, Histochemical, and Electron Microscopical Findings

Michael C. Fishbein, MD; Victor J. Ferrans, MD, PhD; William C. Roberts, MD

The organization of cellular and extracellular components appeared similar and was distinctive in three endocardial papillary elastofibromas studied. Each tumor papilla contained (1) a dense, central core of collagen and elastic tissue, (2) a peripheral, myxomatous layer with deposits of acid mucopolysaccharides, and (3) an overlying, hyperplastic layer of endothelial cells. Ultrastructural study of one tumor showed that the cells in all three zones had numerous cytoplasmic filaments, 100 Angstroms in diameter, and dilated cisterns of endoplasmic reticulum; endothelial cells also had intercellular junctions and numerous pinocytotic vesicles. The myxomatous stroma varied from amorphous to fibrillar, and the collagenous cores showed focal degeneration. The name "endocardial papillary elastofibroma" is suggested to emphasize those features which are most conspicuous and which serve to differentiate this tumor from myxoma.

Accepted for publication Aug 16, 1974.

From the Section of Pathology, National Heart and Lung Institute, National Institutes of Health, Bethesda, Md. Dr. Fishbein is now at the Harbor General Hospital, Torrance, Calif.

Reprint requests to Section of Pathology, National Heart and Lung Institute, National Institutes of Health, Bethesda, MD 20014 (Dr. Ferrans).

Endocardial papillary elastofibroma (also called fibroma, hyaline fibroma, papillary fibroma, fibroelastic hamartoma, fibroangiomyxoma, myxofibroma, myxoma, papillary myxoma, hemangiofibroma, hemangioelastomyxoma, papillary excrescence, giant Lambl excrescence, and papillary endocardial tumor [see Nassar and Parker[1] for review]) is generally believed to be a nonneoplastic proliferation of relatively avascular endocardial connective tissue.[2-5] Endocardial papillary elastofibromas are found on the ventricular surface of the semilunar valves, atrial surface of the atrioventricular valves, chordae tendineae, and atrial and ventricular endocardium.[1-8] These papillary tumors also have been described as resembling sea anemones grossly, with multiple fronds projecting from the endocardial surface.[4] Their histologic appearance can vary somewhat, as evidenced by the various terms used to describe them. They are generally characterized by relatively avascular, acellular collagenous stalks, from which multiple papillae project. Each papilla has a central collagenous core that is surrounded by a loose myxomatous zone and covered by endothelium. Various authors have emphasized the presence of reticulin and elastic fibers within the core and of acid mucopolysaccharide material in the myxoid stroma of endocardial papillary elastofibromas.[1, 3-7] The pathogenesis of this tumor is still uncertain. Since there is much speculation as to its origin but relatively little is known of its detailed morphology, this study was undertaken to examine the histology and ultrastructure of endocardial papillary elastofibroma.

PATIENTS STUDIED

Three cases of solitary endocardial papillary elastofibromas found at necropsy were studied. All three patients had long histories of valvular cardiac disease that eventually required cardiac valve replacement. In none of the three patients were the tumors either suspected or clinically detected during life. Clinical and necropsy data on these three patients are presented in the Table.

MATERIALS AND METHODS

Formalin-fixed tissues were embedded in paraffin, sectioned, and stained by the following methods for histologic study: hematoxylin-eosin, Masson trichrome, Wilder reticulin, elastica-van Gieson, phosphotungstic acid hematoxylin, von Kossa, Alcian blue-PAS, and Rinehart. Part of the formalin-fixed tumor from patient 3 was

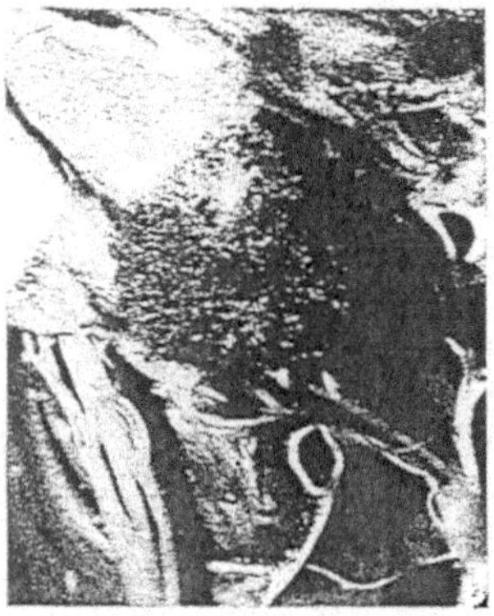

Fig 1.—Tumor on atrial surface of anterior leaflet of tricuspid valve from patient 1. Glistening papillary appearance is characteristic of endocardial papillary elastofibroma (original magnification × 3).

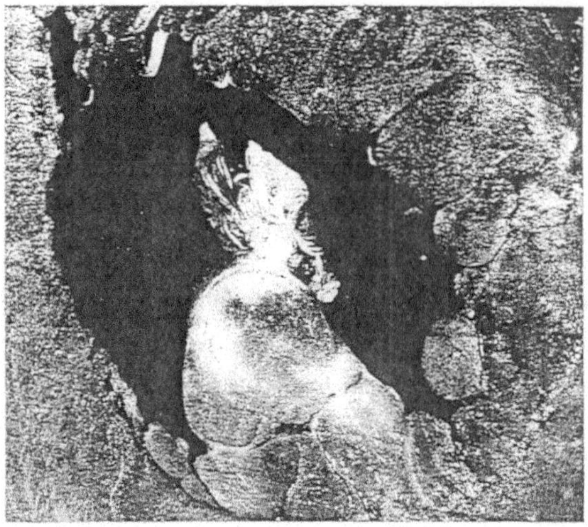

Fig 2.—Transversely cut heart of patient 2 showing tumor arising from two stalks on endocardial surface of left ventricular posteromedial papillary muscle (original magnification × 2.5).

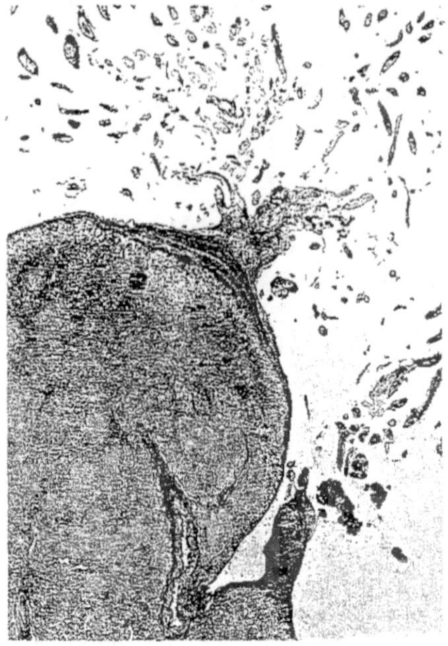

Fig 3.—Section of tumor shown in Fig 2 demonstrating central stalk from which multiple papillae project. Pattern is characteristic of endocardial papillary elastofibroma (elastica-van Gieson, original magnification × 8.5).

refixed with 3% glutaraldehyde in 0.1M phosphate buffer, washed with several changes of 5% sucrose in 0.1M phosphate buffer, pH 7.2, postfixed with 1% osmium tetroxide in Millonig buffer, dehydrated with ethanol and propylene oxide, and embedded in epoxy resin (Maraglas). Semifine (0.5μ thick) sections were stained with alkaline toluidine blue and examined by light microscopy for selection of areas to be studied by electron microscopy. Ultrathin sections were stained with lead citrate and uranyl acetate and examined with the electron microscope. Some ultrathin sections were collected on gold grids, stained with silver tetraphenylporphine sulfonate according to the method of Albert and Fleischer[9] for the demonstration of elastic tissue, and then counterstained with lead citrate and uranyl acetate.

RESULTS

The three tumors ranged from 1.0 to 1.5 cm in largest dimension. In one patient, the tumor was located on the atrial surface of the anterior leaflet of the tricuspid valve (Fig 1). In the other two, the tumors were attached to the mural endocardium of the left ventricle; one tumor had two separate stalks, both of which arose from the surface of the posteromedial papillary muscle (Fig 2 and 3); the other extended between the septal and lateral wall near the apical portion of the ventricle (Fig 4 and 5). All three were glistening papillary masses.

Light Microscopical Observations

Histologically, all three tumors were similar. Three distinctly different areas were present in the papillae of the tumor: (1) a dense central core, (2) a narrow, peripheral, loose, myxomatous region, and (3) an endothelial lining (Fig 6 to 12). The morphology of each individual papilla, which projected from the central collagenous stalk, varied depending on the plane and level of sectioning. True cross-sections, however, showed that these papillae were of variable size, ranging from 0.4 to 2 mm in diameter, and had dense cores in which very few mononuclear cells with round to elongated nuclei and variable amounts of cytoplasm were embedded (Fig 6 to 11). All papillae were covered by a markedly hyperplastic layer of endothelial cells bulging from the surface (Fig 6, 7, and 10). Connective tissue stains showed that the central cores were composed of collagen, reticulin, and granular to finely fibrillar elastic

Clinical and Necropsy Data in Three Patients With Endocardial Papillary Elastofibromas*

Patient/Age, yr/Sex	Clinical Diagnosis	Operation	Heart Weight, gm	Location of Tumor	Size of Tumor, cm (Largest Dimension)
1/46/M	RHD-MS, AS	Age 37-MC Age 46-MVR	550	Apical portion of LV	1.5
2/50/F	RHD-MS, AR, TR	Age 43-MC Age 50-MVR & AVR	500	Posteromedial papillary muscle of LV	1.0
3/62/F	Bicuspid AV-AS	Age 62-AVR	320	Atrial surface of anterior leaflet of TV	1.3

* AR is aortic regurgitation; AS, aortic stenosis; AV, aortic valve; AVR, aortic valve replacement; LV, left ventricle; MC, mitral commissurotomy; MR, mitral regurgitation; MS, mitral stenosis; MVR, mitral valve replacement; RHD, rheumatic heart disease; TR, tricuspid regurgitation; TV, tricuspid valve.

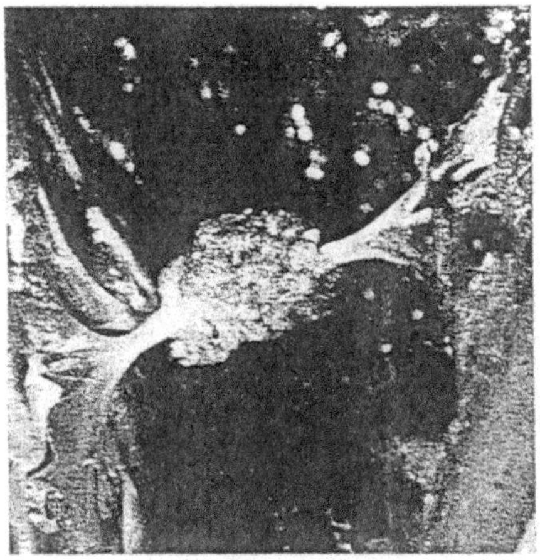

Fig 4.—Tumor in patient 3 extends from left ventricular free wall (right) to septum (left) (original magnification × 2).

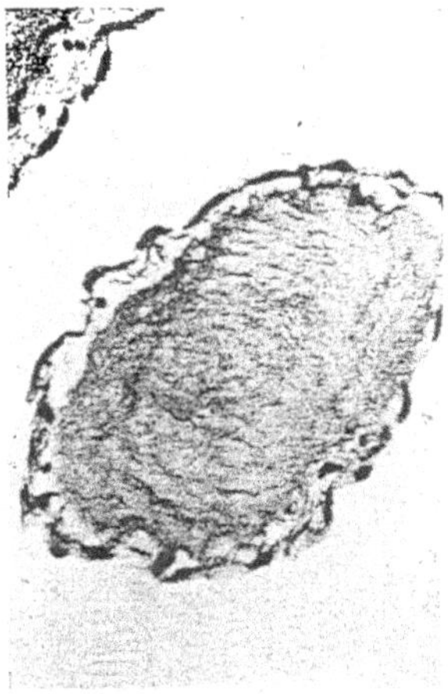

Fig 6.—Papilla from tumor of patient 2 is composed of dense collagenous core surrounded by narrow peripheral zone of loose, myxomatous tissue, and is covered by hyperplastic layer of endothelial cells (hematoxylin-eosin, original magnification × 225).

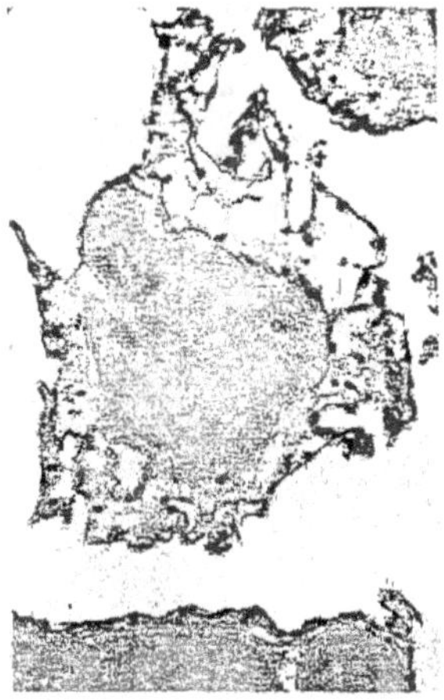

Fig 7.—Section of papilla from tumor of patient 3 shows markedly hyperplastic endothelial cells, loose, vacuolated, myxomatous zone, and dense central core (Masson trichrome, original magnification × 225).

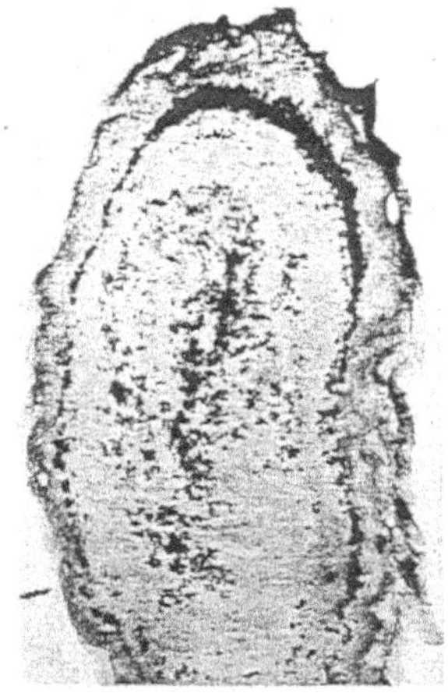

Fig 8.—Oblique section of papilla from tumor of patient 2 showing abundant, particulate elastic tissue within central core (elastica-van Gieson original magnification × 225).

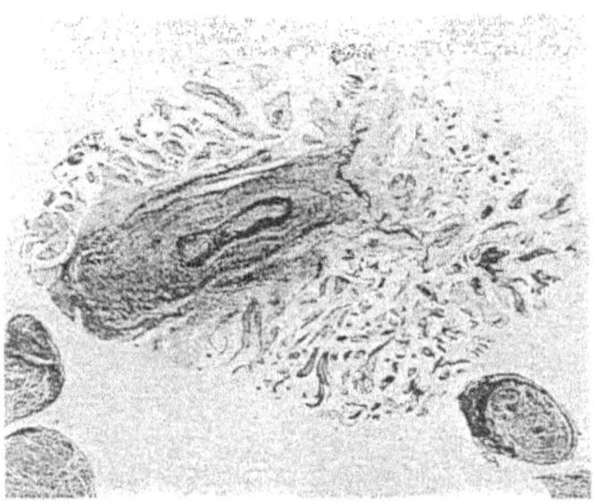

Fig 5.—Section of tumor shown in Fig 4. Stalk contains collagenous and elastic tissue; morphology of papillae varies depending on plane of sectioning (elastica-van Gieson, original magnification × 6.5).

tissue arranged in concentric layers (Fig 8 and 9). Each core was surrounded by a loose, vacuolated, myxomatous-appearing, basophilic stroma in which cells similar to those of the central core were found (Fig 12). Some of the papillae had extravasated erythrocytes within this myxomatous stroma (Fig 10). No vascular structures were identified, and the spaces containing the erythrocytes were not lined by endothelial cells. The loose, peripheral stroma had amorphous deposits of acid mucopolysaccharides (Fig 11).

Electron Microscopical Observations

The endothelial cells covering the tumor papillae had plump, oval to elongated nuclei with peripherally condensed chromatin and indented nuclear membranes (Fig 13). In some cells, the nucleoli were prominent. The cytoplasm of endothelial cells contained numerous filaments, 100 Angstroms in diameter; a few dilated cisterns of endoplasmic reticulum; numerous pinocytotic vesicles; and a few electron-dense lysosomes measuring from 0.1μ to 1μ in diameter. The 100-A filaments (Fig 14) were wavy, nonbranching, and appeared randomly oriented, although many of them tended to align parallel to the nuclear membranes. Attenuated, finger-like projections of cytoplasm extended over the surface of the tumor. Intercellular junctions of the zonula adherens type were present where these cytoplasmic processes joined adjacent endothelial cells (Fig 13). The quality of the preservation of the tissue did not permit a more detailed analysis of junctional structures. Mitochondria showed severe changes of postmortem autolysis. Basement membranes were absent in some areas but well developed in others. Some of the cells immediately beneath the endothelial cells were morphologically indistinguishable from those at the surface and were connected to them by intercellular junctions. Such images were considered to result from tangential planes of sectioning through areas of endothelial cell hyperplasia.

The peripheral, myxomatous zones of the papillae were characterized by a loose matrix of slight to moderate electron density. This matrix consisted of finely granular to fibrillar material (Fig 14). Only an occasional collagenous or elastic fiber was observed in this zone. A few oval to elongated cells occurring individually were found in this zone, usually in close proximity to the layer of endothelial cells. These cells were not connected to each other by intercellular junctions and were ultrastructurally identical to those in the central core.

The central cores of the papillae contained a few oval to elongated cells embedded in a dense stroma composed of collagen fibrils, elastic fibers, and clumped amorphous material. These cells had round to elongated nuclei with irregular wavy borders, occasional deep indentations of the nuclear membranes, and peripheral condensation of chromatin (Fig 15). The cytoplasmic components varied from one cell to another. In some cells (Fig 15), the major elements were 100-A thick filaments similar to those in the endothelial cells. In other cells, the most conspicuous cytoplasmic organ-

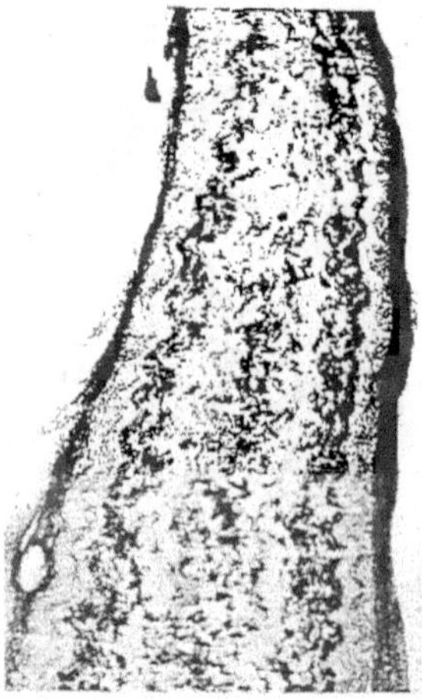

Fig 9.—Longitudinal section of papilla from tumor of patient 2 showing particulate to fibrillar elastic tissue arranged in layers (elastica-van Gieson; original magnification × 225).

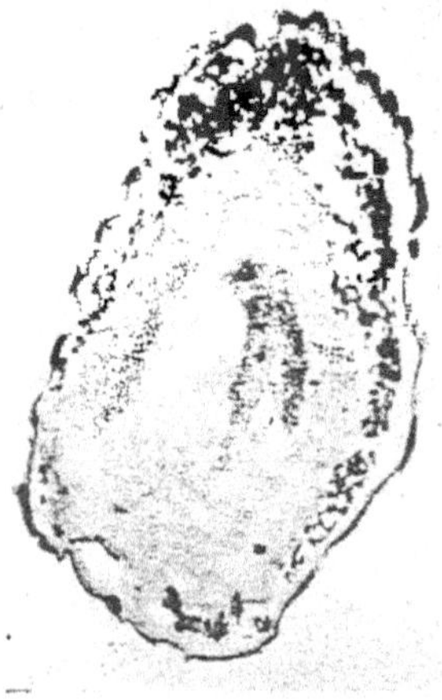

Fig 10.—Section of papilla from tumor of patient 2 showing numerous erythrocytes within peripheral myxomatous zone. These erythrocytes probably enter tumor as result of trauma and damage to covering endothelium (Masson trichrome, original magnification × 225).

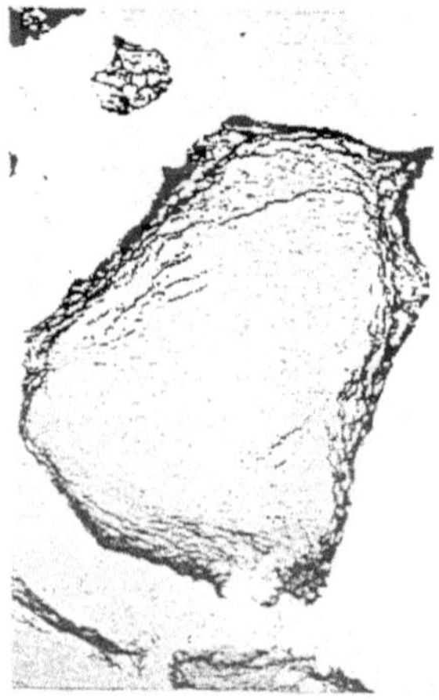

Fig 11.—Section of papilla from tumor of patient 1 showing presence of acid mucopolysaccharides in myxomatous peripheral zone (Rinehart, original magnification × 200).

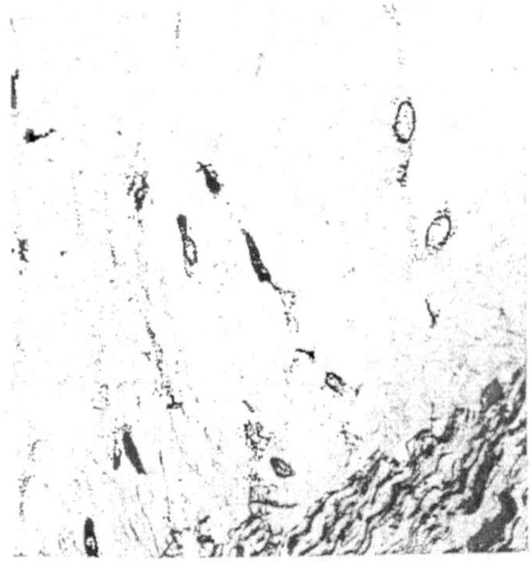

Fig 12.—Semifine (0.5μ thick) section of epoxy-embedded tissue from tumor of patient 3, showing round to elongated mesenchymal cells in loose, myxomatous stroma of peripheral zone of papilla (alkaline toluidine blue, original magnification × 300).

elles were dilated cisterns of rough-surfaced endoplasmic reticulum. Golgi complexes and free ribosomes also were present in these cells. Mitochondria were relatively sparse, and basement membranes were absent. The collagen fibrils measured from 300 to 600 A in diameter and usually were arranged in small bundles. In some areas the collagenous fibrils appeared fragmented and were associated with large amounts of clumped, amorphous material. The elastic fibers were small, approximately 1,000 A in diameter, and poorly organized. They were composed of amorphous material that showed a high affinity for silver tetraphenylporphine sulfonate (Fig 16) and were surrounded by numerous microfibrils measuring approximately 150 A in diameter.

COMMENT

This study confirms previous observations[1-4, 6-8] showing that endocardial papillary elastofibroma is a distinct morphologic entity characterized by the following gross and histologic features: (1) occurrence primarily on cardiac valves, but also on chordae tendineae and mural endocardium; (2) papillary appearance with multiple villus-like projections extending from a central collagenous stalk; and (3) distinct architectural pattern consisting of three zones—a central core (with focal hyalinization) composed of collagen, reticulin and elastic fibers; a peripheral myxomatous zone with deposits of acid mucopolysaccharides; and an overlying layer of hyperplastic endothelium. Electron microscopic studies of this tumor confirmed these findings and also disclosed that the cells of all three regions were ultrastructurally similar in many respects, including their content of cytoplasmic filaments. Endothelial cells were distinguished by their location, intercellular junctions, numerous pinocytotic vesicles, and variably developed basement membranes.

Cytoplasmic filaments of the type described in this report also have been observed in a variety of normal cells, including striated and smooth muscle, endothelial, myoepithelial, glomerular, chondrogenic, glial, epidermal, intestinal epithelial and melanocytic cells, and in numerous types of neoplastic cells (see Ferrans and Roberts[10] for review). Although considerable importance has been attributed to the presence of cytoplasmic filaments in endocardial papillary elastofibroma[7] and in cardiac myxomas, similar filaments have been found in cells of other tumors having a myxomatous stroma, such as fibromyxosarcoma[11] and extraskeletal myxoid chondrosarcoma,[12] as well as in normal cells of Wharton jelly in umbilical cord.[13] The 100 A class of filaments is generally believed to have a cytoskeletal function. Obviously, their presence does not constitute a basis for identification of cell type.

We regard the cells of the endocardial papillary elastofibroma as primitive mesenchymal cells with multipotential capabilities for cellular differentiation. Similar cells have been observed in aorta of swine[14] and chick,[15] theca externa of rat ovarian follicles,[16] various arteriosclerotic lesions,[17-19] granulation tissue,[20] thickened endocardium of the right ventricular outflow tract of patients with tetralogy of Fallot,[21] and cardiac myxomas.[7, 10] The observations in this study suggest that the myxomatous part of the stroma is synthesized by the cells in the surface and that the elastic and collagenous components of the cores are formed by the mesenchymal cells therein. Although this elastic tissue had a peculiar appearance by light microscopy, ultrastructural study showed that it had the usual components (amorphous material and microfibrils) of elastic tissue and that it stained with silver tetraphenylporphine sulfonate as did elastic fibers in endocardium in endocardial fibroelastosis. It should be noted, however, that areas of endocardial thickening in endocardial fibroelastosis contain not only undifferentiated mesenchymal cells (which are few in number) but also typical smooth muscle cells (the predominant cell type) and cells in various stages of differentiation toward either fibroblasts or smooth muscle cells (unpublished observations).

Endocardial papillary elastofibroma often has been compared to the myxoma because of its intracardiac location and its myxomatous stroma. The unique architecture of the individual papillae of endocardial elastofibromas clearly distinguishes them from myxomas. Actually, this architecture is more reminiscent of that of polyps formed by various types of epithelial cells. Except for the endothelial cells on the surface, the cells of the endocardial papillary elastofibroma show no tendency to associate with each other or to undergo morphological differentiation into several varieties of cells. Endocardial papillary elastofibromas do not contain cords of cells, networks of stellate-shaped cells, or primitive blood vessels such as those observed in myxomas.[10] The cells in endocardial papillary elastofibroma contain cytoskeletal filaments, 100 A in diameter, but not the actin-like filaments, 60 to 80 A in diameter, or the patches of Z-band-like material that have been observed together with 100-A filaments in myxoma cells.[10] The cells in endocardial papillary elastofibroma resemble more closely the undifferentiated myxoma cells, which contain only the 100-A type of filaments.[10] Because emphasis has been placed on various different components of the endocardial papillary elastofibroma, this lesion has been, and is, referred to by numerous terms. Since the dense central fibroelastic core is the most conspicuous component of these tumors, and since this feature is not found in the other endocardial tumor, the myxoma, the term "endocardial papillary elastofibroma" seems appropriate for this lesion.

The pathogenesis of endocardial papillary elastofibroma is still uncertain. Many[1,3-5] accept the view of Pomerance[2] that these are giant Lambl excrescences formed by organization of successive layers of fibrin deposits on endothelium.[22] Few authors, however, mention finding fibrin in or on these tumors. Heath and Thompson[3] observed fibrin within the papillae of one tumor. Pomerance[2] mentioned finding small subendothelial zones of fibrin in only one of six tumors. Other reports[5-8,23,24] have not described fibrin deposits associated with the tumors. We found no histologic or ultrastructural evidence of fibrin in, or attached to, the tumors of our three patients. One might expect that, if these tumors indeed grew by

Fig 13.—Electron micrograph of area of surface showing endothelial cell with 100-A filaments, dilated cisterns of endoplasmic reticulum, pinocytotic vesicles, and discrete basement membranes. Underlying stroma consists of finely granular to fibrillar material (original magnification × 7,500). Inset, Zonula adherens type of junction between two endothelial cells (× 15,000).

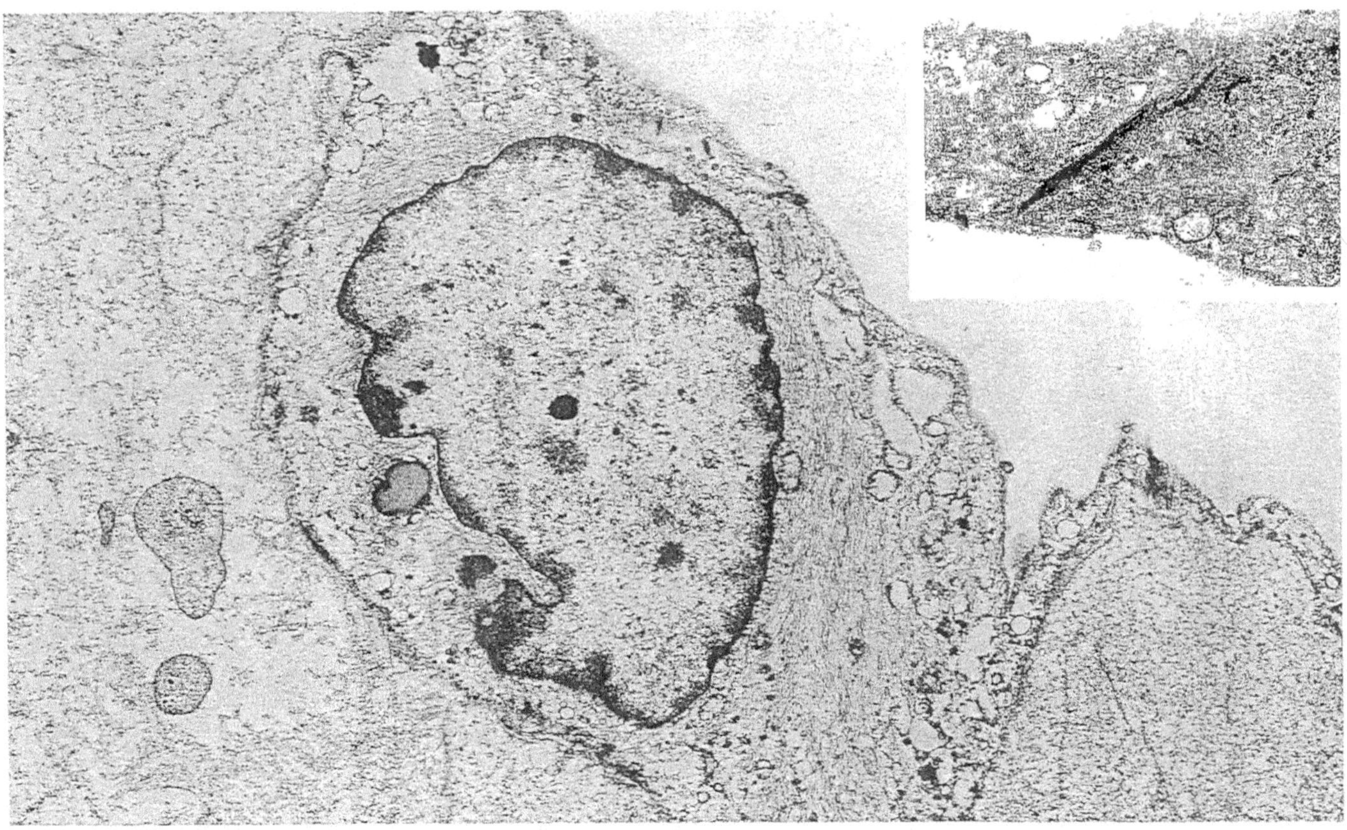

organization of successive layers of fibrin, such fibrin deposits would be an almost constant finding. We consider that the connective tissue cores of the papillae are extensions of the stalk, which is continuous with the subendocardial connective tissue, and that the myxomatous peripheral zones probably represent extensions of the thin, acid mucopolysaccharide-rich subintimal layer of the endocardium. The stroma in these peripheral zones is ultrastructurally similar to that in cardiac myxomas.[10] Regarding the surface layer, we believe that the proliferation of endothelial cells is important in the pathogenesis of endocardial papillary elastofibromas, and that fibrin deposition, if it indeed occurs, is a secondary phenomenon. We observed marked hyperplasia of endothelial cells not only on the surfaces of the tumors but also in foci in adjacent areas of mural endocardium. An increase in the population density of endothelial cells occurs in those areas of the arterial tree where flow is most turbulent.[25] Because of their papillary structure, the surface area of these tumors is extremely large with re-

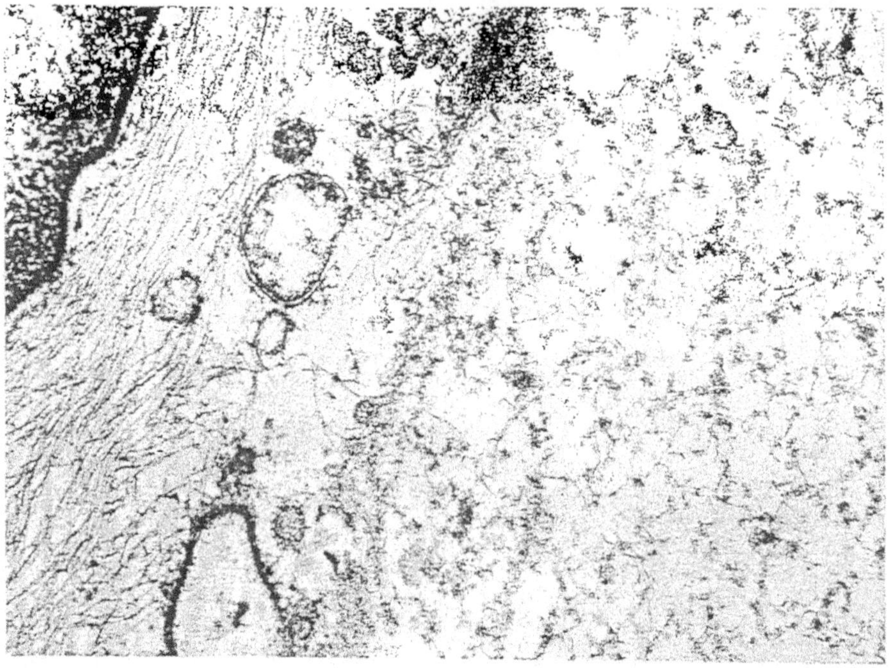

Fig 14.—High magnification view of part of endothelial cell showing 100 A filaments, few pinocytotic vesicles, and adjacent fibrillar and granular stroma (× 45,000).

Fig 15.—Cell in central core of tumor papilla is surrounded by collagenous and elastic fibers. This cell contains 100-A filaments and rough-surfaced endoplasmic reticulum and is very similar to those in peripheral zone and in endothelial layer (× 15,000).

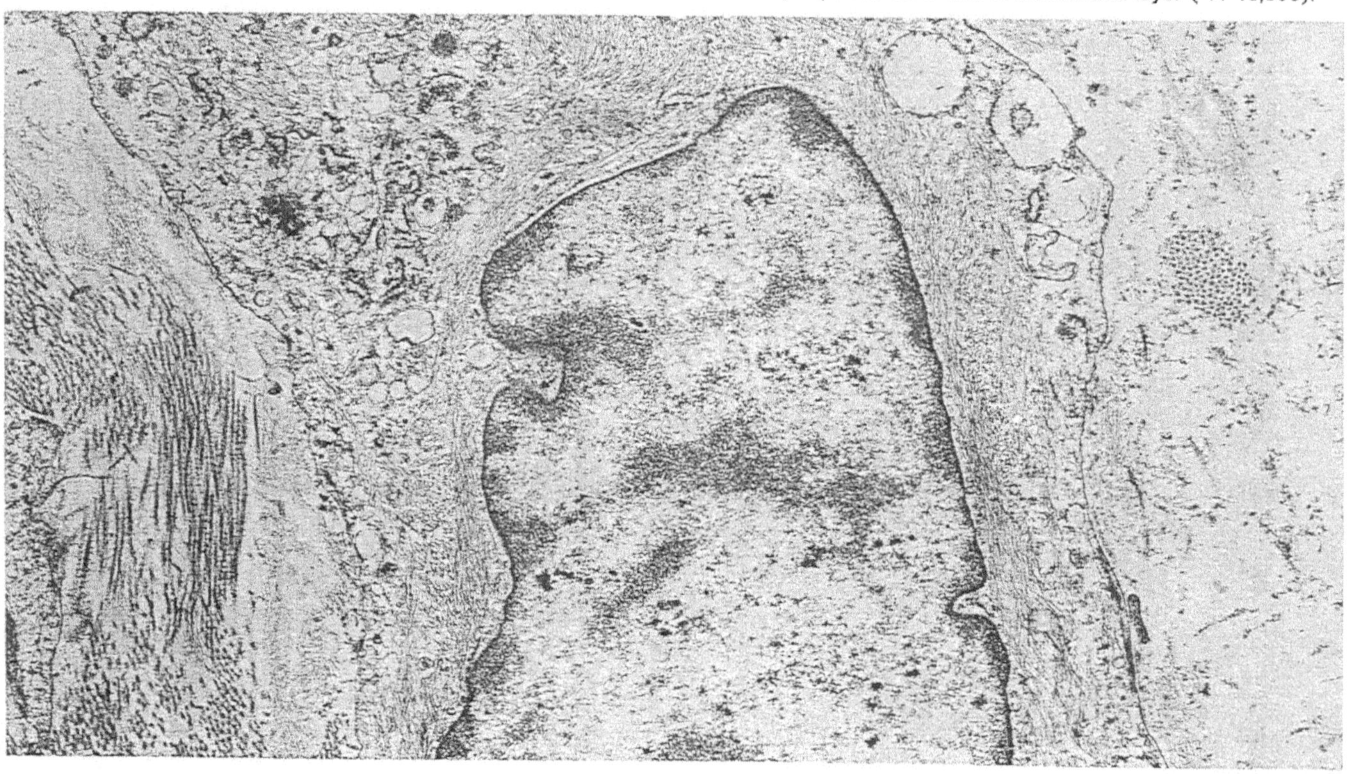

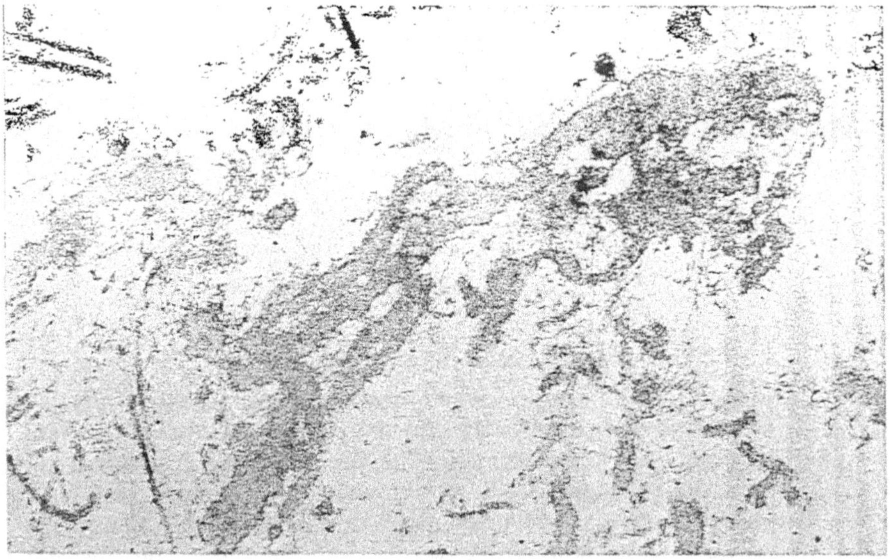

Fig 16.—Central core region stained with silver tetraphenylporphine sulfonate and counterstained with lead citrate and uranyl acetate shows electron-dense appearance characteristic of elastic fibers (× 25,000).

spect to their mass. Thus, from the quantitative standpoint, endothelial cells constitute by far the most important cellular component of endocardial papillary elastofibromas.

The primary event leading to the proliferation of the cells in the endothelial surface and to the formation of the papillae remains unknown. Chronic trauma to endocardium appears important in the pathogenesis of endocardial papillary elastofibroma; the majority of patients reported to have this lesion, and the three patients described herein, had longstanding cardiovascular disease (valvular, pulmonary, or hypertensive) or were old. Turbulent blood flow and its associated mechanical trauma may contribute to the endothelial cell hyperplasia and may be responsible for the degenerative changes in the connective tissue in the stalk and in the cores of the papillae. Although this possibility cannot be excluded completely on the basis of available evidence, a neoplastic nature of endocardial papillary elastofibroma seems unlikely.

References

1. Nassar SGA, Parker JC Jr: Incidental papillary endocardial tumor: Its potential significance. *Arch Pathol* 92:370-376, 1971.
2. Pomerance A: Papillary "tumours" of the heart valves. *J Pathol* 81:135-140, 1961.
3. Heath D, Thompson IM: Papillary "tumours" of the left ventricle *Br Heart J* 29:950-954, 1965.
4. Heath D: Pathology of cardiac tumors. *Am J Cardiol* 21:315-327, 1968.
5. Schiller AL, Schantz A: Papillary endocardial excrescence of the right atrium: Report of two cases. *Am J Clin Pathol* 53:617-621, 1970.
6. Heath D, Best PV, Davis BT: Papilliferous tumours of the heart valves. *Br Heart J* 23:20-24, 1961.
7. Stovin PGI, Heath D, Khaliq SU: Ultrastructure of the cardiac myxoma and the papillary tumour of heart valves. *Thorax* 28:273-285, 1973.
8. Raeburn C: Papillary fibro-elastic hamartomas of the heart valves. *J Pathol* 65:371-373, 1953.
9. Albert EN Fleischer E: A new electron-dense stain for elastic tissue. *J Histochem Cytochem* 18:697-708, 1970.
10. Ferrans VJ, Roberts WC: Structural features of cardiac myxomas: Histology, histochemistry, and electron microscopy. *Hum Pathol* 4:111-146, 1973.
11. Leak LV, Caulfield JB, Burke JF, et al: Electron microscopic studies on a human fibromyxosarcoma. *Cancer Res* 27:261-285, 1967.
12. Enzinger FM, Shiraki M: Extraskeletal myxoid chondrosarcoma: An analysis of 34 cases. *Hum Pathol* 3:421-435, 1972.
13. Parry EW: Some electron microscope observations on the mesenchymal structures of full-term umbilical cord. *J Anat* 107:505-518, 1970.
14. Lee KT, Lee KJ, Lee SK, et al: Poorly differentiated subendothelial cells in swine aortas. *Exp Mol Pathol* 13:118-129, 1970.
15. Moss NS, Benditt EP: Spontaneous and experimentally induced arterial lesions: I. An ultrastructural survey of the normal chicken aorta. *Lab Invest* 22:166-183, 1970.
16. O'Shea JD: An ultrastructural study of smooth muscle-like cells in the theca externa of ovarian follicles in the rat. *Anat Rec* 167:127-140, 1970.
17. Haust MD, More RH, Movat HZ: The role of smooth muscle cells in the fibrogenesis of arteriosclerosis. *Am J Pathol* 37:377-389, 1960.
18. Thomas WA, Jones R, Scott RF, et al: Production of early atherosclerotic lesions in rats characterized by proliferation of "modified smooth muscle cells". *Exp Mol Pathol* (suppl 1):40-61, 1963.
19. Parker F, Odland GF: A correlative histochemical, biochemical and electron microscopic study of experimental atherosclerosis in the rabbit aorta with special reference to the myointimal cell. *Am J Pathol* 48:197-239, 1966.
20. Gabbiani G, Ryan GB, Majno G: Presence of modified fibroblasts in granulation tissue and their possible role in wound contraction. *Experientia* 27:549-550, 1971.
21. Stein AA, Mauro J, Thibodeau L, et al: The histogenesis of cardiac myxomas: Relation to other proliferative diseases of subendothelial vasoform reserve cells, in Sommers SC (ed): *Pathology Annual*. New York, Appleton-Century Crofts, 1969, vol 4, pp 293-312.
22. Magarey FR: On the mode of formation of Lambl's excrescences and their relation to chronic thickening of the mitral valve. *J Pathol* 61:203-208, 1949.
23. Burn CG, Bishop MB, Davies JNP: A stalked papillary tumor of the mural endocardium. *Am J Clin Pathol* 51:344-346, 1969.
24. Dudley HR, Goodale F Jr, O'Neal RM: Fibro-elastic hamartomas of heart valves. *Am J Pathol* 32:35-39, 1956.
25. Flaherty JT, Pierce JE, Ferrans VJ, et al: Endothelial nuclear patterns in the canine arterial tree with particular reference to hemodynamic events. *Circ Res* 30:23-33, 1972.

Coronary Heart Disease After Mediastinal Irradiation for Hodgkin's Disease

RICHARD A. McREYNOLDS, M.D.*
G. LENNARD GOLD, M.D.
WILLIAM C. ROBERTS, M.D.
Bethesda, Maryland

Attention is called to the development of coronary heart disease in two patients several years after they received mediastinal irradiation for Hodgkin's disease. One patient, a 33 year old man, died suddenly eight years after irradiation; necropsy disclosed marked narrowing of all three major coronary arteries. In addition to severe intima fibrous thickening, there also was considerable adventitial scarring of the coronary arteries. This type of coronary sclerosis is different from that seen in the usual patient with coronary heart disease. The second patient, a 42 year old man, had an acute myocardial infarction on two occasions, the first six years after mediastinal irradiation. Observations in previously described patients with coronary heart disease almost surely induced by therapeutic irradiation for Hodgkin's disease are reviewed.

"Radiation always produces injury, and repair of that injury may cause (intimal) proliferation." SHIELDS WARREN, *1961 [1]*

It is well known that ionizing irradiation may damage the heart, and changes in pericardium, myocardium and endocardium have been described [2–4]. Of the three portions of the heart, the epicardium is the one most severely damaged by irradiation [4–6]. Contained within the epicardium are the coronary arteries. Thus, mediastinal irradiation, such as given to many patients with Hodgkin's disease, might be expected to damage the arteries contained in the pericardium. In this report we describe coronary heart disease after irradiation in two patients and review previous reports describing lethal coronary arterial changes after mediastinal irradiation.

DESCRIPTION OF PATIENTS

Case 1. A 33 year old white man (CC No. 06-43-50-6), on routine chest roentgenogram at age 24 (1965), was found to have bilateral hilar masses. Shortly thereafter several anterior mediastinal lymph nodes were excised via a midline sternal splitting incision; histologic examination disclosed Hodgkin's disease (nodular sclerosing type; stage IIa without laparotomy). Neither the pericardial sac nor the pleural spaces were entered at operation. Radiotherapy was instituted, with total dosages as follows: mediastinum, administered exclusively via an anterior port, 5,000 rads (r); left axilla, 3,095 r; right axilla, neck and periaortic areas, 3,000 r each; and spleen, 2,000 r. Following this therapy, lymphadenopathy was no longer present and the patient thereafter was believed to be free of Hodgkin's disease. His blood pressure during his last eight years of life was

From the Section of Pathology, National Heart & Lung Institute, and the Division of Cancer Treatment, National Cancer Institute, National Institutes of Health, Bethesda, Maryland. Requests for reprints should be addressed to Dr. William C. Roberts, Bldg. 10A, Rm 3E-30, NIH, Bethesda, Maryland 20014. Manuscript accepted July 24, 1975.

* Present address: University of Alabama School of Medicine, Birmingham, Alabama 35294.

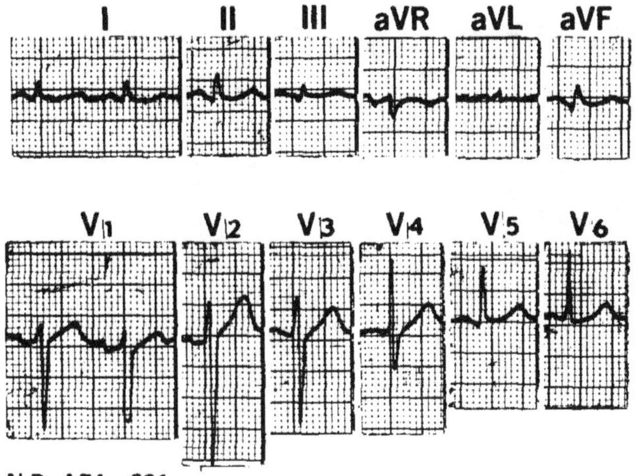

N.B. A74 - 291
5/31/74

Figure 1. *Case 1. Electrocardiogram.*

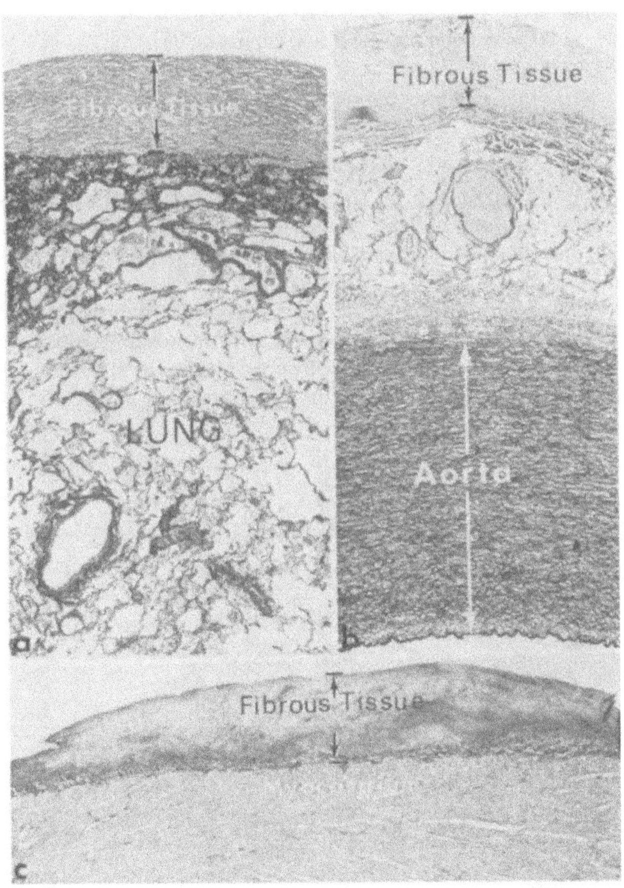

Figure 2. *Case 1. Fibrous thickening of pleura (**a**), adventitia of ascending aorta (**b**) and epicardium (**c**). The thickening in these sites almost certainly resulted from the mediastinal irradiation. Hematoxylin-eosin stain (**a**), Movat stain (**b**) and elastic van Gieson stain (**c**); magnification × 22 (**a** and **b**), × 14 (**c**), reduced by 23 per cent.*

usually 120 to 130 mm Hg systolic and 55 to 80 mm Hg diastolic. Three total serum cholesterol determinations were 179, 290 and 302 mg/100 ml, respectively. He smoked approximately 20 cigarettes daily for 15 years. His heart was always of normal size by chest roentgenogram. An electrocardiogram (Figure 1), recorded 10 weeks before death, disclosed low voltage (sum of QRS complexes in leads I, II and III = <15 m volts) and Q waves in leads III and aVF. He had no symptoms of cardiac dysfunction until 2 1/2 hours before death when he had the onset of severe substernal chest pain. On admission to a hospital, he was hypotensive, had severe rhythm disturbances and shortly thereafter had fatal cardiac arrest.

Necropsy (A74-291) included examination of all body organs. The heart weighed 340 g and the parietal pericardium was adherent by fibrous adhesions in several sites to the visceral pericardium. The epicardium in a number of different sites was thickened by fibrous tissue. The four cardiac chambers were of normal size and their walls were of normal thickness. The four cardiac valves were normal, but the mural endocardium of both ventricles was focally thickened. No gross foci of myocardial necrosis or fibrosis were present.

Histologically, collections of lymphocytes and plasma cells were present in the epicardium, which was focally thickened by dense fibrous tissue (Figures 2 and 3). Focal perivascular fibrosis was observed in sections of left ventricular free wall, ventricular septum and papillary muscles. In addition, a healed microinfarct was observed in the immediate subepicardial portion of the left ventricle, and considerable focal interstitial myocardial fibrosis was observed in the anterior wall of the right ventricle (Figure 3), primarily in areas adjacent to the ventricular septum. No foci of myocardial necrosis were observed histologically.

Three histologic sections were prepared from each of 15 segments of the major epicardial coronary arteries. Each segment was 5 mm long, and consequently approximately 7.5 cm of the epicardial coronary tree was examined microscopically. Every section of major coronary artery showed severe thickening of its wall by both intimal and adventitial fibrous proliferation (Figures 4 to 6). The adventitial scarring was often contiguous with epicardial scarring (Figure 5). In several segments, collections of plasma cells and lymphocytes were present in the adventitia of the coronary arteries (Figure 6). The intimal proliferation consisted primarily of fibrous tissue. Only a rare foam cell, cholesterol cleft or extracellular lipid deposit was observed. The lumens of each of the three major coronary arteries were narrowed: right, >75 per cent; left anterior descending, 51 to 75 per cent; and left circumflex, >75 per cent. The media in several segments was focally compressed, occasionally to the point of total atrophy, by the adventitial and intimal fibrous tissue (Figure 5). No residual Hodgkin's disease was found.

Case 2. A 42 year old white man (Holy Cross Hospital of Silver Spring No. 2129-75) noted a nodule in his inguinal region when 33 years of age. One year later, this nodule was excised; histologic examination showed it to be a lymph node almost totally involved by Hodgkin's disease (mixed-cellularity type). A lymphangiogram disclosed ex-

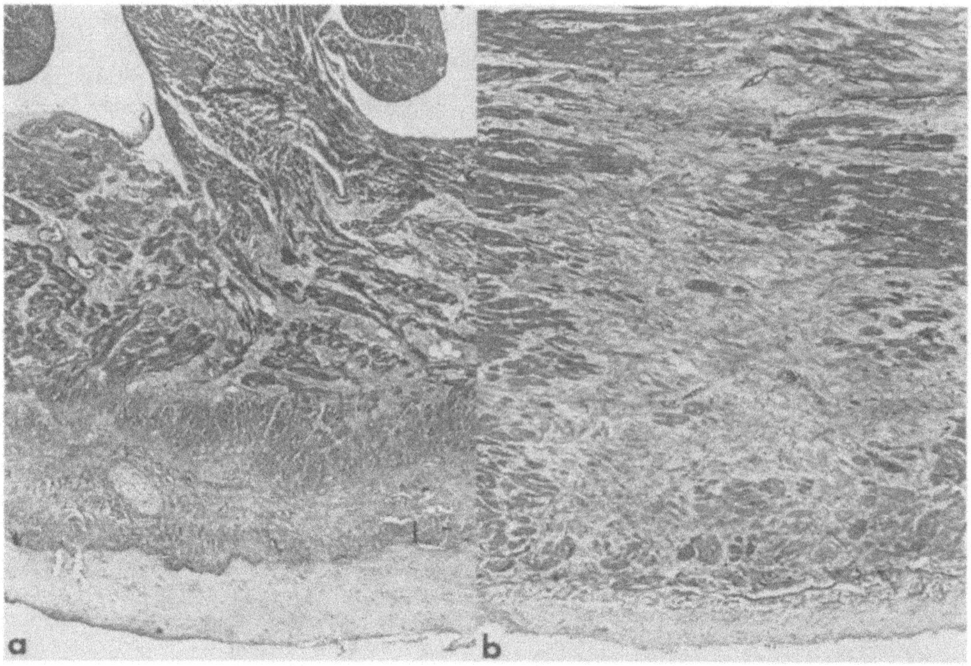

Figure 3. *Case 1. Myocardial scars and epicardial fibrous tissue.* ***a,*** *Transmural scar in right ventricles.* ***b,*** *Subepicardial scar in left ventricle. Movat stain (****a****) and hematoxylin and eosin stain (****b****); magnification × 34 (****a****), × 54 (****b****), reduced by 23 per cent.*

tensive involvement of the retroperitoneal and pelvic lymph nodes. Irradiation was given through large anterior and posterior inverted Y-shaped ports extending from the level of the diaphragm to just below the inguinal regions. The total tissue dose was 6,300 rads. At age 35, a swelling was noted in the region of his left parotid gland, and biopsy again showed Hodgkin's disease. He then was given 4,079 rads via a mantle field which included mediastinum through both anterior (2,143 r) and posterior (1,936 r) ports. At age 36 he received a course of combination chemotherapy. At age 40 (July 1974), he underwent total replacement of the head of the left femur because of aseptic necrosis, almost certainly the result of radiation damage.

At age 41 (February 1974), substernal chest pain developed with radiation down the left arm, for which the patient was hospitalized. Serial electrocardiograms and serum enzymes disclosed classic acute myocardial infarction ("infe-

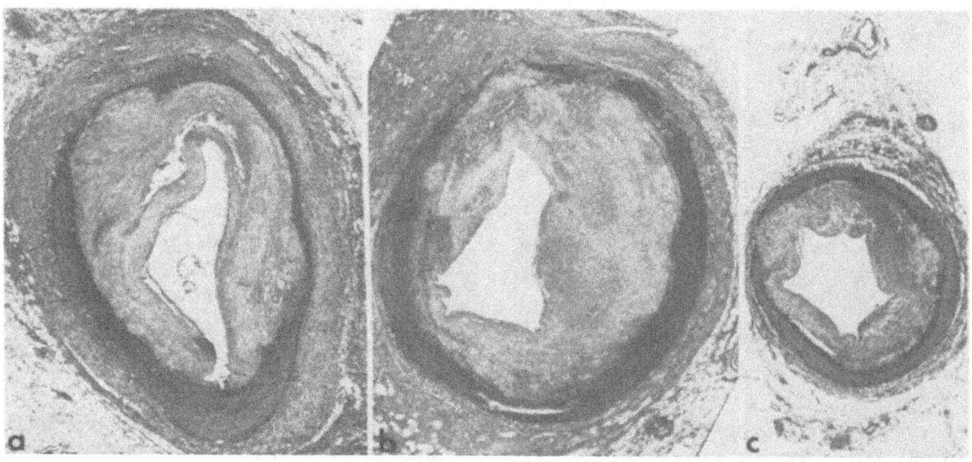

Figure 4. *Case 1. Coronary arteries showing severe luminal narrowing by intimal fibrous tissue, extensive but focal medial atrophy, and adventitial fibrosis.* ***a,*** *Right;* ***b,*** *Left anterior descending; and* ***c,*** *Left circumflex coronary arteries. Movat stains; magnification of each × 16, reduced by 23 per cent.*

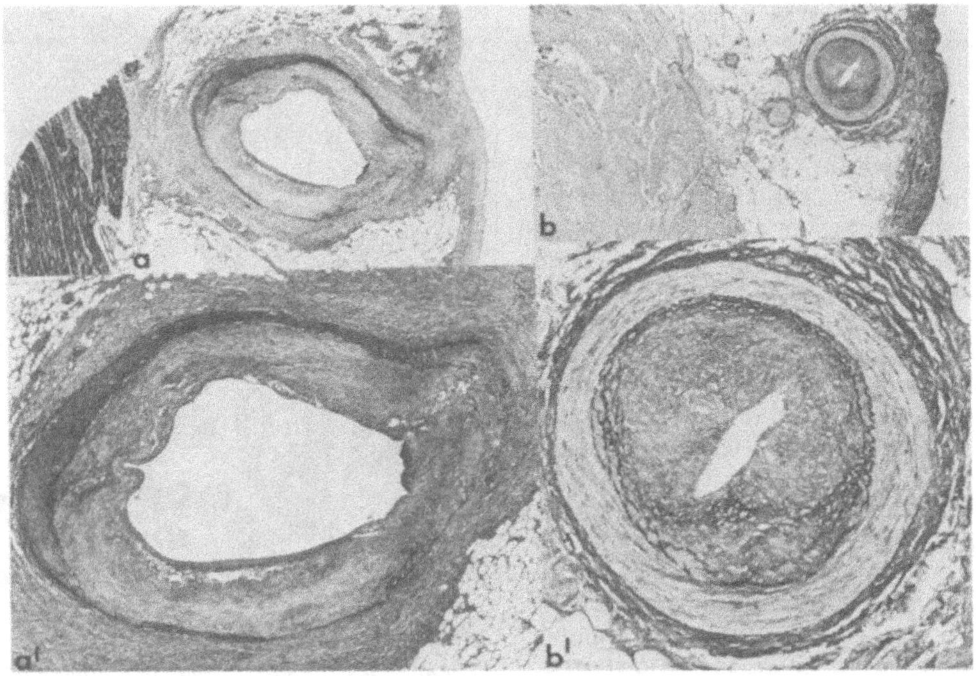

Figure 5. *Case 1. Coronary arteries and epicardium showing continuity of thickened adventitial fibrous tissue with thickened epicardial fibrous tissue.* ***a*** *and* ***a'****, Left anterior descending coronary artery also showing extensive atrophy of media.* ***b*** *and* ***b'****, Right coronary artery with severe luminal narrowing. Movat stains; magnification × 22 (****a****); × 27 (****a'****); × 20 (****b****); × 80 (****a'****), reduced by 28 per cent.*

rior" wall). He recovered from this acute myocardial infarction without complication, and was subsequently free of chest pain and had no evidence of congestive heart failure. He returned to work as an accountant, and remained well until age 42 (June 1975) when he had a second acute myocardial infarction, again well documented by typical electrocardiographic and serum enzyme changes. Coronary angiography is planned after convalescence from this second myocardial infarction.

This patient had been examined on many occasions since age 34. His heart by chest roentgenogram was always of normal size and there was never evidence of ventricular hypertrophy by electrocardiogram. His blood pressure levels were usually less than 140/90 mm Hg, often 110/70 mm Hg. During hospitalization for repair of his hip fracture, a blood pressure of 180/130 mm Hg was recorded. He had smoked about 40 cigarettes daily for 20 years. There was no family history of early coronary heart dis-

TABLE I Clinical and Necropsy Observations in Patients with Coronary Heart Disease After Mediastinal Irradiation

						Time (mo) Irradiation to:		Irradiation		Cardiac Symptoms		
Case	Source	Age at Death (yr)	Sex	Neoplasm	Age at Irradiation (yr)	Cardiac Symptoms	Death	Dose (rads)	Port	Age at First Cardiac Symptom	Age at AMI	First Cardiac Symptom
1	Cohn et al. (1963) [2] & Fajardo et al. (1968) [4]	15	M	HD	14	16	16	4,400*	. . .	15	15	AMI
2	Prentice (1965) [11]	19	M	HD	15	36	50	3,250	Thorax	18	19	AP
3	Dollinger et al. (1966) [12]	41	M	HD	31	2	120	3,910	Med	31	31	AMI
4	Huff, Sanders (1972) [13]	21	M	HD	20	8.5	9	3,500	Mantle	21	21	AMI
5	McReynolds et al. (1976) (present study)	33	M	HD	25	100	100	5,000 (3,095 (3,000	Med L Ax.) R Ax.)	33	. . .	SCD

NOTE: + = present; 0 = absent; — = no data; AMI = acute myocardial infarction; AP = angina pectoris; APn = acute pneumonia; Ax. = axilla; C = serum cholesterol level in mg/100 ml; cardiac symptoms = symptoms of cardiac disease; CHF = congestive heart failure; HD = Hodgkin's disease; HT = hypertension; L = left; LAD = left anterior descending; LC = left circumflex; LM = left main; Med = mediastinum; MI = myocardial infarction; R = right; SCD = sudden coronary death.

ease. During the hospitalization for his first acute myocardial infarction, the total serum cholesterol level was 220 mg/100 ml, and the triglyceride level 81 mg/100 ml.

COMMENTS

Several factors support the view that the coronary disease in Case 1 was the result of mediastinal irradiation rather than the result of atherosclerosis of the usual type: (1) The patient had received large doses of irradiation to the mediastinal tissues eight years earlier. (2) He was young (age 33 years) at the time of sudden coronary death. (3) The patient had other lesions which were readily attributable to the effects of irradiation, including pericardial adhesions and thickening, interstitial myocardial fibrosis of the right ventricle and focal thickening of the mural endocardium of both ventricles. (4) The patient had coronary arterial lesions of a type uncommonly observed in the usual type of coronary atherosclerosis, including severe coronary adventitial fibrosis, usually in continuity with overlying epicardial fibrous tissue, and marked paucity of lipid in the intimal lesions. In our experience [7–10] the dominant component of atherosclerotic plaques large enough to be fatal is fibrous tissue (collagen), but lipid, primarily extracellular, is present in most plaques and constitutes a significiant proportion of them (at least 25 per cent, occasionally much more). In the present patient, the amount of lipid in the plaques examined was minute, and this probably is particularly unusual for such a young patient. Furthermore, the collection of cells in the adventitia of the coronary arteries included large numbers of plasma cells and fewer lymphocytes. In the usual type of coronary atherosclerosis, lymphocytes are dominant and plasma cells are infrequent ("adventitial lymphocytosis"). (5) The patient had relatively "low level" risk factors to the development of accelerated atherosclerosis. Although he did have a slightly elevated blood cholesterol level, smoked cigarettes and was above ideal body weight, he had a normal blood pressure, no cardiomegaly and no family history of coronary disease. (6) He had virtually no atherosclerosis in other systemic arteries, including the aorta.

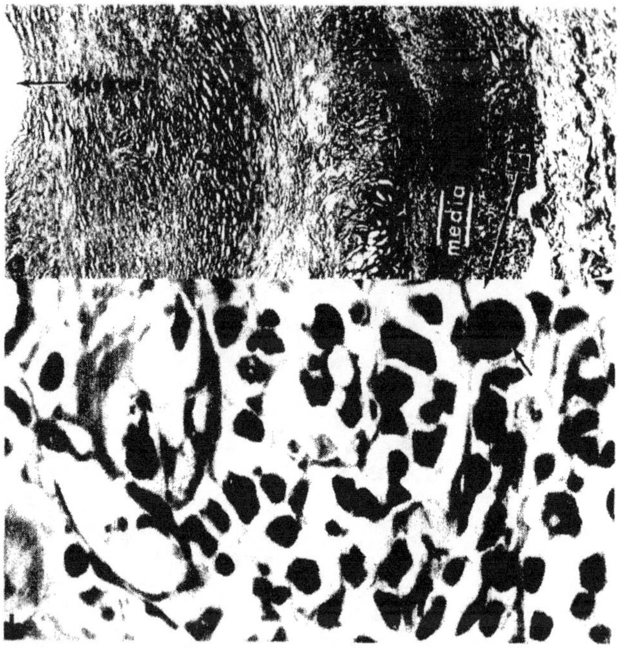

Figure 6. *Case 1. Portion of coronary artery showing severe intimal fibrosis **(a)** and adventitial inflammation **(b)**. The latter consists primarily of plasma cells, and a Russell body (short solid arrow) is visible. Movat stain **(a)** and hematoxylin and eosin stain **(b)**; original magnification × 54 **(a)** and × 860 **(b)**, reduced by 30 per cent.*

In addition to our necropsy patient, at least four

						Necropsy Data							
							Heart Weight		Coronary Arteries: Per cent of Luminal Narrowing				
AP	AMI	CHF	HT	↑C	Cause of Death	HD	(g)	MI	R	LM	LAD	LC	Atherosclerosis of Aorta
0	+	0	–	†	AMI	–	–	+	"Severe intimal proliferation"				0
+	+	+	–	†	AMI	–	–	+	"Typical atherosclerosis"				0
+	+	+	–	205	APn	+	330	+	>75	← widely patent →			"minimal"
?	+	+	0	≤265	AMI	0	–	+	"mild"	"mild"	100‡	"mild"	–
0	0	0	0	≤302	SCD	0	340	0	>75	–	51–75	>75	0

* = calculated dose to heart.
† = no values available.
‡ = thrombus.

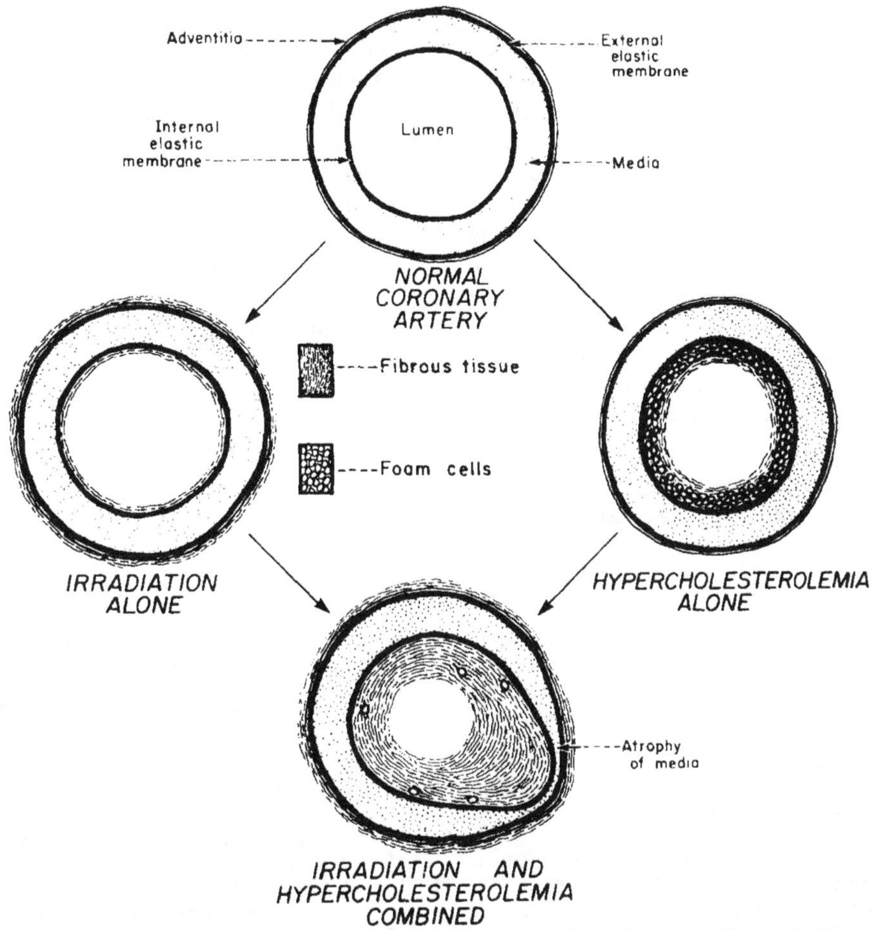

Figure 7. *Diagram showing the synergistic effect of irradiation and hyperlipidemia to cause intimal proliferation of the coronary arteries.*

necropsy patients have been described previously with coronary heart disease occurring after receiving large dose, therapeutic irradiation to the mediastinum (Table I) [11–13]. Each had had Hodgkin's disease and each had received from 3,250 to 5,000 rads (average 4,200 rads) to the mediastinum. All four had had acute myocardial infarcts, all almost surely transmural, when very young (aged 15 to 31 years [average 21 years]). All four had severely narrowed coronary arteries at necropsy. None of the four patients had known risk factors to the development of accelerated atherosclerosis: none had a family history of premature symptomatic or fatal atherosclerosis; none had known systemic hypertension; none had known serum total cholesterol levels above 265 mg/100 ml. Furthermore, all four had minimal or absent atherosclerosis in arteries outside the chest. In addition, each of the four patients had fibrotic changes in the chest other than in the coronary arteries, namely, pericarditis, pericardial adhesions, epicardial fibrosis, pleural adhesions and pulmonary parenchymal fibrosis, all recognized side effects of therapeutic irradiation [14,15]. Thus, it is likely that the coronary atherosclerosis in these four previously described patients was the result of mediastinal irradiation.

Our second patient similarly received large dose mediastinal irradiation to fields which included the heart. His only known predisposing factor to the development of early coronary heart disease was heavy cigarette smoking.

In addition to our one living patient, three other patients with nonfatal acute myocardial infarcts after therapeutic mediastinal irradiation have also been briefly mentioned in previous reports [16–18]. All three were women: one was 35 years of age, and each of the other two were "under 50" years of age at the time of the acute myocardial infarction. The amount of irradiation received was given for only one of the three patients, and she received 5,075 rads to the mediastinum for Hodgkin's disease; post-infarction coronary angiography showed severe narrowing of the left anterior descending and left circumflex arteries and a "small" right coronary artery.

Experimental studies also support the thesis that therapeutic levels of irradiation can produce or hasten coronary atherosclerosis [19–22]. The effects of the irradiation alone, however, are minimal, but when irradiation is given to animals (rabbits or rats) on high cholesterol diets, severe coronary atherosclerosis results, far more severe degrees of atherosclerosis than that resulting from the hypercholesterolemia alone [17,19] (Figure 7). Irradiation and hypercholesterolemia appear to act synergistically to produce considerably more atherosclerosis than that produced by either irradiation or hypercholesterolemia alone. Our patient did have hypercholesterolemia, and although considered "normal" by us, two of the four previously described patients had serum cholesterol levels of 205 and 265 mg/100 ml. (We believe that truly normal serum cholesterol levels are <200 mg/100 ml; what is considered normal in the Western World more likely represents "average.") Possibly, the mechanism of the development of atherosclerosis in these patients is as follows: irradiation damages arterial endothelium; this damage is repaired by platelet aggregation and fibrin deposition, and ultimately by fibrous tissue or collagen [1,23,24]. The associated hypercholesterolemia may act by overstimulating the repair process through its effect on platelet aggregation which eventuates in excessive intimal fibrous proliferation with luminal narrowing.

ACKNOWLEDGMENT

We thank Dr. Costan W. Berard, Head, Hematopathology Section, Laboratory of Pathology, National Cancer Institute, National Institutes of Health, for kindly reviewing the manuscript and for providing helpful suggestions.

REFERENCES

1. Warren S: The Pathology of Ionizing Radiation. Charles C Thomas, Springfield, Ill., 1961, p 24.
2. Cohn KE, Stewart JR, Fajardo LF, Hancock EW: Heart disease following radiation. Medicine (Baltimore) 46: 281, 1963.
3. Roberts WC, Glancy DL, DeVita VT Jr: Heart in malignant lymphoma (Hodgkin's disease, lymphosarcoma, reticulum cell sarcoma and mycosis fungoides). A study of 196 autopsy cases. Am J Cardiol 22: 85, 1968.
4. Fajardo LF, Stewart JR, Cohn KE: Morphology of radiation-induced heart disease. Arch Pathol 86: 512, 1968.
5. Morton DL, Kagan AR, Roberts WC, O'Brien KP, Holmes EC, Adkins PC: Pericardiectomy for radiation-induced pericarditis with effusion. Ann Thorac Surg 8: 195, 1969.
6. Ruckdeschel JC, Chang P, Martin RG, Byhardt RW, O'Connell MJ, Sutherland JC, Wiernik PH: Radiation-related pericardial effusions in patients with Hodgkin's disease. Medicine (Baltimore) 54: 245, 1975.
7. Roberts WC, Buja LM: The frequency and significance of coronary arterial thrombi and other observations in fatal acute myocardial infarction. A study of 107 necropsy patients. Am J Med 52: 425, 1972.
8. Roberts WC: Does thrombosis play a major role in the development of symptom-producing atherosclerotic plaques? Circulation 48: 1161, 1973.
9. Roberts WC: Coronary thrombosis and fatal myocardial ischemia. Circulation 49: 1, 1974.
10. Roberts WC: The status of the coronary arteries in fatal ischemic heart disease. Cardiovasc Clin, vol. 6, 1975.
11. Prentice RTW: Myocardial infarction following radiation. Lancet 2: 388, 1965.
12. Dollinger MR, Lavine DM, Foye LV Jr: Myocardial infarction due to postirradiation fibrosis of the coronary arteries. Case of successfully treated Hodgkin's disease with lower esophageal involvement. JAMA 195: 316, 1966.
13. Huff H, Sanders EM: Coronary-artery occlusion after radiation. N Engl J Med 286: 780, 1972.
14. Berdjis CG: The cardiovascular system, chap 17. Pathology of Irradiation (Berdjis CG, ed), Baltimore, Williams & Wilkins, 1971.
15. van den Brenk HAS: Radiation effects on the pulmonary system, chap 22. Pathology of Irradiation (Berdjis CG, ed), Baltimore, Williams & Wilkins, 1971.
16. Pearson HES: Coronary occlusion following thoracic radiotherapy, 2 cases. (Cases demonstrated before the Royal Society of Medicine.) Proc R Soc Med 50: 516, 1957.
17. Pearson HES: Incidental dangers of X-ray therapy. Lancet 1: 222, 1958.
18. Tracy GP, Brown DE, Johnson LW, Gottlieb AJ: Radiation-induced coronary artery disease. JAMA 228: 1660, 1974.
19. Gold H: Production of arteriosclerosis in the rat. Effect of X-ray and a high-fat diet. Arch Pathol 71: 268, 1961.
20. Gold H: Atherosclerosis in the rat. Effect of X-ray and a high-fat diet. Proc Soc Exp Biol Med 111: 593, 1962.
21. Amromin GD, Gildenhorn HL, Solomon RD, Nadkarni BB, Jacobs ML: The synergism of x-irradiation and cholesterol-fat feeding on the development of coronary artery lesions. J Atheroscler Res 4: 325, 1964.
22. Lamberts HB, de Boer WGRM: Contributions to the study of immediate and early X-ray reactions with regard to chemoprotection. IX. X-ray induced coronary occlusion leading to heart damage in rabbits. Int J Radiat Biol 8: 359, 1964.
23. Warren S: Effects of radiation on normal tissues. VI. Effects of radiation on the cardiovascular system. Arch Pathol 34: 1070, 1942.
24. Fajardo LF, Stewart JR: Pathogenesis of radiation-induced myocardial fibrosis. Lab Invest 29: 244, 1973.

THE CARCINOID ENDOCARDIAL PLAQUE

An Ultrastructural Study

Victor J. Ferrans, M.D., Ph.D., and William C. Roberts, M.D.†*

Abstract

Ultrastructural studies disclosed that the plaque-like endocardial thickenings in three patients with the carcinoid syndrome were composed of smooth muscle cells embedded in a stroma that was rich in acid mucopolysaccharides, collagen, and microfibrils, but devoid of elastic fibers. The smooth muscle cells contained variable numbers of myofilaments and cisterns of rough surfaced endoplasmic reticulum, and their basement membranes were greatly thickened, reduplicated, and arranged in layers. The endocardial plaques appeared histologically and ultrastructurally similar regardless of their location in the heart. The smooth muscle cells in these plaques appear to have been derived from primitive mesenchymal cells, which normally are present in the subendocardial endothelial space. These observations are interpreted as indicating that the plaques develop as a result of healing of a superficial endocardial injury, which may be initiated by release of bradykinin from hepatic metastases of a carcinoid tumor.

The carcinoid syndrome is caused by a metastasizing carcinoid tumor, which is located usually in the small intestine, occasionally in the stomach or bronchus, and rarely elsewhere.[1,2] Carcinoid tumors originate from enterochromaffin cells, which belong to the family of neuroectodermal cells known as APUD cells.[3] Cells in the APUD family share a number of properties, including the presence of secretory granules in their cytoplasm and the ability to synthesize various amines or polypeptide hormones.[3] The spectrum of APUD cell tumors includes neoplasms that produce clinical manifestations related to the secretion of gastrin (tumors of gastric G cells or pancreatic D cells), glucagon (tumors of pancreatic A cells), insulin (pancreatic B cell adenomas), calcitonin (tumors of thyroid C cells), and adrenocorticotrophin (pituitary corticotroph adenomas and oat cell carcinomas of the lung) or even two or more of these highly active polypeptides, as in various adenomas with multiple endocrine secretions.[3] Among APUD cell tumors that produce biologically active amines are pheochromocytomas, which secrete epinephrine and norepinephrine, and carcinoids, which produce serotonin

---

*Senior Investigator, Section of Pathology, National Heart and Lung Institute, National Institutes of Health, Bethesda, Maryland.

†Chief, Section of Pathology, National Heart and Lung Institute, National Institutes of Health, Bethesda, Maryland.

(5-hydroxytryptamine).[3-6] A few gastric carcinoids produce 5-hydroxytryptophan and histamine, presumably because they are deficient in aromatic L-amino acid decarboxylase.[7]

Diagnosis of the carcinoid syndrome usually is established on the basis of increased urinary excretion of 5-hydroxyindoleacetic acid, a metabolite of serotonin.[2] Secretion of a specific type of low molecular weight polypeptide has been demonstrated only very rarely in serotonin secreting carcinoid tumors,[8-11] but hepatic metastases of these tumors are known to contain large amounts of kallikrein.[12,13] Release of kallikrein from these sites (by adrenergic stimulation, alcohol ingestion, or other factors) results in the proteolytic conversion of plasma kininogen to lysyl-bradykinin, which in turn is rapidly hydrolyzed by plasma aminopeptidase to bradykinin, a polypeptide with powerful vasodilating and bronchoconstricting properties.[12,13] The clinical manifestations of the carcinoid syndrome are distinctive: diarrhea and dermal flushing occur in almost all patients, bronchospasm occurs in approximately one third, and peculiar but specific cardiac lesions are present in over one half.[14] The diarrhea in patients with the carcinoid syndrome is believed to be caused by serotonin, since it can be inhibited by serotonin antagonists.[15] The dermal flushes and the bronchospasm are related, at least in a majority of patients, to the release of kinin peptides.[12,13]

The cardiovascular lesions associated with the carcinoid syndrome are pathognomonic, are not associated with tumors of other cells of the APUD family, and bear little resemblance to those in other types of heart disease.[16,17] The carcinoid lesions, herein referred to as "carcinoid plaques," are characterized by the formation of plaque-like thickenings composed of an unusual type of fibrous tissue, which is superimposed on the endocardium of the valvular cusps and cardiac chambers, and on the intima of the great veins, coronary sinus, and occasionally the great arteries. These lesions are most extensive on the right side of the heart and typically result in tricuspid regurgitation and pulmonic stenosis. In contrast to this, left sided cardiac lesions are less frequent and result in little or no valvular dysfunction.[14,16-21] Because little is known of their detailed morphology, we have undertaken light and electron microscopic studies of carcinoid plaques. These studies form the basis for the present communication.

MATERIALS AND METHODS

Tissues for light and electron microscopic studies were obtained at the time of necropsy from three patients with the carcinoid syndrome. Pertinent clinical and pathologic findings in these patients are presented in Table 1.

Tissues for histologic and histochemical study were fixed with phosphate buffered formalin and embedded in paraffin. Sections of these tissues were stained with hematoxylin and eosin, Masson's trichrome, phosphotungstic acid–hematoxylin, elastica–van Gieson, the periodic acid–Schiff (PAS) method with and without predigestion of the sections with amylase, and the alcian blue (pH 1.0 and 2.5) method for acid mucosubstances.

For ultrastructural study, tissues were fixed with cold 3 per cent glutaraldehyde in 0.1 M phosphate buffer, pH 7.2, washed with several changes of 5 per cent sucrose in 0.1 M phosphate buffer, pH 7.2, postfixed with 1 per cent osmium tetroxide in Millonig's phosphate buffer, dehydrated in a graded series of ethanol and propylene oxide, and embedded in Maraglas.[22] Tissues from patients 1 and 2 (carcinoid plaques in the right atrium) had been previously fixed with phosphate buffered formalin; these tissues were refixed with glutaraldehyde and processed further as already described. Tissues from patient 3 (carcinoid plaques involving the right atrial and right ventricular wall, tricuspid valve, and pulmonic valve and uninvolved areas of all four cardiac chambers) were obtained within three hours after death and were fixed directly with glutaraldehyde.

All tissue blocks were embedded using flat embedding molds in order to maintain proper orientation of the endocardial surfaces with respect to the plane of

TABLE 1. Clinical and Pathologic Features in Three Patients with Carcinoid Heart Disease

Pt. no.	*Age (years) Race/sex*	*Duration of illness (years)**	*Diarrhea*	*Flushing*	*Broncho-spasm*	*Cardiac murmur*	*Urinary 5-HIAA excretion†*	*Site of primary tumor*	*Hepatic metast.*	*Heart weight (grams)*	*Distribution of cardiac plaques*
1	32 WF	9	+	+	0	+	580	Ileum	+	250	RA, TV, PV
2	52 WM	2	+	0	0	+	--	Ileum	+	350	RA, TV, PV
3	61 WF	1	+	+	0	+	285	Ileum	+	240	RA, TV, RV, PV, CS, MV, SVC

* = from time of onset of symptoms.
† = maximal recorded values (in mg./24 hr.).
+ = present.
0 = absent.
-- = data not available; diagnosis made at necropsy.
5-HIAA = 5-hydroxyindoleacetic acid.
CS = coronary sinus.
MV = mitral valve.
PV = pulmonic valve.
RA = right atrium.
RV = right ventricle.
SVC = superior vena cava.
TV = tricuspid valve.

sectioning. Semithin (0.5 μ thick) sections of Maraglas embedded tissues were stained with alkaline toluidine blue and examined with a light microscope to select areas for ultrathin sectioning. Ultrathin sections were stained with lead citrate and uranyl acetate and examined with the electron microscope. Selected sections were stained with silver tetraphenylporphin sulfonate, according to the method of Albert and Fleischer,[23] for the ultrastructural demonstration of elastic tissue.

RESULTS

Gross and Light Microscopic Observations

The carcinoid lesions consisted of white, plaque-like endocardial thickenings, which measured up to 2 mm. in thickness (Figs. 1, 2), were superimposed on normal mural or valvular endocardium (Figs. 3 to 5), and were covered by a single layer of endothelial cells. The endothelium overlying carcinoid plaques often appeared hypercellular. Cellular elements were present in moderate numbers in carcinoid plaques (Figs. 6 to 9). Other than rare macrophages and lymphocytes, these elements consisted of a single type of cell, which was elongated, attenuated, occasionally branched or stellate shaped, and always arranged in layers parallel to the surface of the plaque (Figs. 6, 7, 9). These cells had single, narrow, elongated nuclei. Their cytoplasm was eosinophilic; it stained red with Masson's trichrome and blue-black with phosphotungstic acid–hematoxylin. These staining characteristics were interpreted as indicating that the cellular components of carcinoid plaques were smooth muscle cells. The basement membranes of these cells stained intensely by the PAS method (Fig. 9), either with or without predigestion with amylase, and frequently appeared greatly thickened and reduplicated. The stroma in which these cells were embedded was faintly eosinophilic and PAS positive,

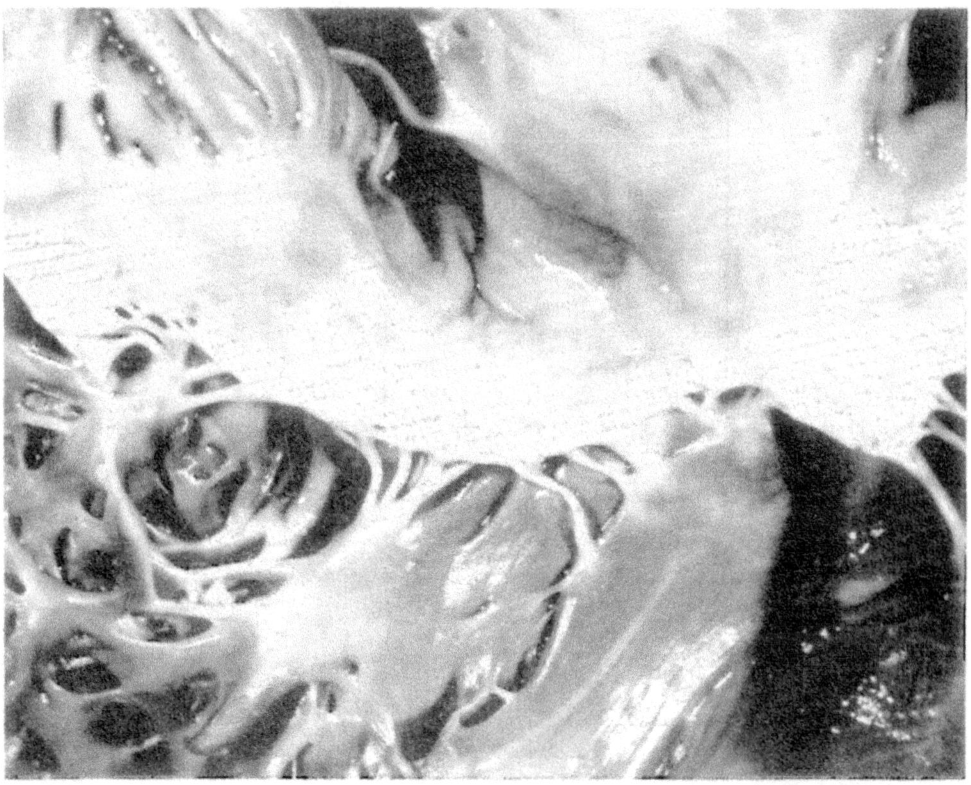

Figure 1. View of opened tricuspid valve of patient 3, showing thickening and contraction of the leaflets and chordae tendineae and thickening of the right atrial endocardium.

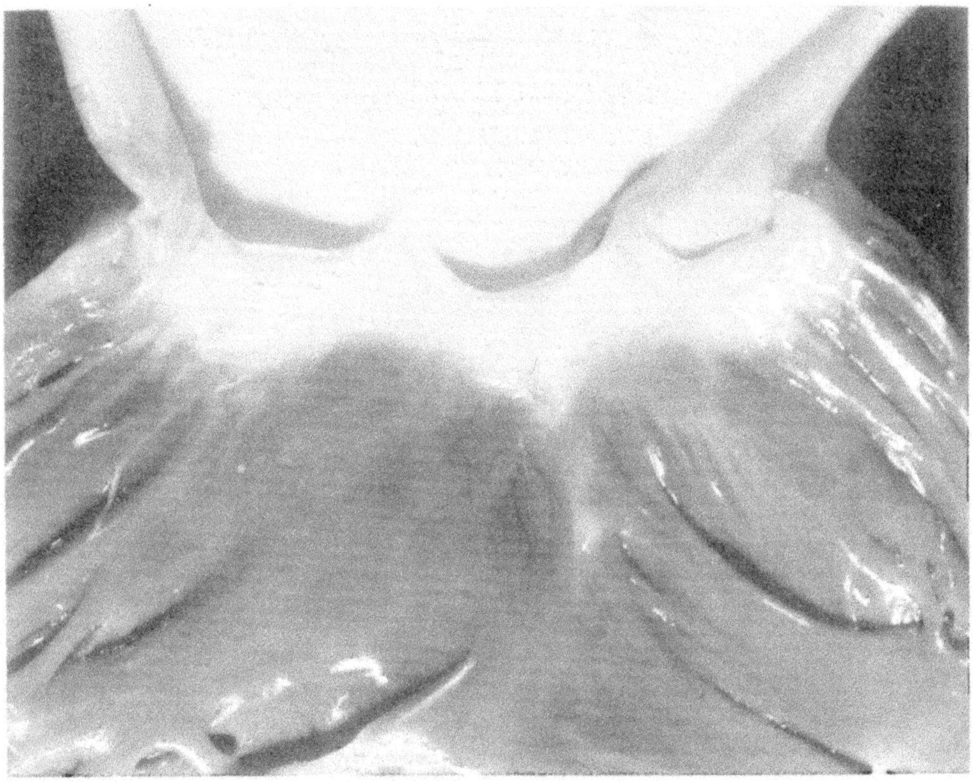

Figure 2. View of opened right ventricular outflow tract (bottom), pulmonic valve (center), and pulmonary trunk (top) of patient 3. The valve cusps are thickened and retracted, and the valvular ring is constricted.

strongly metachromatic, and intensely and diffusely stained by the alcian blue method (at both pH 1.0 and 2.5). Collagen was present in moderate amounts, but no elastic tissue was found in any of the carcinoid plaques examined. A normal appearing internal elastic lamina separated the carcinoid plaques from mural or valvular subendocardium (Fig. 8).

Ultrastructural Observations

The ultrastructure of carcinoid plaques in the three patients studied was remarkably similar, regardless of their location in the right atrium, right ventricle, tricuspid valve, and pulmonic valve. As expected from the conditions of tissue fixation, ultrastructural preservation was much better in tissues from patient 3 than in tissues from the other two patients. For this reason all the electron micrographs of carcinoid plaques shown in this communication are of tissues from patient 3.

As an introduction to the presentation of our observations on the ultrastructure of carcinoid plaques, and as the basis for comparisons, the ultrastructural characteristics of normal human endocardium will be described first. These characteristics vary from one area of the heart to another according to corresponding regional changes in the overall thickness of the endocardium.[24–26] In the ventricles, and particularly in the right ventricular outflow tract,[25] the endocardium is thin (less than 100 μ in thickness) and is composed of a single layer of endothelial cells and of a subendothelial layer that contains collagenous fibrils, acid mucopolysaccharides, a few microfibrils, and a thin elastic tissue lamella (Fig. 10).

In endocardium of normal thickness the endothelial cells are greatly flattened and thin, with centrally located nuclei, variable numbers of pinocytotic vesicles, and thin (200 to 400 Å in thickness) basement membranes; their cytoplasm contains a few small mitochondria, sparse cisterns of rough surfaced endoplasmic

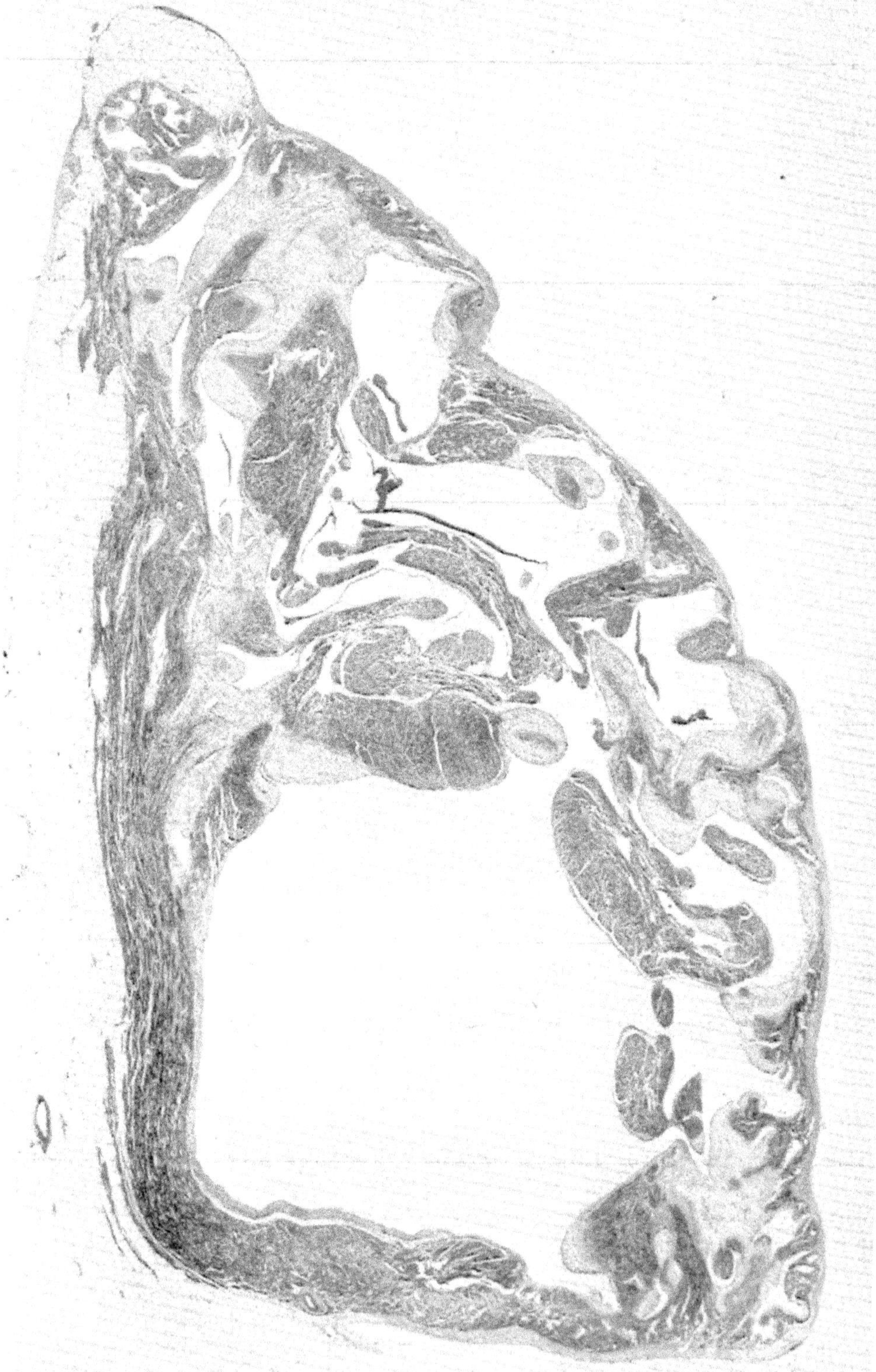

Figure 3. Histologic section through entire right atrial appendage of patient 3. Multiple plaque-like areas of endocardial thickening, which appear pale gray, are present throughout and contrast with the darkly stained muscle of the atrial wall. (Masson's trichrome stain. × 8.)

mucopolysaccharide-rich ground substance of the subendothelial layer appears as material that is amorphous or finely granular in some areas and forms spicules (up to 1000 Å in length) in others.

Cellular elements in the subendothelial space of nonthickened endocardium are few in number and consist of poorly differentiated mesenchymal cells, occasional histiocytes, smooth muscle cells, fibroblast-like cells, unmyelinated nerves and their Schwann cells, and rare mast cells. The poorly differentiated mesenchymal cells are oval or stellate and have single large nuclei, scanty cytoplasm, and no basement membranes. Cytoplasmic organ-

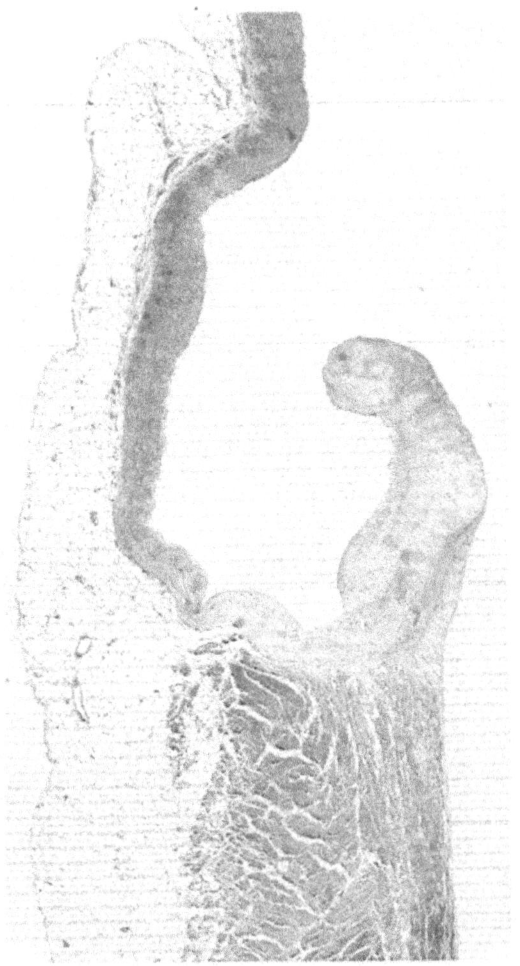

Figure 4. Section through right ventricular wall (bottom), pulmonic valve (center), and pulmonary trunk (top) of patient 3, showing marked thickening of the valve leaflet. This thickening involves the side of the leaflet that faces the pulmonary trunk. (Hematoxylin and eosin stain. × 7.)

reticulum, occasional Weibel-Palade bodies, small Golgi complexes in the perinuclear zones, and variable numbers of filaments measuring 100 Å in diameter (Fig. 10). The edges of endothelial cells overlap slightly with those of their neighbors, to which they are attached by intercellular junctions bearing specialized junctional components similar to those of endothelial cells elsewhere. The collagenous fibrils in the subendothelial space course parallel to the endothelial surface, forming a cross-woven network. Some microfibrils are associated with elastic tissue fibrils, whereas others are arranged into small bundles that were not associated with other structures. The acid

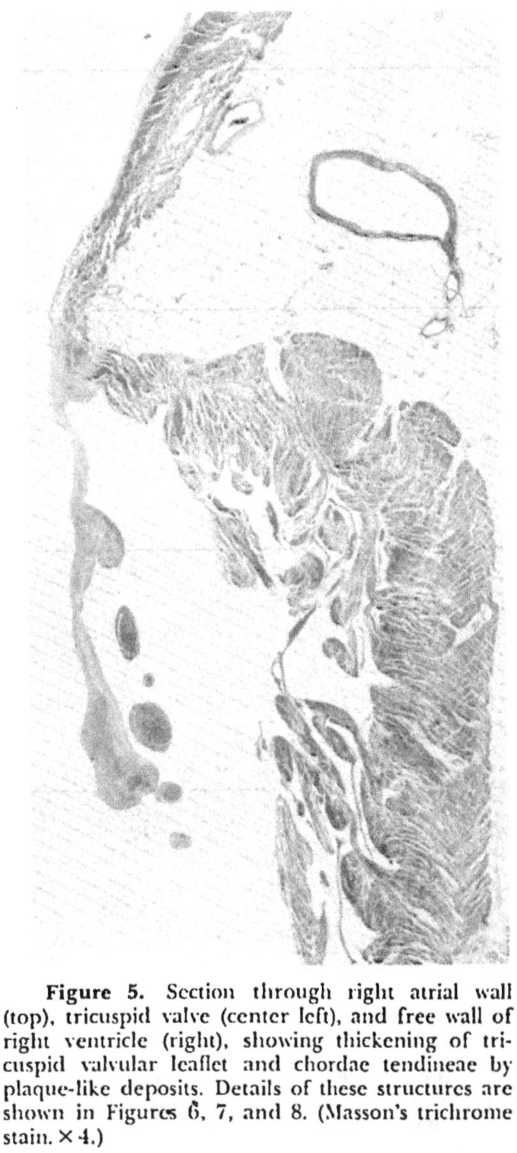

Figure 5. Section through right atrial wall (top), tricuspid valve (center left), and free wall of right ventricle (right), showing thickening of tricuspid valvular leaflet and chordae tendineae by plaque-like deposits. Details of these structures are shown in Figures 6, 7, and 8. (Masson's trichrome stain. × 4.)

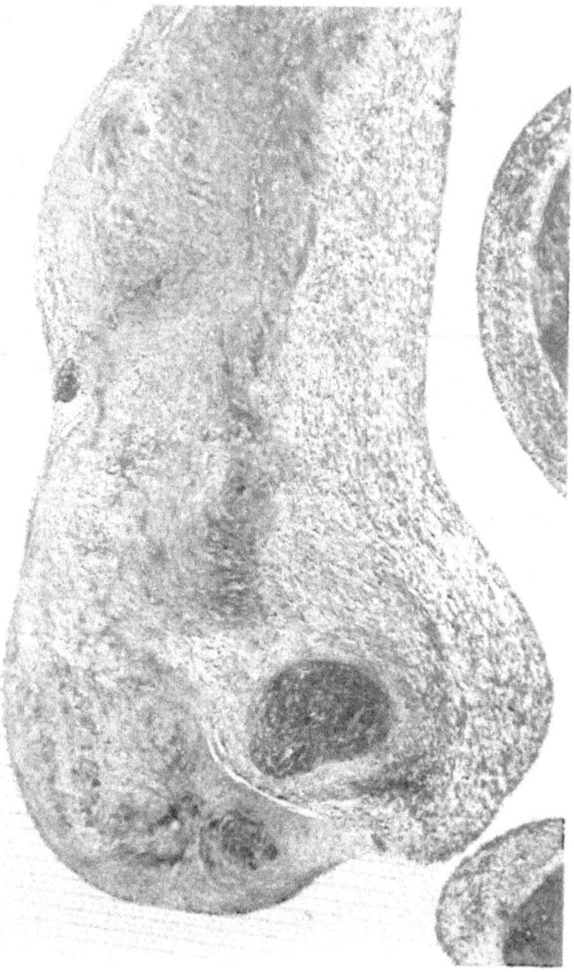

Figure 6. Free edge of tricuspid valve leaflet and parts of two chordae tendineae are sites of formation of carcinoid plaque tissue. Involvement of the valve leaflet is limited to surface facing right ventricular wall. (Masson's trichrome stain. × 100.)

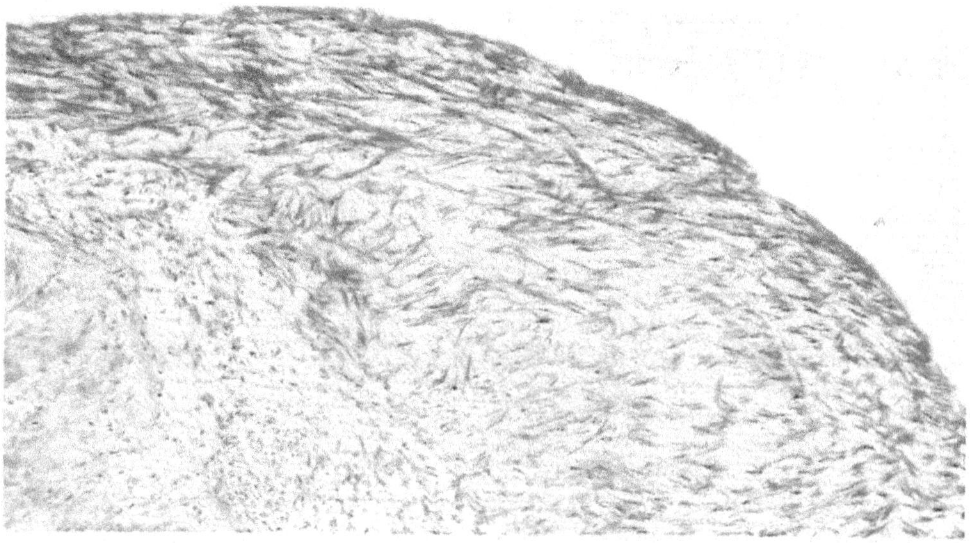

Figure 7. Part of carcinoid plaque (shown at lower magnification in Figure 6) in tricuspid valve. The plaque contains slender, elongated cells aligned parallel to the surface and embedded in a pale staining stroma. (Masson's trichrome stain. × 250.)

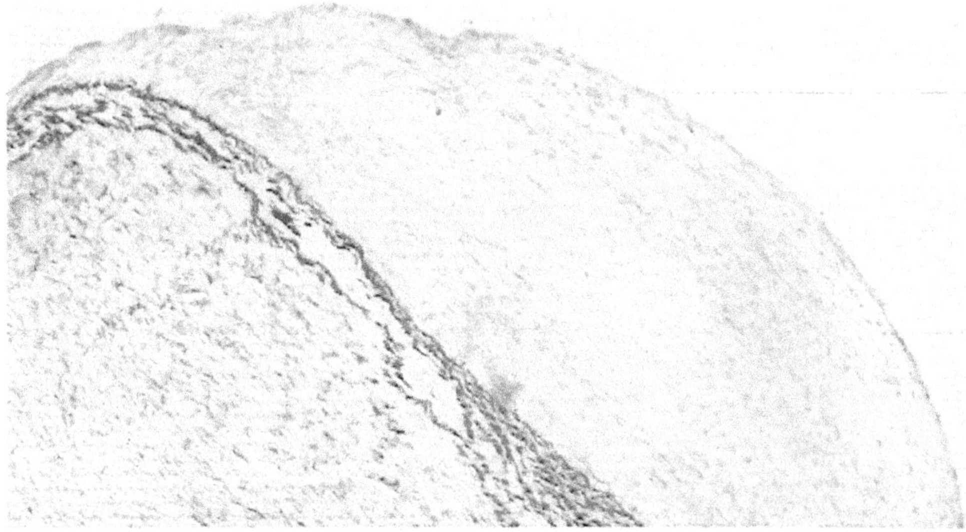

Figure 8. Plaque on right atrial endocardium of patient 3 is similar to that shown in Figure 8, lacks elastic tissue, and is separated from underlying structures by elastic lamellae. (Elastica–van Gieson stain. × 250.)

elles are few and consist of a few small mitochondria and cisterns of rough surfaced endoplasmic reticulum; a few 100 Å thick filaments; small to moderate numbers of free cytoplasmic ribosomes; and loosely clumped, finely granular to amorphous material of moderate electron density, which occupies most of the cytoplasm. Histiocytes are recognizable by their prominent lysosomes and Golgi

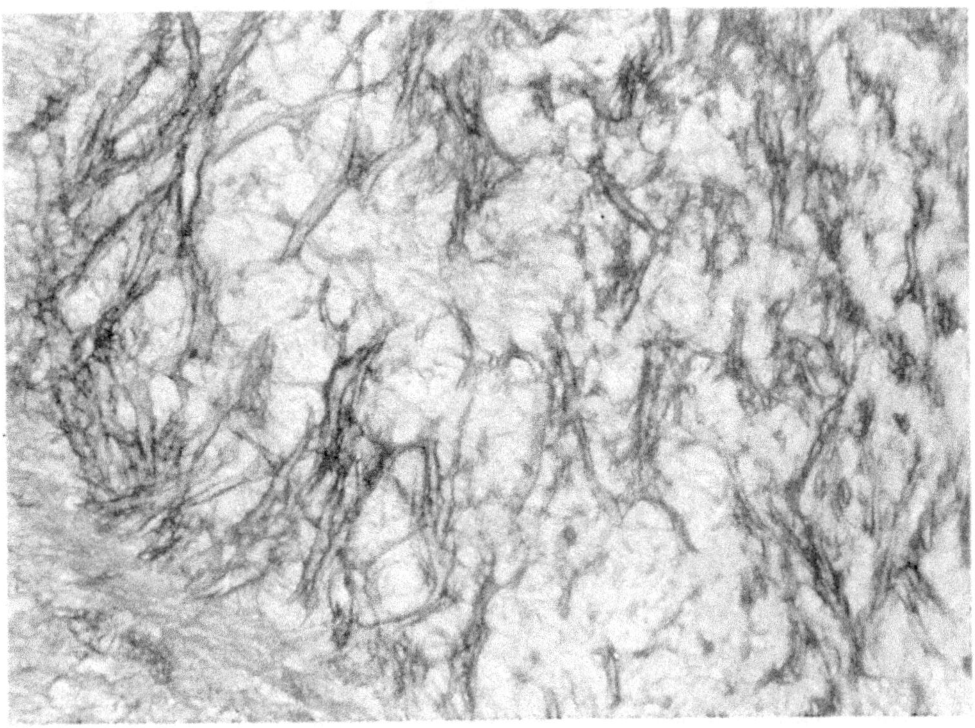

Figure 9. Basement membranes of smooth muscle cells in carcinoid plaque in right atrium of patient 3 are thickened and intensely stained. (Periodic acid–Schiff reaction. × 750.)

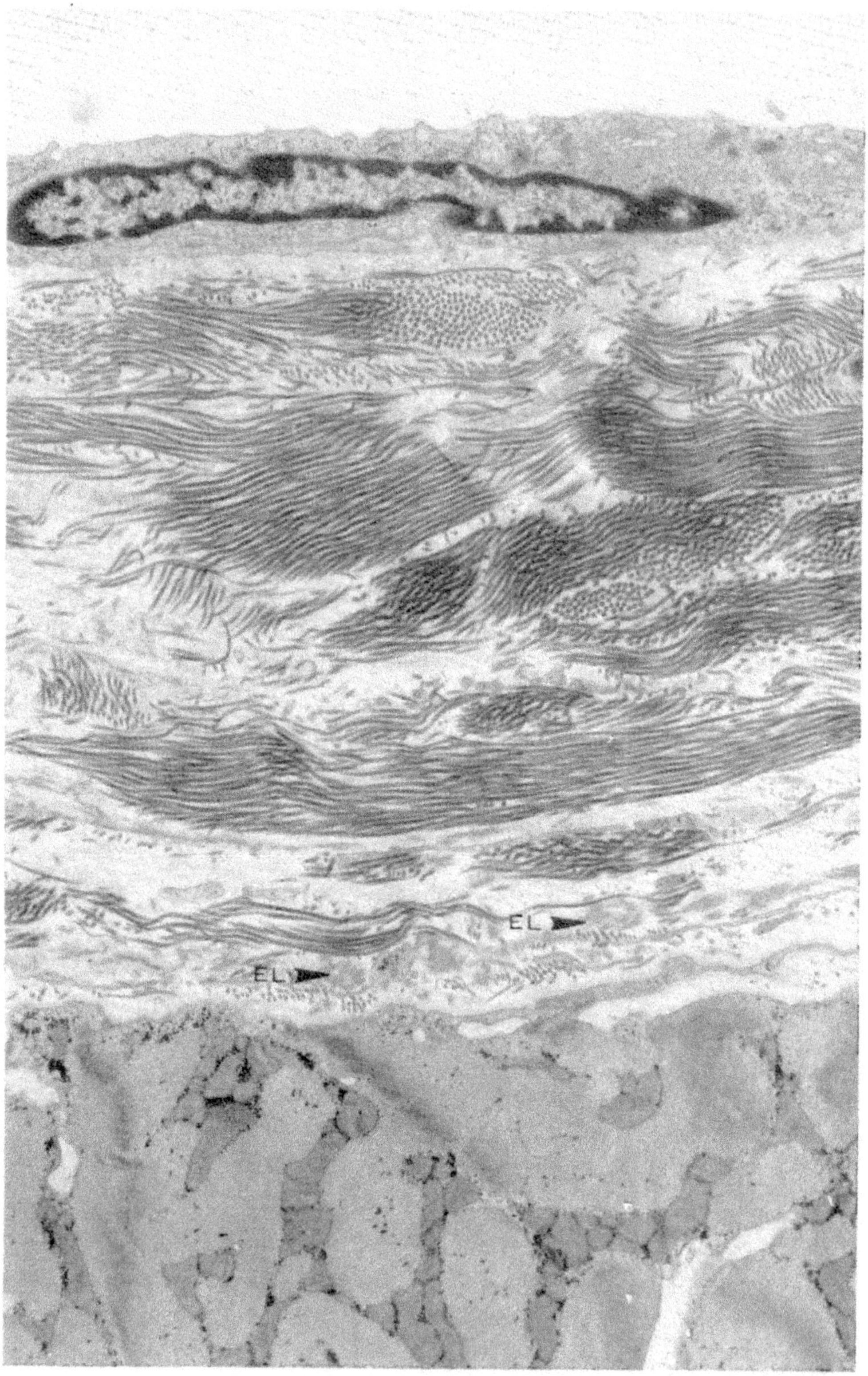

Figure 10. Electron micrograph of endocardium of normal thickness (10 μ) investing crista supraventricularis muscle of 16 year old boy with double outlet right ventricle and infundibular stenosis. Note surface endothelium, subendothelial layer containing collagen fibrils and microfibrils, deeper, discontinuous layer of small elastic fibrils (EL), and part of the innermost layer of cardiac muscle cells. The collagen fibrils are oriented parallel to the surface and form a cross weaving network. (Lead citrate and uranyl acetate stain. × 13,200.)

cisterns. Fibroblasts are characterized by large cisterns of rough surfaced endoplasmic reticulum, which often are filled with electron dense material, and by absent or poorly developed basement membranes.

The basic pattern of organization described for human ventricular mural endocardium is similar to that observed in the endocardium of the canine mitral valve and rat ventricle.[27–29] This pattern is modified in various regions of the heart, particularly in the left atrium where the endocardium is thickest and contains several well developed layers of smooth muscle cells.[24–26, 30] These cells are closely associated with collagenous and elastic fibrils. The elastic tissue in normal and in thickened endocardium from patients with congenital heart disease stains intensely with the silver tetraphenylporphin sulfonate method of Albert and Fleischer (Fig. 11).

Ultrastructural study of carcinoid plaques confirmed the light microscopic observations that they contained smooth muscle cells and appeared devoid of elastic tissue (Fig. 12). Carcinoid plaques also contained cells that shared features of fibroblasts (abundant rough surfaced endoplasmic reticulum) and of smooth muscle cells (filaments measuring 40 to 80 Å in diameter, and peripherally located dense bodies).

The smooth muscle cells in carcinoid

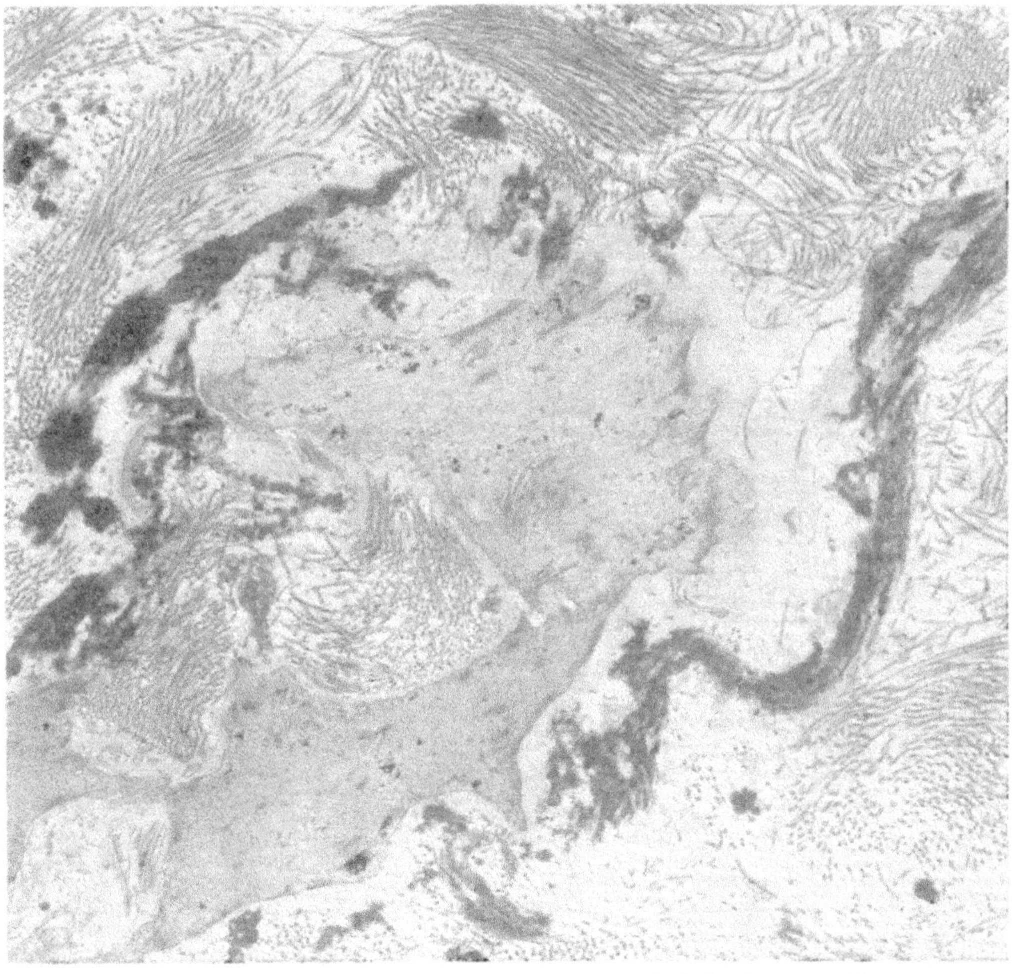

Figure 11. Thickened endocardium overlying crista supraventricularis of 23 year old woman with ventricular septal defect contains smooth muscle cells, collagen fibrils, and abundant, intensely stained elastic fibrils. (Silver tetraphenylporphin sulfonate, lead citrate, and uranyl acetate stains. × 11,500.)

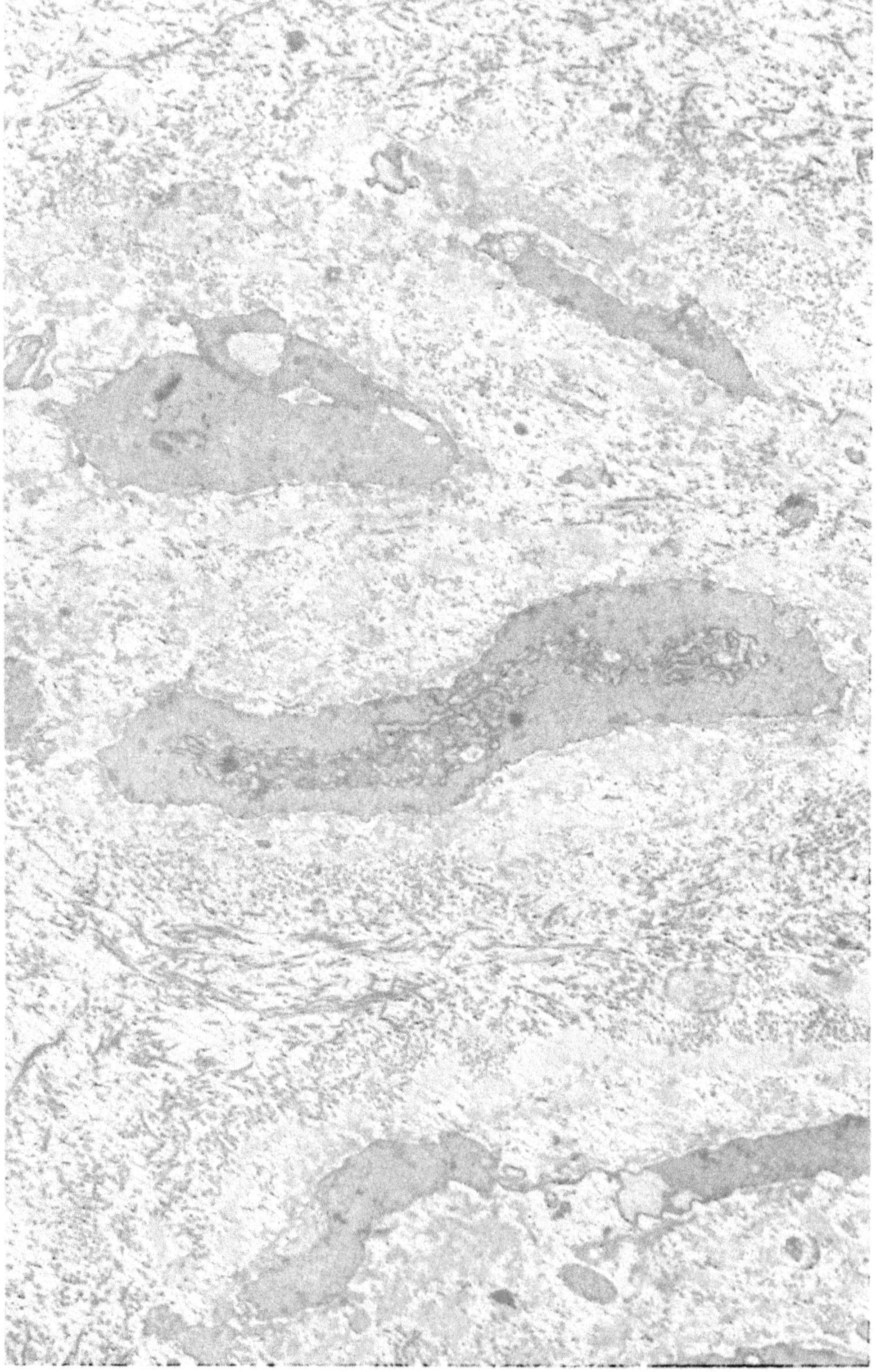

Figure 12. View of several smooth muscle cells in carcinoid plaque in right atrium. Each cell is surrounded by layered basement membrane material and by loosely arranged collagen fibrils. (Lead citrate and uranyl acetate stain. × 14,300.)

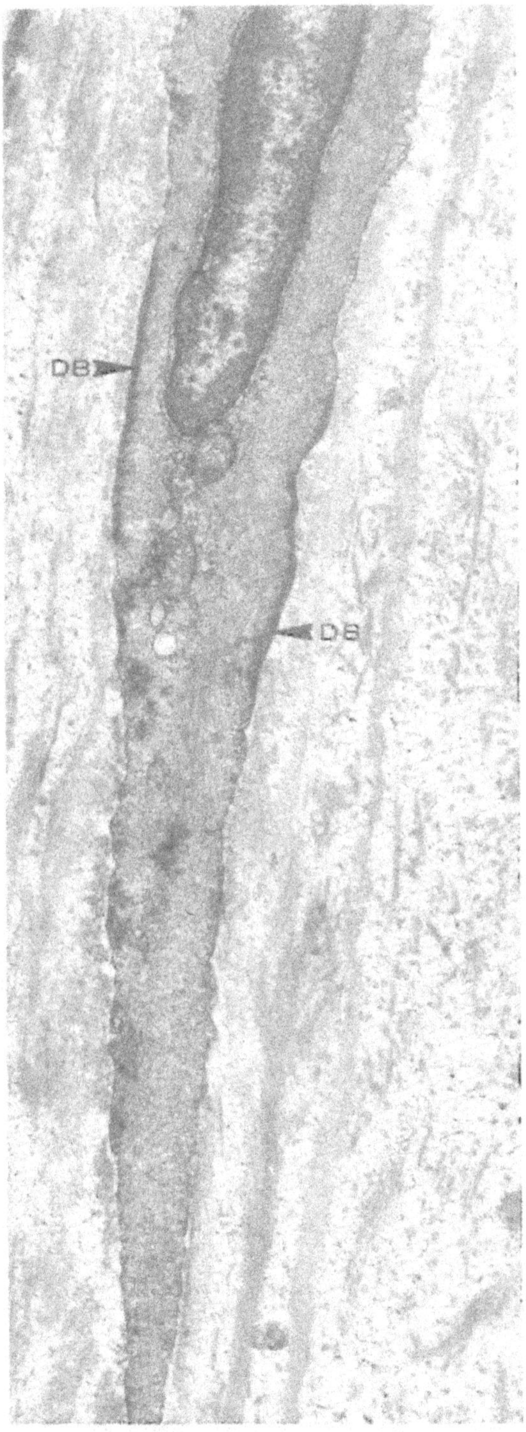

Figure 13. Longitudinal section through part of mature appearing smooth muscle cell in carcinoid plaque in right atrium, showing myofilaments, peripherally located dense bodies (KB) or attachment sites for myofilaments, a few mitochondria, and a single elongated nucleus. The cell is surrounded by layered basement membrane material, collagen fibrils, and spicules and star shaped particles, which are presumed to represent deposits of acid mucopolysaccharides. (Lead citrate and uranyl acetate stain. × 25,500.)

plaques were highly elongated and had single, centrally located nuclei (Figs. 13, 14). The nuclear membranes often appeared indented. The plasma membranes were smooth and had few or no associated pinocytotic vesicles. The cytoplasm was almost completely filled with filaments and contained few mitochondria, inconspicuous Golgi complexes, few lysosomes, and sparse small cisterns of rough surfaced endoplasmic reticulum. Two size classes of cytoplasmic filaments were distinguishable (Fig. 14). Filaments of the first class measured 40 to 80 Å in diameter, were closely packed, constituted by far the predominant class, and were considered to be actin filaments. These filaments were associated with the peripherally located dense bodies. Filaments of the second class measured 100 Å in diameter, were present in small numbers in most cells, and were regarded as morphologically similar to the cytoskeletal filaments present in endothelial cells, in smooth muscle cells, and in a large variety of other types of normal and abnormal cells (see ref. 31 for review). Filaments that morphologically corresponded to those of myosin (130 to 160 Å in diameter) were not observed in these cells. No areas of specialized cellular contact between closely apposed smooth muscle cells in carcinoid plaques were observed; however, the possibility could not be excluded that such areas had existed but had been disrupted by postmortem autolysis. Most of the smooth muscle cells in carcinoid plaques were isolated from each other and were surrounded by relatively large amounts of stroma (Fig. 12).

The most striking and most distinctive feature of smooth muscle cells in carcinoid plaques was the thickening and reduplication of their basement membranes, which were composed of layered filamentous material of moderate electron density (Figs. 12 to 14). The layers of filamentous material often were discontinuous, irregular, and apparently fragmented, but always were associated with smooth muscle cells. The thickness of the individual layers of basement membrane-like material ranged from 1000 to 5000 Å. Some of these layers surrounded smooth muscle cells that appeared to have undergone necrosis. The pattern of distribution of the layers of basement membrane-like

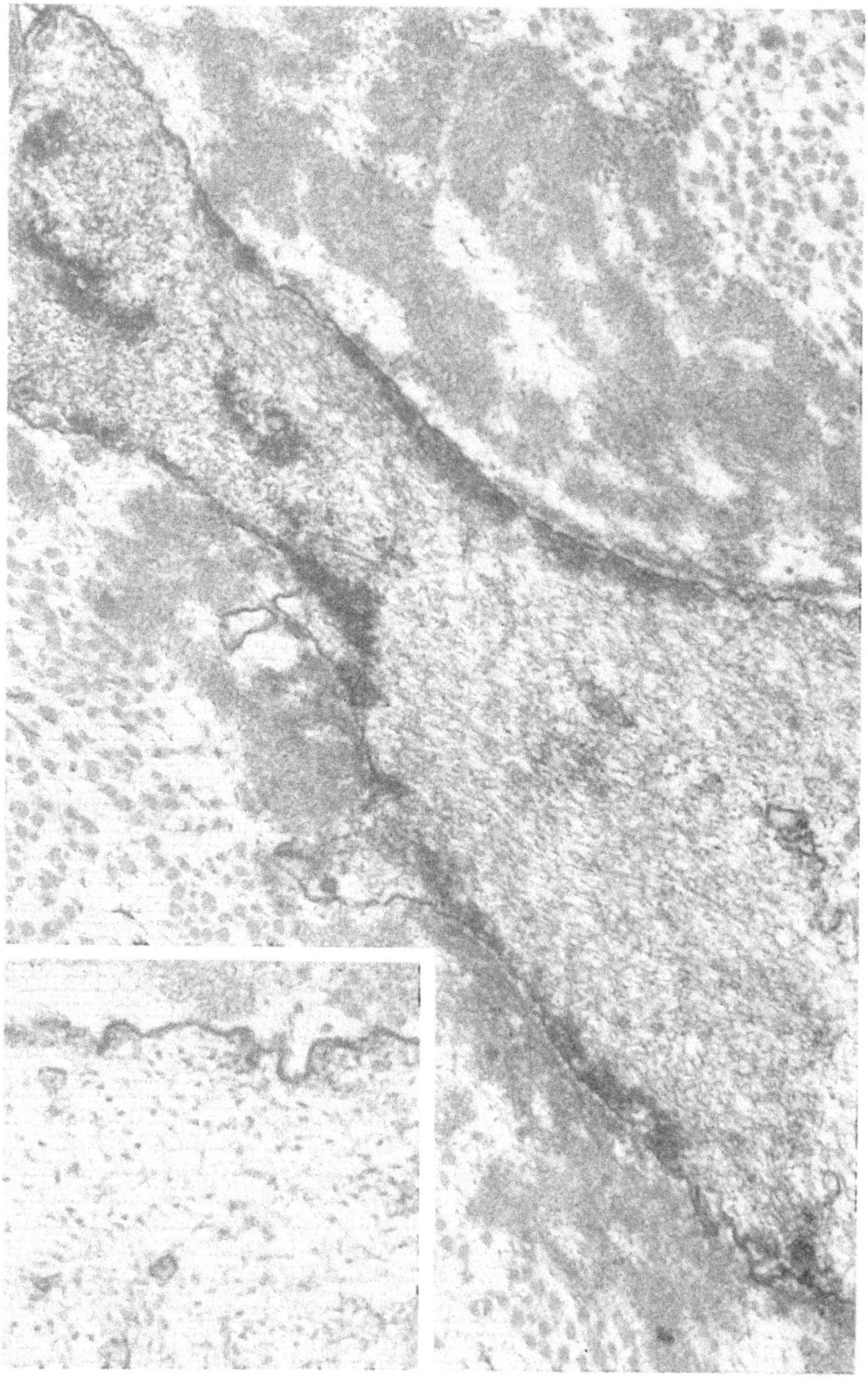

Figure 14. High magnification view of part of well developed smooth muscle cell in right atrial carcinoid plaque, showing peripheral dense bodies and thin myofilaments, which measure 40 to 80 Å in diameter. Note irregular layers of basement membrane material surrounding the cell, and small bundles of microfibrils at upper right. Inset shows cytoplasmic filaments, 100 Å in diameter, in another smooth muscle cell from same area. (Lead citrate and uranyl acetate stain. × 54,000. Inset, × 74,000.)

material corresponded to that of the PAS positive material observed in histologic preparations.

Certain smooth muscle cells in carcinoid plaques differed from the mature smooth muscle cells just described in that they exhibited large elongated perinuclear zones, which were free of cytoplasmic filaments and associated dense bodies (Figs. 15 to 17). These zones contained numerous cisterns of rough surfaced endoplasmic reticulum, but only a few Golgi cisterns, free ribosomes, mitochondria, and elements of smooth surfaced endoplasmic reticulum. Some of the cisterns of rough surfaced endoplasmic reticulum were flattened, but the majority were dilated and filled with fibrillar material resembling that in basement membranes. The number of cisterns of rough surfaced endoplasmic reticulum in these cells was inversely proportional to the number of cytoplasmic filaments. The extent to which these variations in content of reticulum and filaments occurred in smooth muscle cells is illustrated in Figures 12 to 17. No cells in carcinoid plaques were found to be completely free of cytoplasmic filaments or of their associated dense bodies. Cells that were richest in rough surfaced endoplasmic reticulum also contained appreciable numbers of cytoplasmic filaments and dense bodies (Fig. 17).

In addition to the layers of basement membrane material described, the extracellular components of carcinoid plaques consisted of collagen fibrils (Fig. 12), microfibrils (Fig. 14), and spicules and star shaped particles of electron dense material

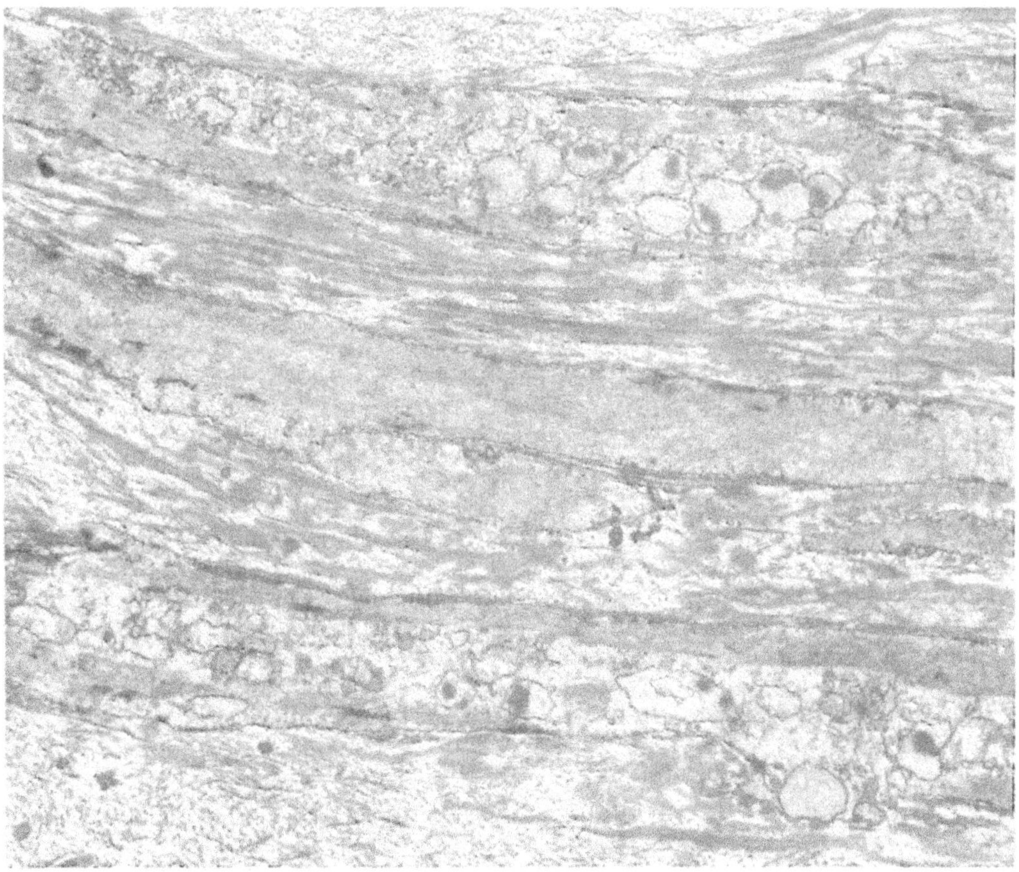

Figure 15. Several adjacent smooth muscle cells in carcinoid plaque in right atrium show considerable variation in their content of myofilaments and of cisterns of rough surfaced endoplasmic reticulum. Some of the latter are filled with electron dense material resembling that in the basement membranes. As in other areas of carcinoid plaques, the basement membranes are thickened, reduplicated, and layered. (Lead citrate and uranyl acetate stain. × 10,000.)

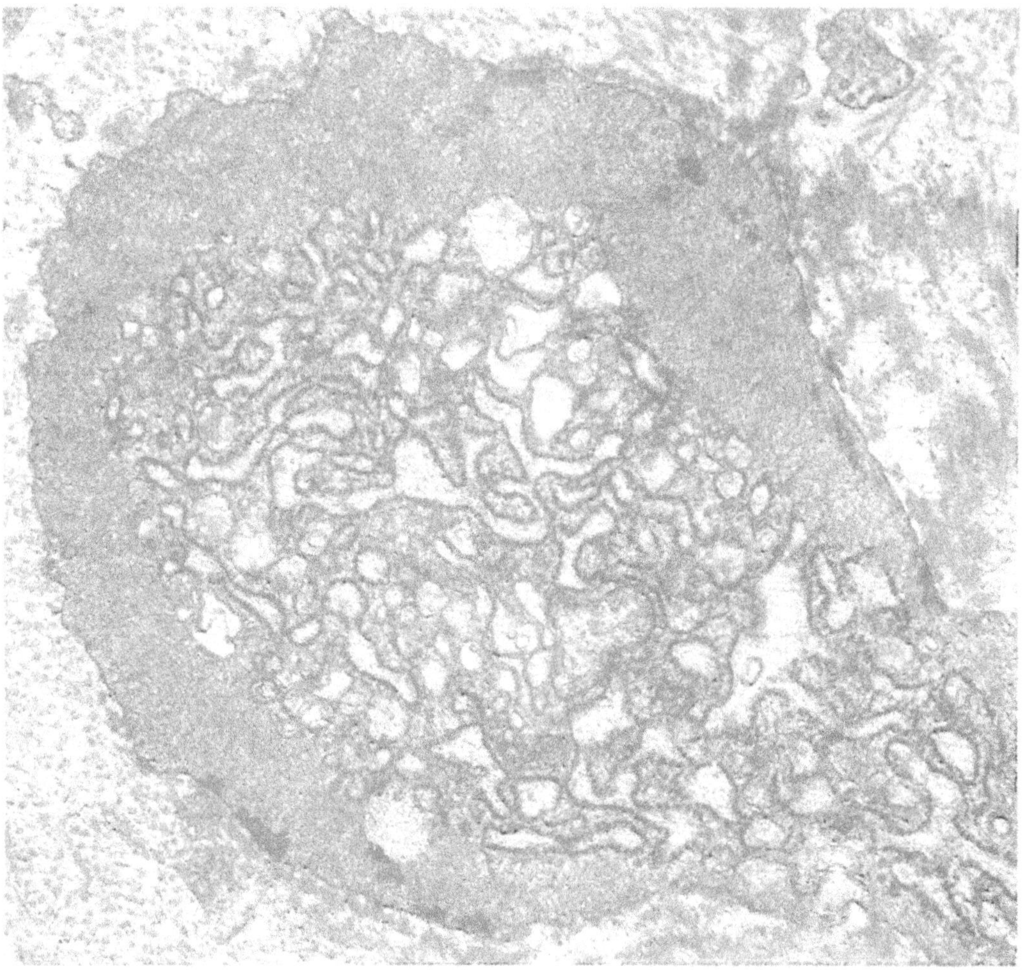

Figure 16. Cross section through smooth muscle cell, which is composed of a peripheral zone containing closely packed myofilaments, and a central zone filled with numerous cisterns of rough surfaced endoplasmic reticulum and a few smooth walled vesicles. (Lead citrate and uranyl acetate stain. × 22,500.)

(Fig. 14). The collagen fibrils ranged in size from 500 to 700 Å and for the most part coursed parallel to the surface, forming a cross-weaving pattern. They were associated with microfibrils, which measured 100 to 150 Å in diameter, occurred in much smaller numbers, and often formed small bundles in the vicinity of the basement membranes of the smooth muscle cells. The electron dense spicules measured approximately 800 Å in length and 200 Å in width, whereas the star shaped particles ranged from 1500 to 2000 Å in overall diameter. Both these types of structures were considered to represent clumped precipitated deposits of acid mucopolysaccharides because their distribution corresponded to that of the alcian blue positive material in the histochemical preparations and because they were morphologically similar to acid mucopolysaccharide deposits observed in other tissues.[31]

DISCUSSION

Morphology of Carcinoid Plaques

Our study shows that the plaque-like thickenings in mural and valvular endocardium of patients with the carcinoid syndrome are composed of smooth muscle cells embedded in a stroma that is rich in

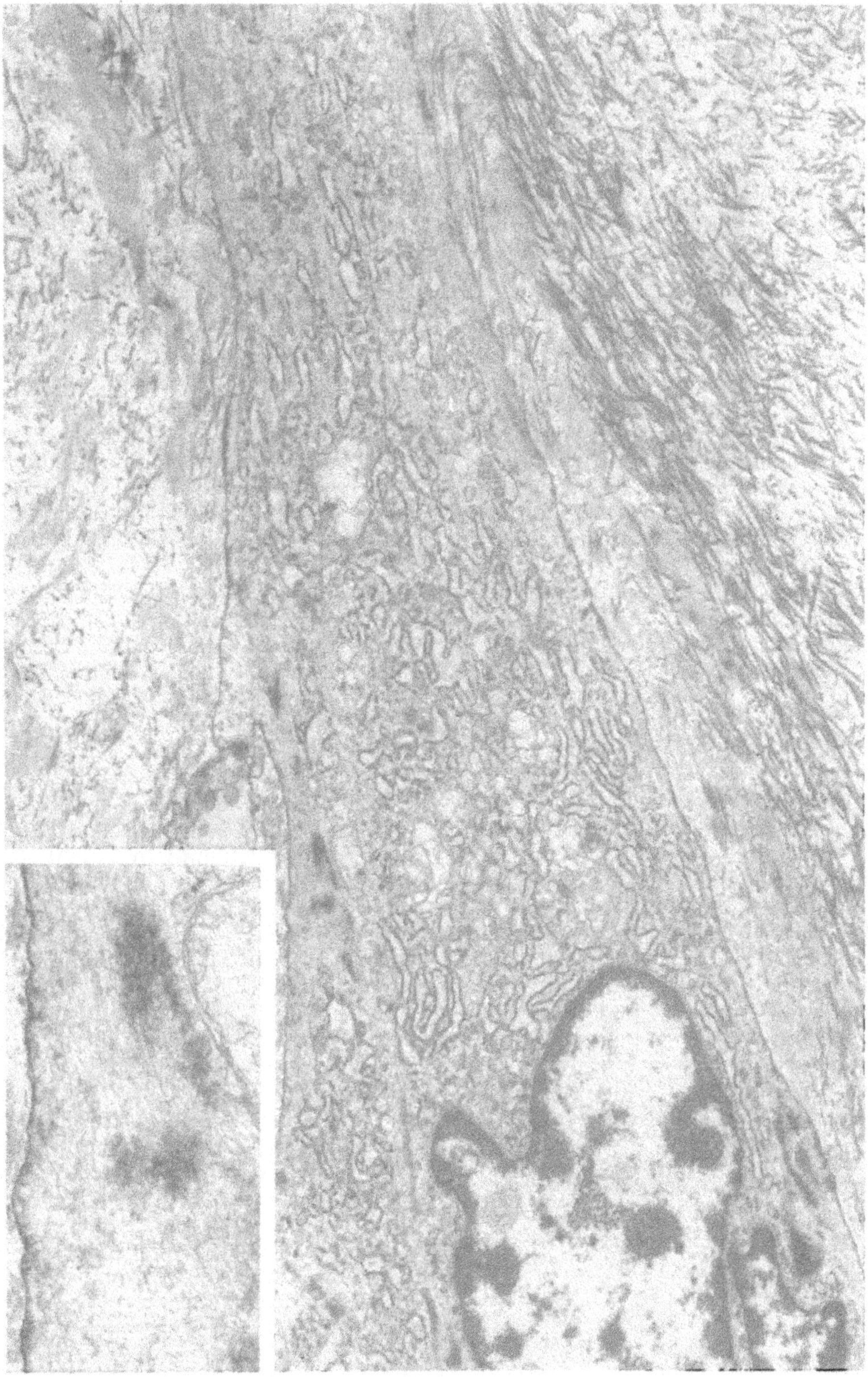

Figure 17. View of cell that contains a large perinuclear zone filled with cisterns of rough surfaced endoplasmic reticulum, and a narrow peripheral zone that contains only a few myofilaments and dense bodies. Note again the layering of the basement membrane material and the more peripherally located collagen fibrils. Inset shows the insertion of thin myofilaments into the dense bodies. (Lead citrate and uranyl acetate stain. × 15,000. Inset, × 54,000.)

acid mucopolysaccharides, basement membrane-like material, collagen fibrils, and microfibrils but lacks elastic fibers (Table 2). The stromal components we observed in ultrathin sections of carcinoid plaques corresponded to those previously found by Cosh and associates[18] in their electron microscopic study of chromium shadowed preparations of mechanically fragmented plaques from the right atrial walls of three patients with the carcinoid syndrome. Cosh et al. described thin jagged lamellae composed of finely granular, amorphous material, which corresponded to the layered basement membrane material found in our study, and fibrils of various sizes, which corresponded to the microfibrils and the immature or young collagen fibrils observed by us. They also described a few dense, square ended fibers and fragments thereof, and interpreted them as possibly representing abnormal elastic fibers. Such structures were not present in the plaques we examined. The preparative techniques used by Cosh et al. did not permit identification of acid mucopolysaccharide deposits.

Our observations on cellular components of carcinoid plaques are similar to those of Himbert et al.[19] and Boutet et al.[21] Each of these groups of investigators studied the ultrastructure of plaques from one patient with the carcinoid syndrome. Although Himbert et al.[19] concluded that fibroblasts were the predominant cell type, their published illustrations show smooth muscle cells and myofibroblast-like cells. These types of cells also were found in the patient studied by Boutet et al.[21] and in each of our three patients. Thus, studies show that carcinoid plaques contain the usual type of smooth muscle cell and also another type of smooth muscle cell large areas of whose cytoplasm are occupied by cisterns of rough surfaced endoplasmic reticulum. Cells with the latter characteristics have been called "myofibroblasts" because they share morphologic features of smooth muscle cells (i.e., cytoplasmic filaments, dense bodies, and prominent basement membranes) and of fibroblasts (i.e., abundant rough surfaced endoplasmic reticulum). Such cells occur in granulation tissue,[32,33] plantar fibromatosis,[34] Dupuytren's contracture,[34] normal interstitial pulmonary tissue,[35] renal interstitium of rabbits with experimentally induced obstructive nephropathy,[36] and the capsule that develops around blood clots implanted into rat peritoneal cavity.[37] It has been postulated that myofibroblasts in the tissues just cited are formed by a process of "activation" of fibroblasts.[32–37] Conversely, smooth muscle cells can develop morphologic features resembling those of fibroblasts.[38] From these observations Gabbiani et al.[31] concluded that "smooth muscle cells and fibroblasts are much more closely related than classical histology would have allowed one to suppose, and [that] either cell may be capable of modulating towards an intermediate cell type."

We were not able to show that the endoplasmic reticulum-rich smooth muscle cells in carcinoid plaques were derived from pre-existing fibroblasts, since we did not find typical fibroblasts in these lesions. It is possible that the reticulum rich smooth muscle cells in carcinoid plaques simply showed evidence of synthetic activity rather than of transformation from one distinct type of cell into another. Such synthetic activity may have been directed toward the formation of basement membrane-like material and of other stromal components of carcinoid plaques. In support of this concept are the observations of Ross,[39] who showed that smooth muscle cells grown in tissue culture develop abundant cisterns of rough surfaced endoplasmic reticulum and synthesize collagen fibrils, microfibrils, elastic fibrils, and basement membrane material. We were not able to make a more direct study of the origin of the smooth muscle cells in carcinoid plaques because we did not observe early lesions. Indeed, "early" lesions have not been observed in other

TABLE 2. Structural Components of Carcinoid Endocardial Plaques

Cellular components
Smooth muscle cells
Myofibroblast-like cells
Overlying layer of endothelial cells
Extracellular components
Collagen fibrils
Microfibrils
Acid mucopolysaccharides
Layered basement membrane material

studies of carcinoid plaques,[14, 16–21] and all carcinoid plaques thus far examined are morphologically similar. This observation suggests that these lesions develop relatively rapidly and become quiescent quickly.

The smooth muscle cells in carcinoid plaques may have originated either from pre-existing smooth muscle cells in endocardium or from primitive undifferentiated mesenchymal cells, which also are normally present in subendothelial areas of endocardium and vascular intima.[40] These primitive mesenchymal cells have been considered to be reserve cells with multipotential capabilities for differentiation into other types of cells, including endothelial cells, smooth muscle cells, and fibroblasts (see ref. 40 for review). The studies of Stein et al.[40] have provided evidence for the occurrence of these various lines of differentiation of mesenchymal cells in thickened endocardium investing right ventricular outflow tract muscle and stenotic aortic and pulmonic valves. This evidence suggests that the connective tissue components of carcinoid plaques are likely to be synthesized by the smooth muscle cells therein, and that such cells are derived from primitive mesenchymal cells in the endocardial subendothelial spaces. The apparent inability of smooth muscle cells in carcinoid plaques to synthesize the amorphous central core material of elastic fibers—even though they do synthesize microfibrils—remains a major unexplained feature of carcinoid heart disease.

Pathogenesis of Carcinoid Plaques

A number of hypotheses, most of which relate to the effects of serotonin release from tumor metastases, have been proposed to explain the pathogenesis of carcinoid plaques. These plaques have been variously considered to result from (1) deposition of some material from blood and not from underlying endocardium or myocardium;[14] (2) liberation of serotonin with endocardial alterations and reparative fibroblastic activity;[16] (3) subendocardial edema and tissue damage by serotonin, with deposition of fibrin in injured endocardium followed by "tanning" of fibrin, layering of fibrin deposits, and plaque formation;[41] (4) combined effects of hyperserotoninemia, hepatic injury, and deficiency of tryptophan or niacin;[42] (5) effects of serotonin on cardiac lymphatics;[43] (6) serotonin leading to the development of systemic or pulmonary arteriovenous fistulas;[44, 45] and (7) release of bradykinin, leading to endothelial damage and subsequent healing by subendothelial proliferation of connective tissue.

Obstruction of cardiac lymphatics produces morphologic changes, including subendocardial hemorrhages and fibroelastotic endocardial thickening, which we consider clearly different from those in carcinoid heart disease.[43] Also different from carcinoid plaques are the endocardial lesions that develop in animals with experimentally induced arteriovenous fistulas.[46] It seems unlikely, therefore, that either of these mechanisms can account for the formation of carcinoid plaques.

A direct pathogenetic effect of substances produced by carcinoid tumors has been the subject of considerable speculation, particularly since acute exposure of endothelial cells to high concentrations of serotonin is known to produce cellular contraction, disruption of intercellular junctions, formation of gaps between adjacent cells, increase in vascular permeability, and leakage and exudation of plasma proteins.[47, 48] Two observations that should be noted with respect to these changes are that the effects of bradykinin on endothelium are morphologically similar to those of serotonin,[47, 48] and that different areas of the vasculature differ in their sensitivities to the disruptive effects of bradykinin and serotonin on endothelium.[48] The effects of these two agents on endocardial endothelium have not been determined. Nevertheless, the observations just reviewed lend substance to the concepts that long term exposure to high concentrations of serotonin, bradykinin, or other, still unidentified peptides can disrupt endocardial endothelium; that the resulting process of plasma protein leakage and endothelial repair leads to plaque formation; and that endothelial damage may be aggravated in certain regions of the heart by hydromechanical forces of turbulent blood flow.[49]

This hypothesis is in accord with the observations that carcinoid plaques are superimposed on normal valvular or endocardial tissue, that they are sharply limited by a normal endocardial elastic tissue lamella, and that they do not involve deeper layers of tissues. These features indicate that the basic injury, which occurs in repeated bouts and eventually leads to connective tissue proliferation and plaque formation, is superficial and involves only the endocardial endothelium and immediately subjacent areas. Such a process of superficial injury and healing is similar to that involved in the repair of aortic endothelial injury and denudation induced by the intra-aortic balloon technique.[50]

The hypothesis just outlined would explain the observations of Clark and Bates,[41] who demonstrated, by means of immunofluorescence techniques, the presence of fibrin and fibrinogen in carcinoid plaques. Although we did not find any material with the typical periodicity of fibrin in carcinoid plaques, these negative findings do not exclude the possibility of the leaking of fibrin or fibrinogen into carcinoid plaques. Under certain circumstances fibrin deposits without periodicity can occur in tissues (see ref. 51 for review). Furthermore, transendothelial passage of various plasma proteins has been shown to occur in normal arteries[52] and in atherosclerotic plaques,[53] and horseradish peroxidase has been demonstrated to pass through the intercellular junctions of endothelial cells in the ventricular endocardium of normal rats.[54] Nevertheless, our observations do not support the concept that carcinoid plaques are formed by the deposition of successive layers of fibrin from the circulating blood plasma, or that layers of organizing fibrin constitute the bulk of the plaques. The layered material that these plaques contained had the characteristics of basement membrane material.

It is uncertain that serotonin is the agent that produces cardiac lesions in patients with the carcinoid syndrome. In a study of patients with carcinoid syndrome, Roberts and Sjoerdsma[17] showed that the quantity of hepatic metastases, the distribution of metastases, the maximal levels of serotonin in plasma, and the maximal levels of 24 hour urinary excretion of 5-hydroxyindoleacetic acid were similar in patients with and in patients without cardiac lesions. The predominant distribution of carcinoid lesions on the right side of the heart was initially attributed to exposure of the right side of the heart to high concentrations of serotonin and to presumed inactivation of serotonin by monoamine oxidase in the lungs. Subsequent studies, however, showed no significant difference in concentrations of serotonin in arterial and venous blood of patients with the carcinoid syndrome.[17]

Spatz[42] found it necessary to combine the long term administration of serotonin with induction of hepatic damage and deficiency of tryptophan or niacin in order to produce endocardial alterations. These alterations consisted only of intravalvular edema and focal fibroblastic endocardial proliferation, changes that differed from those in the carcinoid syndrome. Although these studies were made on guinea pigs, which are relatively insensitive to the pharmacologic effects of serotonin,[47] attempts to produce carcinoid plaques in other species by administering serotonin also have failed (see ref. 42 for review). It remains to be shown that long term administration of serotonin produces cardiac lesions identical to those in patients with the carcinoid syndrome.

The possibility, first suggested by Oates and associates,[12] that the release of bradykinin or related peptides from hepatic metastases is responsible for the cardiac lesions in the carcinoid syndrome deserves further consideration. It is known that bradykinin is inactivated in the lungs through hydrolysis of peptide bonds by enzymes presumed to be located in pulmonary vascular endothelium.[55-57] This inactivation is extremely rapid and efficient, because bradykinin can undergo hydrolysis of up to five of its eight peptide bonds during the three to four seconds required for blood to pass from the pulmonary artery to the pulmonary vein in the rat, and because hydrolysis of any peptide bond of bradykinin reduces its biologic activity by at least 99.5 per cent.[56,57] It would appear therefore that the properties of bradykinin conform to those required to explain the pathogenesis of carcinoid plaques in the heart, namely: release from hepatic metastases, a high degree of toxicity to endothelium, and inactivation by passage through the lungs so that the left side of the heart and the systemic circulation are exposed only to very low concentrations. It remains to be determined whether serotonin and bradykinin are capable of directly stimulating proliferation of smooth muscle cells and their synthesis of connective tissue stromal components. It is well known that many of the pharmacologic actions of both serotonin and bradykinin are exerted through effects on smooth muscle cells. It already has been shown that bradykinin stimulates mitotic activity and DNA synthesis in thymocytes and that this effect is mediated through cyclic AMP.[58] It has been further suggested that bradykinin also acts as a local "wound hormone," which has a mitogenic effect in damaged tissues, where it is released by the action of kallikrein on protein kininogens.[57, 58]

In conclusion, the observations in the present study show that the endocardial plaques in the hearts of patients with the carcinoid syndrome are composed of smooth muscle cells embedded in a stroma that is rich in acid mucopolysaccharides, collagen, and microfibrils but that does not contain elastic fibers. The smooth muscle cells in the plaques probably are derived from primitive mesenchymal cells, which normally are present in the endocardial subendothelial space. It is postulated that these plaques develop as the result of healing of repeated bouts of endothelial cell injury, with a resultant increase in the permeability of the endothelial barrier, and that this damage is aggravated in regions of turbulent blood flow, thus accounting for the localization of plaques in such regions. Although both serotonin and bradykinin are capable of producing endothelial cell damage, available evidence suggests that release of bradykinin from hepatic metastases is responsible for the formation of carcinoid plaques.

REFERENCES

1. Thorson, A., Björk, G., Björkman, G., and Waldenström, J.: Malignant carcinoid of the small intestine with metastases to the liver, valvular disease of the right side of the heart (pulmonary stenosis and tricuspid regurgitation without septal defects), peripheral vasomotor symptoms, bronchoconstriction, and an unusual type of cyanosis. Amer. Heart J., *47*:795–817, 1954.
2. Sjoerdsma, A., Weissbach, H., and Udenfriend, S.: A clinical, physiologic and biochemical study of patients with malignant carcinoid (argentaffinoma). Amer. J. Med., *20*:520–532, 1956.
3. Pearse, A. G. E.: The APUD cell concept and its implications in pathology. *In* Sommers, S. C. (Editor): Pathology Annual. New York, Appleton-Century Crofts, 1974, pp. 27–41.
4. Hosoda, S.: Carcinoid tumors—review of the literature with special reference to sites of origin and humoral substances produced. Acta Pathol. Jap., *22*:533–540, 1972.
5. Friesen, S. R., Hermreck, A. S., and Mantz, F. A.: Glucagon, gastrin and carcinoid tumors of the duodenum, pancreas and stomach: polypeptide "apudomas" of the foregut. Amer. J. Surg., *127*:90–101, 1974.
6. Hajdu, S. I., Winawer, S. J., and Myers, W. P. L.: Carcinoid tumors. A study of 204 cases. Amer. J. Clin. Path., *61*:521–528, 1974.
7. Oates, J. A., and Sjoerdsma, A.: A unique syndrome associated with secretion of 5-hydroxytryptophan by metastatic gastric carcinoids. Amer. J. Med., *32*:333–342, 1962.
8. Schmid, M., Wenzl, H., and Uehlinger, E.: B-inselzell-Adenom des Pankreas mit Hypoglykämie, kombiniert mit multiplen Karzinoidtumoren des Ileum. Schweiz. Med. Wochenschr., *93*:444–446, 1963.
9. Gloof, F., Pletscher, A., and Hardmeier, T.: Metastasierendes Inselzelladenom des Pancreas mit 5-Hydroxytryptamin und Insulinproduktion. Schweiz. Med. Wochenschr., *94*: 1476–1480, 1964.
10. Shames, J. M., Dhurandhar, N. R., and Blackard, W. G.: Insulin-secreting carcinoid tumor with widespread metastases. Amer. J. Med., *44*: 632–637, 1968.
11. Appleyard, N., and Losowsky, M. S.: A pancreatic tumor with carcinoid syndrome and hypoglycemia. Postgrad. Med. J., *46*:159–162, 1970.
12. Oates, J. A., Melmon, K., Sjoerdsma, A., Gillespie, L., and Mason, D. T.: Release of a kinin peptide in the carcinoid syndrome. Lancet, *1*:514–517, 1964.
13. Oates, J. A., Pettinger, W. A., and Doctor, R. B.: Evidence for the release of bradykinin in carcinoid syndrome. J. Clin. Invest., *45*:173–178, 1966.
14. Roberts, W. C., Dangel, J. C., and Bulkley, B. H.: Nonrheumatic valvular cardiac disease: a clinicopathologic survey of 27 different conditions causing valvular dysfunction. Cardiovasc. Clin., *5*:333–446, 1973.
15. Sjoerdsma, A., Lovenberg, W., Engelman, K., Carpenter, W. T., Wyatt, R. J., and Gessa, G. L.: Serotonin now: clinical implications of inhibiting its synthesis with para-chlorphenylalanine. Ann. Int. Med., *73*:607–629, 1970.
16. MacDonald, R. A., and Robbins, S. L.: Pathology of the heart in the carcinoid syndrome. A comparative study. A. M. A. Arch. Path., *63*:103–112, 1957.
17. Roberts, W. C., and Sjoerdsma, A.: The cardiac

disease associated with the carcinoid syndrome (carcinoid heart disease). Amer. J. Med., *36*: 5–34, 1964.
18. Cosh, J., Cates, J. E., and Pugh, D. W.: Carcinoid heart disease. Brit. Heart J., *21*:369–380, 1959.
19. Himbert, J., Even, P., Grosgogeat, Y., and Letac, B.: Cardiopathie carcinoïde (nouvelle observation clinique, hémodynamique, biologique et anatomique). Arch. Mal. Coeur, *58*:1638–1656, 1965.
20. Amoury, R. A.: Heart disease and the malignant carcinoid syndrome. A case report and review of pathophysiologic and pathogenetic mechanisms. Amer. J. Surg., *119*:585–594, 1970.
21. Boutet, M., Lagacé, R., and Delage, C.: Les lésions du coeur droit dans le syndrome carcinoïdien. Étude histochimique et ultrastructurale. Union Med. Canada, *103*:844–849, 1974.
22. Freeman, J., and Spurlock, B. O.: A new epoxy embedment for electron microscopy. J. Cell Biol., *13*:437–443, 1962.
23. Albert, E. N., and Fleischer, E.: A new electron-dense stain for elastic tissue. J. Histochem. Cytochem., *18*:697–708, 1970.
24. Nagayo, M.: Zur normalen und pathologischen Histologie des Endocardium parietale. Beitr. Path. Anat., *45*:283–305, 1909.
25. Domenici, A.: Il comportamento dell'endocardio parietale (in particolare delle sue fibrocellule muscolari liscie) in condizioni cardiache normali e patologiche. Pathologica, *41*:35–44, 1949.
26. Davies, J. N. P., and Coles, R. M.: Some considerations regarding obscure diseases affecting the mural endocardium. Amer. Heart J., *59*:600–631, 1960.
27. Fenoglio, J. J., Pham, T. D., Wit, A. L., Bassett, A. L., and Wagner, B. M.: Canine mitral complex. Ultrastructure and electromechanical properties. Circ. Res., *31*:417–430, 1972.
28. Candiollo, L.: The fine structure of the endocardial endothelium. Z. Zellforsch. Mikroskop. Anat., *61*:486–492, 1963.
29. Melax, H., and Leeson, T. S.: Fine structure of the endocardium in adult rats. Cardiovasc. Res., *1*:349–355, 1967.
30. Lannigan, R. A., and Zaki, S. A.: Ultrastructure of the normal atrial endocardium. Brit. Heart J., *28*:785–795, 1966.
31. Ferrans, V. J., and Roberts, W. C.: Structural features of cardiac myxomas. Histology, histochemistry and electron microscopy. Hum. Path., *3*:111–146, 1973.
32. Hirschel, B. J., Gabbiani, G., Ryan, G. B., and Majno, G.: Fibroblasts of granulation tissue: immunofluorescent staining with antismooth muscle serum. Proc. Soc. Exp. Biol. Med., *138*: 466–469, 1971.
33. Gabbiani, G., Hirschel, B. J., Ryan, G. B., Statkov, P. R., and Majno, G.: Granulation tissue as a contractile organ. A study of structure and function. J. Exp. Med., *135*:719–734, 1972.
34. Gabbiani, G., and Majno, G.: Dupuytren's contracture: fibroblast contraction? An ultrastructural study. Amer. J. Path., *66*:131–147, 1972.
35. Kapanci, Y., Assimacopoulos, A., Irle, C., Zwahlen, A., and Gabbiani, G.: "Contractile interstitial cells" in pulmonary alveolar septa: a possible regulator of ventilation/perfusion ratio? Ultrastructural, immunofluorescence, and in vitro studies. J. Cell Biol., *60*:375–392, 1974.
36. Nagle, R. B., Kneiser, M. R., Bulger, R. E., and Benditt, E. P.: Induction of smooth muscle characteristics in renal interstitial fibroblasts during obstructive nephropathy. Lab. Invest., *29*:422–427, 1973.
37. Ryan, G. B., Cliff, W. J., Gabbiani, G., Irle, C., Statkov, P. R., and Majno, G.: Myofibroblasts in an avascular fibrous tissue. Lab. Invest., *29*:197–206, 1973.
38. Ross, R., and Klebanoff, S. J.: The smooth muscle cell. I. In vivo synthesis of connective tissue proteins. J. Cell Biol., *50*:159–171, 1971.
39. Ross, R.: The smooth muscle cell. II. Growth of smooth muscle in culture and formation of elastic fibers. J. Cell Biol., *50*:172–186, 1971.
40. Stein, A. A., Mauro, J., Thibodeau, L., and Alley, R.: The histogenesis of cardiac myxomas: relation to other proliferative diseases of subendothelial vasoform reserve cells. *In* Sommers, S. C. (Editor): Pathology Annual. New York, Appleton-Century Crofts, 1969, Vol. 4, pp. 293–312.
41. Clark, R. F., and Bates, H. R., Jr.: Endocardial fibrin in carcinoid heart disease. An immunofluorescent demonstration. Arch. Path., *76*: 211–214, 1963.
42. Spatz, M.: Pathogenetic studies of experimentally induced heart lesions and their relation to the carcinoid syndrome. Lab. Invest., *13*:288–300, 1964.
43. Miller, A. J., Pick, R., and Katz, L. N.: Ventricular endomyocardial pathology produced by chronic cardiac lymphatic obstruction in the dog. Circ. Res., *8*:941–947, 1960.
44. McKusick, V. A.: Carcinoid cardiovascular disease. Bull. Johns Hopkins Hosp., *98*:13–36, 1956.
45. Sparks, G. H., and Tombridge, T. L.: Five-hydroxytryptamine (serotonin) and its relationship to the carcinoid cardiovascular syndrome and Rendu-Osler-Weber syndrome. J. Thorac. Surg., *33*:401–411, 1957.
46. Lillehei, C. W., Bobb, T. R. R., and Vischer, M. B.: The occurrence of endocarditis with valvular deformities in dogs with arterio-venous fistulas. Ann. Surg., *132*:577–590, 1950.
47. Movat, H. Z.: The acute inflammatory reaction. *In* Movat, H. Z. (Editor): Inflammation, Immunity and Hypersensitivity. New York, Harper & Row, 1971, pp. 1–130.
48. Majno, G., Shea, S. M., and Leventhal, M.: Endothelial contraction induced by histamine-type mediators. An electron microscopic study. J. Cell Biol., *42*:647–672, 1969.
49. Fryd, D. L.: Certain histological and chemical responses of the vascular interface to acutely induced mechanical stress in the aorta of the dog. Circ. Res., *24*:93–108, 1969.
50. Stemerman, M. B., and Ross, R.: Experimental atherosclerosis. I. Fibrous plaque formation in

primates, an electron microscopic study. J. Exp. Med., *136*:769–789, 1972.

51. Buja, L. M., Ferrans, V. J., and Graw, R. G., Jr.: Cardiac pathologic findings in patients treated with bone marrow transplantation. Hum. Path., 7:17–45, 1976.
52. Duncan, L. E., Jr., Buck, K., and Lynch, A.: The effect of pressure and stretching on the passage of labeled albumin into canine aortic wall. J. Atheroscler. Res., *5*:69–79, 1965.
53. Shimamoto, T., Kobayashi, M., and Numano, F.: Infiltration of γ-globulin, fibrinogen and β-lipoprotein into blood vessel wall by atherogenic stress visualized by immunofluorescence. Proc. Japan Acad., *48*:336–341, 1972.
54. Anversa, P., Giacomelli, F., Wiener, J., and Spiro, D.: Permeability properties of ventricular endocardium. Lab. Invest., *28*:728–734, 1973.
55. Ryan, J. W., Roblero, J., and Stewart, J. M.: Inactivation of bradykinin in the pulmonary circulation. Biochem. J., *110*:795–797, 1968.
56. Ryan, J. W., Roblero, J., and Stewart, J. M.: Inactivation of bradykinin in rat lung. Adv. Exp. Med. Biol., *8*:263–271, 1970.
57. Dorer, F. E., Ryan, J. W., and Stewart, J. M.: Hydrolysis of bradykinin and its higher homologues by angiotensin-converting enzyme. Biochem. J., *141*:915–917, 1974.
58. Whitfield, J. F., MacManus, J. P., and Gillan, D. J.: Cyclic AMP mediation of bradykinin-induced stimulation of mitotic activity and DNA synthesis in thymocytes. Proc. Soc. Exp. Biol. Med., *133*:1270–1274, 1970.
59. Rixon, R. H., Whitfield, J. F., and Bayliss, J.: The stimulation of mitotic activity in the thymus and bone marrow of rats by kallikrein. Horm. Metab. Res., *3*:279–284, 1971.

Primary Sarcoma of the Pulmonary Trunk and/or Right or Left Main Pulmonary Artery—A Rare Cause of Obstruction to Right Ventricular Outflow

Report on Two Patients and Analysis of 35 Previously Described Patients

BARRY M. SHMOOKLER, M.D.
H. BRANDIS MARSH, M.D.
Washington, D. C.
WILLIAM C. ROBERTS, M.D.
Bethesda, Maryland

Clinical and morphologic observations are described in two women with primary sarcoma of the pulmonary trunk, and observations in 35 previously described patients with primary sarcoma involving a major extrapulmonary pulmonary artery are summarized. The neoplasm produces symptoms by causing obstruction to right ventricular outflow or by dislodging tumor fragments to the smaller intrapulmonary pulmonary arteries with or without pulmonary infarction. The sarcoma nearly always arises from the pulmonary trunk to which it is firmly attached. Although it grows to a large size within the lumen, it infrequently, despite its highly malignant histologic pattern, extends through the wall of the pulmonary trunk or metastasizes outside the pulmonary circulation. It may mimic a variety of more common disorders. Diagnosis can be achieved by angiography and treatment starts with total excision.

Obstruction to right ventricular outflow may be due to stenosis within the right ventricle itself, at the level of the pulmonic valve, or at the level of the major pulmonary arteries or their branches. Among the causes of *supravalvular* pulmonic stenosis are pulmonary emboli, disease of the small pulmonary arteries and capillaries, congenital narrowings of the major pulmonary arteries and fibrosing mediastinitis. Although a neoplasm originating proximal to or within the right atrium or right ventricle may extend into the pulmonary trunk or right or left main pulmonary artery, a primary neoplasm arising from the pulmonary artery is infrequently considered as a cause of right ventricular outflow obstruction. We have studied two patients with sarcoma of the pulmonary trunk and each had severe obstruction to right ventricular outflow. Described here are observations in them and in previously described patients with sarcoma of a major extrapulmonary pulmonary artery.

From the Departments of Pathology and Medicine, Washington Hospital Center, Washington, D.C., and the Pathology Branch, National Heart, Lung, and Blood Institute, National Institutes of Health, Bethesda, Maryland 20014. Requests for reprints should be addressed to Dr. William C. Roberts, Building 10A, Room 3E-30, National Institutes of Health, Bethesda, Maryland 20014. Manuscript accepted October 18, 1976.

DESCRIPTIONS OF PATIENTS

Patient 1. A 54 year old white woman (PGGH No. 0791670), who died on August 18, 1970, apparently was well until August 1969 (12 months before death) when she began to note a variety of symptoms including exertional dyspnea, chest pain, palpitations, exertional dizziness, headache, difficulty in concentration and making decisions, restlessness, anxiety, emotional liability, change in sleeping habits, inability to relax, tremor, frequent night-

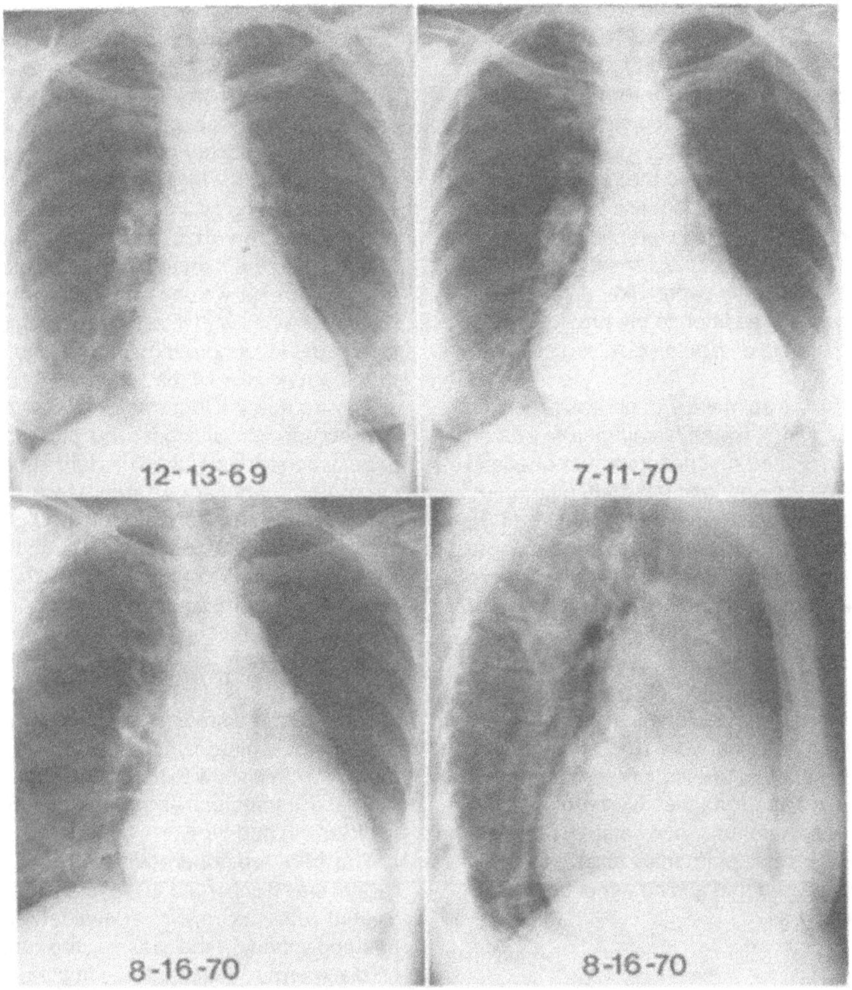

Figure 1. *Patient 1. Chest roentgenograms taken on the dates shown. The cardiac silhouette progressively enlarges. The pulmonary trunk is prominent, particularly on the lateral view.*

mares, nausea and vomiting, weight loss and one syncopal episode. In October 1969, she noted low grade fever, chills, malaise, myalgias, nonproductive cough and pain in the posterolateral portion of the left side of the chest made worse by movement. She was believed to have flu and was treated with antibiotics. These symptoms persisted, and she had another episode of syncope; therefore, on December 13, 1966, she was hospitalized. On examination, her face was puffy and she appeared anxious. A faint "blowing" systolic murmur was audible along the left sternal border. The cardiac sounds were of good quality. The lungs were clear. No abdominal organs were palpable. Subcutaneous edema was absent. A chest roentgenogram (Figure 1) disclosed mild cardiomegaly and clear lungs. An electrocardiogram showed low voltage (sum of QRS in leads I, II and III = 9 mv), nonspecific ST-T wave changes and lack of development of an R wave larger than the S wave until lead V_6. The electrocardiographic changes were interpreted as showing extensive anteroseptal myocardial infarction of uncertain age. The echocardiogram showed no abnormalities. The triosorbin test result was normal. The blood hematocrit value was 33 per cent. The patient was afebrile during her 11 days in the hospital. Her diagnosis on discharge was psychoneurotic depressive reaction.

During the following seven months, marked weakness and episodes of dizziness persisted, she fainted two more times and was retired from her employment because of disability. Dyspnea and chest pain, however, did not recur. She was rehospitalized on July 11, 1970, for reevaluation. The blood pressure was 95/50 mm Hg. There was no neck vein distention. A loud third heart sound was present and the pulmonic component of the second heart sound was loud. A grade 1/6 "scratchy" systolic murmur was audible along the left sternal border. The lungs were clear. The electrocardiogram was unchanged. A chest roentgenogram showed an increase in the size of the cardiac silhouette (Figure 1). Although she told a consulting psychiatrist during this hospitalization that what she needed was a "heart shrinker," not a "head shrinker," the diagnosis at discharge on July 21, again was psychoneurotic depressive reaction.

Following discharge, the severe weakness persisted. Four days before death, severe nausea and vomiting, dizziness and diaphoresis developed. The patient was readmitted one day before death appearing critically ill, dizzy and sweating profusely; her blood pressure was 80/40 mm Hg, rising to 95/50 mm Hg with vasopressors. The precordial murmur was unchanged. The chest roentgenogram (Figure 1) showed considerable enlargement compared to the previous films. The pulmonary "segment" was prominent and the peripheral pulmonary vascularity appeared reduced. A left pleural effusion was present. The electrocardiogram showed nodal or junctional rhythm with wandering pacemaker and frequent ventricular premature beats in addition to the previously described changes. When turning on her left side she suddenly had cardiac arrest.

At necropsy (A70-240), the pulmonary trunk was filled with a large tumor (Figures 2 and 3) which histologically was an undifferentiated sarcoma (Figure 4). The tumor was attached to the pulmonary trunk, to the right and left main pulmonary arteries and to the pulmonic valve cusp (Figures 2 and 3). Both right ventricle and right atrium were dilated, but no myocardial foci of fibrosis or necrosis or tumor implants were present. The pericardial surface, including the adventitia of the major extrapulmonary pulmonary arteries and aorta, was smooth and glistening, and less than 25 ml of serous fluid was present in the pericardial space. The right ventricular wall measured up to 0.5 cm in thickness. The heart weighed 390 g. The epicardial coronary arteries were free of significant luminal narrowing. A small effusion was present in the left pleural space. Although no abnormalities were noted in the lungs on gross inspection, histologic study disclosed tumor in the lumens of numerous small pulmonary arteries (Figure 5). No other metastases were noted and no tumor was found in the pulmonary parenchyma.

Patient 2. A 34 year old white woman (WHC No. 879378) was well until February 5, 1976, when she suddenly experienced severe substernal chest pain with radiation to both arms, associated with dyspnea and nausea while climbing stairs. A minute or so later she fainted; she awoke about 15 minutes later lying on the floor in a pool of urine. Shortly thereafter she was hospitalized. On examination, she appeared healthy. An a wave was noted in the neck veins. The second heart sound at the base was paradoxically split and the pulmonic component was loud. A grade 3/6 systolic, ejection-type precordial murmur, loudest in the pulmonic area, was present. The murmur also was well heard in the right interscapular area. The lungs were clear. No abdominal organs were palpable. Subcutaneous edema was absent.

The blood hematocrit value was 33 per cent, serum iron 30 μg/100 ml, total iron-binding capacity 338 μg/100 ml with 9 per cent saturation. (Anemia had been present since childhood, it was normochromic and normocytic, but its cause was never precisely determined.) Except for a heart rate of 100 beats/min, the electrocardiogram was within normal limits. The chest roentgenogram (Figure 6) showed enlargement of the "pulmonary segment" and slight diminution of the pulmonary markings in the left lung. A phonocardiogram confirmed the accentuation of the pulmonic sound. The maximal intensity of the systolic murmur was recorded in the pulmonic area. An echocardiogram disclosed dilatation of the right ventricle (2.5 cm). At cardiac catheterization, the following pressures (in mm Hg) were recorded: pulmonary arterial wedge mean, 11; distal right pulmonary artery, 20/10; right main pulmonary artery, 50/25; pulmonary trunk, 60/25; right ventricle, 60/18; right atrium, mean 7, a wave 8, v wave 7; and ascending aorta, 100/60 (mean 80). The cardiac index was 3.3 liters/min/m^2. Angiography, with injection of contrast material into the right ventricle, disclosed large filling defects in the pulmonary trunk and in both right and left main pulmonary arteries with total lack of filling of arteries to the lower lobe of the left lung and marked diminution of filling of arteries to the upper lobe of the left lung (Figure 7).

Thoracotomy (Doctors Jorge Garcia and Luis Mispireta) on February 25 disclosed no pericardial abnormalities or excess pericardial fluid. The right atrium, right ventricle and the major pulmonary arteries were quite dilated, and their exterior surfaces were smooth and glistening. Incision into the pulmonary trunk disclosed a large tumor completely filling it and extending into both right and left main pulmonary arteries. The tumor was attached to the intima of the pulmonary trunk over a broad base, but it was unattached to the intima of either the right or left main pulmonary artery. The entire tumor was excised intact (Figure 7) including most or all of the wall of the pulmonary trunk from whence it arose. After closing the pulmonary trunk and discontinuing cardiopulmonary bypass, flow to both lungs via these arteries appeared normal. Histologically (Figure 8), the tumor was a sarcoma, undifferentiated type.

The early postoperative course was unremarkable; the patient was discharged 10 days after operation and thereafter treated with adriamycin. At evaluation in May (three months postoperatively), she was asymptomatic and had no precordial murmur; the pressures in the pulmonary arteries, right ventricle and right atrium were within normal limits, and right ventricular angiography showed no filling defects in any of the pulmonary arteries and normal flow to both lungs. Although still asymptomatic, examination on August 23, however, disclosed a grade 3/6 systolic ejection murmur, loudest along the left upper sternal border, and repeat right ventricular angiogram disclosed a single round filling defect attached to the anterior wall of the pulmonary trunk. The pressures in the right ventricle and pulmonary trunk were identical, 27/7 mm Hg. Because of the reappearance of a filling defect in the pulmonary trunk, repeat thoracotomy was performed on September 15. At thoracotomy (Doctors Jorge Garcia and Luis Mispireta), a small tumor nodule, which histologically was an undifferentiated sarcoma, was found in the pulmonary trunk at the site of the previous suture line. The nodule, including the wall of the pulmonary trunk to which it was attached, was excised and the portion of the pulmonary trunk excised was replaced with a patch. The pulmonic valve cusps were normal, and no tumor was observed in either the right or left main pulmonary artery, lung or mediastinum. The patient's early postoperative course was uneventful.

2

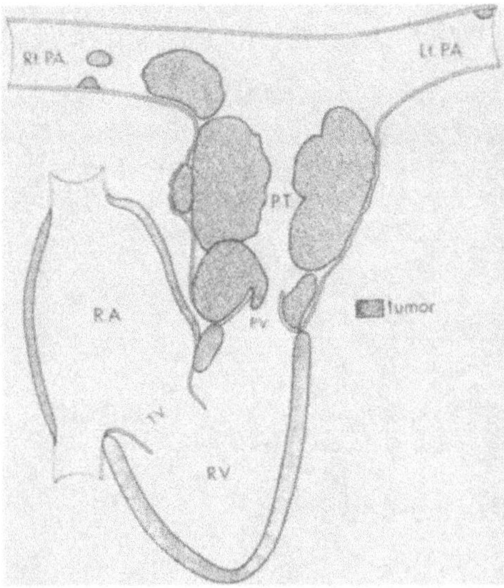

3

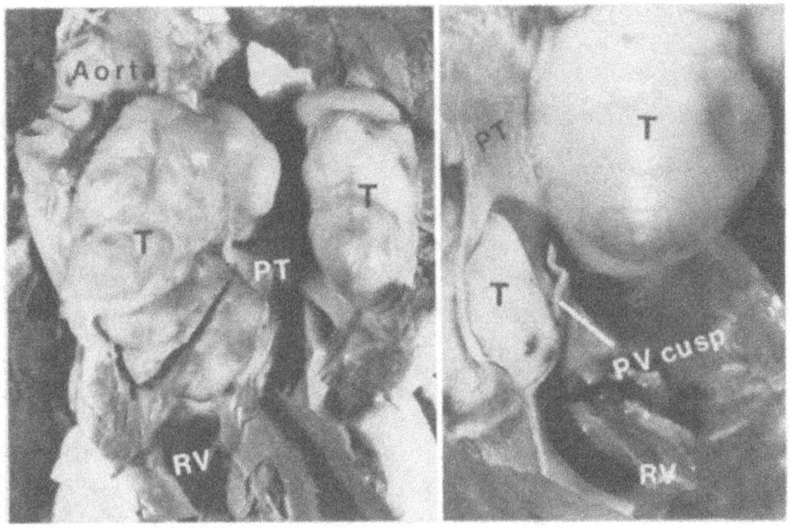

__Figure 2.__ Patient 1. Diagram showing the huge tumor in the pulmonary trunk (PT) with satellite nodules in both right (Rt PA) and left (Lt PA) main pulmonary artery. The sarcoma is firmly attached to the pulmonic valve (PV) cusps and "overhangs" one cusp. RA = right atrium; RV = right ventricle; TV = tricuspid valve.

__Figure 3.__ Patient 1. Photographs of the primary sarcoma which fills nearly the entire pulmonary trunk (PT). T = tumor; RV = right ventricular outflow tract. A close-up of the tumor (T) in a pulmonic valve (PV) sinus is shown on the right.

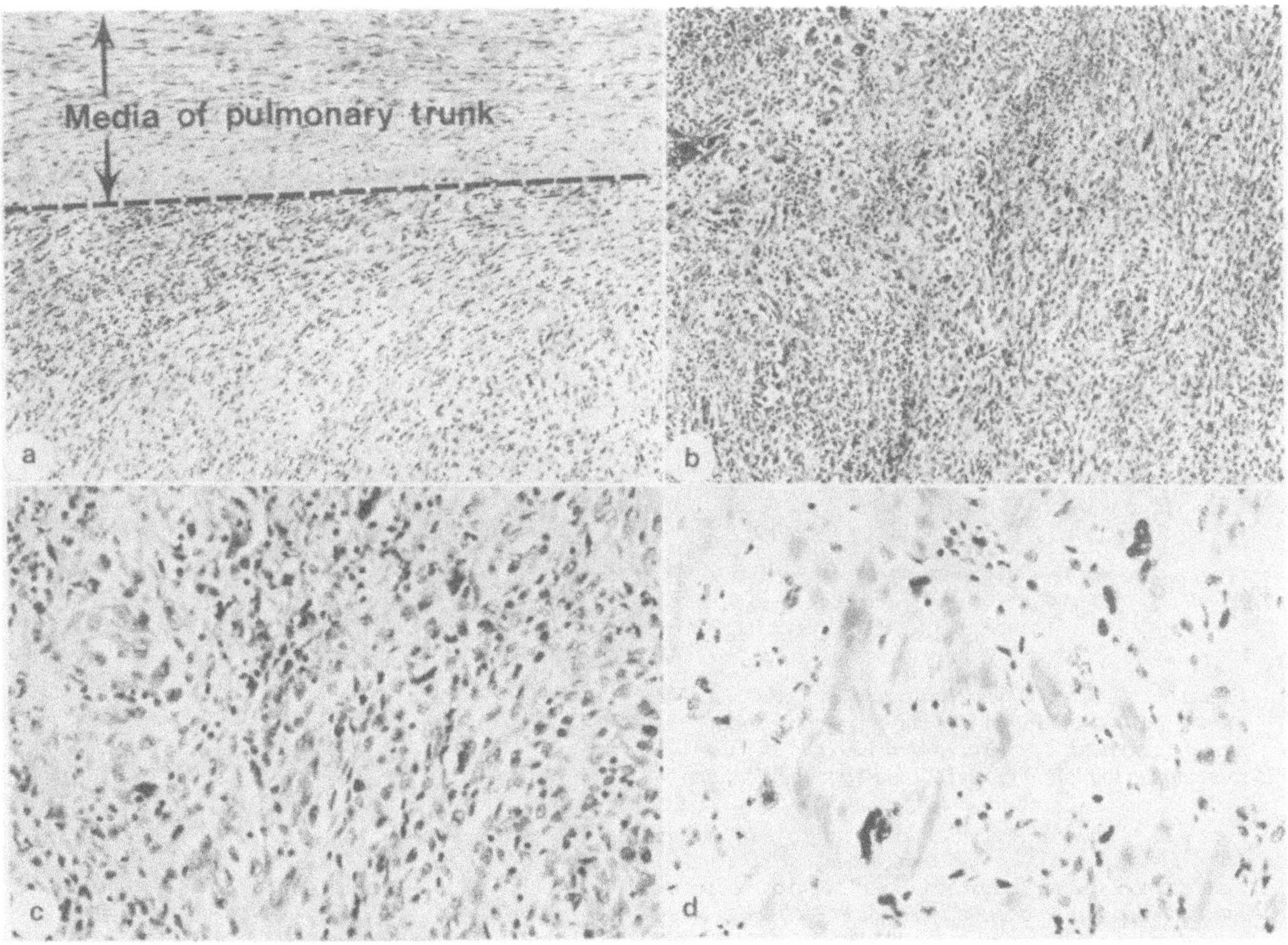

__Figure 4.__ Patient 1. Photomicrographs of the primary sarcoma of pulmonary trunk. __a,__ the upper portion shows the neoplasm attached to the wall of pulmonary trunk. __b, c__ and __d,__ various areas of the primary sarcoma. Tumor giant cells are frequent. Hematoxylin and eosin stains; original magnification × 100 (a and b), × 250 (c and d), reduced by 18 per cent.

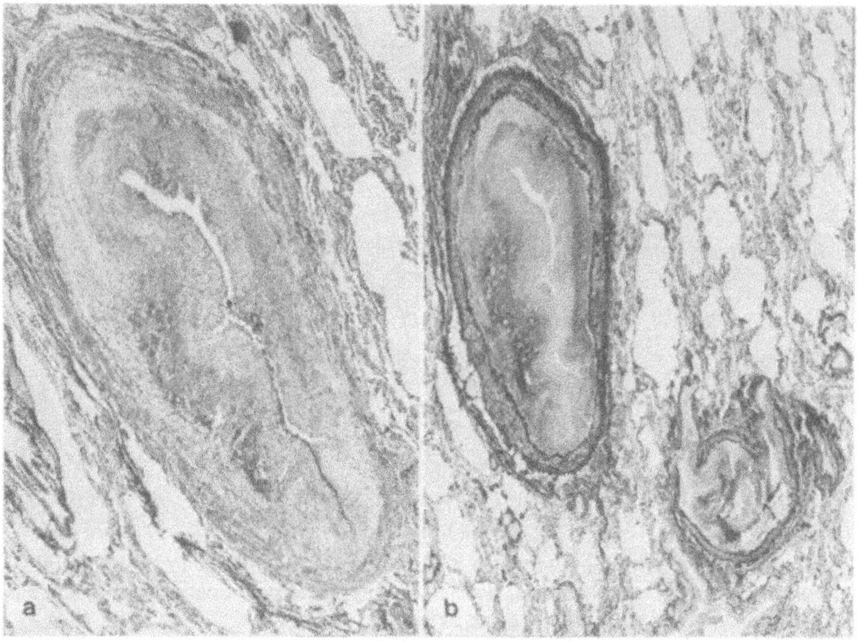

Figure 5. *Patient 1. Tumor emboli in small pulmonary arteries without pulmonary infarction. Hematoxylin and eosin stain (**a**) and elastic van Gieson stain (**b**); original magnification × 40 (a) and × 27 (b), reduced by 27 per cent.*

6

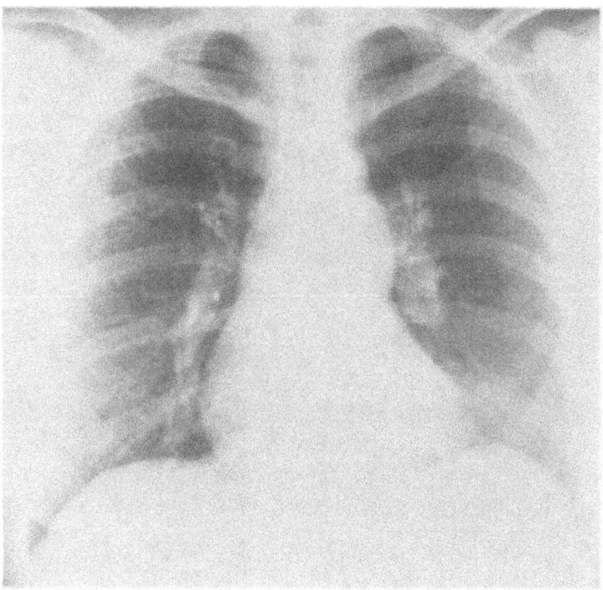

7

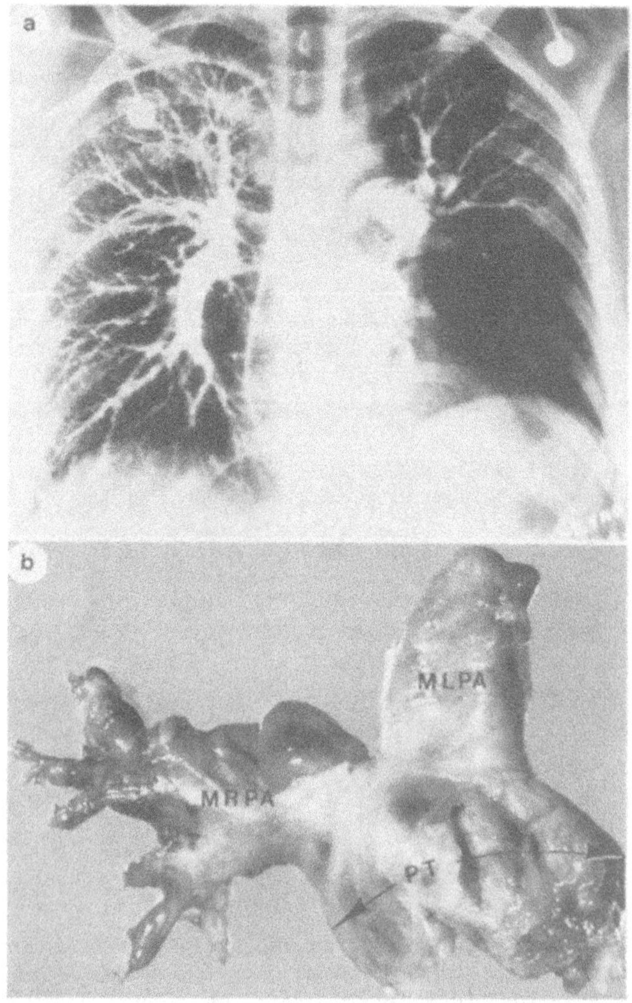

Figure 6. *Patient 2. Chest roentgenogram taken one week before the first operation showing a very prominent "pulmonary segment," and some diminution in the vascular markings in the left lung field compared to the right one.*

Figure 7. *Patient 2. **a,** right ventricular angiogram showing filling defects in the pulmonary trunk and in both right and left main pulmonary arteries and absence of filling of most of the intrapulmonary pulmonary arteries of the left lung. **b,** the operatively excised tumor in the pulmonary trunk (PT) and right (MRPA) and left (MLPA) main pulmonary arteries.*

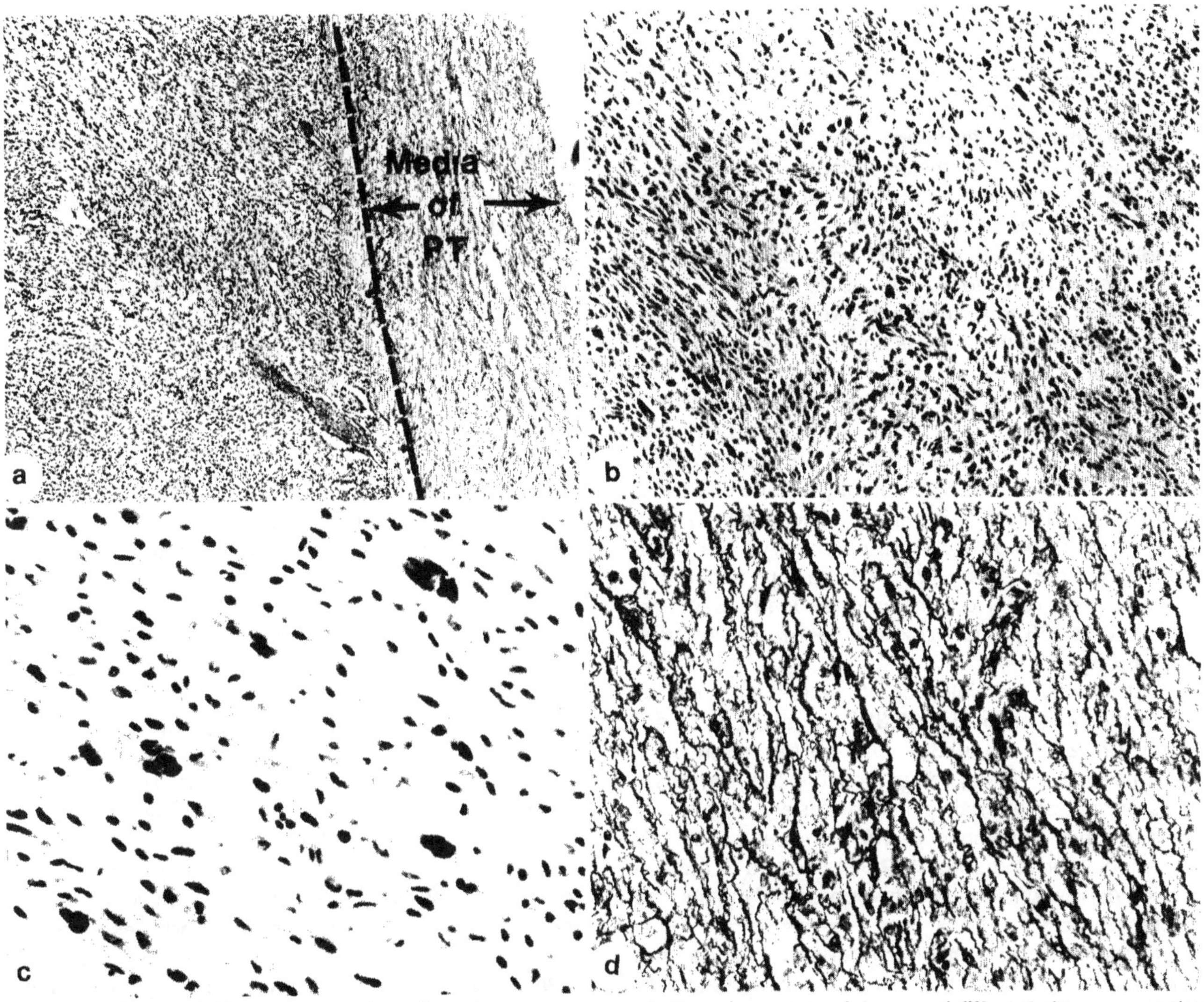

Figure 8. Patient 2. Photomicrographs of the pulmonary sarcoma in the pulmonary trunk in several different sites. ***a,*** *a portion of wall of pulmonary trunk (PT) is shown.* ***b*** *and* ***c,*** *many giant cells are seen.* ***d,*** *reticulin stain showing lining of individual and clusts of tumor cell. Hematoxylin and eosin stain (a, b, c); original magnification × 55 (a), × 140 (b and c), × 350 (d), reduced by 15 per cent.*

SUMMARY OF PREVIOUS REPORTS OF PULMONARY ARTERIAL SARCOMA

Certain clinical and morphologic features in 35 previously described patients with sarcoma arising from a major extrapulmonary pulmonary artery are summarized in Table I. Of the 35 patients, 34 are dead: necropsies were performed in 32 [1–30] and not in two [31,32]: one patient was alive at the time of the report [33]. Diagnosis of sarcoma was confirmed by histologic examination in all 35 patients. The 35 patients ranged in age from 22 to 81 years (average 52); 20 were women and 15 were men. Symptoms included dyspnea, 63 per cent (19 of 30); chest pain, 40 per cent (12 of 30); cough without hemoptysis, 40 per cent (12 of 30); hemoptysis, 30 per cent (nine of 30); and syncope, 23 per cent (seven of 30). The major physical findings included precordial systolic murmur, 64 per cent (18 of 28); cyanosis, 50 per cent (13 of 26); subcutaneous edema, 38 per cent (10 of 26); weight loss, 35 per cent (nine of 26); jugular venous distention, 27 per cent (seven of 26); and basal diastolic murmur (pulmonic area), 11 per cent (three of 28).

The chest roentgenogram, described in 29 of the 35 patients, showed one or more discrete pulmonary parenchymal infiltrates (consistent with, or suspicious of, metastatic neoplasm) in 14 patients (48 per cent), hilar or mediastinal mass in 11 (38 per cent), enlarged cardiac silhouette in 11 (38 per cent), decreased peripheral pulmonary vascular markings in seven (24 per cent) and enlarged pulmonary trunk and/or right or left main pulmonary artery in six (21 per cent). The electrocardiogram, described in 18 of the 35 patients, showed right ventricular hypertrophy in nine.

Hemodynamic information was reported in six [20,25,26,29,32,33] of the 35 patients. The pulmonary trunk could not be entered by the catheter in two patients [25,32]; in the other four, the pulmonary arterial systolic pressure was normal (27 mm Hg) in one [33], and increased in three (62, 70 and 95 mm Hg, respectively). Right ventricular pressures were recorded in five patients: in one patient it was normal [25]; in the other four, the peak systolic pressures ranged from 62 to 110 mm Hg (average 96 mm Hg). Only three patients had both right ventricular and pulmonary arterial pressures recorded: one had no peak systolic pressure gradient [29]; one had a 9 mm Hg gradient [26] and one had a 79 mm Hg gradient [33]. In only one patient was a gradient reported between the pulmonary trunk and a distal pulmonary artery [26]. Of the four patients in whom it was reported, the cardiac index was normal in one [33] and markedly decreased in three [25,26,29].

Angiography, with injection of contrast material into either the right ventricle [29,32] or major pulmonary artery [20,22,23,26,30,33], was performed in eight patients. A large filling defect involving the pulmonary trunk or right or left main pulmonary artery or both was observed in all eight patients. The filling defects usually were lobulated and some [29,32] showed to and fro motion corresponding to the two phases of the cardiac cycle.

Diagnosis of pulmonary arterial sarcoma was not considered until necropsy in 25 of the 32 necropsy patients; in the remaining seven necropsy patients and in the other three patients (Table I), the diagnosis of pulmonary arterial sarcoma was established at thoracotomy. The total duration of symptoms attributable to pulmonary arterial sarcoma from onset to death was available in 30 of the 34 fatal cases; it ranged from one to 39 months (average 12 months).

In all 32 necropsy patients, the sarcoma was located in the pulmonary trunk or main pulmonary artery or both: pulmonary trunk, 31 patients (97 per cent); right main pulmonary artery, 20 patients (63 per cent); left main pulmonary artery, 18 patients (56 per cent). In addition, the sarcoma was attached to the pulmonic valve cusp in 16 patients (50 per cent) and extended below the pulmonic valve into the right ventricular outflow tract in nine (28 per cent). Tumor emboli were found in peripheral intrapulmonary pulmonary arteries in 21 patients (66 per cent). Metastases to organs outside the lung were infrequent. Sarcoma was found in either mediastinal or hilar lymph nodes in five [4,11,12,15,22] of the 32 necropsy patients (16 per cent); three [4,11,15] of them also had metastases to another organ (adrenal gland in one patient, brain in one and bowel in one). Only one other patient had extrapulmonary metastases: to both adrenal glands and to the pancreas [26].

The type sarcoma diagnosed histologically was described as undifferentiated (spindle cell, pleomorphic, anaplastic) in 13 patients (38 per cent), leiomyosarcoma in nine (26 per cent), fibrosarcoma in four (11 per cent), fibromyxosarcoma in three (9 per cent), malignant mesenchymoma in three (9 per cent) and in one patient each fibroleiomyosarcoma (3 per cent), rhabdomyosarcoma (3 per cent) and myxosarcoma (3 per cent).

COMMENTS

Sarcoma of the major extrapulmonary pulmonary arteries is a rare neoplasm thus far described only in adults, and more commonly in women than in men. The tumor is located nearly always (in 34 of the 35 previously described patients and in both of our patients) in the pulmonary trunk to which it is firmly attached. From there it may extend distally into one or both main pulmonary arteries and proximally onto one or more pulmonic valve cusps or into the right ventricular outflow tract. The neoplasm tends to expand the major extrapulmonary pulmonary arteries and to narrow their lumens. Furthermore, probably because of the to-and-fro movement given to it by the contracting heart, portions of the sarcoma frequently dislodge and migrate as tumor emboli into the smaller pulmonary arteries in one or both lungs. From there the tumor may cause pulmonary infarction or grow in situ to appear as a metastatic nodule(s) on the roentgenogram.

The neoplasm histologically is an undifferentiated sarcoma. Although most investigators have attempted to subclassify this sarcoma, this exercise has not proved useful from a prognostic or clinical standpoint. Despite its highly malignant histologic characteristics, the sarcoma is infrequently found outside the pulmonary circulation and usually does not extend through the wall of the pulmonary trunk. Local metastases to hilar or mediastinal lymph nodes are infrequent and pericardial effusions, uncommon.

Sarcoma of the pulmonary trunk (or other major extrapulmonary pulmonary artery) most commonly manifests itself clinically by producing evidence of right ventricular systolic hypertension. The latter most commonly results from obstruction to the pulmonary trunk or to one or both main pulmonary arteries by the growth of the tumor within the lumen. Evidence of right ventricular systolic hypertension also may result, however, from multiple tumor emboli to the lungs. Ob-

TABLE I Clinical and Necropsy Observations in 35 Previously Described Patients with Sarcoma of the Pulmonary

Patient	Reference	Age (yr) and Sex	Dy	Sy	P	H	C-H	Cy	E	Murmur S	Murmur D
			Necropsy Patients								
1	Mandelstamm 1923 [1]	58,M	+	0	+	0	+	0	+	+	0
2	Eschbach 1928 [2]	58,M	+	+	0	0	0	+	0	+	0
3	Froboese 1928 [3]	64,F	—	—	—	—	—	+	+	+	0
4	Kudlich, Schuh 1934 [4]	27,M	—	—	—	—	—	—	—	—	—
5	Goedel 1935 [5]	47,M	+	0	0	0	0	0	+	0	0
6	Martin et al. 1939 [6]	46,F	+	0	0	0	0	0	+	+	0
7	Haythorn et al. 1941 [7]	51,F	+	0	+	+	0	0	0	0	0
8	van du Linde 1942 [8]	23,F	+	0	0	0	0	0	0	+	0
9	Durgin, Ingleby 1946 [9]	53,F	+	+	+	0	0	+	0	0	0
10	Moegen 1951 [10]	70,F	+	0	0	0	0	0	+	+	0
11	Elphinstone, Spector 1951 [11]	61,M	+	0	+	0	+	+	+	+	+
12	Wolf et al. 1960 [12]	63,F	+	0	+	0	0	+	+	+	0
13	Hagström 1961 [13]	59,F	+	+	+	0	+	—	—	—	—
14	Chatelant 1962 [14]	81,M	—	—	—	—	—	—	—	0	0
15	Kovacs et al. 1962 [15]	55,M	—	—	—	—	—	—	—	—	—
16	Green et al. 1964 [16]	47,M	0	+	0	0	0	+	0	+	0
17	Ali, Lee 1974 [17]	36,F	0	0	0	0	+	0	0	0	0
18	Munk et al. 1965 [18]	50,F	+	0	0	0	+	+	+	+	0
19	Olesky 1967 [19]	23,M	0	0	0	+	0	—	—	+	0
20	Friedman, Smith 1968 [20]	53,F	+	0	+	0	0	+	0	+	+
21	Wackers et al. 1969 [21]	69,M	0	0	0	+	0	0	0	0	0
22	Cain #1 1969 [22]	72,F	+	0	0	0	0	+	0	+	0
23	Cain #2 1969 [22]	62,F	0	0	0	+	0	+	—	—	—
24	Cain #3 1969 [22]	31,M	0	0	+	+	0	—	—	—	—
25	Hirsch et al. 1970 [23]	22, F	0	0	0	+	+	+	0	0	0
26	Sethi 1972 [24]	50,F	+	0	+	+	+	+	0	0	0
27	Thijs 1974 [25]	48,F	+	0	+	+	+	0	+	+	0
28	Rao 1974 [26]	59,M	0	0	+	0	+	+	0	+	+
29	Schott, Reinhold 1974 [27]	70,F	0	0	0	+	0	0	+	0	0
30	Kimura, Namiki 1975 [28]	64, F	—	—	—	—	—	—	—	—	—
31	Killebrew, Gerbode 1976 [29]	62,M	+	+	0	0	+	0	0	+	0
32	Olsson et al. 1976 [30]	52,M	0	0	+	0	0	0	0	0	0
			Dead but No Necropsy								
33	Jacques, Barclay 1960 [31]	54,F	+	0	0	0	+	—	—	—	—
34	Hayes et al. 1974 [32]	52,F	+	+	0	0	+	0	0	+	0
			Alive								
35	DiGilio et al. 1972 [33]	45,M	0	+	0	0	0	0	0	+	0

NOTE: Dy = dyspnea; Sy = syncope; P = chest pain; H = hemoptysis; C-H = cough without hemoptysis; Cy = cyanosis; E = subcutaneous edema; S = systolic; D = Diastolic

struction of the pulmonary trunk alone is not associated with pulmonary hypertension, but dislodgement of tumor fragments from the large extrapulmonary pulmonary arteries into the small intrapulmonary pulmonary arteries may occur without obstruction of the pulmonary trunk and consequently produce pulmonary systolic hypertension as well as right ventricular systolic hypertension. The latter obviously may lead to right ventricular dilatation and failure, which is the most common clinical manifestation of this sarcoma.

Sarcoma of the pulmonary trunk is commonly not diagnosed until operation, necropsy or, at least, right ventricular angiography. The most likely explanation for the infrequency of proper diagnosis before operation or necropsy is that the condition is so rare that most physicians probably have not heard of it much less included it in a differential diagnosis. The condition has been confused most frequently with pulmonary emboli of the usual sort, with or without pulmonary infarction. Some of its more unusual clinical features, however, have caused it to be confused with a variety of other disorders, listed in Table II. Our Patient 1 was believed to have a psychoneurotic disorder until shortly before death, despite several hospitalizations for diagnostic purposes. The ejection-type precordial systolic murmur in some patients has caused confusion with aortic stenosis, especially when associated with syncope. Two patients presented initially with evidence of dis-

Trunk and/or Right or Left Main Pulmonary Artery

Chest Roentgenogram					RVH	Means of Dx		Duration	Location of Sarcoma						Metastatic Sarcoma		
CE	H/M Mass	Lung Lesions	↑PA	↓Pul Vas	on ECG	O	N	(mo) of Symptoms	PV	PT	RMPA	LMPA	Distal PA	RVOT	Lung	LN	Other
+	0	+	0	0	—	0	+	7	+	+	0	0	0	+	+	0	0
+	0	+	0	0	—	0	+	12	+	+	0	0	+	+	0	0	0
—	—	—	—	—	—	0	+	25	0	+	+	+	0	0	0	0	0
—	—	—	—	—	—	0	+	—	+	+	+	+	+	+	+	+	+
—	—	—	—	—	—	0	+	4	+	+	0	+	+	+	+	0	0
—	—	—	—	—	0	0	+	4	+	+	+	+	0	+	0	0	0
0	+	+	0	0	—	0	+	8	0	+	0	0	+	0	+	0	0
0	0	+	0	0	0	0	+	8	+	+	0	0	0	+	+	0	0
—	—	—	—	—	—	0	+	2	0	+	0	+	0	0	0	0	0
0	0	+	0	0	0	0	+	12	0	+	+	0	0	0	+	0	0
+	+	0	+	+	+	0	+	9	+	+	0	0	+	0	0	+	+
+	0	0	+	0	+	0	+	39	0	+	+	+	+	0	+	+	0
0	+	+	0	0	—	0	+	24	+	+	+	+	+	+	+	0	0
+	+	0	0	0	0	0	+	21	+	+	0	0	+	0	+	0	0
—	—	—	—	—	—	0	+	—	+	+	0	0	0	0	+	+	+
+	0	0	+	+	+	0	+	7	0	+	+	+	+	+	0	0	0
0	0	+	0	0	—	0	+	3	0	+	+	+	+	0	+	0	0
+	0	+	+	+	+	0	+	18	0	+	+	+	+	0	+	0	0
0	0	+	0	0	—	0	+	21	+	+	+	+	+	+	0	0	0
0	+	0	0	+	0	+	+	21	0	0	+	+	0	0	+	0	0
0	+	0	0	0	+	0	+	7	0	+	+	0	+	0	+	0	0
0	+	+	0	0	0	0	+	10	+	+	+	0	+	0	+	0	0
0	0	0	0	0	—	0	+	12	0	+	+	+	0	0	+	0	0
0	+	0	0	0	—	+	+	18	+	+	+	0	+	0	+	+	0
0	+	0	0	0	0	+	+	11	0	+	+	0	+	0	+	0	0
0	+	0	0	0	+	+	+	13	0	+	+	+	+	0	+	0	0
+	0	0	0	0	+	+	+	7	+	+	+	+	+	0	+	0	0
+	0	0	0	+	+	0	+	4	+	+	0	+	+	0	+	0	+
+	0	+	0	0	—	0	+	10	0	+	+	+	+	0	+	0	0
0	0	+	0	0	—	0	+	—	+	+	0	0	0	0	0	0	0
+	0	0	0	0	0	+	+	3	0	+	0	+	0	0	0	0	0
0	0	+	0	+	—	+	+	1	0	+	+	0	+	0	+	0	0
0	+	+	0	+	—	+	0	"yrs"	0	+	0	+	0	0	+	+	
0	0	0	+	0	0	+	0	31	+	+	+	+	—	—	—	—	—
0	0	0	+	0	+	+	0	—	+	+	+	+	—	—	—	—	—

NOTE: CE = cardiac enlargement; H/M = hilar or mediastinal; PA = pulmonary artery; Pul Vas = pulmonary vascularity; RVH = right ventricular hypertrophy; Dx = diagnosis; O = operation; N = necropsy; PV = pulmonic valve; PT = pulmonary trunk; RMPA = right main pulmonary artery; LMPA = left main pulmonary artery; LN = lymph node; RVOT = right ventricular outflow tract; 0 = absent or negative; + = present or positive; — = no information available.

seminated intravascular coagulation [21,27]. The patient described by Wolf and associates [12] presented with features typical of pheochromocytoma, including a postitive Regitine® test. A large cardiac silhouette on a chest roentgenogram may indicate extension of the sarcoma through the wall of the pulmonary trunk leading to pericardial effusion. Such was the case in the patient described by Thijs and associates [25].

Although a highly malignant sarcoma, operative resection of sarcoma of the pulmonary trunk may prove highly beneficial as exemplified by our Patient 2 and by the patient described by DiGilio and associates [33]. Both our Patient 2 and the latter patient have undergone

TABLE II Differential Diagnosis of Sarcoma of the Pulmonary Trunk

1. Pulmonary embolism
2. Metastatic pulmonary neoplasm
3. Idiopathic (primary) pulmonary hypertension
4. Aortic stenosis
5. Psychosomatic disorder
6. Pheochromocytoma
7. Hematologic disorder
8. Pericardial effusion
9. Idiopathic dilated cardiomyopathy
10. Fibrosing mediastinitis

thoracotomy twice within a year, but both patients continue to be symptom-free without tumor implants in the lung. Our Patient 2 had recurrence of sarcoma at the suture line in the pulmonary trunk but was symptom-free at the time of the second operation. Whether chemotherapeutic agents or irradiation will prove useful in treating patients with pulmonary arterial sarcoma is unknown because of the rarity of the neoplasm.

ACKNOWLEDGMENT

We thank Dr. James E. Hutchinson, formerly, Pathologist at Prince Georges General Hospital, Cheverly, Maryland, for allowing us to study Patient 1. We thank members of the Department of Radiology, Washington Hospital Center, for allowing us to reproduce the roentgenograms shown in Figures 6 and 7.

REFERENCES

1. Madelstamm M: Ueber Primaere Neubildungen des Herzens. Virchows Arch Pathol Anat 245: 43, 1923.
2. Eschbach H: Ueber ein malignes Leiomyom des Endocords mit Verstopfung der Lungenschlagader. Beitr Z Pathol Anat 80: 672, 1928.
3. Froboese C: Emboliformes Sarkom des Hauptstammes der Pulmonalasterie. Zentralbl Allg Pathol 44: 148, 1928.
4. Kudlich H, Schuh W: Ein Beitrag zum myoplastischen Sarkom der Lungenschlagader. Virchows Arch [Pathol Anat] 294: 113, 1934.
5. Goedel A: Zur Kenntnis des primaeren Lungenschlagadersarkom. Frankfurt Z Pathol 49: 1, 1935.
6. Martin W, Tuohy E, Will C: Primary tumor of the heart (entrance of the pulmonary artery). Am Heart J 17: 728, 1939.
7. Haythorn SR, Ray WB, Wolff RA: Primary fibromyxosarcomas of the heart and pulmonary artery. Am J Pathol 17: 261, 1941.
8. van du Linde HM: Sarcoom van de Longslagader. Ned Tijdschr Geneeskd 86: 1049, 1942.
9. Durgin B, Ingleby H: Primary sarcoma of the pulmonary artery. Clinics 5: 182, 1946.
10. Moegen P: Veber einen primoeren sarkomatoesen Tumor des Pulmonalartesie mit ausgedehuten Metastasen in der rechten Lunge. Z Kreislaufforsch 40: 150, 1951.
11. Elphinstone R, Spector R: Sarcoma of the pulmonary artery. Thorax 14: 333, 1951.
12. Wolf P, Dickenman R, Langston J: Fibrosarcoma of the pulmonary artery, masquerading as a pheochromocytoma. Am J Clin Pathol 34: 146, 1960.
13. Hagström L: Malignant meserchymoma in pulmonary artery and right ventricle. Report of a case with unusual location and histological picture. Acta Pathol Microbiol Scand 51: 87, 1961.
14. Chatelant F: Fibromyxosarcome des valvules pulmonaires et son extension dans les poumons. Pathol Microbiol (Basel) 25: 366, 1962.
15. Kovács K, Illýes E, Szabo K, et al.: Primary sarcoma of the pulmonary artery. Orv Hetil 103: 841, 1962 (abstract 132 in Excerpta Medica, sec 5, vol 16, 1963).
16. Green J, Crevasse L, Sharklin D: Fibromyxosarcoma of the pulmonary artery. Associated with syncope, intractable heart failure, polycythemia and thrombocytopenia. Am J Cardiol 13: 547, 1964.
17. Ali MY, Lee GS: Sarcoma of the pulmonary artery. Cancer 17: 1220, 1974.
18. Munk J, Griffel B, Kogan J: Primary mesenchymoma of the pulmonary artery: radiologic features. Br J Radiol 38: 104, 1965.
19. Olesky J: Pierwotny miesniak zlosliwy tetnicy plucnej. Pol Arch Med Wewn 38: 663, 1967.
20. Friedman H, Smith C: Leiomyosarcoma of the pulmonary artery. JAMA 203: 809, 1968.
21. Wackers FJ, Van Der Schoot JB, Hampe JF: Sarcoma of the pulmonary trunk associated with hemorrhagic tendency. Cancer 23: 339, 1969.
22. Cain H: Veber primaere Sarkome des Hauptstammes der Arteria Pulmonalis. Dtsch Med Wochenschr 94: 1607, 1969.
23. Hirsch A, Chrétien J, Renault P, et al.: Sarcome primitif de l'àrtère pulmonaire chez une jeune femme. Récidive rapide après èxérèse. Déséès. J Fr Med Chir Thorac 24: 147, 1970.
24. Sethi G, Slaven J, Kepes J, et al.: Primary sarcoma of the pulmonary artery. J Thorac Cardiovasc Surg 63: 587, 1972.
25. Thijs LG, Kroon TAJ, Leeuwen Th M Van: Leiomyosarcoma of the pulmonary trunk associated with pericardial effusion. Thorax 29: 490, 1974.
26. Rao W, Krishnaswami S, Cherian G, et al.: Sarcoma of the pulmonary artery with metastases to pancreas and adrenal glands. Chest 66: 459, 1974.
27. Schott G, Reinhold F: Chronische Verlaufsform einer Verbrauchskoagulopathie beim Sarkom der A. pulmonalis. Z Gesamte Inn Med 29: 257, 1974.
28. Kimura M, Namiki M: A case of sarcoma arising from the pulmonary artery valve, presenting multiple tumor-like shadows. Jap J Thorac Dis 13: 111, 1975.
29. Killebrew E, Gerbode F: Leiomyosarcoma of the pulmonary artery diagnosed preoperatively by angiocardiography. Replacement with composite graft. J Thorac Cardiovasc Surg 71: 469, 1976.
30. Olsson H, Spitzer R, Erston W: Primary and secondary pulmonary artery neoplasia mimicking acute pulmonary embolism. Radiology 118: 49, 1976.
31. Jacques J, Barclay R: The solid sarcomatous pulmonary artery. Br J Dis Chest 54: 217, 1960.
32. Hayes W, Farha S, Brown R: Primary leiomyosarcoma of the pulmonary artery. Am J Cardiol 34: 615, 1974.
33. DiGilio M, Lee H, Tatooles C, et al.: Myxosarcoma of the pulmonary valve. Chest 62: 639, 1972.

Electrocardiogram in Neoplastic and Hematologic Disorders

Joseph Lindsay, Jr., M.D., Samuel D. Goldberg, M.D., and William C. Roberts, M.D.

ELECTROCARDIOGRAM IN NEOPLASMS

Metastatic tumor to the heart is present at necropsy in about 10 percent of patients dying of malignant tumors.[1-4] Primary tumors of the heart are rare. Their frequency is about one-sixteenth that of secondary cardiac tumors.[5]

Clinical findings resulting from neoplastic disease of the heart depend upon the size and location of the tumor. Involvement of the pericardium, either parietal or visceral or both, may result in pericardial effusion with or without cardiac tamponade. The effusion may be serous, hemorrhagic, or even pyogenic.[6] Cardiac arrhythmias may result from interference by the tumor with the generation or transmission of the electrical activity of the heart. Extensive replacement of myocardium by tumor (or, in the case of leukemia, hemorrhage) may result in an enlarged cardiac silhouette, an abnormal ECG, and the clinical syndrome of cardiac failure attendant upon altered myocardial contractility or compliance. In addition to pericarditis, pyogenic or fungal infections produce myocardial abscess particularly in patients with leukemia or lymphoma.[6] Obstruction to flow of blood by an intracavitary tumor may result in vena caval obstruction or valvular stenosis with or without resulting syncope.[7,8] Less specific findings suggestive of altered cardiac function, e. g., systolic precordial murmurs, edema, and dyspnea, are common, but, particularly in metastatic tumors, may be consequences of altered serum electrolytes, anemia, hypoxia, hypoproteinemia, pulmonary metastases, or radiation effects.

The ECG is often abnormal in patients with either primary or secondary tumors of the heart. Nonspecific abnormalities such as low voltage, sinus tachycardia, and nonspecific ST-T changes are particularly frequent, but these abnormalities appear equally frequently in patients with similar neoplasms but without cardiac metastases.[6,9,11] Furthermore, it may be difficult to be sure that even a dramatic ECG abnormality is attributable to cardiac metastases and is not due to associated disease processes or to the cardiotoxicity of antineoplastic therapeutic agents.[12,13]

Primary Cardiac Neoplasms

Among these rare tumors only myxomas, which constitute about a half, sarcomas, a fifth, and so-called rhabdomyomas, another fifth, occur with sufficient frequency to allow collection of a substantial series of patients.[5]

Myxoma

Myxomas may obstruct blood flow across a cardiac valve, may be the source of systemic or pulmonary emboli, and may be associated with fever, weight loss, an elevated erythrocyte sedimentation rate, or abnormal serum proteins. Three quarters are located in the left atrium, and most of the remainder are in the right atrium.[8, 14, 15] They are least frequent in the left ventricle and, rarely, they may occur in more than one chamber.

Various electrocardiographic abnormalities, based on previous reports,[16-20] in patients with myxomas are summarized in Table 1. Valvular obstruction produced by the tumor appears to account for most of the ECG abnormalities. Thus, left atrial overload is often present in left atrial myxoma and right atrial overload in right atrial myxoma, reflecting the blockade at the associated atrioventricular valve (Figs. 1, 2, 3, 4, 5). In left atrial myxoma, as in mitral stenosis, right axis deviation and, in severe cases, right ventricular hypertrophy are encountered (Figs. 4 and 5). The QRS complex is of low amplitude in many patients with right atrial myxoma. The electrical signal possibly is dampened by the tumor mass in the right atrium which may prolapse into the right ventricle during systole. Obstruction to right ventricular outflow probably accounts for the right ventricular hypertrophy seen electrocardiographically in patients with right ventricular myxoma. Right bundle branch block (RBBB) may occur with myxoma of the right atrium or ventricle (Fig. 2 and 3); perhaps the RBBB is a consequence of impingement by the tumor mass against the ventricular septum.

Atrial arrhythmias are encountered in atrial myxoma involving either atrium, but they are less common in myxoma than in mitral stenosis (Fig. 1).

It has been postulated that coronary embolism arising from a left atrial myxoma produces the ECG evidence of acute myocardial infarction which is occasionally seen. In the 45 patients described by Campeau and David,[21] two had anterior myocardial infarction patterns. However, all such patients do not have infarcts at necropsy (Fig. 6). A similar number of Goodwin's series of patients with left atrial myxomas had chest pain and signs of coronary occlusion.[14] Kroopf and Peterson[22] reported a patient with electrocardiographic findings suggesting acute anterior myocardial infarction, and necropsy disclosed external compression of the left circumflex coronary artery and no significant intrinsic disease of the artery.

Rhabdomyoma

Congenital nodular glycogenic infiltration of the myocardium, probably a form of cardiac glycogen storage disease, was formerly termed rhabdomyoma.[25] Although they

Table 1. Electrocardiographic findings in myxoma

	Left atrial[17-19]	*Right atrial*[20]	*Right ventricular*[16]
Total patients	30	35	16
Atrial fibrillation	4 (13%)	4 (11%)	0
First degree AV block	0	3 (9%)	0
Atrial abnormality	19 (63%)*	19 (54%)†	2 (13%)
Right axis deviation	16 (53%)	8 (23%)	8 (50%)
Right ventricular hypertrophy	6 (20%)	0	5 (31%)
Incomplete RBBB	0	0	5 (31%)
Complete RBBB	0	11 (31%)	3 (19%)
Low voltage QRS	0	18 (51%)	0

*Usually suggestive of left atrial overload.
†Usually suggestive of right atrial overload.

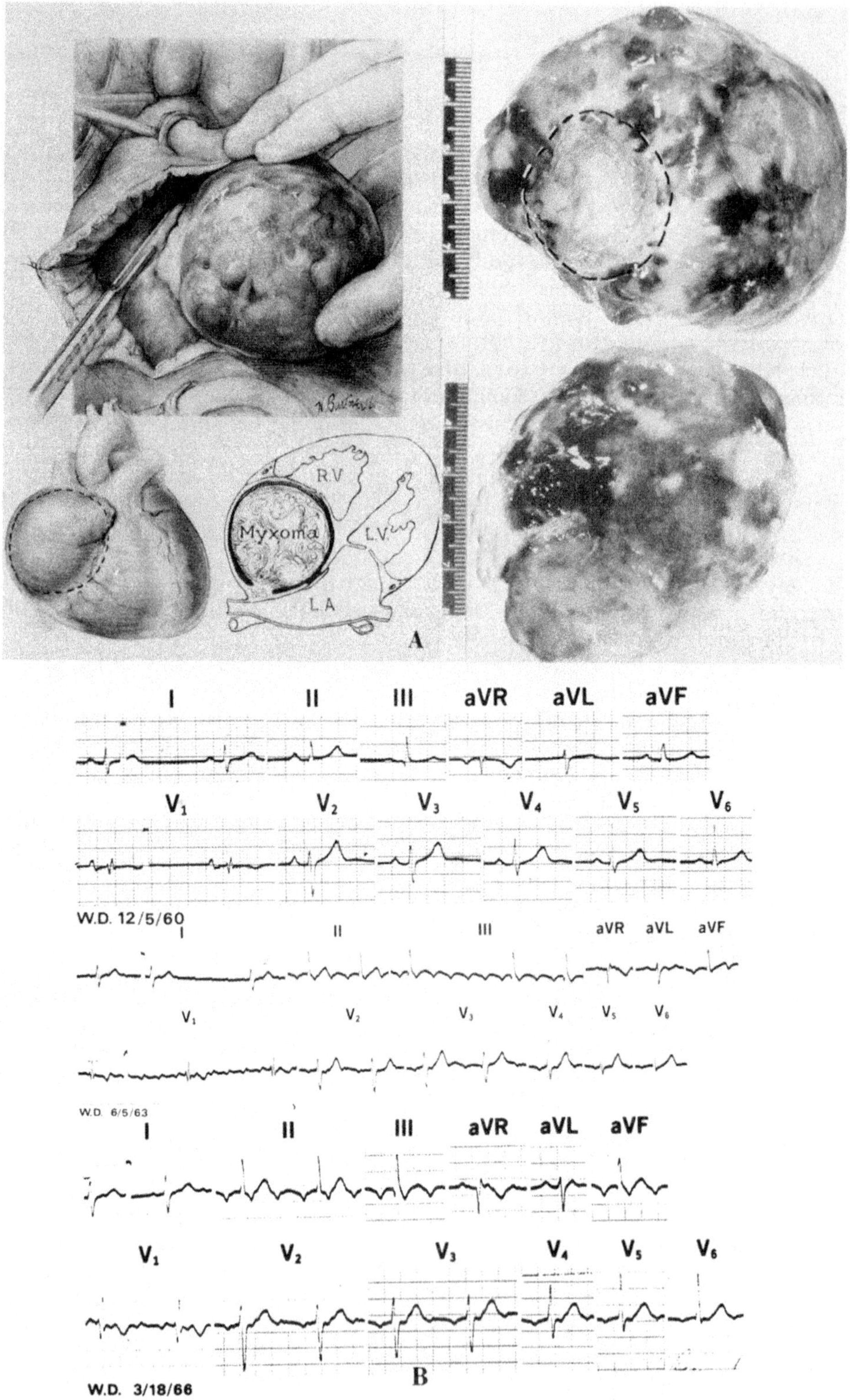

Figure 1. Right atrial myxoma.(A) A 46-year-old man (S61-980) who had congestive cardiac failure, dizzy spells, and chest pain for 12 years before excision of a 142 gm. right atrial myxoma (left) on May 17, 1961. The stump of the tumor is surrounded by the dashed circle in the upper right photograph. The lower right is a cut section of the tumor. A 5 mm. Hg mean diastolic gradient was recorded preoperatively between right atrium and right ventricle. The preoperative electrocardiogram (B) dated December 5, 1960, shows incomplete right bundle branch block and an abnormal P wave consistent with right atrial enlargement. The postoperative electrocardiograms show development of atrial tachycardia with a considerable degree of atrioventricular block. Neither an atrial arrhythmia nor a conduction defect had been present preoperatively.

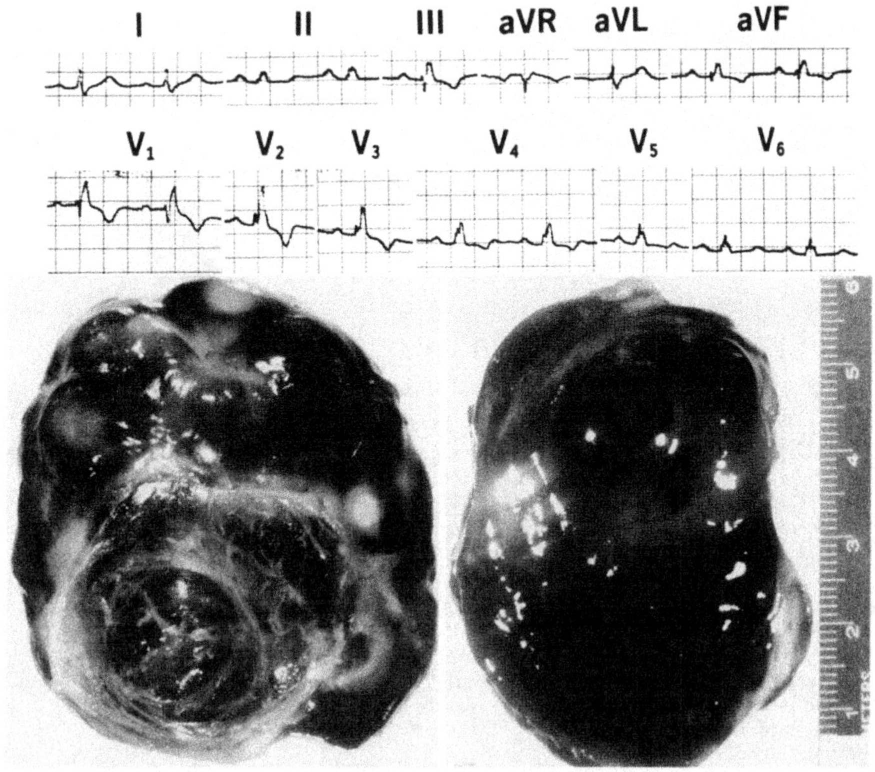

Figure 2. Right atrial myxoma. This 51-year-old woman (S71-560) had congestive cardiac failure, dizziness, and chest pain for 19 months before excision of a 60 gm. right atrial myxoma. Preoperatively, the right atrial mean pressure was 14, A wave 24, and V wave 12 mm. Hg. The electrocardiogram recorded immediately preoperatively shows right bundle branch block. The lower photographs show external surfaces of the myxoma. Attachment stump is on the left.

are not true neoplasms, rhabdomyomas are the most common "tumors" in infants and the ones most frequently associated with abnormal cardiac rhythms. The tumors are usually located in the left ventricular free wall or in the ventricular septum. Paroxysmal supraventricular tachycardia and ventricular tachycardia are the most common cardiac manifestations. Intraventricular conduction disturbances are frequent and complete atrioventricular block can occur.[25]

Fibroma

Among the rare benign primary tumors of the heart, only fibromas have been the subject of a substantial review.[26] Histologically benign and most likely congenital, these tumors may be associated with sudden death in childhood. The clinical features suggest subaortic stenosis, endocardial fibroelastosis, or anomalous origin of a coronary artery. Eight of 28 cases of intramural fibroma reviewed by Hoen and Ellis had ECGs.[26] Ectopic rhythms were found in two, right bundle branch block in one, other forms of intraventricular conduction delay in two, left ventricular hypertrophy in two, and nonspecific ST-T changes in three instances. In one case, a pattern of old myocardial infarction was present.

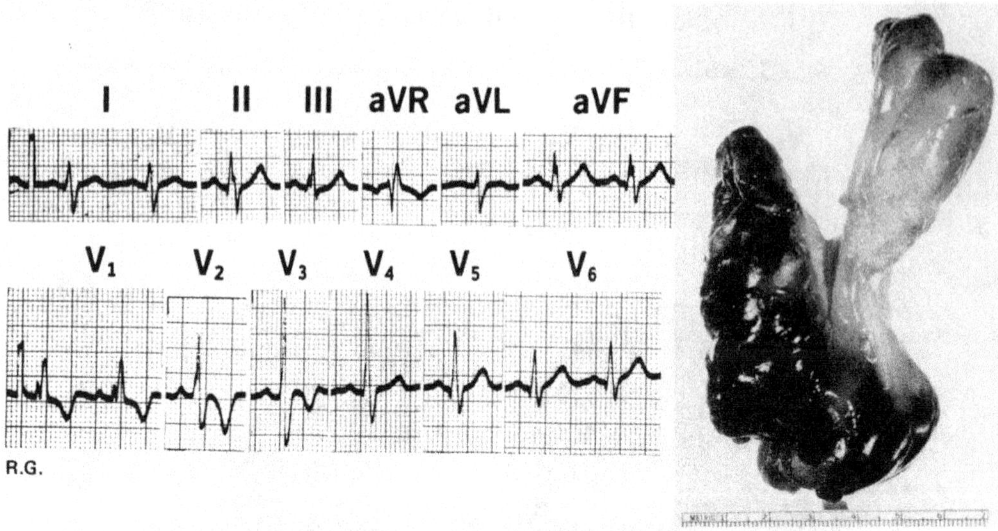

Figure 3. Right ventricular myxoma. A 21-year-old man (S64-478) had three syncopal episodes with exertion during ten months preceding the excision of the 82 gm. right ventricular myxoma illustrated here. A precordial murmur was detected for the first time after his initial episode of syncope. When examined shortly before cardiac operation, a grade 4/6 holosystolic murmur was loudest along the left sternal border. Catheterization showed the right ventricular pressure to be 63/5 mm. Hg and the pulmonary arterial pressure to be 15/7 mm. Hg, yielding a 48 mm. Hg peak systolic pressure gradient. Angiography disclosed a large filling defect in the right ventricle. The electrocardiogram exhibits right bundle branch block. During each ventricular systole, the tumor extended out the outflow tract to contact the bifurcation of the pulmonary trunk. Note the resulting Y-shaped deformity of the tumor.

Sarcoma

Sarcomas, the only primary malignant neoplasms of the heart, account for more than 20 percent of all primary cardiac tumors. Most are angiosarcomas; the remainder are fibrosarcomas, lymphosarcomas, or rhabdomyosarcomas. These tumors usually originate within the right side of the heart and often obstruct inflow into the right atrium or

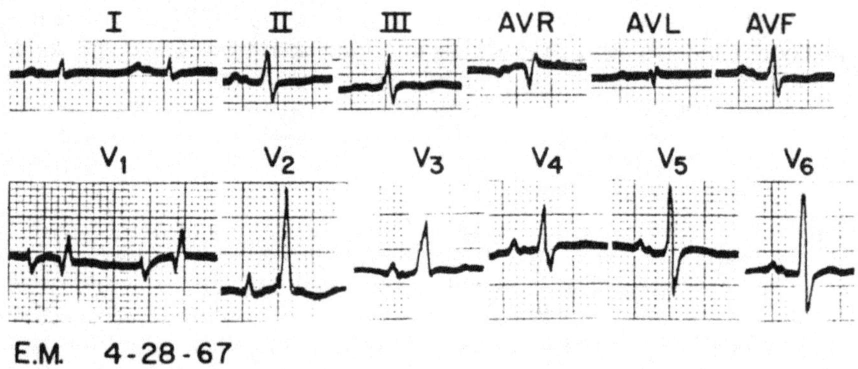

Figure 4. Left atrial myxoma. A 71-year-old woman (67A-297) had progressive congestive cardiac failure for seven months prior to the excision of a 70 gm. myxoma. Preoperatively, the pulmonary arterial pressure was 68/30 mm. Hg. The electrocardiogram, recorded two days preoperatively, shows evidence of biatrial enlargement and right ventricular hypertrophy.

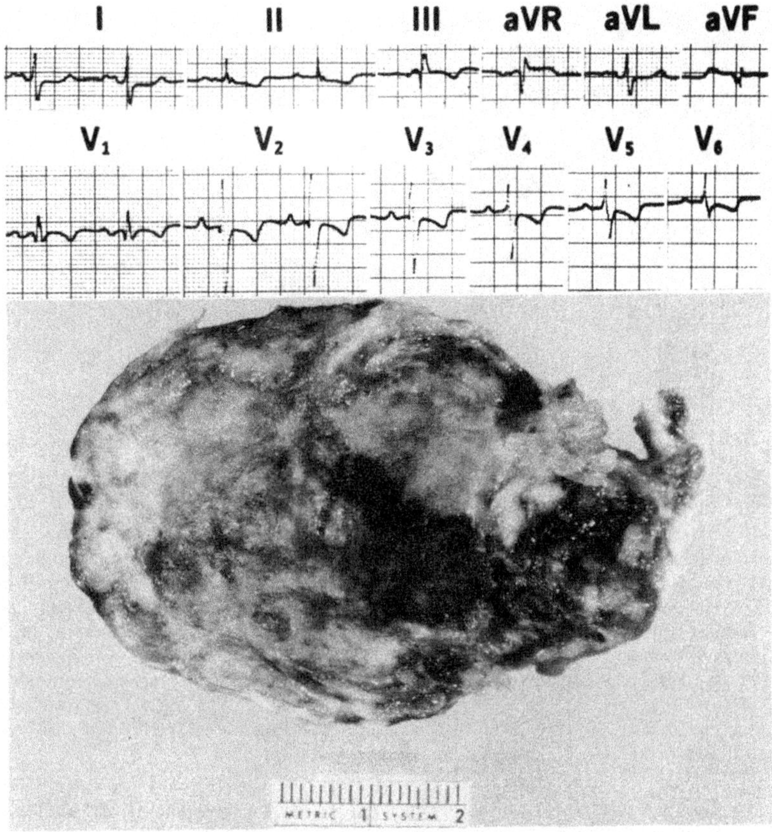

Figure 5. Left atrial myxoma. A 60-year-old woman (S74-1556) had the onset of exertional dyspnea and cardiomegaly at age 37. At age 45, a 24 hour period of severe chest pain associated with sweating occurred and two weeks later an electrocardiogram was "compatible with myocardial infarction." From age 55 to 60, congestive cardiac failure progressively worsened. At age 60, the above electrocardiogram was recorded demonstrating left atrial enlargement and right ventricular hypertrophy. At catheterization, the pressures (in mm. Hg) were: pulmonary artery 80/30; right ventricle 80/16; mean pulmonary arterial wedge 27 with a V of 38; left ventricle 120/8; and aorta 120/80. A filling defect was observed within the left atrium and at operation a 65 gm. myxoma was excised from that chamber. Coronary angiography revealed severe (>75 percent) luminal narrowing of the left anterior descending, left circumflex, and right coronary arteries and, at operation, aortocoronary bypass grafts were placed to the right and left anterior descending coronary arteries.

ventricle. They also frequently involve pericardium producing pericardial effusion, which is often hemorrhagic.

Glancy and associates[27] reviewed certain clinical and morphologic features in 41 patients with angiosarcoma of the heart. Of the 24 patients in whom ECG findings were described, 23 were abnormal: ST-T wave changes, usually non-specific but typical of pericarditis, in 15; low QRS voltage in 13; right axis deviation in 5; supraventricular arrhythmias in 4; right bundle branch block in 2; changes consistent with an old myocardial infarction in 2; and changes suggesting recent myocardial infarction in 2.

Rhabdomyosarcoma[28] and fibrosarcoma[29] have been reported to obstruct right ventricular outflow. ECG findings of right ventricular overload or right bundle branch block were noted.

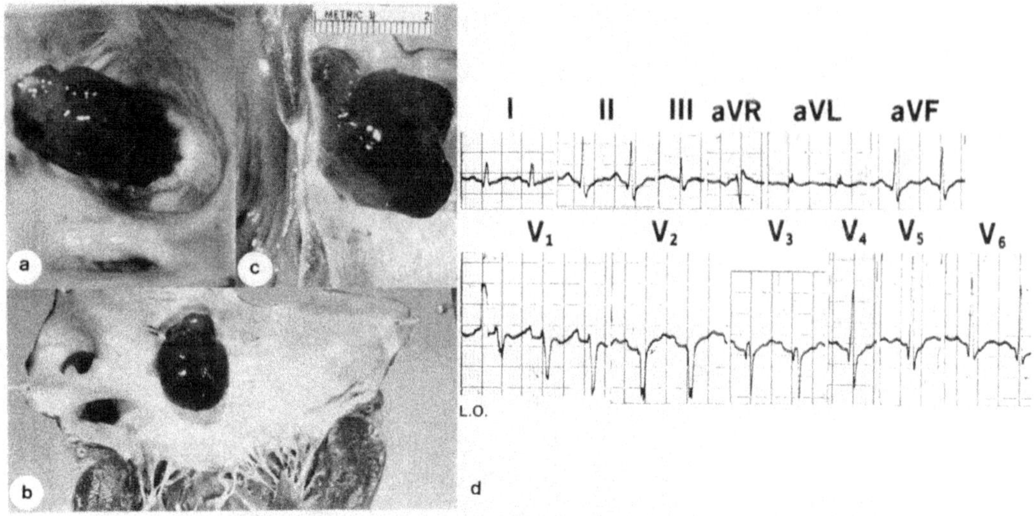

Figure 6. Left atrial myxoma. This tumor, an incidental necropsy finding in a 60-year-old man, (A69-275) never caused evidence of cardiac dysfunction during life because it was not large enough to obstruct the mitral orifice. (a) Myoxoma from above. (b) Opened left atrium and mitral valve. (c) Longitudinal section of the myxoma. (d) Electrocardiogram recorded in last month of life. The heart weighed 450 gm. and the left ventricle was hypertrophied but not dilated. The patient had had mild systemic hypertension. There were no myocardial foci of fibrosis or necrosis. The electrocardiographic finding of anterior myocardial infarction is thus unexplained. The diagnosis of coronary embolization with infarction could have been erroneously inferred during life.

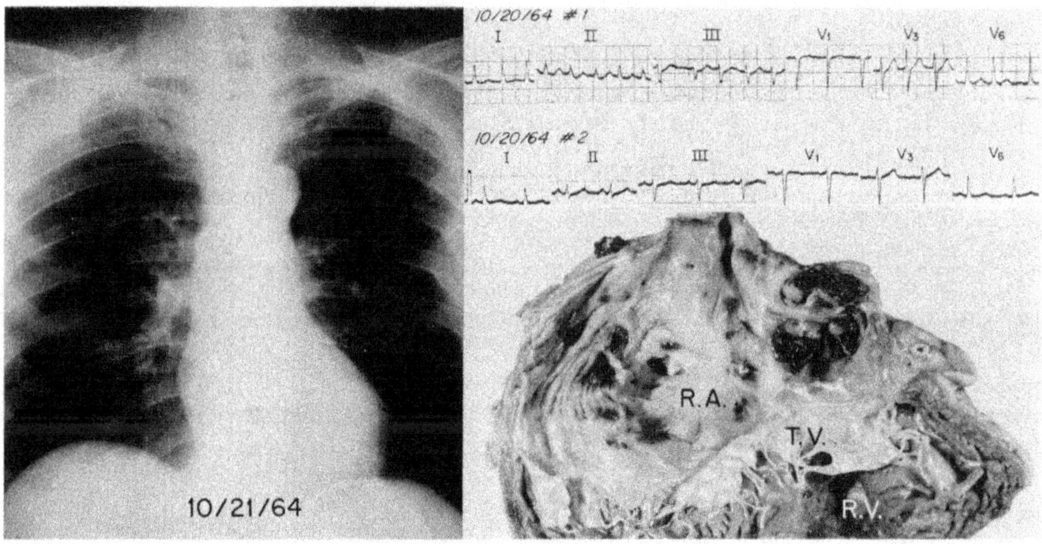

Figure 7. Metastatic melanoma. Chest roentgenogram, electrocardiograms, and heart in a 58-year-old man (A64-213) who died on December 8, 1964, of widespread melanoma 20 months after excision of a melanoma in the chest. He developed atrial fibrillation seven weeks before death (ECG #1), but reverted to sinus rhythm the same day after being given digitalis (ECG #2). He had no further evidence of cardiac dysfunction. At necropsy, the heart weighed 400 gm., and all cardiac chambers were invaded by tumor. Shown in the lower right is the opened right atrium (RA), tricuspid valve (TV), and right ventricle (RV). There are numerous black tumor nodules ("tumor thrombi") projecting from the right atrial endocardium.

Secondary Cardiac Neoplasms

Although almost every primary tumor has been reported to invade the heart, carcinoma of the lung and breast account for the largest number of patients with secondary tumor of the heart.[2,4] Each of these tumors is common and each is close to the heart. Although uncommon in terms of total number of secondary tumors to the heart, melanoma (Figs. 7 and 8) metastasizes to the heart in a higher percentage, namely 70 percent, than any other tumor.[10] Leukemia (Fig. 9) and lymphoma (Fig. 10) also involve the heart with great frequency. Leukemic infiltrates have been found at necropsy in nearly

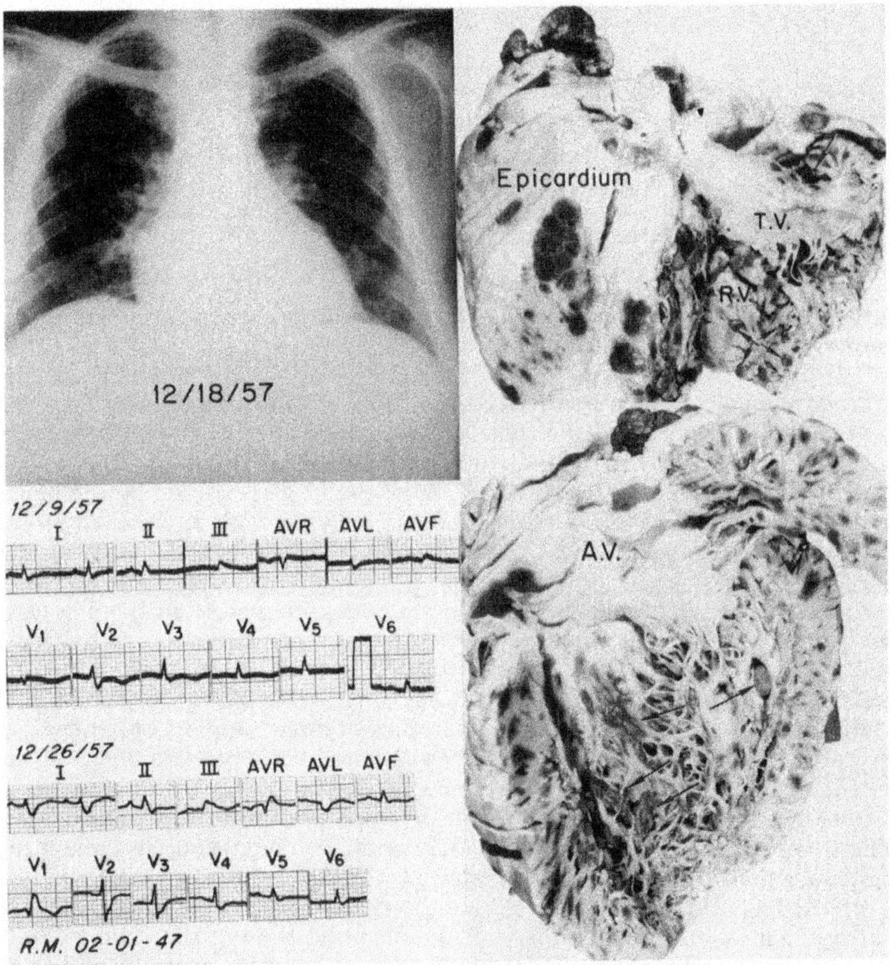

Figure 8. Metastatic melanoma. Chest roentgenogram, electrocardiograms, the opened right atrium, tricuspid valve (TV), and right ventricle (RV) *(upper right)* in a 33-year-old man (A57-260), who died of metastatic melanoma on December 27, 1957, three years after removal of a melanoma from the scalp. During the last month of life, a ventricular gallop, pulsus alternans, and orthostatic hypotension developed. Diabetes insipidus, the result of pituitary metastasis, and Addison's disease, the result of adrenal metastasis, prevented the congestive phenomena of cardiac failure. The cardiac silhouette was enlarged by chest roentgenogram on December 18, 1957. Electrocardiograms showed sinus tachycardia, low QRS voltage, and inverted T waves in leads V1-4 and, during the last week of life, right bundle branch block (December 26, 1957). At necropsy, a pericardial effusion (350 ml.) was present. The heart weighed 320 gm. Extensive melanoma metastases were present in the epicardium, myocardium, and endocardium of all four cardiac chambers, and numerous small tumor thrombi (arrows) projected from the right atrial, right ventricular, and left ventricular endocardium.

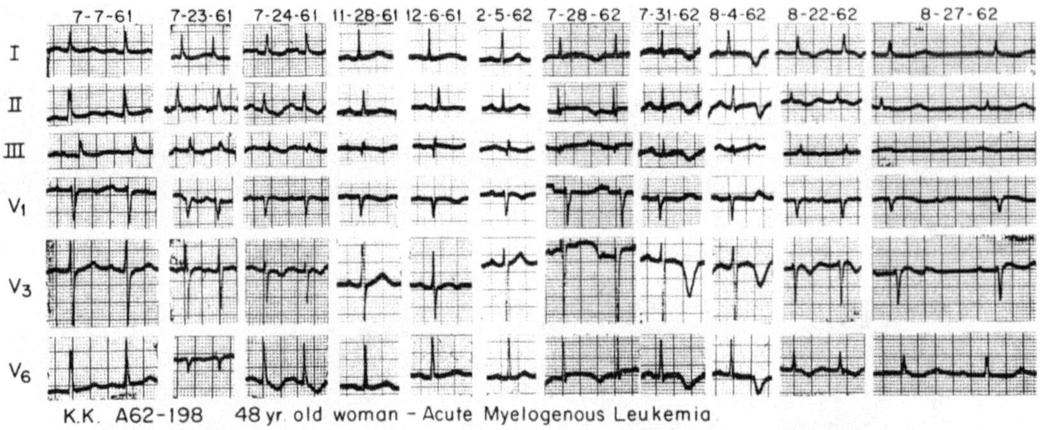

Figure 9. Acute myelogenous leukemia. Several electrocardiograms depicted changes in the heart rate, T waves and QT intervals in a 48-year-old woman with acute myelogenous leukemia. These alterations were attributed to anterior wall ischemia since correction of the serum potassium, calcium, and magnesium abnormalities failed to reverse these changes. No abnormalities were observed on anatomic study of the heart.

40 percent of patients, and cardiac hemorrhages, particularly in acute leukemia, are equally as frequent.[6] Lymphoma involves the heart in about 25 percent of patients.[6, 11, 30, 31]

The true frequency with which ECG aberrations result from metastatic cardiac neoplasm is unknown. This is true because no systematic attempt to obtain serial records has been made, and many patients do not have ECGs recorded in close proximity to their death. Therefore, retrospective analysis of the ECG recorded before death in patients found at necropsy to have cardiac metastases cannot be interpreted as providing such information. Changes appear to be equally frequent in patients dying of cancer who have no cardiac metastases.[5, 9-11] Table 2, modified from that published by Roberts and associates,[11] highlights this problem in patients with malignant lymphoma. Nevertheless, certain relatively infrequent abnormalities seem clearly related to cardiac neoplasm.

Atrial arrhythmias may result from cardiac metastases (Fig. 7). Atrial flutter and atrial fibrillation are reported in nearly all studies of large numbers of patients with secondary cardiac tumors. James and Carrera suggested three possible mechanisms: "Involvement of atrial sympathetic nerve fibers by the tumor; invasion of an atrial coronary artery by the tumor with production of atrial infarction; and presence of tumor invading noninfarcted areas of atrial myocardium."[32] They report a patient in whom these phenomena were demonstrated histologically. Subsequently, James and his associates reported a patient with chronic granulocytic leukemia with intractable multifocal atrial arrhythmias caused by extensive leukemic infiltration of the sinus node.[33] Thus, failure of sinus node function consequent to tumor invasion may constitute a fourth pathogenetic mechanism. The sick sinus syndrome, including marked sinus bradycardia and atrial arrhythmias, has been observed in a patient with reticulum cell sarcoma involving the heart.[34] Extensive tumor infiltration of the sinoatrial node and conduction system seemed to account for these findings as well as for the right bundle branch block and incomplete AV block which also were present.

Metastatic cancer may produce ECG findings of myocardial infarction. Q waves may result from electrical "dead zones" produced by tumor invasion of the myocardium.[35] Altered QRS forces may be accompanied by ST-T abnormalities quite characteristic of ischemia (Figs. 8 through 11). These latter abnormalities may occur alone and are prob-

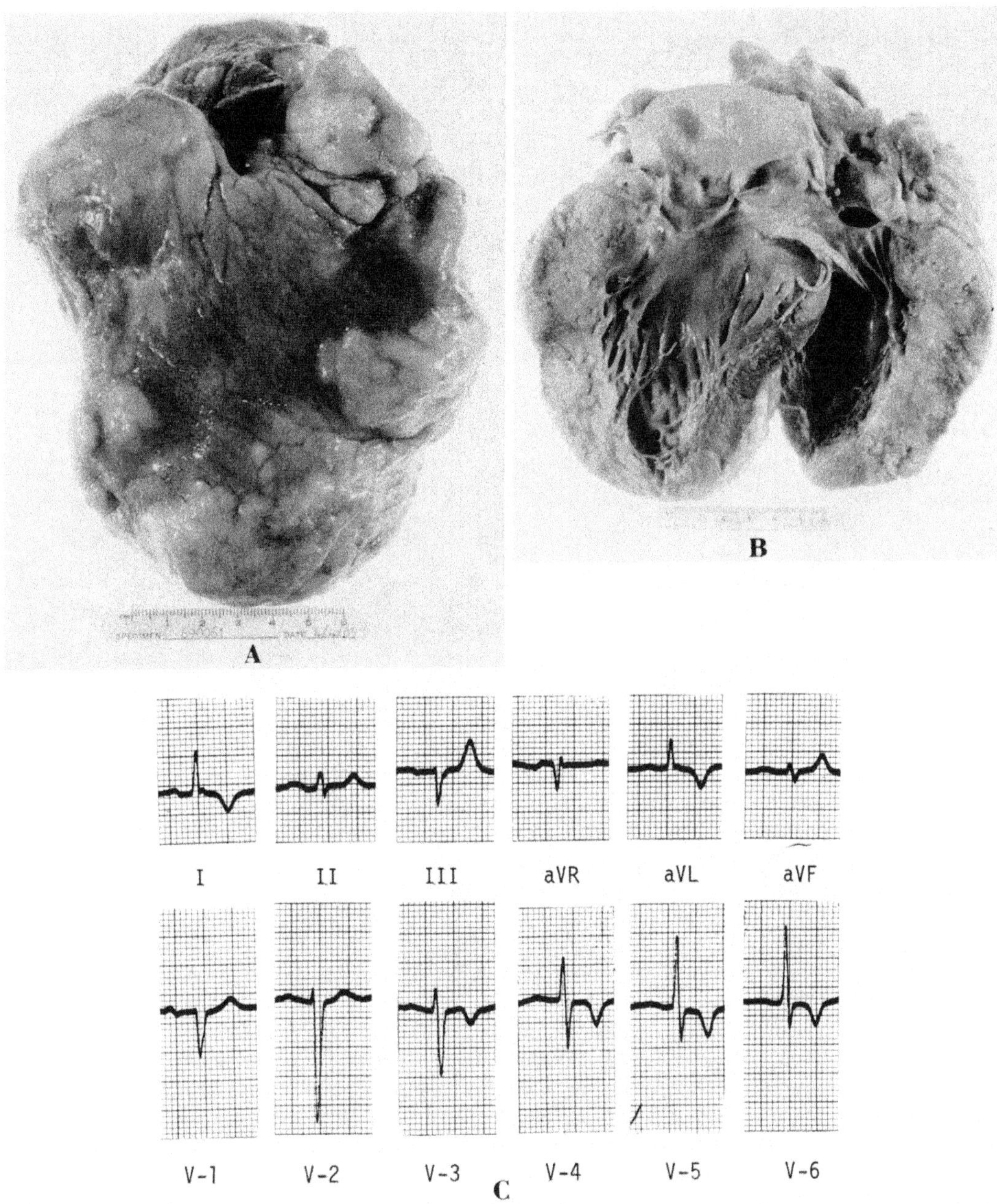

Figure 10. Lymphosarcoma. Lymphosarcoma involving the myocardium in a 35-year-old man. Tumor masses may be seen on the external view (A) and involve the full thickness of the left ventricle (B). "Ischemic" T waves are present on the electrocardiogram (C) recorded one month prior to death.

ably more common.[36] One interesting report attributes a fatal inferior myocardial infarction with typical ECG findings to occlusion by a tumor nodule of the circumflex branch of the left coronary artery.[29] In yet another patient, the classic triad of atrial infarction (abnormal P waves, atrial arrhythmias, and deviation of the P-Ta segment) has been reported to result from metastatic bronchogenic carcinoma.[37]

Table 2. Electrocardiographic abnormalities in lymphoma

	Patients with cardiac lymphoma (no.)	*Patients without cardiac lymphoma (no.)*	*Totals*
Electrocardiograms	33	104	137
Abnormal tracing	20 (61%)	64 (62%)	84
Normal tracing*	13	40	53
Low voltage (Sum of QRS in I, II, III < 1.5 mv.)	10	23	33
Ectopic tachycardia			
Atrial fibrillation	1	1	2
Atrial flutter	1	0	1
Atrial tachycardia	2	1	3
Atrioventricular block			
Prolonged PR interval (>0.20 sec.)	1	3	4
Second degree	2	0	2
Complete AV dissociation	1	1†	2
Premature contractions			
Nodal	0	2	2
Atrial	1	6	7
Ventricular	7	7	14
Left axis deviation	2	7	9
Right axis deviation	0	3	3
Right bundle branch block	1	0	1
ST-T wave changes			
Nonspecific	8	17	25
Ischemic	2	7	9
Digitalis effect	1	7	8
Potassium disturbance	0	8	8
Pericarditis type	2	1	3
P wave abnormality	1	5	6

*Normal except for sinus tachycardia.

†Lasted only one day on each of two occasions. Last tracing was entirely normal.

Atrioventricular block may result from tumor invasion of the heart.[38-40] Histologically, neoplastic involvement of the AV nodal region has been documented.[38] His bundle electrograms in the case of Conde and associates revealed block at the AV nodal level.[40] Redwine was able to collect sixteen instances of complete heart block from the literature and add one of his own.[39] Seven were attributable to carcinoma of the lung and several others to leukemic infiltrates. Incomplete atrioventricular block seems somewhat more common and is reported in several large collections of secondary cardiac neoplasms.[1, 11] A small benign primary tumor of the atrial septum, a mesothelioma or coelothelioma, may produce complete heart block by invading the AV node.[41] It is rare and we are not aware of any reports of antemortem diagnosis.

Pericardial involvement by neoplasm may be manifest electrocardiographically; the abnormalities of the ST segment and T wave, however, may not be sufficiently diagnostic to allow distinction from more nonspecific causes. In tamponade, electrical alternans, i.e., alternation in the amplitude of all components of the ECG complex, may occur.

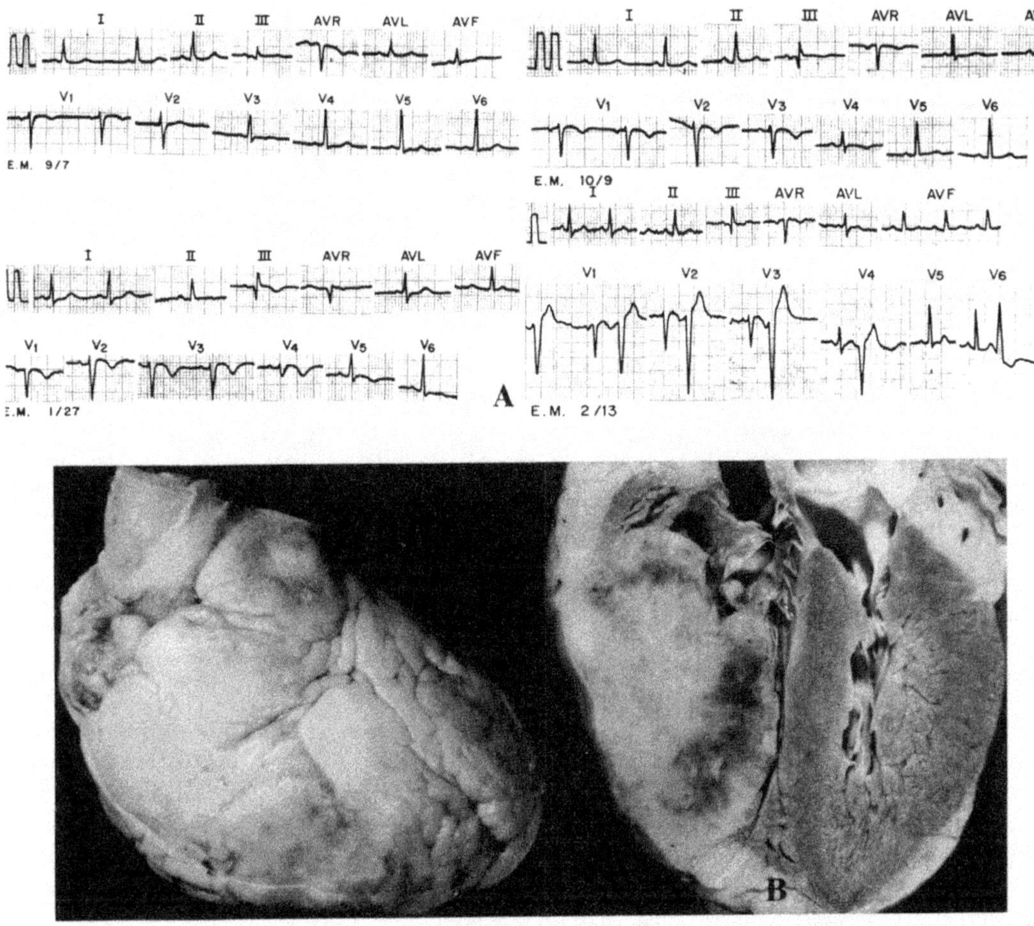

Figure 11. Metastatic adenocarcinoma. Electrocardiograms (A) and necropsy specimen (B) from a 70-year-old woman (73A-145) with widespread metastases from adenocarcinoma of the colon. At necropsy, the right ventricle was filled with neoplasm which extended through the full thickness of right ventricular wall. No symptoms of cardiac dysfunction occurred during life. The electrocardiograms were recorded two to eight months before her death on April 21, 1973. Abnormal T waves suggesting anterior ischemia appear as do premature ventricular beats. Exterior view of the heart and longitudinal section of the ventricles demonstrate the tumor mass occupying most of the right ventricle.

Extracardiac Neoplasms with Humoral Cardiac Effects

Pheochromocytoma

Systemic hypertension consequent to the excessive catecholamine production by a pheochromocytoma results in left ventricular overload and produces thereby ECG evidence of left ventricular hypertrophy. Secondary repolarization abnormalities and evidence of left atrial overload often attend the ventricular hypertrophy.

Rare patients with pheochromocytoma have been described whose presentation resembles that of individuals with cardiomyopathy.[42-46] Hypertension is not a prominent feature of their illness. Ectopic arrhythmias and electrocardiographic evidence of ischemia have been observed in such patients.[42, 45] It is thought that in these patients, epinephrine production is predominant and that myocardial necrosis consequent to that

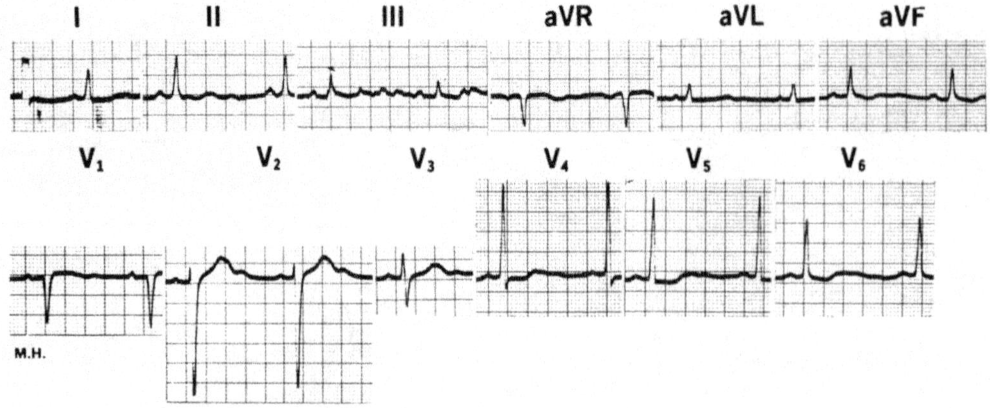

Figure 12. Aldosterone secreting adrenal tumor. Electrocardiogram in a 47-year-old woman (S61-1522) with systemic hypertension (240-170/140-110 mm. Hg) secondary to primary hyperaldosteronism. The urinary aldosterone levels were elevated and the serum potassium was 2.6 mEq./L. The electrocardiogram shows prominent U waves and prolonged QU interval typical of hypokalemia. At laparotomy, a large adenoma was found in the right adrenal gland.

hormone is responsible. Administration of excessive exogenous catecholamines to patients or to experimental animals has been shown to result in such necrosis.

Adrenocortical Adenoma

Aldosterone secreting adenomas of the adrenal cortex produce hypertension and thus left ventricular hypertrophy. They are also noteworthy since hypokalemia, a hallmark of these neoplasms, may distort the electrocardiogram (Fig. 12).

Carcinoid Heart Disease

About 50 percent of patients with metastatic carcinoid tumors, primary in the small bowel or, rarely, elsewhere, exhibit a pathognomonic cardiac lesion.[46] Focal or diffuse collections of a peculiar variety of fibrous tissue are observed on the endocardium of valvular cusps, of the cardiac chambers, of the great veins, and occasionally of the great arteries. The deposition is most common and most extensive in the right heart chambers and valves in the majority of instances. Functionally, pulmonic stenosis and tricuspid regurgitation are produced most frequently.[46] These fibrous deposits are believed to be due to a humoral secretion by the tumor. Serotonin was originally suspected, but a bradykinin is now considered a more likely possibliity.[47] (Figs. 13 and 14.)

The electrocardiographic features of this rare disorder have not been uniform. Among the nine patients reported by Roberts and Sjoerdsma, low voltage of the QRS was most common.[46] Right axis deviation and right bundle branch block were each present in one patient. Abnormalities of repolarization were also encountered. Right ventricular hypertrophy was notable for its absence, although the ST-T abnormalities in one instance were diagnosed as right ventricular strain.

Electrocardiographic Abnormalities Due to Cancer Chemotherapy

Cardiac toxicity is a major side effect of certain recently introduced antineoplastic drugs. Adriamycin, an agent producing demonstrable therapeutic benefit in both hematologic and solid tissue neoplasms, has attracted the greatest attention,[12, 13] but other related agents have been indicted as well.[48]

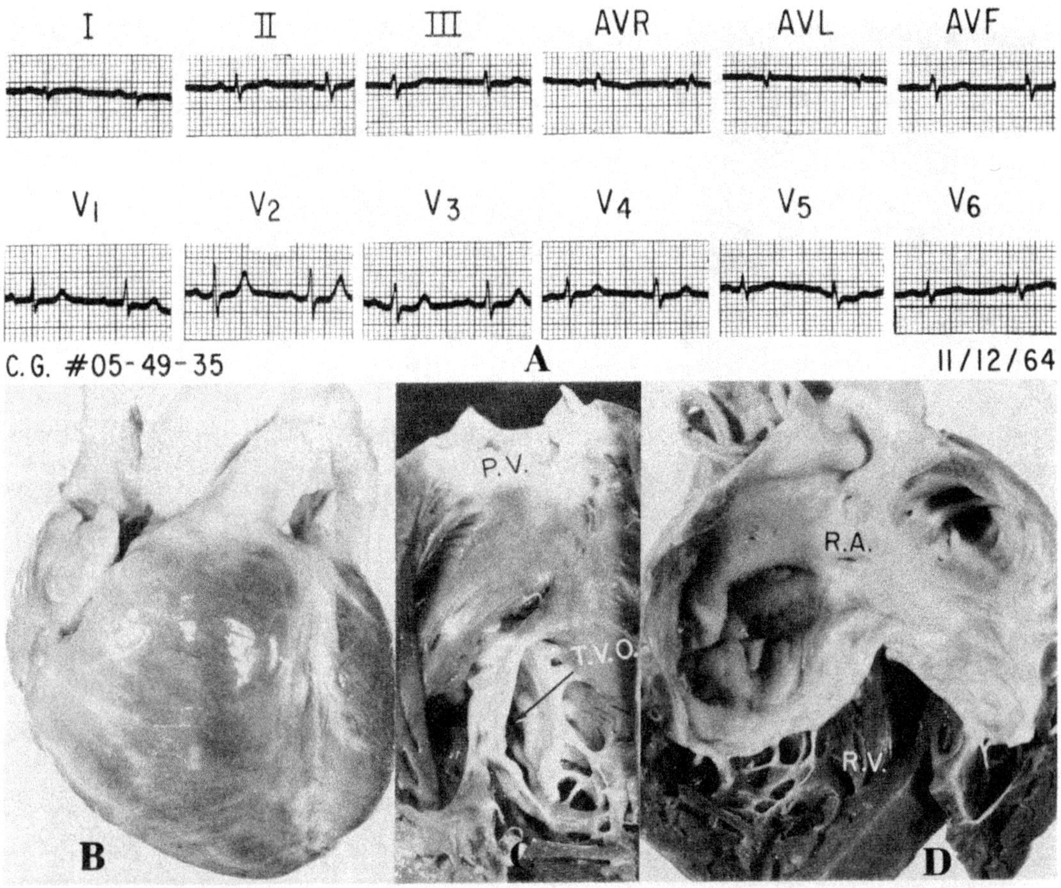

Figure 13. Metastatic carcinoid. (A) Electrocardiogram and heart in a 32-year-old woman (A64-211) with clinical evidence of the carcinoid syndrome for 9 years. She developed clinical evidence of pulmonic stenosis and tricuspid regurgitation. At cardiac catheterization performed eight months before death, the pressures (in mm. Hg) were: Pulmonary artery 20/8; right ventricle 45/13; and right atrium, A wave 18, V wave 23, mean 15. The cardiac index was 3.2 L./min./m.^{2} The electrocardiogram shows low voltage, which is the most common electrocardiographic abnormality observed in patients with carcinoid heart disease. (B) Intact heart showing considerable dilatation of the right ventricle and atrophy of the subepicardial adipose tissue. (C) Opened right ventricle showing thickened tricuspid and pulmonic valves (PV). (TVO) = tricuspid valve orifice. (D) Opened right atrium (RA), tricuspid valve, and right ventricle (RV) showing diffuse thickening of the endocardium of the right atrium (carcinoid plaquing).

Among 399 patients treated with adriamycin by one group, eleven patients developed sudden severe congestive failure apparently attributable to the myocardial toxicity of the agent.[12] Eight died of their heart failure within three weeks. The effect seems to be dose related, since ten of these eleven and all of the fatal cases were among the 33 patients who received more than 550 mg. of adriamycin per square meter of body surface area. Thus, of patients receiving more than this amount almost one third developed congestive heart failure and one fourth died because of decompensation.

The ECG features of adriamycin toxicity are not specific. Progressive diminution in the QRS amplitude was common in the cardiotoxic patients but was also observed in others.[12] Moreover, transient ECG abnormalities are often associated with the administration of the drug regardless of the total dose.[12, 13] Sinus tachycardia, supraventricular tachyarrhythmias, premature ventricular contractions, and repolarization abnormalities have been noted.

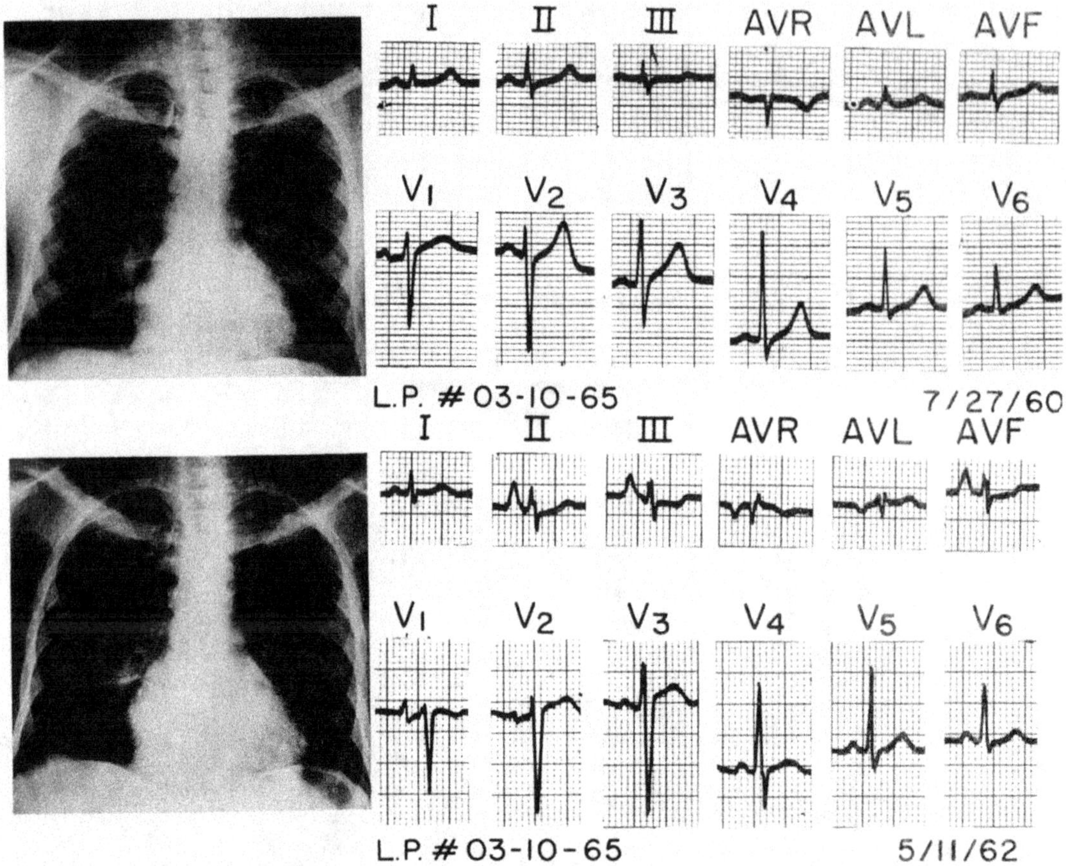

Figure 14. Metastatic carcinoid. Chest roentgenograms and electrocardiograms in a 40-year-old man (A63-96) who died in April 1963, of widespread carcinoid metastases and typical features of the carcinoid syndrome. A pansystolic blowing murmur typical of tricuspid regurgitation developed between the upper and lower roentgenograms and electrocardiograms shown here, as did peaked P waves characteristic of right atrial enlargment. At necropsy, there was typical carcinoid fibrosis involving the tricuspid, pulmonic, and mitral valves, and endocardium of right atrium.

ELECTROCARDIOGRAPHIC ABNORMALITIES IN ANEMIA

No ECG abnormalities characteristic of anemia are known.[49] Moreover, the frequency with which abnormalities are found in anemic patients has varied from 19[50] to 80 percent.[51] The lower prevalence is probably more applicable in the western world. Nineteen of 100 patients with a hemoglobin less than 8 gm. per 100 ml. had abnormalties, but eight had additional processes which may have accounted for the changes. The records of the eleven in whom anemia seemed the sole significant process exhibited ST-T abnormalties, often quite minor in character.[50]

It is noteworthy that more severe and chronic anemia is associated more frequently with ECG abnormalities. Of 100 patients seen in India with chronic anemia and an average hemoglobin of 3.6 gm. per 100 ml., 72 had abnormal repolarization, often quite striking.[51] Left ventricular hypertrophy was diagnosed in 15. Arrhythmia was uncommon even in such severely ill patients. Six had premature atrial and five had premature ventricular beats. One instance of atrial tachycardia was detected.

Sickle cell disease is a distinct problem. In addition to the chronic volume overload imposed by lifelong severe anemia, increased pulmonary vascular resistance attribut-

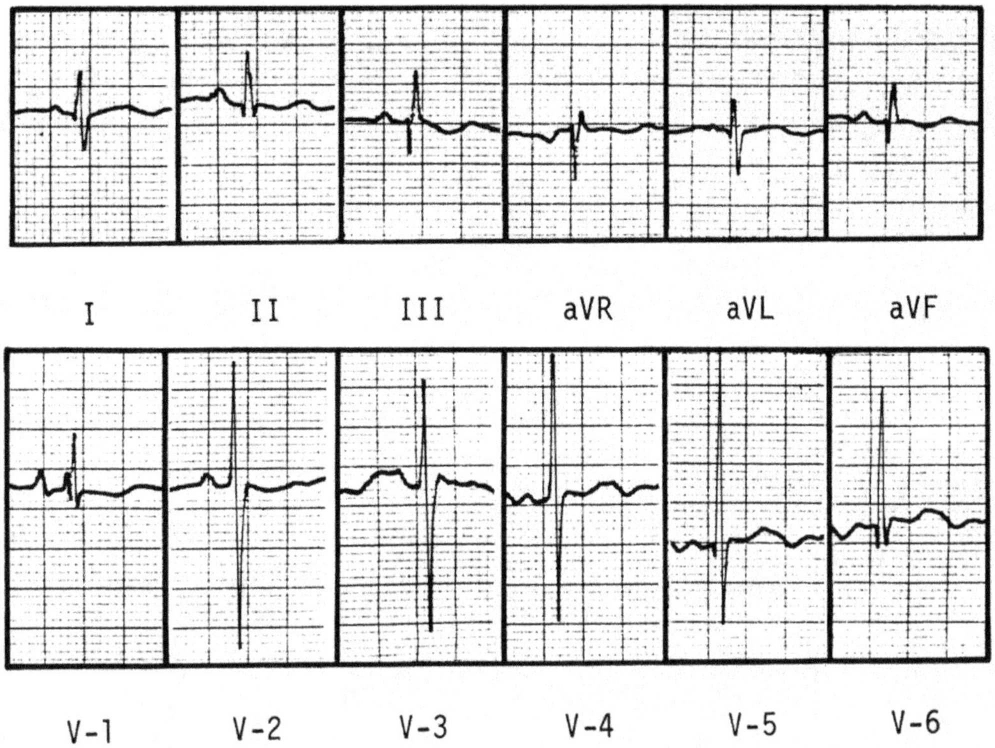

Figure 15. Sickle cell anemia. Electrocardiogram from a 38-year-old man with sickle cell anemia and pulmonary hypertension. Pulmonary artery pressure was 48/14 mm. Hg at catheterization. His right ventricle was 0.9 cm. thick at necropsy. There is evidence of right atrial and right and left ventricular enlargment.

able to thrombo-occlusive disease adds an additional load for the right ventricle in some patients (Fig. 15). Myocardial ischemia due to occlusive disease in the coronary circulation has been postulated but never clearly established since histologic evidence of ischemic necrosis has been difficult to document in these patients.[52]

For these reasons, electrocardiographic abnormalities are common. Evidence of left ventricular hypertrophy is seen in half such patients and combined ventricular hypertrophy in 10 to 15 percent. Isolated right ventricular hypertrophy is infrequent, as is evidence of atrial enlargement.[53, 54] Arrhythmias are rarely reported. Uzsoy found one instance of atrial fibrillation in 148 patients.[53] First degree AV block is observed in approximately 10 percent.

ECG evidence for myocardial ischemia is not convincing. T wave abnormalities and ST depression are common but tend not to be characteristic of ischemia. Uzsoy found electrocardiographic evidence of myocardial infarction in two patients. One had an infarction at autopsy. His report does not make it clear that sickle cell disease was in fact responsible.[53]

REFERENCES

1. Bisel, H. F., Wroblewski, F., and LaDue, J. S.: *Incidence and clinical manifestations of cardiac metastases.* JAMA 153:712, 1953.
2. Gassman, H. S., Meadows, R., Jr., and Baker, L. A.: *Metastatic tumors of the heart.* Am. J. Med. 19: 357, 1955.
3. Hanfling, S. M.: *Metastatic cancer to the heart.* Circulation 22:474, 1960.

4. KLINE, I. W.: *Cardiac lymphatic involvement by metastatic tumor.* Cancer 29:799, 1972.
5. GRIFFITHS, G. C.: *A review of primary tumors of the heart.* Prog. Cardiovasc. Dis. 7:465, 1965.
6. ROBERTS, W. C., BODEY, G. P., AND WERTLAKE, P. T.: *The heart in acute leukemia.* Am. J. Cardiol. 21: 388, 1968.
7. FREIMAN, A. H.: *Cardiovascular disturbances associated with cancer.* Med. Clin. North Am. 50:733, 1966.
8. HARVEY, W. P.: *Clinical aspects of cardiac tumors.* Am. J. Cardiol. 21:328, 1968.
9. BERGE, T., AND SIEVERS, J.: *Myocardial metastases—a pathological and electrocardiographic study.* Br. Heart J. 30:383, 1968.
10. GLANCY, D. L., AND ROBERTS, W. C.: *The heart in malignant melanoma.* Am. J. Cardiol. 21:555, 1968.
11. ROBERTS, W. C., GLANCY, D. L., AND DEVITA V. T.: *The heart in malignant lymphoma (Hodgkin's disease, lymphosarcoma, reticulum cell sarcoma, and mycosis fungoides)—a study of 196 autopsy cases.* Am. J. Cardiol. 22:85, 1968.
12. LEFRAK, E. A., PITHA, J., ROSENHEIM, S., ET AL.: *A clinicopathologic analysis of adriamycin cardiotoxicity.* Cancer 32:302, 1973.
13. BLUM, R. H., AND CARTER, S. K.: *Adriamycin—a new anticancer drug with significant clinical activity.* Ann. Intern. Med. 80:249, 1974.
14. GOODWIN, J. F.: *Diagnosis of left atrial myxoma.* Lancet 1:464, 1963.
15. GREENWOOD, W. F.: *Profile of atrial myxoma.* Am. J. Cardiol. 21:367, 1968.
16. SNYDER, S. N., SMITH, D. C., LOU, F. Y. K., ET AL.: *Diagnostic features of right ventricular myxoma.* Am. Heart J. 91:240, 1976.
17. ALDREDGE, H. E., AND GREENWOOD, W. F.: *Myxoma of the left atrium.* Br. Heart J. 22:189, 1960.
18. GOODWIN, J. F., STANFIELD, C. A., STEINER, R. E., ET AL.: *Clinical features of left atrial myxoma.* Thorax 17:91, 1962.
19. NASSER, W. K., DAVIS, R. H., DILLON, J. L., ET AL.: *Atrial myxoma.* Am. Heart J. 83:694, 1972.
20. HANSEN, J. F., LYNBORG, K., ANDERSEN, M., ET AL.: *Right atrial myxoma.* Acta Med. Scand. 186:165, 1969.
21. CAMPEAU, L., AND DAVID, P.: *Myxoma of the heart.* Canad. Med. Arch. 82:586, 1960.
22. KROOPF, S. S., AND PETERSON, C. A.: *Anaplastic myxoma of left atrium.* Arch. Intern. Med. 100:819, 1957.
23. SANNERSTEDT, R., VARNAUSKAS, E., PAULIN, S., ET AL.: *Right atrial myxoma—report of a case and review of the literature.* Am. Heart J. 64:243, 1962.
24. MORRISSEY, J. F., CAMPETI, F. L., MAHONEY, E. B., ET AL.: *Right atrial myxoma—report of two cases and review of the literature.* Am. Heart J. 66:4, 1963.
25. WENGER, N. K.: *Cardiac glycogenosis,* in Hurst, J. W. (ed.): *The Heart.* McGraw-Hill Book Co., New York, 1974, p. 1356.
26. HOEN, A. G., AND ELLIS, E. J.: *Intramural fibroma of the heart.* Am. J. Cardiol. 17:579, 1966.
27. GLANCY, D. L., MORALES, J. B., AND ROBERTS, W. C.: *Angiosarcoma of the heart.* Am. J. Cardiol. 21: 413, 1968.
28. O'REILLY, M. V., MCDONALD, R. T., AND FORNASIER, V. L.: *Clinical presentation of a myocardial rhabdomyosarcoma.* Br. Heart J. 37:672, 1975.
29. GOLDSTEIN, S., AND MAHONEY, E. B.: *Right ventricular fibrosarcoma causing pulmonary stenosis.* Am. J. Cardiol. 17:570, 1966.
30. JAVIER, B. V., YOUNT, W. J., CROSBY, D. J., ET AL.: *Cardiac metastases in lymphoma and leukemia.* Dis. Chest 52:481, 1967.
31. SUMNERS, J. E., JOHNSON, W. W., AND AINGER, L. E.: *Childhood leukemic heart disease.* Circulation 40:575, 1969.
32. JAMES, T. N., AND CARRERA, G. M.: *Pathogenesis of arrhythmias associated with metastatic tumors of the heart.* N. Engl. J. Med. 260:869, 1959.
33. SURYAPRASAD, A. G., VAN SLYCK, E. J., AND JAMES, T. N.: *The sinus node in chronic granulocytic leukemia.* Chest 61:494, 1972.
34. METZGER, A. L., GOLDBARG, A. N., AND HUNTER, R. L.: *Sick sinus node syndrome as the presenting manifestation of reticulum cell sarcoma.* Chest 60:602, 1971.
35. HARRIS, T. R., COPELAND, G. D., AND BRODY, D. A.: *Progressive injury current with metastatic tumor of the heart.* Am. Heart J. 69:392, 1965.
36. BAGBY, G. C., GOLDMAN, R. D., NEWMAN, H. C., ET AL.: *Acute myocardial infarction due to childhood lymphoma.* N. Engl. J. Med. 287:338, 1972.

37. Rothfield, E. L., and Zirken, R. M.: *Unusual ECG evidence of metastatic cardiac tumor resembling atrial infarction.* Am. J. Cardiol. 10:881, 1962.

38. James, T. N.: *Metastases of hypernephroma to atrioventricular node.* N. Engl. J. Med. 266:705, 1962.

39. Redwine, D. B.: *Complete heart block caused by secondary tumors of the heart.* Texas Med. 70:59, 1974.

40. Conde, C. A., Meller, J., Pantazopoulos, J., et al.: *Reticulum cell sarcoma with intracardiac metastases.* Am. J. Cardiol. 36:357, 1975.

41. Lafargue, R. T., Hand, A. M., and Lev, M.: *Mesothelioma (coelothelioma) of the AV node.* Chest 59:570, 1971.

42. Wiswell, J. G., and Crago, R. M.: *Reversible cardiomyopathy with pheochromocytoma.* Trans. Am. Clin. Climat. Assoc. 80:185, 1968.

43. Garcia, R., and Jennings, J. M.: *Pheochromocytoma masquerading as a cardiomyopathy.* Am. J. Cardiol. 29:568, 1972.

44. Baker, G., Zeller, N. H., Weitzner, S., et al.: *Pheochromocytoma without hypertension presenting as cardiomyopathy.* Am. Heart J. 83:688, 1972.

45. Pelkonen, R., and Pitkanen, E.: *Unusual electrocardiographic changes in pheochromocytoma.* Acta Med. Scand. 173:41, 1963.

46. Roberts, W. C., and Sjoerdsma, A.: *The cardiac disease associated with the carcinoid syndrome.* Am. J. Med. 36:5, 1964.

47. Grahame-Smith, D. G.: *The carcinoid syndrome.* Am. J. Cardiol. 21:376, 1968.

48. Ainger, L. E., Bushore, J., Johnson, W. W., et al.: *Daunomycin—a cardiotoxic agent.* J. Natl. Med. Assoc. 63:261, 1971.

49. Varat, M. A., Adolph, R. J., and Fowler, N. O.: *Cardiovascular effects of anemia.* Am. Heart J. 83: 415, 1972.

50. Gonzalez-de-Cossio, A., Sanchez-Medal, L., and Smyth, J. F.: *Electrocardiographic modifications in anemia.* Am. Heart J. 67:166, 1964.

51. Sanghvi, L. M., Misra, S. N., Bannerji, K., et al.: *ECG in chronic severe anemia.* Am. Heart J. 56; 79, 1958.

52. Baroldi, G.: *High resistance of the human myocardium to shock and red cell aggregation (sludge).* Cardiology 54:271, 1969.

53. Uzsoy, N. K.: *Cardiovascular findings in patients with sickle cell anemia.* Am. J. Cardiol. 13:320, 1964.

54. Ng, M. L., Liebman, J., Anslovar, J., et al.: *Cardiovascular findings in children with sickle cell anemia.* Dis. Chest 52:788, 1967.

CARDIAC CANDIDIASIS IN CANCER PATIENTS

DANIEL C. IHDE, MD,* WILLIAM C. ROBERTS, MD,§ KENDALL C. MARR, MD,† HARMAR D. BRERETON, MD,† WILLIAM P. MCGUIRE, MD,* ARTHUR S. LEVINE, MD,‡ AND ROBERT C. YOUNG, MD*

Histologically proven infection of the heart by *Candida* organisms occurred in 17 (10%) of 168 cancer patients with candidiasis studied at necropsy. All 17 patients were among the 85 patients with disseminated *Candida* infection; none of the 83 patients with localized candidiasis had involvement of the heart. Abscesses in the myocardium were present by histologic examination in all 17 patients and in 8 were evident on gross inspection as well. The mural endocardium was also affected in 5 patients from direct extension of a myocardial abscess. The valves were uninvolved. Pericardial infection was detected in 2 patients. The 17 patients with cardiac *Candida* infection had a higher frequency of positive premortem blood and cerebrospinal fluid cultures and of presence of *Candida* in the heart's blood than did the 68 patients with disseminated candidiasis but without involvement of the heart. Symptoms or signs of cardiac dysfunction resulting from the cardiac *Candida* infection were not readily detected in any patient. The clinical and pathologic features of cardiac candidiasis in cancer patients are distinct from those observed in *Candida* endocarditis.

Cancer 41:2364–2371, 1978.

CANDIDIASIS IS THE MOST COMMON FUNGAL INfection in patients with cancer,[3,9] yet despite increasing awareness of the setting in which invasive candidiasis is likely to occur, the majority of these infections elude diagnosis until biopsy of tissue or necropsy examination is obtained.[3,8,13] We have reviewed the case records and autopsy protocols of 168 of our cancer patients with candidiasis[4] in an attempt to elucidate the clinical features which are associated with disseminated infection and infection of specific organs. In the course of this study information on cardiac involvement with this fungus was sought.

Endocarditis is the manifestation of *Candida* infection of the heart most often discussed in recent medical literature. Although *Candida* endocarditis does rarely occur in the patient with malignant neoplastic disease,[17] disseminated candidiasis, in which the bulk of cardiac lesions are myocardial rather than endocardial,[2,6,8,11] is the usual presentation of widespread infection with this fungus in the cancer patient. Clinically apparent cardiac dysfunction produced by invasion of the heart by systemic malignancy[15,16] or infection [16] is often minimal. Similarly, the functional import of cardiac candidiasis has been stated to be uncertain,[19] although a high frequency of electrocardiographic abnormalities and otherwise unexplained hypotension have recently been ascribed to such fungal invasion.[6]

The present report describes our experience with cardiac candidiasis in a group of patients with fatal cancer. Particular emphasis is placed on the cardiac pathology and its differences from the changes observed in the heart in *Candida* endocarditis,[1] the clinical and necropsy correlates predictive of cardiac involvement, and the functional significance of invasion of the heart by this fungus. Three of our 17 cases have previously been reported.[5]

MATERIALS AND METHODS

The clinical records and final autopsy reports of all patients dying at the Clinical Center of the National Institutes of Health between 1965 and 1972 with necropsy diagnoses of candidiasis and malignant neoplastic disease were reviewed. The diagnosis of *Candida* infection was considered established only in cases and specific organs in which the organism was noted to be present on microscopic examination. Data were

From the * Medicine Branch, † Radiation Oncology Branch, and ‡ Pediatric Oncology Branch, National Cancer Institute, and the § Pathology Branch, National Heart, Lung, and Blood Institute, National Institutes of Health, Bethesda, Maryland.

Address for reprints: Dr. D. C. Ihde, NCI-VA Medical Oncology Branch, Veterans Administration Hospital, 50 Irving St., N.W., Washington, D.C. 20422.

Accepted for publication September 26, 1977.

abstracted from the hospital chart of the patient's final admission and from the autopsy report. Age, sex, and underlying neoplasm; signs and symptoms of illness; the type and hematologic side effects of cancer treatment; the duration and type of antimicrobical therapy; the number and type of clinically diagnosed and culturally confirmed premortem infections; biochemical, roentgenographic, electrocardiographic, and microbiological laboratory examinations; the presence of persistent malignant neoplasia, microorganisms recorded from the heart's blood, and histologically documented infections at necropsy were recorded.

After review of all pertinent available information on each patient, the clinical significance of each infectious process present at death was retrospectively assigned. A major infectious cause of death was defined as an infection which was though to have directly contributed to or to have been the sole cause of death.

Gross and microscopic cardiac pathology was reviewed in all patients in whom *Candida* organisms were observed on histologic examination of the heart. An average of 8 sections of heart was examined in each of these cases, and each section included the full thickness of myocardial wall from epicardium to endocardium. Of the 8 sections, only 1 was of the atrial wall and the other 7, of ventricular wall.

Disseminated *Candida* infection was considered to be present when organisms were observed in the tissues of the gastrointestinal (GI) tract and 1 or more non-GI organs, or in 2 or more non-GI organs in the absence of GI involvement. All other infections were considered to be localized. The results of premortem and postmortem blood cultures were not used to assess the extent of infection. Among the 168 patients with diagnoses of both cancer and candidiasis, 85 had disseminated and 83, localized infections.

The frequencies with which various clinical and pathologic factors occurred were compared in patients with localized and disseminated candidiasis, and in patients with *Candida* infection of the heart compared to those with disseminated candidiasis not involving the heart. The Chi-square test of statistical association, with Yates' correction, was utilized for these comparisons, using 2-tailed tests of significance.

Results

Clinical Observations

Of the 168 patients dying with candidiasis, 17 (10%) had *Candida* infection of the heart. Nine of these 17 patients were male, and 6 were less than 20 years of age. Nine had acute leukemia; 3, the terminal phase of chronic leukemia; 4, lymphoma, and 1, carcinoma of the cervix.

All patients with cardiac candidiasis died with extensive, disseminated fungal infection. Counting the GI tract as a single organ, *Candida* was demonstrated in each patient in a median of seven organs (range 2-13) at necropsy. The kidney contained *Candida* organisms in 15 patients, the GI tract in 14, the lung in 13, the liver in 12, and the central nervous system (CNS) in 10. Renal candidiasis was always accompanied by infection of either the CNS, the liver, or both. Infections with multiple microorganisms were common. Bacterial or non-*Candida* fungal infections were documented either premortem or postmortem or both in all but 2 patients. Five patients, however, died without postmortem evidence of any infection other than *Candida*.

A past history of cardiac disease was absent in all 17 patients. During the last month of life, systolic ejection murmurs were heard in 5 patients and third heart sounds in 4. Evidence of congestive heart failure was present in 4 cases, once in association with bacterial sepsis and daunomycin administration, and once with sepsis alone. In 2 instances the heart failure was transient and unexplained. Persistent refractory hypotension was noted in 4 patients, 3 of whom had documented bacterial sepsis and one of whom had major hemorrhage. Increased size of the cardiac silhouette was noted during the final month of life on chest X-rays of 4 of the 17 patients. In 5 patients no electrocardiogram (ECG) was recorded in the last month of life. In 4 others the ECG was either normal or unchanged from a previous tracing, while in the remaining 8 cases new ECG abnormalities were noted.

These changes included atrial premature contractions in 2 cases and ventricular premature contractions in 1, low voltage in 1, T wave abnormalities in 3 and ST segment-T wave abnormalities, often in association with tachycardia, in 5. None had bradycardia.

This frequency of abnormal cardiac symptoms, signs, and findings was not considered remarkable for a cohort of dying patients, and did not accurately distinguish those with cardiac infection from other patients with disseminated candidiasis without cardiac lesions.

Factors associated with disseminated candidiasis are listed in Table 1. All of these 22 items were more frequently present in patients with cardiac candidiasis than in those without

Table 1. Factors Occurring more often in Disseminated than in Localized Candidiasis

Premortem	
Hematologic malignancy†	Administration of iv antibiotics more than 50% of last admission**
Length of final hospital admission >1 month*	*Candida* in blood culture*
Neutrophil count >1,500/mm³ less than 50%† or <100/mm³ more than 50%* of last admission	Serum gamma-globulin <0.7 g/dl†
Administration of iv fluids more than 50% of last admission†	Administration of oral nystatin†
	Infection with *E. coli**
Postmortem	
Cancer in remission at autopsy*	*Candida* involvement of liver,† stomach,† small bowel,† large bowel,† heart,† central nervous system (CNS),† kidney,† or lung†
Candida cultured from heart's blood†	*Candida* infection a major cause of death†
Infection with *Aspergillus**	

* $p < 0.05$, † $p < 0.01$.

it. This reflects the fact that all cases with cardiac involvement had disseminated infection. Parameters distinguishing the patients with cardiac involvement from those with disseminated disease not affecting the heart are enumerated in Table 2. Among the cases with heart infection, 41% with premortem blood and 33% with premortem cerebrospinal fluid cultures submitted had one or more of these cultures positive for *Candida*. At autopsy, the heart's blood contained *Candida* in 76%. These factors probably reflect extensive hematogenous dissemination of *Candida* organisms rather than cardiac involvement *per se*, since 8 of the 10 parameters listed in Table 2, including premortem and postmortem blood cultures, were also significantly more common in the presence of renal or CNS infection or both, compared to patients with disseminated infection not involving the latter two organs. Factors that were not significantly associated with dissemination of *Candida* infection in our patients included treatment with cytotoxic chemotherapy and corticosteroids, duration and degree of lymphocytopenia, major surgery, persistent fever despite administration of antibiotics, hyperglycemia, positive *Candida* cultures from sputum, throat, urine, or stool, and detection of a *Candida* species other than *C. albicans*. Although some of these characteristics are considered to predispose to systemic candidiasis, we presumably failed to detect such correlations because we studied a relatively homogenous population of patients without other major illnesses intensively treated for cancer.

Table 2. Factors Occurring more often in Cardiac Candidiasis than in Disseminated Disease not Involving the Heart

Premortem
Candida in blood culture*
Candida in cerebrospinal fluid culture†
Clinical diagnosis of candidiasis*
Postmortem
Candida cultured from heart's blood†
Infection with fungus other than *Candida* or *Aspergillus**
Candida involvement of liver,† CNS,† or kidney†
Candida infection a major cause of death†
Lack of major infectious cause of death other than *Candida**

* $p < 0.05$, † $p < 0.01$.

Cardiac Pathology

Left ventricular hypertrophy was present at necropsy in 3, and ventricular chamber dilation in 2 of the 17 patients. Two patients had significant coronary arterial luminal narrowing.

The gross manifestations of *Candida* infection were most evident in the myocardium. Millimeter-sized abscesses were seen in 8 patients (Fig. 1). Among the 8 cases, abscesses were noted in the left ventricular myocardium in all, and in right ventricular myocardium in 3. Mural endocardial abscesses, from direct extension of myocardial infection, were seen in 4 patients (Fig. 2).

The cardiac valves were normal in all 17 patients. Gross cardiac hemorrhage was observed in 9 cases, in the left ventricular myocardium in 7 (5 of whom also had gross left ventricular abscesses), the right ventricular myocardium in 4, the ventricular endocardium in 5, the atrial myocardium in 3, and the pericardium in 1. Gross myocardial necrosis or fibrosis was absent in all patients. Diffuse obliterative fibrinous pericarditis was noted in a single case.

On microscopic examination myocardial abscesses containing *Candida* organisms (Figs. 2–5) were present in all 17 patients. Numerous myocardial abscesses were observed in 5 patients, two to 10 abscesses in 7, and a single focus in 5. In 16 patients these abscesses occurred in the left ventricle, with biventricular involvement in 8. The remaining patient had isolated right ventricular abscesses. Atrial abscesses were identified in 3 of 10 and left ventricular papillary

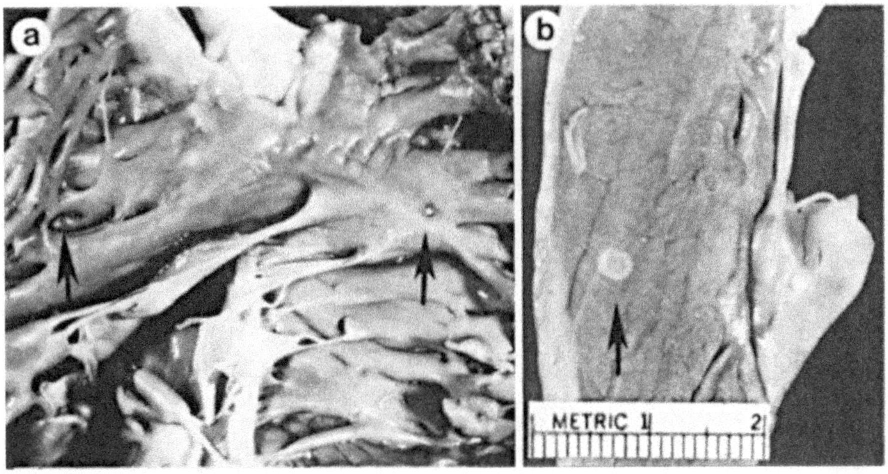

FIG. 1A–B *Candida* abscesses in right ventricle A) and in left ventricular free wall B) (arrows) in a 26-year-old man (A66-159) with chronic myelocytic leukemia. During life there was no evidence of cardiac dysfunction.

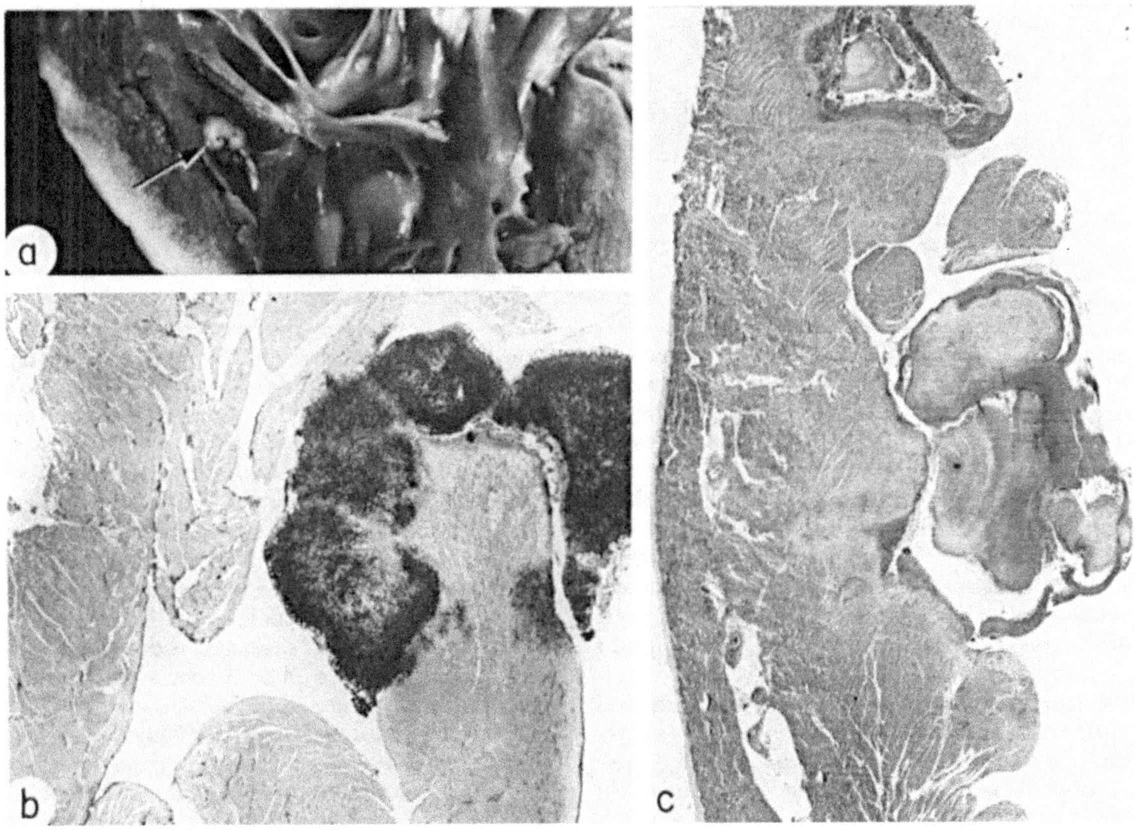

FIG. 2A–C *Candida* abscesses in mural endocardium representing an extension of myocardial *Candida* abscesses in 2 patients. A and B): Gross appearance A) of a ventricular endocardial vegetation (arrow) in a 65-year-old man (A66-180) with chronic myelocytic leukemia for one year; microscopically B), the right ventricular wall reveals an endocardial vegetation containing massive numbers of *Candida* organisms. C) Right ventricular wall showing 2 large abscesses in mural endocardium and in adjacent myocardium in a 29-year-old man (A66-159) with chronic myelocytic leukemia for 4 years. Three months before death pleural effusion developed from which *Candida* organisms were cultured. Methenamine silver stain:×14 B); H&E ×7 C).

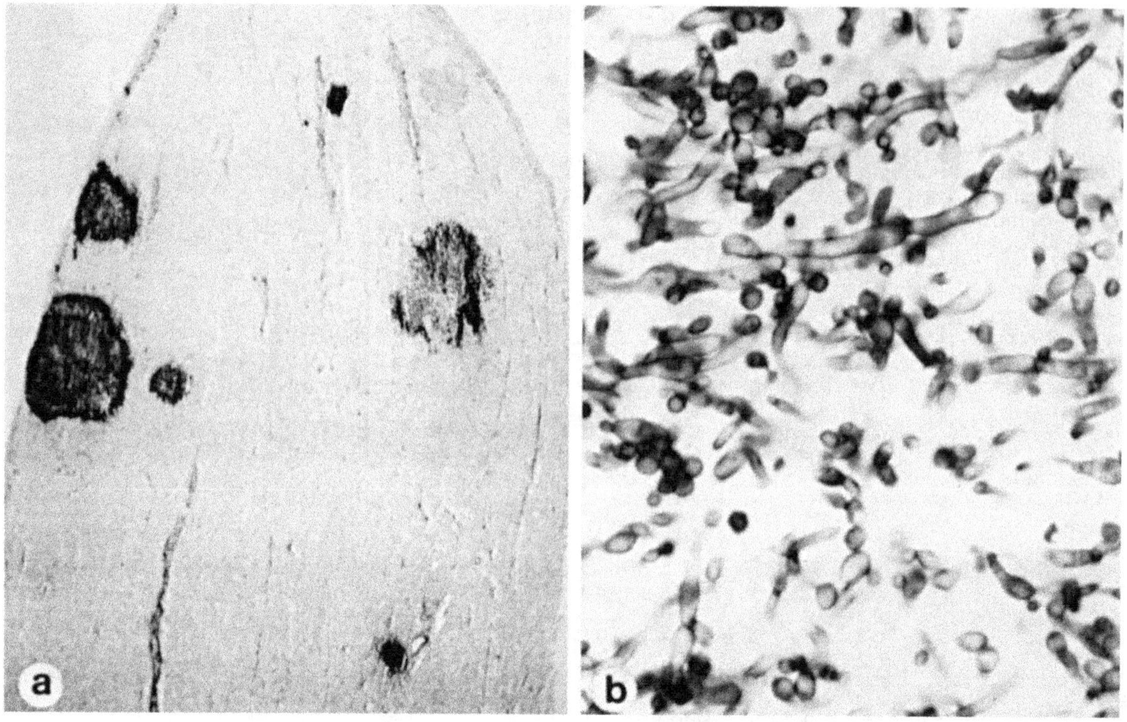

FIG. 3A–B *Candida* abscesses in a left ventricular papillary muscle A) and close-up of the *Candida* organisms B) in a 20-year-old man (A72-151) with acute myeloblastic leukemia. Gross myocardial abscesses were present in the left and right ventricular free walls and ventricular septum in addition to the papillary muscles. No precordial murmur was heard. Periodic acid-Schiff stains: ×12 A), ×860 B).

muscle abscesses (Fig. 3) in 7 of 14 cases with sections of these structures available for examination. Five patients had mural endocardial abscesses (Fig. 2), while valvular surfaces were always normal.

Three of the 5 patients with endocardial abscesses also had blood vessel wall invasion with *Candida*, and in 2 of the 5 pericardial invasion with the fungus was observed. An inflammatory cellular infiltrate was associated with the areas of abscess formation in 8 of the 17 cases, and a giant-cell reaction in 2 (Fig. 5). Myocarditis in the absence of organisms was not observed. In 2 patients hemorrhage was present within an abscess, while in only 2(1 with acute and 1 with chronic leukemia) was tumor invasion of the heart detected.

Discussion

Louria[11] has described the differing clinical manifestations of *Candida* endocarditis and disseminated candidiasis in a general hospital population. The disseminated disease runs a more acute course with less frequent embolic phenomena, is more often accompanied by *Candida* funguria and previous antibiotic administration, and is less frequently caused by *Candida* species other than *C. albicans*. Our data suggest congestive heart failure is less common than in endocarditis. *Candida* endocarditis most often occurs after cardiac surgery and therapy for subacute bacterial endocarditis or in narcotic addicts and patients with valvular heart disease.[1,11] Disseminated candidiasis is associated with debilitating illness such as cancer, diabetes, indwelling catheters, administration of antibiotics and corticosteroids,[11] and major surgery.[2]

Pathologic examination of the heart in *Candida* endocarditis reveals vegetations on one or more usually previously abnormal valves and occasionally on the mural endocardium.[1] Myocardial abscesses containing *Candida* organisms and *Candida* abscesses in other body organs are uncommon.[1,18] Mycotic emboli in coronary arteries rarely lead to myocardial infarction. Acute and chronic myocarditis in areas devoid of organisms may occur frequently.[1] On prosthetic valves, the nidus of infection may arise in areas of host neoendocardium.[14] In a report on infective endocarditis in cancer patients,[17] 2 of the 4 patients with *Candida* infection had preexisting valvular abnormalities.

Cardiac pathology in disseminated candidiasis differs in several respects from that observed in endocarditis. The usual cardiac finding at necropsy in patients with disseminated infection is the presence of myocardial *Candida* abscesses, often (over 50% in our hands) visible only by microscopic examination.[2,6,10,11] The abscesses are most common in the wall of left ventricle, presumably because its mass is the greatest. Involvement of the papillary muscles may be particularly common, possibly because these structures are end organs in terms of blood supply. Mural endocardial involvement occurred in nearly a third of our patients and always represented extension of a myocardial abscess, while valvular endocardial involvement was absent. Pericardial extension occurs in a minority of cases.[2,6,8,10]

Microscopically, an inflammatory-cell response to the *Candida* cardiac abscesses may be absent or present. This variation appears to result from differing responses to the myelosuppression from cytotoxic chemotherapy. Myocarditis in the absence of *Candida* organisms was not observed in our patients and neither was it seen by Franklin *et al.*[6] Blood-vessel invasion by the *Candida* organisms occurred in 3 of our patients and also was observed in patients studied by Franklin *et al.*[6] We did not observe cardiac necrosis due to *Candida* but others[6,11] occasionally have. The high incidence of cardiac hemorrhage in this series is similar to what one of us[15] found in leukemic patients at autopsy.

Cardiac candidiasis is part of a systemic infectious process; the heart alone is rarely afflicted.[6,8,9,11] Cardiac involvement in disseminated candidiasis has been reported to occur in half or more of cases,[2,10–12] but we and others[3,7–9,13] have observed it in only 7–25% of such patients. This discrepancy appears to result from different case detection methods and definitions of disseminated disease, and studies of different patient populations. In series[3,9] such as this one composed exclusively of cancer patients, the frequency of cardiac infection is low.

Premortem diagnosis of *Candida* infection of the heart or even of disseminated candidiasis is difficult.[8,20] In our data only positive blood and cerebrospinal fluid cultures were useful premortem in distinguishing patients with cardiac candidiasis from other cases with disseminated infection without involvement of the heart. These positive cultures appeared to reflect wide-

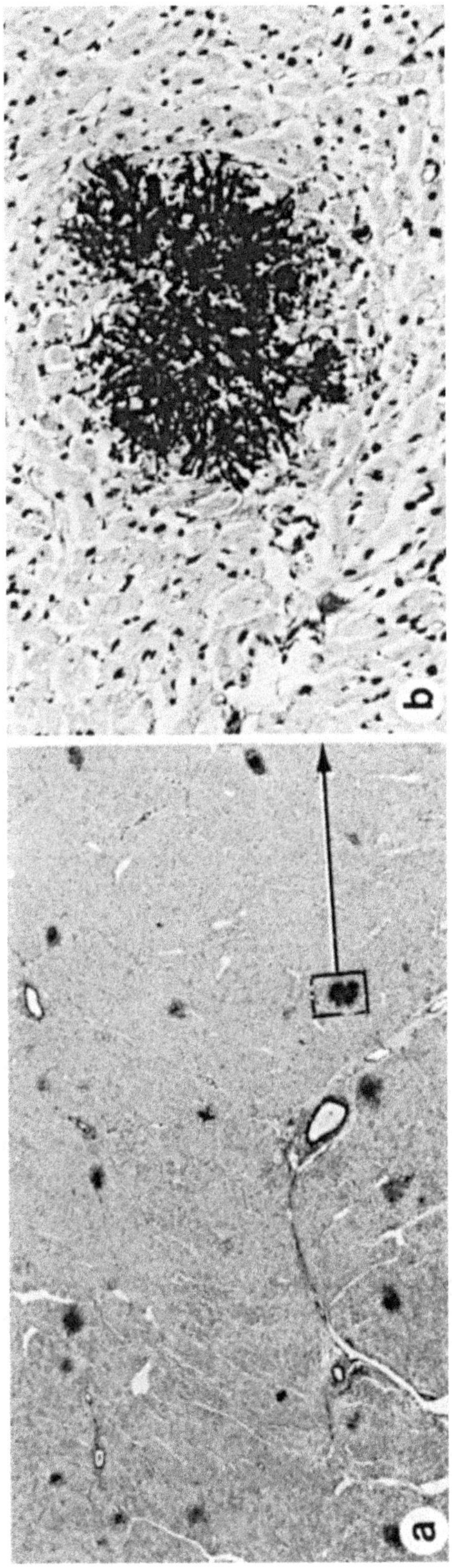

FIG. 4A–B Photomicrographs showing *Candida* abscesses in myocardium A) and B) of a 14-year-old boy (A68–309) with the leukemic phase of lymphocytic lymphoma. Numerous *Candida* abscesses were present in most body organs. Periodic acid-Schiff stains: ×16 A), ×182 B).

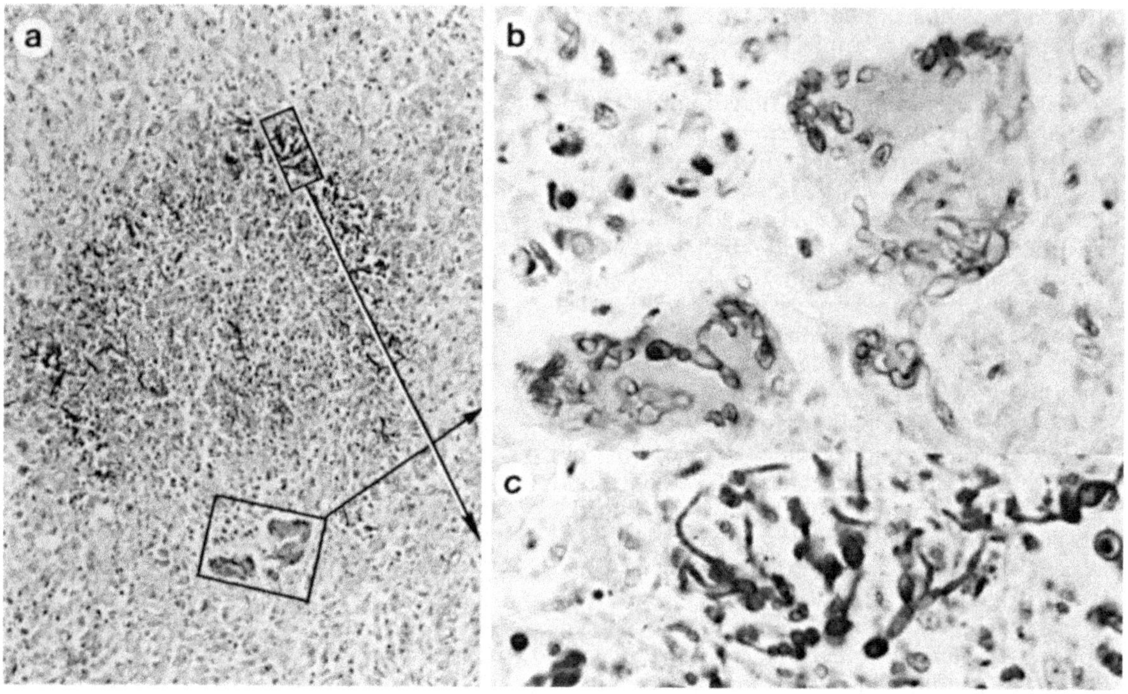

FIG. 5. Myocardial *Candida* species abcess A) showing a giant cell reaction B) to the fungal organisms in an 8-year-old boy (A66–75) with acute myeloblastic leukemia. Giant-cell reaction to the *Candida* organisms was observed in only 2 (12%) of our 17 patients with cardiac candidiasis but immunosuppression by chemotherapeutic agents was considerable in most of the patients. A close-up of the *Candida* organisms is shown in C). Periodic acid-Schiff stains: ×150 A), ×860 B and C).

spread hematogenous extension of infection, particularly to the kidney, heart, and CNS, rather than predicting for cardiac invasion alone. Cultures of other sites considered alone were not useful in detecting disseminated infection. Law *et al.*[10] found that 75% of their patients had premortem blood cultures containing *Candida*. This was independent of whether the heart was infected at autopsy, but all of these cases had extensive candidiasis.

In cancer patients, especially in the presence of immunosuppression, leukopenia, and positive *Candida* cultures from three or more other sites and in the absence of a contaminated intravenous catheter, candidemia is most often associated with disseminated infection.[20]

The functional importance of the cardiac lesions in disseminated candidiasis is difficult to ascertain. Van Kirk *et al.*[19] reported complete heart block in a patient found to have *Candida* invasion of the conducting system at necropsy. It is likely, however, that cardiac candidiasis is of little clinical significance since the myocardial lesions are small, being grossly visible in only 8 of 17 of our cases and in 7 of 31 of the patients of Franklin *et al.*[6] Consequently only a small fraction of functioning myocardium is replaced. Little evidence of major cardiac impairment could be detected in our patients, although such signs could have been obscured by frequently coexisting sepsis and overwhelming disease in other organs.

Franklin *et al.*[6] found a high incidence of ECG abnormalities and unexplained hypotension in their closely monitored patients with cardiac candidiasis, but speculated that the latter may have been due to candidemia itself[11] rather than to loss of myocardial tissue. Insufficient ECG observations are available in our patients to contradict the former findings, but all patients with prolonged hypotension associated with cardiac infection in this series had other major medical problems.

Little other pertinent data are available. Law *et al.*[10] noted congestive heart failure requiring administration of digitalis in over half of their patients dying with disseminated candidiasis, but their data reveals that this occurred independently of whether the heart was infected. Cardiovascular causes of death were equally uncommon in the patients of Parker *et al.*[12] who died with superficial or deep candidiasis. At this point, it appears most reasonable to assume that fungal infection of the heart in the patient with disseminated candidiasis is not the most likely cause of any cardiovascular deterioration.

REFERENCES

1. Andriole, V. T., Kravetz, H. M., Roberts, W. C., and Utz, J. P.: Candida endocarditis: Clinical and pathologic studies. *Am. J. Med.* 32:251–285, 1962.

2. Bernhardt, H. E., Orlando, J. C., Benfield, J. R., Hirose, F. M., and Foos, R. Y.: Disseminated candidiasis in surgical patients. *Surg. Gynecol. Obstet.* 134:819–825, 1972.

3. Bodey, G. P.: Fungal infections complicating acute leukemia. *J. Chron. Dis.* 19:667–687, 1966.

4. Brereton, H. D., Ihde, D., Levine, A. S., and Young, R. C.: Candida infections: Clinical and pathologic correlations in 168 consecutive autopsy proven cases in cancer patients. *Proc. Am. Assoc. Cancer Res.* 18:19, 1977 (Abstract).

5. Buchbinder, N. A., and Roberts, W. C.: Active infective endocarditis confined to mural endocardium: A study of six necropsy patients. *Arch. Pathol.* 93:435–440, 1972.

6. Franklin, W. G., Simon, A. B., and Sodeman, T. M.: Candida myocarditis without valvulitis. *Am. J. Cardiol.* 38:924–928, 1976.

7. Hart, P. D., Russell, E., Jr., and Remington, J. S.: The compromised host and infection: II. Deep fungal infection. *J. Infect. Dis.* 120:169–191, 1969.

8. Hughes, J. M., and Remington, J. S.: Systemic candidiasis, a diagnostic challenge. *Calif. Med.* 116:8–17, June, 1972.

9. Hutter, R. V. P., and Collins, H. S.: The occurrence of opportunistic fungus infections in a cancer hospital. *Lab. Invest.* 11:1035–1045, 1962.

10. Law, E. J., Kim, O. J., Stieritz, D. D., and MacMillan, B. G.: Experience with systemic candidiasis in the burned patient. *J. Trauma* 12:543–552, 1972.

11. Louria, D. B., Stiff, D. P., and Bennett, B.: Disseminated moniliasis in the adult. *Medicine* 41:307–337, 1962.

12. Parker, J. C., Jr., McCloskey, J. J., and Knauer, K. A.: Pathobiologic features of human candidiasis: A common deep mycosis of the brain, heart, and kidney in the altered host. *Am. J. Clin. Pathol.* 65:991–1000, 1976.

13. Rifkind, D., Marchioro, T. L., Schneck, S. A., and Hill, R. B., Jr.: Systemic fungal infections complicating renal transplantation and immunosuppressive therapy. *Am. J. Med.* 43:28–38, 1967.

14. Robboy, S. J., and Kaiser, J.: Pathogenesis of fungal infection on heart valve prostheses. *Hum. Pathol.* 6:711–715, 1975.

15. Roberts, W. C., Bodey, G. P., and Wertlake, P. T.: The heart in acute leukemia: A study of 420 autopsy cases. *Am. J. Cardiol.* 21:388–412, 1968.

16. Roberts, W. C., Glancy, D. L., and DeVita, V. T.: Heart in malignant lymphoma (Hodgkin's disease, lymphosarcoma, reticulum cell sarcoma, and mycosis fungoides): A study of 196 autopsy cases. *Am. J. Cardiol.* 22:85–107, 1968.

17. Rosen, P., and Armstrong, D.: Infective endocarditis in patients treated for malignant neoplastic diseases: A postmortem study. *Am. J. Clin. Pathol.* 60:241–250, 1973.

18. Seelig, M. S., Speth, C. P., Kozinn, P. J., Taschdjian, C. L., Toni, E. F., and Goldberg, P.: Patterns of Candida endocarditis following cardiac surgery: Importance of early diagnosis and therapy (an analysis of 91 cases). *Prog. Cardiovasc. Dis.* 17:125-160, 1974.

19. Van Kirk, J. E., Simon, A. B., and Armstrong, W. R.: Candida myocarditis causing complete atrioventricular block. *JAMA* 227:931–933, 1974.

20. Young, R. C., Bennett, J. E., Geelhoed, G. W., and Levine, A. S.: Fungemia with compromised host resistance: A study of 70 cases. *Ann. Intern. Med.* 80:605–612, 1974.

Cardiac Sarcoma Causing "ASH" and Simulating Coronary Heart Disease

JEFFREY M. ISNER, M.D.
Bethesda, Maryland

M. WAYNE FALCONE, M.D.
Waco, Texas

RENU VIRMANI, M.D.
WILLIAM C. ROBERTS, M.D.
Bethesda, Maryland

A patient is described in whom primary cardiac sarcoma preferentially infiltrated the ventricular septum while essentially sparing the left ventricular free wall, resulting in striking echocardiographic and morphologic asymmetry between septum and free wall (ASH). No reports have appeared previously of a patient with an intramural cardiac neoplasm demonstrated by echocardiogram. Additionally, the patient clinically had features typical of coronary heart disease, yet at necropsy the extramural coronary arteries showed insignificant (<75 per cent) cross-sectional area luminal narrowing by atherosclerotic plaques.

The majority of malignant neoplasms involving the heart are located within a cardiac wall and these intramural neoplasms are extremely difficult to diagnose clinically. Echocardiography has been helpful in the diagnosis of neoplasms located within a cardiac cavity, but diagnosis of an intramural cardiac neoplasm by this technic has not been reported. Recently, we studied a patient in whom cardiac sarcoma by echocardiography simulated asymmetric septal hypertrophy (ASH). In addition, the patient had typical clinical evidence of coronary heart disease, a rare manifestation of a cardiac neoplasm. A description of these unusual clinical and morphologic observations in this patient are described in this report.

CASE REPORT

A 48 year old cattleman/blacksmith who died in June 1977 was hospitalized for the first time in June 1972 because of the sudden onset of crushing substernal chest pain while roping a cow. The chest pain radiated to the neck and to both arms, and was associated with pallor, diaphoresis and dyspnea. Serial electrocardiograms and enzyme measurements including serum creatinine phosphokinase >5,000 IU, were consistent with an acute myocardial infarct, anterior wall. Congestive heart failure and recurrent ventricular tachycardia also occurred transiently.

Because of recurrent exertional chest pain usually relieved by the ingestion of nitroglycerin, cardiac catheterization was performed a year later. The intracardiac pressures were normal; the left ventricular end-diastolic pressure was 12 mm Hg. The lumen of the left anterior descending coronary artery proximal to its first diagonal branch was reduced about 50 per cent in diameter, the circumflex branch contained trivial irregularities, and the right coronary artery was small but otherwise normal. In December 1974 (**Figure 1**), and in January and April 1975, he was rehospitalized because of severe substernal chest pain unrelieved by nitroglycerin. The electrocardiogram on each occasion

From the Pathology Branch, National Heart, Lung, and Blood Institute, National Institutes of Health, Bethesda, Maryland; and the Department of Cardiopulmonary Medicine, Providence Hospital, Waco, Texas. Requests for reprints should be addressed to Dr. William C. Roberts, Building 10A, Room 3E-30, National Institutes of Health, Bethesda, Maryland 20014. Manuscript accepted September 27, 1978.

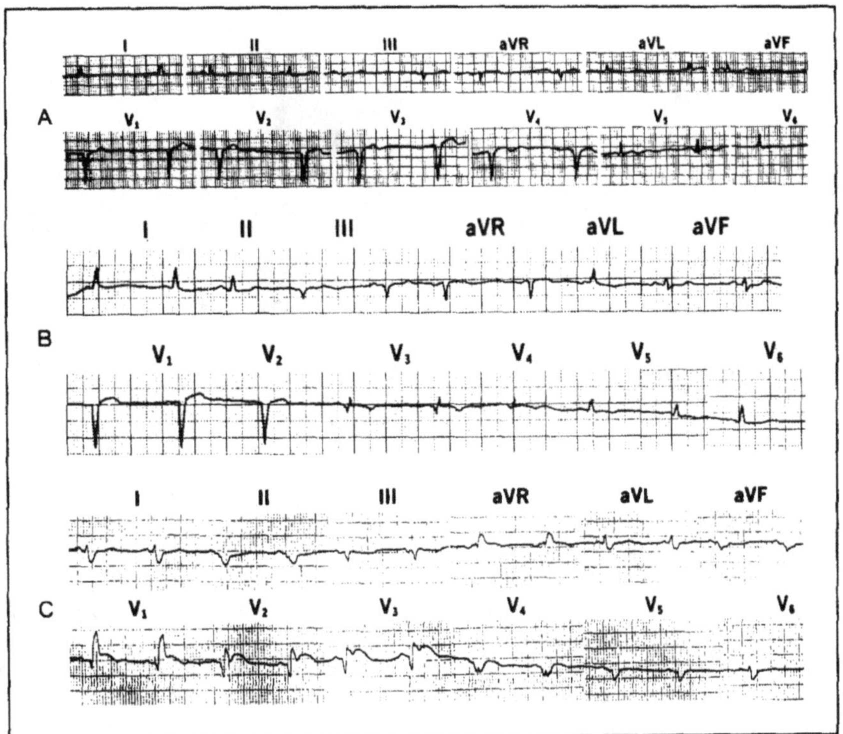

Figure 1. Electrocardiograms. **A,** this was recorded in December 1974 during one of several admissions for angina pectoris. Remarkable features include loss of R waves associated with persistent S-T segment elevations and T-wave inversion in leads V_1-V_4, and low voltage (sum of QRS in leads I, II and III <1.5 mv). **B,** recorded on November 26, 1975, is fairly similar. **C,** recorded on May 14, 1977, four weeks before death, shows a new right bundle branch block.

failed to show evidence of acute myocardial infarction and the serum enzymes remained normal. Except for an elevated (20 mm Hg) left ventricular end-diastolic pressure, the intracardiac pressures again were normal. Angiography showed a 50 per cent diameter reduction of the lumen of the left anterior descending artery and a 75 per cent diameter reducton of the lumen of the left circumflex coronary artery. The right coronary artery appeared small but normal. Lung scan in April 1975 showed a perfusion defect of the upper lobe of the right lung and warfarin sodium therapy was begun.

From August 1975 until March 1977, chest pain recurred about once every two months but hospitalization was not required. In March 1977, however, the patient noted fever (temperatures to 101°F), sweats, dysphagia, hoarseness and pain in the sternal and clavicular areas made worse on inspiration. In May 1977, examination revealed new murmurs of mitral and tricuspid regurgitation, an electrocardiogram (Figure 1) showed a new right bundle branch block, and a chest roentgenogram showed marked enlargement of the cardiac silhouette and an infiltrate in the lower lobe of the left lung. An echocardiogram (**Figure 2**) showed a striking difference in the thickness of the ventricular septum and left ventricular free wall. Lung scan demonstrated perfusion defects, and barium swallow disclosed posterior and rightward displacement of the esophagus. On May 31, 1977, the patient underwent pericardiocentesis and pericardial biopsy. Histologic examination suggested an undifferentiated neoplasm. His condition deteriorated rapidly thereafter, and he died on June 13.

At necropsy, the parietal pericardium was focally adherent to the visceral pericardium by tumor; the amount of fluid in the pericardial sac was not increased. The heart with the tumor (Figure 2 and **Figure 3**) (histologically, an undifferentiated sarcoma (**Figure 4**)) weighed 1,300 g. Neoplasm virtually replaced the ventricular septum whereas the left ventricular free wall contained few tumor deposits (Figure 3). The maximal thickness of ventricular septum and the left ventricular free wall were 3.2 and 1.9 cm, respectively. Tumor surrounded the left anterior descending, and right and left circumflex coronary arteries at many sites (**Figure 5**). Of the fifty-six 5-mm segments of extramural coronary artery examined histologically, 19 showed tumor completely surrounding the coronary artery, and in three segments there was collapse of the wall due to tumor compression (**Table I,** Figure 5). Other than two small metastases in the lungs, the noncardiac organs were free of tumor.

COMMENTS

In the first necropsy description of "asymmetric hypertrophy of the heart," Teare [1] classified the massive hypertrophy of the ventricular septum as a "tumor of the

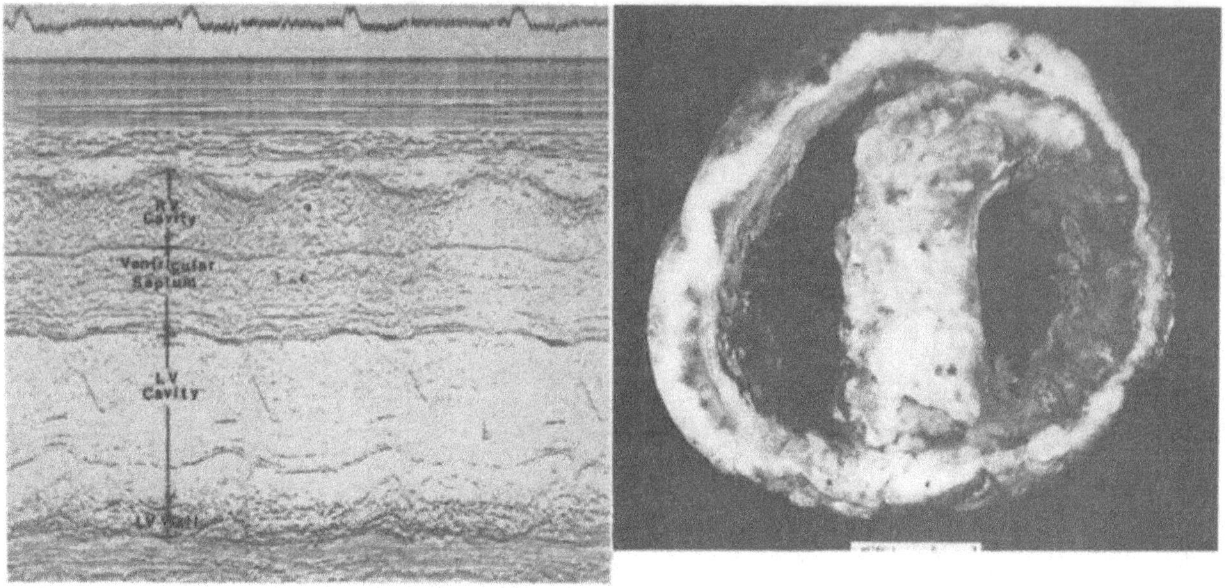

Figure 2. Echocardiogram (left) and transverse cut of cardiac ventricles at approximate level of the echo beam on the patient described. The ventricular septum by echo measures 3.0 cm in thickness and at necropsy (on this slice), 3.2 cm in maximal thickness; the left ventricular (LV) free wall by echo measures about 1.3 cm and at necropsy the left ventricular myocardial wall measures 1.6 cm in maximal thickness.

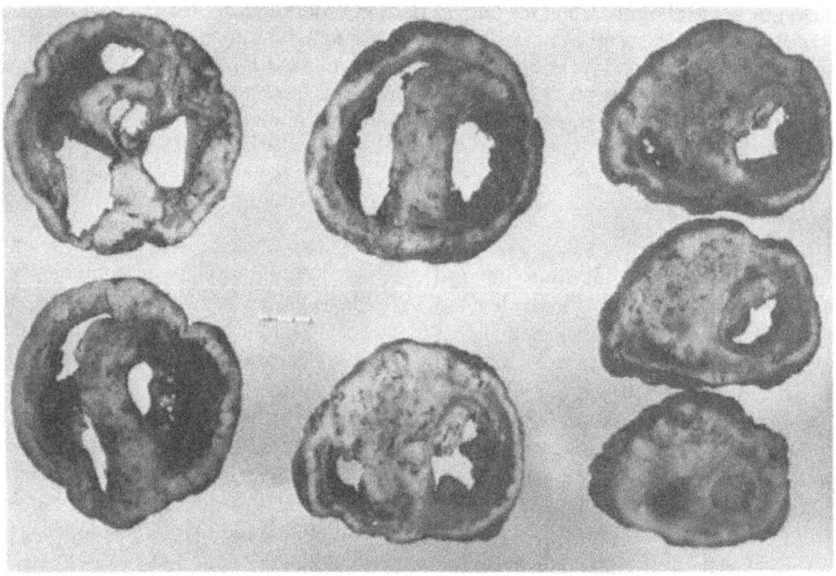

Figure 3. The heart at necropsy. Composite of transverse sections showing neoplastic replacement of myocardium, particularly of the septum. The tumor is white. The upper left is the most basal section, and the lower right is the most apical section.

heart." Although there is as yet no universally accepted terminology for the entity originally reported by Teare, most would agree that it is not a neoplasm. Our patient appears to be the first described with "asymmetric hypertrophy of the heart," or left ventricular asymmetry, resulting from a true neoplasm.

Echocardiographic identification of cardiac tumors has been limited previously to those tumors located within a cavity. The prototype is the left atrial myxoma. Interruption of the normally echo "silent" cardiac chambers by reflections from echo-dense tumors allowed initial ultrasound recognition of this neoplasm by Effert and Domanig in 1959 [2]. Subsequently, primary cardiac neoplasms were identified in other cardiac chambers [3–6]. *Intramural* tumors, in contrast to intracavitary tumors, do not produce a differential echo

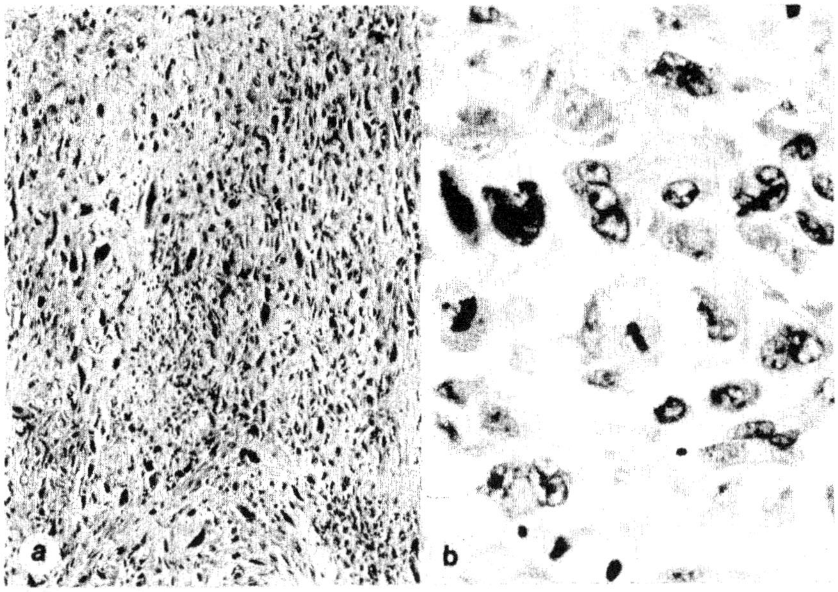

Figure 4. Photomicrographs of the sarcoma. The cells are large and spindle shaped. Mitotic figures are present. Hematoxylin and eosin stains, magnification × 130 (**a**) and 860 (**b**), reduced by 33 per cent.

density relative to normal myocardium, and they have escaped echocardiographic detection. Distortion of the normal cardiac architecture (e.g., increase in wall thickness) by tumor infiltration would appear to be a prerequisite for echocardiographic detection of an intramural tumor. Asymmetric distortion, as occurred in our patient, enhanced the possibility of ultrasound recognition.

Asymmetric septal hypertrophy (ASH) is the echocardiographic hallmark of the condition described by Teare and now most commonly called hypertrophic cardiomyopathy. Although ASH is a highly sensitive marker for hypertrophic cardiomyopathy [7,8], it is not specific for this disorder. Thus, ventricular septums thicker than left ventricular free walls, i.e., ASH, have been reported in conditions causing thinning of the left ventricular free wall relative to the septum or in conditions causing thickening of the septum relative to the free wall. The most common cause of preferential free wall thinning certainly is myocardial infarction, and the most common cause of preferential septal thickening appears to be right ventricular systolic hypertension from any of a variety of conditions. Cardiac neoplasm must now be added to this list of causes of ASH. The septal-free wall asymmetry in our patient resulted from a primary *increase* in septal thickness due to tumor infiltration; it did not occur as the result of free wall thinning.

Three features of the echocardiogram in our patient suggested that he did not have hypertrophic cardiomyopathy. First, the end-diastolic left ventricular cavity size (5.6 cm) was at the upper limits of normal for this patient's body surface area, atypical for patients with hypertrophic cardiomyopathy in whom the left ventricular cavity size is typically normal to small [9]. Second, the E to F slope of the anterior mitral leaflet was clearly within normal limits (>80 mm/sec), a finding that would be highly unusual for a patient with symptomatic hypertrophic cardiomyopathy [7]. Third, the position of the anterior mitral valve leaflet at the onset of systole was not displaced anteriorly, another finding at variance with typical hypertrophic cardiomyopathy [9]. Surprisingly, although the amplitude of septal motion was diminished, the normal vector of septal motion was preserved despite near total replacement of the septum by tumor.

A second unique feature of our patient was that his clinical features simulated those of patients with symptomatic coronary atherosclerosis. We are unaware of any previously described patient in whom angiographic coronary arterial narrowing indistinguishable from coronary atherosclerosis resulted from external compression of the coronary artery by a cardiac neoplasm. Furthermore, our patient experienced an "acute myocardial infarction" that was classic in terms of symptoms, electrocardiographic evolution and enzyme elevation, despite the absence at necropsy five years later of significant (>75 per cent cross-sectional area [10,11]) coronary luminal narrowing by atherosclerotic plaques. Although the lumen of one 5 mm segment of the distal left anterior descending coronary artery was compressed by neoplasm, there was no myocardial necrosis in the area distal to the site of narrowing, or, for that matter, in any other area of myocardium. We can only presume, however, that the clinical evidence of myocardial necrosis resulted from tumor replacement of myocardium. The conduction abnormality which appeared one month before death almost certainly resulted from the massive infiltration of the heart by tumor. Frolich and associates [12], Javier et al. [13], and Cera, Karlinsky and Rodin [14] each described a patient with obstruction of the lumen of a coronary artery by tumor emboli or metastases, whereas Kroopf and Peterson [15] described a patient with electrocardiographic evidence of acute myocardial infarction related to compression of a coronary artery. Harris and his asso-

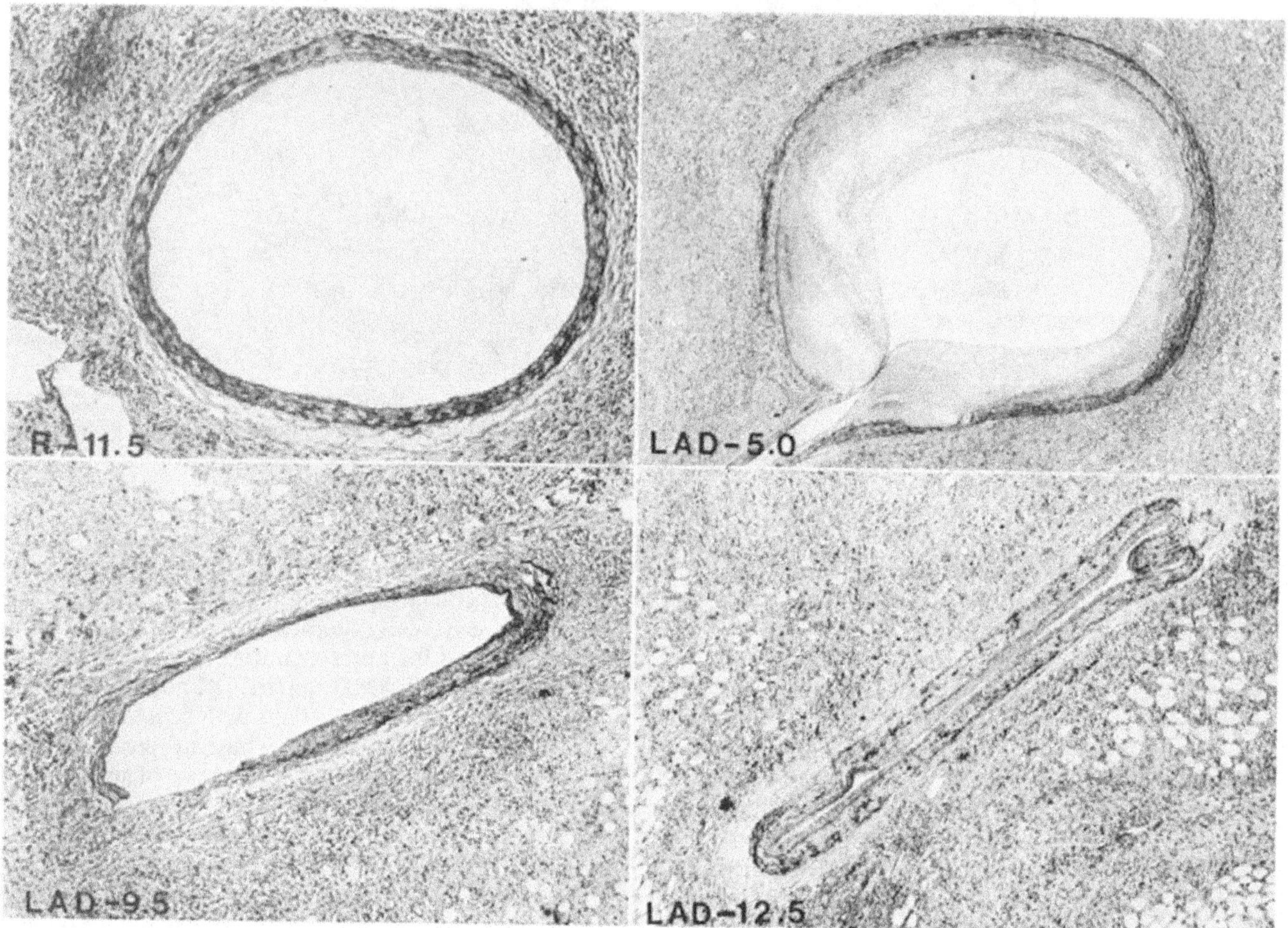

Figure 5. Epicardial coronary arteries, all surrounded by tumor. The numbers indicate the distances from respective coronary ostia to the sites where the section was taken. The right (R) one is surrounded but not compressed by tumor. The lumen of the left anterior descending (LAD) is narrowed by atherosclerotic plaque at 5.0 cm. At 9.5 cm, the wall of the left anterior descending is totally replaced at one point by tumor. At 12.5 cm, despite the absence of significant intimal thickening, tumor compression results in a slit-like lumen. Movat stains: R–11.5, magnification × 13; LAD–5.0, magnification × 26; LAD–9.5, magnification, × 43; LAD–12.5, × magnification 43; all reduced by 25 per cent.

TABLE I Number of Coronary Segments (0.5 cm) of the Four Major Coronary Arteries Showing Various Degrees of Cross-Sectional Area Luminal Narrowing and Number Surrounded by Tumor and Compressed by Tumor

Coronary Artery	Total No. 0.5 cm Segments	No. Segments Surrounded by Tumor	No. Segments Lumen Compressed >75% by Tumor	No. of 0.5 cm Segments Showing % of Cross-Sectional Area Narrowing by Atherosclerotic Plaque			
				0–25	26–50	51–75	76–100
Right	16	4	0	11	5	0	0
Left main	4	0	0	4	0	0	0
Left anterior descending	21	17*	2	12	6	3	0
Left circumflex	15	2	1*	7	5	3	0
Total	56	23	3	34	16	6	0

* In one section, tumor invaded the wall of the artery.

ciates [16] described a patient with bronchogenic carcinoma in whom necropsy revealed myocardial necrosis without apparent coronary arterial involvement; the necrosis was attributed to direct invasion by tumor metastases. Finally, Franciosa and Lawrinson [17] described a patient with anterolateral and posterior left ventricular wall necrosis secondary to compression of the lumen of the left anterior descending and left circumflex coronary arteries by metastatic bronchogenic carcinoma. This last patient is the only other patient (that we are aware of) in whom tumor-related myocardial necrosis simulated clinical and laboratory evolution of acute transmural myocardial infarction. And finally, rapid growth of the sarcoma itself within the heart may have caused relative "cardiac" ischemia, i.e., the increased metabolic rate of the cardiac sarcoma may have "outstripped" the ability of the coronary arteries, despite their insignificant narrowing, to perfuse adequately both the sarcoma and the myocardium. Certainly, much of the tumor in the heart was necrotic, suggesting that the latter mechanism may have been operative.

REFERENCES

1. Teare D: Asymmetrical hypertrophy of the heart in young adults. Br Heart J 20: 1, 1958.
2. Effert S, Domanig E: The diagnosis of intra-atrial tumors and thrombi by the metrasonic echo method. Ger Med Mon 6: 1, 17, 1959.
3. Waxler EB, Kawai N, Kasparian H: Right atrial myxoma: echocardiographic, phonocardiographic and hemodynamic signs. Am Heart J 83: 251, 1972.
4. Nanda NC, Barold SS, Gramiak R, et al.: Echocardiographic features of right ventricular outflow tumor prolapsing into the pulmonary artery. Am J Cardiol 40: 272, 1977.
5. Farooki ZQ, Adelman S, Green EW: Echocardiographic differentiaton of a cystic and a solid tumor of the heart. Am J Cardiol 39: 107, 1977.
6. Meller J, Teichholz LE, Pichard AD, et al.: Left ventricular myxoma. Echocardiographic diagnosis and review of the literature. Am J Med 63: 816, 1977.
7. Abbasi AS, MacAlpin RN, Eber LM, et al.: Echocardiographic diagnosis of idiopathic hypertrophic cardiomyopathy without outflow obstruction. Circulation 46: 897, 1972.
8. Henry WL, Clark CE, Epstein SE: Asymmetric septal hypertrophy. Echocardiographic identification of the pathognomonic abnormality of IHSS. Circulation 47: 225, 1973.
9. Henry WL, Clark CE, Griffith JM, et al.: Mechanism of left ventricular outflow obstruction in patients with obstructive asymmetric septal hypertrophy (idiopathic hypertrophic subaortic stenosis). Am J Cardiol 35: 337, 1975.
10. Roberts WC, Buja LM: The frequency and significance of coronary arterial thrombi and other observations in fatal acute myocardial infarction. Am J Med 52: 425, 1972.
11. American Heart Association Committee Report: A reporting system on patients evaluated for coronary artery disease. Circulation 51: 7, 1975.
12. Frolich ED, Shnider BI, Leonard JJ: Antemortem diagnosis of metastatic sarcoma to the heart: a case report. Am Heart J 57: 623, 1959.
13. Javier BV, Yount WJ, Crosby DJ, et al.: Cardiac metastasis in lymphoma and leukemia. Dis Chest 52: 482, 1967.
14. Cera I, Karlinsky W, Rodin A: Tumor embolism of the left coronary artery. Am Heart J 53: 472, 1957.
15. Kroopf SS, Peterson CA: Anaplastic myxoma of left atrium. Arch Intern Med 100: 819, 1957.
16. Harris T, Copeland G, Brody D: Progressive injury current with metastatic tumor of the heart. Am Heart J 69: 392, 1965.
17. Franciosa JA, Lawrinson W: Coronary artery occlusion due to neoplasm. A rare cause of acute myocardial infarction. Arch Intern Med 128: 797, 1971.

The "Charcoal Heart"*

Melanoma to the Cor

Bruce F. Waller, M.D.; John S. Gottdiener, M.D.; Renu Virmani, M.D.; and William C. Roberts, M.D., F.C.C.P.

Dr. William C. Roberts: Herein we will discuss the findings in a woman with fatal melanoma to the heart. She manifested certain cardiopulmonary problems of patients with cardiac metastases. Dr. Waller will describe the patient.

Dr. Bruce F. Waller: A 38-year-old white woman who died on May 19, 1979, had noted a mole on her left thigh at the age of 24 years. After excision at that time, histologic examination disclosed the mole to be a superficial spreading-type melanoma. No metastases were found, and no other therapy was given. At the age of 36 years (January 1977; 28 months before death), the patient noted a "lump" in her groin, and excision again disclosed melanoma. The results of a chest roentgenogram (Fig 1), gallium scan, and cardiopulmonary physical examination were normal. In April 1977, the aortocaval, left superficial, and deep inguinal lymph nodes were excised. In July 1977, the patient started chemotherapy (methyl CCNU).

In March 1979 (two months before death), the patient noted exertional dyspnea, subcutaneous edema in the right leg, weakness, and a black "lump" on her back. Examination revealed a "quiet" precordium and faintly audible cardiac sounds. The systemic arterial blood pressure was 130/70 mm Hg, and the systolic systemic pressure fell 6 mm Hg with inspiration. On the chest roentgenogram the cardiac

*From the Pathology and Cardiology Branches, National Heart, Lung, and Blood Institute, National Institutes of Health, Bethesda, Md.
Reprint requests: Dr. Roberts, National Institutes of Health, Bldg 10A, Room 3E30, Bethesda 20205

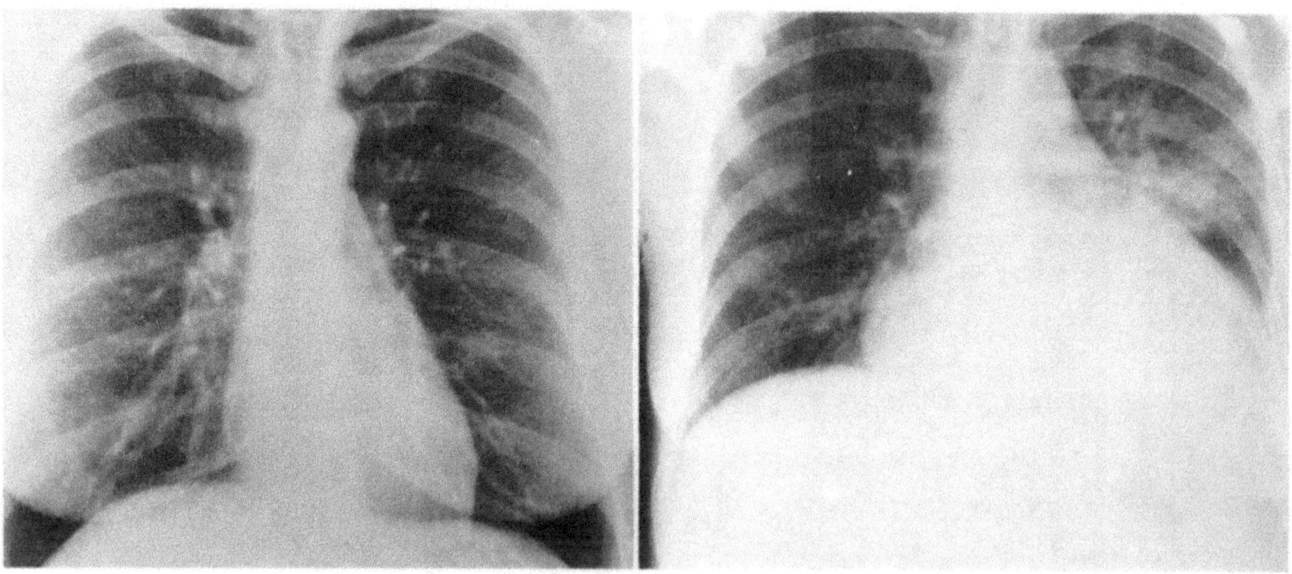

FIGURE 1. Posteroanterior chest roentgenograms. A (*left*), Normal findings (Jan 15, 1977). B (*right*), Chest roentgenogram taken on April 15, 1979 shows markedly enlarged cardiac silhouette, with bilateral pleural effusions and prominent pulmonary vascular markings, and none of these findings were present on earlier roentgenograms.

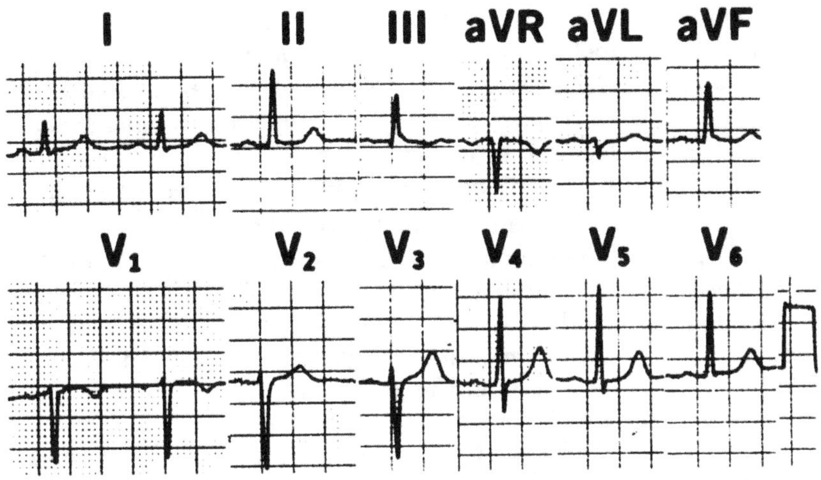

FIGURE 2. Electrocardiogram obtained two months before death shows sinus tachycardia, nonspecific changes in S-T segments and T waves, and low voltages.

silhouette was enlarged, and a large left-sided pleural effusion was present. The electrocardiogram (Fig 2) showed sinus tachycardia and nonspecific changes in the S-T segment and T wave; and the sum of the QRS complexes in leads 1, 2, and 3 was less than 15 mV.

By April 1979, the dyspnea was present at rest, and the patient coughed frequently. The systemic blood pressure was 110/75 mm Hg, and the systolic pressure fell 7 mm Hg with inspiration. The jugular veins were distended, and a "scratchy" systolic precordial murmur was present. On the chest roentgenogram (Fig 1), the cardiac silhouette was larger and echo-free spaces surrounded the heart on the echocardiogram (Fig 3). On cardiac catheterization, the pressures (in mm Hg) were as follows: right atrium, a 8 and v 10 (mean 9); right ventricle, 40/8; pulmonary artery, 40/16 (mean 22); and pulmonary arterial wedge, a 14 and v 16 (mean 24). Pericardiocentesis on April 27, 1979 yielded 200 ml of clear fluid. A pericardial drain was left in place and it yielded 2,200 ml of fluid over the next 11 days. The drain was then removed, and the patient went home. Nine days later (two days before death), she was

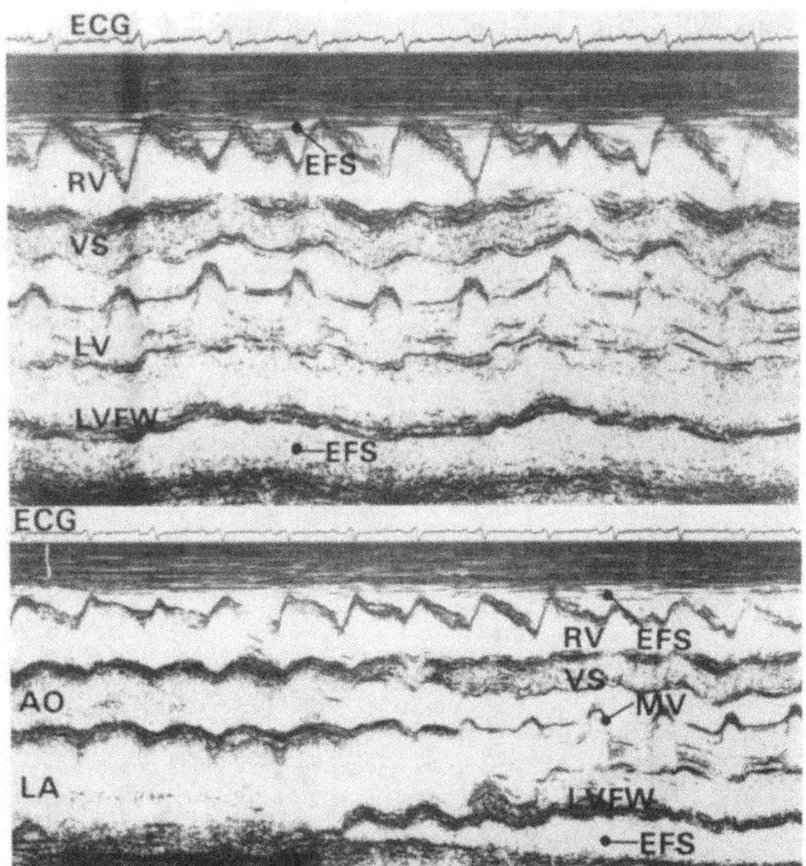

FIGURE 3. Echocardiogram obtained one month before death. Large echo-free spaces (EFS) are seen anterior to right ventricle (RV) and posterior to left ventricle (LV), and both spaces persist throughout systole and diastole, while posterior echo-free space disappears posterior to left atrium (LA). There is exaggerated anteroposterior movement of ventricles (so-called "swinging heart"). VS, Ventricular septum; LVFW, left ventricular free wall; AO, aorta; and MV, mitral valve.

again hospitalized because of progressively diminishing cerebral function. No clinical evidence of cardiac dysfunction was present on reexamination.

Dr. Roberts: Dr. Virmani, what was found at necropsy?

Dr. Renu Virmani: At necropsy, the pericardial sac contained about 200 ml of serous fluid. The heart weighed 440 gm, and the walls of all four cavities were extensively replaced by pigmented and nonpigmented melanoma (Fig 4 and 5), which also was present in the lungs, pleura, liver (2,100 gm, with about 80 percent replacement by tumor), kidneys (100 gm each, with over 90 percent replacement by tumor), adrenal glands, gastrointestinal tract, peritoneum, breast, skin, and spleen (histologically only).

Dr. Roberts: The patient had a small melanoma removed from the leg, and she remained free of clinical evidence of local recurrence or metastases until 14 years later (28 months before death). At necropsy, virtually every organ of the body was riddled with melanoma.

During the 1930s, many reports, primarily studies of individual cases, described patients with cardiac metastases from a variety of cancers. In more recent years, when large series of patients with various types of cardiac metastases were collected, it became apparent that from a percentage standpoint, melanoma was the most frequent neoplasm metastasizing to the heart. *Of 100 necropsies of patients with each type of malignant neoplasm,* the incidence of metastases to the heart is highest in melanoma (about 65 percent),[1] followed by leukemia (about 37 percent),[2] lymphoma (about 25 percent)[3] and then lung and breast (each about 10 percent).[4,5] If this frequency of cardiac metastases is looked at in another way, *ie, of 100 necropsies in patients with cardiac metastases of all types,* the secondary tumor most frequent in the heart is lung (in men) and breast (in women), each about 10 percent, and the incidence of the other metastatic cancers is considerably less than 10 percent.

Not only is melanoma the most frequent tumor metastasizing to the heart on a percentage basis, again assuming 100 cases of each type of cancer, but also the absolute amount of tumor deposited in the heart in melanoma is, on the whole, far greater than with any other cancer;[1] for example, in the present patient the percentage of right and left ventricular myocardium replaced by melanoma was enormous (Fig 5), yet despite the huge size and numbers of deposits of tumor in the heart, there was no clear clinical evidence of cardiac dysfunction. About 60 days before death, the patient complained of dyspnea, but a large pleural effusion was present, metastases to the lung were apparent, and only 200 ml of pericardial fluid was found, not enough to

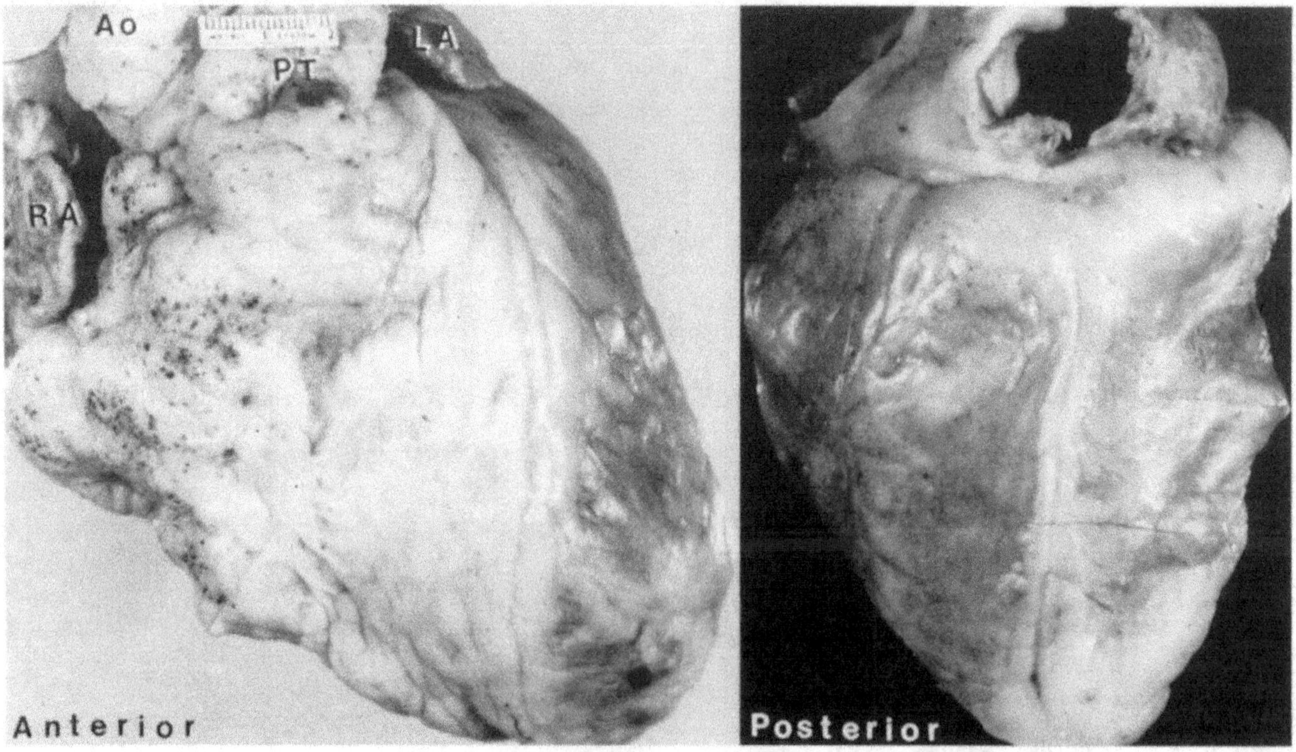

FIGURE 4. Anterior and posterior external views of heart, showing pigmented epicardial melanotic implants. Ao, Aorta; PT, pulmonary trunk; LA, left atrium; and RA, right atrium.

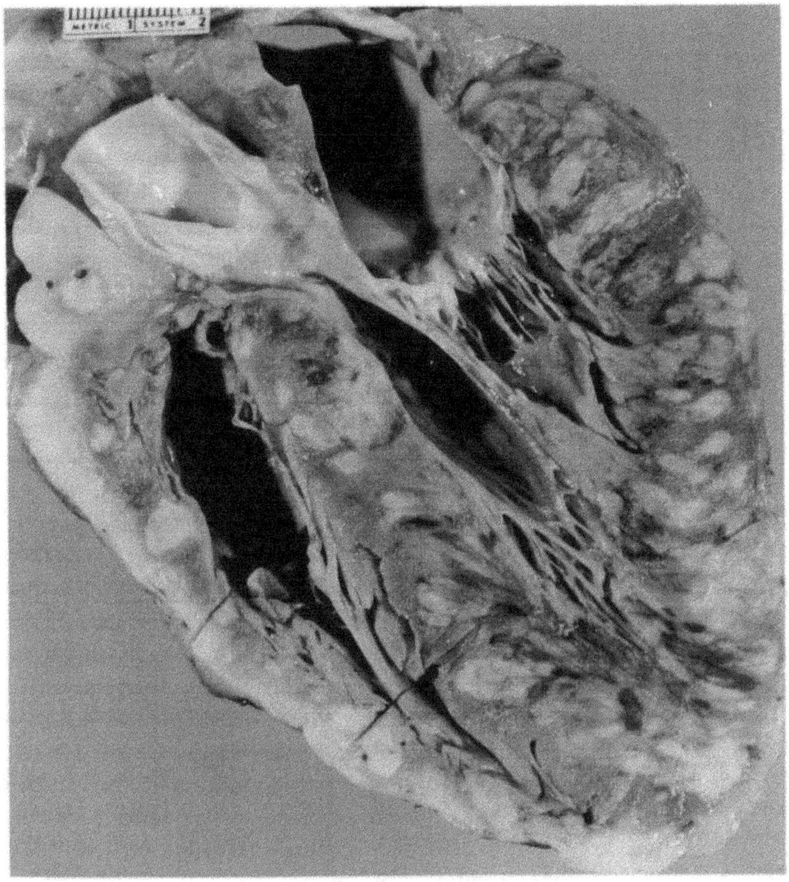

FIGURE 5. Longitudinal section of heart, showing massive myocardial replacement by pigmented and nonpigmented melanoma.

cause myocardial compression. The distended veins in the neck and the quiet heart sounds could easily have resulted from the pulmonary problems. Cardiac catheterization, performed about a month before death, ruled out the presence of cardiac tamponade by the finding of much higher pulmonary arterial mean wedge and pulmonary arterial diastolic pressures than the right atrial mean and right ventricular end-diastolic pressures. Pericardiocentesis, which was done 22 days before death, yielded about 200 ml of serous fluid, and a pericardial drain was left in place for the following 11 days, but only an average of 200 ml of clear fluid was drained from the pericardial space during each of the 11 days. The tube was then removed, pericardiocentesis was never repeated, and at necropsy, only about 200 ml of fluid was found. After the pericardial drain was removed, evidence of cardiac dysfunction did not appear.

The patient's final few days were characterized by diminishing cerebral function. The acta scan disclosed no evidence of metastases to the brain, and at necropsy the brain was normal. Thus, the possibility that the cerebral symptoms were due to inadequate arterial profusion of the brain due to poor myocardial function must be considered. The presence of the large deposits of melanoma in the walls of the cardiac ventricles suggests that the ventricles did not function normally; however, despite these deposits of tumor, neither ventricle became dilated.

Dr. Gottdiener, could you summarize the expected M-mode echocardiographic findings in patients with pericardial effusions and point out the usefulness or the lack thereof of the echocardiogram in differentiating pericardial effusion with tamponade from that without tamponade?

Dr. John S. Gottdiener: Detection of pericardial effusion was one of the first applications of echocardiography and still remains the most sensitive and reliable method for establishing this diagnosis.[6,7] The diagnosis of pericardial effusion by M-mode echocardiographic studies is suggested by the presence of an echo-free space between the epicardium of the left ventricular free wall and the parietal pericardium. With large effusions an echo-free space also may be present anterior to the right ventricular epicardium. While an isolated continuous (systolic and diastolic) posterior echo-free space generally indicates pericardial effusion, an isolated anterior echo-free space may occur without an effusion. Other echocardiographic consequences of a large accumulation of fluid in the pericardial sac include (1) an exaggerated anteroposterior movement of the ventricles (so-called "swinging heart"); (2) parallel movement of the left and right ventricular free walls and ventricular septum, rather than movement in opposite directions; (3) varying distances from the anterior wall of the chest to the epicardial surface of the right ventricle with each heartbeat (the equivalent of electrical alternans); (4) pseudomitral valve prolapse; and (5) beat-to-beat variation in the excursion of the anterior mitral leaflet in ventricular diastole (D to E points).

Although highly sensitive and specific in detecting pericardial effusions, ultrasound is less useful in detecting the presence of cardiac tamponade, which remains primarily a *clinical* judgment; however, recently, the following two echocardiographic patterns[8,9] suggestive of tamponade have been reported: (1) an increase in the end-diastolic right ventricular dimension during inspiration, with a simultaneous decrease in the dimension of the left ventricular cavity; and (2) an alternation of the E-to F slope (mitral valvular closing velocity). Both findings disappear after relief of the tamponade. Thus, while it is very helpful in diagnosing pericardial effusion, echocardiographic study currently is of limited value in diagnosing cardiac tamponade.

Dr. Roberts: The composition of the pericardial fluid in the present patient was serous and virtually devoid of erythrocytes. It is well appreciated that hemorrhagic effusions suggest the possibility of cancer. In our patient the heart could hardly have had more metastatic implants, some of which were epicardial in location (Fig 4), and yet the fluid in the pericardial space was clear. In a study of necropsies of patients with lymphoma,[3] it was shown that pericardial, pleural, and peritoneal effusions were more commonly related to the presence of severe hypoalbuminemia in the serum than to the presence of deposits of tumor on the serosal surfaces. The present patient had a serum level of albumin of 2.4 gm/100 ml during the last month of life.

Dr. Waller, what clinical or laboratory findings are most helpful in diagnosing secondary metastases to the heart?

Dr. Waller: A wide variety of clinical, electrocardiographic, and roentgenographic findings have been used to diagnose cardiac dysfunction due to cardiac metastases. Some clinical features have little or no correlation with the presence or extent of cardiac metastases; for example, sinus tachycardia, which has frequently been suggested as a criterion for clinically determining the presence of cardiac metastases, is found during the last weeks of life in at least half of the patients dying of malignant melanoma who have no cardiac metastases. Nevertheless, the presence of cardiac metastases can often be determined before death. The development of cardiac dysfunction without other apparent cause in a patient known to have a malignant tumor suggests cardiac metastases; however, the problem is being certain that the clinical findings really indicate cardiac dysfunction, rather than their being the result of associated anemia, hypoproteinemia, or pulmonary metastases. Dyspnea, tachypnea, tachycardia, systolic precordial murmurs, edema, effusions into body cavities, or any of several electrocardiographic abnormalities may occur in patients with malignant tumors but without cardiac metastases. On the other hand, one or more of the following clinical findings in a patient with a malignant tumor and without previous heart disease strongly suggests the presence of cardiac metastases: *(1) acute pericarditis; (2) cardiac tamponade or constriction; (3) rapid increase in the size of the heart on the roentgenogram; (4) onset of an ectopic tachycardia; (5) development of second-degree or third-degree atrioventricular block; and (6) onset of unequivocal congestive cardiac failure.* Cytologic examination of pericardial fluid and angiocardiograms obviously will increase the accuracy of diagnosing cardiac metastases. When the tumor is metastatic melanoma, the clinical diagnosis of cardiac metastases is aided by the knowledge that two of three patients will develop tumor of the heart before death.

Dr. Roberts: If a person lost as much myocardium as our patient through myocardial infarction from coronary heart disease, the ECG almost certainly would have indicated "myocardial damage." In the present patient, in whom probably over half of the ventricular myocardium had been replaced by tumor, evidence of myocardial damage on the ECG was lacking. Why the ECG is so useful in myocardial necrosis but so unhelpful in myocardial replacement due to secondary tumor is unclear. There has been only one study, to my knowledge, in which patients with a specific cancer with metastases to the heart have had their ECGs analyzed and compared to patients with the same neoplasm but without metastases to the heart.[3] When this control type of electrocardiographic analysis is performed on patients with specific cancers, the frequency of electrocardiographic abnormalities is identical in the patients with compared to those without cardiac metastases but with the same malignant tumor of the body.[3,10]

References

1 Glancy DL, Roberts WC: The heart in malignant melanoma: A study of 70 autopsy cases. Am J Cardiol 21:555-571, 1968

2 Roberts WC, Bodey GP, Wertlake PT: The heart in acute leukemia: A study of 420 autopsy cases. Am J Cardiol 21:388-412, 1968

3 Roberts WC, Glancy DL, DeVita VJ Jr: Heart in malignant lymphoma (Hodgkin's disease, lymphosarcoma, reticulum cell sarcoma and mycosis fungoides). A study of 196 autopsy cases. Am J Cardiol 22:85-107, 1968
4 Onuigbo WI: The spread of lung cancer to the heart, pericardium, and great vessels. Jpn Heart J 15:234-238, 1974
5 Kline IK: Cardiac lymphatic involvement by metastatic tumor. Cancer 29:799-808, 1972
6 Feigenbaum H, Waldhausen JA, Hyde LP: Ultrasound diagnosis of pericardial effusion. JAMA 191:107-112, 1965
7 Horowitz MS, Schultz CS, Stinson EB, et al: Sensitivity and specificity of echocardiographic diagnosis of pericardial effusion. Circulation 50:239-247, 1974
8 D'Cruz IA, Cohen HC, Prabhu R, et al: Diagnosis of cardiac tamponade by echocardiography. Circulation 52: 460-465, 1975
9 Settle HP, Adolph RJ, Fowler NO, et al: Echocardiographic study of cardiac tamponade. Circulation 56:951-959, 1977
10 Lindsay J Jr, Goldberg SD, Roberts WC: Electrocardiogram in neoplastic and hematologic disorders. Cardiovasc Clin 8:225-242, 1977

Radiation Heart Disease

Analysis of 16 Young (Aged 15 to 33 Years) Necropsy Patients Who Received Over 3,500 Rads to the Heart

FRANK C. BROSIUS, III, M.D.*
BRUCE F. WALLER, M.D.
WILLIAM C. ROBERTS, M.D.
Bethesda, Maryland

Certain clinical and necropsy findings are described in 16 young (aged 15 to 33 years) patients who received >3,500 rads to the heart five to 144 months before death. All 16 had some radiation-induced damage to the heart: 15 had thickened pericardia (five of whom had evidence of cardiac tamponade); eight had increased interstitial myocardial fibrosis, particularly in the right ventricle; 12 had fibrous thickening of the mural endocardium and 13 of the valvular endocardium. Except for valvular thickening, the changes were more frequent in the right side of the heart than in the left, presumably because of higher radiation doses to the anterior surface of the heart. In six of the 16 study patients and in one of 10 control subjects, one or more major epicardial coronary arteries were narrowed from 76 to 100 percent in cross-sectional area by atherosclerotic plaque; one patient had a healed myocardial infarct at necropsy and one died suddenly. In 10 patients and in the 10 control subjects, the four major epicardial coronary arteries were examined quantitatively: 6 percent of the 469 five millimeter segments of coronary artery from the patients were narrowed from 76 to 100 percent (controls = 0.2 percent, p = 0.06) and 22 percent were narrowed from 51 to 75 percent (controls = 12 percent). The proximal portion of the arteries in the patients had significantly more narrowing than the distal portions. The arterial plaques in the patients were largely composed of fibrous tissue; the media were frequently replaced by fibrous tissue, and the adventitia were often densely thickened by fibrous tissue. In five patients, there was focal thickening (with or without luminal narrowing) of the intramural coronary arteries. Thus, radiation to the heart may produce a wide spectrum of functional and anatomic changes but particularly damage to the pericardia and the underlying epicardial coronary arteries.

In the early part of this century, the heart was considered a "radioresistant" organ [1,2]. With the introduction of megavoltage radiotherapy for treatment of neoplasms, however, it became apparent that the heart could, indeed, be damaged by high-dose radiation. The nature and extent of the damage, however, in both human subjects and in nonhuman experimental animals are still debated. Pericardial thickening with or without effusion or constriction has been confirmed from several centers [3-28]. In several "case reports" clinical or necropsy evidence of myocardial ischemia and coronary arterial narrowing has been described in young persons who had received high-dose mediastinal radiation [10,29-41]. Increased myocardial fibrosis

From the Pathology Branch, National Heart, Lung, and Blood Institute, National Institutes of Health, Bethesda, Maryland. Requests for reprints should be addressed to Dr. William C. Roberts, Building 10A, Room 3E-30, National Institutes of Health, Bethesda, MD 20205. Manuscript accepted September 11, 1980.

* Present address: Department of Medicine, University of Michigan Medical Center, Ann Arbor, MI 48104.

has been described as a consequence of high-dose mediastinal irradiation [3,10,11,16,25,42–46]. The effect of high-dose radiation on the mural and valvular endocardium has received virtually no attention. Furthermore, the extensiveness of the coronary disease has not been described previously in young necropsy patients who received megavoltage therapy to the mediastinum. In the report which follows, the effect of high-dose irradiation in 16 young necropsy patients is described. Particular attention is given to the mural and valvular endocardial damage and to the extent of the coronary narrowing that were found.

PATIENTS STUDIED AND FINDINGS

To be included in this study, patients had to be under 35 years of age at death, had to have had an autopsy, had to have received a total of more than 3,500 rads to the heart, and the heart specimens had to be examined by at least one of us. Sixteen patients fulfilled these criteria. Certain clinical and necropsy observations in them are summarized in **Table I.** The patients ranged in age from 15 to 33 years (mean 26 years) at death; 13 were men and three were women (Patients 6, 10, and 13, Table I). Thirteen had Hodgkin's disease; two (Patients 8 and 15), carcinoid; and one (Patient 10), histiocytic lymphoma. The number of rads administered to the anterior surface of the heart ranged from 3,987 to 8,769 (mean 5,592), and to the posterior surface, from 3,000 to 5,000 (mean 3,932). (The method for calculating the radiation dose is described in the Appendix.) In 15 patients the apical portion of the heart was excluded from the direct radiation field. The interval from the end of the irradiation period to death ranged from five to 144 months (mean 55 months). Ten patients received one or more chemotherapeutic agents, including six who received prednisone (for one to 12 six-week periods) and three who received doxorubicin. None had cushingoid features at any time. No patient had clinical evidence of chronic congestive cardiac failure and none had chest pain which could have been interpreted as evidence of myocardial ischemia. Six patients smoked cigarettes (10 to 20 daily). Electrocardiograms, recorded in 14 patients (all after irradiation), disclosed sinus rhythm in all, nonspecific S-T segment or T wave changes in nine, low (sum of QRS complexes in leads I, II and III ≤15 mv) voltage in five (four had pericardial effusions) and complete right bundle branch block in one.

Five patients had large cardiac silhouettes on chest roentgenograms (**Figure 1**), and five had clinical findings (distended neck veins, subcutaneous edema, paradoxical pulse and Kussmaul's sign) of cardiac tamponade. Four of the five patients with clinical features of tamponade had pericardiocentesis with removal of large quantities of fluid (Figure 1), and two patients (Patients 9 and 12, Table I) subsequently had partial pericardiectomies because of recurring signs of cardiac tamponade.

Blood hematocrit values about one month before death ranged from 20 to 48 percent (mean 33 percent); serum total protein, 3.5 to 7.5 g/dl (mean 5.5 g/dl); and serum albumin, from 1.3 to 4.9 g/dl (mean 2.8 g/dl). The highest total serum

TABLE I Clinical and Necropsy Findings in 16 Patients with Radiation Heart Disease

Patient	Age (yr)	Age (yr) at Dx	Calculated Rad to Heart		Mo. from Rad to Death	CT	TC*	Hct† (%)	HW (g)	PE	TE		IMF			No. 5-mm S CAs	No. 5-mm S >75% XSA	TICA	
			Ant	Post							M	V	RV	VS	LV			RV	LV
1	15	12	5,202	3,000	34	0	129	43	170	300‡	+	+	+	0	0	...	...	+	0
2	19	16	5,648	3,600	35	0	139	20	270	0	+	+	+	0	0	...	...	0	0
3	24	23	5,842	3,500	22	+	140	39	245	100	0	+	+	+	+	50	0	+	0
4	24	20	5,295	3,600	42	+	120	29	190	260	+	+	+	0	0	54	0	+	0
5	25	22	5,186	3,092	39	0	172	30	290	75	0	+	0	...	0	44	2	0	0
6	25	23	4,100	4,000	11	0	176	37	250	0	+	+	+	+	...	55	0	+	0
7	26	19	4,185	3,000	78	0	146	21	250	200	+	+	+	0	+	...	...	0	0
8	26	24	3,987	3,600	5	0	250	34	290	0	+	+	0	0	0	50	8	0	0
9	27	20	7,047	4,000	53	+	198	...	370	0	+	+	0	...	0	44	0	0	0
10	29	27	4,932	4,200	20	0	168	31	155	0	+	+	+	0	0	42	0	0	0
11	29	17	4,054	4,000	144	0	168	27	240	0	0	0	0	...	0	37	1	0	0
12	29	21	4,341	4,025	84, 62§	+	...	27	225	0	+	+	0	0	0	43	12	0	0
13	30	25	5,419	4,495	44	0	187	35	170	0	+	+	0	0	0	...	...	0	0
14	30	27	8,769	4,800	27,2§	+	130	31	...	375	+	0	0	0	0	...	...	0	0
15	33	20	6,600	5,000	137	0	170	45	230	0	0	0	0	0	0	50	5	0	0
16	33	24	8,866	5,000	104	0	308	48	350	0	+	+	+	0	+	13	5	+	+

NOTE: + = present; 0 = absent or none; . . . = no data; CA = coronary artery; CT = cardiac tamponade; Dx = diagnosis; ECG = electrocardiogram; Hct = hematocrit; HW = heart weight; IMF = interstitial myocardial fibrosis; LV = left ventricle; M = mural; PE = pericardial effusion; RV = right ventricle; S = segments; TC = total serum cholesterol; TE = grossly thickened endocardium; TICA = thickened intramural coronary artery; V = valve; VS = ventricular septum; XSA = cross-sectional area.
* Highest recorded value.
† Value about one month before death.
‡ Number of milliliters.
§ Received two courses of radiotherapy.

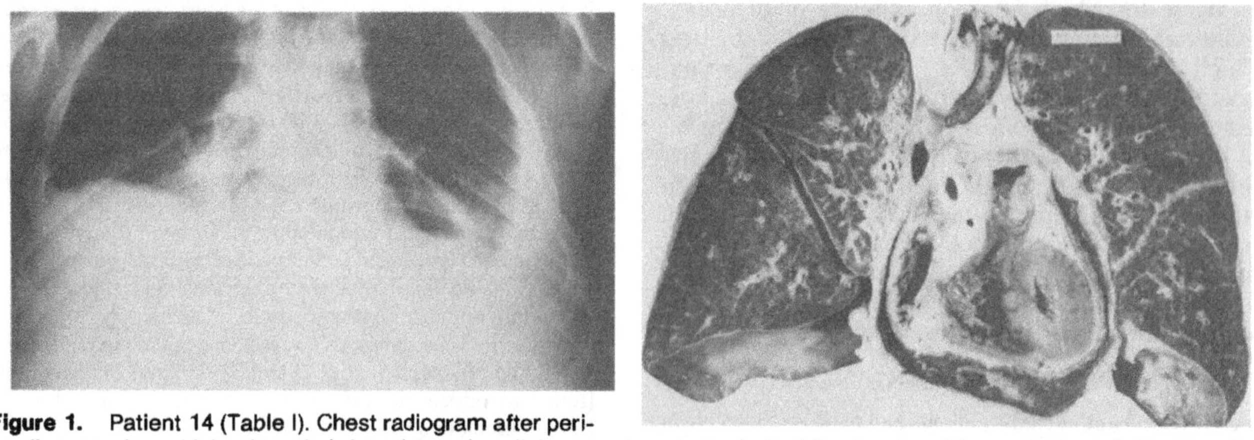

Figure 1. Patient 14 (Table I). Chest radiogram after pericardiocentesis and injection of air into the pericardial sac and posterior half of the heart and lungs (**left**), and after they had been sectioned longitudinally (**right**). The pericardia are thickened primarily by fibrous tissue.

cholesterol values (15 patients) ranged from 120 to 308 mg/dl (mean 173 mg/dl); this value was >180 mg/dl in four patients.

An additional 10 patients matched closely for age and sex to the study patients were used as control subjects. Certain characteristics of them are shown in **Table II.** None received therapeutic mediastinal irradiation, none ever had symptoms of cardiac dysfunction, all died from noncardiac conditions, and seven received one or more chemotherapeutic agents, including six who received prednisone (for one or more six-week periods) and one who received doxorubicin.

At necropsy, *fluid* was present in the *pericardial* sacs in 12 of the 16 study patients: in six, the amount was <50 ml; in the other six, 75 to 375 ml. The remaining four patients (Patients 9, 10, 12 and 13, Table I) had pericardial *fibrous* adhesions which obliterated the pericardial spaces, but two had had partial pericardiectomies. Four patients had *fibrinous* pericardial adhesions (**Figure 2**). In all but one patient the epicardial surface was thickened by fibrous tissue (Figure 2). The hearts ranged in weight from 155 to 370 g (mean 246 g). None of the 16 patients had grossly visible or histologically discernible foci of myocardial coagulation necrosis. Only one patient (Patient 12, Table I, **Figure 3**) had a grossly visible scar on the ventricular wall at necropsy; in him it involved the posterior wall of the left ventricle, and the three major (right, left anterior descending and left circumflex) epicardial coronary arteries were severely narrowed. On histologic examination of at least one histologic section from the wall of each cardiac ventricle (mean 2.5 sections per ventricle), increased *interstitial myocardial fibrosis* was observed in the right ventricular free wall in eight patients (**Figure 4**), in the left ventricular free wall in three patients and in the ventricular septum in two patients. In one of the 10 control subjects, mild interstitial myocardial fibrosis was observed (Table II). Unequivocal damage to individual myocardial cells was not detected in any study patient or in any control subject by histologic study.

The *mural endocardium* of one or more chambers was

TABLE II **Clinical and Necropsy Findings in 10 Control Subjects**

Control Subjects	Age (yr)	Dx	Age at Dx (yr)	TC (mg/dl)	Hct (%)	TSP (g/dl)	Alb (g/dl)	HW (g)	IMF RV	IMF VS	IMF LV	No. 5-mm Segments of 4 Major CAs	No. Narrowed >75%
1	19	U*	19	...	...	...	...	370	0	0	0	63	0
2	21	AML	18	86	35	7.1	4.0	280	0	0	0	22	0
3	22	ALL	20	200	31	3.8	1.6	500	0	0	0	56	0
4	23	ALL	19	178	19	7.1	4.7	430	0	0	0	62	0
5	26	CML	21	154	30	3.9	1.2	220	0	0	0	42	1
6	28	HL	28	147	34	4.4	2.3	360	0	0	0	37	0
7	29	Ch	28	...	27	6.7	2.7	200	0	0	0	28	0
8	29	BT	28	212	34	6.5	2.8	270	0	0	0	46	0
9	33	MM	30	182	...	6.1	3.1	280	0	0	0	48	0
10	36	HS	...	...	...	...	...	...	+	...	+	34	0

NOTE: + = present; 0 = absent or none; . . . = no data; Alb = albumin; ALL = acute lymphocytic leukemia; AML = acute myelocytic leukemia; BT = brain tumor; CA = coronary artery; Ch = choriocarcinoma; CML = chronic myelocytic leukemia; Dx = diagnosis; Hct = hematocrit; HL = histiocytic lymphoma; HS = heat stroke; HW = heart weight; IMF = interstitial myocardial fibrosis; MM = malignant melanoma; TC = total serum cholesterol; U = unknown.

* Idiopathic sudden death.

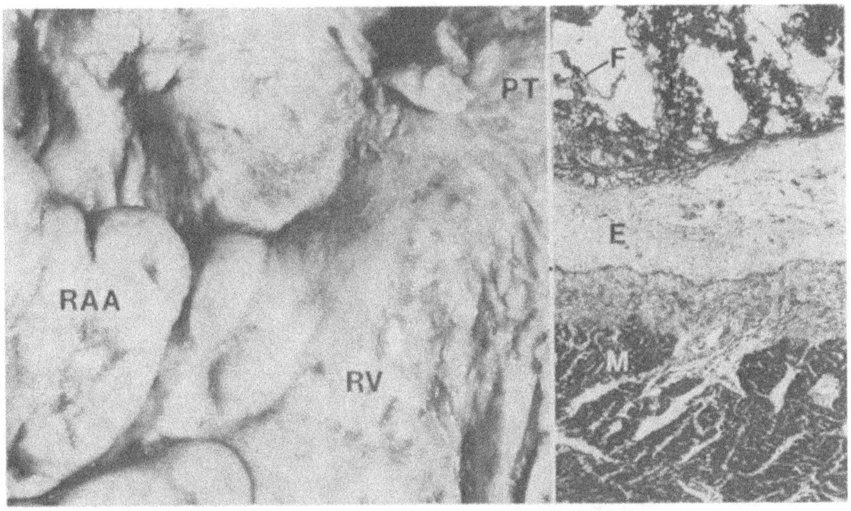

Figure 2. *Fibrinous pericarditis.* **a,** Patient 7 (Table I). Close-up of the epicardial surface of the right atrial appendage (RAA), right ventricle (RV) and pulmonary trunk (PT) demonstrating thickened epicardium and fibrinous deposits. **b,** Patient 12 (Table I). Photomicrograph of a portion of right ventricular surface showing thickened epicardium (E) and overlying fibrinous deposits (F). M = myocardium. Movat stain; magnification × 35, reduced by 16 percent.

thickened in 12 patients: right atrium in eight; right ventricle in 10 (**Figure 5**); left atrium in none and left ventricle in three. This thickening resulted from proliferation of fibrous tissue, containing some elastic fibers. One or more *cardiac valves* were focally thickened by fibrous tissue (often with substantial numbers of elastic fibers) in 13 patients; tricuspid in eight; pulmonic in two, mitral in 13 (**Figure 6**) and aortic in eight. The thickening in all patients was relatively mild and not sufficient

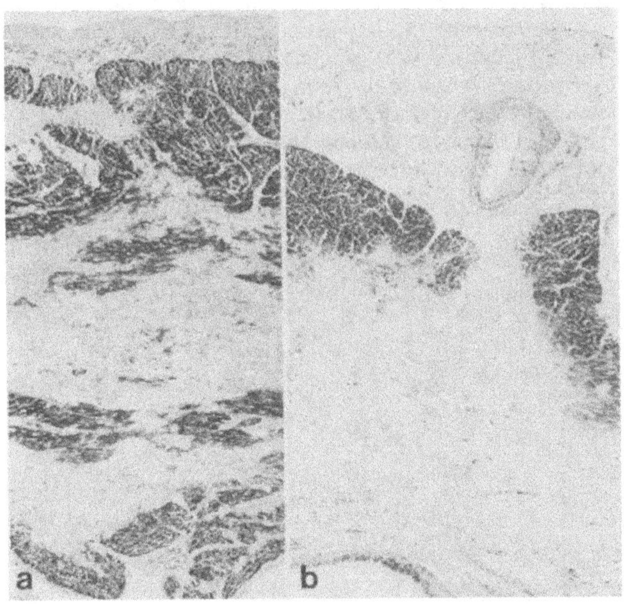

Figure 3. Patient 12 (Table I). Transmural replacement fibrosis of the right ventricle (a) and of the left ventricle (b). The left ventricle is abnormally thinned. Movat stains; magnification each × 21, reduced by 32 percent.

to produce valvular dysfunction. Neither of the two patients with the carcinoid syndrome had carcinoid heart disease [46].

Six of the 16 study patients had one or more of their four major (right, left main, left anterior descending, left circumflex) *epicardial* (extramural) *coronary arteries* narrowed >75 percent in cross-sectional area by atherosclerotic plaque (**Figures 7 and 8**): only one of the four major arteries was so narrowed in one patient, two arteries in one patient; three arteries in three patients; and four arteries in one patient. Thus, of the 64 major coronary arteries in the 16 study patients, the lumens in 16 (25 percent) were narrowed from 76 to 100 percent in cross-sectional area, an average of one of four major coronary arteries per patient. Of the 40 major coronary arteries in the 10 control subjects, only one was narrowed from 75 to 100 percent in cross-sectional area by atherosclerotic plaque.

In 10 of the 16 patients and in all 10 control subjects, the four major epicardial coronary arteries were examined in detail as follows. Each was excised intact, roentgenographed and cut transversely (to its longitudinal axis) into 5-mm long segments. Each segment was labelled sequentially from either its aortic ostium or from its origin from the left main artery. The 5-mm segments were labeled, dehydrated (alcohol and xylene), embedded in paraffin, and two histologic sections were cut and stained from each paraffin block. The Movat stain was used on one histologic section, and all determinations of luminal narrowing were based on examination of the Movat-stained sections. The degrees of narrowing were based on histologic examination by two of us of each cross-section magnified 25 to 50 times. The judgment regarding the degree of luminal narrowing of each 5-mm segment was based on the degree of luminal obliteration within the luminal circle bordered by the internal elastic membrane. The circle was visually subdivided into four equal-sized quadrants, and the percent of cross-

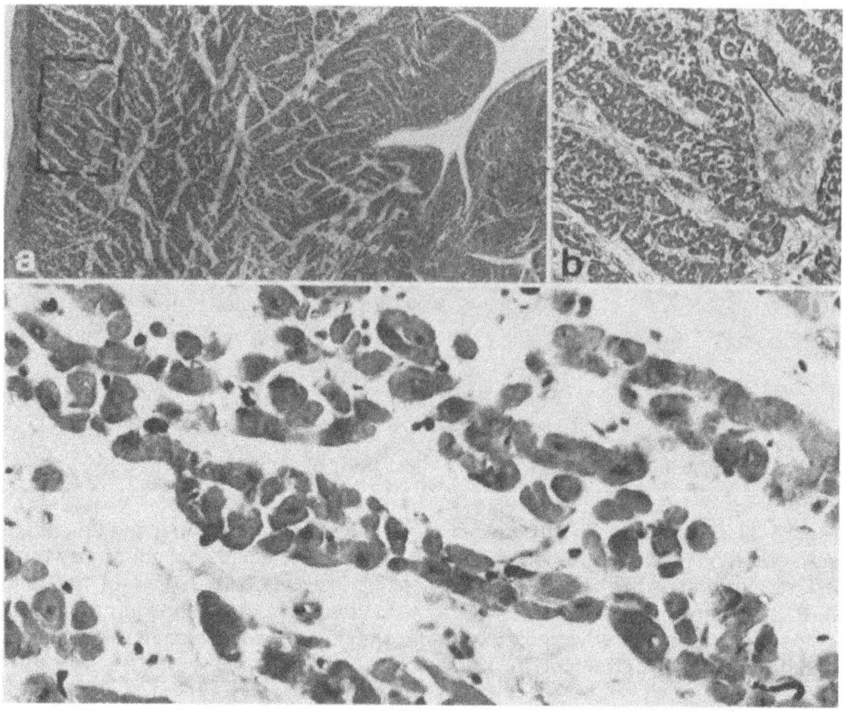

Figure 4. Photomicrographs (**a** and **b** [boxed-portion of **a**]) of the right ventricular free wall in Patient 3 (Table I). The amount of interstitial fibrous tissue is increased. An intramural coronary artery (CA) is thickened and narrowed by fibrous tissue. **Lower,** close-up of a portion of right ventricular myocardium in Patient 6 (Table I) showing increased interstitial fibrous tissue. Hematoxylin and eosin stains, magnification × 11 (**a**), × 55 (**b**); and Movat stain; magnification × 256 (**lower**), reduced by 14 percent.

sectional area luminal narrowing in each 5-mm segment was determined as follows: 0 to 25, 26 to 50, 51 to 75 and 76 to 100. Reliability of such assessment in comparison to values obtained by video-planimetry has been shown to be very high [47]. Of the 469 five-mm long segments of major coronary artery examined in the 10 study patients, 28 (6 percent) were narrowed from 76 to 100 percent in cross-sectional area by atherosclerotic plaque (controls = 0.2 percent); 103 (22 percent) were narrowed from 51 to 75 percent (controls = 12 percent); 207 (44 percent) were narrowed from 26 to 50 percent (controls = 67 percent) and 131 (28 percent) were narrowed from 0 to 25 percent (controls = 21 percent) (**Figure 9**). The amount of narrowing in each of the four categories of narrowing was similar for each of the four major coronary arteries in the study patients (**Figure 10**); similarly, in the control subjects (Figure 10). A significantly ($p < 0.02$) higher percent of 5-mm segments

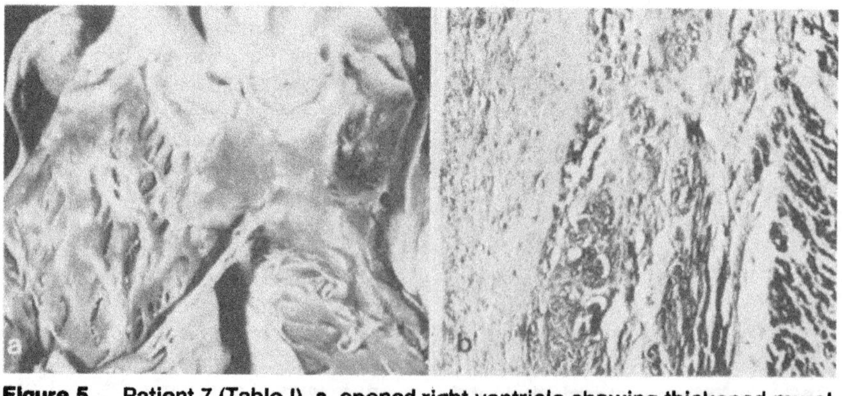

Figure 5. Patient 7 (Table I). **a,** opened right ventricle showing thickened mural endocardium; the pulmonic valve cusps are also mildly thickened. **b,** photomicrograph of the thickened right ventricular endocardium and interstitial myocardial fibrosis. Movat stain; magnification × 55, reduced by 41 percent.

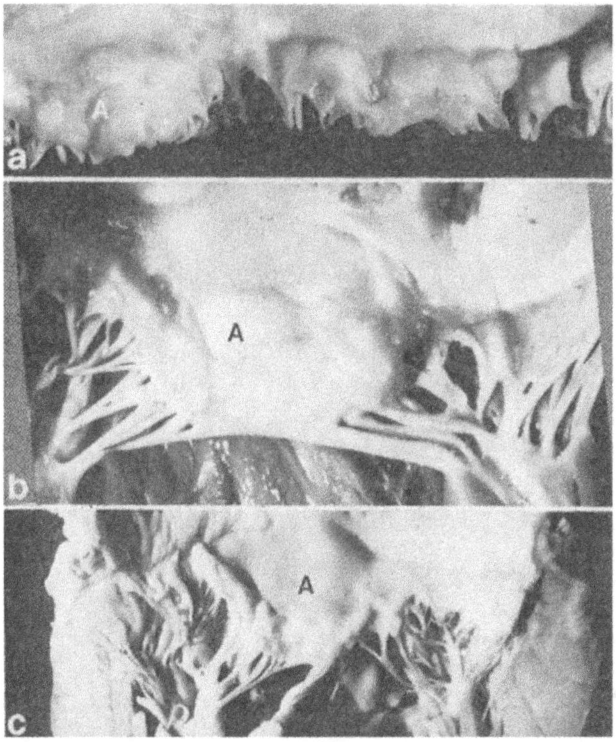

Figure 6. Mitral valves in Patients 12 (**a**), 13 (**b**) and 3 (**c**) (Table I). Each valve, especially the anterior (A) leaflet, is focally thickened by fibrous tissue.

in the proximal halves of the right and left anterior descending coronary arteries in the study patients were narrowed >50 percent in cross-sectional area than in the distal halves of these arteries (**Figure 11**).

In each of the 469 histologic sections of major coronary artery in the 10 study patients (plus 13 sections in Patient 16; total 482), and in each of the 438 sections of coronary artery in the 10 control subjects, the composition of intimal, medial and adventitial lesions was determined (**Figure 12**). Of the 482 sections of coronary artery examined in the 11 study patients, the intimal lesions in all consisted mainly of fibrous tissue: in 339 sections (70 percent), entirely of fibrous tissue (controls = 365 sections [83 percent]); in four sections (1 percent), of fibrous tissue plus calcific deposits (controls = 0); in 120 sections (25 percent), of fibrous tissue plus lipid deposits (controls = 68 sections [16 percent]); and in the remaining 19 sections (4 percent), of fibrous tissue, lipid and calcific deposits (controls = five sections [1 percent]). Thus, 100 percent (482 sections) of the intimal lesions contained fibrous tissue, 29 percent (134 sections) contained lipid, usually both intracellular ("foam cells") and extracellular (controls = 18 percent of sections contained lipid), and 5 percent (23 sections) contained calcific deposits (controls = 1 percent). The internal elastic membrane was disrupted in 187 (39 percent) of 482 sections in the study patients and in 148 (34 percent) of the 438 sections in the control subjects.

The media of the coronary arteries in the 482 sections in the 11 study patients was partially replaced by fibrous tissue in 364

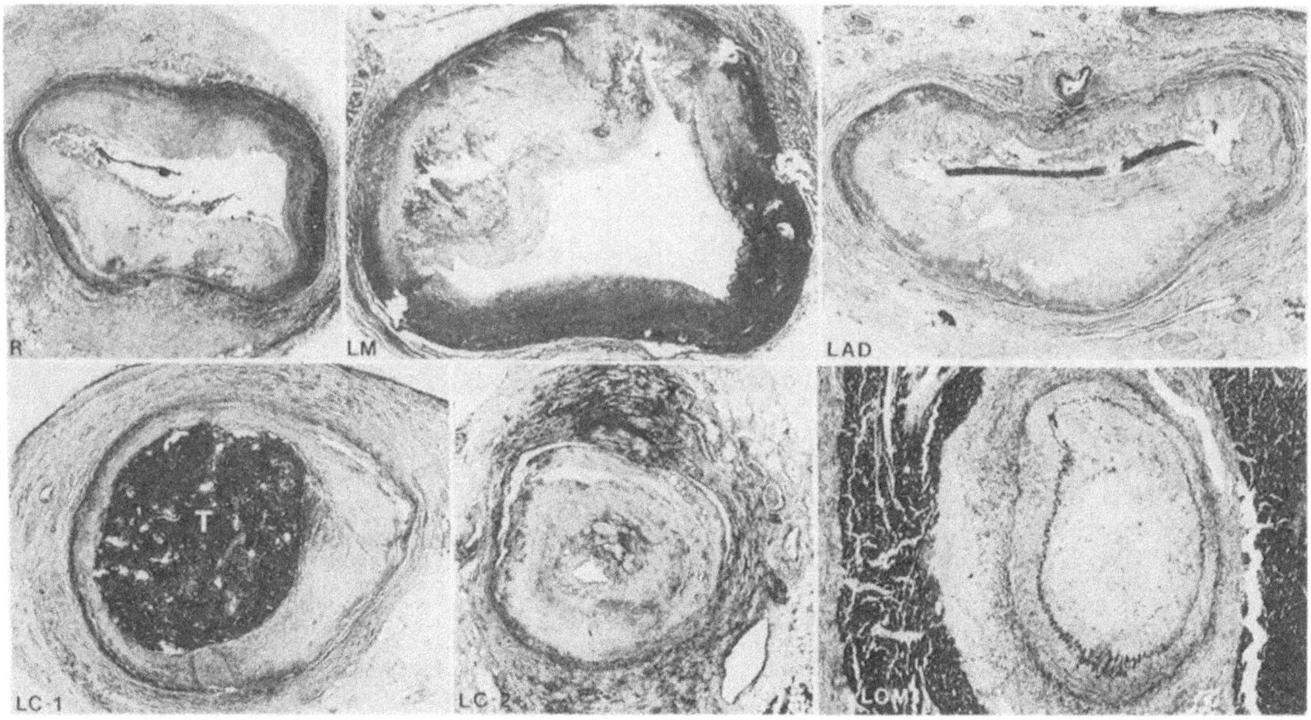

Figure 7. Patient 12 (Table 1). Major epicardial coronary arteries showing severe luminal narrowing by atherosclerotic plaques and medial and adventitial fibrosis. R = right; LM = left main; LAD = left anterior descending; LC = left circumflex; and LOM = left obtuse marginal coronary arteries. The proximal portion of the left circumflex artery (LC-1) contains an organized thrombus (T), just distal to which the artery is narrowed >95 percent in cross-sectional area by atherosclerotic plaque. The left oblique marginal artery is totally occluded as it tunnels into left ventricular myocardium. Movat stains; magnification × 27 (R, LM, LAD, LC-1 and LC-2); and × 35 (LOM), reduced by 38 percent.

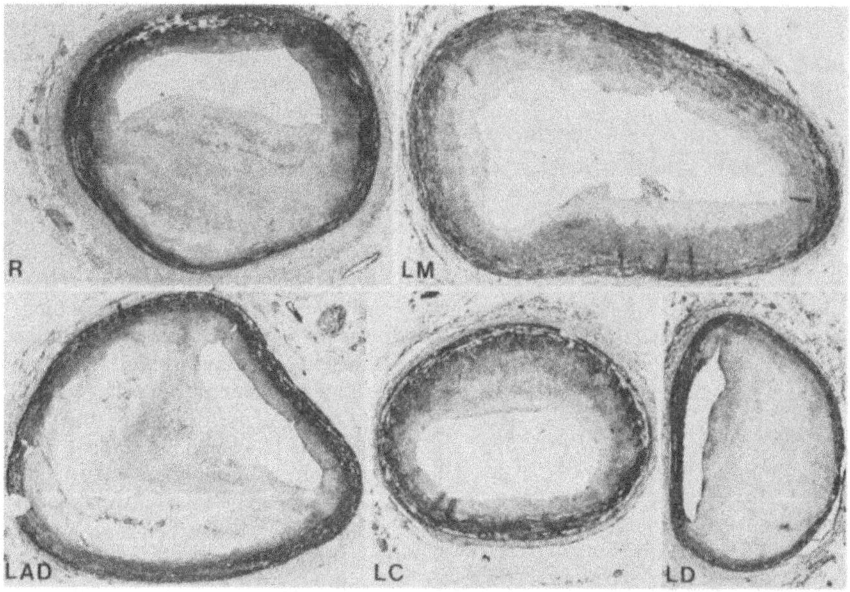

Figure 8. Patient 8 (Table I). Major epicardial coronary arteries at sites of maximal luminal narrowing. R = right; LM = left main; LAD = left anterior descending; LC = left circumflex; and LD = left diagonal coronary arteries. Movat stains; magnification each × 20, reduced by 30 percent.

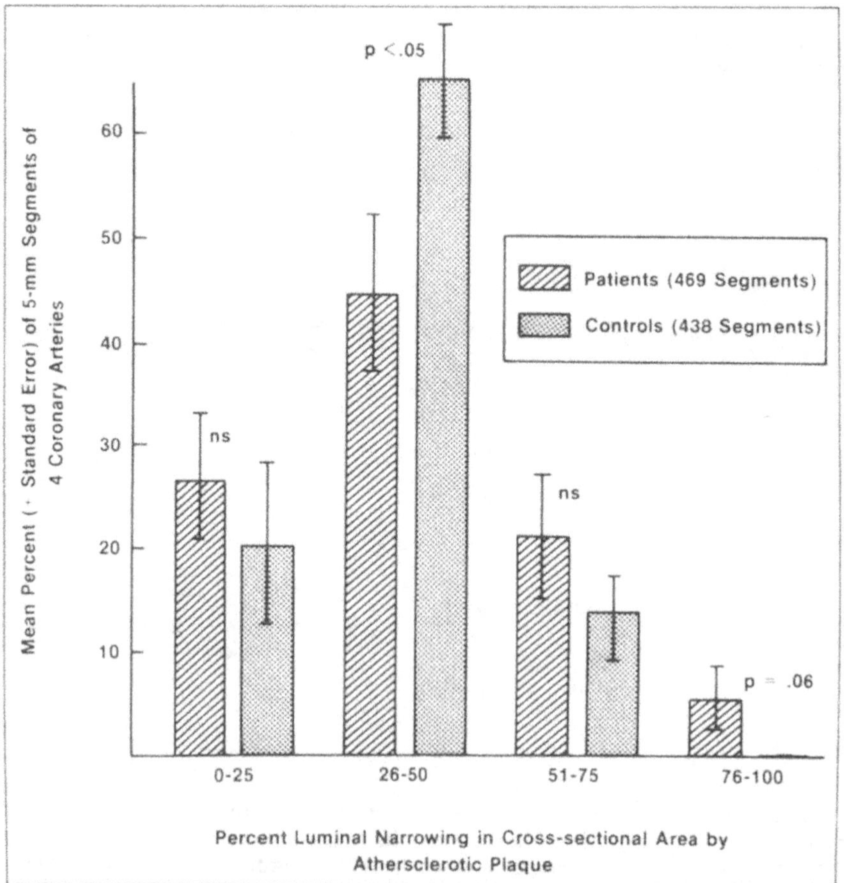

Figure 9. Percent of 5 mm segments of all four major coronary arteries narrowed to various degrees in 10 patients with radiation heart disease and 10 control subjects.

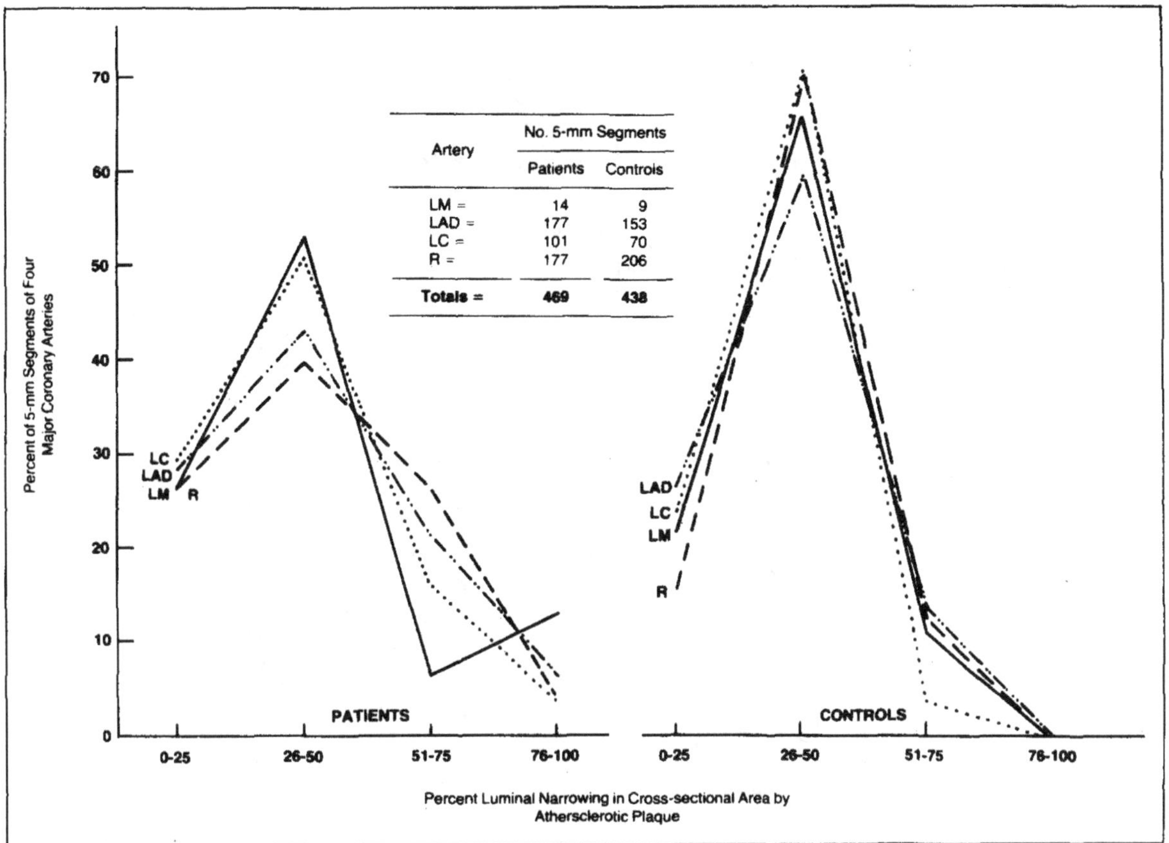

Figure 10. Percent of 5 mm segments of the right (R), left main (LM), left anterior descending (LAD) and left circumflex (LC) coronary arteries narrowed to four categories of narrowing in 10 patients with radiation heart disease and in 10 control subjects.

sections (76 percent) (controls = 43 of 438 sections [10 percent]; p <0.001). In addition, the medial wall was thinned in 84 (17 percent) of 482 sections (controls = 53 [12 percent] of 438 sections).

The coronary arterial adventitial fibrous tissue was clearly increased in 234 (49 percent) of 482 sections in the 11 study patients and in 14 (3 percent) of the 438 sections in the 10 control subjects (p <0.01).

Each section of myocardial wall from both study patients and control subjects was examined to determine the status of the *intramural coronary arteries.* Five of the 16 study patients and none of the 10 control subjects had one or more abnormal intramyocardial coronary arteries (**Figures 3 and 4**). In all five patients, the abnormal intramural arteries were located in the right ventricular free wall; one patient had similar, abnormal arteries in the left ventricular free wall. The arteries involved in each patient were few in number and located near the epicardial surface, very close to overlying thickened epicardium. No abnormalities were observed in the intramural coronary arteries located in the subendocardial half of the myocardial wall. The abnormalities consisted of intimal fibrous thickening with or without luminal narrowing, medial thickening and usually periadventitial fibrous thickening. The changes in all patients were focal, i.e., most arteries were normal, and few were involved with the changes described.

COMMENTS

Each of the 16 study patients described herein was young (aged 15 to 33 years [mean 26 years]), each had received >3,500 rads to the heart from five to 144 months before death for therapy of a malignant neoplasm, and the heart in each was studied in detail at necropsy. During life, five had clinical evidence of myocardial constriction from excessive pericardial fluid (tamponade), requiring pericardiocentesis in four and pericardiectomy in two; an additional patient, who during life never had evidence of cardiac disease, died suddenly and necropsy disclosed his death to be the result of severe coronary arterial narrowing. Thus, six of the 16 patients had clinical evidence of cardiac dysfunction.

Although only six of our 16 patients had clinical evidence of cardiac dysfunction, at necropsy all had anatomic evidence of cardiac abnormality. All but one had fibrous thickening of the pericardium, two had fibrous pericardial adhesions, and eight had excessive pericardial fluid. The mural or valvular endocardium or both also was thickened focally by fibrous tissue in 14 of the 16 patients, and the fibrous tissue located between myocardial cells (interstitial myocardial fibrosis) was

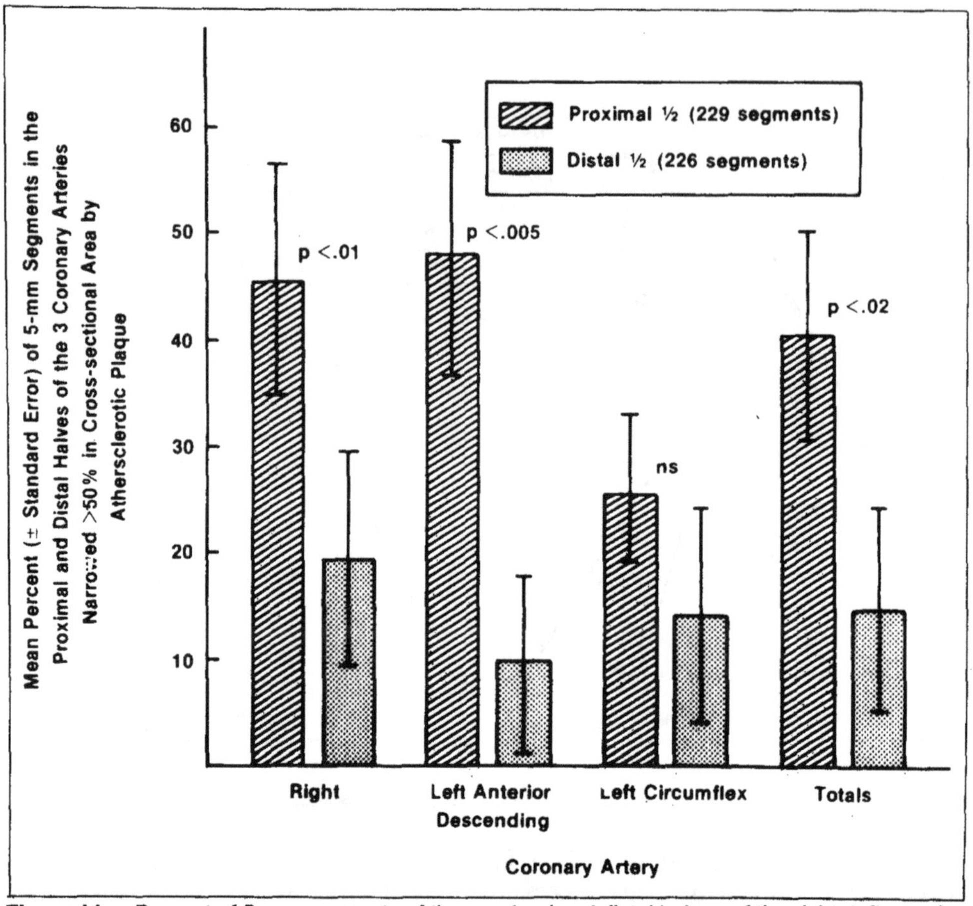

Figure 11. Percent of 5 mm segments of the proximal and distal halves of the right, left anterior descending and left circumflex coronary arteries in the 10 study patients with radiation heart disease.

increased in amount in half the patients. The increase in fibrous tissue in all three layers of the ventricular wall (epicardium, myocardium and endocardium) was much more extensive and much more frequent in the right ventricle than in the left ventricle presumably because of higher radiation doses to the anterior surface of the heart. Although the increase in the fibrous tissue in the myocardial wall and mural endocardium caused no apparent clinical evidence of cardiac dysfunction in our patients, it is conceivable that the ventricular walls would have become more rigid or less compliant as the young patients aged. Likewise, the focal fibrous thickening of the cardiac valves in our patients produced no apparent valvular dysfunction, but had they lived for several decades longer, valvular dysfunction may have been the consequence. Indeed, in at least four patients mitral or aortic regurgitation or both have been reported to have developed after high-dose irradiation to the heart [9,10,22]. Although the increase in fibrous tissue in epicardium, myocardium and mural endocardium in our patients was far more extensive in the right ventricle than in the left ventricle, the fibrous thickening of the valves on the left side of the heart was decidedly greater than that on the right-side. The fibrous thickening of both the mural and valvular endocardium, however, in our patients was relatively mild and could have been overlooked had not it been looked for specifically. Thickening of mural endocardium after high-dose irradiation has been described only once previously [16]. Although mild, it was unequivocal in our patients.

The most important contribution of the present study is the detailed information regarding the epicardial coronary arteries. Damage to these vessels by high-dose irradiation has been reported previously [10,29–41], but the extent of, and the type of, damage to these arteries have not been described. It is now clear that high-dose irradiation can cause damage to the epicardial coronary arteries and allow intimal proliferation of mainly fibrous tissue to produce luminal narrowing. Of our 16 patients, 16 of the 64 major (right, left main, left anterior descending and left circumflex) epicardial coronary arteries were narrowed >75 percent in cross-sectional area, primarily by fibrous plaques. In contrast, of 10 control subjects of similar age and sex, only one of 40 major epicardial coronary arteries were similarly nar-

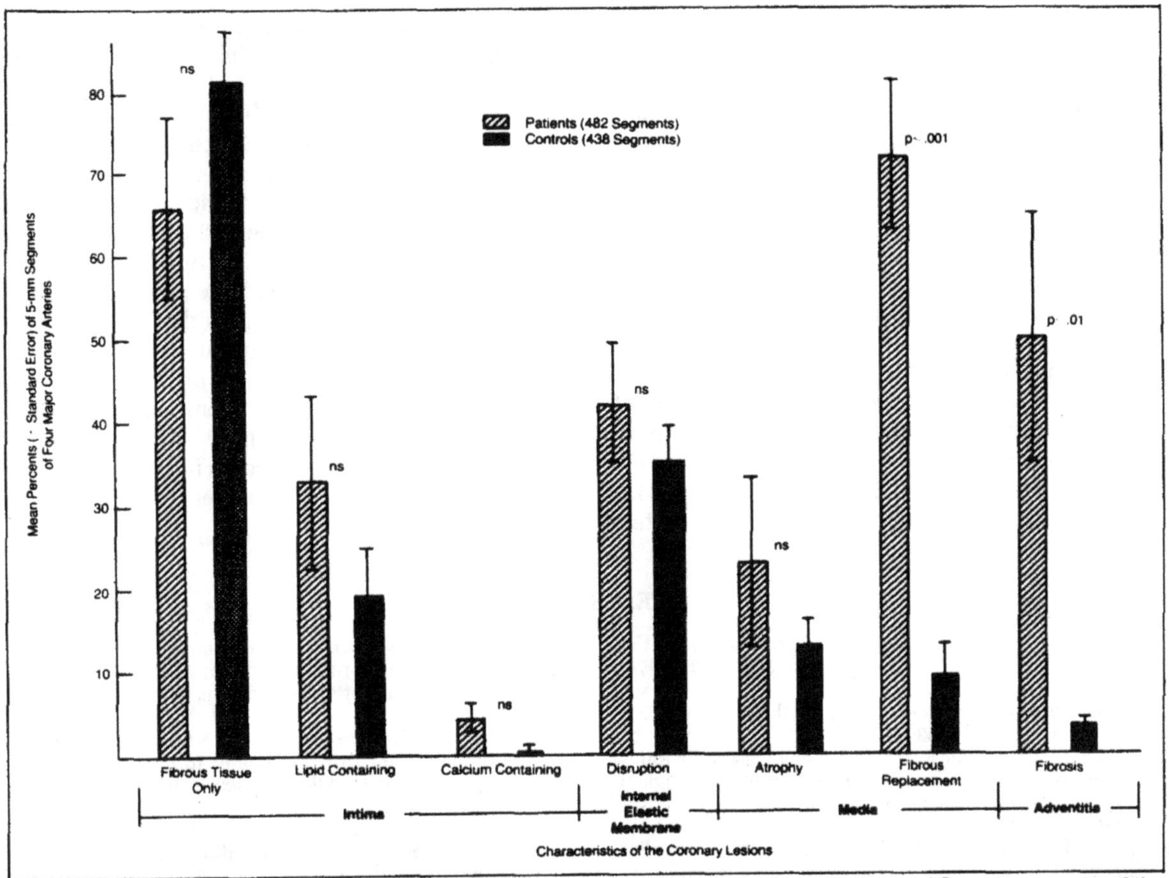

Figure 12. Morphology of coronary arterial lesions in radiation heart disease: percent of 5 mm segments of the four major epicardial coronary arteries showing various changes in the intima, media and adventitia in 11 study patients and 10 control subjects.

rowed. Of 469 five-milliliter segments of the four major epicardial coronary arteries in 10 study patients, 28 (6 percent) were narrowed >75 percent in cross-sectional area (controls = one of 438 sections [p = 0.06]) and another 22 percent were narrowed 51 to 75 percent (controls = 13 percent). Thus, our study patients clearly had more coronary narrowing than did the control subjects, and none had pronounced recognized risk factors to premature atherosclerosis.

The dominant component of the atherosclerotic plaques in both our study patients and in the control subjects was fibrous tissue; very little lipid was present in either. The study patients, however, had a striking loss of smooth muscle cells from the media (76 percent of sections versus 10 percent of sections in the controls). Furthermore, adventitial fibrosis was noted in 49 percent of the coronary sections in the study patients and in only 3 percent of the sections in the control subjects. Thus, high dose radiation causes coronary luminal narrowing, particularly in the proximal portions of the major coronary arteries (possibly because they receive more rads than the distal portions), adventitial scarring and damage to the smooth muscle cells in the media.

The minor abnormalities in the intramural coronary arteries, mainly in the right ventricular wall, in the study patients do not appear sufficient to produce functional abnormality.

Finally, a number of the 16 study patients were irradiated with techniques now considered unacceptable by most modern radiotherapists (viz., anterior-only ports, tumor doses >4,000 rads, 2 megavoltage radiation sources, multiple courses of radiotherapy). Indeed, many centers now utilize a "sub-carinal block" to shield the heart from radiation, after a total tumor dose of 3,000 rads is reached [26]. Thus, it might be argued that the types of radiation damage herein demonstrated, will be diminished or eliminated through use of modern techniques. Although such a trend is to be hoped for, in four of the 16 patients radiation doses to both the anterior and posterior surfaces of the heart were <4,200 rad: radiation levels considered acceptable by modern therapists. Therefore, it still seems likely that at least in some young people who receive radiation to the heart, cured of their primary tumor, anatomic and functional cardiac abnormalities will ultimately develop due to the radiation therapy.

ACKNOWLEDGMENT

We are grateful to A. S. Lichter, M.D., National Cancer Institute, Bethesda, Maryland, for assistance in calculating radiation doses and interpreting radiotherapy techniques.

APPENDIX

The radiation doses to the anterior and posterior surfaces of the heart were determined as follows: (1) The posterior surface was considered to be at the mid-plane of the mediastinum (8 to 11 cm posterior to the chest surface) and, hence, to have absorbed the dose denoted in the patient's records as the "midplane" or "tumor" dose. (2) The anterior surface was considered to be 3 cm posterior to the chest surface. (3) The fractional doses for both the posterior and anterior surfaces were determined by matching the "equivalent area" of each of the radiation ports with the distance from the radiation source on a standard fractional depth dose data table for a 6 megavoltage photon beam source (Radiation Oncology Branch, National Cancer Institute). (4) The absolute radiation dose to the anterior surface thus equaled the fractional dose to the anterior heart surface divided by the fractional dose to the posterior heart surface times the absolute dose to the posterior heart surface (or "mid-plane dose"). (5) For nine patients who had been treated with a 2 megavoltage radiation source, the dose calculated for the anterior surface of the heart was multiplied (for anterior ports) or divided (for posterior ports) by a factor of 1.2 to compensate for the lower penetrance of x-rays from this source compared to those from a 6 megavoltage source. The doses thus calculated were considered to represent maximum possible dose.

REFERENCES

1. Desjardins AU: Action of roentgen rays and radium on the heart and lungs. Am J Roentgenol 1932; 27: 153–176, 303–335, 477–495.
2. Leach JE: Effect of roentgen therapy on the heart; clinical study. Arch Int Med 1943; 72: 715–745.
3. Fried JR, Goldberg H: Post-irradiation changes in the lungs and thorax. A clinical, roentgenological and pathological study, with emphasis on late and terminal stages. Am J Roentgenol 1940; 43: 877–895.
4. Blumenfeld H, Thomas SF: Chronic massive pericardial effusion following roentgen therapy for carcinoma of the breast. Radiology 1945; 44: 335–340.
5. Tricot R, Baillet J, Helmke G: La péricardite constrictive post-radiotherapique (à propos d'un cas personnel). Arch Mal Coeur 1954; 47: 922–940.
6. Gimlette TMD: Constrictive pericarditis. Br Heart J 1959; 21: 9–16.
7. Hurst DW: Radiation fibrosis of pericardium with cardiac tamponade. Can Med Assoc J 1959; 81: 377–380.
8. Connolly DC, Burchell HB: Pericarditis: a 10 year survey. Am J Cardiol 1961; 7: 7–13.
9. Steinberg I: Effusive-constrictive radiation pericarditis. Two cases illustrating value of angiocardiography in diagnosis. Am J Cardiol 1967; 19: 434–439.
10. Cohn KE, Stewart JR, Fajardo LF, Hancock EW: Heart disease following radiation. Medicine (Baltimore) 1967; 46: 281–298.
11. Stewart JR, Cohn KE, Fajardo LF, Hancock EW, Kaplan HS: Radiation-induced heart disease. Radiology 1967; 89: 302–310.
12. Teng CY, Nemickas R, Tobin JR Jr, Szanto PB, Gunnar RM: Pericardial effusion following radiation to the chest. Report of a case. Dis Chest 1967; 52: 549–552.
13. Muggia FM, Cassileth PA: Constrictive pericarditis following radiation therapy. Am J Med 1968; 44: 116–123.
14. Roberts WC, Glancy DL, DeVita VT: Heart in malignant lymphoma (Hodgkin's disease, lymphosarcoma, reticulum cell sarcoma and mycosis fungoides). A study of 196 autopsy cases. Am J Cardiol 1968; 22: 85–107.
15. Masland DS, Rotz CT Jr, Harris JH Jr: Postradiation pericarditis with chronic pericardial effusion. Ann Intern Med 1968; 69: 97–102.
16. Fajardo LF, Stewart JR, Cohn KE: Morphology of radiation-induced heart disease. Arch Pathol 1968; 86: 512–519.
17. Morton DL, Kagan AR, Roberts WC, O'Brien KP, Holmes EC, Adkins PC: Pericardiectomy for radiation-induced pericarditis with effusion. Ann Thorac Surg 1969; 8: 195–208.
18. Haas JM: Symptomatic constrictive pericarditis developing 45 years after radiation therapy to the mediastinum. A review of radiation pericarditis. Am Heart J 1969; 77: 88–95.
19. Pierce RH, Hafermann MD, Kagan AR: Changes in the transverse cardiac diameter following mediastinal irradiation for Hodgkin's disease. Radiology 1969; 93: 619–624.
20. Lawson RAM, Ross WM, Gold RG, Blesovsky A, Barnsley WC: Post-radiation pericarditis. Report on four more cases with special reference to bronchogenic carcinoma. J Thorac Cardiovasc Surg 1972; 63: 841–847.
21. Kagan AR, Hafermann M, Hamiton M, Pierce R, Morton D, Johnson R: Etiology, diagnosis, and management of pericardial effusion after irradiation. Radiol Clin Biol 1972; 41: 171–182.
22. Morton DL, Glancy DL, Joseph WL, Adkins PC: Management of patients with radiation-induced pericarditis with effusion: a note on the development of aortic regurgitation in two of them. Chest 1973; 64: 291–297.
23. Martin RG, Ruckdeschel JC, Chang P, Byhardt R, Bouchard RJ, Wiernik PH: Radiation-related pericarditis. Am J Cardiol 1975; 35: 216–220.
24. Byhardt R, Brace K, Ruckdeschel J, Chang P, Martin R, Wiernik PH: Dose and treatment factors in radiation related pericardial effusion associated with the mantle technique for Hodgkin's disease. Cancer 1975; 35: 795–802.
25. Ruckdeschel JC, Chang P, Martin RG, et al.: Radiation-related pericardial effusions in patients with Hodgkin's disease. Medicine (Baltimore) 1975, 54: 245–259.
26. Carmel RJ, Kaplan HS: Mantle irradiation in Hodgkin's disease. Cancer 1976; 37: 2813–2825.
27. Green B, Zornoza J, Ricks JP: Eccentric pericardial effusion after radiation therapy of left breast carcinoma. Am J Roentgenol 1977; 128: 27–30.
28. Schneider JS, Edwards JE: Irradiation-induced pericarditis. Chest 1979; 75: 560–564.
29. Pearson HES: Coronary occlusion following thoracic radiotherapy, 2 cases. Proc R Soc Med 1957; 50: 516.
30. Dollinger MR, Lavine DM, Foye LV Jr: Myocardial infarction following radiation (letter to the editor). Lancet 1965; 2: 246.
31. Prentice RTW: Myocardial infarction following radiation (Letter to the Editor). Lancet 1965; 2: 388.
32. Dollinger MR, Lavine DM, Foye LV Jr: Myocardial infarction due to post-irradiation fibrosis of the coronary arteries.

Case of successfully treated Hodgkin's disease with lower esophageal involvement. JAMA 195: 316–319, 1966.

33. Huff H, Sanders EM: Coronary-artery occlusion after radiation. N Engl J Med 1972; 286: 780.
34. Tracy GP, Brown DE, Johnson LW, Gottlieb AJ: Radiation-induced coronary artery disease. JAMA 1974; 228: 1660–1662.
35. Ringrose, TL: Radiation-"induced" coronary artery disease. JAMA 1974; 230: 960–961.
36. McReynolds RA, Gold GL, Roberts WC: Coronary heart disease after mediastinal irradiation for Hodgkin's disease. Am J Med 1976; 60: 39–45.
37. Ali MK, Khalil KG, Fuller LM, et al.: Radiation-related myocardial injury: management of two cases. Cancer 1976; 38: 1941–1946.
38. Rodgers DL: Precocious myocardial infarction after radiation treatment for Hodgkin's disease. Chest 1976; 70: 675–677.
39. Murphy GK: Cancer and the coroner. JAMA 1977; 237: 786–788.
40. Iqbal SM, Hanson EL, Gensini GG: Bypass graft for coronary artery stenosis following radiation therapy. Chest 1977; 71: 664–666.
41. Rasmussen S, Døssing M, Walbom-Jørgensen S: Coronary heart disease—a possible risk in mega voltage therapy? Acta Med Scand 1978; 203: 237–239.
42. Hartman FW, Bollinger A, Doub HP, Smith FJ: Heart lesions produced by deep x-rays. An experimental and clinical study. Bull Johns Hopkins Hosp 1927; 41: 36–67.
43. Fajardo LF, Stewart JR: Pathogenesis of radiation-induced myocardial fibrosis. Lab Invest 1973; 29: 244–257.
44. DiMatteo J, Vacheron A, Heulin A, et al.: Complications cardiques de la radiotherapie thoracique. Arch Mal Coeur 1978; 71: 447–452.
45. Bouvrain Y, Roujeau J, Rogard JM: Myocardite post-radiotherapique. Sem Hop Paris 1977; 53: 433–436.
46. Roberts WC, Sjoerdsma A: The cardiac disease associated with the carcinoid syndrome (carcinoid heart disease). Am J Med 1964; 36: 5–34.
47. Isner JM, Wu M, Virmani R, Jones AA, Roberts WC: Comparison of degrees of coronary arterial luminal narrowing determined by visual inspection of histologic sections under magnification among three independent observers and comparison to that obtained by video planimetry. An analysis of 559 five-mm segments of 61 coronary arteries from eleven patients. Lab Invest 1980; 68: 831–838.

Carcinoma of the Lung Causing Pulmonary Arterial Stenosis*

Bruce F. Waller, M.D., F.C.C.P.; Ross D. Fletcher, M.D.; and William C. Roberts, M.D., F.C.C.P.

A patient is described in whom carcinoma of the lung caused compression and obstruction of the left and right main pulmonary arteries and auscultatory features of peripheral pulmonary arterial stenosis.

Herein we describe findings in a man with carcinoma of the lung causing auscultatory features of peripheral pulmonary arterial stenosis. To our knowledge, such a patient has not been described previously.

Case Report

A 55-year-old man was healthy until January 1977 (11 months before death), when left anterior chest pain and dyspnea first appeared. He had smoked a package of cigarettes daily for 30 years. The mean jugular venous pressure was equivalent to about 6 cm of water, and a prominent A wave was visible. The carotid arterial pulse was normal. The breath sounds were decreased, and the percussion note was dull over the left chest. A right ventricular impulse was easily palpable. The second heart sound at the base was widely split on inspiration, and never became single during expiration (Fig 1). The pulmonary component of the second heart sound was increased in intensity. A third heart sound, S_3, was present over the right sternal border. A grade 3/6 systolic ejection murmur was heard over the precordium, both axillae and back, loudest over the second right and left intercostal spaces, and the murmur increased in intensity with inspiration, especially along the right sternal border and in the right axilla. No diastolic murmurs were heard. An ECG showed prominent left ventricular voltage and nonspecific ST segment and T wave changes. His chest roentgenogram (Fig 2) disclosed complete opacification of the left lung field. An echocardiogram was consistent with pulmonary hypertension.

Tissue obtained from the left main stem bronchus showed small-cell carcinoma. At right-sided cardiac catheterization, the pressures (in mm Hg) were as follows: right atrium, a = 8, v = 7); right ventricle, 55/10; pulmonary trunk, 55/10; proximal right pulmonary artery, 55/10, and distal right pulmonary artery, 22/10 (Fig 1). Right atrial angiogram (Fig 2) disclosed normal right atrial and ventricular cavities and pulmonary trunk, but severe narrowing of the left main and moderate narrowing of the right main pulmonary arteries.

The patient received chemotherapy and local irradiation, and a chest roentgenogram four weeks later showed considerable clearing of the left lung field. Moreover, the intensity of the systolic ejection murmur had decreased to grade 1/6.

*From the Pathology Branch, National Heart, Lung, and Blood Institute, National Institutes of Health, Bethesda, Md, and the Division of Cardiology, Department of Medicine, Veterans Administration Hospital, Washington, D.C.
Reprint requests: Dr. Roberts, Building 10A, Room 3E30, National Institutes of Health, Bethesda 20205

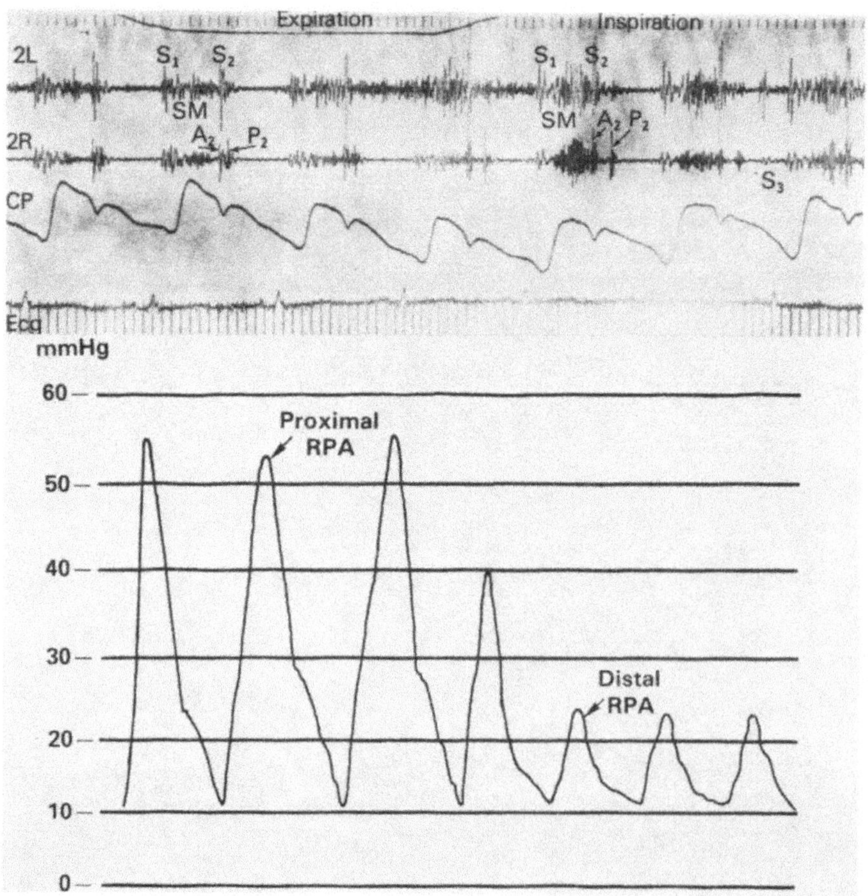

FIGURE 1. Phonocardiogram *(upper)* recorded at second left (2L) and right (2R) intercostal spaces showing systolic murmurs (SM) and a persistently split second heart sound (S_2). A_2= aortic component of S_2, CP=external carotid pulse; P_2=pulmonic component of S_2; S_1=first heart sound; S_3=third heart sound. Pressure tracing *(lower)* with pullback from distal to proximal right main pulmonary artery (RPA).

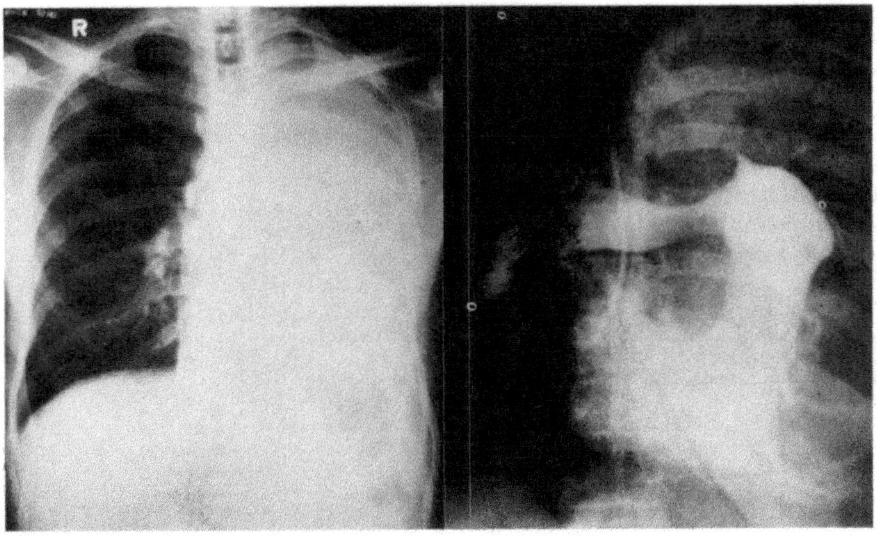

Figure 2. Posteroanterior chest roentgenogram *(left)* showing opacification of left lung field and angiogram *(right)* with injection into right atrium demonstrating severe luminal narrowing of left main and moderate narrowing of right main pulmonary arteries. Roentgenograms done 11 months before death.

He slowly deteriorated, however, and died ten months later (November 1977). His only evidence of right-sided congestive heart failure at any time was the presence of a third heart sound, which varied with respiration.

At necropsy, both right and left lung parenchyma and pleura were extensively replaced by carcinoma (Fig 3). The left main bronchus and pulmonary artery were severely compressed by tumor. The right main pulmonary artery was partially compressed by surrounding tumor. A large cavity filled with necrotic tumor was present in the upper left lobe. Histologic sections showed tumor invasion of the walls of the right and left main pulmonary arteries and intrapulmonary arteries. The heart weighed 420 g, and the right ventricle was dilated.

Discussion

Although many reports have described exterior compression of one or more major extrapulmonary pulmonary arteries by neoplasm, auscultatory evidence of obstruction to one or more major pulmonary arteries has not been documented previously. In our patient, total obstruction to the left main pulmonary artery and partial obstruction to the right main pulmonary artery was documented by both angiography (during life) and

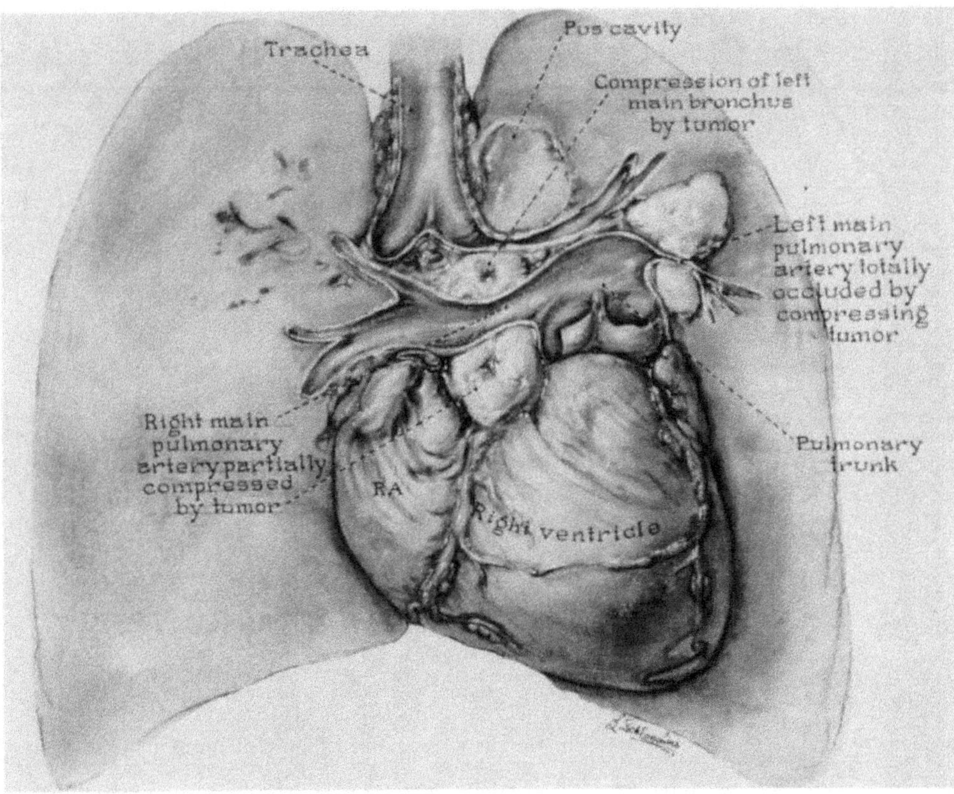

Figure 3. Drawing of heart and lungs at necropsy. Lumen of left main pulmonary artery totally occluded by carcinoma, compressing it externally, and lumen of right main pulmonary artery partially obstructed by similar mechanism. Both right ventricle and right atrium are dilated.

necropsy, and a 33 mm Hg peak systolic pressure gradient between proximal and distal right main pulmonary artery was found at catheterization. The wide splitting of the second heart sound at the cardiac base in our patient can be attributed to the peripheral pulmonary stenosis. There was not enough right ventricular failure (only a third heart sound) in the presence of the pulmonary hypertension in our patient to account for the wide splitting of the second heart sound.

ACKNOWLEDGMENT: The authors thank W. Proctor Harvey, M.D., Chief, Division of Cardiology, Department of Medicine, Georgetown University, Washington, D.C., for reviewing the manuscript and for making useful suggestions.

Cardiac lymphoma mimicking hypertrophic cardiomyopathy

Henry Scott Cabin, M.D., Ralph M. Costello, M.D., Gopalan Vasudevan, M.D., Barry J. Maron, M.D., and William C. Roberts, M.D. *Bethesda, Md., and Greensburg, Pa.*

Among patients with lymphoma, about 25% at autopsy have the neoplasm in the heart.[1] The cardiac involvement, however, infrequently causes cardiac dysfunction, and when cardiac dysfunction does occur it rarely is the initial manifestation of the lymphoma.[1, 2] Such was the case, however, in a 62-year-old man who had been well until 6 weeks before death when exertional dyspnea and substernal discomfort appeared, followed in several days by subcutaneous edema and nonexertional (nocturnal) dyspnea. Examination 19 days before death disclosed overt evidence of congestive cardiac failure (CHF), a blood pressure of 130/180 mm Hg, and a grade 1/6 systolic murmur at the left sternal border and apex. ECG (Fig. 1) disclosed changes consistent with posterior wall damage and chest roentgenogram (Fig. 2) showed an enlarged cardiac silhouette and pleural effusions. Despite treatment with digoxin and furosemide, CHF worsened and the intensity of the precordial systolic murmur increased to grade 4/6. On echocardiogram (Fig. 3), the left ventricular (LV) cavity was not dilated, the mitral leaflets moved anteriorly during ventricular systole (SAM), the ventricular septum and LV free wall were thickened, and the left

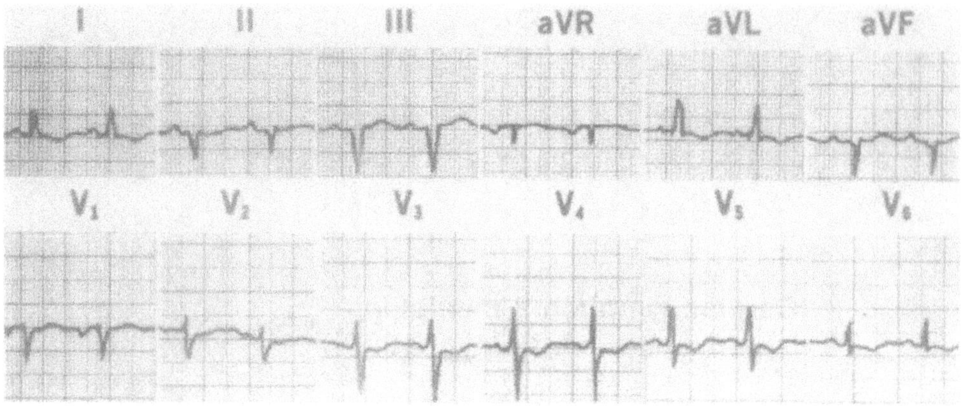

Fig. 1. ECG obtained 12 days before death. Pathologic Q waves are present in leads II, III, and aV_F and the ST segments and T waves in several leads are abnormal.

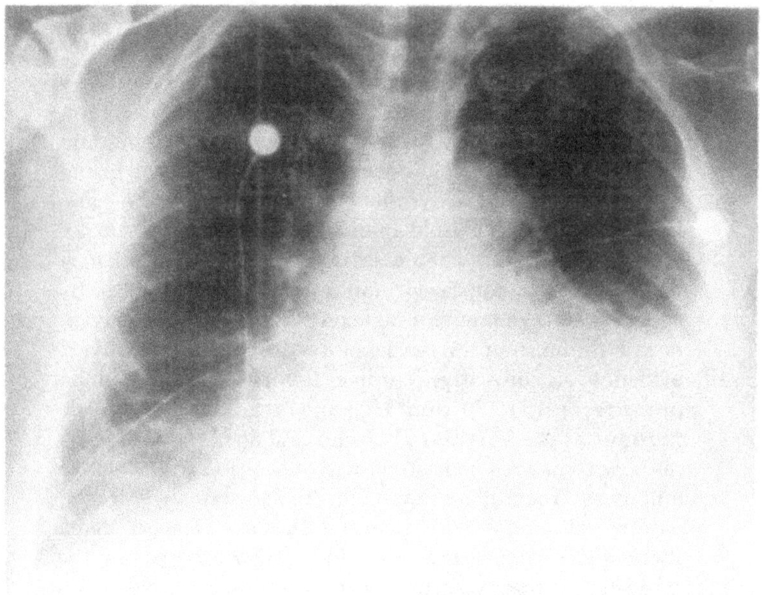

Fig. 2. Anteroposterior chest radiograph obtained 15 days before death. The cardiac silhouette is enlarged, pleural effusions are present, the pulmonary vessels are prominent, and the interstitial markings are abnormally prominent.

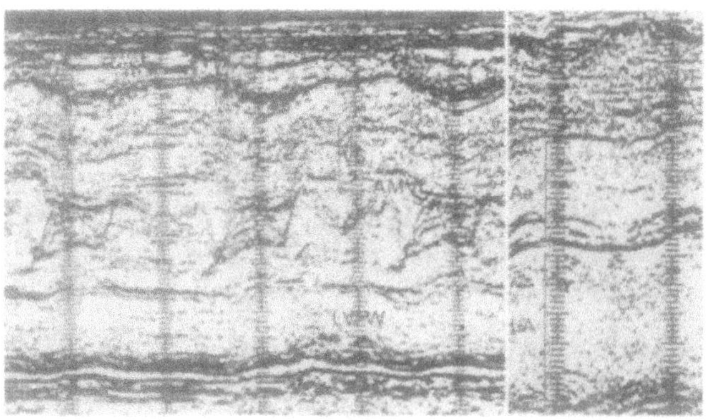

Fig. 3. M-mode echocardiograms obtained 18 days before death. The left ventricular free wall *(LVFW)* and ventricular septum *(VS)* are thickened. The LV cavity is of normal or less than normal size, the mitral leaflets move anteriorly during ventricular systole *(open arrow)*, and the left atrium *(LA)* is dilated. *AMVL* = anterior mitral valve leaflet; *Ao* = aorta; *RVOT* = right ventricular outlfow tract.

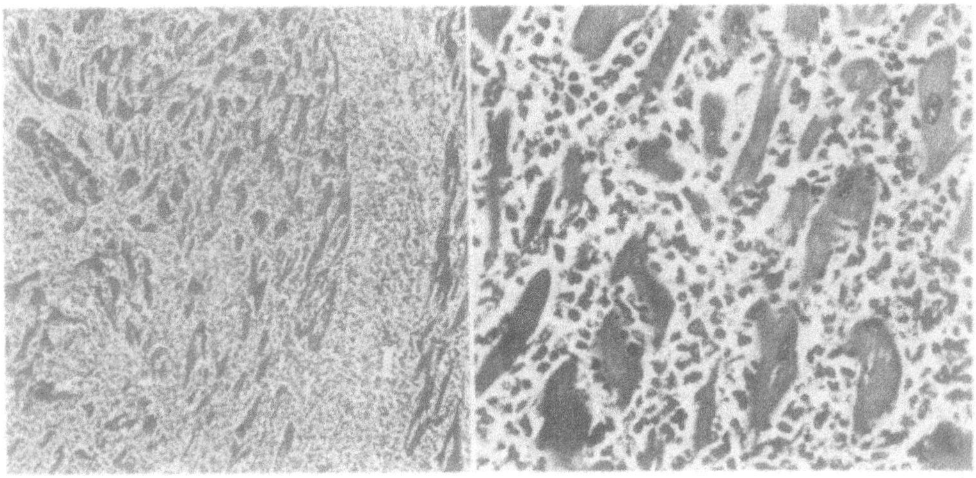

Fig. 4. Photomicrographs of lymphoma in the left ventricular wall. (Hematoxylin and eosin stains; original magnifications ×80 [*left*], ×330 [*right*].

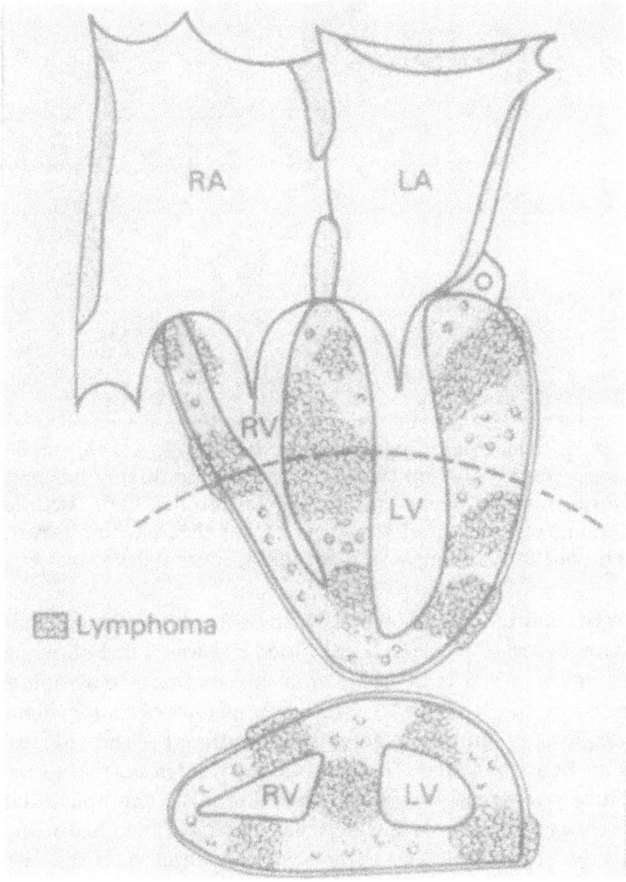

Fig. 5. Diagram showing locations of grossly visible lymphomatous nodules in the heart. *LA* = left atrium; *LV* = left ventricle; *RA* = right atrium; *RV* = right ventricle.

atrial cavity was dilated. With discontinuation of digoxin and furosemide and with institution of propranolol, CHF and intensity of the precordial murmur lessened. Three days later, however, cardiac arrest occurred. Although successfully resuscitated, he became comatose the next day and died 12 days later.

Necropsy disclosed diffuse fibrinous pericardial adhesions and extensive replacement of the cardiac ventricular walls by lymphoma (undifferentiated non-Burkitt's type) (Figs. 4 and 5). The thickening of the ventricular walls was entirely the result of neoplastic infiltration. The heart plus the infiltrating tumor weighed 910 gm. The lumina of the epicardial coronary arteries were free of significant narrowing and the four cardiac valves were normal. No myofiber disorganization was present in the ventricular septum. The only other site of lymphoma was in a mesenteric lymph node.

The above-described patient with lymphoma is unusual for the following reasons: (1) the neoplasm was limited to the heart, except for a small focus in a mesenteric lymph node; (2) the cardiac lymphoma caused cardiac dysfunction which was the initial and the only clinical manifestation of the lymphoma; (3) lymphoma was never suspected clinically; and (4) the cardiac involvement by the lymphoma mimicked hypertrophic cardiomyopathy (HC) (worsening of CHF and intensification of precordial systolic murmur by digitalis and diuretics and lessening of both by propranolol, and compatible echocardiographic findings). Although sarcoma primarily involving the ventricular septum has mimicked HC,[3] we have found no reports of other primary or secondary cardiac neoplasms simulating clinically HC.

We thank Dr. Elaine S. Jaffe, Chief, Hematopathology, Laboratory of Pathology, National Cancer Institute, National Institutes of Health, Bethesda, Maryland, for reviewing the histologic sections of the lymphoma and for classifying it for us.

REFERENCES

1. Roberts WC, Glancy DL, DeVita VT Jr: Heart in malignant lymphoma (Hodgkin's disease, lymphosarcoma, reticulum cell sarcoma and mycosis fungoides). A study of 196 autopsy cases. Am J Cardiol **22**:85, 1968.
2. Levitt LJ, Ault KA, Pinkus GS, Sloss LJ, McManus BM: Pericarditis and early cardiac tamponade as a primary manifestation of lymphosarcoma cell leukemia. Am J Med **67**:719, 1979.
3. Isner JI, Falcone MW, Virmani R, Roberts WC: Cardiac sarcoma causing "ASH" and simulating coronary heart disease. Am J Med **66**:1025, 1979.

Fatal catecholamine crisis in pheochromocytoma: Curable cause of cardiac arrest

Bruce M. McManus, M.D., Ph.D.,
Thomas A. Fleury, M.D., and William C. Roberts, M.D.
Bethesda, Md., and Washington, D.C.

When a 56-year-old person presents in the emergency room with chest pain, cold clammy skin, nausea with or without vomiting, hypotension, and either tachy- or bradycardia, the most likely diagnosis is acute myocardial infarction (AMI). Such a symptom complex occurred in patient F.C. but the coronary arteries at necropsy were normal and the cause of "cardiogenic" shock was noncardiac in origin. She had been well until age 43 years (1967) when syncope occurred, and thereafter she fainted as often as once weekly and as infrequently as bimonthly, always unrelated to exertion but frequently related to psychologic stress. Loss of consciousness was never longer than a few seconds and unassociated with seizure activity, urination, defecation, or cranial trauma. Between syncopal attacks she had frequent severe headaches (throbbing, often extending to the neck), usually associated with nervousness, palpitations, nausea and, occasionally, vomiting. With the headaches, she occasionally also had pain in the anterior chest and/or upper abdomen. At age 44 years (1969), she was hospitalized for evaluation, but no specific abnormalities were found. Blood pressure (BP) was 120/70 mm Hg, hematocrit 45%, fasting blood glucose 122 mg/dl, and postprandial blood glucose 64 mg/dl, 5-hour glucose tolerance was normal, and ECG was normal (Fig. 1, *upper panel*). In 1971 while visiting a hospital emergency room because of palpitations, nausea, and vomiting and severe headache, her heart stopped but she was resuscitated. She then remained in the intensive care unit for 10 days and ECG (Fig. 1, *middle panel*) and serum enzymes showed no evidence of AMI. Chest pain in April, 1980, required hospitalization but serial ECG and serum enzymes again were normal.

Approximately 18 hours before death in October, 1980, at age 56 years, she again had an episode of throbbing headache, palpitations, severe fatigue, nausea and vomiting, and anterior chest pain. When seen 5 hours before death she was pale, cold, and clammy. ECG 4 hours before death showed heart rate (HR) 140 beats/min and right axis deviation (Fig. 1, *bottom panel*). On arrival 1 hour later at the hospital, BP was 85/70 mm Hg, she was severely cyanotic, and had bibasilar pulmonary rales. The WBC count was 10,500 mm^3 with 64% polymorphonuclear leukocytes, and the arterial blood pH was 7.0. Following decrease in HR to 30 beats/min unresponsive to atropine, asystole occurred. At necropsy a ***pheochromocytoma*** weighing 15 gm involved the right adrenal gland (Fig. 2). The heart weighed 275 gm and the ventricular myocardium was grossly normal. The lumina of the epicardial coronary arteries were widely patent (Fig. 3). On histologic study, numerous foci of contraction band necrosis and interstitial inflammatory cells, mainly polymorphonuclear leukocytes, were observed in both left and right ventricular walls (Fig. 4).

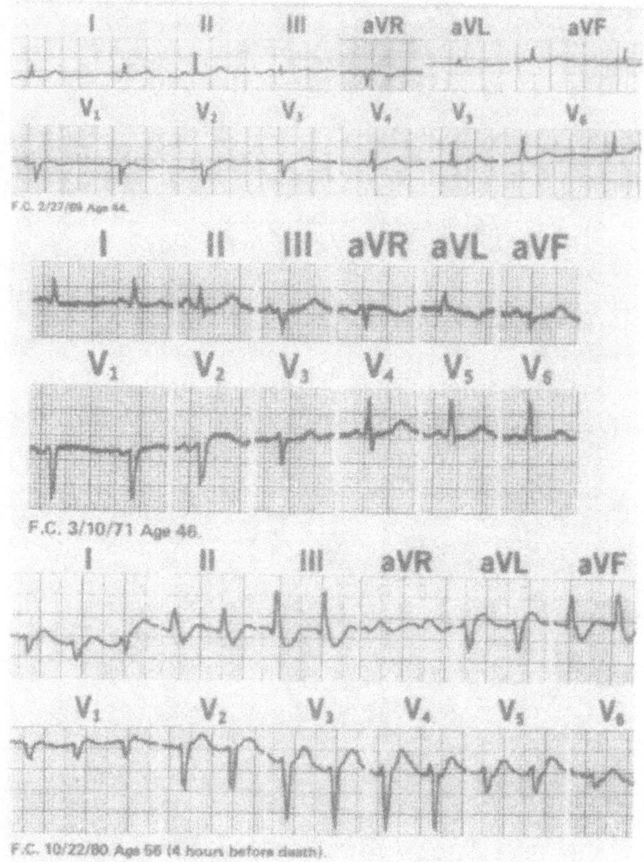

Fig. 1. Electrocardiograms recorded at ages 44, 46, and 56 years of age. The ***top*** tracing was recorded during her first workup for syncope and other symptoms. The ***middle*** tracing was recorded 4 days after her first cardiac arrest. The ***bottom*** tracing was recorded 4 hours before death.

The above described patient had clinical features of periodic epinephrine hypersecretion for 13 years and died during a catecholamine crisis. She had an adrenal gland pheochromocytoma, widely patent coronary arteries, acute myocarditis and contraction band necrosis, the latter two abnormalities being typical morphologic features resulting from catecholamine hypersecretion.[1] The unusual features of her illness included syncope (reported

From the Pathology Branch, National Heart, Lung and Blood Institute, National Institutes of Health; and the Department of Pathology, Sibley Memorial Hospital.

Received for publication June 11, 1981; accepted June 24, 1981.

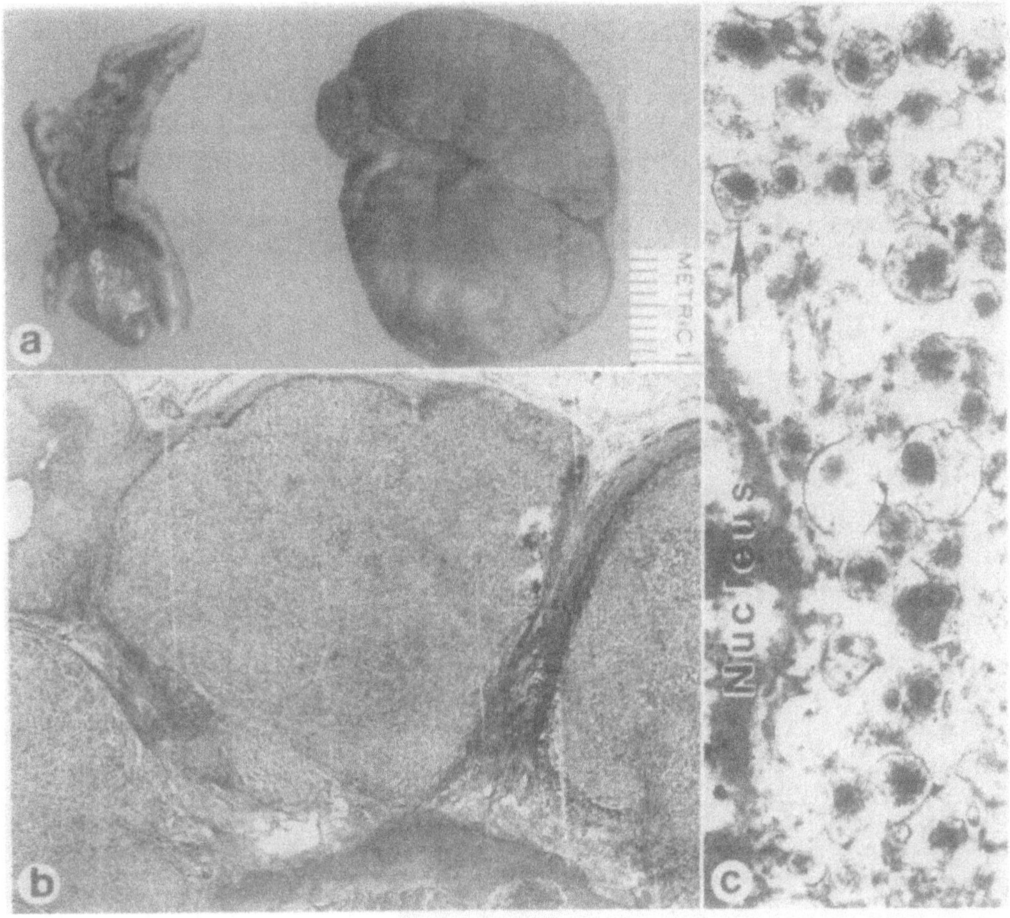

Fig. 2. Pheochromocytoma. *a,* Tumor in right adrenal gland and near-normal left adrenal gland. *b,* Tumor showing broad fibrous bands separating nodules and a small amount of residual adrenal cortex *(upper left)* (Hematoxylin-eosin stain; original magnification ×11). *c,* Electron micrograph of tumor showing a portion of a tumor cell with several characteristic cytoplasmic catecholamine-containing granules (*arrow*) (original magnification ×52,000). (Electron micrograph courtesy of Drs. Hung Chiang and Timothy Triche, Ultrastructural Pathology Section, Laboratory of Pathology, NCI)

in only one previous patient),[2] lack of systemic hypertension (normal-sized heart at necropsy), and unexpected cardiac arrest, once with successful resuscitation. Cardiac arrest in patients with pheochromocytoma is exceedingly rare in the absence of systemic hypertension, chronic congestive heart failure, and of operative manipulation of the neoplasm.[3-6] Thus pheochromocytoma or hypercatecholamine states need to be added to the list of causes of cardiac arrest. In our patient, her first cardiac arrest occurred 9 years before death. Coronary angiography in persons with coronary disease who are successfully resuscitated after cardiac arrest most commonly discloses severe fixed narrowing of one or more of the major epicardial coronary arteries.[7] Had this procedure been done in our patient, her coronary arteries would have been devoid of fixed narrowings and, consequently, causes of cardiac arrest in the presence of normal coronary arteries would have been sought. Pheochromocytoma is a *curable* cause of unexpected cardiac arrest.

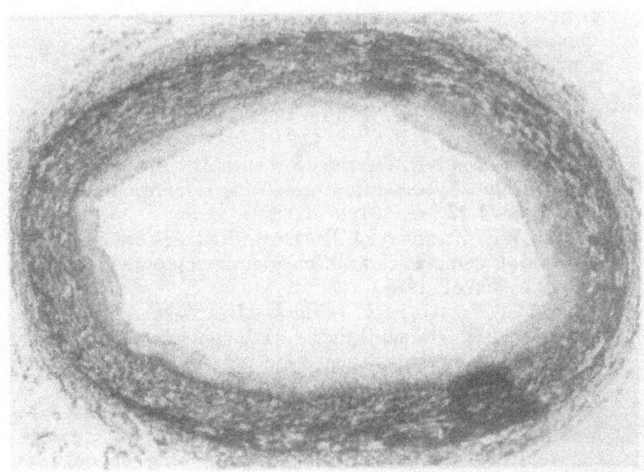

Fig. 3. Transverse section of normal right coronary artery. All major coronary arteries were similar to this. (Movat stain; original magnification ×27).

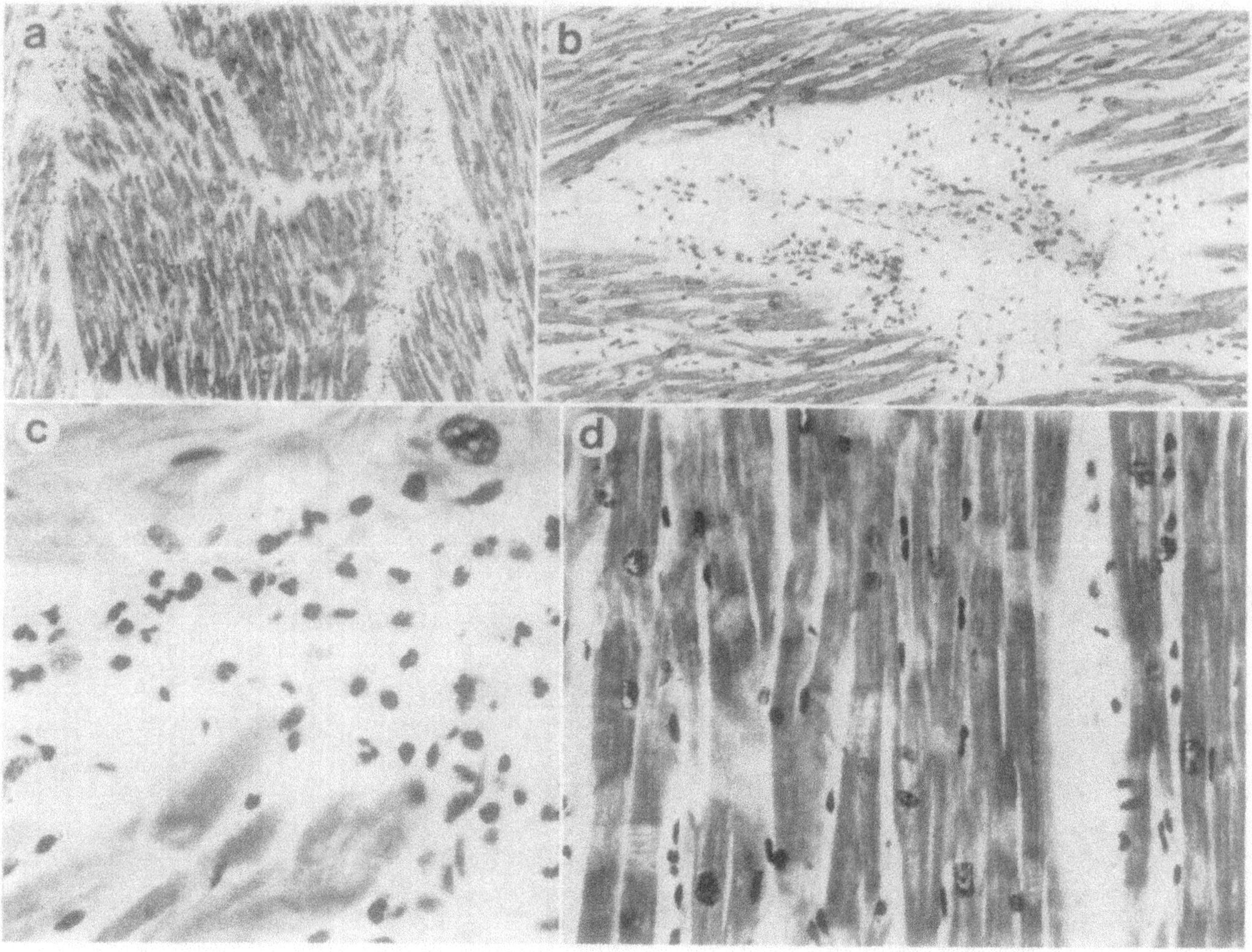

Fig. 4. Left ventricular myocardium with acute myocarditis and contraction band necrosis. *a,* Diffuse infiltration by inflammatory cells through myocardium. *b,* Perivascular inflammation. *c,* Close-up of the inflammatory infiltrate. *d,* Contraction-band necrosis of myocytes. (Hematoxylin and eosin stains; original magnification ×20 (*a*), ×45 (*b*), ×540 (*c*), ×330 (*d*)).

REFERENCES

1. Van Vliet PD, Burchell HB, Titus JL: Focal myocarditis associated with pheochromocytoma. N Engl J Med **274:**1102, 1966.
2. Thomas JE, Rooke ED, Krale WF: The neurologist's experience with pheochromocytoma. JAMA **197:**754, 1966.
3. Page LB, Raker JW, Berberick FR: Pheochromocytoma with predominant epinephrine secretion. Am J Med **47:**648, 1969.
4. Baker G, Zellen NH, Weitzner S, Leach JK: Pheochromocytoma without hypertension presenting as cardiomyopathy. Am Heart J **83:**688, 1972.
5. Radtke WE, Kazmier FJ, Rutherford BD, Sheps SG: Cardiovascular complications of pheochromocytoma crisis. Am J Cardiol **35:**701, 1975.
6. Aronoff SL, Passamani E, Borowsky BA, Weiss AN, Roberts R, Cryer PE: Norepinephrine and epinephrine secretion from a clinically epinephrine-secreting pheochromocytoma. Am J Med **69:**321, 1980.
7. Myerburg RJ, Conde CA, Sung RJ, Mayorga-Cortes A, Mallon SM, Sheps DS, Appel RA, Castellanos A: Clinical, electrophysiologic and hemodynamic profile of patients resuscitated from prehospital cardiac arrest. Am J Med **68:**568, 1980.

Osteogenic Sarcoma Metastatic to the Heart

KATHERINE A. SEIBERT, M.D., Ph.D.
CARL W. RETTENMIER, M.D.
BRUCE F. WALLER, M.D.
WILLIAM E. BATTLE, M.D.
ARTHUR S. LEVINE, M.D.
WILLIAM C. ROBERTS, M.D.
Bethesda, Maryland

Of 20 patients with fatal osteogenic sarcoma who underwent postmortem examination, four had metastases to the heart. One had recurrent ventricular tachycardia, one had anatomic evidence of aortic regurgitation due to massive periaortic neoplastic infiltration that prevented coaptation of the aortic cusps during ventricular diastole, one had massive invasion of the peri-superior vena caval tissues and typical clinical features of the superior vena caval syndrome, and one had neoplastic obstruction of the inferior vena cava as it entered the thorax. Among patients with either primary or secondary neoplasms to the heart, osteogenic sarcoma is unique because the metastases contain bone and, therefore, may be *radiographically visible;* they are usually *large* and often *intracavitary.*

Metastases to the heart occur in about 10 percent of patients with fatal cancer, but only about 10 percent of them have evidence of cardiac dysfunction during life [1–5]. Although many isolated case reports of various sarcomas metastatic to the heart are available, groups of patients with various sarcomas to the heart studied at postmortem examination are rare. Recently, we studied a patient with osteogenic sarcoma metastatic to the heart both clinically and morphologically. The unusual nature of her clinical course stimulated us to review other necropsy subjects with osteogenic sarcoma studied in the National Cancer Institute. Of 20 patients with this bone neoplasm who underwent postmortem examination, four had metastases to the heart at necropsy. This report describes the nature of their cardiovascular involvement.

PATIENTS STUDIED

Certain clinical and morphologic observations in the four patients are summarized in **Table I** and illustrated in **Figures 1 to 6.** Radiographic features in Patient 4 have been described briefly elsewhere [6]. The primary osteosarcoma was located in a leg bone in two and the pelvis in two. The interval from diagnosis of osteogenic sarcoma to death varied from three to 48 months (mean 26). Only one (Patient 4) had unequivocal evidence of cardiac dysfunction. This 39 year old woman fainted while hospitalized for chemotherapy 10 months before death and a 24-hour Holter monitor recording disclosed 32 separate episodes of ventricular tachycardia (Figure 4). She was treated thereafter with quinidine daily and was free of syncopal episodes or arrhythmias (as determined by three more 24-Holter monitorings) until one week before death when syncope recurred and several episodes of ventricular tachycardia were again documented. At the time of the first documented episode of ventricular tachycardia, chest radiography, bone scan, and computerized tomography disclosed a calcified mass within the right side

From the Pediatric, Medicine and Pathology Branches, National Cancer Institute, and the Pathology and Cardiology Branches, National Heart, Lung and Blood Institute, National Institutes of Health, Bethesda, Maryland. Requests for reprints should be addressed to Dr. William C. Roberts, Building 10A, Room 3E-30, National Institutes of Health, Bethesda, Maryland, 20205. Manuscript accepted on November 6, 1981.

TABLE I **Certain Observations in Our Four Necropsy Subjects with Osteogenic Sarcoma (OS) Metastatic to the Heart**

Patient No.	Necropsy No.	Age (yr)	Sex	Interval Dx OS to Death (mo)	Site of Primary OS	Location of OS in Heart E	RV W	RV C	LV W	LV C	Size OS in Heart (1+ to 4+)	Obstruction SVC	Obstruction IVC
1	A70–185	15	M	25	Femur	+	0	0	0	0	4+	0	+
2	A75–290	24	M	48	Tibia	+	0	+	0	+	4+	+	0
3	A79–74	28	F	11	Ilium	+	0	0	+	0	1+	0	0
4	A80–81	39	F	20	Ilio-Sacrum	0	+	+	0	0	4+	0	0

C = cavity; Dx = diagnosis; E = epicardium; F = female; IVC = inferior vena cava; LV = left ventricle; RV = right ventricle; SVC = superior vena cava; W = wall.

of the heart (Figures 5 and 6). The abnormal QRS complexes during the episodes of ventricular tachycardia were of the left bundle block pattern, suggesting that they originated from the right ventricular free wall or from the right ventricular portion of the septum.

Although two of the four patients had dyspnea at rest, each of the four had numerous pulmonary metastases. Only one (Patient 4, Table I) had a third heart sound and that was observed only during fluid challenge. Two patients had subcutaneous edema; Patient 1 had external compression of the inferior vena cava by tumor and edema of the legs and abdomen, and Patient 2 had external compression of the superior vena cava (Figures 2 and 3) with edema limited to the head and neck. Thus, none of the four patients had overt evidence (except during fluid overload) of congestive heart failure or chest pain.

Electrocardiography, in the three adults, showed only nonspecific changes, except for the patient with ventricular tachycardia.

Chest radiography (Figures 1, 2 and 6) in all four patients disclosed numerous pulmonary metastases in each and unequivocal bony metastases in the heart in Patient 4 (Figure 5).

At necropsy, mediastinal and pulmonary metastases completely encased the heart and great vessels in Patient 1 (Figure 1). The tumor encasing the great arteries prevented the aortic valve cusps from coapting during ventricular diastole, and although a murmur of aortic regurgitation was not recorded, the extensiveness of the mediastinal neoplasm may have prevented its being heard. The systemic arterial pressure was 100/60 mm Hg. A grade 2/6 systolic murmur, loudest over the second right intercostal space, had been recorded. Patient 2 had huge metastases in the right lung and they extended into the pericardial space and into both atrial

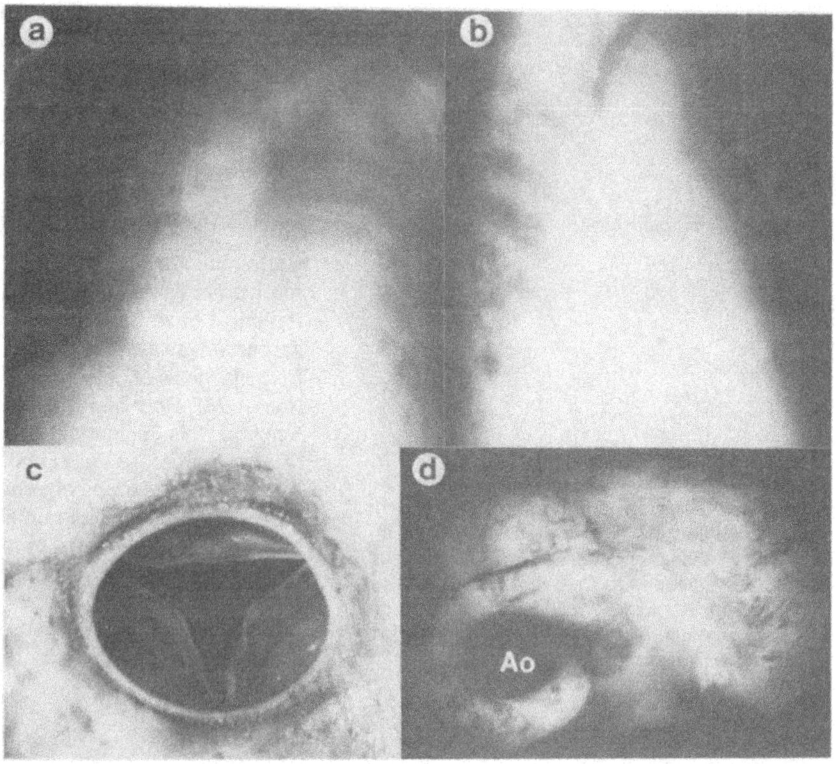

***Figure 1. Patient 1, Table I. A** and **B**, chest radiographs one month before death showing extensive mediastinal and left pulmonary radiodensities. **C**, view of aortic valve from above. The cusps are unable to close completely because the walls of aorta are encased in bone. **D**, postmortem radiograph of the basal portion of the heart and ascending aorta (Ao) showing massive calcium that completely encircled the aorta and much of the heart.*

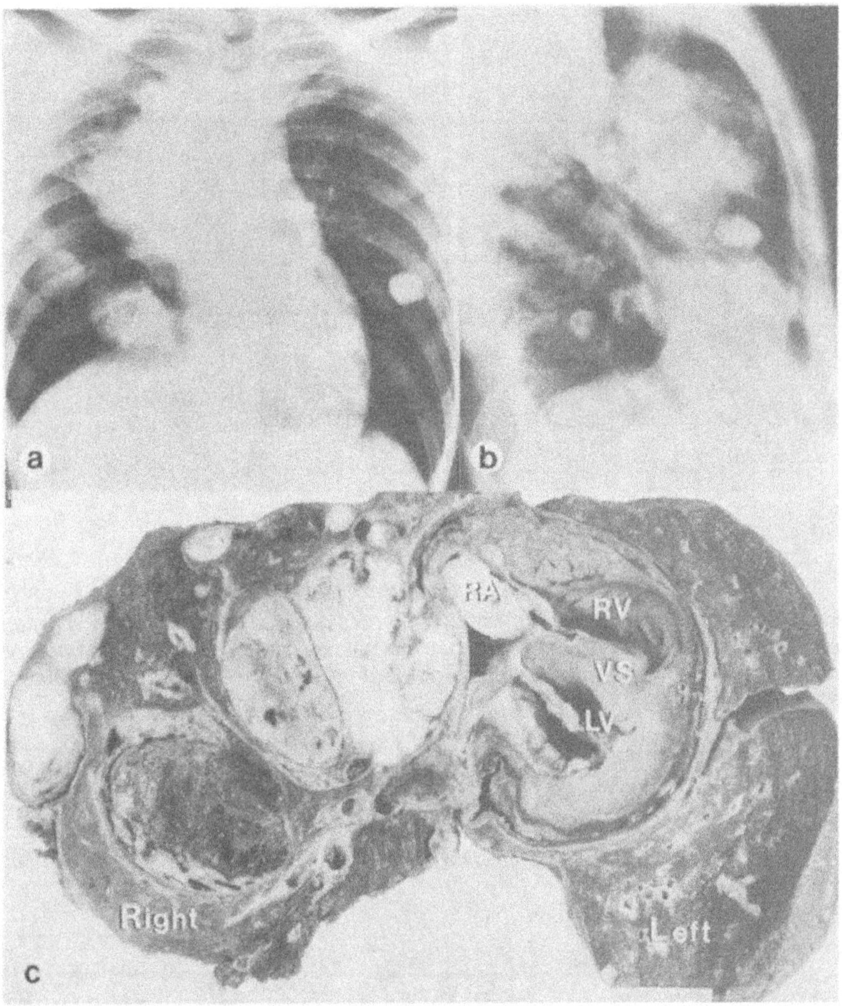

***Figure 2. Patient 2, Table I. A** and **B,** posteroanterior and lateral chest radiographs showing metastatic masses in the lungs and mediastinum. **C,** transverse cut of the lungs and heart showing multiple metastatic masses in the right lung and within the right atrium (RA). LV = left ventricle; RV = right ventricle; VS = ventricular septum.*

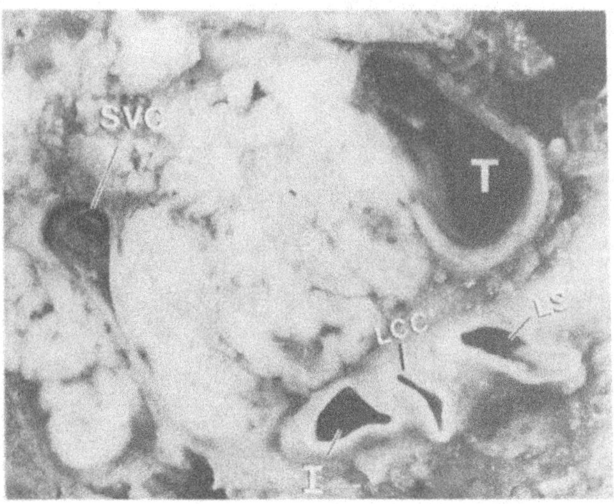

***Figure 3. Patient 2, Table I.** External compression by metastatic sarcoma causing severe narrowing of the superior vena cava (SVC) with a thrombus within the residual lumen. I = innominate artery; LCC = left common carotid artery; LS = left subclavian artery; T = trachea.*

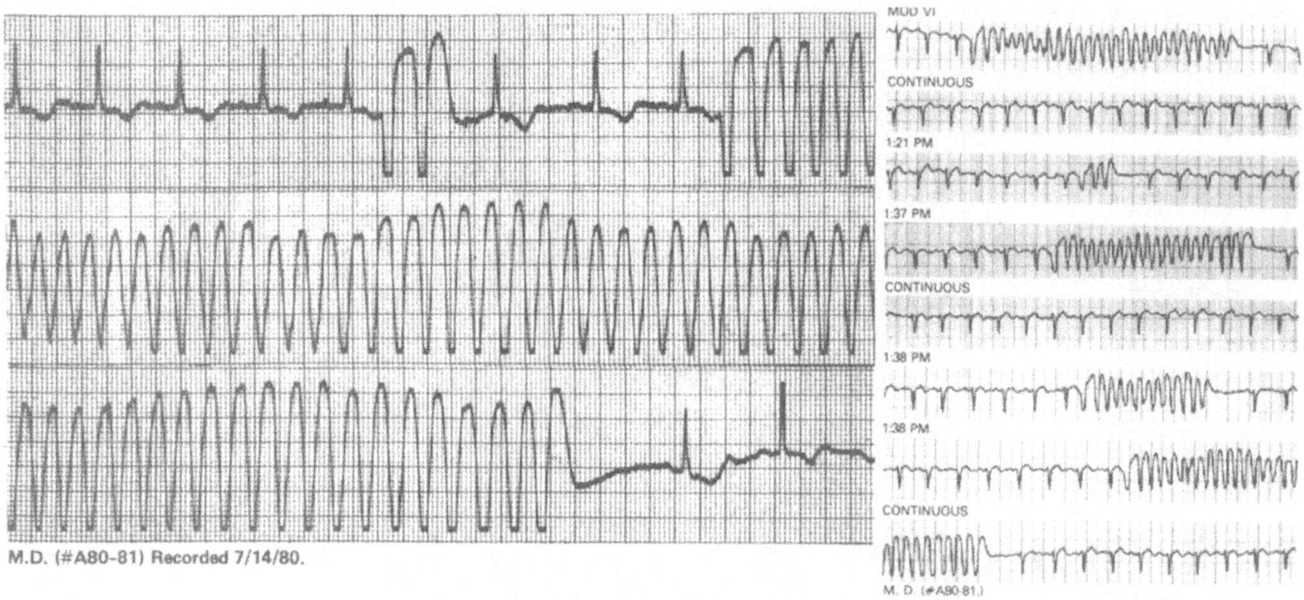

Figure 4. Patient 4, Table I. *Portion of Holter monitor recording (lead V_5) (**left**) before onset of quinidine sulfate therapy showing a 10-second run of ventricular tachycardia and back-to-back ventricular premature complexes recorded 10 months before death. Monitor rhythm strips (modified lead V_1 [mod V1]) (**right**) recorded one week before death showing frequent bursts of ventricular tachycardia.*

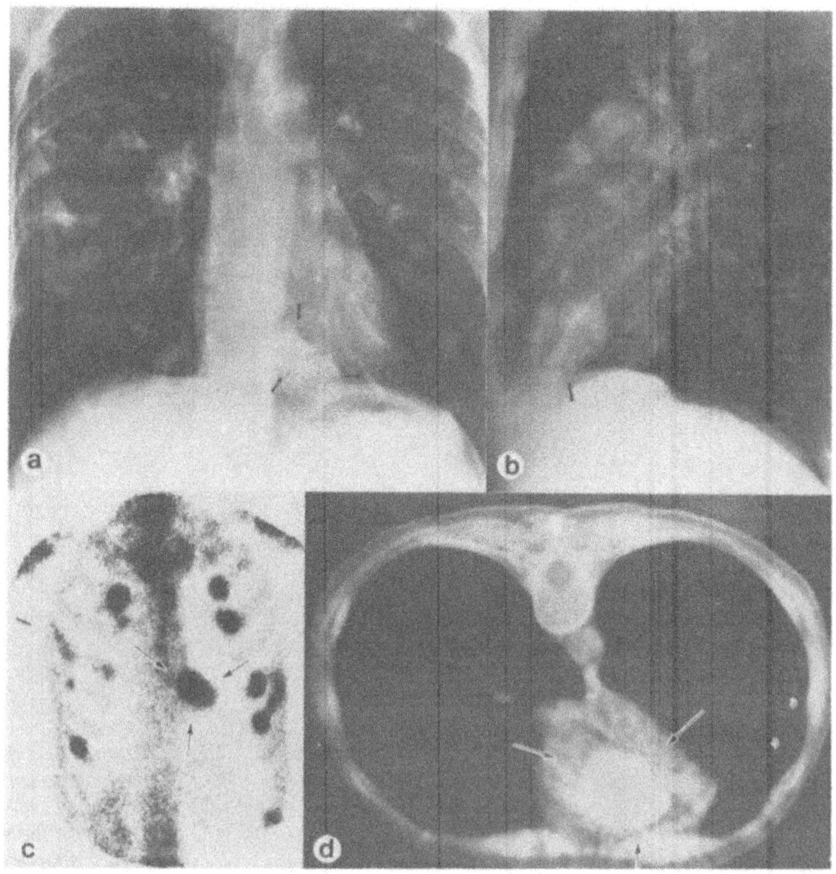

Figure 5. Patient 4, Table I. *Chest radiographs (**A** and **B**), bone scan (**C**), and computerized tomogram (**D**) showing multiple metastatic nodules in the lung, and one (**arrows**) within the right ventricle (Reproduced, with permission from Dunnick et al. [6]).*

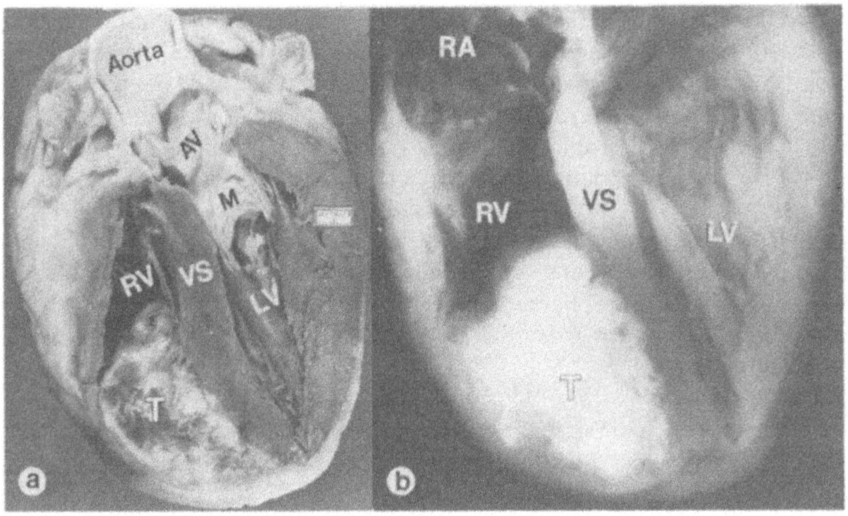

Figure 6. Patient 4, Table I. *Longitudinal view of heart (**A**) showing a large tumor (T) mass within the right ventricle (RV) and radiograph of heart at necropsy (**B**). AV = aortic valve; LV = left ventricle; VS = ventricular septum; RA = right atrium (Photograph by Margaret M. M. Moore).*

cavities (Figures 2 and 3). Patient 3 had only a 1.5 cm metastatic nodule within the posterior left ventricular wall. Patient 4 had a large tumor deposit in the right ventricular cavity, and it extended into the adjacent right ventricular free wall and ventricular septum (Figure 6).

COMMENTS

Of the four patients just described with osteogenic sarcoma metastatic to the heart, three had widespread cardiac metastases at postmortem examination and one had symptoms of cardiac dysfunction due to ventricular tachycardia. Her ventricular arrhythmia became apparent 10 months before death and was suppressed by quinidine for nearly 10 months despite evidence that the right ventricular tumor mass continued to grow. Two other patients, however, had vena caval obstruction and one had anatomic evidence of aortic valve regurgitation.

Limited reported data are available in other necropsy subjects with osteogenic sarcoma metastatic to the heart [7,8]. In **Table II** are summarized data in seven such reports in which findings are specifically described [9–15]. Although one of the seven patients had syncope, venricular tachycardia was not documented in any. Engle and associates [16], however, described ventricular tachycardia resulting from a resectable cardiac tumor in a child, and Caldwell and colleagues [17] have suggested that ventricular tachycardia in a child should warrant angiocardiography to search for a cardiac tumor. Four of the seven patients whose findings are summarized in Table II had severe dyspnea without pulmonary metastases, and this symptom may have represented evidence of congestive heart failure. A neoplasm was located within a cardiac cavity in all seven: in one or both right-sided cardiac cavities in all seven and in one or both left-sided cavities as well in

TABLE II Observations in Seven Previously Reported Necropsy Subjects with Osteogenic Sarcoma Metastatic to the Heart

First Author [Reference]	Year of Publication	Age at Death (yr)	Race	Sex	Site of Primary	Interval Dx to Death (mo)	Metastases to Organs Other Than Heart: Lungs	Other	Symptoms and Signs: D	S	C	E	ECG: LV	BBB	IC	Location of Metastases in Heart*: Right Side: Wall	Right Side: Cavity	Left Side: Wall	Left Side: Cavity	Epicardium
Hektoen [9]	1893	12	–	M	Tibia	8	+	0	+	0	0	0	–	–	–	+	+	0	0	0
Laurian [10]	1957	13	W	F	Tibia	7	+	0	+	0	+	0	–	0	+	0	+	0	0	0
Dorfman [11]	1966	12	W	M	Femur	5	0	0	+	0	0	0	–	+†	+	0	+	0	0	0
Dalal [12]	1978	21	W	M	Tibia	60	0	0	+	0	0	+	+	0	+	+	+	0	0	+
Takatsu [13]	1979	41	W	F	Rib	2	0	+	+	0	0	0	0	0	+	+	+	+	+	0
Magovern [14]	1980	23	W	F	Arm	54	+	0	0	+	0	0	–	+§	–	+	+‡	0	0	0
Wise [15]	1980	30	W	F	Arm	21	0	0	+	0	+	0	+	+§	–	–	+‡	0	0	0

* Large in all seven patients.
† Indeterminate type.
‡ Operatively excised.
§ Right.
BBB = bundle branch block; C = peripheral cyanosis; D = dyspnea; Dx = diagnosis; E = subcutaneous edema; ECG = electrocardiogram; IC = ischemic changes; LV = low voltage; S = syncope.

one. Two of our four patients had intracavitary locations of the cardiac metastases. Although it was absent in our three patients who had electrocardiography, bundle branch block of the right or indeterminate type was present in three of the six patients (in Table II) in whom electrocardiographic findings were reported.

The most unique feature of osteogenic sarcoma involving the heart is that the metastases may be *radiologically visible*. This situation occurred in our Patient 4 in whom a metastastic mass was identified in the right ventricle by radiography 10 months before death. Although the cardiac metastases were not identified within the heart by radiography during life in the other three patients, retrospective examination of the radiographs with knowledge of the location of metastases found at necropsy allowed their identification on radiographs posthumously. Of course, echocardiography, particularly two-dimensional (apical view) [18], is also useful for identifying intracavitary tumors and even intramural tumors [19]. Our Patient 4 had M-mode echocardiography that gave normal results, and, although two-dimensional echocardiography was performed, an apical four-chamber view was not obtained. Tumors located in the inflow and body portion of the right ventricle are usually not detected by one-dimensional echocardiography, which discerns the outflow portion of this chamber.

ACKNOWLEDGMENT

We thank Mr. Ted Crump and Dr. Nobuyuki Shitara who provided translations for two articles used in the preparation of this manuscript.

REFERENCES

1. Roberts WC, Bodey GP, Wertlake PT: The heart in acute leukemia. A study of 420 autopsy cases. Am J Cardiol 1968; 21: 388–412.
2. Glancy DL, Morales JB, Roberts WC: Angiosarcoma of the heart. Am J Cardiol 1968; 21: 413–419.
3. Glancy DL, Roberts WC: The heart in malignant melanoma. A study of 70 autopsy cases. Am J Cardiol 1968; 21: 555–571.
4. Roberts WC, Glancy DL, DeVita VT Jr: Heart in malignant lymphoma (Hodgkin's disease, lymphosarcoma, reticulum cell sarcoma and mycosis fungoides). A study of 196 autopsy cases. Am J Cardiol 1968; 22: 85–107.
5. Lindsay J Jr, Goldberg SD, Roberts WC: Electrocardiogram in neoplastic and hematologic disorders. In: Rios JC, ed. Clinical electrocardiographic correlations. Philadelphia: FA Davis, 1977; 225–242 (Cardiovasc Clinics 1977; 8: 225–242).
6. Dunnick NR, Seibert K, Cramer H: Cardiac metastasis from osteosarcoma. J Comput Assist Tomog 1981; 5: 253–255.
7. Jeffree M, Price CH, Sissons HA; The metastatic patterns of osteosarcoma. Br J Cancer 1975; 32: 87–106.
8. Uribe-Botero G, Russell W, Sutow W, Martin R: Primary osteosarcoma of bone—a clinicopathologic investigation of 243 cases, with necropsy studies in 54. Am J Clin Pathol 1977; 67: 427–435.
9. Hektoen L: Three specimens of tumors of the heart: metastatic carcinomatous nodule in the myocardium, implantation-sarcoma of the right ventricle, primary round-celled sarcoma of the epicardium. Medical News 1893; 63: 571–574.
10. Laurain AR: Intracardial tumor culture of osteogenic sarcoma with fatal tumor embolism. Am J Clin Pathol 1957; 27: 664–671.
11. Dorfman HD, Michaels GL: Cardiac metastases in osteogenic sarcoma. Bull Hosp Joint Dis 1966; 27: 1–8.
12. Dalal BI, Raju BS, Datta BN, Khatri HN: Metastatic osteosarcoma of heart: report of a case and review of literature. Ind J Cancer 1978; 15: 84–86.
13. Takatsu T, Kino M, Sawada K, et al.: Metastatic osteosarcoma in heart: diagnostic problem of osteosarcoma metastasized to the heart [in Japanese]. Nippon Rinsho 1979; 37: 402.
14. Magovern GJ, Yusuf MF, Liebler GA, Pugh RP, Joyner CR: The surgical resection and chemotherapy of metastatic osteogenic sarcoma of the right ventricle. Ann Thorac Surg 1980; 29: 76–80.
15. Wise NK, Peter RH, Wechsler AS, Moore JO, Saltzman HA: Right ventricular obstruction secondary to intracardiac metastatic osteosarcoma. Clin Cardiol 1980; 3: 200–203.
16. Engle MA, Ebert P, Redo SF: Recurrent ventricular tachycardia due to resectable cardiac tumor. Circulation 1974; 50: 1052–1057.
17. Caldwell P, Ricketts H, Dillard D, Guntheroth W: Ventricular tachycardia in a child: an indication for angiocardiography? Am Heart J 1974; 88: 777–781.
18. Jaffe C, Kelley M, Taunt K: Two-dimensional echocardiographic identification of a right ventricle tumor. Radiology 1978; 129: 471–472.
19. Isner JM, Falcone MW, Virmani R, Roberts WC: Cardiac sarcoma causing "ASH" and simulating coronary heart disease. Am J Med 1979; 66: 1025–1030.

Clinical and Morphologic Cardiac Findings After Anthracycline Chemotherapy

Analysis of 64 Patients Studied at Necropsy

JEFFREY M. ISNER, MD, VICTOR J. FERRANS, MD, PhD, STEVEN R. COHEN, MD, BRUCE G. WITKIND, MD, RENU VIRMANI, MD, JOHN S. GOTTDIENER, MD, J. ROBERT BECK, MD, and WILLIAM C. ROBERTS, MD

The relation between clinical evidence of and histologic signs of anthracycline cardiotoxicity was evaluated by reviewing the clinical and morphologic findings in 64 patients studied at necropsy, all of whom had received doxorubicin or daunorubicin chemotherapy during life. Of the 64 patients, 20 (31%) had documented clinical toxicity consisting of impaired left ventricular systolic performance; in 7 (35%) of these 20 patients, histologic signs of toxicity were absent. In the remaining 13 patients with clinical toxicity, histologic signs of toxicity ranged from mild to severe. Of the 44 (69%) patients without clinical signs of drug toxicity, 21 (48%) had no histologic sign of cardiotoxicity; in 23 (52%) of the patients without clinical toxicity, however, morphologic signs of cardiotoxicity were nevertheless present—mild in most patients, but extensive in 4. Signs of extensive histologic toxicity (19 [30%] of 64 patients) were associated with large doses (>450 mg/m²) of the drug, mediastinal irradiation, and age >70 years. This study suggests that attempts to monitor cardiotoxicity by serial evaluation of cardiac histology in patients undergoing anthracycline chemotherapy may be seriously limited by the fact that clinical evidence of toxicity may be present without histologic signs of toxicity; likewise, histologic signs of anthracycline toxicity may be present without clinical evidence of toxicity.

The anthracycline drugs doxorubicin (Adriamycin™) and daunorubicin (Daunomycin™) are 2 of the most effective chemotherapeutic agents presently available for treatment of patients with solid tumors and leukemias.[1] Cardiac toxicity is a well-recognized complication of these agents and is frequently the dose-limiting factor in their administration.[2,3] Although endomyocardial biopsy has been used in several centers to monitor patients receiving anthracycline chemotherapy,[4] limited information is available regarding the results of necropsy examination of patients who have received these drugs.[5–7] The present study was designed to determine (1) the extent of morphologic cardiotoxicity at necropsy in patients treated with anthracycline compounds, and (2) the degree to which the results of morphologic examination of necropsy hearts correlated with clinical evidence of cardiac dysfunction.

From the Pathology and Cardiology Branches, National Heart, Lung, and Blood Institute, National Institutes of Health, Bethesda, Maryland. Manuscript received January 5, 1983, accepted January 6, 1983.

Address for reprints: Jeffrey M. Isner, MD, Tufts-New England Medical Center, 171 Harrison Avenue, Box 70, Boston, Massachusetts 02111.

Methods

Review of the clinical records of all patients with malignant neoplasms who died and underwent necropsy examination at the National Cancer Institute, Bethesda, Maryland, between January 1, 1970, and June 30, 1979, revealed 93 patients who had been treated with anthracyclines. In 11 patients, the gross and/or histologic material available for review was inadequate; in 18 additional patients, interpretation of both clinical and morphologic cardiac findings was complicated by medical problems such as severe anemia, renal failure, hemosiderosis, and myxedema. These 29 patients, therefore, were eliminated from further study. The remaining 64 patients form the basis of the present study. Review of gross and histologic findings and reexamination of the hearts from these 64 patients were performed without knowledge of the clinical cardiac findings.

The hearts of all 64 patients were evaluated grossly for pericardial disease, chamber dilatation, mural thrombus, and foci of fibrosis or necrosis. Histologic sections from the left ventricular free wall, ventricular septum, and right ventricular free wall were stained with hematoxylin-eosin and phosphotungstic acid hematoxylin. Each section was examined by 3 observers, who, by consensus, assigned to it a histologic score. Two characteristics were used to score the extent of histologic cardiotoxicity: vacuolization of cardiac muscle cells (Fig. 1a)

TABLE I Clinical and Morphologic Findings in 20 Patients With Clinical Evidence of Anthracycline Toxicity

Age (yr) & Sex	Interval Onset Sx to Death	Physical Examination			CXR		Echo		Hemodynamic Data		Cardiac Therapy		
		JVD	Rales	S_3	CE	PVH	LVd	FS	CVP	PAOP	Dig	Diur	Improved
Patients Without Histologic Signs of Anthracycline Toxicity													
5F	18 d	0	+	+	0	+	—	—	—	—	+	+	+
15M	1 d	+	+	+	+	+	50	0.16	20	—	+	+	0
18M	7 d	+	+	+	+	+	—	—	20	—	+	+	0
26F	1 d	0	+	+	0	+	—	—	18	—	+	+	0
37F	2 mo	+	+	+	+	+	—	—*	—	—	+	+	+
61M	7 mo	0	0	+	+	+	—	—	—	—	+	+	+
61M	14 mo	+	+	0	+	+	65	0.28	15	—	+	+	+
Patients with Histologic Signs of Anthracycline Toxicity													
13M	6 d	+	0	+	+	+	47	0.16	—	—	+	+	0
39M	4 mo	0	+	+	+	+	51	0.18	9	18	+	+	+
21M	15 d	+	+	+	+	0	58	0.19	20	20	+	0	0
22F	5 wk	0	+	0	+	0	52	0.19	18	—	+	+	+
35F	11 mo	+	+	+	+	+	54	0.19	—	22	+	+	+
78M	2 d	+	+	+	+	+	—	—	—	—	+	+	0
12M	9 d	+	+	0	+	+	46	0.30	17	—	+	+	+
15F	3 mo	0	0	+	+	0	61	0.10	—	18	+	+	+
29F	7 d	+	+	+	+	+	55	0.27	16	20	+	+	0
49F	1 mo	0	0	0	+	0	52	0.08	—	26	+	+	0
5M	17 d	+	0	+	0	0	—	—	—	—	+	+	+
33F	2 mo	+	0	+	0	0	44	0.23	—	—	+	+	+
11F	4 wk	+	+	+	+	+	46	0.13	—	—	+	+	+

* Preejection period/left ventricular ejection time = 0.61.
CE = cardiac enlargement; CVP = central venous pressure; DA = daunorubicin; DO = doxorubicin; DIG = digitalis; Diur = diuretic; FS = fractional shortening; Histo Tox = histologic toxicity; JVD = jugular venous distention; LVd = left ventricular end-diastolic dimension; Med Irrad = mediastinal

and myofibrillar dropout (Fig. 1b). The severity of each of these 2 histologic features was assessed for each section of the myocardium according to the following scale: 0 = none, 1 = mild, 2 = moderate, and 3 = extensive. The final score of histologic cardiotoxicity for a particular patient was arrived at by adding the highest grade for vacuolization and the highest grade for myofibrillar dropout observed on any of the various sections of myocardium from the patient. For example, a patient who received a score of 2+ for vacuolization and 1+ for myofibrillar dropout would receive a final score of 3+ for histologic cardiotoxicity.

The hospital records of all 64 patients were reviewed without knowledge of the necropsy findings. Echocardiograms performed in 26 patients also were reevaluated without knowledge of necropsy findings or of the original interpretation of the study.

Statistical significance regarding characteristics of groups with and without clinical or histologic toxicity was assessed by the chi-square test.

Results

Patients with clinical evidence of drug toxicity: Of the 64 patients, 20 (31%) had clinical evidence of cardiotoxicity (Table I). These 20 patients included 10 males and 10 females, aged 5–78 years (average 29). Their total dose of anthracycline drug ranged from 85 to 900 mg/m^2 (average 450), administered over a period of 4 to 156 weeks (average 41). Four patients also received mediastinal irradiation to a total dose of 4,000, 9,450, 12,450, and 12,600 rads, respectively. In 16 of these 20 patients, evidence of cardiotoxicity included hemodynamic documentation (12 patients) (elevated central venous pressure or elevated pulmonary capillary wedge pressure, or both) and/or echocardiographic documentation of decreased fractional shortening (11 patients); in the remaining 4 patients, the diagnosis of a drug-induced cardiomyopathy was based on a combination of physical signs of cardiac decompensation (jugular venous distention, inspiratory rales, S_3 gallop sound) and radiographic signs of pulmonary venous hypertension and cardiomegaly. All 20 patients with clinical signs of drug toxicity received digoxin and 10 also received diuretics.

In 7 of the 20 patients with clinical signs of drug toxicity, the pericardial sac contained >50 ml of fluid (average 186, range 80 to 300). Two of these 7 patients had received mediastinal irradiation, and in 1 the pericardial fluid was grossly hemorrhagic; in the remaining 6 the fluid was serosanguinous. None of the 7 patients had cardiac metastases. The average heart weight in the 17 adult patients with clinical signs of drug toxicity was 358 g (range 240 to 500) (Table I). In 18 of the 20 patients, the heart weight observed exceeded that predicted according to body weight[8] by an average of 106 g. In 11 of the 20 patients, both ventricular cavities were dilated, while in 4 other patients the left ventricle alone was dilated; in the remaining 5 patients, neither ventricular cavity was dilated. The presence or absence of cavity dilatation at necropsy was *not* a function of the interval between the onset of clinical signs of toxicity and death. In 2 patients, the dilated ventricular cavities contained mural thrombus (Fig. 2); neither patient had a history of peripheral embolic events.

Histologic signs of cardiotoxicity were observed in 13 of the 20 patients with clinical signs of drug toxicity (Tables I and II): these 13 patients included 10 of the 15 patients with and 3 of the 5 without cavity dilatation. The combined histologic scores for toxicity among these 13 patients ranged from 1 to 5 (average 2.3).

TABLE I (Continued)

Age (yr) & Sex	Oncologic Therapy: Total Anthracycline (mg/m^2)	Oncologic Therapy: Duration Rx (wks)	Oncologic Therapy: Total Rads Med Irrad	Gross Findings: Heart Wt (g) Obs (Pred)	Gross Findings: Dilated Ventricles	Histologic Findings: Myocyte Vacuoles	Histologic Findings: Myofibrillar Dropout	Histologic Findings: Histo Tox score
Patients Without Histologic Signs of Anthracycline Toxicity								
5F	345(DA)	26	0	150(99)	+	0	0	0
15M	530(DA)	32	0	450(253)	+	0	0	0
18M	630(DA)	32	0	295(297)	0	0	0	0
26F	330(DA)	12	0	320(258)	+	0	0	0
37F	550(DO)	88	0	270(260)	+	0	0	0
61M	210(DO)	4	0	396(350)	0	0	0	0
61M	250(DO)	8	0	500(352)	+	0	0	0
Patients With Histologic Signs of Anthracycline Toxicity								
13M	490(DA)	60	0	450(129)	+	0	1+	1
39M	180(DO)	4	4,000	350(300)	+	1+	0	1
21M	600(DO)	156	12,600	450(390)	+	1+	1+	2
22F	570(DO)	12	0	380(283)	0	0	2+	2
35F	900(DO)	60	12,450	240(249)	+	2+	0	2
78M	280(DO)	10	0	300(245)	0	2+	0	2
12M	195(DO)	3	0	300(253)	+	1+	2+	3
15F	510(DO)	20	0	380(155)	+	2+	1+	3
29F	550(DO)	28	0	280(189)	+	1+	2+	3
49F	550(DO)	42	0	310(249)	+	2+	1+	3
5M	500(DO)	12	0	90(54)	+	2+	2+	4
33F	85(DO)	16	9,450	270(258)	0	2+	2+	4
11F	750(DO)	132	0	200(120)	+	3+	2+	5

irradiation; Obs = observed; PAOP = pulmonary artery occlusion pressure; Pred = predicted; PVH = pulmonary vascular hypertension; Rx = treatment; Sx = symptoms; + = present; 0 = absent.

In contrast to the previous 13 patients, histologic signs of cardiotoxicity were absent from multiple sections of myocardium in 7 of the 20 patients with clinical signs of drug toxicity (Table I). These 7 patients included 5 patients with and 2 without cavity dilatation. The 7 patients in whom clinical evidence of anthracycline cardiotoxicity was *not* associated with histologic abnormalities ranged in age from 5 to 61 years. Four received up to 630 mg/m^2 of daunorubicin, while 3 received 210 to 500 mg/m^2 of doxorubicin. All had evidence on physical examination of congestive heart failure. On chest radiograms, signs of pulmonary venous hypertension were present in all, and 5 of 7 had an enlarged cardiac silhouette. Two patients had abnormal echocardiograms, 1 had abnormal systolic time intervals, and 4 had elevated venous pressures.

Patients without clinical evidence of drug toxicity: Of the 64 patients, 44 (69%) had no clinical signs of cardiotoxicity. These patients (23 males, 21 females) ranged in age from 2 to 70 years (average 44).

Three of these 44 patients had >50 ml of fluid in the pericardial sac (500, 400, and 100), while in 3 others the pericardial space was obilterated by dense, fibrous adhesions. One of the former 3 patients and all of the latter 3 had received >4,900 rads of mediastinal irradiation. The average heart weight, excluding 2 children, was 278 g (range 105 to 450). In 29 patients, the observed heart weight exceeded the predicted heart weight by an average of 65 g. Biventricular dilatation was observed in 4 patients, and mild left ventricular enlargement in 2. Left ventricular mural thrombus was found in 1 patient with no history of peripheral embolic events.

Histologic signs of cardiotoxicity were observed in 23 (52%) of the 44 patients, despite the fact that none of these 44 patients had clinical evidence of anthracycline cardiotoxicity (Table II). In 15 of the 23 patients, the histologic findings were limited to a mild degree (combined score 1/6) of vacuolization (14 patients) or myofibrillar dropout (1 patient). In the remaining 8 patients, however, more extensive morphologic changes were noted: 4 patients received combined scores of 2/6 for histologic cardiotoxicity.

TABLE II Relation of Clinical Toxicity to Type and Extent of Morphologic Toxicity

Clinical Toxicity	Patients (n)	Myocardial Vacuoles 0	Myocardial Vacuoles 1	Myocardial Vacuoles 2	Myocardial Vacuoles 3	Myofibrillar Loss 0	Myofibrillar Loss 1	Myofibrillar Loss 2	Myofibrillar Loss 3
+	20	9	4	6	1	10	4	6	0
0	44	22	17	3	2	37	7	0	0
Totals									
n	64	31	21	9	3	47	11	6	0
%	. . .	48	33	14	5	74	17	9	0

(Type and Extent of Morphologic Toxicity)

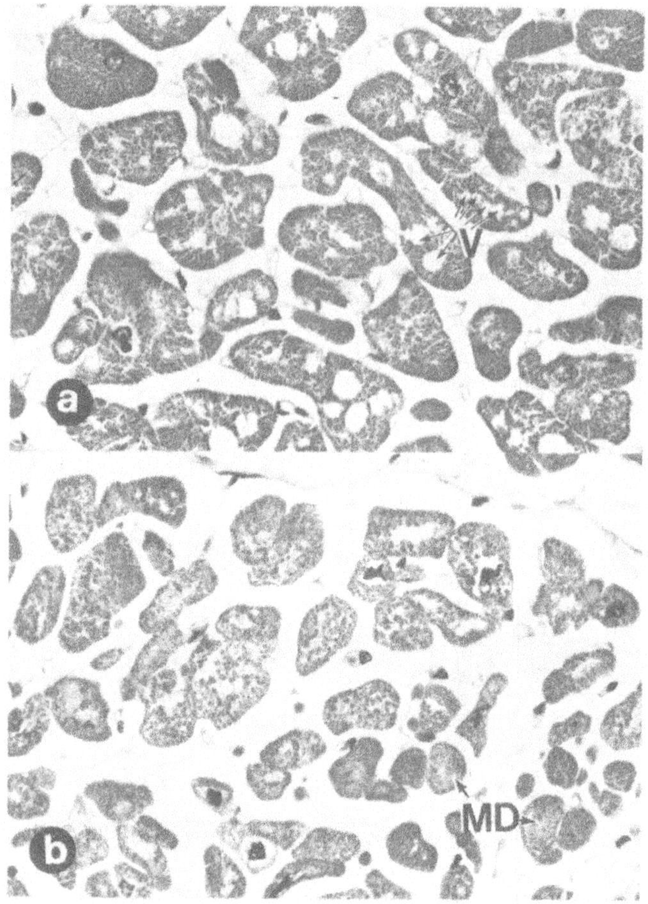

FIGURE 1. Findings used to score the extent of histologic cardiotoxicity: (a) vacuolization (V) of cardiac muscle cells, and (b) myofibrillar dropout (MD). This patient (15-year-old girl, Table I) received a histologic toxicity score of 3 (2+ vacuolization, 1+ myofibrillar dropout). (Hematoxylin and eosin stain; magnification ×500, reduced 33%.)

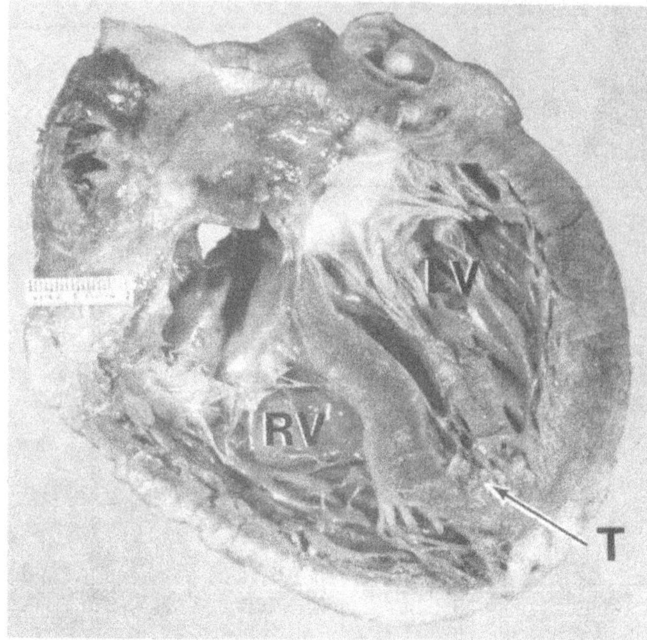

FIGURE 2. Biventricular cavity dilatation in 15-year-old girl (Table I) with clinical and histologic evidence of anthracycline cardiotoxicity. The apical portion of the dilated left ventricle (LV) contains antemortem thrombus (T). RV = right ventricle.

Patients grouped according to final (combined) scores for histologic cardiotoxicity (Fig. 3): The entire study group of 64 patients was analyzed from the standpoint of the combined score for histologic toxicity. Twenty-eight patients had a combined score of 0; 7 had clinical signs of toxicity while 21 did not. Seventeen patients received a histologic score of 1; clinical toxicity was present in 2 patients and absent in 15. Eight patients received a histologic score of 2; clinical toxicity was present in 4 and absent in 4. Seven patients received a histologic score of 3; 4 had clinical toxicity and 3 did not. Three patients received a histologic score of 4; 2 had clinical toxicity and 1 did not. Only 1 patient had a histologic score of 5 and this patient had overt clinical cardiotoxicity.

Relation between clinical cardiotoxicity and gross and histologic signs of toxicity (Fig. 4): Of the total 64 patients, 18 had neither clinical or structural evidence of cardiotoxicity. In 36 patients, histologic signs of toxicity were observed. Of these, 23 had no clinical evidence of toxicity, including 4 with dilated ventricles. Three patients had both clinical and histologic signs of toxicity unassociated with ventricular cavity dilatation. A complete "triad" of clinical, gross anatomic, and histologic signs of cardiotoxicity was observed in only 10 patients.

Of the remaining 10 patients of the study group of 64, 3 had ventricular cavity dilatation without histologic or clinical evidence of cardiotoxicity, 5 had clinical toxicity and cavity dilatation without histologic evidence of toxicity, and 2 had clinical signs of toxicity unassociated with either gross or histologic signs of toxicity. Thus, in 8 patients, cavity dilatation was not associated with histologic abnormalities.

Finally, in the entire study group of 64 patients, 20 had clinical signs of toxicity, and 2 of these patients showed no evidence of either cavity dilatation or histologic abnormalities. In 1, clinical evidence of toxicity consisted of jugular venous distention, inspiratory rales, and an S_3 gallop sound on physical examination; cardiomegaly and pulmonary venous hypertension on chest radiogram; and a central venous pressure of 20 mm Hg. The second patient also had an S_3 gallop sound, and cardiomegaly and pulmonary venous hypertension on chest radiogram. Both patients received treatment with digoxin and diuretics and 1 improved. Neither patient had pericardial fluid at necropsy.

The sensitivity of the histologic necropsy examination was calculated as follows: Patients with clinical and histologic toxicity/(patients with cardiotoxicity and histologic toxicity) + (patients with clinical toxicity without histologic toxicity) = 13/(13 + 7) = 0.65. The specificity of histologic necropsy examination was calculated as follows: Patients without clinical toxicity and without histologic toxicity/(patients without clinical toxicity and without histologic toxicity) + (patients with histologic toxicity without clinical toxicity) = 21/(21 + 23) = 0.48. The predictive value of the finding of his-

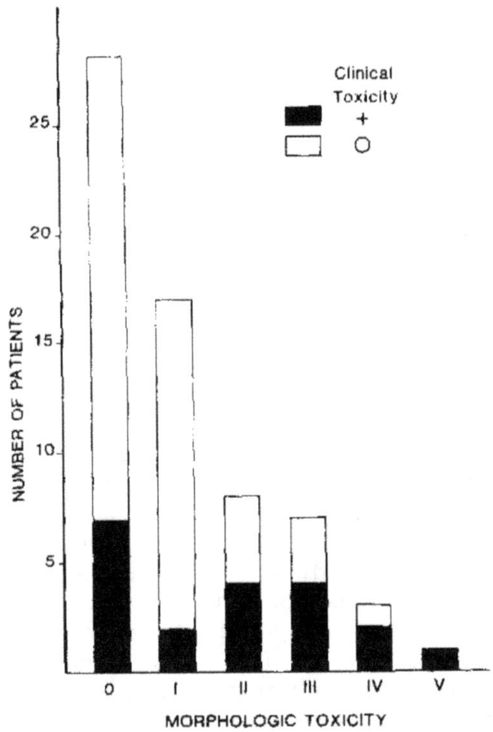

FIGURE 3. Number of patients with and without clinical evidence of cardiac toxicity in each category of histologic toxicity (see text for histologic toxicity grading system).

tologic toxicity was calculated as follows: Patients with clinical and histologic toxicity/(patients with clinical and histologic toxicity) + (patients with histologic toxicity without clinical toxicity) = 13/(13 + 23) = 0.36. This predictive value when tested proved not significantly different from random variation in toxicity (chi-square = 0.91, p >0.30).

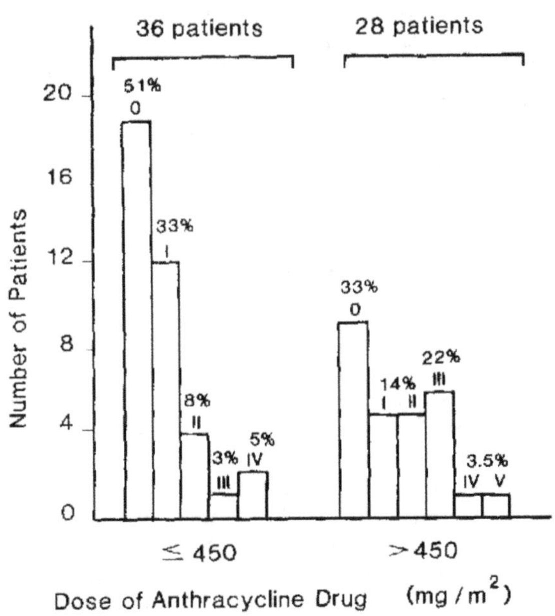

FIGURE 5. Scores for histologic toxicity grouped according to cumulative dose of anthracycline drug administered (≤450 or >450 mg/m²).

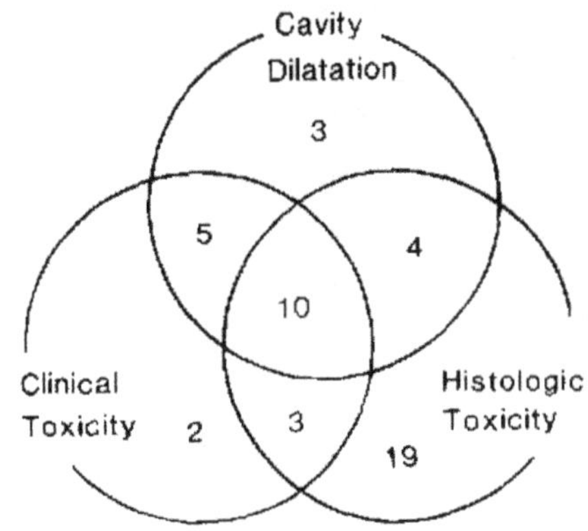

FIGURE 4. Relation of clinical cardiotoxicity to gross and histologic signs of cardiotoxicity. (Of the total 64 patients, 18 had neither clinical toxicity, cavity dilatation, nor morphologic toxicity and are not represented in this figure.)

Histologic toxicity as a function of cumulative dose of anthracycline drug: The relation between the extent of histologic signs of cardiotoxicity and the cumulative dose in mg/m² of anthracycline is illustrated in Figure 5. Of the 28 patients who received anthracycline therapy >450 mg/m², 13 (46%) had histologic scores of 2 to 5; in contrast, of 36 patients who received anthracycline therapy <450 mg/m², only 6 (17%) had histologic scores of ≥2 (p = 0.0097). Nevertheless, extensive histologic abnormalities were not limited to patients treated with >450 mg/m² of drugs: One patient treated with 100 mg/m² received a histologic toxicity score of 4 and had clinical signs of toxicity; 3 patients

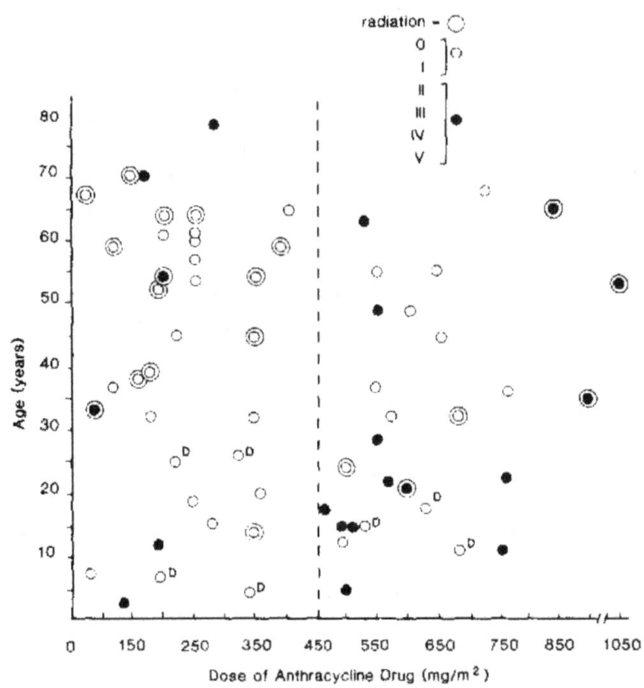

FIGURE 6. Morphologic toxicity as a function of cumulative dose of anthracycline drug, mediastinal irradiation, and age. All but 2 of the patients with scores of II to V received >450 mg/m², mediastinal irradiation, or were ≥70 years of age.

TABLE III Distribution of Histologic Changes (Morphologic Toxicity) in the Ventricular Walls of the Heart in 64 Necropsy Patients

Portion of Heart	Sections Examined (n)	Final Grade of Morphologic Toxicity 0	I	II	III	IV	V	Nonrepresentative Sections
Left ventricular free wall	62	26	14	8	7	3	1	3
Ventricular septum	36	12	7	6	5	0	1	5
Right ventricular free wall	50	22	7	3	5	3	1	9
Totals								
n	148	60	28	17	17	6	3	17
%	...	41	19	11	11	4	1	12

treated with 100 to 200 mg/m^2 received histologic toxicity scores of 2, 3, and 4, respectively, and 1 had clinical signs of toxicity; 2 patients treated with 200 to 300 mg/m^2 received a histologic toxicity score of 2.

Histologic toxicity as a function of cumulative drug, dose, age, and mediastinal irradiation: The effects of increasing age and mediastinal irradiation, in combination with cumulative drug dose, are illustrated in Figure 6. Of the 19 patients with combined histologic scores of 2 through 5, 13 received anthracycline therapy >450 mg/m^2. Of the 6 patients with extensive histologic changes who received <450 mg/m^2 of drug, 2 were treated with mediastinal irradiation (5,800 and 9,450 rads, respectively), and 2 were ≥70 years of age. Thus, all but 2 patients, in whom extensive histologic signs of anthracycline cardiotoxicity were recognized at necropsy, received >450 mg/m^2 of anthracycline therapy, or received combined mediastinal irradiation, or were ≥70 years of age.

Distribution of histologic abnormalities: The distribution of the histologic changes representing anthracycline cardiotoxicity is shown in Table III. Of 62 sections of left ventricular free wall from 64 patients, only 3 sections (5%) demonstrated histologic toxicity of lesser severity than was recognized in sections from either the ventricular septum or right ventricular free wall. Of 36 sections of ventricular septum taken from the 64 patients, only 5 (14%) were not representative of histologic lesions observed in sections taken from other sites of the myocardium. Of 50 sections taken from the right ventricular free wall, 9 (18%) were nonrepresentative. In those cases in which histologic toxicity was most extensive (histologic toxicity scores of 3, 4, and 5), these lesions were seen on sections taken from all 3 sites, that is, the right and left ventricular free walls and ventricular septum. The lesions corresponding to a histotoxicity score of 1 or 2 were more variable in distribution: In patients receiving a score of 1 or 2, the histologic abnormality was present in the left ventricle in 82 and 100%, respectively; in the ventricular septum in 64 and 64%; and in the right ventricular free wall in 54 and 50%.

Electrocardiographic findings in patients with and without clinical signs of drug toxicity: Electrocardiograms recorded between the time of onset of symptoms and the time of death were available in 9 of the 20 patients with clinical evidence of anthracycline toxicity. Two of the 9 patients had diminished amplitude of the QRS complex ("low voltage": ΣQRS amplitude [leads I, II, and III] ≤15 mm); in 1 of these 2 patients plus 1 other of the 9 patients, serial recordings demonstrated >30% diminution of the summated amplitude of the QRS complex in the limb leads. Pericardial heart disease was responsible for low voltage in only 1 of these patients. The mean cardiac weight of the 3 patients with reduced electrocardiographic QRS voltage was 248 g; the mean cardiac weight of the remaining 6 patients was 345 g.

Of the total group of 40 patients without clinical evidence of drug toxicity, 35 had electrocardiograms that were available for review: 11 (13%) had low voltage, including 1 with >30% diminution of the summated limb lead QRS amplitude on serial recordings. Their mean heart weight was 286 g, and none had pericardial heart disease, myxedema, cardiac amyloidosis, or hemochromatosis.

As a group, the 14 patients with low voltage and/or serial diminution in summated QRS amplitude did not differ significantly from the 30 patients with normal amplitude QRS complexes in terms of histologic findings: Vacuolar lesions were seen in 30% of the patients with and in 58% of the patients without low voltage; myofibrillar dropout in 20% of those with and in 28% of those without low voltage; interstitial fibrosis in 15% of those with and in 17% of those without low voltage; and attenuated myocytes ("fiber thinning") in 45% of the patients with versus 47% of those without low voltage.

Discussion

Anthracycline-induced cardiomyopathy was first reported by Tan et al[9] in 1967 in a 16-year-old girl treated with daunorubicin. Subsequent reports[10–14] confirmed the potential cardiotoxicity of daunorubicin and its derivative compound, doxorubicin. In the first detailed account of the morphologic findings of anthracycline-induced cardiomyopathy, Lefrak et al[5] described 2 patients in whom necropsy examination disclosed gross anatomic findings of biventricular dilatation with cavitary thrombus and histologic findings consisting of cytoplasmic hyaline transformation and cytoplasmic vacuolization. In both patients, clinical signs of a dilated cardiomyopathy had developed after they had received 720 and 825 mg/m^2 of doxorubicin.

Cortes et al[7] subsequently studied at necropsy 51 patients with doxorubicin, 17 (33%) of whom had signs of "toxic cardiopathy," defined as a combination of "intracellular edema, intracellular vacuolization, and myocardial fibrosis"; 5 had had congestive heart failure before death, and the remaining 12 never had overt cardiac failure.

Subsequent to these early necropsy observations, most published information regarding morphologic findings in patients receiving anthracycline drugs has been derived from analysis of myocardial biopsy specimens obtained from patients undergoing anthracycline chemotherapy.[4] Interest in this technique developed principally from 2 observations: (1) Although the development of anthracycline cardiotoxicity in general correlated with cumulative drug dose, in certain patients serious cardiotoxicity developed at relatively low doses,[15–19] while others, clearly in need of continuing chemotherapy, tolerated higher doses of the drug without adverse effects.[20] (2) Noninvasive methods contemporary to the early 1970s (electrocardiography, systolic-time intervals, echocardiography) proved unreliable for detecting latent, subclinical cardiac toxicity.[21–26] Thus, it was hoped that evaluation of serial biopsies might detect signs of potential cardiotoxicity before the time when cardiotoxicity became inevitable, and furthermore that biopsy analysis might predict how much longer a given patient could safely tolerate continued administration of anthracycline therapy.

The present study was designed to evaluate the correlation between clinical and morphologic signs of anthracycline cardiac toxicity in patients studied at necropsy. Examination of necropsy specimens eliminates the potential pitfalls posed by biopsy specimens, particularly the small size of tissue specimen,[27,28] limitation of sampling to subendomyocardial myocardium, and access to only 1 cardiac ventricle.[29] In addition, we hoped to extend the experience of Cortes et al[7] by (1) evaluating the pathologic material without knowledge of the clinical history, and (2) by establishing more rigid criteria for the definition of clinical and histologic signs of cardiotoxicity.

The present investigation suggests that prediction of clinical anthracycline cardiotoxicity on the basis of histologic changes is uncertain, because correlation between morphologic and functional changes is imperfect. Histologic signs of anthracycline cardiotoxicity may be absent, despite unequivocal clinical signs of a dilated cardiomyopathy: this situation was observed in 7 (35%) of our 20 patients. This finding has 3 important implications. The first, regarding therapy, is that in these 7 patients, an endomyocardial biopsy performed before the development of overt congestive heart failure would have suggested that treatment with anthracycline drugs could be continued safely. The second is that at least some of the "false-negative" results described in patients studied by the biopsy technique[22] are unlikely to have resulted simply from sampling errors. The third is that myofibrillar dropout and dilatation of the sarcoplasmic reticulum are not the only factors involved in the pathogenesis of anthracycline-induced cardiac failure. The concept that such failure is simply the result of structural damage to tissue represents an oversimplification of a very complex series of morphologic and biochemical changes.

The counterpart of the foregoing findings is that histologic signs of cardiotoxicity may be present without clinical signs of cardiac dysfunction: this situation was observed in 23 (52%) of 44 patients in the present report. Histologic signs of toxicity unassociated with clinical toxicity have been observed frequently in patients studied by endomyocardial biopsy, and, if extensive, have been interpreted as a contraindication to continued administration of anthracycline chemotherapy in these patients. The finding of morphologic toxicity in an asymptomatic patient—in the biopsy and, now, necropsy experience—suggests that such subclinical morphologic alteration may be the basis for the development of latent cardiac dysfunction described in long-term survivors of anthracycline therapy.[30,31] In nonhuman animal models of anthracycline toxicity, delayed development of cardiomyopathy has been observed as long as 6 months after discontinuation of therapy, and has been interpreted as evidence that the myocardial effects of anthracycline compounds are cumulative and irreversible.[32]

The serious discrepancies between morphologic and clinical evidence of toxicity found in the present investigation suggests that morphologic monitoring of patients receiving anthracycline drugs is of limited value for predicting the development of anthracycline cardiomyopathy. In contrast, physiologic evaluation of the cardiac response to exercise[26,31,33] or increased afterload[34] may improve the sensitivity of monitoring such patients for clinical evidence of latent cardiotoxicity. Long-term follow-up of such patients will determine whether such latent toxicity ultimately progresses to overt congestive heart failure.

Because this was a retrospective study and necropsy material from these patients had not been routinely preserved in glutaraldehyde fixative, examination of material was by necessity limited to gross anatomic and light microscopic studies. Nevertheless, as has been pointed out before, the morphologic lesions of anthracycline toxicity are evident by light microscopy.[27]

Electrocardiographic changes (low voltage or serial reduction ≥30% in limb lead voltage) previously proposed as evidence of anthracycline cardiotoxicity[35] correlated poorly with signs of morphologic toxicity in our patients, a finding noted previously by others.[23,36] The finding of low voltage was related to cardiac atrophy in patients with systemic cachexia, rather than to drug toxicity. The finding that cardiac atrophy frequently forms the morphologic basis for diminished QRS amplitude in such patients[37] makes this electrocardiographic feature particularly unsuitable for monitoring patients likely to be cachectic by virtue of their systemic illness.

Finally, our findings confirm observations made previously by Von Hoff,[2] Bristow,[33] and Billingham[38] regarding "risk factors" for anthracycline cardiotoxicity. Extensive morphologic toxicity was observed, with 2 exceptions, only in patients treated with >450 mg/m^2 of drug, or in patients in whom a smaller dose was administered in association with mediastinal irradiation or to a patient ≥70 years of age. These findings support the concept of empiric limitation of total dose of drug, if possible, to <450 mg/m^2, and to an even smaller total in patients likely to receive mediastinal irradiation and in patients ≥70 years of age. Nevertheless, the finding of clinical or morphologic toxicity in patients treated with lower total doses of drug unassociated with mediastinal irradiation or advanced age suggests that empiric limitation of total dose of anthracycline is not by itself adequate to protect against the cardiotoxic effects of these drugs and mandates some form of associated monitoring.

References

1. **Young RC, Ozols RF, Myers CE.** The anthracycline antineoplastic drugs. N Engl J Med 1981;305:139–153.
2. **Von Hoff DD, Layard MW, Basa P, Davis HL Jr, Von Hoff AL, Rozencweig M, Muggia FM.** Risk factors for doxorubicin-induced congestive heart failure. Ann Intern Med 1979;91:710–717.
3. **Von Hoff DD, Rozencweig M, Layard M, Slavik M, Muggia FM.** Daunomycin-induced cardiotoxicity in children and adults. A review of 110 cases. Am J Med 1977;62:200–206.
4. **Bristow MR, Mason JW, Billingham ME, Daniels JR.** Doxorubicin cardiomyopathy: evaluation of phonocardiography, endomyocardial biopsy, and cardiac catheterization. Ann Intern Med 1978;88:168–175.
5. **Lefrak EA, Pitha J, Rosenheim S, Gottlieb JA.** A clinicopathologic analysis of Adriamycin cardiotoxicity. Cancer 1973;32:302–314.
6. **Buja LM, Ferrans VJ, Mayer RJ, Roberts WC, Henderson ES.** Cardiac ultrastructural changes induced by daunorubicin therapy. Cancer 1973;32: 771–788.
7. **Cortes EP, Lutman G, Wanka J, Wang JJ, Pickren J, Wallace J, Holland JF.** Adriamycin (NSC-123127) cardiotoxicity: a clinicopathologic correlation. Cancer Chermother Rep 1975;6:215–225.
8. **Smith HL.** Relation of the weight of the heart to the weight of the body and of the weight of the heart to age. Am Heart J 1928;4:79–93.
9. **Tan CL, Tasaka H, Yu KP, Murphy ML, Karnofsky D.** Daunomycin, an anti-tumor antibiotic, in the treatment of neoplastic disease. Clinical evaluation with specific reference to childhood leukemia. Cancer 1967;20: 333–353.
10. **Malpas JS, Bodley Scott R.** Rubidomycin in acute leukemia in adults. Br Med J 1968;3:227–229.
11. **Bonadonna G, Monfardini S.** Cardiac toxicity of daunorubicin. Lancet 1969;1:837.
12. **Smith B.** Damage to the intrinsic cardiac neurones by rubidomycin (daunorubicin). Br Heart J 1969;31:607–609.
13. **Alnger LE, Bushore J, Johnson WW, Ito J.** Daunomycin: a cardiotoxic agent. J Natl Med Assoc 1971;63:261–267.
14. **Middleman E, Luce J, Frei E III.** Clinical trials with Adriamycin. Cancer 1971;28:844–850.
15. **Rinehart JJ, Lewis RP, Balcerzak SP.** Adriamycin cardiotoxicity in man. Ann Intern Med 1974;81:475–478.
16. **Starkebaum GA, Durack DT.** Early onset of daunorubicin (Daunomycin) cardiotoxicity. Lancet 1975;2:711–712.
17. **Ippoliti G, Casirola G, Marini, Invermizzi R.** Daunorubicin cardiotoxicity (letter). Lancet 1976;1:430.
18. **Harrison DT, Sanders LA.** Pericarditis in a case of early daunorubicin cardiomyopathy. Ann Intern Med 1976;85:339–341.
19. **Bristow MR, Thompson PD, Martin RP, Mason JW, Billingham ME, Harrison DC.** Early anthracycline cardiotoxicity. Am J Med 1978;65:823–832.
20. **Blum RH, Carter SK.** Adriamycin. A new anticancer drug with significant clinical activity. Ann Intern Med 1974;80:249–250.
21. **Minow RA, Benjamin RS, Gottlieb JA.** Adriamycin (NSC-123127) cardiomyopathy: an overview with determination of risk factors. Cancer Chemother Rep 1975;6:195–201.
22. **Mason JW, Bristow MR, Billingham ME, Daniels JR.** Invasive and noninvasive methods of assessing adriamycin cardiotoxic effects in man: superiority of histopathologic assessment using endomyocardial biopsy. Cancer Treat Rep 1978;62:857–864.
23. **Fulkerson PK, Talley R, Kleinman D, Weaver SK, Leier CV, Balcerzak SP, Lewis RP.** Noninvasive profile in the prospective monitoring of Adriamycin cardiomyopathy. Cancer Treat Rep 1978;62:881–886.
24. **Hutchinson RJ, Bailey C, Wood D, Donaldson MH.** Systolic time intervals in monitoring for anthracycline cardiomyopathy in pediatric patients. Cancer Treat Rep 1978;62:907–910.
25. **Henderson IC, Sloss LJ, Jaffe N, Blum RH, Frei E III.** Serial studies of cardiac function in patients receiving Adriamycin. Cancer Treat Rep 1978;62:923–929.
26. **Alexander J, Dainiak K, Berger HL, Goldman L, Johnstone D, Reduto L, Duffy T, Schwartz P, Gottschalk A, Zaret BL.** Serial assessment of doxorubicin cardiotoxicity with quantitative radionuclide angiocardiography. N Engl J Med 1978;300:278–283.
27. **Billingham ME, Mason JW, Bristow MR, Daniels JR.** Anthracycline cardiomyopathy monitored by morphologic changes. Cancer Treat Rep 1978;62:865–872.
28. **Isner JM, Maron BJ, Roberts WC.** Comparison of amount of myocardial cell disorganization in operatively excised septectomy specimens with amount observed at necropsy in 18 patients with hypertrophic cardiomyopathy. Am J Cardiol 1980;46:42–47.
29. **Ferrans VJ, Roberts WC.** Myocardial biopsy: a useful diagnostic procedure or only a research tool? Am J Cardiol 1978;41:965–967.
30. **Gottlieb SL, Edmiston WA Jr, Haywood LJ.** Late, late doxorubicin cardiotoxicity. Chest 1980;78:880–882.
31. **Gottdiener JS, Mathisen DJ, Borer JS, Bonow RO, Myers CE, Barr LH, Schwartz DE, Bacharach SL, Green MV, Rosenberg SA.** Doxorubicin cardiotoxicity: assessment of late left ventricular dysfunction by radionuclide cineangiography. Ann Intern Med 1981;94:430–435.
32. **Jaenke RS.** Delayed and progressive myocardial lesions after Adriamycin administration in the rabbit. Cancer Res 1976;36:2958–2966.
33. **Bristow MR, Mason JW, Billingham ME, Daniels JR.** Dose-effect and structure-function relationships in doxorubicin cardiomyopathy. Am Heart J 1981;102:709–718.
34. **Borow KM, Keane JF, Castaneda AR, Freed MD.** Systemic ventricular function in patients with tetralogy of Fallot, ventricular septal defect and transposition of the great arteries repaired during infancy. Circulation 1981;64:878–885.
35. **Minow RA, Benjamin RS, Lee ET, Gottlieb JA.** QRS voltage change with Adriamycin administration. Cancer Treat Rep 1978;62:931–934.
36. **Weaver SK, Fulkerson PK, Lewis RP, Leier C.** A paucity of chronic electrocardiographic changes with Adriamycin therapy. J Electrocardiog 1978;11:233–238.
37. **Isner JM, Fortin RV, Oliphant LH, Crisciticllo MG.** Cardiac atrophy is a frequent etiology for the electrocardiographic finding of low voltage (abstr). Circulation 1982;66:Suppl II:II-127.
38. **Billingham ME, Bristow MR, Glatstein E, Mason JW, Masek M, Daniels JR.** Adriamycin cardiotoxicity: endomyocardial biopsy evidence of enhancement by irradiation. Am J Surg Pathol 1977;1:17–23.

The Carcinoid Syndrome: Comparison of 21 Necropsy Subjects with Carcinoid Heart Disease to 15 Necropsy Subjects without Carcinoid Heart Disease

ELIZABETH M. ROSS, M.D.
WILLIAM C. ROBERTS, M.D.
Bethesda, Maryland

Carcinoid heart disease is a morphologically specific type of cardiac disorder that involves the mural and valvular endocardium on the right side of the heart. Twenty-one subjects (57 percent) (Group I) with carcinoid heart disease and 15 subjects (43 percent) (Group II) without carcinoid heart disease were studied at necropsy. The two groups were similar in mean age (54 years versus 55 years), duration of clinical illness (4.7 years versus 6.3 years), body weight (50 kg versus 52 kg), systemic blood pressure (117/77 mm Hg versus 128/77 mm Hg), blood hematocrit levels (37 percent versus 36 percent), total serum protein levels (6.0 g/dl), and serum albumin levels (2.2 g/dl versus 2.6 g/dl). The two groups were different in the frequency of the presence of precordial murmurs consistent with tricuspid regurgitation and/or pulmonic stenosis (95 percent versus 13 percent), cardiomegaly by chest radiography (38 percent versus 0), low voltage on electrocardiography (47 percent versus 0), and location of the primary site of the carcinoid tumor. Total electrocardiographic 12-lead QRS voltage was similar in each group (105 mm versus 132 mm) (10 mm = 1 mV). Of Group I subjects, 43 percent died of cardiac causes; none of the Group II subjects died of cardiac causes. Of the 21 subjects with carcinoid heart disease, seven had left-sided cardiac involvement, but in none was it of functional significance. Thus, although carcinoid heart disease frequently is the cause of death in patients with the carcinoid syndrome, the development of carcinoid heart disease is not related to the duration of symptoms of the carcinoid syndrome.

In 1964, Roberts and Sjoerdsma [1] reported clinical and necrospy findings in 17 subjects with the carcinoid syndrome, nine with and eight without carcinoid heart disease. Since that date, we have studied both clinically and at necropsy an additional 19 subjects with this syndrome. This report summarizes findings in the entire group of 36 subjects, specifically seeking clues to distinguish clinically those subjects with carcinoid heart disease from those without carcinoid heart disease, and it evaluates the effect of carcinoid heart disease on prognosis.

SUBJECTS AND METHODS

Definitions. *Carcinoid syndrome*—the presence of histologically proved carcinoid tumor in a site other than the appendix with metastases to both local lymph nodes and to one or more other sites, and the presence of diarrhea, wheezing, and/or cutaneous flushing. *Carcinoid heart disease*—the presence of grossly visible, focal, uniform fibrous lesions on the mural endocardium of the right atrium, right ventricle, or left ventricle and the presence of diffuse or focal thickening of the cusps of tricuspid and/or pulmonic valves with or without involvement of the mitral and/or aortic valves; histologic examination

From the Pathology Branch, National Heart, Lung and Blood Institute, National Institutes of Health, Bethesda, Maryland. Requests for reprints should be addressed either to Dr. Elizabeth M. Ross, Washington Hospital Center, 110 Irving Street, NW, Room 3B-44B, Washington, D.C. 20010, or to Dr. William C. Roberts, Building 10A, Room 3E-30, National Institutes of Health, Bethesda, Maryland 20205. Manuscript accepted December 28, 1984.

TABLE I Clinical and Morphologic Findings in 21 Subjects with Carcinoid Heart Disease

Subject	Necropsy Number	Age (years) and Sex	Length of Illness (years)	SAP (mm Hg)	Site of Primary Carcinoid	Precordial Murmur (grade 0-6) TR	PS	Other	CT Ratio >0.5	Hct (percent)	TP (g/dl)	Alb (mg/dl)
1	A-63-222	28F	1.5	120/70	SI	0	+	PR	0	34	—	—
2	A-64-217	32F	9	95/70	Ileum	+	+	TS	0	39	5.0	1.4
3	A-63-96	39M	3	90/70	SI	+	0	PR	0	39	7.3	0.6
4	A-57-49	41M	3	110/70	Ileum	0	+	0	0	36	6.6	2.2
5	A-65-180	42M	5	125/80	Ileum	+	0	0	+	43	7.6	1.9
6	A-66-165	47M	13	100/70	Ileum	0	+	0	0	30	4.8	2.5
7	A-57-238	50F	12	100/70	Ileum	0	+	PR	0	37	4.7	2.6
8	A-62-9	52F	1.5	120/80	Jejunum	0	+	0	0	30	5.1	2.0
9	A-70-214	52M	4	—	Ileum	0	0	0	0	29	—	2.2
10	A-65-93	53M	3.5	100/65	Ileum	+	+	0	+	35	6.5	2.8
11	A-61-68	57F	4	140/90	Ileum	0	+	PR	+	37	6.6	3.3
12	A-61-266	57F	4	110/65	Ileum	+	+	0	0	35	5.7	2.5
13	A-68-49	57F	8	120/76	Ileum	+	0	TS	0	40	5.3	2.3
14	A-59-223	59M	6	100/60	Ileum	+	0	PR	+	43	6.5	2.2
15	A-72-96	61F	1	110/80	Ileum	+	0	0	0	45	6.9	3.0
16	A-61-193	64M	1.5	130/80	Jejunum	+	+	TS/PR	+	43	4.9	1.4
17	A-65-127	64F	1	110/75	Ileum	0	+	0	+	37	5.1	1.8
18	A-59-192	67M	7	110/70	Ileum	0	+	0	0	35	5.0	2.8
19	A-76-210	68M	9	130/80	—	+	0	0	0	38	7.2	3.8
20	A-62-34	69M	1	120/80	Ileum	+	+	0	+	33	6.7	3.3
21	83-A-94	72M	0.5	180/130	Ileum	+	0	0	+	—	—	2.3

* Zero indicates amount of pericardial fluid to be less than 50 ml.
† Zero indicates amount of pleural fluid to be less than 100 ml on either side.
‡ Zero indicates amount of peritoneal fluid to be less than 100 ml.
A = ascites; Alb = serum albumin; BW = body weight; CT = cardiothoracic; Hct = hematocrit; HIAA = hydroxyindole acetic acid; HW = heart weight; MV = mitral valve; Pe = pericardial; Pl = pleural; PR = pulmonic regurgitation; PS = pulmonic stenosis; PV = pulmonic valve; RA = right atrium; RV = right ventricle; SAP = systemic artery pressure; SE = subcutaneous pitting edema; SI = small intestine; TP = total protein; TR = tricuspid regurgitation; TS = tricuspid stenosis; TV = tricuspid valve; VC = vena cava.

of the thickened valvular cusps and thickened mural endocardium discloses uniform-appearing fibrous tissue devoid of elastic fibrils. These specific mural and valvular endocardial lesions will be referred to herein as *carcinoid plaques*.

Methods. The medical records of cases coded as "carcinoid syndrome" in the files of the Pathology Branch, National Heart, Lung, and Blood Institute, were retrieved and examined, and pertinent clinical and morphologic data (to be summarized later) recorded. The 19 hearts studied since 1964 were re-examined by both of us. (The hearts in the first 17 cases had been examined earlier by one of us [W.C.R.].) The necropsy records of all 36 cases were examined. At least two histologic sections of one or more grossly visible carcinoid plaques were examined in each subject; the range was two to 37 sections (average 12) per subject. Data were analyzed using the Student t test. A p value of 0.05 was accepted as indicating a significant difference between the groups.

HW (g)	BW (kg)	Highest Urinary 5-HIAA (mg/24 hours)	Hepatic Weight (g)	Location of Carcinoid Plaque						Effusion (amount in ml)			
				RA	TV	RV	PV	MV	VC	Pe*	Pl†	A‡	SE
250	—	263	—	+	+	0	+	+	+	—	—	—	+
250	37	288	1,950	+	+	+	+	0	0	0	+ (500)	+ (350)	+
280	48	432	2,900	+	+	0	+	+	0	0	0	+ (1,950)	+
220	42	890	7,400	+	+	0	+	0	0	0	0	+ (200)	0
420	55	450	2,130	+	+	+	+	+	0	0	0	+ (500)	+
250	67	§	4,000	+	0**	0	+	0	0	0	+ (200)	+ (1,500)	0
250	38	1,270	4,500	+	+	+	+	0	0	+ (100)	+ (2,500)	+ (20)	+
200	43	220	2,800	+	+	+	+	+	+	0	0	+ (4,600)	+
350	50	—	3,000	+	+	+	+	0	0	0	+ (600)	+ (3,000)	+
320	40	350	2,150	+	+	0	+	0	+	0	+ (250)	0	+
270	60	283	2,300	+	+	+	+	0	+	0	0	0	+
210	50	274	1,800	+	+	+	+	+	+	0	+ (750)	+ (525)	+
290	45	§	1,800	+	+	+	+	0	0	+ (50)	+ (1,100)	+ (500)	+
350	56	580	1,800	+	+	0	+	0	+	+ (150)	0	+	+
240	46	285	1,700	+	+	0	+	0	+	0	0	+ (750)	+
400	50	524	1,600	+	+	+	+††	+	0	0	0	0	+
250	47	135	2,150	+	+	0	+	0	+	0	0	+ (1,500)	+
280	62	—	2,500	+	+	+	+	0	0	+ (50)	+ (1,000)	+ (700)	+
480	67	500	5,700	0	+	+	+	+	0	0	0	+ (500)	+
475	52	120	2,600	0	+	0	+††	0	0	0	0	+	+
370	—	—	1,800	+	+	+	+	0	0	0	0	+	+

§ Markedly positive.
** Grossly normal; histologically abnormal.
†† Pulmonary trunk involved also.

RESULTS

Of the 36 subjects with the carcinoid syndrome, 21 (57 percent) at necropsy had carcinoid heart disease (Group I) and 15 (43 percent) did not (Group II). Certain findings in the subjects with carcinoid heart disease are summarized in **Table I,** and in those without in **Table II.**

Morphologic Findings. All 36 subjects had histologically proved carcinoid tumors with local lymph node involvement and metastases to one or more distant sites. Only one subject did not have hepatic metastases (Subject 15, Group II). Metastases to organs other than the liver occurred in 14 (67 percent) of 21 subjects in Group I and in 11 (73 percent) of 15 subjects in Group II. Pulmonary metastases occurred in five subjects in Group I and in eight in Group II. Bone metastases oc-

TABLE II Clinical and Morphologic Findings in 15 Subjects with Carcinoid Syndrome but without Carcinoid Heart Disease

Subject	Necropsy Number	Age (years) and Sex	Length of Illness (years)	SAP (mm Hg)	Site of Primary Carcinoid	Precordial Systolic Murmur	CT Ratio >0.5	Hct (percent)	TP (g/dl)	Alb (mg/dl)	HW (g)	BW (kg)	Highest Urinary 5-HIAA (mg/24 hours)	Hepatic Weight (g)	Effusion (amount in ml)			
															Pe*	Pl†	A‡	SE
1	A-67-232	28F	1	130/80	Stomach	+	0	34	7.5	2.9	150	39	—	5,660	0	+ (1,450)	+ (2,000)	+
2	A-62-75	40F	4	90/50	Ileum	0	0	34	4.8	1.4	230	42	60	3,500	0	+ (130)	0	+
3	A-72-43	42M	25	170/110	Bronchus	+	—	29	5.9	3.8	570	75	119	6,400	0	0	+ (1,000)	+
4	A-70-29	43M	20	110/60	Ileum	0	0	36	6.1	2.1	335	59	153	4,700	0	+ (800)	0	+
5	A-59-44	45M	5	120/80	Bronchus	0	0	37	6.6	3.1	450	75	588	6,100	0	0	0	0
6	A-56-199	47M	3	135/90	Cecum	0	0	47	—	—	300	68	124	2,100	+ (70)	0	0	0
7	A-64-118	51F	3.5	125/60	Ileum	+	0	28	5.6	1.8	250	41	§	2,100	0	0	0	+
8	A-72-139	59M	8	130/85	Ileum	0	0	34	7.0	2.7	240	47	196	1,300	0	0	+	+
9	A-69-275	60M	2	160/80	Bronchus	+	0	39	6.5	3.8	430	60	14.3	3,600	0	0	0	+
10	A-63-67	65F	3	95/60	Ileum	0	0	28	5.6	1.8	250	28	23	510	0	+ (450)	0	+
11	A-60-46	67M	8	130/80	Ileum	0	0	38	7.4	3.3	300	55	43	2,100	0	0	+ (4,000)	+
12	A-60-68	67F	1	170/90	Ileum	0	0	33	6.6	2.3	270	48	§	1,650	0	0	0	0
13	A-57-219	69M	9	120/80	Meckel's	+	0	43	5.2	2.7	270	59	854	3,800	+ (50)	+ (700)	0	+
14	A-58-166	74M	1.5	100/80	SI	0	0	27	5.4	1.9	290	31	400	2,500	0	0	0	+
15	A-58-32	75M	1	130/75	Ileum	0	0	38	—	—	320	57	73	1,700	0	0	+ (2,000)	0

* Zero indicates amount of pericardial fluid to be less than 50 ml.
† Zero indicates amount of pleural fluid to be less than 100 ml on either side.
‡ Zero indicates amount of peritoneal fluid to be less than 100 ml.
§ Markedly positive.
Abbreviations as in Table I.

curred in nine Group I subjects and in six Group II subjects.

Carcinoid plaques were present on tricuspid and pulmonic cusps in all 21 Group I subjects (**Figures 1** to **6**). Carcinoid plaques also were present on one or both left-sided cardiac valves in seven subjects: mitral valve only in six and both mitral and aortic valves in one. The thickening of the tricuspid and pulmonic leaflets was diffuse and uniform in 19 of the 21 subjects (Figures 3, 5, and 6). In the other two patients (Subjects 6 and 8, Group I), the thickening on both right-sided valves was focal. In contrast, the thickening of the mitral leaflets, except for one subject (Subject 16, Group I), was focal and to far less degree than the involvement of either tricuspid or pulmonic cusps (Figure 2). The involvement of the aortic valve in the one subject consisted of a small fibrous plaque on one of the three aortic valve cusps. Carcinoid plaques were present on the mural endocardium of the right atrium in 19 subjects, on the mural endocardium of the right ventricle in 13, and on the mural endocardium of the left ventricle in seven. The mural endocardial plaques of the right atrium were always thicker and covered a larger area than those in the right ventricle; mural plaques in the left ventricle always were small. In several subjects, focal carcinoid plaques also were observed in the coronary sinus, inferior and superior caval veins, brachiocephalic vein, and pulmonary trunk. In one subject, a small carcinoid plaque was present in the ascending aorta.

Histologically, carcinoid plaques consisted of fibrous tissue, devoid of elastic fibrils, deposited on the endocardial surfaces of the valve cusps and the cardiac chambers and on the intima of the vessels (Figures 1 to 6). The underlying endocardium and intima were not involved and were delineated by an elastic membrane. The fibrotic process was located on the ventricular aspect of the posterior and septal tricuspid valve leaflets, usually causing them to adhere to the underlying ventricular wall. The fibrotic process involved both atrial and ventricular aspects of the anterior tricuspid valve leaflet. The fibrotic process involved the pulmonic valve cusps on their arterial or downstream aspects, causing infolding of the distal third or so of the cusps toward the sinuses. As with the tricuspid septal and posterior leaflets, the carcinoid involvement of the mitral leaflets was also entirely on their ventricular aspects.

The tricuspid valve was usually fixed in an open position, producing regurgitation with or without some degree of stenosis (Figure 3). The left side of the heart never had lesions severe enough to cause dysfunction. The carcinoid plaques on the pulmonic valve cusps caused relative rigidity of the cusps and relative constriction of the circumference of the pulmonary trunk at the level of the valve sinuses. (Figures 3, 5, and 6). The result was usually a pulmonic valve orifice that was

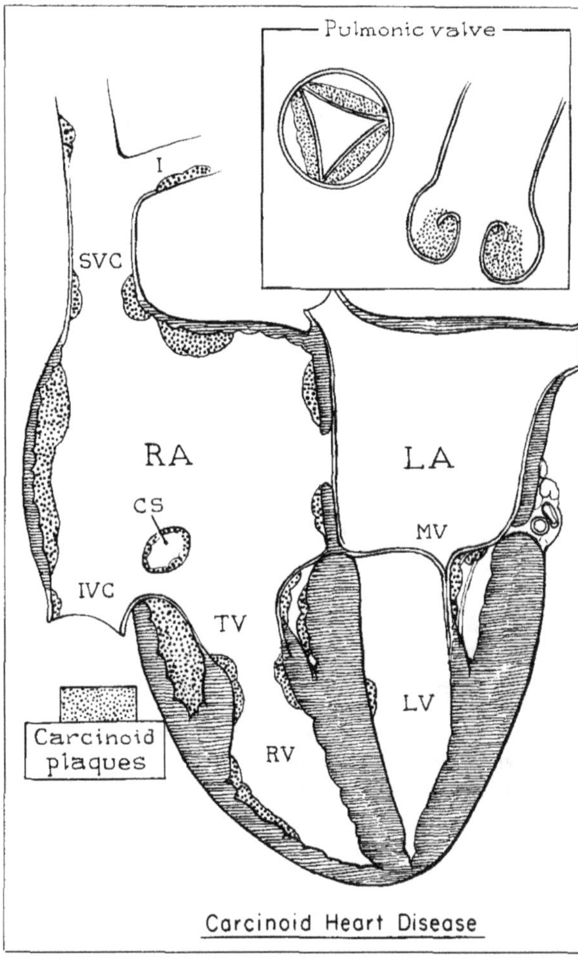

Figure 1. *Illustration of location and distribution of carcinoid plaques. CS = ostium of coronary sinus; I = innominate (brachiocephalic) vein; IVC = inferior vena cava; LA = left atrium; LV = left ventricle; MV = mitral valve; RA = right atrium; RV = right ventricle; SVC = superior vena cava; TV = tricuspid valve.*

smaller than normal, thus producing some degree of stenosis. Because the cusps were thickened and relatively immobile, they were not able to appose one another during ventricular diastole, and pulmonic regurgitation was the usual result.

Clinical Findings. No significant differences were observed between the subjects with carcinoid heart disease and those without carcinoid heart disease in sex (57 percent men versus 67 percent men); mean age (54 years versus 55 years); frequency of diarrhea (100 percent versus 93 percent); flushing (81 percent versus 93 percent); pericardial effusion (25 percent versus 13 percent); pleural effusions (40 percent versus 33 percent); and subcutaneous edema (90 percent versus 73 percent). Both groups had similar mean body weights (50 kg versus 52 kg) and mean heights (169 cm versus 168 cm); systemic blood pressures (117/77 mm Hg

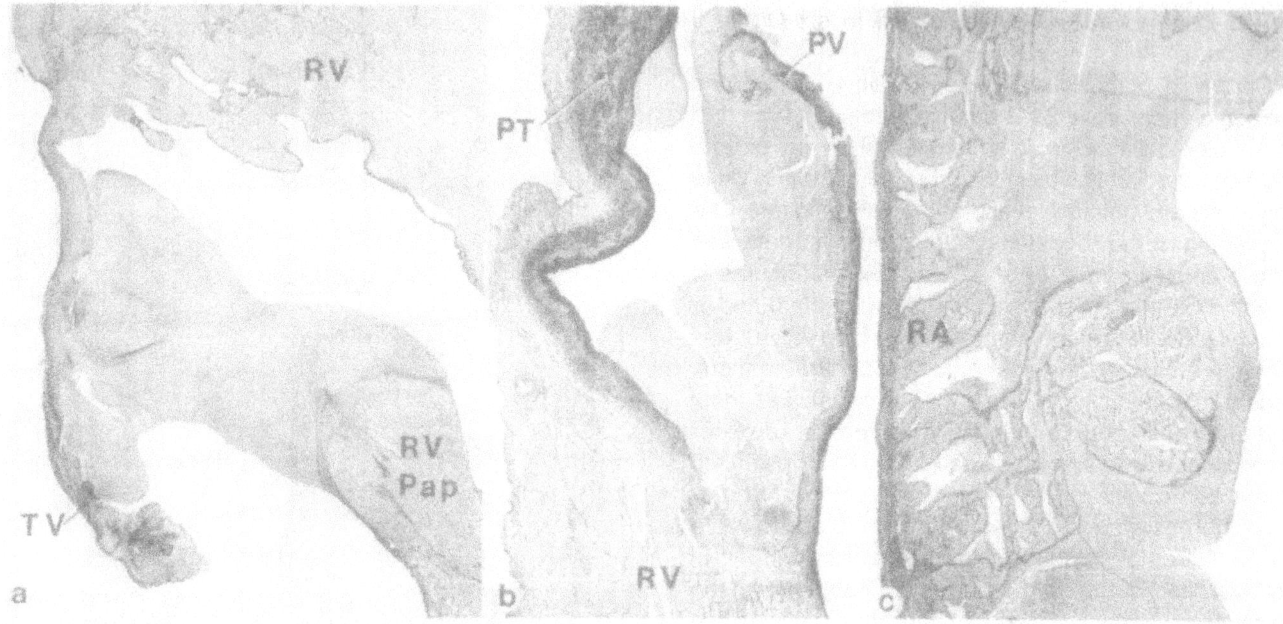

Figure 2. *(Subject 2, Table I)* ***A,*** *photomicrograph of tricuspid valve (TV) cusp with underlying right ventricular (RV) wall and papillary (Pap) muscle. The cusp is adherent to the papillary muscle by carcinoid plaque.* ***B,*** *photomicrograph of pulmonic valve (PV) cusp, wall of pulmonary trunk (PT), and right ventricle. Carcinoid plaque is present in the pulmonic sinus and on the endothelium of the pulmonary trunk. The distal portion of the cusp is folded inward.* ***C,*** *photomicrograph of a portion of the wall of the right atrium (RA) showing deposit of carcinoid plaque on the endocardium. The plaque is thicker than the original atrial wall (Verhõeff-van Gieson elastic tissue stains; original magnification × 15 [****A*** *and* ***B****], × 19 [****C****], reduced by 35 percent).*

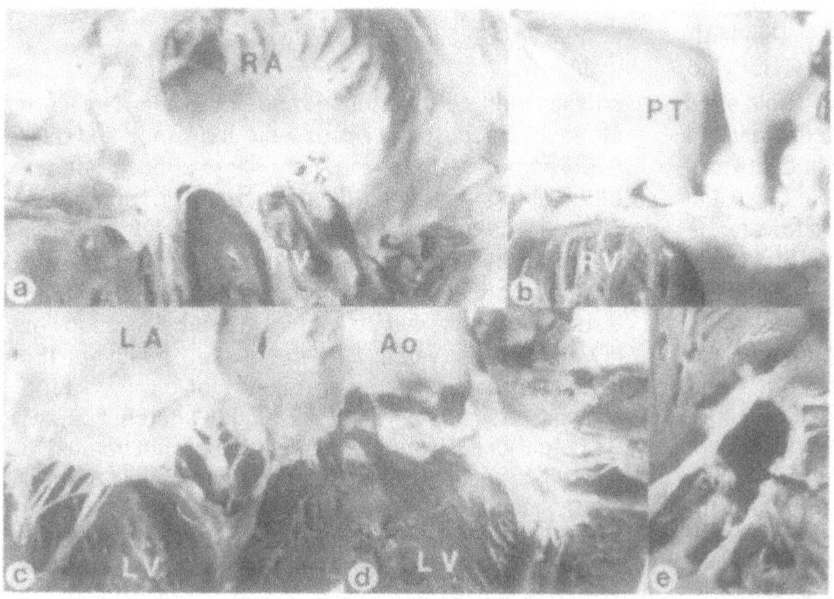

Figure 3. *(Subject 5, Table I)* ***A,*** *opened right atrium (RA) and right ventricle (RV) showing carcinoid plaque; the tricuspid valve leaflets and attached chordae are thick and shortened.* ***B,*** *opened pulmonic valve showing diffuse involvement by carcinoid plaque resulting in marked shortening and retraction of the cusps. The wall of the pulmonary trunk (PT) is folded at the level of the valve.* ***C,*** *opened left atrium (LA), mitral valve, and left ventricle (LV) showing focal plaque deposits on the leaflets.* ***D,*** *opened aorta (Ao), aortic valve, and left ventricle showing focal plaque deposits.* ***E,*** *tricuspid valve seen from the right ventricle showing a fixed and incompetent orifice.*

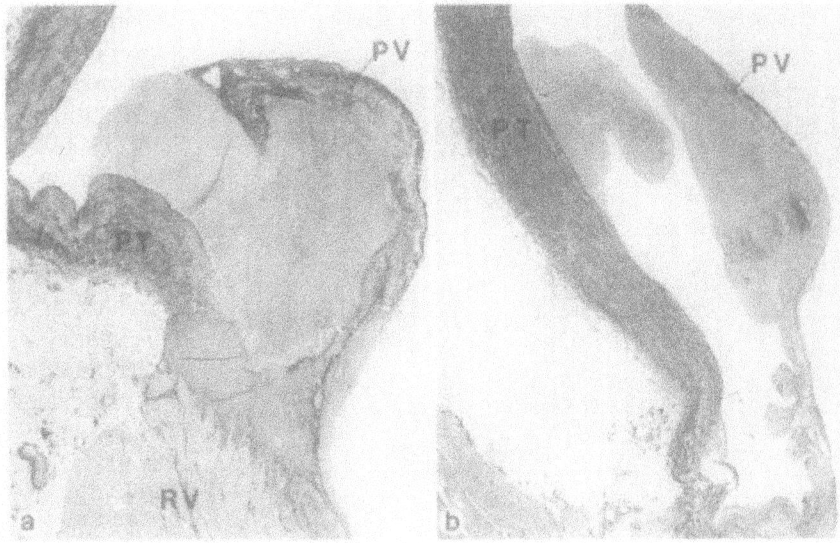

Figure 4. *(Subject 5, Table I)* ***A,*** *photomicrograph of a pulmonic valve (PV) cusp showing infolding of its distal portion and complete obliteration of the sinus by carcinoid plaque. PT = pulmonary trunk; RV = right ventricle.* ***B,*** *photomicrograph of another pulmonic valve cusp showing carcinoid plaque on one side of the cusp and on the pulmonary trunk but no fixation of the cusp (Verhoeff-van Gieson elastic tissue stain; original magnification each × 11, reduced by 43 percent).*

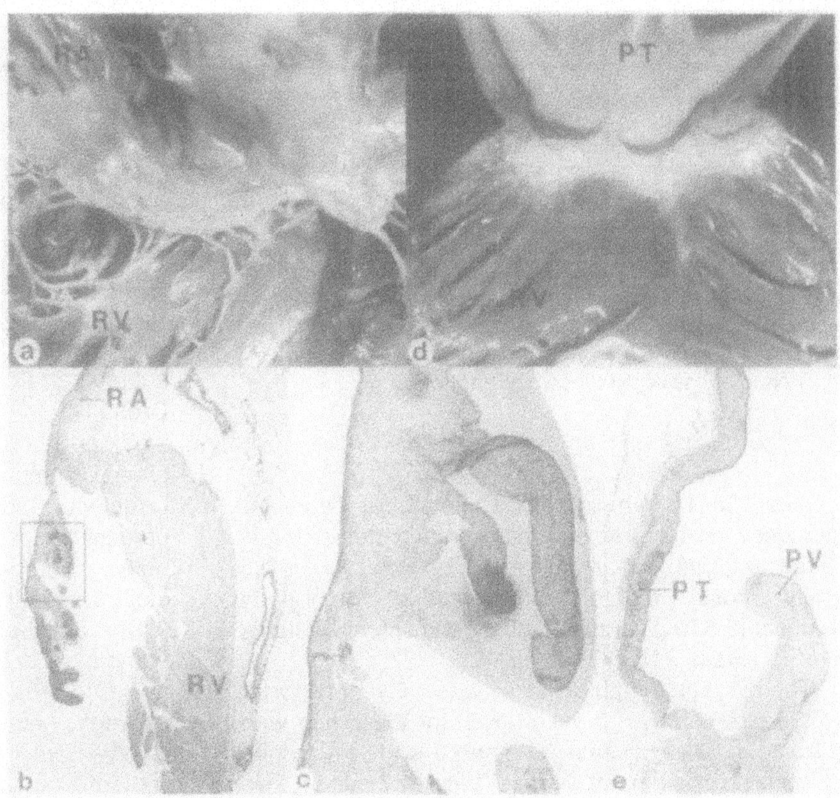

Figure 5. *(Subject 15, Table I)* ***A,*** *opened right atrium (RA), tricuspid valve, and right ventricle (RV) showing a thickened valve and atrial carcinoid plaques.* ***B,*** *photomicrograph of a portion of the right atrium, tricuspid valve, and right ventricle showing carcinoid plaque involving the leaflet and chordae.* ***C,*** *photomicrograph of the leaflet and chordae of the tricuspid valve indicated by a* ***box*** *in* ***B. D,*** *opened pulmonary trunk (PT), pulmonic valve, and right ventricle showing diffusely thickened and retracted valve cusps.* ***E,*** *photomicrograph of a pulmonic valve (PV) cusp and pulmonary trunk showing carcinoid plaque primarily on the "downstream" aspect of the cusp (Verhoeff-van Gieson elastic tissue stains; original magnification × 6[****B****], × 25 [****C****], × 8 [****E****], reduced by 45 percent).*

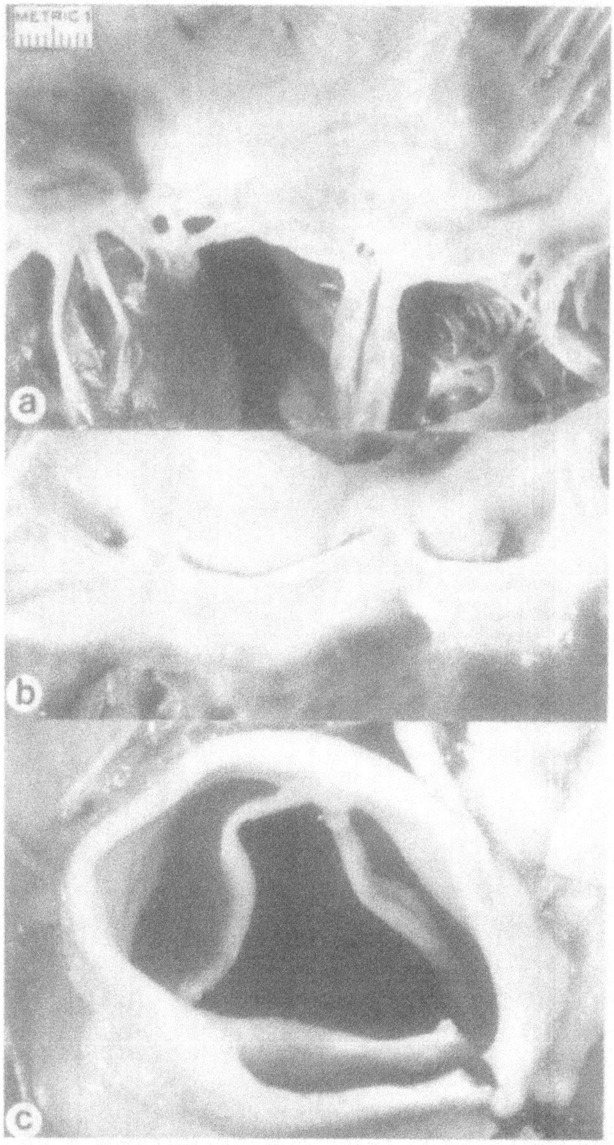

Figure 6. *(Subject 21, Table I)* ***A,*** *opened right atrium, tricuspid valve, and right ventricle showing thickened leaflets and chordae.* ***B,*** *opened pulmonic valve showing diffusely thickened cusps.* ***C,*** *nearly intact pulmonic valve showing thickened cusps and an incompetent orifice.*

versus 128/77 mm Hg); blood hematocrit levels (37 percent versus 35 percent); total serum protein (6.0 g/dl versus 6.0 g/dl) and albumin levels (2.3 g/dl versus 2.6 g/dl); cardiac weights (305 g versus 304 g); hepatic weights (2,830 g versus 3,180 g); and splenic weights (155 g versus 245 g).

The average length of illness was 1.6 years shorter (4.7 years versus 6.3 years) (NS) for the group with carcinoid heart disease compared with the group without carcinoid heart disease (**Figures 7** and **8**). Two subjects without carcinoid heart disease had extraordinarily long survivals (20 years and 25 years) from onset of symptoms attributable to carcinoid syndrome. The range of survival from onset of symptoms to death in the group with heart disease was 0.5 to 13 years. Of the 21 subjects with carcinoid heart disease, seven lived less than two years from onset of symptoms and seven lived longer than five years. The range of survival from onset of symptoms to death in the group without heart disease was one to 25 years; of the 15 subjects, five survived less than two years and five lived longer than five years.

Of the 28 subjects that had urinary 5-hydroxyindole acetic acid levels measured, the average was insignificantly higher in the group with carcinoid heart disease compared with the group without carcinoid heart disease (429 mg/dl versus 221 mg/dl). The duration of symptoms did not correlate with the level of 5-hydroxyindole acetic acid.

The two groups differed from each other in the location of the primary tumor. In Group I, the small intestine was the site of the primary tumor in 20 (95 percent) subjects, whereas it was the site of the primary tumor in 10 (67 percent) of the 15 subjects in Group II ($p < 0.05$).

The two groups differed in the frequency of precordial murmurs. Systolic murmurs were recorded in 20 of 21 subjects with carcinoid heart disease and in five of 15 subjects without carcinoid heart disease. A murmur consistent with tricuspid regurgitation (systolic, over left sternal border with increase in intensity during inspiration) was heard in 12 (57 percent) of the 21 subjects in Group I and in two (13 percent) of 15 subjects in Group II. A murmur consistent with pulmonic valve stenosis was described in 13 (62 percent) of 21 subjects in Group I, and a flow murmur was noted in three (20 percent) of 15 subjects in Group II. A diastolic murmur consistent with pulmonic regurgitation was described in six of 21 subjects in Group I, and in no subject in Group II. A diastolic murmur consistent with tricuspid valve stenosis was heard in three (14 percent) of the 21 subjects in Group I and in none of the 15 subjects in Group II.

Other features also helped differentiate the two groups. Compared with the Group II subjects, the Group I subjects had a higher frequency of wheezing (48 percent versus 20 percent) and peritoneal effusions (75 percent versus 33 percent); a higher percent of cardiothoracic ratios of more than 0.5 (38 percent versus 0); and a higher frequency of low voltage (sum of QRS complexes in leads I to III 15 mm or less) (10 mm = 1 mV) (9 of 19 [47 percent] versus 0 of 15). Death appeared to be attributable at least in part to the cardiac involvement in nine (43 percent) of the 21 Group I subjects, but in none of the 15 Group II subjects.

Electrocardiographic Findings. Electrocardiograms

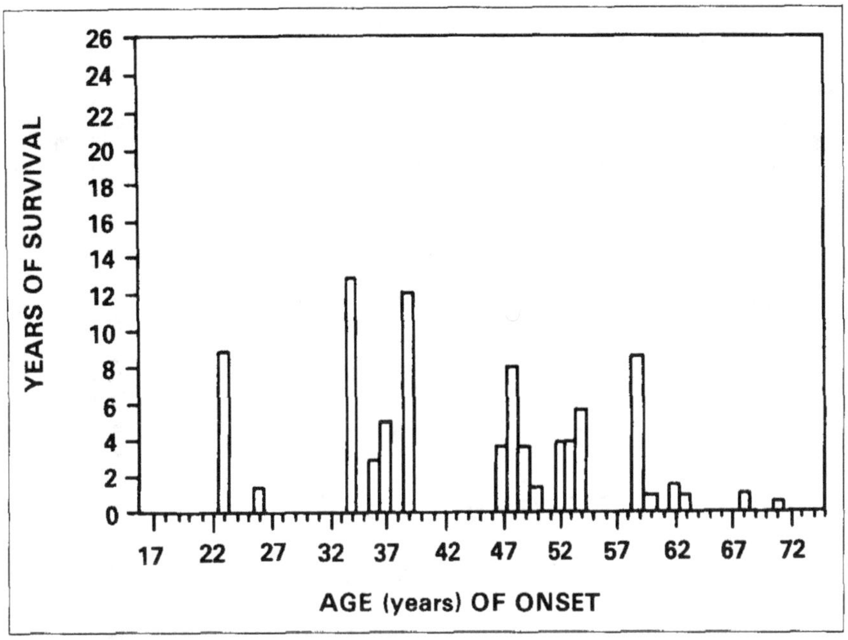

Figure 7. *Graph showing years of survival from onset of symptoms of carcinoid syndrome for individual subjects with carcinoid heart disease (Table I).*

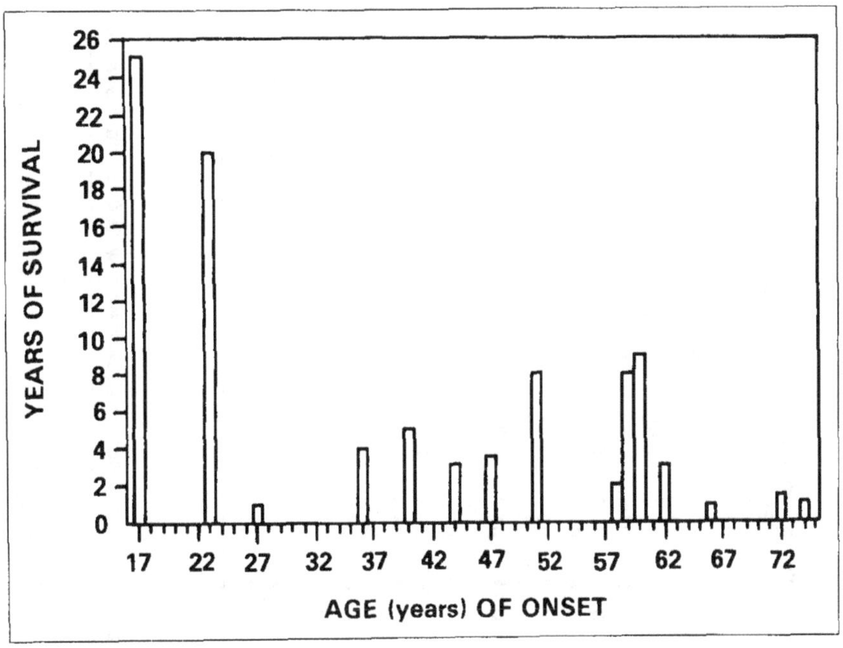

Figure 8. *Graph showing years of survival from onset of symptoms of carcinoid syndrome for individual subjects without carcinoid heart disease (Table II).*

were re-examined in 34 of the 36 subjects, and the findings are recorded in each subject in **Tables III** and **IV (Figures 9** and **10**). The interval from the electrocardiographic recording to death ranged from seven to 186 days (mean 69) in the 19 Group I subjects with electrocardiograms and from 11 to 232 days (mean 73) in the 15 Group II subjects.

The ventricular rates were similar in Groups I and II (88 beats per minute versus 91 beats per minute). One subject had premature atrial beats (Subject 19, Group I) on a resting electrocardiogram and two subjects had ventricular premature complexes (Subjects 8 and 13, Group II). The duration of the P-R, QRS, and Q-T intervals was similar in both groups.

The QRS voltage in each of the 12 leads was measured in 34 subjects. In the 19 Group I subjects, it ranged from 58 to 227 mm (mean 105), and in the 15 Group II subjects total 12-lead QRS voltage ranged from 89 to

TABLE III **Electrocardiographic Findings in 19 Subjects with Carcinoid Heart Disease**

Subject	Interval ECG to Death (days)	VR (beats/minute)	Intervals (seconds) P-R	QRS	Q-T	Voltage (mm) I	II	III	aVR	aVL	aVF	V_1	V_2	V_3	V_4	V_5	V_6	Total QRS 12-Lead Voltage (mm)	Axis
2	34	85	0.16	0.08	0.28	3	6	5	3	3	5	6	9	7	6	5	4	59	120°
3	10	83	0.16	0.08	0.30	3	5	4	3	2	4	15	13	10	7	6	7	79	60°
4	104	120	0.16	0.06	0.32	4	7	4	5	3	5	21	37	23	28	17	13	167	0°
5	7	110	0.18	0.10	0.30	7	9	7	7	5	7	8	9	11	11	15	15	104	110°
6	115	52	0.20	0.08	0.42	6	7	6	7	6	5	4	13	15	16	20	14	119	30°
7	33	100	0.13	0.06	0.28	2	4	4	3	3	4	5	12	12	6	7	6	68	90°
8	186	110	0.14	0.08	0.32	7	5	2	5	3	3	10	15	13	13	11	7	94	0°
10	13	100	0.16	0.08	0.30	3	7	6	4	5	6	5	13	20	20	16	12	117	110°
11	28	65	0.20	0.08	0.48	5	7	5	5	3	6	6	19	17	14	10	7	104	30°
12	47	80	0.14	0.08	0.26	4	5	7	3	4	6	5	10	17	13	8	5	87	90°
13	107	100	0.18	0.08	0.30	4	10	8	8	5	9	9	23	20	11	10	11	128	0°
14	16	73	0.20	0.06	0.36	3	3	4	2	3	3	4	8	10	6	6	6	58	110°
15	42	85	0.16	0.08	0.36	4	4	4	4	2	4	3	8	6	7	6	6	58	60°
16	59	100	0.14	0.08	0.36	6	5	3	6	4	4	13	22	24	16	17	8	129	30°
17	39	80	0.12	0.08	0.36	7	5	7	4	6	5	5	12	6	4	8	7	76	30°
18	105	82	0.19	0.06	0.36	3	7	5	6	3	6	16	22	18	6	8	6	106	60°
19	160	75	0.16	0.08	0.36	3	3	2	3	2	2	2	16	18	18	18	9	96	60°
20	35	90	0.16	0.10	0.36	4	6	9	3	6	8	9	13	24	17	11	6	116	−60°
21	180	75	0.24	0.08	0.36	13	9	10	11	10	7	15	30	38	39	30	15	227	−30°
Mean	69	88	0.17	0.07	0.34	5	6	5	5	4	5	8	16	16	14	12	9	105	

ECG = electrocardiography; VR = ventricular rate.

TABLE IV **Electrocardiographic Observations in 15 Subjects with Carcinoid Syndrome but without Carcinoid Heart Disease**

Subject	Interval ECG to Death (days)	VR (beats/minute)	Intervals (seconds) P-R	QRS	Q-T	Voltage (mm) I	II	III	aVR	aVL	aVF	V_1	V_2	V_3	V_4	V_5	V_6	Total QRS 12-Lead Voltage (mm)	Axis
1	134	90	0.16	0.08	0.38	4	8	8	6	2	7	5	8	9	19	24	16	116	60°
2	232	110	0.13	0.09	0.38	7	7	3	6	3	4	11	23	30	21	13	7	135	30°
3	65	75	0.18	0.08	0.36	8	8	3	7	5	5	5	22	14	24	17	14	132	45°
4	67	110	0.16	0.06	0.35	5	11	6	8	3	8	9	19	16	15	12	10	122	60°
5	31	92	0.15	0.07	0.36	6	9	5	6	3	7	10	11	13	21	18	10	119	30°
6	35	80	0.16	0.08	0.37	10	9	4	10	6	5	19	36	37	23	15	9	183	30°
7	71	80	0.20	0.08	0.36	8	8	5	7	6	6	8	15	11	8	12	8	102	30°
8	35	55	0.14	0.08	0.44	2	16	15	8	8	16	16	28	22	30	19	12	192	30°
9	106	133	0.16	0.06	0.36	5	12	9	6	3	10	8	20	13	25	23	18	152	60°
10	45	71	0.11	0.07	0.39	2	9	9	4	3	9	8	17	20	15	10	9	115	90°
11	102	75	0.16	0.08	0.32	6	7	5	6	3	6	6	14	17	15	8	6	99	30°
12	24	100	0.12	0.06	0.34	13	9	9	10	9	6	13	15	15	15	12	9	135	0°
13	35	78	0.14	0.09	0.36	3	9	8	5	3	9	6	6	9	13	11	7	89	60°
14	95	120	0.12	0.08	0.34	6	16	13	12	4	15	26	29	8	18	15	13	175	60°
15	11	98	0.16	0.10	0.36	4	12	16	5	9	13	5	6	11	9	9	8	107	−60°
Mean	73	91	0.15	0.08	0.36	6	10	8	7	5	8	10	18	16	18	14	10	132	

Abbreviations as in Table III.

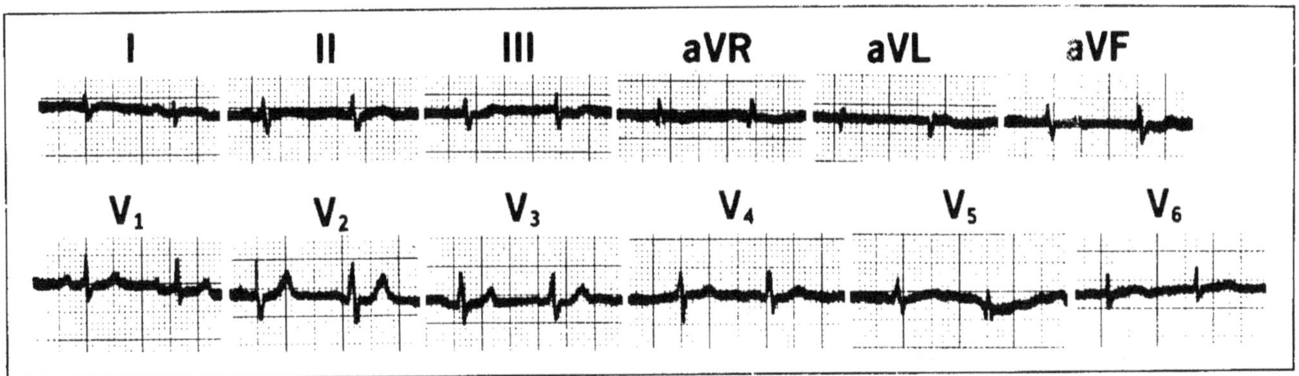

Figure 9. *(Subject 2, Table I) Electrocardiogram showing low QRS voltage in limb leads and an R wave that is greater than the S wave in V_1 to V_6.*

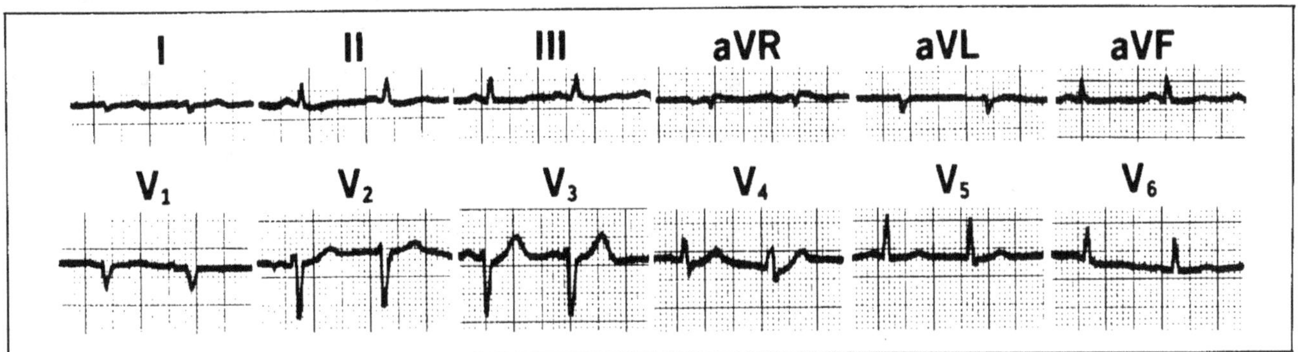

Figure 10. *(Subject 7, Table I) Electrocardiogram showing low QRS voltage in limb leads, vertical axis, T wave changes, and delayed precordial transition.*

192 mm (mean 132) (NS). Total 12-lead QRS voltage was 175 mm or less in 20 (95 percent) of 21 subjects with carcinoid heart disease and in 12 (80 percent) of 15 subjects without carcinoid heart disease. Of the 34 subjects with electrocardiograms, six (18 percent) had hearts weighing more than 400 g (clearly above normal). The total 12-lead QRS voltage in the six subjects with hearts of increased weight ranged from 96 to 152 mm (mean 120), and in the 28 subjects with normal-sized hearts it ranged from 58 to 227 mm (mean 116) (NS).

Of the 36 subjects, cardiac catheterization data are available in three. Right-sided pressure tracings in Subject 2, Group I, are shown in **Figures 11** and **12**.

COMMENTS

Examination of the hearts in our 36 subjects with the carcinoid syndrome disclosed that over half (58 percent) had carcinoid heart disease. Why carcinoid heart disease occurs in some patients with the carcinoid syndrome and not in others remains unexplained. Our data refute the earlier suggestions that patients with carcinoid heart disease have longer symptomatic illnesses compared with those without carcinoid heart disease [2–5]. The mean survival after onset of dermal flushing or diarrhea or wheezing (whichever symptom came first) was 4.7 years in our 21 subjects with carcinoid heart disease and 6.3 years in the 15 subjects without carcinoid heart disease (NS). Another proposal explaining the presence of carcinoid heart disease in some but not in other patients with the carcinoid syndrome is differing blood serotonin levels between the two groups. The mean urinary 5-hydroxyindole acetic acid levels in 16 subjects with carcinoid heart disease was 429 mg per 24 hours, and 221 mg per 24 hours (NS) in the 12 subjects without carcinoid heart disease.

Although its cause and mechanism of formation is unclear, carcinoid heart disease is a unique form of heart disease. It consists of the deposition of a peculiar type of fibrous tissue devoid of elastic fibrils within which are smooth muscle cells and mucopolysaccharide material on the mural and valvular endocardium, primarily on the right side of the heart [6]. A fascinating feature of the deposits (carcinoid plaques) is that by histologic and electron microscopic examination they all look alike. In other words, the deposits do not appear to go through various developmental stages—there are no early and late stages, only one stage. This morpho-

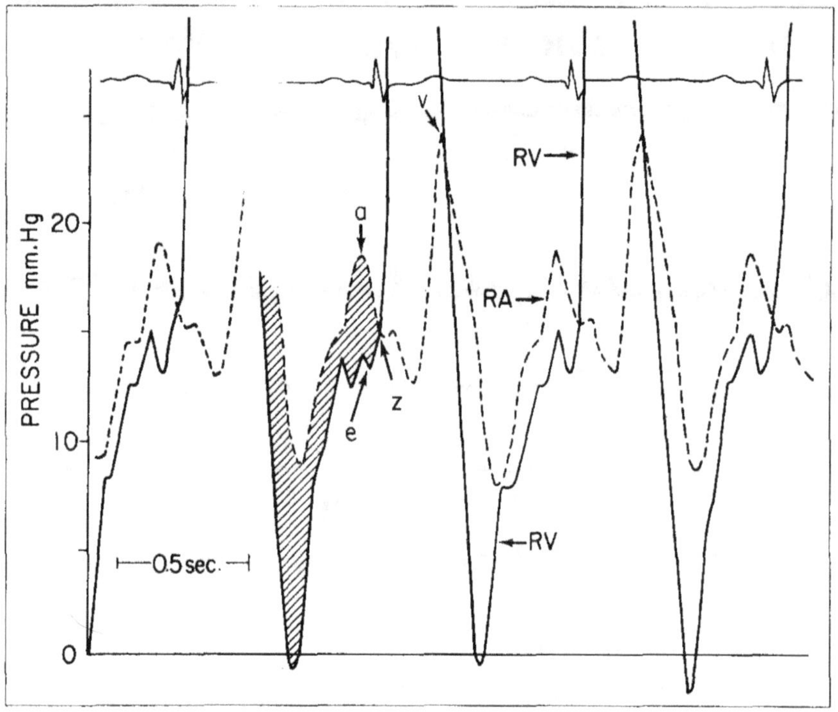

Figure 11. *(Subject 2, Table I) Right-sided pressure tracing in a patient with tricuspid regurgitation and stenosis. The* ***hatched*** *area indicates the pressure gradient between right atrium (RA) and right ventricle (RV). a = A wave; e = E point; v = v wave; z = Z point. Lead II of the electrocardiogram is at the* ***top.*** *(Reproduced with permission from Roberts WC, Mason DT, Wright LD Jr: The non-distensible right atrium of carcinoid disease of the heart. Am J Clin Pathol 1965; 44: 627–631.)*

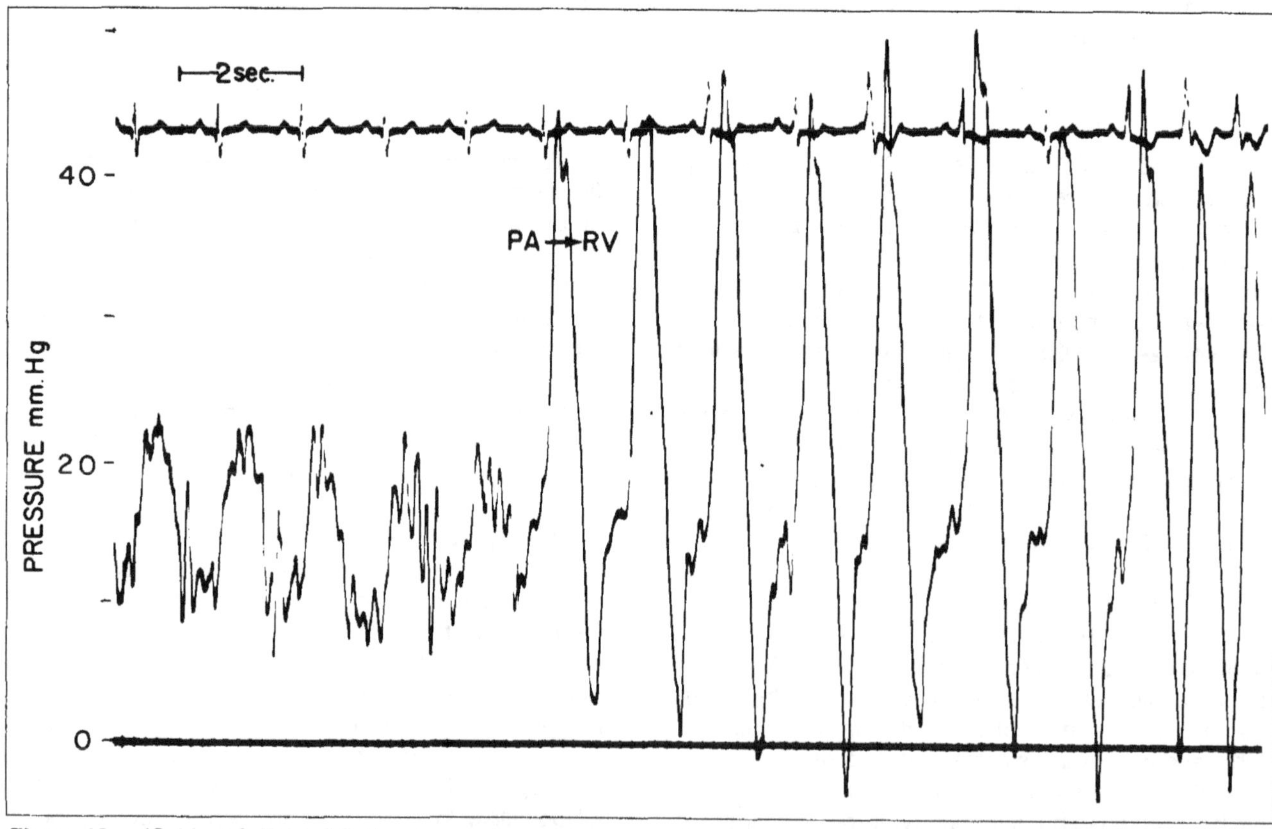

Figure 12. *(Subject 2, Table I) Pullback pressure tracing from pulmonary trunk (PA) to right ventricle (RV) showing a 20 mm Hg peak systolic pressure gradient. The lead II electrocardiogram is shown at the* ***top.*** *(Reproduced with permission from Roberts WC, Mason DT, Wright LD Jr: The non-distensible right atrium of carcinoid disease of the heart. Am J Clin Pathol 1965; 44:*

logic observation supports the view that the carcinoid endocardial plaque results from the deposit of a substance from the blood.

Not only is the composition of the carcinoid endocardial plaque unique [1,2], but the site of its occurrence in the heart is unique. The plaques are far more common on the right side of the heart than on the left, and even when present on the left, the right-sided plaques are always more extensive and larger. Among our 21 subjects with carcinoid heart disease, the carcinoid plaques were limited to the right side of the heart in 15 (71 percent).

All of our 21 subjects with carcinoid heart disease had involvement of both tricuspid and pulmonic valves by carcinoid plaques, and 19 of them also had carcinoid plaques on the mural endocardium of the right atrium and usually also on the mural endocardium of the right ventricle. The number of subjects with right-sided valvular dysfunction as a consequence of the carcinoid plaques on the valvular leaflets is less certain because of the relative difficulty in diagnosing by auscultation mild degrees of tricuspid and pulmonic valve dysfunction. In two of the 21 subjects with right-sided carcinoid heart disease, the degree of morphologic involvement of both valves was minimal and valvular function clearly was not affected. Of the remaining 19 subjects, 18 had precordial systolic and/or diastolic murmurs of grade 2/6 or greater intensity. The carcinoid deposits on the left-sided valve(s) in the six subjects did not appear extensive enough to cause valvular dysfunction.

Although the composition and location of the carcinoid plaques on both right-sided cardiac valves are similar, the functional consequences of the carcinoid plaques are different. The deposits occur nearly entirely on the downstream side of the valvular leaflets, i.e., on the ventricular aspects of the septal and posterior tricuspid leaflets and on the pulmonary arterial side of the pulmonic valve cusps. On the anterior tricuspid valve leaflet, the deposits can be on both sides. The consequences of the "downstream" deposition is an adherence of the leaflet to the underlying mural endocardium (tricuspid septal and posterior leaflets) or to the underlying pulmonary arterial endothelium (pulmonic valve) via the carcinoid plaques. The fibrous tissue of the carcinoid plaque acts as a constricting substance such that the "ring" of both right-sided cardiac valves is made smaller than normal and at the same time leaflet mobility is diminished. The consequence is tricuspid regurgitation with or without some degree of stenosis. Nearly all patients with pure tricuspid regurgitation (no element of stenosis) have dilated valve rings, but patients with some degree of stenosis in addition to regurgitation do not have dilated anuli. Patients with carcinoid heart disease follow this principle. Thus, patients with carcinoid heart disease have much more tricuspid regurgitation than stenosis, but usually there is some degree of stenosis, albeit small.

In contrast to the tricuspid valve, the dominant functional pulmonic valve lesion is stenosis, although all patients with stenosis have some degree of pulmonic regurgitation. The reason for the difference—compared with the tricuspid valve—is that the orifice of the normal pulmonic valve is much smaller initially than the orifice of the tricuspid valve. Thus, the constriction by deposition of carcinoid plaques within the pulmonic sinuses causes constriction of the pulmonic root with the production of pulmonic stenosis. Because the distal portions of the pulmonic cusps are inverted toward the sinuses and the mobility of the cusps is lost, some degree of regurgitation is inevitable in all patients with carcinoid who have any degree of pulmonic stenosis.

Although combined lesions of both mitral and aortic valves are fairly common as a consequence of either rheumatic heart disease or infective endocarditis or both, combined lesions of both tricuspid and pulmonic valves are rare, and carcinoid is the only condition in which uniformly both—not just one—right-sided valves are involved together. The two dominant functional consequences of right-sided carcinoid heart disease are pulmonic stenosis and tricuspid regurgitation. These two lesions in the same patient are particularly unfavorable because the pulmonic stenosis increases the degree of tricuspid regurgitation. A commonly employed method of producing chronic congestive heart failure in experimental animals is by banding the pulmonary trunk to create pulmonic stenosis, and excising or destroying one or more tricuspid valve cusps to make the valve purely regurgitant. Thus, right-sided carcinoid heart disease in essence creates this experimental model. If a patient with carcinoid heart disease had only dysfunction of the pulmonic or the tricuspid valve, probably the functional consequence would be insignificant. It is the combination of both right-sided valvular lesions—namely pulmonic stenosis and tricuspid regurgitation—that has the potential of being devastating.

Clinical diagnosis of carcinoid heart disease can usually be established by noninvasive means. Auscultation, of course, is the first clue. In 20 (95 percent) of our 21 subjects with carcinoid heart disease and in five (33 percent) of our 15 subjects without carcinoid heart disease, one or more precordial murmurs were recorded ($p < 0.05$). Of the 20 subjects with precordial murmurs and carcinoid heart disease, eight had both systolic and diastolic murmurs and 12 had only systolic murmurs; of the five subjects with precordial murmurs but without carcinoid heart disease, the murmurs in all were systolic only. Thus, nearly all patients with carcinoid heart disease have precordial murmurs, and when the murmur has a diastolic component, diagnosis

TABLE V Observations in 15 Previously Reported Patients with Carcinoid Heart Disease and Right-Sided Cardiac Operation

Reference	Age (years) at Time of Operation and Sex	Interval (years) First Carcinoid Symptom to Surgery	Operation (type)		Interval (months) Cardiac Symptoms to Cardiac Operation	Interval (months) Cardiac Operation to Death	Preoperative Catheterization				Murmurs				Type (size) Prosthesis or Bioprosthesis
			TV	PV			RA-RV MDG (mm Hg)	TR	RV-PA PSG (mm Hg)	PR	TR	TS	PR	PS	
[2]	35F	19	+ (A)	+ (C)	5	Died postop	12	+	32	0	+	+	0	+	0
[9]	50M	15	+ (R)	+ (C)	60	72	24	+	48	0	+	+	+	+	Starr-Edwards (3 M)
[11]	31M	7	0	+ (E)	—	1	10	+	40	0	+	0	0	+	0
[10]	26F	9	+ (R)	+ (C)	5	132*	6	+	45	0	+	+	0	+	Kay-Shiley (6)
[3]	57M	3	+ (R)	0	18	4	0	+	3	0	+	0	+	+	Bjorck-Shiley (27)
[4]	46F	33	+ (R)	0	6	21*	4	—	10	0	0	+	0	+	Bjorck-Shiley (31)
[12]	24F	<0.5	+ (R)	+ (R)	4	24	4	+	32	0	+	0	0	+	Porcine(—)
[14]	64F	10	+ (R)	+ (R)	3	1	—	+	18	+	+	0	0	+	Bioprosthesis (—)
[16]	34M	5	+ (R)	+ (C)	12	96*	11	0	50	0	0	0	0	+	Starr-Edwards (3 M)
[13]	30F	18	+ (R)	+ (C)	12	4*	22	+	45	0	+	+	0	+	Porcine (27)
[15]	60F	<1	+ (R)	0	15	12*	5	+	—	0	+	0	0	0	Carpenter-Edwards (27)
[5]	53M	4.5	+ (R)	0	18	8	0	+	0	0	+	0	0	0	Porcine (27)
[17]	62M	25	+ (R)	+ (R)	—	24*	5	+	20	+	+	+	0	+	Porcine (—)
[18]	63F	1.5	+ (R)	+ (C)	18	2	4	+	8	0	+	0	0	+	Porcine (—)
[19]	56F	3	+ (R)	0	<8	23*	4	+	0	—	—	—	—	—	St. Jude (31)

* Alive.

A = annuloplasty; C = commissurotomy; E = excision; MDG = mean diastolic gradient; PA = pulmonary artery; postop = postoperatively; PR = pulmonic regurgitation; PS = pulmonic stenosis; PSG = peak systolic gradient; PV = pulmonic valve; R = replacement; RA = right atrium; RV = right ventricle; TR = tricuspid regurgitation; TS = tricuspid stenosis; TV = tricuspid valve; — = no information available.

of carcinoid heart disease can be made with confidence.

The systemic arterial blood pressure is not helpful in either diagnosing carcinoid syndrome or distinguishing those with carcinoid heart disease from those without carcinoid heart disease. Only three of our 36 subjects had indirect systolic systemic arterial pressures of more than 140 mm Hg and/or diastolic arterial pressures of more than 90 mm Hg: one of the 21 with carcinoid heart disease and two of the 15 without carcinoid heart disease. The average peak systolic pressure was 117 mm Hg in the 21 subjects with carcinoid heart disease, and 128 mm Hg in the 15 subjects without carcinoid heart disease; the average diastolic pressure in both groups was 77 mm Hg.

Chest radiography was helpful in diagnosing carcinoid heart disease. The cardiothoracic ratio was more than 0.50 in eight (38 percent) of 21 subjects with carcinoid heart disease and in none of 15 subjects without carcinoid heart disease. Thus, the cardiothoracic ratio is not a very sensitive test for carcinoid heart disease, but it is specific.

Resting electrocardiography was somewhat useful in distinguishing the subjects with carcinoid heart disease from those without carcinoid heart disease. The sum of the QRS voltage in leads I, II, and III was 15 mm or less in nine of the 21 subjects with carcinoid heart disease and in none of the 15 subjects without carcinoid heart disease ($p < 0.05$). The sum of the total 12-lead QRS voltage ranged from 58 to 227 mm (10 mm = 1 mV) in 34 subjects, and the mean values were not significantly different between the two groups (105 mm versus 132 mm). In only three subjects (one with carcinoid heart disease) was this total 12-lead QRS voltage more than 175 mm. Evidence of right ventricular hypertrophy was rare. The R wave was greater than the S wave in either lead V_1 or V_2 in only four of the 19 subjects with carcinoid heart disease and in none of the 15 subjects without carcinoid heart disease. Right axis deviation (more than 90 degrees) was present in only 4 of the 19 subjects with carcinoid heart disease and in none of the 15 subjects without carcinoid heart disease. Despite right atrial dilatation in most of the subjects with carcinoid heart disease, all 19 with carcinoid heart disease and all 15 without carcinoid heart disease had sinus rhythm. The P-R interval was normal (0.20 second or less) in 18 of 19 subjects with carcinoid heart disease and in 14 of 15 subjects without carcinoid heart disease. The width of the QRS complex was normal (0.12 second or less) in all subjects, irrespective of whether or not they had carcinoid heart disease. Thus, other than the higher frequency of low voltage in the subjects with carcinoid heart disease, electrocardiography was not helpful in distinguishing those subjects with carcinoid heart disease from those without carcinoid heart disease.

Although not performed in any of our 36 subjects, echocardiography, particularly cross-sectional, is helpful in diagnosing carcinoid heart disease. Two reports have described echocardiographic features in relatively large groups of patients with carcinoid heart disease. Callahan and associates [7] described retrospectively echocardiographic features in 20 patients with the carcinoid syndrome. By physical examination, 15 patients had a diagnosis of carcinoid heart disease and the other five did not. Both M-mode and cross-sectional examinations in the latter five patients disclosed no abnormal findings. Of the 15 patients with auscultatory evidence of carcinoid heart disease, five had normal M-mode and cross-sectional echocardiographic findings. The other 10, all of whom had tricuspid regurgitation by physical examination, had dilated right ventricular cavities, abnormal motion of the ventricular septum, and of the nine in whom the tricuspid valve leaflets were visualized by cross-sectional echocardiography, strikingly abnormal tricuspid leaflets (thickened and retracted with fixed orifice). The pulmonic valve cusps were not visualized in any patient by M-mode echocardiography, but in the four in whom they were visualized by cross-sectional echocardiography, the pulmonic valve cusps were abnormal in each.

Howard and associates [8] prospectively examined by cross-sectional echocardiography 14 patients with the carcinoid syndrome, and eight had definite abnormalities of one or both right-sided cardiac valves. Clinically, five had auscultatory evidence of tricuspid regurgitation and all five had diffusely thickened and retracted tricuspid valve leaflets; the other nine patients had normal tricuspid valves by echocardiography. Four patients by auscultation had evidence of pulmonic stenosis with or without pulmonic regurgitation. The pulmonic valve cusps were visualized by echocardiography in seven patients: two had retracted pulmonic cusps with decreased systolic motion (one of whom had pulmonic stenosis by auscultation) and five had normal cusps (none of whom had auscultatory evidence of pulmonic stenosis).

Although none of our 21 subjects with carcinoid heart disease had an operative procedure performed on either the tricuspid or pulmonic valve or both, right-sided cardiac valve excision with or without valve replacement or valve commissurotomy or annuloplasty has been carried out in at least 15 patients [2–5,9–20]. The findings in these patients are summarized in **Table V.** At operation, the patients ranged in age from 26 to 64 years (mean 46); three were women and six were men. The interval from onset of symptoms and signs of congestive heart failure to cardiac valve operation ranged from three to 60 months (mean 14) and the interval from onset of symptoms of the carcinoid syndrome to cardiac valve operation ranged from 0.5 to 33 years (mean 10). Preoperatively, at least 12 of the 15 patients had hemodynamic evidence of tricuspid valve stenosis with mean diastolic pressure gradients between right atrium and right ventricle ranging from 4 to 24 mm Hg (mean 9). Of 15 patients, 14 had tricuspid regurgitation, which was graded as severe at angiography in at least seven patients. Pullback pressures between pulmonary artery and right ventricle were recorded in 14 patients, 12 of whom had peak systolic pressure gradients ranging from 3 to 50 mm Hg (average 29). The presence or absence of pulmonic regurgitation as determined by pulmonary angiography was noted in 12 patients, and only two apparently had regurgitation into the right ventricle during ventricular diastole. Of the 15 patients, 14 had tricuspid valve procedures: replacement in 13 and anuloplasty in one; 10 patients had pulmonic valve procedures: commissurotomy in six, replacement in three, and excision only in one. Of the 15 patients, eight had died at the time of the report: four within two months of operation, and one each four, eight, 24, and 72 months after operation. The other seven patients were alive 4 to 132 months (median 23) after operation.

REFERENCES

1. Roberts WC, Sjoerdsma A: The cardiac disease associated with the carcinoid syndrome (carcinoid heart disease). Am J Med 1964; 36: 5–34.
2. Wright PW, Mulder DG: Carcinoid heart disease. Report of a case treated by open heart surgery. Am J Cardiol 1963; 12: 864–868.
3. Lund HG, Cleveland RJ, Greenberg LH, Lippmann M, Dollinger MR: Tricuspid valve replacement in carcinoid heart disease. West J Med 1974; 120: 412–415.
4. Honey M, Paneth M. Carcinoid heart disease: successful tricuspid valve replacement. Thorax 1975; 30: 464–469.
5. Schoen FJ, Hausner RJ, Howell JF, Beazley HL, Titus JL: Porcine heterograft valve replacement in carcinoid heart disease. J Thorac Cardiovasc Surg 1981; 81: 100–105.
6. Ferrans VJ, Roberts WC: The carcinoid endocardial plaque. An ultrastructural study. Hum Pathol 1976; 7: 387–409.
7. Callahan JA, Wroblewski EM, Reeder GS, Edwards WD, Seward JB, Tajik AJ: Echocardiographic features of carcinoid heart disease. Am J Cardiol 1982; 50: 762–768.
8. Howard RJ, Drobac M, Rider WD, et al: Carcinoid heart disease: diagnosis by two-dimensional echocardiography, Circulation 1982; 66: 1059–1065.
9. Aroesty JM, DeWeese JA, Hoffman MJ, Yu PN: Carcinoid heart disease. Successful repair of the valvular lesions under cardiopulmonary bypass. Circulation 1966; 34: 105–110.
10. Carpena C, Kay JG, Mendex AM, Redington JV, Zubiate P, Zucker R: Carcinoid heart disease. Surgery for tricuspid and pulmonary valve lesions. Am J Cardiol 1973; 32: 229–233.
11. Garcia E, Taboada CF, Hall RJ, Cooley DA: Carcinoid heart disease: cardiac surgery for intractable heart failure. Cardiovasc Dis Bull Texas Heart Institute 1974; 1: 408–412.
12. McGuire MR, Pugh DM, Dunn MI: Carcinoid heart disease. Restrictive cardiomyopathy as a late complication. J Kans Med Soc 1978; 79: 661–665.
13. Okada RD, Ewy GA, Copeland JG: Echocardiography and surgery in tricuspid and pulmonary valve stenosis due to carcinoid syndrome. Cardiovasc Med 1979; 4: 871–881.
14. Nielsen MS, Manners JM: Valve replacement in carcinoid syndrome. Anaesthesia 1979; 34: 494–499.
15. Sworn MJ, Edlin GP, McGill GA, Mousley JS, Monro JL: Tricuspid valve replacement in carcinoid syndrome due to ovarian primary. Br Med J 1980; 280: 85–86.
16. Hendel N, Leckie B, Richards J: Carcinoid heart disease: eight-year survival following tricuspid valve replacement and pulmonary valvotomy. Ann Thorac Surg 1980; 30: 391–395.
17. Gutierrez FR, McKnight RC, Jaffe AS, Ludbrook PA, Biello D, Weldon CS: Double porcine valve replacement in carcinoid heart disease. Chest 1982; 81: 101–103.
18. Come PC, Come SE, Hawley CR, Gwon N, Riley MF: Echocardiographic manifestations of carcinoid heart disease. J Clin Ultrasound 1982; 10: 233–237.
19. Miller BR, Vohr FH, Christian FV, Singh AK: Cardiac valvular replacement in carcinoid heart disease. Am J Med 1983; 75: 896–898.
20. Kay JH: Eleven-year follow-up after tricuspid valve replacement and pulmonic valvulotomy in the carcinoid syndrome (letter). Am J Cardiol 1984; 53: 651.

Embryonal Botryoid Rhabdomyosarcoma of the Mitral Valve

RACHEL HAJAR, MD
WILLIAM C. ROBERTS, MD
GORDON M. FOLGER, Jr., MD

Primary neoplasms arising within the heart are rare, especially in childhood.[1,2] Origin of a primary neoplasm from cardiac valvular endocardium is especially rare.[3,4] Such was the case, however, in the child described in this report.

An 8-year-old boy had been considered healthy until he collapsed suddenly during play. He had been found to have a precordial systolic murmur 4 weeks earlier but its cause was not investigated. After the collapse, he was aphasic and had a right hemiparesis. A palpable thrill and grade 3/6 systolic ejection murmur were present in the suprasternal notch and a grade 2/6 systolic murmur was audible over the cardiac apex. The electrocardiogram was consistent with left ventricular hypertrophy and chest radiogram disclosed slight cardiomegaly. Two-dimensional echocardiogram (Fig. 1) disclosed a mobile, polypoid mass attached to the ventricular aspect of the anterior mitral leaflet. With ventricular systole the mass entered the left ventricular outflow tract, its tip crossing the aortic valve orifice. Emergency mitral valve replacement was carried out. At surgery, the tumor was pink, multilobulated and botryoid (Fig. 1). During its removal, several lobules dislodged from the main body of the tumor. Histologically, the tumor was consistent with embryonal botryoid rhabdomyosarcoma. After surgery, the child became decerebrate and died 48 hours after operation.

The botryoid appearance of this unusual tumor allowed its diagnosis by echocardiography. The occurrence of this sarcoma arising from a cardiac valve has not been previously reported.[3-6] At least 9 patients have been described in whom a true neoplasm arose from a cardiac valve.[2-5,7] When involving a semilumar valve, the usual hemodynamic consequence is stenosis, and when involving an atrioventricular valve, regurgitation. Our patient had auscultatory evidence of both left ventricular outflow obstruction and mitral regurgitation. Dislodgement of fragments of a neoplasm arising from a cardiac leaflet is common because of the leaflet's movement.

From the Departments of Medicine and Pediatrics, Hamad General Hospital, Doha, Qatar, and the Pathology Branch, National Heart, Lung, and Blood Institute, National Institutes of Health, Bethesda, Maryland 20205. Manuscript received May 31, 1985, accepted June 7, 1985.

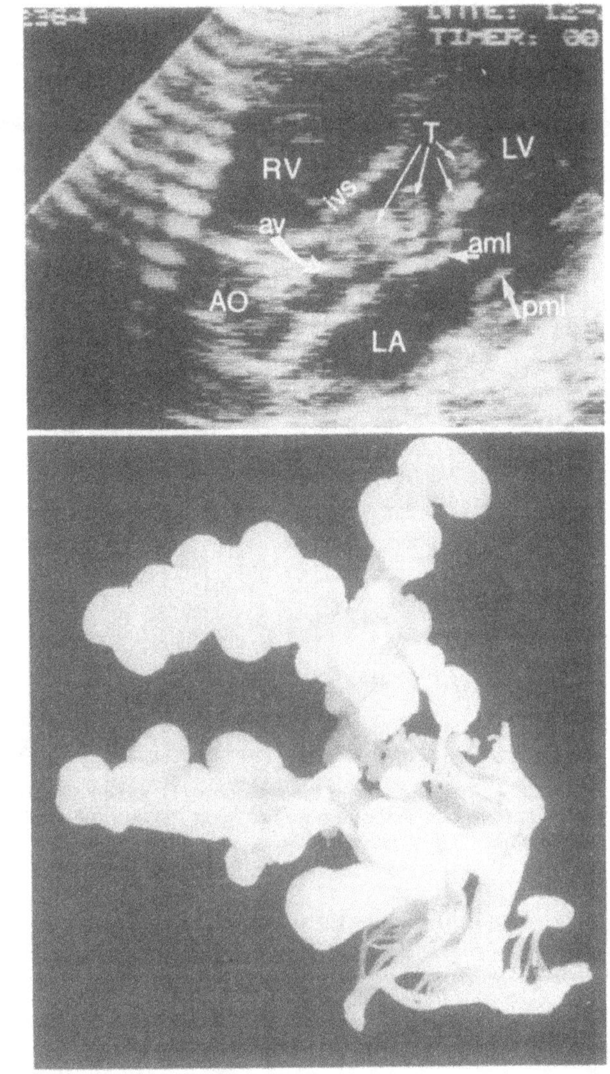

FIGURE 1. ***Top,*** **echocardiogram in modified subcostal projection. Early ventricular diastole. Note the multilobulated tumor (T) (*arrows* from the T) having attachment to the anterior mitral leaflet (aml). The lobulations extend from the body of the left ventricle (LV) to the level of the aortic valve (av) (*curved arrow*). *Bottom,* gross appearance of the tumor and anterior mitral leaflet with attachments oriented to correlate with the tumor position in the echocardiogram. The botryoid appearance of this mass is nearly identical to that seen on the echocardiogram. AO = aortic root; LA = left atrium; RV = right ventricle; lvs = ventricular septum; pml = posterior mitral leaflet.**

References

1. Nadas AS, Ellison RC. Cardiac tumors in infancy. *Am J Cardiol 1968;21:363–366.*
2. Reece IJ, Cooley DA, Frazier OH, Hallman GL, Powers PL, Montero CG. Cardiac tumors. *Clinical spectrum and prognosis of lesions other than classical benign myxoma in 20 patients. J Thorac Cardiovasc Surg 1984;88:439–446.*
3. Barberger-Gateau P, Paquet M, Desaulniers D, Chenard J. *Fibrolipoma of the mitral valve in a child. Clinical and echocardiographic features. Circulation 1978;58:955–958.*
4. Sandrasagra FA, Oliver WA, English TAH. *Myxoma of the mitral valve. Br Heart J 1979;42:221–223.*
5. Fine G. *Primary tumors of the pericardium and heart. Cardiovasc Clin 1973;5:208–238.*
6. Hardin NJ, Wilson JM III, Gray GF, Gay WA Jr. *Experience with primary tumors of the heart. Clinical and pathological study of seventeen cases. Johns Hopkins Med J 1974;134:141–155.*
7. Catton RW, Guntheroth WG, Reichenbach DD. *A myxoma of the pulmonary valve causing severe stenosis in infancy. Am Heart J 1963;66:248–252.*

Cardiac-Compressing Intrapericardial Teratoma at Birth

Katrina R. Brabham, BA, and William C. Roberts, MD

Intrapericardial teratomas are rare and generally seen in infants and young children.[1-10] They may cause respiratory distress, pericardial effusion and cardiac compression. Several case reports have described children with this neoplasm in whom operative excision was life saving.[5-7,9] We present a stillborn infant with a massive intrapericardial teratoma that caused fatal cardiac compres-

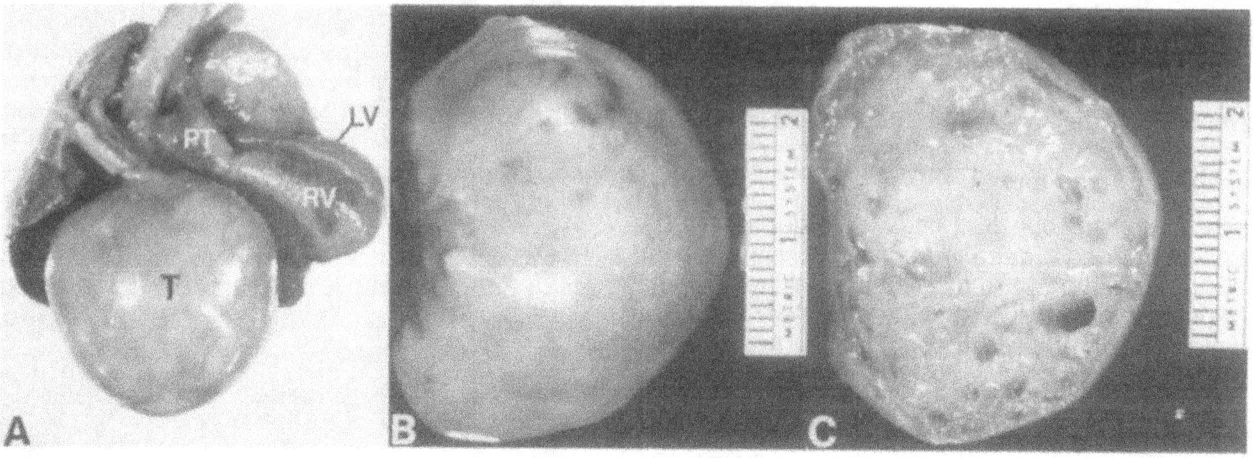

FIGURE 1. Photographs of the teratoma (T), which displaced the heart cephalad and to the left (*A*), view of the smooth surfaced teratoma after its excision from the heart (*B*) and cut section of the teratoma (*C*) showing cysts. LV = left ventricle; PT = pulmonary trunk; RV = right ventricle.

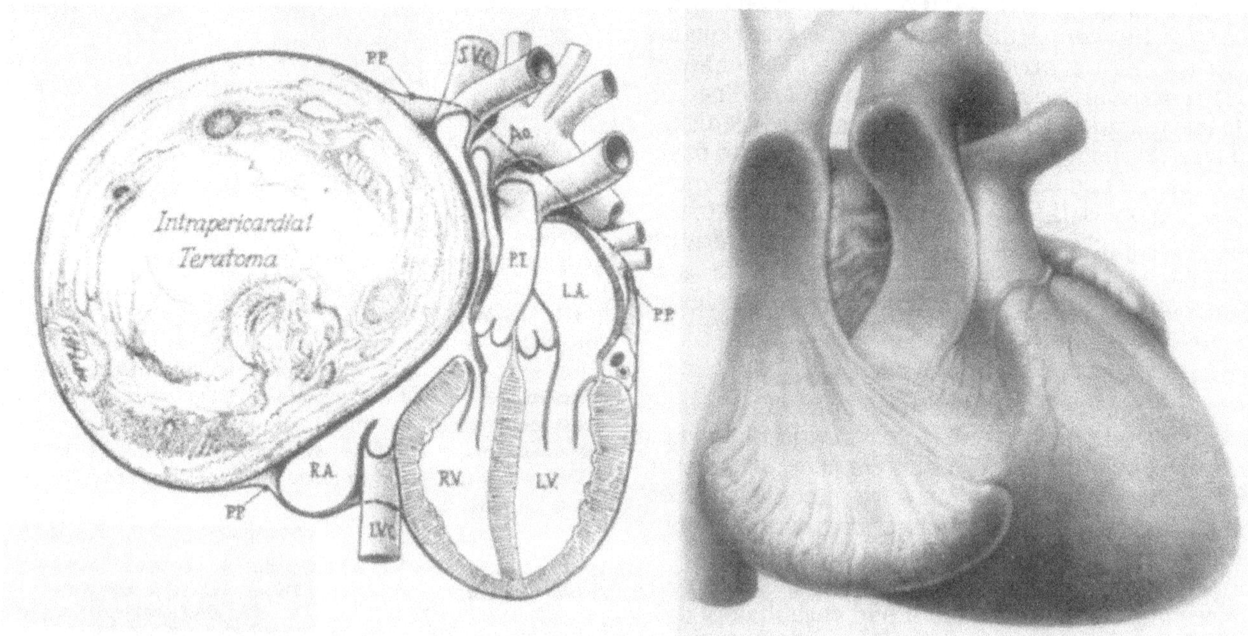

FIGURE 2. Drawings of cut surface of the teratoma and heart (*left*) and of the right side of the heart (*right*) showing where the teratoma had compressed the superior vena cava (SVC), right atrium (RA), right ventricle (RV) and ascending aorta (Ao). IVC = inferior vena cava; LA = left atrium; LV = left ventricle; PP = parietal pericardium; PT = pulmonary trunk.

sion. Its occurrence in a stillborn has been previously reported only once.[10]

An 1,800-g macerated boy was born to a 23-year-old gravida 1, para 0 healthy woman. She had no complications until the twenty-ninth week of pregnancy when she developed marked polyhydramnios. The last fetal movements were felt 4 days before delivery. On the day of her delivery, the mother developed signs consistent with placental abruption. The infant was born breech. At autopsy, the heart weighed 8 g. It was displaced cephalad and to the left. Otherwise, the heart was anatomically normal. Attached to the epicardium by loose connective tissue was a 20-g mass measuring 3.5 × 3.0 × 3.0 cm. The right atrium, right ventricle and ascending aorta were severely compressed by the mass (Figures 1 and 2). The tumor was easily separated from the heart; its cut surface contained numerous small cysts. Histologically, the tumor was composed of smooth muscle, and glial, cartilage and epithelial cells in a matrix of undifferentiated mesochymal tissue.

Teratomas are neoplasms that contain endodermic, mesodermic and neuroectodermic germinal layers. They occur in the testes, ovaries, sacroccygeal area, retroperitoneally, intracranially and in the neck and thorax. Teratomas within the pericardial sac and attached to the ascending aorta or epicardium, as in our patient, are the second most frequent tumors in infancy.[8] Carachi et al[9] collected 44 cases of intrapericardial teratoma, and Sumner et al[5] found 50 cases. Only 6 previous infant deaths were found.[2,8,10] Death generally resulted from hemorrhage during operative removal of the tumor, cardiac compression or malignancy.[8]

From the Pathology Branch, National Heart, Lung and Blood Institute, National Institutes of Health, Bethesda, Maryland 20892. Manuscript received September 6, 1988, and accepted October 1.

1. Willis RA. An intrapericardial teratoma in an infant. *J Pathol 1946;58:284–286.*
2. Claireaux AE. An intrapericardial teratoma in a newborn infant. *J Pathol Bacteriol 1951;63:743–745.*
3. Legnami FA, Corwin RD. Intrapericardial teratoma. *Am Heart J 1963;65:674–677.*
4. McConaghie RJ, Friedman IJ. Intrapericardial teratoma. *Am J Dis Child 1965;110:683–685.*
5. Sumner TE, Crowe JE, Klein A, McKone RC, Weaver RL. Intrapericardial teratoma in infancy. *Pediatr Radiol 1980;10:51–53.*
6. Arciniegas E, Hakimi M, Farooki Z, Green E. Intrapericardial teratoma in infancy. *J Thorac Cardiovasc Surg 1980;79:306–311.*
7. Zerella JT, Halpe DCE. Intrapericardial teratoma—neonatal cardiorespiratory distress amenable to surgery. *J Pediatr Surg 1980;15:961–963.*
8. Agozzino L, Vosa C, Arciprete P, de Leva F, Cotrufo M. Intrapericardial teratoma in the newborn. *Int J Cardiol 1984;5:21–28.*
9. Carachi R, Campbell PE, Chow CW, Mee BB. Alpha-feto-protein-(AFP)-secreting intra-pericardial teratoma—report of a case diagnosed on CT scanning. *Z Kinderchir 1986;41:369–370.*
10. Cyr DR, Guntheroth WG, Nyberg DA, Smith JR, Nudelman SR, Ek M. Prenatal diagnosis of an intrapericardial teratoma. *J Ultrasound Med 1988;7:87–90.*

Growth Rate of Left Atrial Myxoma

Sonya Malekzadeh, BA, and William C. Roberts, MD

How fast do left atrial (LA) myxomas grow? To attempt to answer this question we examined publications describing patients in whom myxoma recurred in the left atrium after earlier excision of a similar tumor from this chamber.

Although many publications have described recurrence of myxoma in the left atrium after previous operative excision, most did not provide either the weight or the dimensions of the myxoma excised at the second operation.[1-14] At least 10 publications (9 patients) have described either the dimensions or weight of a recurrent myxoma in the left atrium and these 9 cases are summarized in Table I.[15-24] Of the 7 patients in whom the information was provided, the largest dimension of the recurrent LA myxoma ranged from 1.5 to 10.0 cm (mean 5.1), and the interval from the first operative excision to the operation for excision of the recurrent LA myxoma ranged from 11 to 76 months (mean 33). Thus, the recurrent myxoma in these 7 patients increased in size an average of 0.15 cm/month or 1.8 cm/year between the 2 operations. In 3 of the 9 patients with recurrent LA myxoma, the weight of the recurrent tumor was provided: the recurrent tumor weighed 19, 30 and 58 g and the interval between the 3 operations was 24, 30 and 36 months, respectively. Thus, the recurrent LA myxoma in these 3 patients grew an average of 1.2 g/month or 14 g/year.

Whether or not the original LA myxoma grew as rapidly as the recurrent LA myxoma in the aforementioned patients is, of course, unknown. Two echocardiographic reports, however, also have attempted to determine how fast or slowly the initial LA myxoma grew. Roudaut et al[25] described a 45-year-old man with an echocardiographically normal LA cavity and mitral valve at the time of coronary artery bypass grafting, but echocardiogram 8 months later disclosed an LA mass that at operation was 5.5 × 4.0 cm in size. Marinissen et al[26] described a 65-year-old man who had an echocardiographically normal LA cavity and mitral valve at the time of coronary artery bypass grafting, but echocardiogram 18 months later disclosed an LA mass that at operation was 6.0 × 4.0 cm in size. Thus, in these 2 patients the original LA myxoma may have grown as rapidly as 0.44 cm/month or over 5 cm/year. Whatever their exact growth rate may be, both recurrent and initial LA myxoma appear to grow rather rapidly.

From the Pathology Branch, National Heart, Lung, and Blood Institute, National Institutes of Health, Bethesda, Maryland 20892. Manuscript received June 27, 1989; revised manuscript received and accepted July 17, 1989.

1. Gerbode F, Kerth WJ, Hill JD. Surgical management of tumors of the heart. *Surgery 1967;61:94–101.*

2. Puel P, Castany P, Enjalbert A. Notre expèrience de la chirurgie des myxomes intracardiaques: rapport d'une forme recidivante et reoperee avec succes. *Ann Chir Thorac Cardiovasc 1973;12:293–294.*

3. Chassignolle J-F, Termet H, Age C, Dureau G, Du Gres B, Samuel D, Michaud P. A propos d'une sèrie de 10 myxomes intracardiaques opérés. *Ann Chir Thorac Cardiovasc 1973;12:297–298.*

4. Hardin NJ, Wilson JM III, Gray GF, Gay WA Jr. Experience with primary tumors of the heart. Clinical and pathological study of seventeen cases. *Johns Hopkins Med J 1974;134:141–155.*

5. Read RC, White HJ, Murphy ML, Williams D, Sun CN, Flanagan WH. The malignant potentiality of left atrial myxoma. *J Thorac Cardiovasc Surg 1974;68:857–868.*

6. Sasaki S, Lin YT, Redington JV, Mendez AM, Zubiate P, Kay JH. Primary intracavitary cardiac tumors. A review of 11 surgical cases. *J Cardiovasc Surg 1977;18:15–21.*

7. O'Neil MB Jr, Grehl TM, Hurley EJ. Cardiac myxomas: a clinical diagnostic challenge. *Am J Surg 1979;138:68–76.*

8. St John Sutton MG, Mercier L-A, Giuliani ER, Lie JT. Atrial myxomas. A review of clinical experience in 40 patients. *Mayo Clin Proc 1980;55:371–376.*

9. Brandt B III, Mijangos J, Easley RM Jr, Sengupta A. Recurrent atrial myxoma. Report of a case. *Am Surg 1980;46:469–470.*

10. Popa IP. Intracardiac myxomas. Report on 28 cases. *Chirurgie 1981;107:701–706.*

11. Fujiwara T, Motochiro K, Kiso A, Katsumura T, Hirota S. Recurrence of a left atrial myxoma. Considerations on the pathogenesis of recurrence. *Kyobu Geka 1982;35:101–104.*

12. Cleveland DC, Westaby S, Karp RB. Treatment of intra-atrial cardiac

TABLE I Pertinent Findings in Eight Previously Reported Patients with Recurrent Left Atrial Myxoma in Which the Dimensions or Weight of the Recurrent Tumor Were Provided

First Author	Publication Year (Ref.)	Pt Age (yrs), Sex	Size of Initial Myxoma (cm)	Weight of Initial Myxoma (g)	Interval Between Operation (months)	Size of Recurrent Myxoma (cm)	Weight of Recurrent Myxoma (g)	Growth Rate of Myxoma	
								cm/mo	g/mo
Bahl	1969[15]	34, F	3.0	—	76	1.5	—	0.02	—
Walton	1972[16]	49, F	7.0 × 3.5	—	23	7.5 × 3.0	—	0.33 × 0.13	—
Maranhao	1973[17,18*]	49, F	5.0 × 4.0	—	44	5.0 × 3.0 × 4.0	—	0.11 × 0.07 × 0.09	—
Kabbani	1973[19]	19, F	—	—	19	10.0 × 2.5†	—	0.53 × 0.13	—
Mussini-Montpellier	1973[20]	7, M	—	31	24	—	19	—	0.79
Zackai	1974[21]	47, M	—	—	11	1.9 × 0.06	—	0.17 × 0.005	—
Jugdutt	1975[22]	46, M	—	80	30	6.5 × 3.0 × 2.0	30	0.22 × 0.108 × 0.07	1
Attar	1980[23]	57, M	—	76	36	—	58	—	1.6
Markel	1986[24]	18, F	4.0 × 3.0 × 2.0	22	30	3.0 × 1.5 × 0.4	—	0.1 × 0.05 × 0.01	—

* This case was reported in 2 different journals.
† This patient actually had 4 separate myxomas recurrent in the left atrium. This dimension is the largest of the 4 tumors.

tumors. *JAMA 1983;249:2799–2802.*
13. Grauer K, Grauer MC. Familial atrial myxoma with bilateral recurrence. *Heart Lung 1983;12:600–602.*
14. Gray IR, Williams WG. Recurring cardiac myxoma. *Br Heart J 1985;53: 645–649.*
15. Bahl OP, Oliver GC, Ferguson TB, Schad N, Parker BM. Recurrent left atrial myxoma. Report of a case. *Circulation 1969;40:673–676.*
16. Walton JA Jr, Kahn DR, Willis PW III. Recurrence of a left atrial myxoma. *Am J Cardiol 1972;29:872–876.*
17. Maranhao V, Gooch AS, Yang SS, Goldberg H. Regrowth of a left atrial myxoma. *Chest 1973;63:98–100.*
18. Maranhao V, Fernandez J, Gooch AS, Morse D, Nichols HT, Goldberg H. Resection of regrowth of a left atrial myxoma complicated by complete heart block three years following its primary resection. *J Cardiovasc Surg 1973;14:338–343.*
19. Kabbani SS, Cooley DA. Atrial myxoma. Surgical considerations. *J Thorac Cardiovasc Surg 1973;65:731–737.*
20. Mussini-Montpellier J, Cornet E, Gillot F, Le Bodic M-F, Michaud J-L, Nomballais M-F. Aspects histologiques d'une recidive de myxome de l'oreillette gauche chez un enfant. *Ann Chir Thorac Cardiovasc 1973;12:239–240.*
21. Zackai AH, Weber DJ, Ramsby G, Wong B. Recurrence of left atrial myxoma. *J Cardiovasc Surg 1974;15:467–471.*
22. Jugdutt BI, Rossall RE, Sterns LP. An unusual case of recurrent left atrial myxoma. *Can Med Assoc J 1975;112:1099–1100.*
23. Attar S, Lee Y-C, Singleton R, Scherlis L, David R, McLaughlin JS. Cardiac myxoma. *Ann Thorac Surg 1980;29:397–405.*
24. Markel ML, Armstrong WF, Waller BF, Mahomed Y. Left atrial myxoma with multicentric recurrence and evidence of metastases. *Am Heart J 1986; 111:409–413.*
25. Roudaut R, Gosse P, Dallocchio M. Rapid growth of a left atrial myxoma shown by echocardiography. *Br Heart J 1987;58:413–416.*
26. Marinissen KI, Essed C, Groot C, Schelling A, Hagemeijer F. Growth rate of left atrial myxoma. Development of a symptomatic left atrial myxoma less than two years after coronary artery bypass grafting. *Chest 1987;92:941–942.*

Pathologic Findings Associated With Interleukin-2–Based Immunotherapy for Cancer: A Postmortem Study of 19 Patients

AMY H. KRAGEL, MD, WILLIAM D. TRAVIS, MD, LAURIE FEINBERG, MD, STEFANIA PITTALUGA, MD, LILIANE M. STRIKER, MD, WILLIAM C. ROBERTS, MD, MICHAEL T. LOTZE, MD, JAMES J. YANG, MD, AND STEVEN A. ROSENBERG, MD

The use of interleukin-2 (IL-2), either alone or in combination with lymphokine-activated killer cells, tumor infiltrating lymphocytes, or other immunotherapeutic agents has added a new list of alternatives to conventional antineoplastic regimens. Little information is available about the pathologic changes occurring in patients treated with these agents. In this study, we reviewed the necropsy materials from 19 patients, 12 men and 7 women, with a variety of malignancies including melanoma, renal cell carcinoma, gastrointestinal and pulmonary adenocarcinoma, and metastatic gastrinoma, who died after receiving IL-2–based immunotherapy. Death occurred at intervals ranging from less than 1 hour to 143 days following the last dose of therapy. All patients dying at or less than 43 days following cessation of therapy had lymphoid infiltrates of varying intensity in residual tumor. At necropsy, the major cause of death unrelated to the presence of metastatic tumor was bacterial sepsis. In addition, we found evidence of significant cardiac and pulmonary toxicity: two patients with acute myocardial infarction, one with and one without significant coronary artery disease, two cases of unexplained lymphocytic myocarditis, and one case of fatal pulmonary capillary plugging following an infusion of lymphokine-activated killer cells. Thus, not unlike other forms of therapy for cancer, IL-2–based immunotherapy does not appear to be without significant toxicity. HUM PATHOL 21:493–502. This is a US government work. There are no restrictions on its use.

The use of interleukin-2 (IL-2) as an immunotherapeutic agent for the treatment of metastatic carcinoma has been under evaluation since the early 1980s when methods for producing recombinant IL-2 were developed.[1,2] Several clinical trials have shown that immunotherapy with IL-2, alone and in combination with other agents including lymphokine-activated killer (LAK) cells, is capable of inducing partial and complete remissions in patients with various types of cancer.[3-5] At the same time, clinical toxicity associated with IL-2 has been recognized, and several publications have described the frequency of various manifestations of IL-2 toxicity.[3-8] Reported side effects have included nausea, vomiting, malaise, altered mental status, somnolence, skin rash, weight gain, hypotension, angina pectoris, cardiac arrhythmias, acute myocardial infarction, myocarditis, increased serum creatinine, decreased urinary output, hyperbilirubinemia, anemia, eosinophilia, thrombocytopenia, serious bacterial infections, and alterations in thyroid gland function.[3-18]

The use of IL-2, either alone or in combination with LAK cells, tumor infiltrating lymphocytes (TILs), or other immunotherapeutic agents has added a new list of alternatives to existing conventional antineoplastic regimens. As the use of these agents increases, it becomes increasingly important to study the effects which IL-2–based immunotherapy has on various organ systems and to develop an understanding of the impact of therapy on the ultimate causes of death in these patients. Little published information is available regarding the pathologic changes in patients who have received IL-2. In this article, we describe morphologic findings at necropsy in 19 patients who had received IL-2 based immunotherapy.

METHODS

Patients Studied

Nineteen consecutive patients were identified in the files of the Laboratory of Pathology, National Cancer Institute, as having received IL-2–based immunotherapy treatment. These included IL-2 alone and IL-2 in combination with either LAK cells (mononuclear cells obtained by leukopheresis and subsequently incubated with IL-2 for 2 to 3 days), alpha interferon, cyclophosphamide, monoclonal antibodies, or TILs.

Materials Examined

The autopsy protocols and clinical records were reviewed. The following items from these records were noted: (1) specific immunotherapy regimen received; (2) interval from the last dose of therapy to death; (3) signs and symptoms of adverse reactions during therapy; and (4) cause of death.

The following organs were studied in detail: heart, lungs, thyroid, liver, kidney and skin. In 16 of the 19 cases, the heart specimen was available for review and was reexamined. In these cases, two to four additional 2 cm sections

From the Pathology Branch, National Heart, Lung, and Blood Institute, the Laboratory of Pathology and Surgery Branch, National Cancer Institute, and Metabolic Disease Branch, National Institute of Diabetes and Digestive and Kidney Diseases, National Institutes of Health, Bethesda, MD; and Mayo Medical School, Mayo Clinic, Rochester, MN. Accepted for publication September 5, 1989.

Key words: myocarditis, acute myocardial infarction, diffuse alveolar damage, thyroiditis, lymphoid infiltrate, lymphokine activated killer cells.

Address correspondence and reprint requests to William D. Travis, MD, Laboratory of Pathology, Building 10, Room 2N212, National Cancer Institute, National Institutes of Health, Bethesda, MD 20892.

0046-8177/90/2105-0005$0.00/0

of both right and left ventricle (including papillary muscle) were taken, fixed in formalin, processed, sectioned, and stained with hematoxylin and eosin. Hematoxylin and eosin-stained sections were available for review in 18 of 19 cases. Formalin-fixed sections of kidney, lung, and liver were reviewed in all cases. In addition, sections of kidney stained by the periodic acid-Schiff method were examined. In 18 of 19 cases, sections of thyroid were reviewed, In three cases, sections of skin were available for review. All other hematoxylin and eosin-stained sections taken at the time of autopsy were reviewed. The extent and location of tumor and the presence or absence of a lymphoid infiltrate within or around that tumor was noted in each case. The lymphoid infiltrate, if present, was graded on a scale of 1 to 3.

RESULTS

Clinical Features

The clinical features of the 19 patients studied are summarized in Table 1. Twelve men and seven women, aged 22 to 67 years (mean 50), with a variety of malignancies, including renal cell carcinoma (eight cases), malignant melanoma (six cases), adenocarcinoma of the lung (two cases), adenocarcinoma of the stomach (one case), colorectal carcinoma (one case), and gastrinoma (one case) were studied. All patients received IL-2. Lymphokine-activated killer cells were included in the treatment protocols of 11 patients, alpha interferon in those of two patients, TILs in those of two patients, cyclophosphamide in that of one patient, and monoclonal antibodies in that of one patient.

Tumor Pathology

Metastatic disease at necropsy was extensive in 18 (95%) patients. Tumor was identified in lungs (18 cases), lymph nodes (10 cases), liver (10 cases), heart (seven cases), adrenal glands (six cases), bone marrow (five cases), brain (five cases), gastrointestinal tract (four cases), spleen (three cases), pancreas (two cases), thyroid gland (two cases), skin (two cases), gall bladder (two cases), urinary bladder (two cases), bone (two cases), testes (two cases), uterus and ovary (one case), breast (one case), and other soft tissue sites in five cases. One patient (patient no. 1, Table 1), who received IL-2 as adjuvent therapy following resection of lymph nodes containing metastatic melanoma, had no detectable tumor at either the initiation of therapy or at necropsy.

Lymphoid infiltrates were identified either at the periphery of or within the tumor in 14 patients (Table 1, Fig 1). All of these 14 patients died within 43 days of the last dose of therapy. The amount of infiltrate varied from 1+ to 3+. No correlation was found between the severity of the infiltrate and the interval between the last dose of therapy and death. No apparent correlation was noted between the type of malignancy and the presence or severity of the lymphoid infiltrate.

Cardiac Findings

The clinical signs and symptoms of cardiac dysfunction or ischemia and the gross and microscopic findings in the hearts of the patients studied are sum-

TABLE 1. Certain Clinical and Necropsy Findings in 19 Patients Receiving Immunotherapy

Case No.	Age/Race/Sex (yr)	Type of Malignancy	Immunotherapy Regimen	Interval From Last Rx to Death (d)	Tumor-associated Lymphocytes at Necropsy (1-3+)	Cause of Death
1	22/W/F	Melanoma	IL2/LAK	0	NA	Respiratory Failure*
2	67/W/M	Renal cell CA	IL2	1	1+	AMI
3	51/W/M	Renal cell CA	IL2	4	2-3+	Sepsis
4	24/W/M	Melanoma	IL2/LAK	4	1+	Sepsis
5	45/W/M	Adeno CA, colorectal	IL2/LAK	4	1+	Sepsis
6	65/W/M	melanoma	IL2/MoAb	6	3+	Metastatic disease
7	55/W/M	Renal cell CA	IL2/aIFN	8	1+	Metastatic disease
8	34/W/F	Melanoma	IL2/TILs	13	1+, focal	Metastatic disease
9	53/W/F	Renal cell CA	IL2/Cytoxan	16	1+, focal	Sepsis, GI bleed
10	59/W/M	Adeno CA, lung	IL2/LAK	17	1+, focal	Sepsis
11	57/W/M	Renal cell CA	IL2/aIFN	20	3+	Anoxic encephalopathy†
12	25/W/M	Melanoma	IL2/TILs	20	1+, focal	Sepsis, metastatic disease
13	58/B/M	Renal cell CA	IL2/LAK	42	1+	Sepsis/multi-system failure
14	59/W/M	Adeno CA, GE jct	IL2/LAK	43	1+	Sepsis, GI bleed
15	58/B/F	Renal cell CA	IL2/LAK	47	0	Metastatic disease
16	67/W/M	Gastrinoma	IL2/LAK	67	0	Metastatic disease
17	53/W/M	Renal cell CA	IL2/LAK	71	0	Cardiac failure secondary to AMI
18	40/W/F	Adeno CA, lung	IL2/LAK	74	0	Metastatic disease
19	43/W/F	Melanoma	IL2/LAK	143	0	Metastatic disease

Abbreviations: aIFN, alpha interferon; AMI, acute myocardial infarction; CA, carcinoma; GE jct, gastroesophageal junction; GI, gastrointestinal; IL-2, interleukin 2; LAK, lymphokine-activated killer cells; MoAb, antimelanoma antibodies; NA, not applicable, no tumor present at necropsy; Rx, immunotherapy; TILs, tumor infiltrating lymphocytes.

* Pulmonary capillary engorgement and interstitital infiltration by lymphocytes.

† Anoxic encephalopathy followed a cardiac arrest after aspiration of gastric contents during a period of altered mental status associated with therapy.

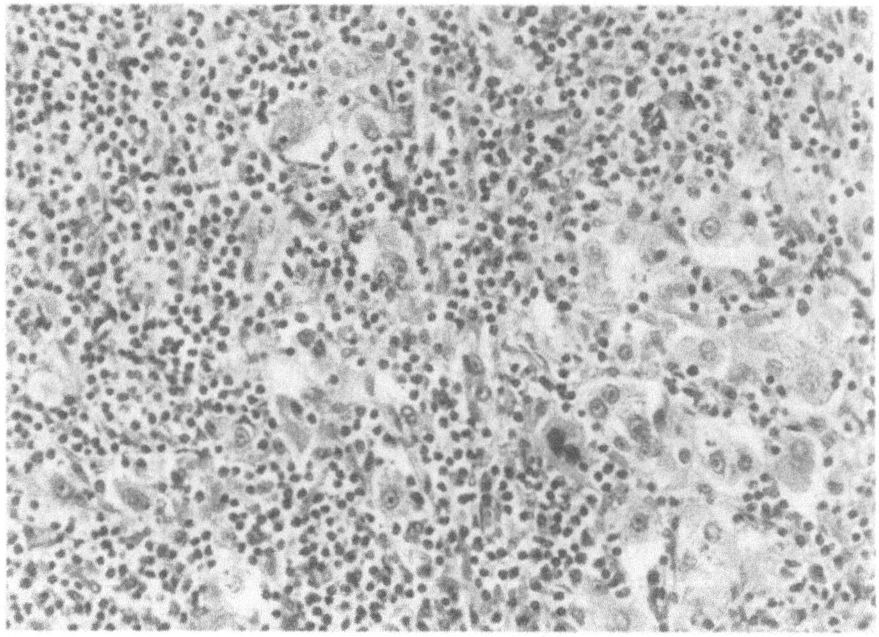

FIGURE 1. Section of liver (case no. 11) entirely replaced by metastatic renal cell carcinoma with dense lymphocytic infiltrate. (Hematoxylin and eosin stain; original magnification × 250.)

marized in Table 2. Significant weight gain during therapy occurred in all 19 patients and varied from 2% to 29% of the admission weight (mean 10%). Significant hypotension occurred in 17 patients (89%) and was severe enough to warrant vasopressor therapy in 13 patients. Arrhythmias (atrial in four and ventricular in eight) were noted in nine patients (47%), eight of whom had some form of right or left ventricular necrosis or fibrosis. The presence of or severity of weight gain, hypotension, or arrhythmias did not correlate with any specific pathologic finding at necropsy.

A lymphocytic myocarditis (Fig 2) was present in two of the four patients dying less than 5 days from the last dose of therapy in whom the heart was available for review. Both of these (patients no. 1 and 3, Table 2) had a patchy inflammatory infiltrate in the walls of both ventricles (predominately lymphocytic, with a few polymorphonuclear leukocytes and eosinophils). There was associated myocyte degeneration and necrosis. No infectious etiology was identified in either case.

Septic myocarditis was observed in three patients who had acute inflammatory infiltrates in the myocardium associated with bacterial sepsis. Patient no. 4 had an acute inflammatory infiltrate and minute abscesses in the myocardium. This patient had evidence of severe and generalized sepsis at necropsy. The other two patients had focal interstitial inflammatory infiltrates without associated necrosis or myocyte degeneration. In patient no. 11, the infiltrate was mixed (polymorphonuclear leukocytes, lymphocytes, and eosinophils) and in the second patient (patient no. 16), it was predominantly polymorphonuclear. Isolated lymphoid aggregates were found in the myocardium of two additional patients (patient nos. 18 and 19).

Acute myocardial infarction was present in one case (patient no. 2) and a healed myocardial infarct was present in a second (patient no. 17). In both cases, the clinically recognized events compatible with acute myocardial infarcts occurred while on therapy or immediately after it was halted. At necropsy, the heart in case no. 2 weighed 520 g and there was > 75% cross-sectional-area narrowing of at least one of the major epicardial coronary arteries. The age of the infarct as evaluated histologically was compatible with the clinical event which occurred less than 24 hours before death. Patient no. 17 had a massive transmural circumferential healed myocardial infarct which extended from the apex to the base of the left ventricle (Fig 3). The major epicardial coronary arteries were virtually devoid of atherosclerotic plaque. The age of the infarct was compatible histologically with a clinically recognized event 71 days before death.

Renal Findings

Selected clinical parameters of renal dysfunction including peak blood urea nitrogen, creatinine, and blood urea nitrogen-to-creatinine ratio while on therapy were tabulated. Virtually all patients had elevated blood urea nitrogen and creatinine during therapy. The peak urea nitrogen/creatinine ratio while on therapy ranged from 8 to 31 (mean 17).

Autolysis was quite pronounced in several cases, and the tubular lesions observed may be largely related to postmortem artifacts. The glomeruli and blood vessels were better preserved. The following tubular lesions were observed: tubular dilation (13 cases), tubular atrophy (eight cases), casts (15 cases), and loss of brush border of the tubular proximal segment (seven cases). Necrosis and regeneration could not be evaluated in the autopsy specimens. No correlation was found between the presence or severity of acute tubular lesions and either the peak blood urea nitrogen/creatinine ratio during therapy or the interval between death and the last dose of therapy. Of the

TABLE 2. Cardiac Findings, Clinical and Anatomic, in 19 Patients Who Received Immunotherapy

Case No.	Interval Last Rx to Death (d)	Signs and Symptoms of Clinical Toxicity While on Therapy: Weight Gain (% of adm wt)	Hypotension*	Ischemia†	Arrhythmias: Atrial‡	Arrhythmias: Ventricular§	Maximum CA % CSA Narrowing	Right or Left Ventricular: Myocytolysis (0-4+)	Contraction Band Necrosis (0-4+)	Nontransmural Fibrosis (0-4+)	Lymphocytic Myocarditis (0-4+)
1	0	9	4+	3+	4+	4+	0-25	0	0	0	2+
2[‖]	1	3	4+	4+	4+	4+	>75	0	1+	1+	0
3	4	3	2+	0	2+	1+	0-25	0	0	1+	1-2+
4	4	7	4+	0	0	4+	0-25	0	3-4+	2+	0
5	4	2	4+	0	0	0	—	—	—	—	—
6	6	10	3+	0	0	0	—	1+	0	0	0
7	8	9	3+	0	1+	0	26-50	1+	1+	1+	0
8	13	25	3+	0	0	0	26-50	0	0	0	0
9	16	7	0	0	0	0	—	1+	0	0	0
10	17	6	3+	0	0	0	—	0	0	0	0
11	20	10	2+	4+	4+	2+	51-75	0	0	1-2+	0
12	20	21	3+	0	0	0	0-25	0	0	0	0
13	42	3	3+	0	0	0	0-25	0	0	1+	0
14	43	3	0	0	0	1+	51-75	0	0	1+	0
15	47	9	3+	0	0	0	0-25	1-2+	0	0	0
16	67	8	3+	0	3+	0	0-25	0	0	1+	0
17[¶]	71	8	4+	4+	0	4+	0-25	1-2+	0	1+	0
18	74	13	3+	0	0	0	0-25	0	0	0	0
19	143	29	2+	0	0	1+	0-25	0	0	0	0

Note: 0 = negative.

Abbreviations: adm wt, admission weight; CA, coronary artery; CSA, cross-sectional area; d, days; RV, right ventricular; LV, left ventricular.

* Hypotension: 1+, hypotension not requiring therapy; 2+, hypotension responding to fluid therapy; 3+, hypotension requiring and responsive to pressors; 4+, hypotension unresponsive to pressors.

† Ischemia: 2+, nonspecific electrocardiographic (ECG) changes, elevated creatinine kinase; 3+, angina, ischemic changes in ECG, elevated MB band, 4+, myocardial infarction.

‡ Atrial arrhythmias: 1+, sinus tachycardia >110 beats per minute; 2+, premature atrial contractions, 3+, atrial fibrillation or sinus tachycardia >150 beats per minute: 4+, atrial arrhythmia with hypotension.

§ Ventricular arrhythmias: 1+, unifocal ventricular premature contractions; 2+, multifocal ventricular premature contractions, bigeminy, trigeminy; 3+, nonsustained ventricular tachycardia (VT); 4+, sustained VT.

‖ Acute transmural myocardial infarct, <24 hours.

¶ Circumferential transmural left ventricular infarct, >6 weeks.

19 patients, six had interstitial lymphoid infiltrates unassociated with glomerular or tubular lesions. No correlation was found between evidence of clinical toxicity while on therapy (peak blood urea nitrogen or creatinine or their ratio) or interval from last dose of therapy to death, and the presence of an interstitial lymphoid infiltrate. Three patients with renal cell carcinoma had other renal lesions including acute pyelonephritis (patient no. 3), increased cellularity within the mesangial areas (patient no. 2), and diffuse severe mesangial sclerosis (patient no. 11). One patient (patient no. 1) with malignant melanoma had focal glomerulosclerosis.

Pulmonary Findings

Clinical and morphologic findings are summarized in Table 3. Pulmonary toxicity was severe enough in 10 patients to necessitate intubation during the course of therapy. Despite this, no correlation was found between the severity of pulmonary toxicity while on therapy and the survival from the last dose of therapy.

Lung weight, reflecting pulmonary edema, congestion, pneumonia, tumor, and other infiltrates, was heavy in the five patients who died less than 5 days from the last dose of therapy, but it was equally heavy in other patients dying at prolonged intervals after therapy was halted and when clinical evidence of pulmonary toxicity was reversed (Table 3).

The lungs disclosed variable histologic changes. The most striking changes were seen in patient no. 1, a 22-year-old white woman who received IL-2 and LAK cells for treatment of melanoma (Fig 4). She died in severe respiratory distress less than 1 hour after an infusion of LAK cells and 1 week following a course of high dose IL-2 treatment. The lungs contained marked numbers of lymphoid cells in the pulmonary capillaries. The cells were mostly large lymphocytes, with a high nuclear-to-cytoplasmic ratio and hyperchromatic nuclei. In addition, a marked perivascular and interstitial lymphoid infiltrate, occasional small fibrin microthrombi, and focal hyaline membranes were found. While perivascular and interstitial lymphoid infiltrates were seen in two patients each, in none was it nearly as prominent as in this patient. Hyaline membranes were seen in two other patients, both with diffuse alveolar damage. No specific pulmonary findings at necropsy seemed to correlate with the degree of clinical toxicity during therapy or with the interval from the last dose of

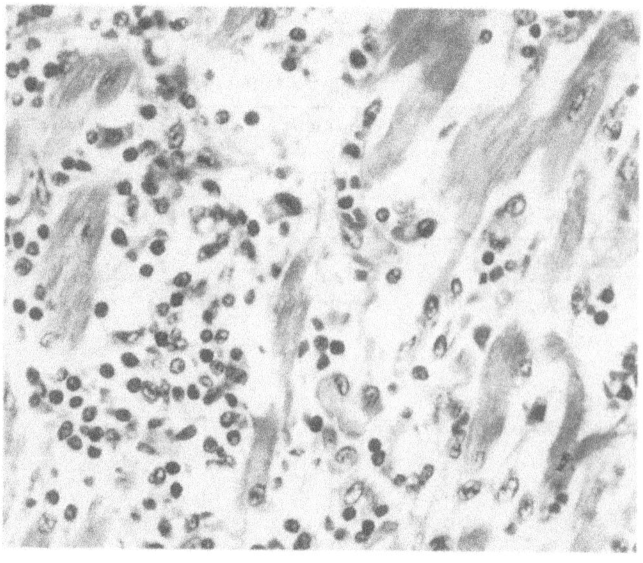

FIGURE 2. Section of left ventricular myocardium (case no. 3) showing a lymphocytic myocarditis. Individual myocytes show degenerative changes. (Hematoxylin and eosin stain; original magnification × 204.)

therapy to death. Bronchopneumonia was found in nine patients and in six it appeared to contribute significantly to the patient's terminal course.

Hepatic Findings

Evidence of hepatobiliary toxicity as reflected in the serum bilirubin and morphologic findings in the liver are outlined in Table 4. Peak serum bilirubin while on therapy ranged from 0.5 to 10.6 mg/dL. No correlation was found between peak bilirubin and the survival from the last dose of therapy. Almost all patients had some degree of centrilobular congestion at necropsy.

All seven patients dying within 8 days of the last dose of therapy had a lymphocytic portal infiltrate, which was more prominent in the two patients dying within 24 hours (Fig 5). Patient no. 2 had extension of this infiltrate beyond the limiting plate with rare foci of associated single-cell hepatocyte necrosis. Patient no. 4 had a mixed lymphocytic, eosinophilic, and polymorphonuclear portal infiltrate and acute cholangitis. Five of the six patients dying within 6 days of the last dose of therapy had lymphocytic sinusoidal infiltrates (Fig 5). Sinusoidal infiltrates were seen in no patients dying later than 6 days from the last dose of therapy.

Three patients dying 20 days or later after cessation of therapy had lymphocytic portal infiltrates. In patients no. 13 and 14 portal fibrosis and extensive metastases also were present. These changes were consistent with chronic biliary obstruction.

At least six patients had other foci of hepatic necrosis, considered to be secondary to either congestion or metastatic tumor.

Steatosis was seen in three patients dying within 5 days of therapy, and in three patients at longer intervals from therapy.

Acute or chronic cholangitis in four patients was either associated with generalized sepsis or extensive hepatic metastases. Severe cholestasis was associated with acute cholangitis in two patients, and with extrahepatic biliary obstruction secondary to tumor in one patient.

A bile duct adenoma and a hemangioma were incidental findings in two patients. Foci of extramedullary hematopoesis were identified in two other patients dying long after cessation of therapy.

Thyroid Gland Findings

Three of the four patients (nos. 1, 2, and 4) dying within 5 days had lymphoid infiltrates in the thyroid

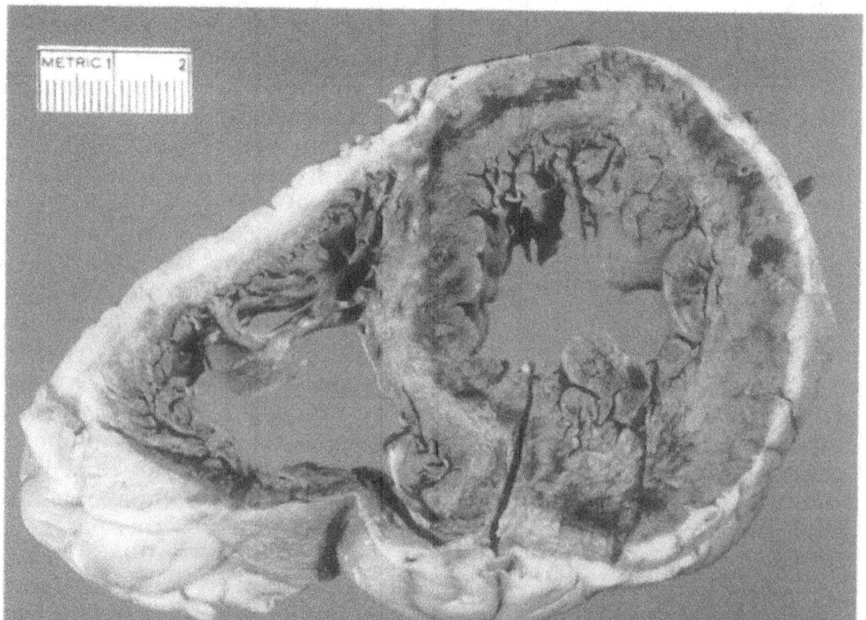

FIGURE 3. Transverse section of the ventricular chambers of the heart (case no. 17) with circumferential left ventricular scarring and biventricular dilatation. The infarct is both subendocardial and transmural. The dark staining of the myocardium corresponds to foci of intracellular calcific deposits. The coronary arteries were essentially devoid of atherosclerotic plaque in this case.

TABLE 3. Pulmonary Findings, Clinical and Anatomic, in Patients Receiving Immunotherapy

Case No.	Interval Last Rx to Death	Clinical Toxicity on Therapy*	Lung Weight (combined, g)	Interstitial Lymphocytes (0-4+)	Perivascular Lymphocytes (0-4+)	Hyaline Membranes (+/−)	Fibrin Microthrombi +/−	Pneumonia +/1
1	0	4+	1,350	3+	3+	focal	+	0
2	1	4+	1,350	0	0	0	+	0
3	4	2+	2,800	0	0	0	0	+
4	4	4+	>1,850	0	0	+	0	+
5	4	4+	2,900	1+ focal	0	0	0	+
6	6	3+	1,100	0	0	0	+	0
7	8	0	1,350	0	0	0	0	0
8	13	4+	700	0	1+	0	0	+
9	16	0	1,410	0	0	0	0	0
10	17	4+	2,000	0	0	0	0	+
11	20	4+	1,450	0	1+	0	+	+
12	20	2+	900	0	0	0	+	+
13	42	4+	2,650	0	0	+	0	0
14	43	0	2,160	0	0	0	0	+
15	47	3+	850	0	0	0	0	0
16	67	0	1,410	0	0	0	0	0
17	71	4+	1,130	0	0	0	0	0
18	74	4+	1,500	1+	0	0	0	0
19	143	0	660	0	0	0	0	+

Abbreviation: Rx, immunotherapy.
* Clinical pulmonary toxicity while on therapy: 1+, Exertional dyspnea; 2+, Dyspnea at rest; 3+, Severe respiratory distress; 4+, Intubation required.

gland, and in one (patient no. 1, Fig 6) they were severe and associated with parenchymal destruction. Two patients (nos. 14 and 17) dying late also had lymphoid infiltrates: several isolated lymphoid aggregates in one patient and moderate lymphoid infiltrates and associated mild parenchymal fibrosis in one patient.

Dermal Findings

Hematoxylin and eosin-stained sections of skin lesions were reviewed in three cases. Subepidermal bullae associated with minimal inflammation were present in one patient, a mild superficial lymphocytic perivascular infiltrate in one patient, and a pustular dermatitis in one patient.

Miscellaneous Findings

With the exception of case no. 1, who in addition to the previously described myocardial, renal, pulmonary, hepatic, and thyroid glandular lesions had lymphoid hyperplasia of ileum, spleen, and lymph nodes, no other significant lesions were noted in sections of the gastrointestinal, reproductive, or hematopoietic organs. (Changes within hematopoietic organs were not assessed systematically because of postmortem changes in these organs.)

Cause of Death

The cause of death (Table 1) was considered the direct result of the presence of metastatic disease in eight patients (one of whom was septic terminally): cerebral metastases (three cases), lung metastases (three cases), lung and liver metastases (one case), and liver and inferior vena cava metastases (one case). In seven other patients, sepsis was considered the cause of death: antemortem blood cultures and/or postmortem cultures of blood and/or lung were positive for *Escherichia coli* and *Klebsiella pneumoniae* in two; *E. coli* and *Enterobacter* sp in one; *Pseudomonas aeruginosa* in one; and *Bacteroides fragilis* in one. In one patient, micro-abscesses containing colonies of gram-positive cocci suggestive of *Staphylococcus* species were identified in multiple organs at necropsy. In one patient, no specific organism was identified as a source of sepsis. In none of these seven patients was a mycobacterium, fungus, or protozoal organism considered responsible for the sepsis. Candida species *fungemia* was seen in one terminal patient (no. 17) who died with severe congestive heart failure secondary to an acute myocardial infarction. The fungemia occurred approximately 6 weeks after cessation of therapy and was not felt to be a consequence of therapy. In eight cases, death was considered directly or indirectly related to the consequences of immunotherapy. Two of these patients died from complications of an acute myocardial infarct (nos. 2 and 17, Table 1); one died with severe respiratory distress and plugging of pulmonary vessels with large atypical lymphoid cells (no. 1, Table 1), three died of sepsis (nos. 3 to 5, Table 1), one died of multisystem failure which developed during therapy and was associated with terminal sepsis (no. 13, Table 1), and one death was secondary to anoxic encephalopathy 20 days after aspiration-induced cardiac arrest (no. 11, Table 1). The latter patient was believed to have aspirated because of an altered mental status associated with therapy.

DISCUSSION

Sepsis was the major cause of death not directly related to the presence of metastatic disease in this

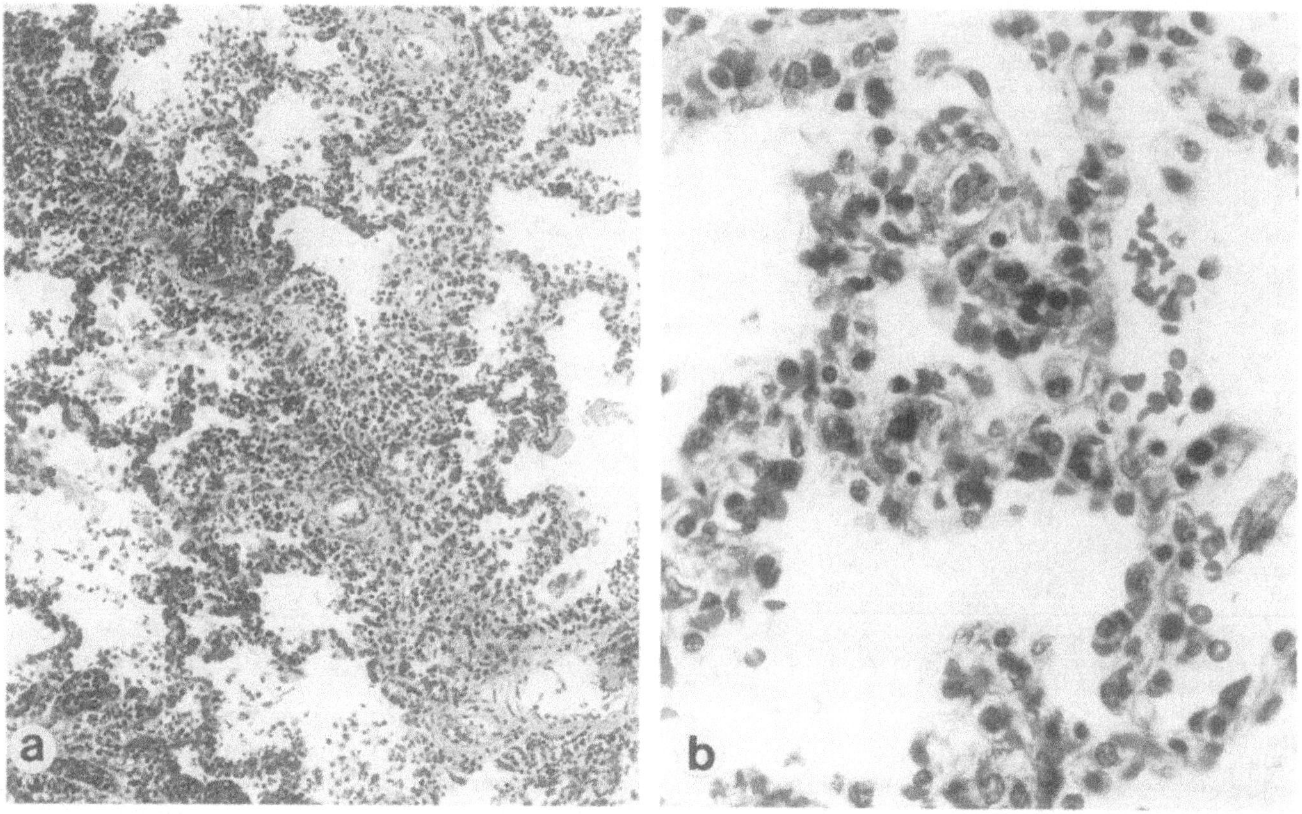

FIGURE 4. Sections of lung (case no. 1) from a 22-year-old female with malignant melanoma who died within 1 hour of infusion of LAK cells and 1 week following high-dose IL-2 therapy. (a) Low-power view showing an extensive interstitial lymphoid infiltrate and congestion of capillaries [original magnification × 125.] (b) High-power view showing engorgement of capillaries with both large and small lymphocytes [original magnification × 500.]

series of 19 patients who received IL-2–based therapy for cancer. It is remarkable that bacterial organisms were responsible for the seven cases of fatal sepsis rather than one of the opportunistic agents associated with conventional chemotherapy and T cell immunosuppression. The paucity of opportunistic infection and the high frequency of serious bacterial infections in patients treated with IL-2 have been previously noted.[11,15,17] Potential explanations for the high frequency of bacterial sepsis may be found in recent evidence that IL-2–based therapy may cause neutrophil dysfunction including depressed Fc receptor expression and decreased chemotactic response.[19] Other recognized alterations in immune function include the development of anergy and decreased proliferative response to soluble antigens.[20] While additional studies are currently underway to further evaluate the immunologic defenses of patients treated with these regimens, it seems clear that the immunologic alterations induced by these agents are not solely directed at the tumor and that they may have serious consequences.

Our study demonstrates the evidence of acute myocardial infarction and lymphocytic myocarditis in patients receiving IL-2–based treatments. Patients receiving IL-2 have been shown to develop a variety of clinical cardiac side effects including profound hypotension, a decrease in systemic vascular resistance, a decrease in ejection fraction, and an increase in heart rate, findings similar to those seen in patients with sepsis.[12,13,16] A small percentage of patients have either atrial or ventricular arrhythmias while on therapy.[3-5] Clinical evidence of acute myocardial infarction or angina pectoris while on therapy has been reported,[3-5,13] and the presence of myocarditis in patients receiving immunotherapy had been documented.[18] Acute myocardial infarction occurred in two of our patients in the face of profound hypotension secondary to immunotherapy. One patient had severe coronary artery disease and the second had widely patent coronary arteries. Two of the four patients dying less than 5 days from the last dose of immunotherapy had a lymphocytic myocarditis without an apparent infectious etiology. All of our patients who had either atrial or ventricular arrhythmias during therapy had either an acute myocardial infarct, a lymphocytic or bacterial myocarditis, or died late with patchy nontransmural fibrosis. Whether or not this nontransmural fibrosis represents a healed myocarditis remains speculative.

Pulmonary toxicity associated with IL-2–based therapy appears primarily to be a consequence of the development of pulmonary edema and to be a transient phenomenon. In a recent review[5] some degree of respiratory distress occurred in 10%, and respiratory distress severe enough to warrant intubation occurred in 4% of 1,039 courses of IL-2–based therapy. The one fatality in this series of 19 patients, which was due to respiratory failure associated with early diffuse alveolar damage and LAK-cell congestion of

TABLE 4. Clinical and Necropsy Findings Pertaining to Liver Pathology

Case No.	Interval Last Rx to Death	Peak Bilirubin on Therapy (mg/dl)	Lymphocytic Portal Inflammation 0-4+	Lymphocytic Sinusoidal Infiltrate 0-4+	Necrosis 0-4+	Cholestasis 0-4+	Steatosis 0-4+	Cholangitis +/−
1	0	2.3	2+	3+	0	0	2+	0
2	1	0.9	2+	1+	1+	0	0	0
3	4	1.1	1+*	2+	0	0	2+	0
4	4	10.6	1+	1+	0	0	2+	+, acute
5	4	0.8	1+	0	0	0	0	0
6	6	0.5	1+	1+	0	0	0	0
7	8	4	1+	0	0	0	0	0
8	13	4.8	0	0	2+	3+	2+	0
9	16	1	0	0	0	0	0	0
10	17	3.8	0	0	0	0	0	0
11	20	5.2	1+	0	0	0	2+	+
12	20	2.6	0	0	0	0	3+	0
13	42	3.8	1+†	0	4+	3+	0	+, acute and chronic
14	43	4.7	2+†	0	3+	0	0	+, chronic
15	47	4.4	0	0	2+	0	0	0
16	67	2.7	0	0	0	0	0	0
17	71	6.5	0	0	focal	3+	0	0
18	74	5.3	0	0	0	0	0	0
19	143	1	0	0	0	0	0	0

Abbreviation: Rx, immunotherapy.
* Eosinophils and polymorphonuclear leukocytes were also present.
† Consistent with chronic biliary obstruction.

pulmonary capillaries, demonstrates the potential for serious pulmonary toxicity associated with administration of LAK cells. The perivascular lymphoid infiltrate which was seen in this patient resembles that which has been observed in rat and mice IL-2 toxicity experiments.[21,22]

The high incidence of portal lymphocytic infiltrates and hepatic sinusoidal infiltrates in patients dying at short intervals after therapy suggests that these findings are directly related to immunotherapy. The accumulation of LAK cells in the liver shortly after infusion of these cells has also been documented by rectilinear scanning.[23] Lymphocytic portal infiltrates, seen in many patients dying shortly after therapy, and the associated necrosis which was seen in one patient have been described in studies of IL-2 toxicity in rats.[21] While reversible cholestasis is a recognized complication of IL-2–based therapy,[8] bile stasis was not appreciated except in patients with other evidence of obstructive jaundice.

Alterations in thyroid function have been reported.[10] We observed a high frequency of lymphoid infiltrates in the thyroid gland of patients dying shortly after cessation of therapy, suggesting that these may be immediate sequelae of therapy. The clinical significance of these findings is not clear, as

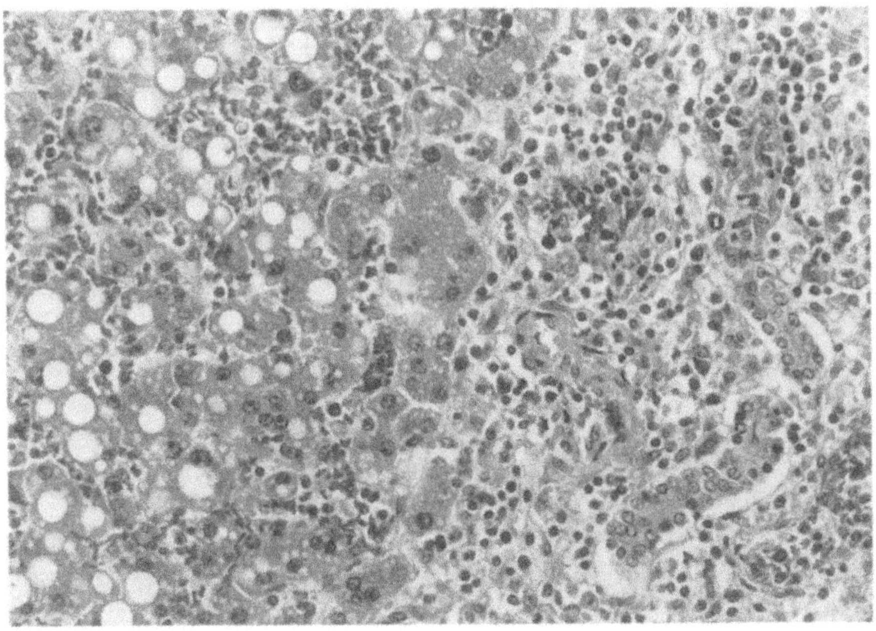

FIGURE 5. Section of liver (case no. 1) from a 22-year-old female who died shortly after an infusion of LAK cells and 1 week following a course of high-dose IL-2. There is a dense portal and sinusoidal lymphoid infiltrate. Hepatocytes show microvesicular steatosis. (Hematoxylin and eosin stain; original magnification × 250.)

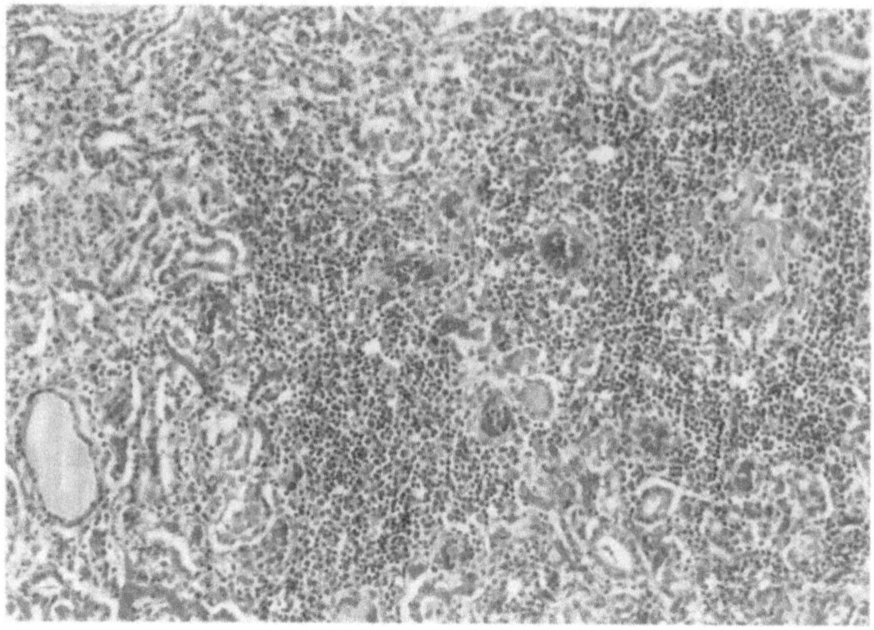

FIGURE 6. Section of thyroid gland (case no. 1) showing a lymphocytic thyroiditis. There is extensive lymphocytic infiltration of the thyroid gland with destruction of follicles. (Hematoxylin and eosin stain; original magnification × 125.)

tests of thyroid function were not available for review in all patients.

Renal dysfunction, attributed to prerenal azotemia,[6] is uniformly present in patients receiving IL-2. No consistent renal findings were present at necropsy which could be related to immunotherapy. Likewise, despite the high frequency of dermal changes[3-5,9] in patients receiving IL-2–based therapies, no pathologic correlates were identified at autopsy.

In summary, in addition to the uniform finding of lymphoid infiltrates in the tumors of patients dying less than 43 days after cessation of therapy which, presumably, is related to its beneficial effects, IL-2–based immunotherapy, not unlike other forms of therapy for the treatment of malignancy, is associated with serious side effects. Despite this, in only 10 of the more than 650 patients who have been treated with these agents at this institution (including eight of the patients described in this report) was death felt to be a direct consequence of therapy. In the 19 patients described in this report there may be an increased frequency of fatal bacterial infections as well as significant cardiac and pulmonary toxicity. As these 19 patients represent a small fraction of the more than 650 patients who have received IL-2–based immunotherapy at this institution,[5] continued follow-up is necessary to document the frequency and confirm the significance of our findings.

REFERENCES

1. Taniguchi T, Matsui H, Fujita T, et al: Structure and expression of a cloned cDNA for human interleukin-2. Nature 302:305-310, 1983

2. Rosenberg SA, Grimm EA, McGrogan M, et al: Biological activity in recombinant human interleukin-2 produced in E coli. Science 223:1412-1415, 1984

3. Rosenberg SA, Lotze MT, Muul LM, et al: A progress report on the treatment of 157 patients with advanced cancer using lymphokine-activated killer cells and interleukin-2 or high dose interleukin-2 alone. N Engl J Med 316:889-897, 1987

4. Fisher RI, Coltman CA, Doroshow JH, et al: Metastatic renal cancer treated with interleukin-2 and lymphokine-activated killer cells. A phase II clinical trial. Ann Intern Med 108:518-523, 1988

5. Rosenberg SA, Lotze MT, Yang JC, et al: Experience with the use of high dose interleukin-2 in the treatment of 652 patients with cancer. Ann Surg 210:474-485, 1989

6. Belldegrun A, Webb DE, Austin HA, et al: Effects of interleukin-2 on renal function in patients receiving immunotherapy for advanced cancer. Ann Intern Med 106:817-822, 1987

7. Marolda R, Belli F, Prada A, et al: A phase I study of recombinant interleukin-2 in melanoma patients. Toxicity and clinical effects. Tumori 73:575-584, 1987

8. Fisher B, Keenan AM, Garra BS, et al: Interleukin-2 induces profound reversible cholestasis: A detailed analysis in treated patients. J Clin Oncol 7:1852-1862, 1989

9. Gaspari AA, Lotze MT, Rosenberg SA, et al: Dermatologic changes associated with interleukin-2 adminsitration. JAMA 258:1624-1629, 1987

10. Atkins MB, Mier JW, Parkinson DR, et al: Hypothyroidism after treatment with interleukin-2 and lymphokine-activated killer cells. N Engl J Med 318:1557-1563, 1988

11. Begley MG, Shawker TH, Robertson CN, et al: Fournier gangrene: Diagnosis with scrotal US. Radiology 169:387-389, 1988

12. Gaynor ER, Vitek L, Sticklin L, et al: The hemodynamic effects of treatment with interleukin-2 and lymphokine-activated killer cells. Ann Intern Med 109:953-958, 1988

13. Nora R, Abrams JS, Tait NS, et al: Myocardial toxic effects during recombinant interleukin-2 therapy. JNCI 81:59-63, 1989

14. Osanto S, Cluitmans FH, Franks CR, et al: Myocardial injury after interleukin-2 therapy. Lancet 2:48-49, 1988

15. Schwartzentruber D, Lotze MT, Rosenberg SA: Colonic perforation. An unusual complication of therapy with high dose interleukin-2. Cancer 62:2350-2353, 1988

16. Lee RE, Lotze MT, Skibber JM, et al: Cardiorespiratory effects of immunotherapy with interleukin-2. J Clin Oncol 7:7-20, 1989

17. Bock SN, Lee RE, Fisher B, et al: A prospective randomized trial evaluating prophylactic antibiotics to prevent catheter-related sepsis in patients treated with immunotherapy. J Clin Oncol 8:161-169, 1990

18. Samlowski WE, Ward JH, Craven CM, et al: Severe myocarditis following high dose interleukin-2 administration. Arch Pathol Lab Med 113:838-841, 1989

19. Jablons D, Bolton E, Mertins S, et al: In vivo administration of interleukin-2 to humans alters circulating neutrophil Fc receptor expression and chemotaxis. J Immunol (in press)

20. Wiebke EA, Rosenberg SA, Lotze MT: Acute immunologic effects of interleukin-2 therapy in cancer patients: Decreased delayed type hypersensitivity response and decreased proliferative response to soluble antigens. J Clin Oncol 6:1440-1449, 1988

21. Matory YL, Chang AE, Lipford EH III, et al: Toxicity of recombinant human interleukin-2 in rats following intravenous infusion. J Biol Response Mod 4:377-390, 1985

22. Puri RK, Travis WD, Rosenberg SA: Decrease in Interleukin-2 induced vascular leakage in the lungs of mice by administration of recombinant Interleukin-1 in vivo. Cancer Res 49:969-976, 1989

23. Rosenberg SA: Adoptive immunotherapy: Accomplishments and prospects. Cancer Treat Rep 68:233-255, 1984

Primary Sarcoma of the Heart Causing Mitral Stenosis

Michael J. Domanski, MD, Thomas F. Delaney, MD, David E. Kleiner, Jr., MD, Mary Goswitz, MD, Arthur Agatston, MD, Eben Tucker, MD, Michael Johnson, MD, and William C. Roberts, MD

Cardiac sarcomas are rare and mitral stenosis caused by this neoplasm in the left atrium is even rarer. Such was the case, however, in the patient to be described herein.

A 46-year-old woman (CC no. 22-72-58-1) who died on January 7, 1990, had been well until April 1989, when she had an episode of dizziness and right eye blindness that resolved spontaneously. In June 1989, she had a transient episode of right lower arm numbness and right eye blindness that resolved spontaneously. In September 1989, she developed orthopnea, dyspnea with walking, syncope and easy fatigability. In October 1989, examination by a cardiologist disclosed a loud first heart sound, a grade 1/6 systolic ejection murmur at the left sternal border and apex that radiated into the axilla and a grade 2/6 systolic murmur at the right sternal border that increased with inspiration. Chest radiograph suggested a dilated left atrium and was consistent with congestive heart failure. An echocardiogram disclosed severe mitral stenosis, mild mitral regurgitation, a dilated right atrium and right ventricle, pericardial effusion and a large mass in the region of the posterior mitral leaflet protruding into and obstructing the mitral orifice (Figure 1). Cardiac catheterization revealed the following pressures (in mm Hg): right atrial mean, 20; right ventricular, 105/18; pulmonary artery wedge mean, 35; left ventricular, 125/18; and aortic, 125/80. The pulmonary artery wedge—left ventricular mean diastolic gradient was 20 mm Hg. The left ventricle contracted normally. By angiography, neither mitral nor aortic valve regurgitation was present and the epicardial coronary arteries were normal. Thoracotomy was performed and a "lemon"-sized mass involving the basal portion of the left ventricular wall was found. Computed tomography after operation localized the mass to the region of the posterior mitral leaflet. Electrocardiogram showed changes of right ventricular hypertrophy, incomplete right bundle branch block and left atrial abnormality. Echocardiogram showed a large mass in the region of the mitral valve and it extended into the left atrium and left ventricle. By Doppler, the estimated mean mitral pressure gradient was 18 mm Hg. Magnetic resonance imaging (Figure 2) confirmed these findings. The patient received radiation therapy, but died suddenly.

At necropsy (A90-2), the heart with the neoplasm weighed 530 g. The visceral and parietal pericardia

---

From the Cardiology and Pathology Branches, National Heart, Lung, and Blood Institute, the Radiation-Oncology Branch and Laboratory of Pathology, National Cancer Institute, Bethesda, Maryland; the Division of Cardiology, Georgetown University Hospital, Washington, D.C.; the Division of Cardiology, Mount Sinai Medical Center, Miami, Florida; and the National Institutes of Health, Building 10, Room 7B15, Bethesda, Maryland 20892. Manuscript received and accepted May 24, 1990.

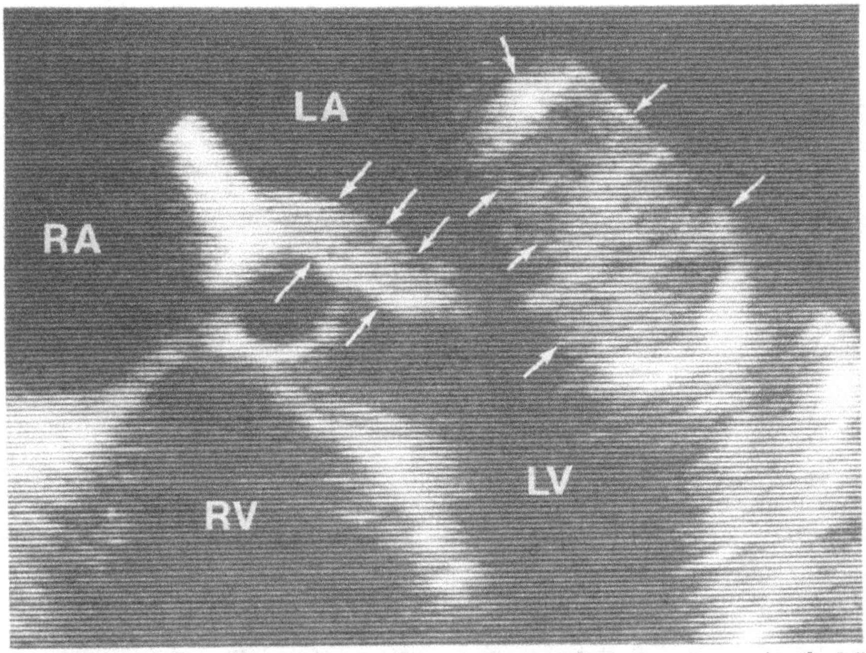

FIGURE 1. Transesophageal echocardiogram showing the tumors *(arrows)* in the left atrial (LA) wall. LV = left ventricle; RA = right atrium; RV = right ventricle.

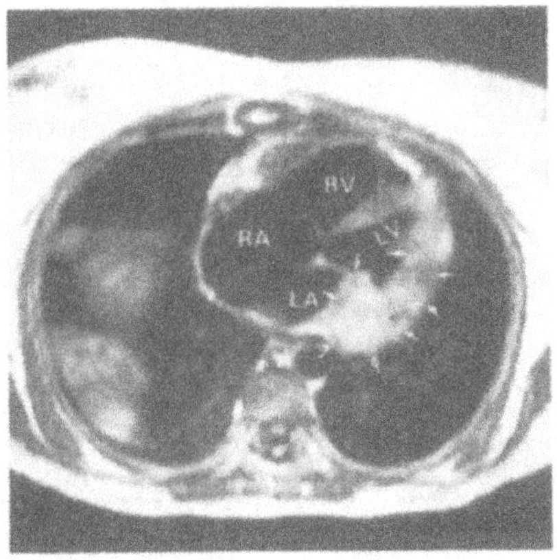

FIGURE 2. Magnetic resonance image of thorax showing the tumor in the walls of left atrium (LA) and left ventricle (LV) and pulmonary infarcts in 1 lung from occlusion of several pulmonary arteries by sarcoma from the right atrium. Abbreviations as in Figure 1.

were adhered to one another by fibrous and neoplastic adhesions. The neoplasm in the wall of the left atrium caused severe obstruction to the mitral orifice (Figure 3) and also to the left pulmonary veins. The neoplasm also invaded the coronary sinus, basal portion of the left ventricular wall and a single tumor deposit was present in the right atrial cavity at the orifice of the coronary sinus. The only body organ containing the neoplasm other than the heart was the lung; a tumor was present in several pulmonary arteries with resulting pulmonary infarcts. Histologically, the neoplasm was a spindle-cell sarcoma. Both pleural spaces (approximately 1,000 ml each) and the peritoneal cavity (1,400 ml) contained dark, amber-colored watery fluid.

The aforementioned patient had sarcoma involving the left atrium and the tumor extended into the mitral orifice producing severe mitral stenosis. We found 7 previously reported cases of left atrial sarcoma causing mitral stenosis and pertinent observations in them are listed in Table I.[1–7] Only 1 of the previously reported cases had the mitral obstruction confirmed by catheterization,

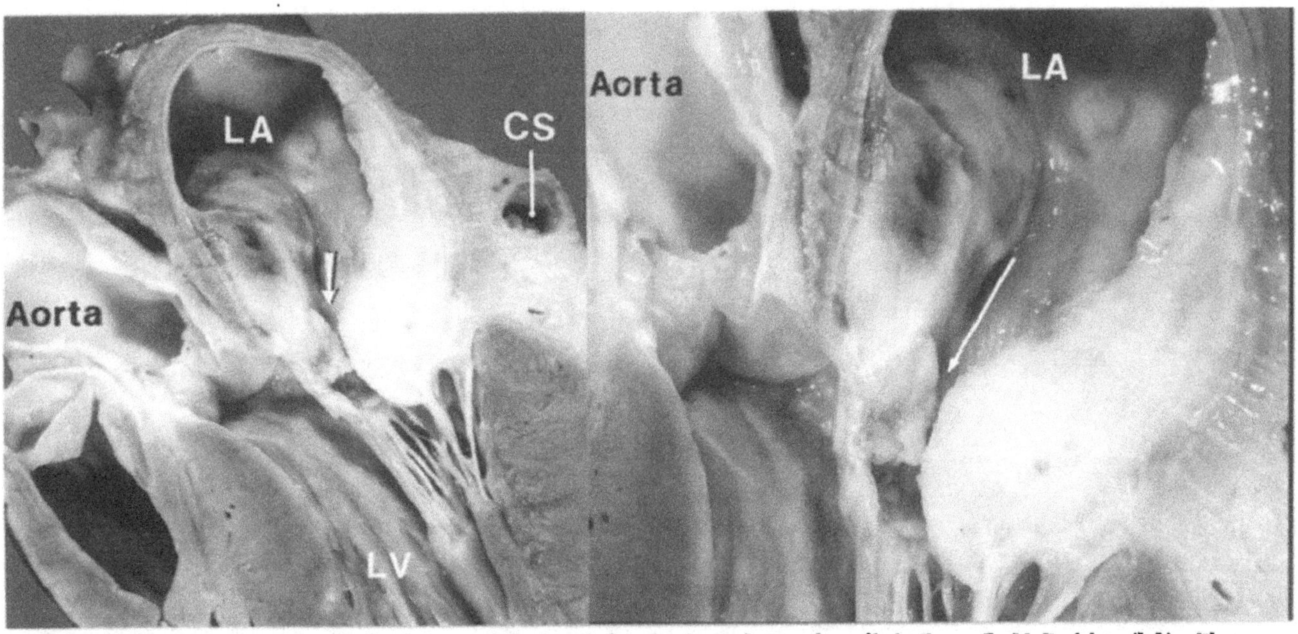

FIGURE 3. Photographs of longitudinal views of the heart showing large tumor deposits in the wall of left atrium (LA) with resulting severe obstruction *(arrows)* to the mitral valve orifice. Tumor also invaded the coronary sinus (CS). Abbreviations as in Figure 1.

TABLE I Observations in Previously Reported Patients with Left Atrial Sarcoma Causing Mitral Stenosis

Case	First Author	Year	Age (yr) & Sex	Duration of Symptoms (months)	DM	OS	P_2	PAW-LV MDG (mm Hg)	Echocardiographic Evidence of MS	Type of Sarcoma
1	Muir	1966	50 F	3	0	—	—	—	—	Chondrosarcoma
2	Dutschmann	1974	39 F	7	+ (4/6)	+	+	—	—	Rhabdomyosarcoma
3	Shuh	1978	37* F		+ (2/6)	+	+	—	—	Fibrous histiocytoma
4	Frendsen	1981	39 F	0.5	+	—	—	—	—	Mesenchymoma
5	Terashima	1983	27 F	5	—	—	—	—	—	Fibrous histiocytoma
6	Ormerod	1984	48 M	"Weeks"	+	—	—	—	+	Angiosarcoma
7	Villasenor	1985	82 F		+ (2/6)	+	—	28	+	Rhabdomyosarcoma

* Only patient still alive at follow-up.
DM = diastolic murmur; LV = left ventricle; MDG = mean diastolic gradient; MS = mitral stenosis; OS = opening snap; PAW = pulmonary arterial wedge; P_2 = pulmonary component of second heart sound; ↑ = increased; + = present; 0 = negative; — = no informatiion.

but all had clear anatomic evidence of mitral obstruction by the neoplasm. Another unusual feature of this sarcoma was invasion of the coronary sinus by the neoplasm and migration (embolization) of the neoplasm from the lumen of the coronary sinus into the right atrium. Portions of the right atrial tumor migrated into several peripheral pulmonary arteries (another embolism), causing neoplastic pulmonary infarcts.

1. Muir CS, Seah CS. Primary chondrosarcomatous mesenchymoma of the mitral valve. *Thorax 1966; 21:254–262.*
2. Dutschmann L, Duarte S, Da Costa JN. Rhabdomyosarcoma of the heart (a case of unusual localization). *Angiology 1974;25:186–196.*
3. Shah AA, Churg A, Sbarbarao JA, Shepard JM, Lamberti J. Malignant fibrous histiocytoma of the heart presenting atrial myxoma. *Cancer 1978;42: 2466–2471.*
4. Frandsen NE, Andersen G, Nielsen JR. Malignant mesenchymoma of the heart presenting as mitral stenosis. *Acta Med Scand 1981;209:235–237.*
5. Terashima T, Aoyama K, Nihei K, Nito T, Imai Y, Takahashi K, Shichibei D. Malignant fibrous histiocytoma of the heart. *Cancer 1983;52:1919–1926.*
6. Omerod OJ, Spratt PM, Lewis NP, Wallwork J. Primary angiosarcoma of the heart mimicking a left atrial myxoma. *Thorax 1984;39:798–799.*
7. Villasenor HR, Fuentes F, Walker WE. Left atrial rhabdomyosarcoma mimicking mitral valve stenosis. *Tex Heart Inst J 1985;12:107–110.*

Myocarditis or Acute Myocardial Infarction Associated With Interleukin-2 Therapy for Cancer

Amy H. Kragel, MD,* William D. Travis, MD,† Ronald G. Steis, MD,‡
Steven A. Rosenberg, MD,§ and William C. Roberts, MD*

The hearts of eight patients aged 22 to 67 years (mean, 41 years) who died during or within 4 days of interleukin-2 (IL-2) based immunotherapy for treatment of renal cell carcinoma or melanoma were studied at necropsy. Death resulted from combined cardiorespiratory failure in two patients, sepsis in four patients, acute myocardial infarction in one patient, and myocarditis in one patient. Transmural left ventricular necrosis was present in one of the two patients with significant atherosclerotic coronary artery narrowing. Noninfectious myocarditis was present in five patients: the inflammatory infiltrate was lymphocytic in four and composed of a mixture of eosinophils and lymphocytes in one. Although treatment-related deaths associated with high-dose IL-2 therapy are uncommon (1.5% in 652 consecutive patients), the potential for significant myocardial ischemia or myocarditis exists, and careful monitoring for arrhythmias or myocardial failure is warranted. *Cancer* 66:1513–1516, 1990.

INTERLEUKIN-2 (IL-2) BASED immunotherapy for the treatment of cancer has been associated with a variety of hemodynamic and cardiac alterations, including hypotension, tachycardia, decreased systemic vascular resistance, decreased ejection fraction, variable changes in pulmonary arterial wedge pressure, and peripheral edema.[1–3] In addition, atrial and ventricular arrhythmias, angina pectoris, myocarditis (noninfectious), and acute myocardial infarction have been reported.[4–8] Some of these abnormalities can be explained by the development of a "capillary leak syndrome" with profound hypotension. We studied the hearts at necropsy of eight patients who died during or within 4 days of cessation of IL-2-based immunotherapy to identify anatomic cardiac abnormalities associated with IL-2 administration.

From the *Pathology Branch, National Heart, Lung, and Blood Institute, and the †Laboratory of Pathology, ‡Clinical Research Branch, Biological Response Modifiers Program, and §Surgery Branch, National Cancer Institute, National Institutes of Health, Bethesda, Maryland.

The authors thank all of the many people involved in the care of the patients included in this study, including Dr. Mario Sznol, Clinical Research Branch, National Cancer Institute, Frederick Memorial Hospital, and the physicians and nurses of the Clinical Center, National Institutes of Health, Bethesda, Maryland.

Address for reprints: Amy H. Kragel, MD, Pathology Branch, National Heart, Lung, and Blood Institute, Building 10, Room 2N258, Bethesda, MD 20892.

Accepted for publication February 22, 1990.

Patients and Methods

The autopsy records of the Pathology Laboratory, National Cancer Institute, were searched for patients in whom IL-2-based immunotherapy had been administered and in whom death had occurred within 5 days of the cessation of therapy. Nine such patients were identified; in one patient, however, neither the heart nor histologic sections were available for review. The remaining eight cases are the subject of this report. In each case, the clinical records, necropsy report, heart specimen, and multiple hematoxylin and eosin stained sections of right and left ventricular myocardium were examined.

Results

The clinical and morphologic features of the five men and three women are summarized in Table 1. Certain features of patients 1, 2, 6, and 8 were reported previously.[8] Therapy was administered for the treatment of melanoma in six patients and for renal cell carcinoma in two. In

TABLE 1. Clinical and Cardiac Necropsy Findings in 8 Patients Receiving Interleukin-2-Based Immunotherapy

Case no.	Age (yr)	Sex	Immunotherapy regimen	Interval treatment to death (days)	Mode of death	Evidence of toxicity while on therapy: Hypotension*	Ischemia†	Arrhythmias: Atrial‡	Arrhythmias: Ventricular§	HW (g)	Dilated cavity: RV	Dilated cavity: LV	CA narrowing (% CSA)	Myocarditis
1	22	F	IL2/LAK	0	CR Failure	4+	3+	4+	4+	295	+	0	0–25	+
2	24	M	IL2/LAK	4	Sepsis	4+	0	0	4+	355	+	0	0–25	+
3	30	M	IL2/TILs/C	4	Sepsis	–	–	–	–	440	+	0	0–25	+
4	34	M	IL2/TILs/C	4	Sepsis	–	–	–	–	430	0	0	0–25	0
5	50	F	IL2/LAK	1	CR Failure	0	0	0	0	330	+	0	0–25	+
6	51	M	IL2	4	Sepsis	2+	0	2+	1+	365	0	0	0–25	+
7	53	F	IL2	1	Sudden Death	1+	0	–	–	415	0	0	76–95	+
8	67	M	IL2	1	AMI	4+	4+	4+	4+	520	0	0	76–95	0

(0): negative; (–): information not available; AMI: acute myocardial infarction; C: cyclophosphamide; CA: coronary artery; CR: cardiorespiratory; CSA: cross-sectional area narrowing; HW: heart weight; IL2: interleukin 2; LAK: lymphokine-activated killer cells; LV: left ventricle, RV: right ventricle; TIL: tumor infiltrating lymphocytes.

* Hypotension: 1+ = hypotension not requiring therapy, 2+ = hypotension responding to fluid therapy, 3+ = hypotension requiring and responsive to pressors, 4+ = hypotension unresponsive to pressors.

† Ischemia: 2+ = nonspecific electrocardiographic changes, elevated CK, 3+ = angina, ischemic changes on electrocardiogram, elevated MB band, 4+ = AMI.

‡ Atrial arrhythmias: 1+ = sinus tachycardia > 110 beats/min, 2+ = premature atrial complexes, 3+ = atrial fibrillation or sinus tacchycardia > 150 beats/min, 4+ = atrial arrhythmia with hypotension.

§ Ventricular arrhythmias: 1+ = unifocal ventricular premature complexes, 2+ = multifocal ventricular premature complexes, bigeminy, trigeminy, 3+ = nonsustained ventricular tachycardia (VT), 4+ = sustained VT.

addition to IL-2, the immunotherapy regimens of three of the patients included lymphokine-activated killer (LAK) cells and two included tumor-infiltrating lymphocytes and cyclophosphamide.

The immediate cause of death varied. Severe combined cardiorespiratory failure immediately following an infusion of LAK cells occurred in two patients. Patient 1 (Table 1) had extensive plugging of pulmonary capillaries and widening of alveolar septae by lymphoid cells with early focal diffuse alveolar damage, and patient 5 (Table 1) had extensive intra-alveolar hemorrhage and early diffuse alveolar damage. Both patients also had a noninfectious myocarditis at necropsy. Patient 7 (Fig. 1) was found dead in bed following LAK therapy; the extent of metastatic disease was not considered sufficient to account for her death, but the left anterior descending coronary artery was narrowed greater than 75% in cross-sectional area by atherosclerotic plaque and a lymphocytic myocarditis also was present. Patient 8 had an acute myocardial infarction while on therapy. The remaining four patients died of consequences of bacterial sepsis, including one with severe renal failure (patient 4).

The heart weight was increased (> 350 g in women and > 400 g in men) in four patients. Two patients with cardiomegaly had coronary artery disease with more than 75% cross-sectional area narrowing by plaque of at least one of the four major epicardial coronary arteries. In one of these two (patient 8, Table 1), gross and microscopic examination of the heart showed transmural myocardial necrosis histologically compatible with a 24-hour-old infarct. Of the remaining seven patients, six had evidence of a diffuse, patchy myocarditis (Fig. 1). In four patients (1, 3, 6, and 7 [Table 1]), the inflammatory infiltrate was predominately lymphocytic; in one (patient 5), the infiltrate was composed of a mixture of eosinophils and lymphocytes; and in one (patient 2), it was composed of a mixture of polymorphonuclear leukocytes, lymphocytes, and eosinophils with microabscess formation. Only in this last patient was the etiology of the myocarditis believed to be infectious: colonies of organisms were identified within the abscesses. In all six of these patients, there was myofiber degeneration and scattered foci of myocyte necrosis. In the two patients dying with severe cardiorespiratory failure and in the one case of sudden death due to myocarditis, the myocarditis was of greater severity than in the other two cases of noninfectious myocarditis.

In no patient was there grossly visible right or left ventricular fibrosis. Microscopic examination of hematoxylin and eosin stained sections disclosed mild interstitial fibrosis in three cases (patients 2, 4, and 6). Foci of contraction-band necrosis were noted in several cases, including one (patient 2) in whom the final resuscitative measures were prolonged and had included open cardiac massage.

Discussion

While death associated with high-dose IL-2 therapy is rare (1.5% in 652 consecutive patients treated with high-dose IL-2-based immunotherapy),[6] we found cardiac morphologic abnormalities in seven of our eight patients who died within 4 days of therapy. These abnormalities

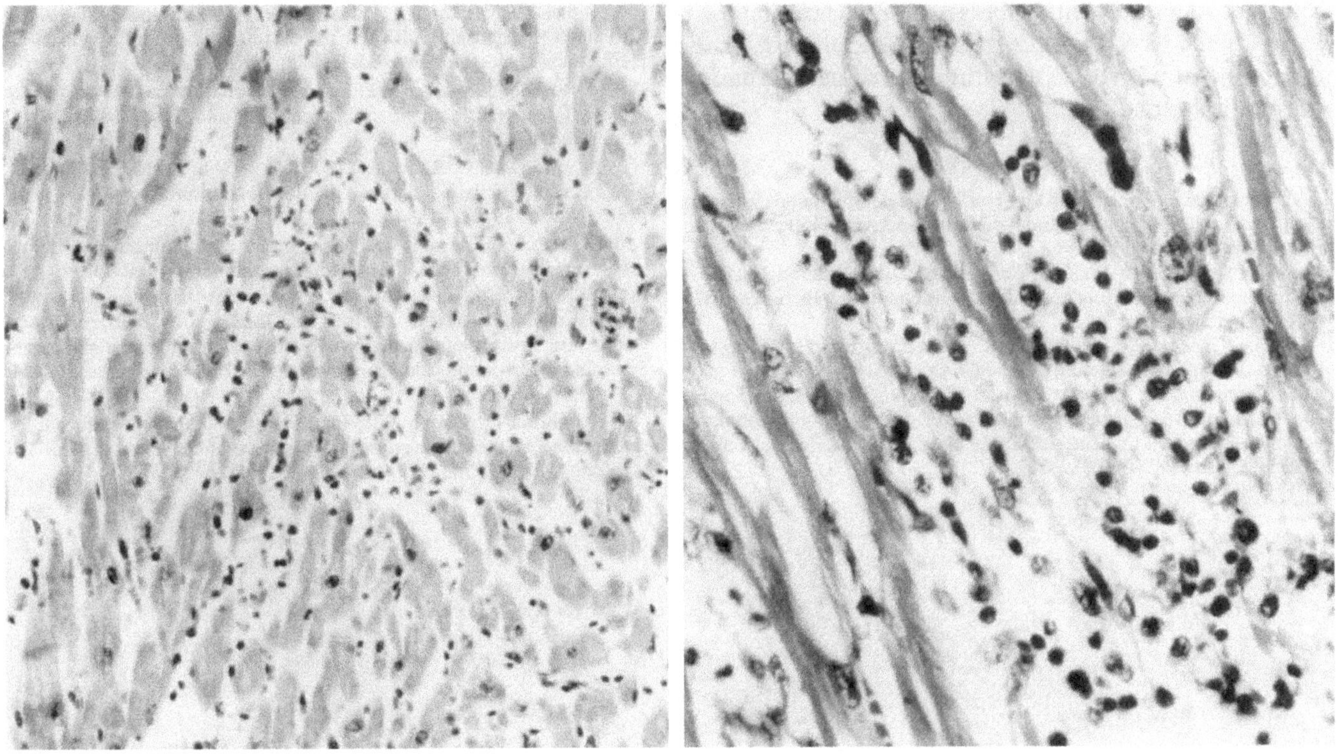

FIG. 1. Hematoxylin and eosin stained sections of left ventricular myocardium showing an interstitial lymphocytic infiltrate with degeneration and necrosis of myocytes. These sections were taken from patient 7, a 53-year-old woman who was found dead in bed, unexpectedly, 1 day after receiving her last dose of IL-2 (left, ×250; right, ×500).

included acute myocardial infarction associated with severe atherosclerotic coronary artery disease in one patient, noninfectious myocarditis in five patients, and bacterial myocarditis in one patient.

Clinical evidence of angina pectoris and acute myocardial infarction has been reported previously in patients receiving IL-2-based immunotherapy for cancer.[2,4–6] In addition to the patient described in this report in whom acute myocardial infarction was associated with severe atherosclerotic coronary artery disease and whose death occurred within 4 days of cessation of IL-2-based therapy, we have seen two additional cases at necropsy in which acute myocardial infarction occurred during therapy in the absence of atherosclerotic coronary artery disease but in whom death did not occur until later. The first patient[8] was a 53-year-old man who died 71 days after cessation of therapy, and necropsy disclosed cardiomegaly, biventricular dilatation, and a large transmural left ventricular circumferential infarct extending from apex to base. The second patient was a 20-year-old woman who died 21 days after therapy was stopped, and necropsy disclosed transmural left ventricular necrosis. In both of these cases, the epicardial coronary arteries were virtually devoid of atherosclerotic plaque. Thus, it appears that the profound hypotension associated with IL-2 therapy can precipitate ischemic myocardial injury even in the absence of underlying atherosclerotic coronary artery disease.

Noninfectious myocarditis associated with IL-2-based immunotherapy has been described previously.[7,8] It is likely that myocarditis is responsible, at least in part, for the arrhythmias and decreased ejection fractions in patients receiving this therapy. The exact role that IL-2 plays in the development of myocarditis, however, is unknown.

The presence of a direct effect of IL-2 on myocardial function has not been identified in humans. Changes in myocyte contractility in response to IL-2, however, have been observed in rat myocyte cell cultures.[9] In addition, interleukin-1 and tumor necrosis factor, whose production may be stimulated by IL-2-based immunotherapy, decrease myocardial contractility in cell culture in response to β-adrenergic stimulation.[10]

We have not observed noninfectious myocarditis in other patients who died at intervals longer than 7 days after the cessation of therapy.[8] This observation suggests that it is either a transient phenomenon or that it occurs in patients who may have an increased susceptibility to IL-2 toxicity and subsequently die shortly after therapy. Because of the high frequency of myocarditis observed in our study and the potential for ischemic myocardial damage, patients receiving IL-2 should be monitored for the development of cardiac arrhythmias and cardiac failure during IL-2-based therapy.

REFERENCES

1. Gaynor ER, Vitek L, Sticklin L *et al.* The hemodynamic effects of treatment with interleukin-2 and lymphokine-activated killer cells. *Ann Intern Med* 1988; 109:953–958.
2. Nora R, Abrams JS, Tait NS, Hiponia DJ, Silverman HJ. Myocardial toxic effects during recombinant interleukin-2 therapy. *J Natl Cancer Inst* 1989; 81:59–63.
3. Lee RE, Lotze MT, Skibber JM *et al.* Cardiorespiratory effects of immunotherapy with interleukin-2. *J Clin Oncol* 1989; 7:7–20.
4. Rosenberg SA, Lotze MT, Muul LM *et al.* A progress report on the treatment of 157 patients with advanced cancer using lymphokine-activated killer cells and interleukin-2 or high dose interleukin-2 alone. *N Engl J Med* 1987; 316:889–897.
5. Fisher RI, Coltman CA, Doroshow JH *et al.* Metastatic renal cancer treated with interleukin-2 and lymphokine-activated killer cells. A phase II clinical trial. *Ann Intern Med* 1988; 108:518–523.
6. Rosenberg SA, Lotze MT, Yang JC *et al.* Experience with the use of high dose interleukin-2 in the treatment of 652 patients with cancer. *Ann Surg* 1989;210:474–485.
7. Samlowski WE, Ward JH, Craven CM, Freedman RA. Severe myocarditis following high dose interleukin-2 administration. *Arch Pathol Lab Med* 1989; 113:838–841.
8. Kragel AH, Travis WD, Feinberg L *et al.* Pathologic findings associated with interleukin-2 based immunotherapy for cancer: A postmortem study of 19 patients. *Hum Pathol* 1990;21:493–502.
9. Fink S, Finiasz M, Sterin-Borda L, Borda E, de Bracco MM. Interleukin 2 stimulates heart contractility in the presence of exogenous arachidonate or the calcium ionophore A 23187. *Immunol Lett* 1988; 17:183–188.
10. Gulick T, Chung MK, Pieper SJ, Lange LG, Schreiner GF. Interleukin 1 and tumor necrosis factor inhibit cardiac myocyte β-adrenergic responsiveness. *Proc Natl Acad Sci* 1989; 86:6753–6757.

Clinically undetected cardiac lymphoma causing fatal congestive heart failure

Charles Stewart Roberts, MD, John S. Gottdiener, MD, and William C. Roberts, MD. *Bethesda, Md.*

Of all metastatic cancers, about 10% involve the heart. In absolute numbers, the most common sources of cardiac metastases are lung and breast cancers. In relative numbers, however, cardiac involvement is most frequent in melanoma (64%),[1] leukemia (37%),[2] and lymphoma (24%).[3] Furthermore, of the few patients with cardiac lymphoma having cardiac dysfunction, the cardiac manifestations are rarely the dominant feature of the patient's illness.[3-13] Such was the case, however, in the patient described herein.

R.A. (CC No. 11-95-95-5), a 64-year-old woman, had been well until 7 months before death, when she developed fever rising to 40.4° C and nausea, which necessitated her hospitalization in 2 weeks. Except for fever, which disappeared several days later, the physical examination yielded no abnormal findings. The blood hematocrit was 29%; the white blood cell count was 2500/mm^3; the platelet count was 78,000/mm^3; the erythrocyte sedimentation rate in 1

From the Surgery, Cardiology, and Pathology Branches, National Heart, Lung, and Blood Institute, National Institutes of Health.

Reprint requests: William C. Roberts, MD, Building 10, Room 2N258, NIH, Bethesda, MD 20892.

4/4/23593

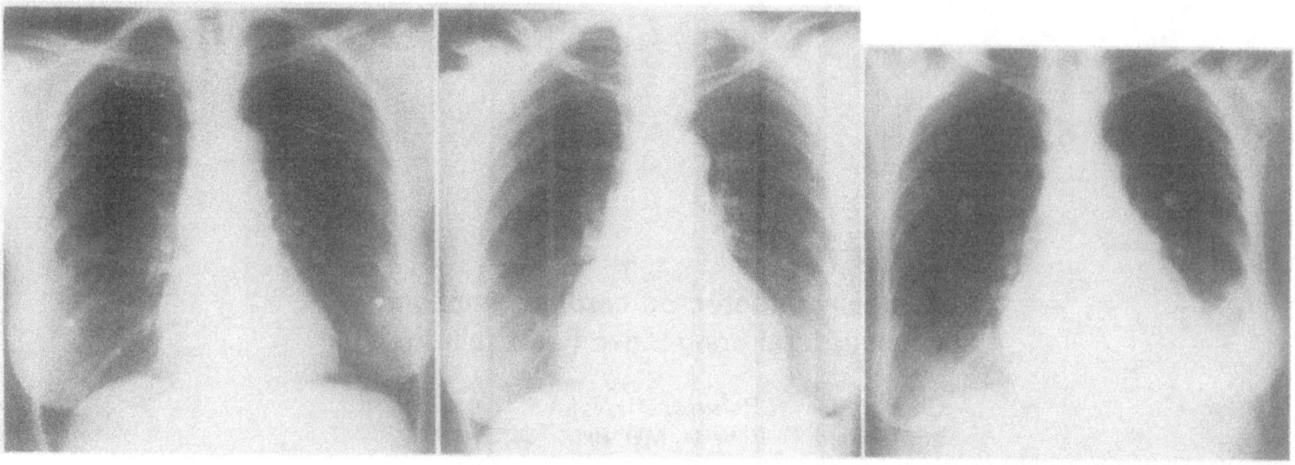

Fig. 1. Posterior-anterior chest radiographs. **Left panel,** Seven months before death, showing no abnormalities. **Middle panel,** Four months before death, showing a large cardiac silhouette. **Right panel,** One month before death, after anterior pericardiectomy, showing new bilateral lower lobe infiltrates and pleural effusions.

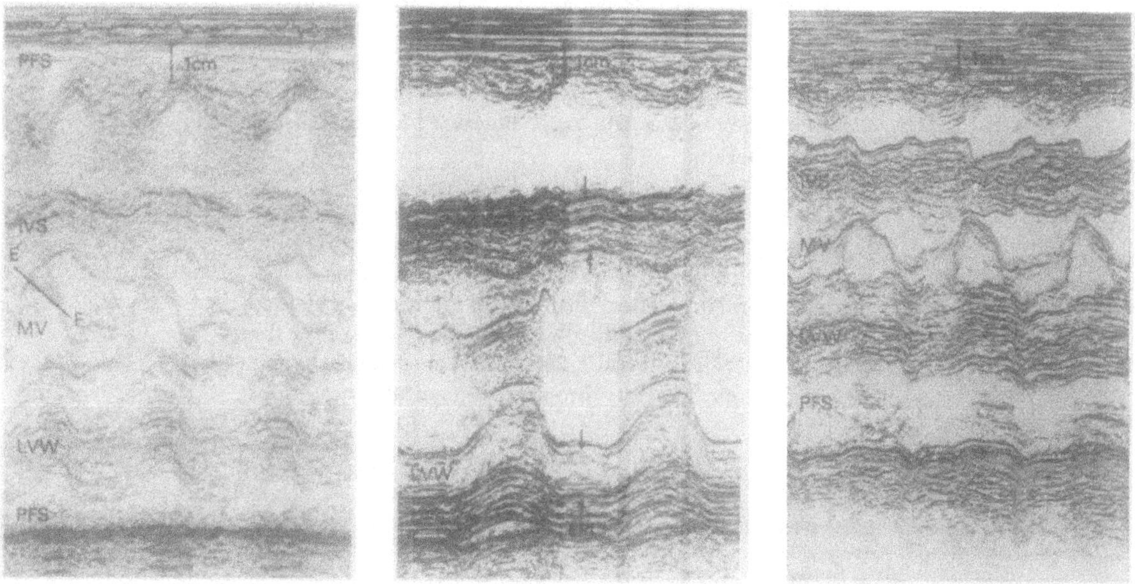

Fig. 2. Echocardiograms, longitudinal axis views. **Left panel,** Four months before death, showing decreased slope *(EF)* of early diastolic mitral valve closure (48 mm/sec; normal $\geq$60 mm/sec), anterior and posterior echo-free space suggestive of moderate-sized pericardial effusion, and preserved systolic left ventricular wall motion. **Middle panel,** Two months before death, after anterior pericardiectomy, showing dense posterior pericardial echoes that have replaced the previously echo-free space and persistent left ventricular wall thickening (interventricular system 1.3 cm, posterior left ventricular wall 1.3 cm; normal 0.6 to 1.1 cm) with intact systolic left ventricular wall motion. **Right panel,** Three weeks before death, showing recurrent posterior pericardial effusion accompanied by a decrease in the left ventricular cavity dimension in diastole in comparison with previous studies. *DPE,* Dense pericardial echoes; *EPI,* epicardium; *IVS,* interventricular septum; *LVW,* posterior left ventricular wall; *MV,* mitral valve; *PFS,* pericardial free space.

hour was 36 mm, and total serum protein was 5.7 gm/dl, with albumin 2.9 gm/dl. The purified protein derivative of tuberculin skin test and hepatitis surface antigen tests were positive; but febrile agglutinins, blood cultures, antinuclear antibody (ANA) and lupus erythematosus (LE) preparations, and sputa cultures for acid-fast organisms were negative. The bone marrow was hypocellular. The chest roentgenogram (Fig. 1) and electrocardiogram were normal. Upper and lower gastrointestinal radiographs were normal. The splenic scan showed mild splenomegaly, and the hepatic scan suggested dilated bile ducts. The cause of the patient's problems was not determined during the 4-week

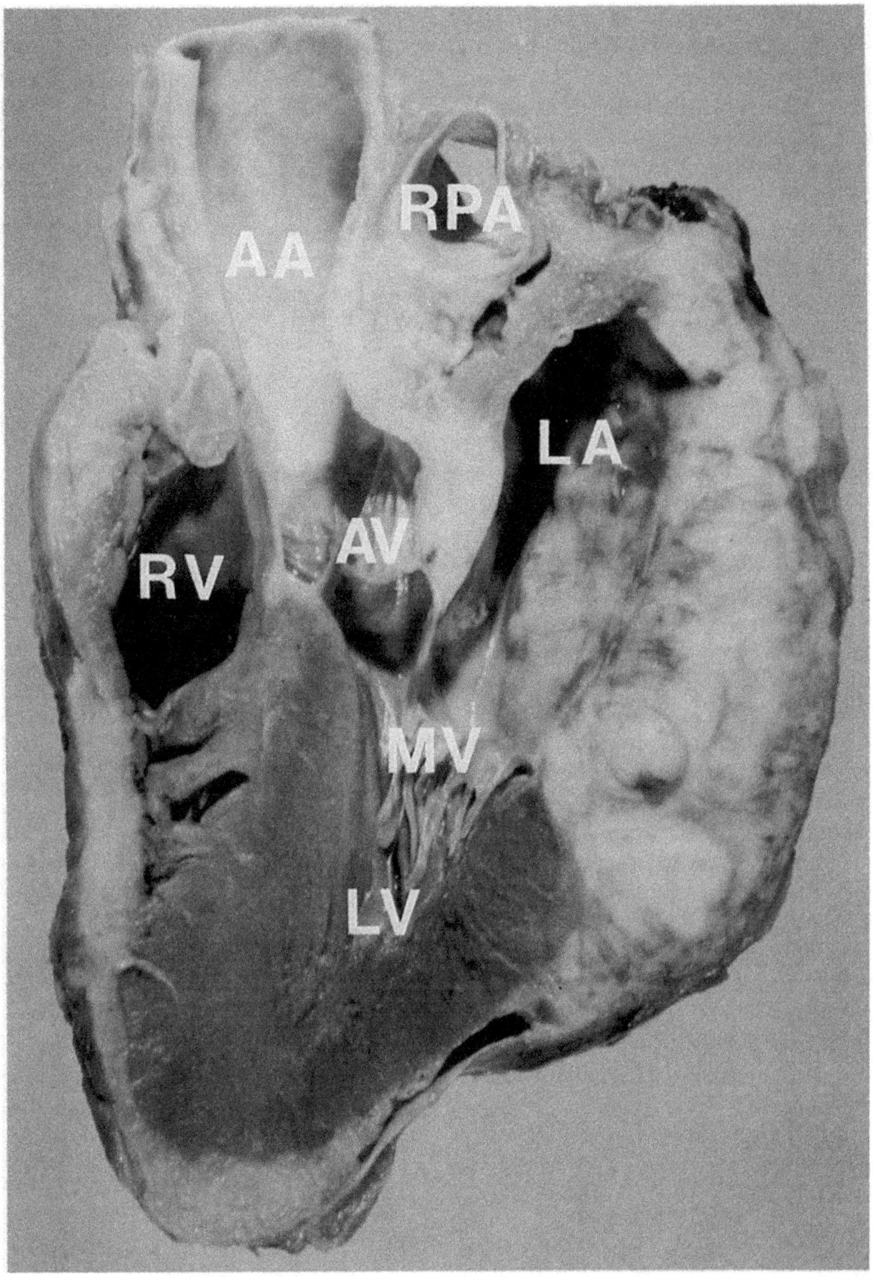

Fig. 3. Photograph of a longitudinal section of the left side of the heart showing tumor in atrial septum and the left atrial and left ventricular free walls posteriorly. *AA*, ascending aorta; *AV*, aortic valve; *LA*, left atrium; *LV*, left ventricle; *MV*, mitral valve; *RPA*, main right pulmonary artery; *RV*, right ventricle.

hospitalization. Six weeks later (4 months before death), examination disclosed a two-component pericardial friction rub and S_4 and S_3 gallop sounds. The physical examination was otherwise normal. The blood hemotocrit was now 40%; white cell count was 4,900/mm^3; platelet count was 160,000/mm^3; erythrocyte sedementation rate was 42 mm in 1 hour; serum glutamic oxaloacetic transaminase was 107, and puruvic transaminase was 101 U/L (normal < 45); total serum proteins were 5.7 gm/dl, albumin was 3.0 gm/100 dl, and cryoprotein and C1q circulating immune complexes were positive. The fever and pericardial rub persisted and the cardiac silhouette increased in size. Echocardiography showed no anterior free space, which was previously present, and dense echoes were posterior to the left ventricular wall. Left ventricular systolic wall motion was normal (Fig. 2). The electrocardiogram now showed low voltage.

Because of enlargement of the cardiac silhouette, anterior pericardectomy was performed 8 weeks before death. The parietal pericardium was thin and the sac contained

830 ml of serous fluid. The posterior walls of both the left atrium and left ventricle were thickened. Histologic examination of the parietal pericardium showed perivascular lymphocytic "cuffing." The pericardial fluid contained no tumor cells, and cultures were negative. Postoperatively, the PR interval was prolonged and complete heart block later developed. Two weeks postoperatively, overt evidence of congestive heart failure was apparent, and 3 weeks postoperatively, abdominal pain and ileus developed. Samples of feces tested positively for occult blood, and the blood hematocrit decreased to 23%. Hemoptysis later developed and a chest roentgenograph disclosed a right lower lobe infiltrate. The echocardiogram now showed reappearance of the posterior free space and marked diminution of the left ventricular cavity size. Pulmonary and abdominal angiograms were normal, and brochoscopy showed inflamed, hemorrhagic bronchi. The congestive heart failure worsened, and at 7 weeks postoperatively catheterization disclosed a pulmonary arterial pressure of 36/18 mm Hg and a pulmonary artery wedge mean pressure of 32 mm Hg. The cardiac index was 2.2 L/min/m^2 and the stroke volume index was 20 ml/m^2. A grade 3/6 systolic blowing apical murmur now was audible. The cardiac silhouette continued to enlarge. Bilateral lower lobe pulmonary infiltrates, pleural effusions and hepatomegaly appeared. About 2 weeks before death, ventricular arrhythmias appeared and the patient died of progressive congestive failure.

At necropsy, the heart, including tumor, weighed 640 gm. Extensive adhesions were evident between visceral and parietal pericardia. Polypoid tumor extended from the inferior vena cava into the right atrial cavity and from there into the right ventricular cavity. The atrial septum and most of the left atrial free wall were infiltrated by tumor, which attached to the posterior wall of both left atrium and left ventricle (Fig. 3). Histologically, the tumor was typical of *histiocytic lymphoma*. Some hilar lymph nodes and both adrenal glands were replaced by the neoplasm. The liver weighed 1340 gm and had diffuse macronodular cirrhosis. The spleen weighed 360 gm. Microscopically, tumor was present in the heart, lungs, liver, spleen, kidneys, adrenal glands, hilar lymph nodes, bone marrow, bowel, and meninges.

The above-described patient spent nearly 5 of the last 7 months of her life in the hospital. Despite numerous and various types of tests performed and anterior pericardiectomy 2 months before death, a definitive diagnosis was never made. The sequence of signs during her illness was fever followed by pericardial rub, then congestive heart failure, and finally conduction disturbances and arrhythmias. Cardiac involvement at initial presentation of malignant lymphoma is rare.[5-13] Primary cardiac lymphoma initially diagnosed by routine cytology of pericardial fluid was recently reported by Castelli et al,[11] who found only two previously published reports of antemortem cytologic diagnosis of primary cardiac lymphoma. The diagnostic difficulties of cardiac involvement by lymphoma were emphasized recently by Coghlan et al.,[12] in whose patient echocardiograms at three different institutions and cytology on two occasions failed to provide the correct diagnosis. Echocardiography generally, however, is the best method for diagnosing cardiac tumors.[7] What is particularly remarkable about our patient is that pericardial fluid cytology, echocardiography, and anterior pericardiectomy failed to reveal the diagnosis apparently because the tumor lay hidden in the posterior wall of the heart.

REFERENCES

1. Glancy DL, Roberts WC. The heart in malignant melanoma. A study of 70 autopsy cases. Am J Cardiol 1968;21:5555-71.
2. Roberts WC, Bodey GP, Westlake PT. The heart in acute leukemia: a study of 420 autopsy cases. Am J Cardiol 1968;21:388-412.
3. Roberts WC, Glancy KL, DeVita VT. Heart in malignant lymphoma (Hodgkin's disease, lymphosarcoma, reticulum cell sarcoma, and mycosis fungoides). A study of 196 autopsy cases. Am J Cardiol 1968;22:85-107.
4. McDonald PJ, Mann RB, Bulkley BH. Involvement of the heart by malignant lymphoma. A clinicopathologic study. Cancer 1982;49:944-51.
5. Chou ST, Arkles LD, Gill DG, Pinkus N, Parkin A, Hicks JD. Primary lymphoma of the heart. A case report. Cancer 1983;52:744-7.
6. Gelman KM, Ben-Ezra JM, Steinschneider M, Dutcher JP, Keefe DL, Factor SM. Lymphoma with primary cardiac manifestations. AM HEART J 1986;111:808-11.
7. Armstrong WF, Buck JD, Hoffman R, Waller BF. Cardiac involvement by lymphoma: detection and follow-up by two-dimensional echocardiography AM HEART J 1986;112:627-36.
8. Gill PS, Chandraratna PA, Meyer PR, Levine AM. Malignant lymphoma: cardiac involvement at initial presentation. J Clin Oncol 1987;5:216-24.
9. Cairns P, Butany J, Fulop J, Radowski H, Hassaram S. Cardiac presentation of non-Hodgkin's lymphoma. Arch Pathol Lab Med 1987;111:80-3.
10. Kuo T, Yang CP, Lin CH, Chang CH. Lymphoblastic lymphoma presenting as a huge intracavitary cardiac tumor causing heart failure. Pediatr Pathol 1987;7:341-9.
11. Castelli MJ, Mihalov ML, Posniak HV, Gattuso P. Primary cardiac lymphoma initially diagnosed by routine cytology. Case report and literature review. Acta Cytol 1989;33:355-8.
12. Coghlan JG, Paul VE, Mitchell AG. Cardiac involvement by lymphoma: diagnostic difficulties. Eur Heart J 1989;10:765-8.
13. Iwase M, Nagura E, Miyahara T, Goto J, Kajita M, Yamanda H. Malignant lymphoma compressing the heart and causing acute left-sided heart failure. AM HEART J 1990;119:968-70.

II Neoplasms of the Heart

WILLIAM C. ROBERTS

Like any organ or tissue, neoplasms involving the heart may be *primary* or *secondary*. The most common primary neoplasm is *myxoma*, which as a neoplasm is benign but which as a tumor may be fatal because it can obstruct the orifice of an atrioventricular valve or the outflow tract of either cardiac ventricle. Most myxomas are attached to the atrial septum, most commonly by a stalk that is smaller than the largest diameter of the tumor. The small attachment site allows the tumor to descend toward the ventricle during atrial emptying, and, if the tumor is large enough, it can descend into the atrioventricular valve orifice, partially obstructing it. Most myxomas attach to the left atrial aspect of the atrial septum, and therefore lie in the left atrial cavity. Attachment to the right side of the atrial septum occurs only 25% as frequently as the left atrial location. The tumor can grow to a much larger size in the low-pressure right atrium before producing symptoms than it can in the left atrium, however. Both the right atrial cavity and the trucuspid valve orifice appear to expand to a much larger size than either the left atrium or mitral orifice before symptoms of cardiac dysfunction appear. About 5% of cardiac myxomas are located in a ventricular cavity, and then usually in the right ventricle. With ventricular systole the tumor may protrude through the pulmonic valve orifice to produce outflow obstruction and possibly pulmonary emboli.

The second most common primary cardiac neoplasm is *sarcoma*. They may be of many varieties, including fibrosarcoma, liposarcoma, rhabdomyosarcoma, and hemangiosarcoma. They can involve any portion of the heart and most are rapidly fatal.

Secondary Neoplasms

The most common neoplasm seen in the heart represents a metastases from a primary site in another body organ or tissue. The frequency of secondary neoplasms in the heart is dependent on whether one is trying to determine the frequency of cardiac metastases among all patients with malignancies, or the frequency of cardiac metastases among patients with a specific type of malignancy. As shown in Figure 66-1, of 1000 patients with noncardiac primary malignancies of all types observed consecutively, about 100 (10%) were found at autopsy to have metastases to the heart. Of the 100 with cardiac metastases, only 10 (10%) will have signs or symptoms of cardiac dysfunction; 9 will be the consequence of pericardial involvement, and only 1 will be the consequence of intracavitary or intramyocardial involvement. Of all patients with secondary cardiac tumors, the most common site of the primary carcinoma will be the *breast* in women and the *lung* in men, because these two tumors are the most common in each sex. The neoplasms with the highest frequency of metastases to the heart will be as follows: melanoma, 70%; leukemia, 37%; lymphoma, 24%; carcinoma of the lung, 8%; and carcinoma of the breast, 8%.

Location of Neoplasms

As shown in Figure 66-1, the *visceral pericardium* (epicardium) is by far the most frequent location of neoplasms

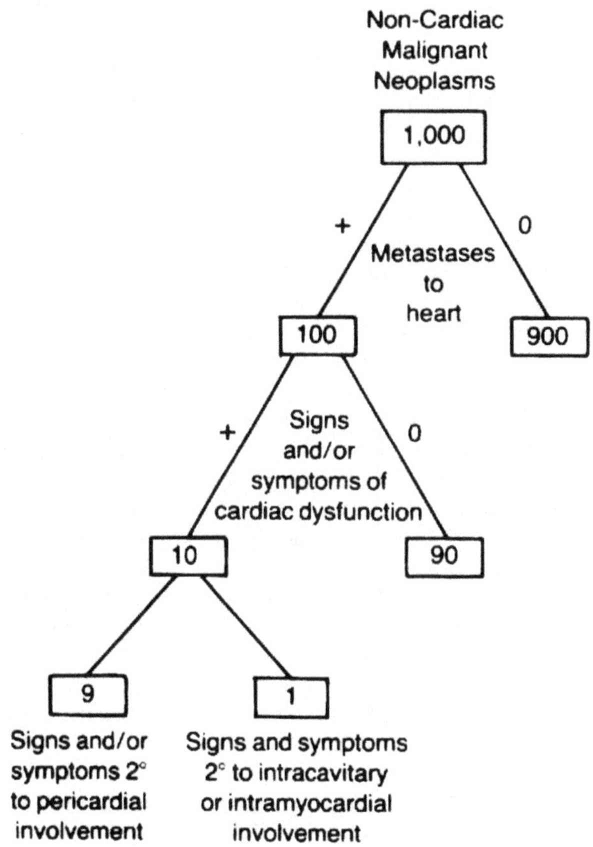

FIGURE 66-1. Location of primary or secondary neoplasms in the heart.

involving the heart. The epicardial deposits may be either focal or diffuse, they may or may not be associated with pericardial effusion, and they may or may not lead to myocardial constriction, to tamponade, or to both. The *endocardium* is the next most frequent location of cardiac neoplasms. The neoplasm in this location may be essentially flat on the mural endocardium, or the neoplasm may protrude into the cavity. Most intracardiac tumors do not produce inflow or outflow obstruction but, if they are strategically located or are large enough, obstruction may result. The *myocardial wall* (intramural) is the least common site of tumor deposition. In this location the tumor usually does not produce evidence of cardiac dysfunction. On occasion, however, an intramyocardial tumor deposit can produce an arrhythmia (either atrial or ventricular) or a conduction disturbance (varying degree of atrioventricular block or bundle branch block).

Cardiac Consequences of Therapy of Malignant Neoplasms

A common consequence of radiation therapy to tumorous involvement of mediastinal lymph nodes (usually by Hodgkin's disease) is the development of *radiation heart disease*. This condition usually occurs only when the heart has received as much as 4000 rads from one or more portals. The most common early consequence of significant numbers of rads to the heart is fibrinous pericardial disease with or without pericardial effusion. At this early stage, the fluid accumulation may be large enough to produce cardiac tamponade. The most common late consequence is fibrous obliterative pericardial disease. In this circumstance, the parietal and visceral pericardia are everywhere adherent to one another by fibrous adhesions, and pericardial fluid (the "oil" of the pericardial sac) is no longer present. The coronary arteries are located within the subepicardial adipose tissue. Sufficient rads to the heart may cause proliferation of fibrous tissue within their lumens. With severe luminal narrowing, the result may be sudden death, angina pectoris, or acute myocardial infarction. Another consequence of excessive rads to the heart is damage to valvular and mural endocardium. This damage, manifested simply by fibrous tissue proliferation, rarely leads to cardiac dysfunction. The final type of radiation damage is to the myocardial walls, particularly the right ventricular wall. This damage usually takes the form of an increase in intramyocardial fibrous tissue and rarely produces, in and of itself, signs or symptoms of cardiac dysfunction.

Another type of cardiac damage resulting from therapy of noncardiac malignancies is that resulting from use of excessive doses of anthracycline-type drugs. These medicines, if given in high enough doses, cause damage directly to myocardial cells. If enough myocardial cells are damaged the ventricles dilate, and ventricular systolic function may be depressed accordingly. The consequence is a dilated heart of increased mass that looks grossly identical to the heart of idiopathic dilated cardiomyopathy.

Lipomatous Hypertrophy of the Atrial Septum

A common finding in older persons, particularly those considerably overweight, is the deposition of fat, not only widespread beneath the epicardium, but also in the atrial septum (except in the area of the fossa ovale membrane). The deposits of fat in the atrial septum may cause it to thicken from its normal 5-mm thickness to as much as 50 mm. This thickening, which is entirely the result of fatty infiltration, is only toward the right atrium. Diagnosis may be made by tomography or cross-sectional echocardiography. The only danger of the excessive fatty infiltration into the atrial septum is that it is commonly associated with various atrial arrhythmias, and can be confused with a malignant neoplasm.

Clinical, Electrocardiographic and Morphologic Features of Massive Fatty Deposits ("Lipomatous Hypertrophy") in the Atrial Septum

JAMSHID SHIRANI, MD, WILLIAM C. ROBERTS, MD, FACC*

Bethesda, Maryland

Objectives. This study examined the morphologic features and the clinical significance of massive fatty deposits in the atrial septum of the heart.

Background. Large deposits of adipose tissue in the atrial septum were first described in 1964 and have been referred to as "lipomatous hypertrophy" of the atrial septum. A relation between these fatty deposits and atrial arrhythmias has been suggested.

Methods. The thickness of the atrial septum cephalad to the fossa ovalis ranged from 1.5 to 6 cm in 91 patients and was ≥2 cm in 80 patients. This report focuses primarily on the latter 80 patients.

Results. The thickness of the atrial septum in the 80 patients correlated with body weight and the thickness of the adipose tissue in the atrioventricular groove and that covering the right ventricle. In 53 patients (67%), one or more of the four major epicardial coronary arteries were narrowed >75% in cross-sectional area by atherosclerotic plaque. Atrial arrhythmias were present in 31 patients (40%). Patients with larger deposits of fat (atrial septal thickness ≥3 cm) had a higher frequency of atrial arrhythmias (60% vs. 34%, $p < 0.01$). The atrial septum was significantly thicker in patients with atrial arrhythmia compared with those without atrial arrhythmias (2.9 vs. 2.3 cm, $p < 0.01$). Of the 28 patients with available electrocardiograms, 20 (71%) showed atrial arrhythmias (nine atrial premature complexes, seven atrial fibrillation, three atrial tachycardia, one ectopic atrial rhythm and one junctional rhythm).

Conclusions. Massive fatty deposits in the atrial septum are associated with large deposits of fat elsewhere in the body and other parts of the heart. They are frequently associated with atrial arrhythmias and atherosclerotic coronary artery disease.

(J Am Coll Cardiol 1993;22:226–38)

In the western world there is an expectation among many that people gain weight with age. The increase in weight is primarily due to the deposition of fat in various locations in the body. The heart is not spared from the fatty deposits. Most often the fat in the heart is in the subepicardial adipose tissue, particularly in the areas where the epicardial coronary arteries are located. Another location for fatty deposits in the heart is the atrial septum. When the fatty deposits in the atrial septum are large, such deposits have been called "lipomatous hypertrophy of the atrial septum." Since the initial description of this entity in 1964 (1), several reports (2–20) describing relatively few cases have appeared. Some reports (2–4) have suggested that some cardiac arrhythmias, particularly those of atrial origin, may be a consequence of this fatty deposition in the atrial septum. This report analyzes a large group of patients with massive infiltration of the atrial septum by fat to discern if there were specific clinical or electrocardiographic features that could be attributed to these fatty infiltrates.

From the Pathology Branch, National Heart, Lung, and Blood Institute, National Institutes of Health, Bethesda, Maryland.

Manuscript received September 3, 1992; revised manuscript received November 20, 1992, accepted December 1, 1992.

*Present address: Baylor Cardiovascular Institute, Baylor University Medical Center, 3500 Gaston Avenue, Dallas, Texas 75246.

Address for correspondence: Jamshid Shirani, MD, Department of Medicine, Division of Cardiology, Medical College of Virginia, MCV Station, Box 123, Richmond, Virginia 23298.

Methods

Sources of patients. The files of the Pathology Branch, which include essentially only cases with cardiovascular disease, were searched for cases coded as "lipomatous hypertrophy of the atrial septum" or "atrial septal lipoma." Although the files include cases entered as early as 1953, the first case of lipomatous hypertrophy of the atrial septum was not coded until 1975. Since that time, 91 cases have been so coded and approximately 7,000 cases >15 years of age were accessioned in the Pathology Branch from 1975 to July 1992.

The hearts from all 91 patients were originally examined and coded by one of the authors (W.C.R.) and subsequently 74 of the 91 hearts were examined by the other author (J.S.). The hearts in the 91 cases were submitted by 19 different medical centers, including 26 from Suburban Hospital (Bethesda, Maryland), 14 from the District of Columbia Veterans Affairs Hospital, 11 from the National Naval Medical Center, 9 from Georgetown University Medical Center, 9 from the District of Columbia Medical Examiners' Office, 5 from the Washington Hospital Center, 3 from Franklin Square Hospital (Baltimore, Maryland), 2 from the Clinical Center of the National Institutes of Health, 2 from Sibley Hospital (Washington, D.C.) and 1 each from each of 10 other medical centers. The medical records from each of the 91 cases were reviewed and the actual electrocardiograms were obtained in 29 cases.

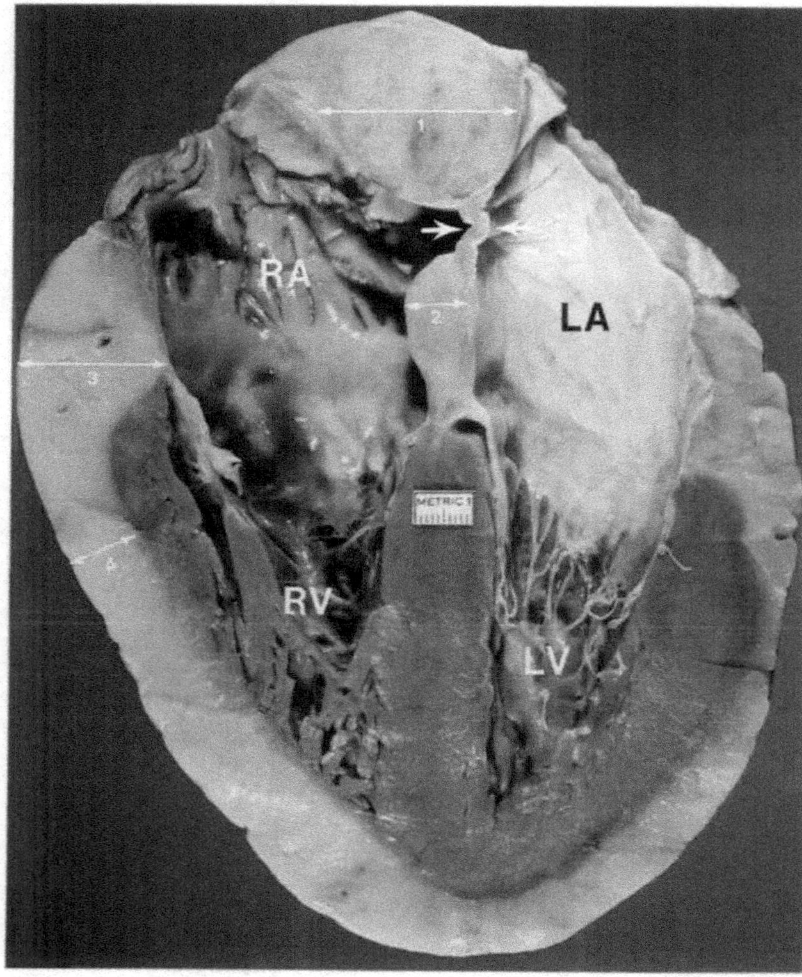

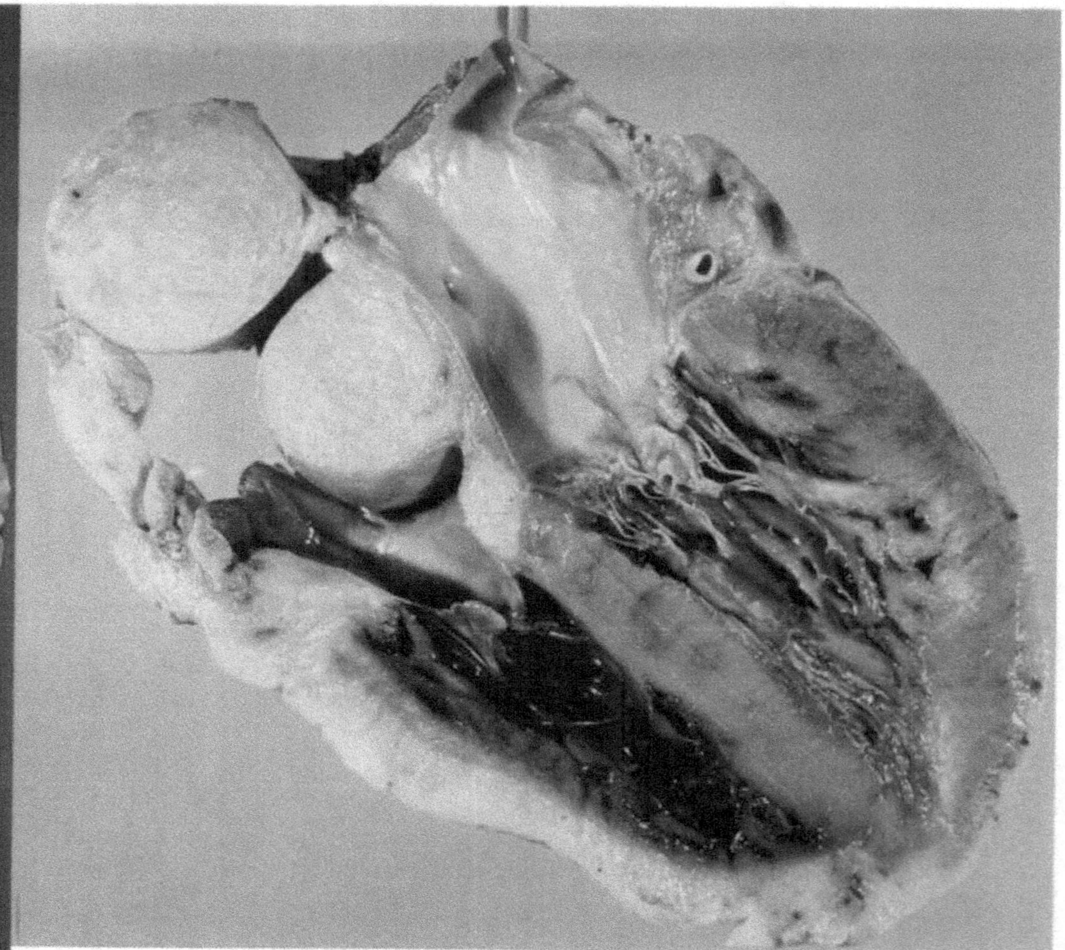

Figure 1 (left). Four-chamber view of the heart of a 70-year old man (NNMC# A86-42), showing the method used to measure the thickness of the cephalad portion of the atrial septum [1], the caudal portion of the atrial septum [2], the fat in the right atrioventricular groove [3] and the fat overlying the right ventricular wall [4]. LA = left atrium; LV = left ventricle; RA = right atrium; RV = right ventricle. The **double arrowheads** point to the fossa ovalis.

Figure 2 (right). Four-chamber view of the heart of a 74-year old woman (GT# 774-42). The caudal portion of the atrial septum is thicker than that in any of the other 90 cases.

Table 1. Clinical and Morphologic Findings in 11 Patients With Fatty Deposits in the Atrial Septum and an Atrial Septal Thickness <2 cm

Pt No.	Age (yr)/ Gender	HD in Life	AP	AMI	AA*	Htn	DM	Fatal CAD	HW (g)	Heart Floats	Thickness of Atrial Septum (cm)	≥1 CA With >75% ↓ in CSA by Plaque	LV Fibrosis	LV Necrosis
1	49/M	+	0	0	0	+	0	0†	580′	0	1.6	0	0	0
2	53/F	0	0	0	0	0	0	0	300‡	+	1.7	0	0	0
3	57/M	0	0	0	0	+	0	+	355	+	1.8	+	0	0
4	67/M	+	+	+	+	+	0	+	530	+	1.8	+	0	+
5	71/M	0	0	0	0	0	0	0	465	+	1.8	+	0	0
6	72/M	+	+	+	+	0	+	+	555	0	1.7	+	+	0
7	76/F	+	0	+	+	0	0	+	610	+	1.8	+	0	+
8	79/M	+	+	+	+	0	0	+	410	+	1.5	+	0	+
9	79/F	0	0	0	0	+	0	0	420	+	1.5	+	0	0
10	80/F	0	0	0	0	+	0	0	425	+	1.5	0	0	0
11	89/F	+	+	+	+	0	+	+	520	+	1.8	+	+	0
Total or mean value	70	6	4	5	5	5	2	6	470	9	1.7	8	2	3

*None had ventricular arrhythmias. †Died of aortic valve infective endocarditis. ‡Patient had cachexia and died of metastatic breast cancer. AA = atrial arrhythmia; AMI = acute myocardial infarction; AP = angina pectoris; CA = coronary artery; CAD = atherosclerotic coronary artery disease; CSA = cross-sectional area; DM = diabetes mellitus; F = female; HD = heart disease; Htn = systemic hypertension; HW = heart weight; LV = left ventricular; M = male; Pt = patient; 0 = absent; + = present; ↓ = decrease.

Methods of examining the hearts. Each heart was weighed on very accurate scales after fixation in formalin from 3 to 14 days and after carefully removing all portions of parietal pericardium and after removing the pulmonary trunk and ascending aorta by transverse incisions approximately 2-cm cephalad to the sinotubular junctions. Hearts received completely intact were placed in a large container of water to see whether or not they floated. (A floating heart is indicative of a very fatty heart [21].)

Each of the four major coronary arteries (right, left main, left anterior descending, left circumflex) was examined by transverse incisions, each about 5 mm apart, and the maximal degrees of cross-sectional area narrowing of each was recorded (0% to 25%, 26% to 50%, 51% to 75%, 76% to 100%). The cardiac ventricles were not opened in an entirely uniform fashion; they were opened by coronal, sagittal or transverse incisions, or a combination of these incisions. The maximal thickness of the fat in the right atrioventricular (AV) groove and that covering the right ventricular myocardium was measured as illustrated in Figure 1.

The atria were opened by a coronal incision, such that the midportion of the fossa ovalis of the atrial septum was incised. Measurements of the maximal thicknesses of the atrial septum both cephalad and caudal to the fossa ovalis were made after the incision through the midportion of the fossa ovalis (Fig. 1).

Statistical analysis. For each variable, the mean value and standard deviation was determined. Correlations were calculated between the thickness of the atrial septum and body weight, 12-lead QRS voltage and thickness of adipose tissue inferior to fossa ovalis, in the AV groove and overlying the right ventricular wall. Statistical analysis of the noncontinuous variables was done by the chi-square method. Continuous data were analyzed by the Student *t* test. A probability < 0.05 was considered significant.

Results

Atrial septal thickness cephalad versus caudal to the fossa ovalis. In all 91 patients, the thickness of the atrial septum cephalad to the fossa ovalis was always greater than that of the atrial septum caudal to the fossa ovalis. Either none or only minimal amounts of adipose tissue were present in the fossa ovalis. The maximal thickness of the cephalad portion of atrial septum ranged from 1.5 to 6 cm (mean 2.4) and that of the caudal portion of septum from 0.3 to 2.4 cm (mean 0.9). The 91 cases were divided into two groups on the basis of the maximal thickness of the cephalad portion of the atrial septum. One group consisted of 11 patients in whom the maximal atrial septal thickness ranged from 1.5 to 1.8 cm, and pertinent clinical and morphologic findings in these patients are detailed in Table 1.

The other group consisted of 80 patients in whom the maximal right to left thickness of the cephalad portion of atrial septum ranged from 2 to 6 cm (mean 2.5). The remainder of this report focuses on these 80 patients. Of the 80 patients, 69 (86%) had an atrial septum with a maximal thickness of 2 to 3 cm and 11 patients (14%) had an atrial septum with a maximal thickness >3 cm. Certain clinicopathologic findings in the patients with an atrial septum ≥2 cm are summarized in Table 2 and illustrated in Figures 1 to 11. The 80 patients (52 men, 28 women) ranged in age from 48 to 91 years (mean 69). Only 1 patient was <50 years of age and only 1 was >90 years of age; 12 patients were aged 51 to 60 years, 5 patients 81 to 90 years and 61 patients (76%) 61 to 80 years of age.

Table 2. Clinical and Morphologic Findings in 80 Patients With Massive Fatty Deposits in the Atrial Septum

	All Patients (n = 80)	Men (n = 52)	Women (n = 28)
Age (yr), range (mean)	48–91 (69 ± 9)	48–91 (68 ± 9)	53–86 (71 ± 9)
White/black	72/8	47/5	25/3
Heart disease in life	47/77 (61%)	30/49 (61%)	17 (61%)
Angina pectoris	19/77 (25%)	16/49 (33%)	3 (11%)
Myocardial infarction	20/77 (26%)	14/49 (29%)	6 (32%)
Congestive heart failure	21/77 (27%)	11/49 (22%)*	10 (36%)*
Sudden death	26/79 (33%)	21/51 (41%)*	5 (18%)*
Arrhythmias			
Supraventricular	31/77 (40%)	18/49 (37%)	13/28 (48%)
Ventricular	6/78 (8%)	6/50 (12%)	0 (0%)
Systemic hypertension	46/77 (60%)	31/49 (63%)	15 (54%)
Habitual alcoholism	10/76 (13%)	9/48 (19%)	1 (4%)
Diabetes mellitus	19/77 (25%)	15/49 (31%)	4 (14%)
Corticosteroid therapy	10/76 (13%)	6/48 (13%)	4 (14%)
Cancer			
All	28/78 (36%)	17/50 (34%)	11 (39%)
Fatal	22/28 (79%)	15/17 (88%)	7/11 (64%)
Body weight (kg), range (mean)†	55–125 (79 ± 14)	57–118 (82 ± 13)	55–125 (75 ± 16)
Height (cm), range (mean)†	145–193 (168 ± 12)	150–193 (173 ± 10)*	145–193 (162 ± 12)*
Cause of death			
Cardiac	37 (46%)	27 (52%)	10 (36%)
Vascular	10 (13%)	6 (11%)	4 (14%)
Noncardiovascular	33 (41%)	19 (37%)	14 (50%)
Death outside hospital	13/75 (17%)	10/47 (21%)	3 (9%)
Heart weight (g), range (mean)	300–915 (545 ± 125)	345–915 (566 ± 118)	300–880 (505 ± 134)
Heart floats in water	52/69 (75%)	35/48 (73%)	17/21 (81%)
No. of coronary arteries with >75% ↓ in CSA by plaque			
4	3 (4%)	2 (4%)	1 (4%)
3	13 (16%) } 53 (67%)	9 (18%) } 41 (80%)*	4 (14%) } 12 (43%)*
2	18 (23%)	16 (31%)	2 (7%)
1	19 (24%)	14 (27%)	5 (18%)
0	27 (33%)	10 (20%)	16 (57%)
Coronary arteries with >75% ↓ in CSA by plaque			
Left main	4 (5%)	2 (4%)	2 (7%)
Left anterior descending	47 (59%)	38 (73%)*	9 (32%)*
Left circumflex	21 (26%)	14 (27%)	7 (25%)
Right	34 (43%)	27 (52%)*	7 (25%)*
Left ventricular fibrosis	22 (28%)	18 (35%)*	4 (14%)*
Left ventricular necrosis	15 (19%)	10 (19%)	5 (18%)
Mitral annular calcium	21 (26%)	14 (27%)	7 (25%)
Thickness of atrial septum (cm), range (mean)			
Cephalad portion	2–6 (2.5 ± 0.7)	2–5 (2.4 ± 0.5)*	2–6 (2.8 ± 0.9)*
Caudal portion	0.3–2.4 (1.0 ± 0.3)	0.4–1.5 (0.9 ± 0.2)	0.3–2.4 (1.0 ± 0.5)
Thickness of fat in atrioventricular groove, range (mean) (cm)	0.7–2.6 (1.7 ± 0.5)	0.7–2.6 (1.6 ± 0.5)	0.7–2.5 (1.8 ± 0.6)
Thickness of fat over the right ventricle, range (mean) (cm)	0.2–1.5 (0.7 ± 0.2)	0.3–1.5 (0.7 ± 0.2)	0.2–1.3 (0.7 ± 0.3)

*p ≤ 0.05. †Data available in 40 patients. Abbreviations as in Table 1.

Small versus large septum. Comparison of the 59 patients with a smaller septum (2 to 2.9 cm) with the 21 patients with a larger septum (≥3 cm) disclosed significant differences in the frequency of male gender (73% vs. 43%), atrial arrhythmias (34% vs. 60%), systemic hypertension (71% vs. 55%), mean heart weight (520 vs. 565 g) (despite the smaller percent of men in the group with a larger heart) and a smaller quantity of cardiac fat overall as evidenced by the percent of hearts that floated in water (70% vs. 94%) (Table 3). Neither diabetes mellitus nor corticosteroid therapy had an effect on the thickness of the atrial septum. The average thickness of the septum in the 19 patients with diabetes mellitus was 2.4 cm and that in the 58 patients without diabetes was 2.6 cm. The mean thickness of the septum was 2.8 cm in the 10 patients on corticosteroid therapy and 2.5 cm in those not receiving corticosteroid therapy.

Coronary artery disease. Comparison of the 53 patients with significant coronary artery disease (one or more major epicardial coronary arteries narrowed >75% in cross-sectional area by atherosclerotic plaque at necropsy) with

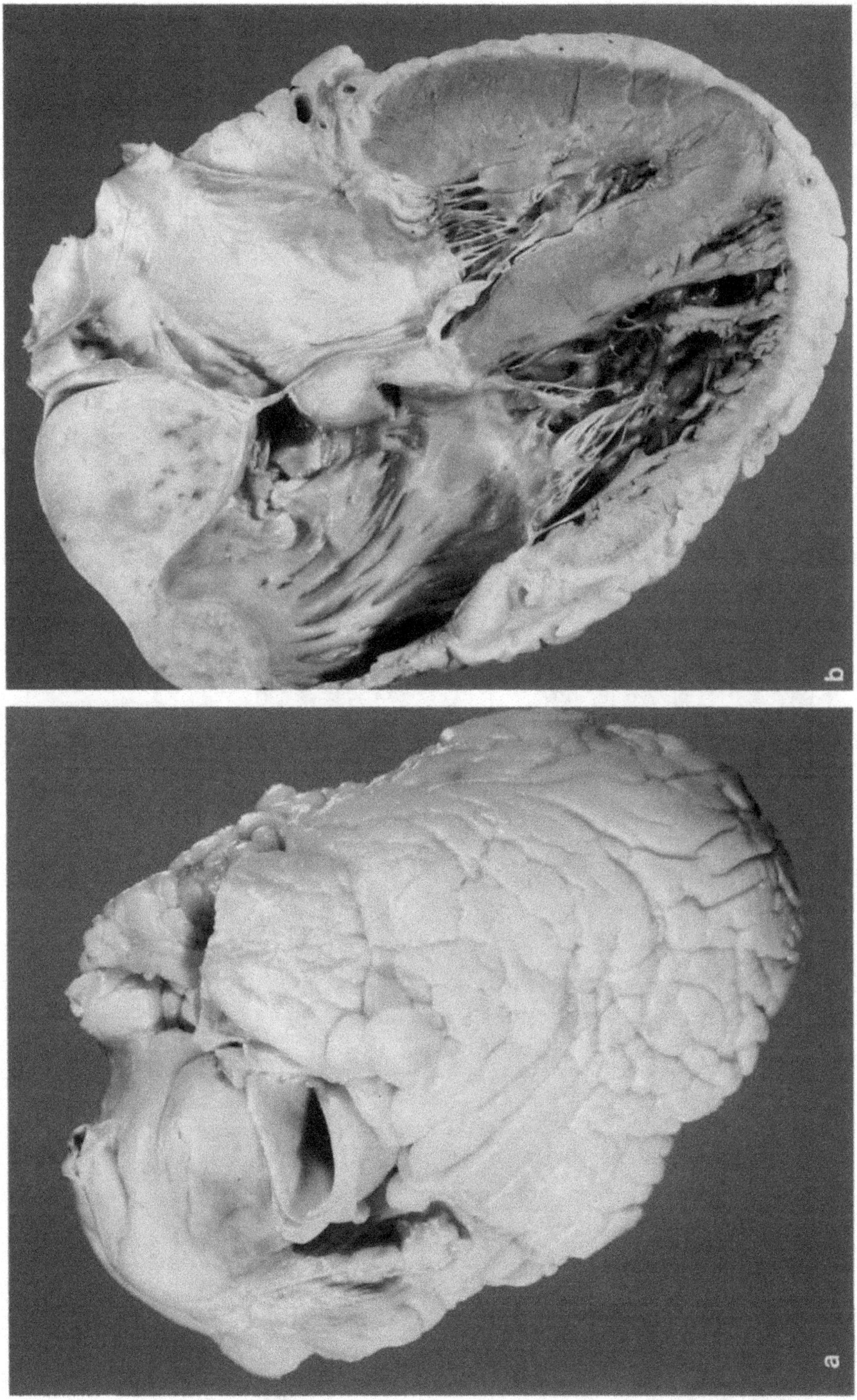

Figure 3. Exterior (a) and four-chamber (b) view of the heart of an 83-year old woman (NNMC# A88-43), showing massive amounts of epicardial adipose tissue covering the entire surface of both ventricles.

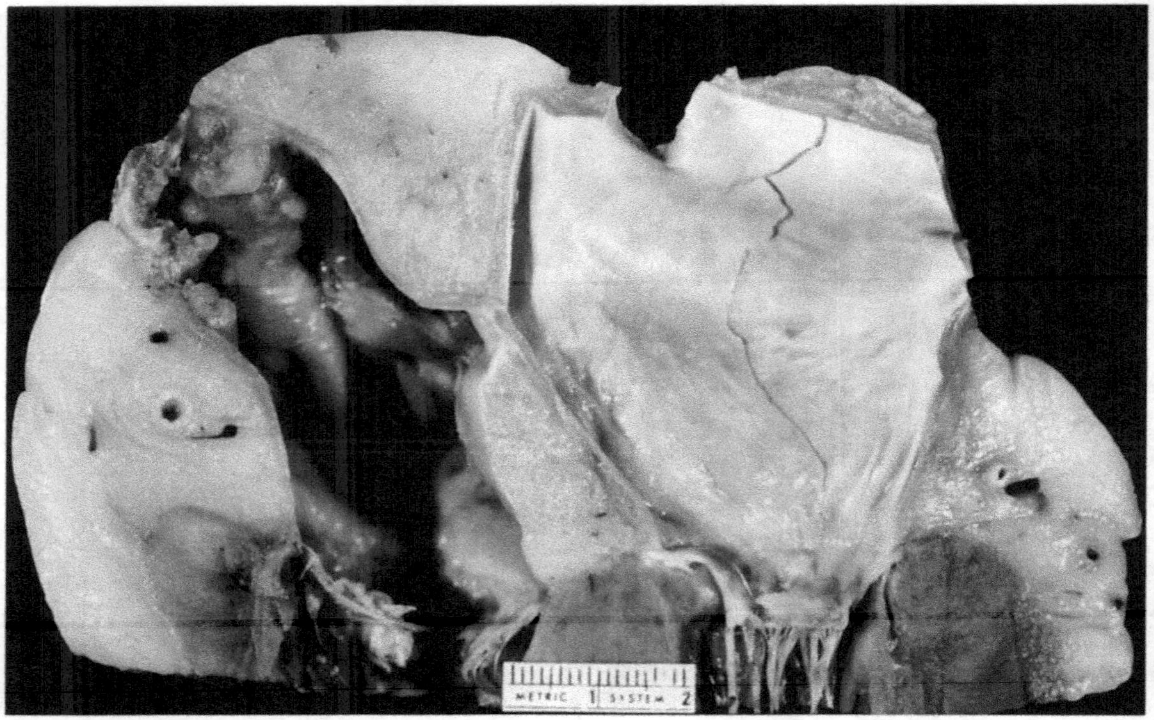

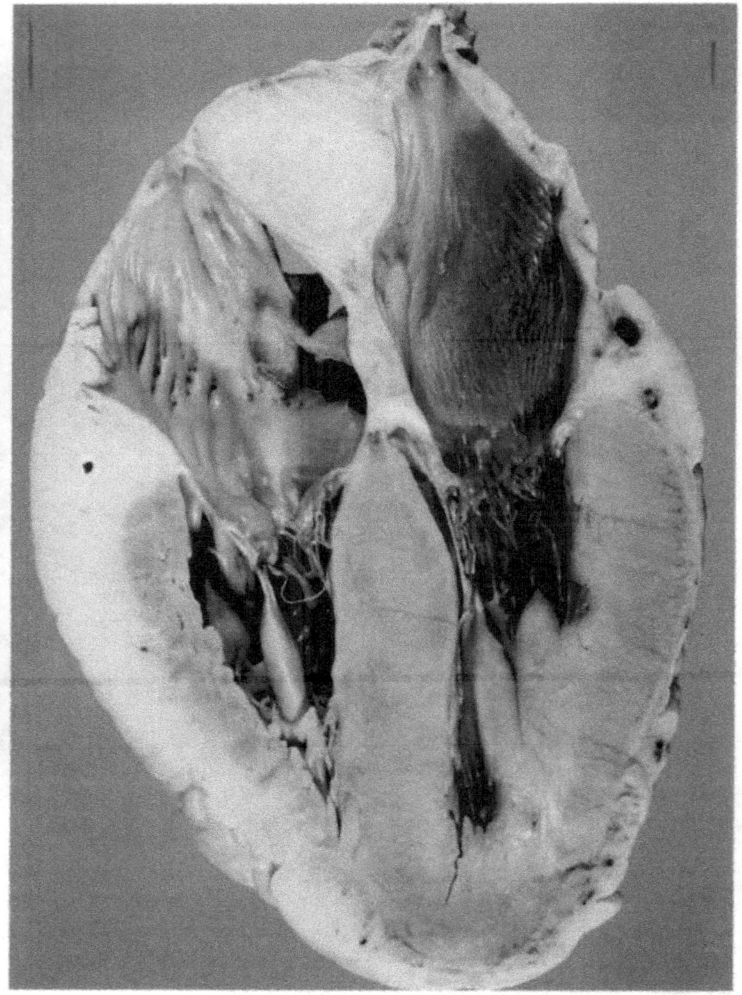

Figure 4 (left). Coronal section of the right and left atria and the atrial septum of the heart of a 71-year old woman (SV# 7/78).

Figure 5 (right). Four-chamber view of the heart of a 77-year old woman (NNMC# A89-33). The coronal section through the atrial septum is made slightly anterior to the fossa ovalis.

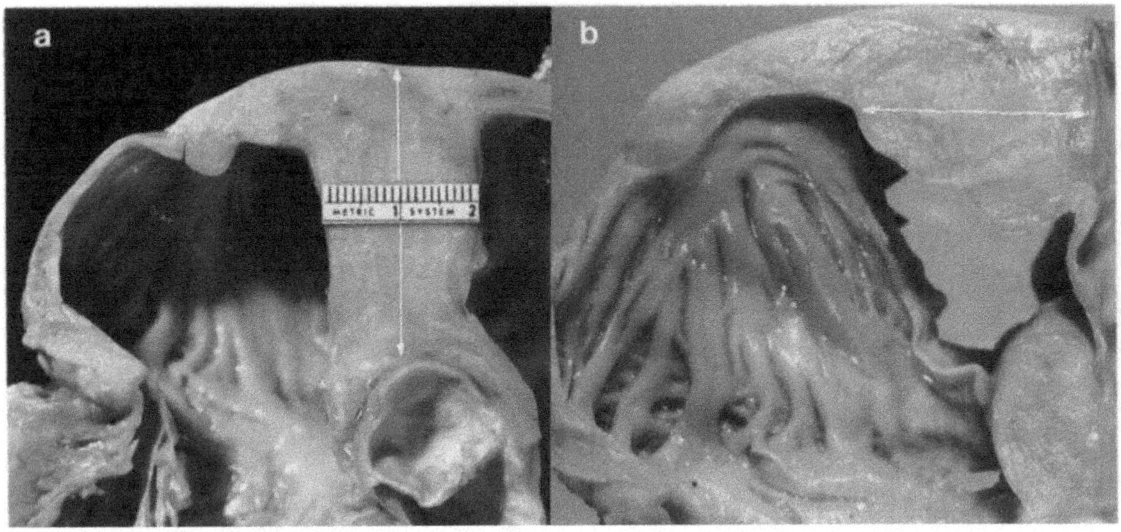

Figure 6. Close-up of the right atrium and atrial septum in a four-chamber view of the heart of a 76-year old woman (NNMC# A75-32). The coronal section is anterior to the fossa ovalis in **a** and at the level of the fossa ovalis in **b**. If the atrial septum is measured from its cephalad to its caudal extension as shown in **a (between the arrows)**, the thickness of the septum would be nearly twice that of the cephalad portion at the level of the fossa ovalis as shown in **b**. Measurements in the present study were all done as shown in **b**.

the 27 patients with insignificant coronary narrowing disclosed a significantly higher proportion of men (77% vs. 41%), a lesser frequency of fatal cancer (21% vs. 42%) and a smaller mean thickness of the atrial septum (2.4 vs. 2.9 cm). No significant difference in the frequency of atrial arrhythmias between the two groups was observed (41% vs. 38%).

Fatal cancer. Comparison of the 22 patients with fatal cancer with the 56 patients without cancer disclosed a significantly lower frequency of coronary artery disease in the cancer group (50% vs. 73%) and a smaller mean heart weight among the women (405 vs. 545 g). The mean thickness of the atrial septum was similar between these two groups (2.5 vs. 2.6 cm).

Atrial arrhythmias and conduction disturbances. Comparison of the 31 patients with atrial arrhythmias with the 46 patients without such arrhythmias disclosed a thicker atrial

Figure 7. Postmortem radiograph (**a**) and four-chamber view (**b**) of the heart of a 73-year old man (SH# A92-12). The needle (enclosed by **perpendicular lines**) in the atrial septum (**arrows**) measures 2.8 cm in length.

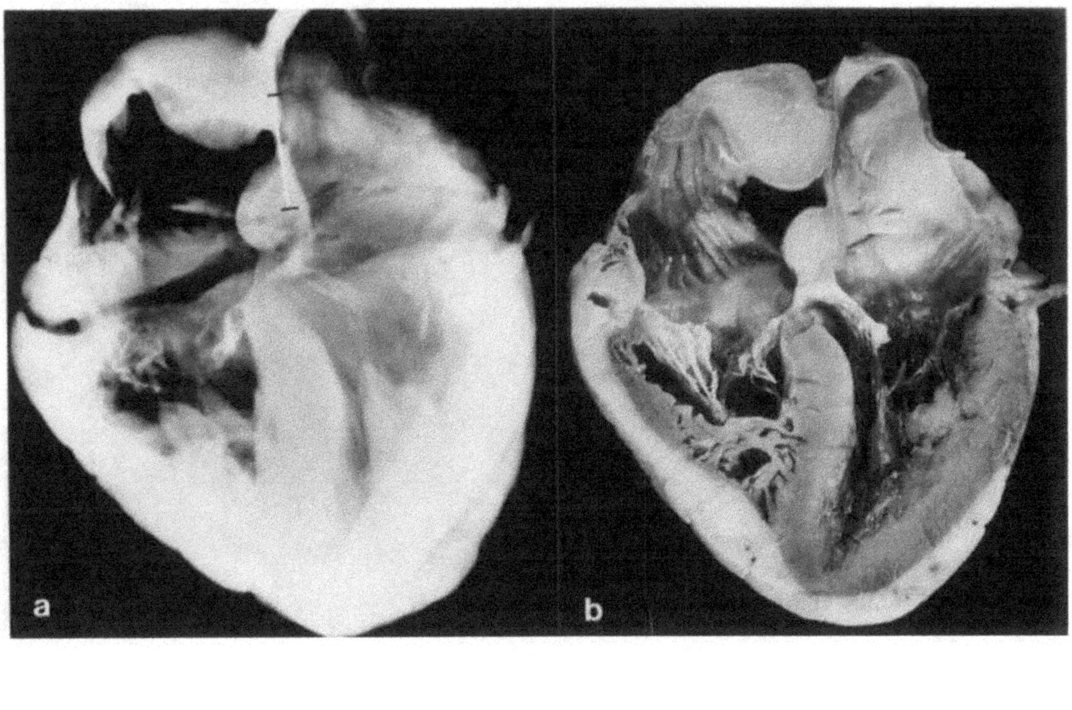

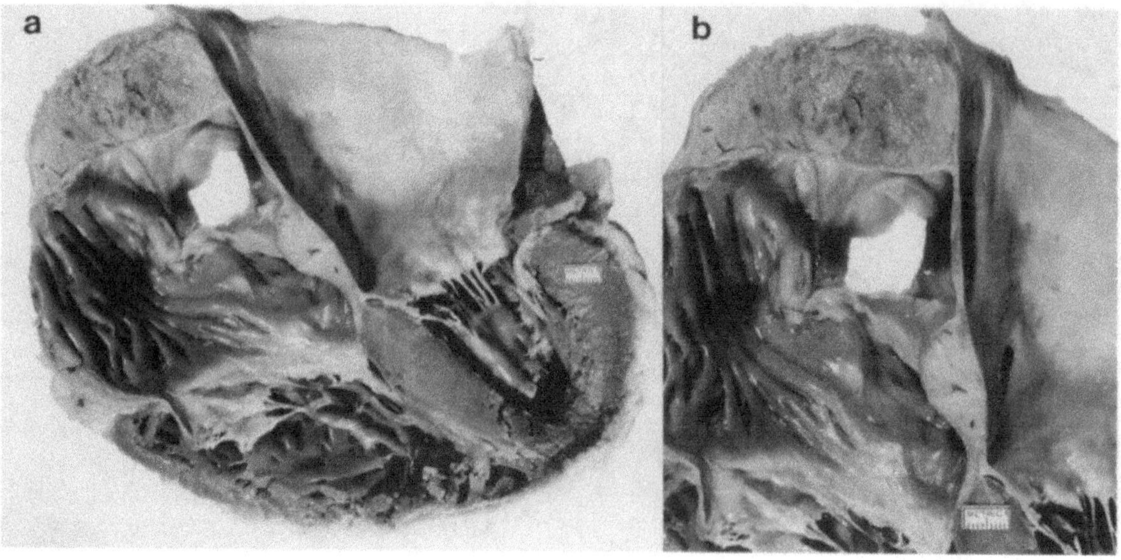

Figure 8. Four-chamber view of the heart of a 71-year old woman (a) and close-up of the right and left atria and atrial septum (b) (FSH# A-4088). Both atria are very dilated. The portion of the atrial septum cephalad to the fossa ovalis is 6 cm thick.

septum in the patients with arrhythmia (2.9 vs. 2.3 cm), a heavier heart in the women (545 vs. 470 g) and a higher frequency of signs and symptoms of congestive heart failure (42% vs. 17%) (Table 4). No significant differences occurred in the frequency of significant coronary artery disease (68% vs. 67%) or of myocardial infarction (45% vs. 37%) (Table 4).

Various electrocardiographic measurements were performed in 28 of the 80 patients with an atrial septum ≥2 cm in thickness (Table 5). Twelve (43%) of the 28 patients with an electrocardiogram had chronic atrial arrhythmias (atrial fibrillation in 8). Of the 18 patients with sinus, junctional or ectopic atrial rhythm, 9 (50%) had atrial premature complexes. Six patients (21%) had major conduction disturbances, but four of them had myocardial infarction. Total

Figure 9. Four-chamber view of the heart of a 78-year old man (a) and close-up of the right atrium and atrial septum (b).

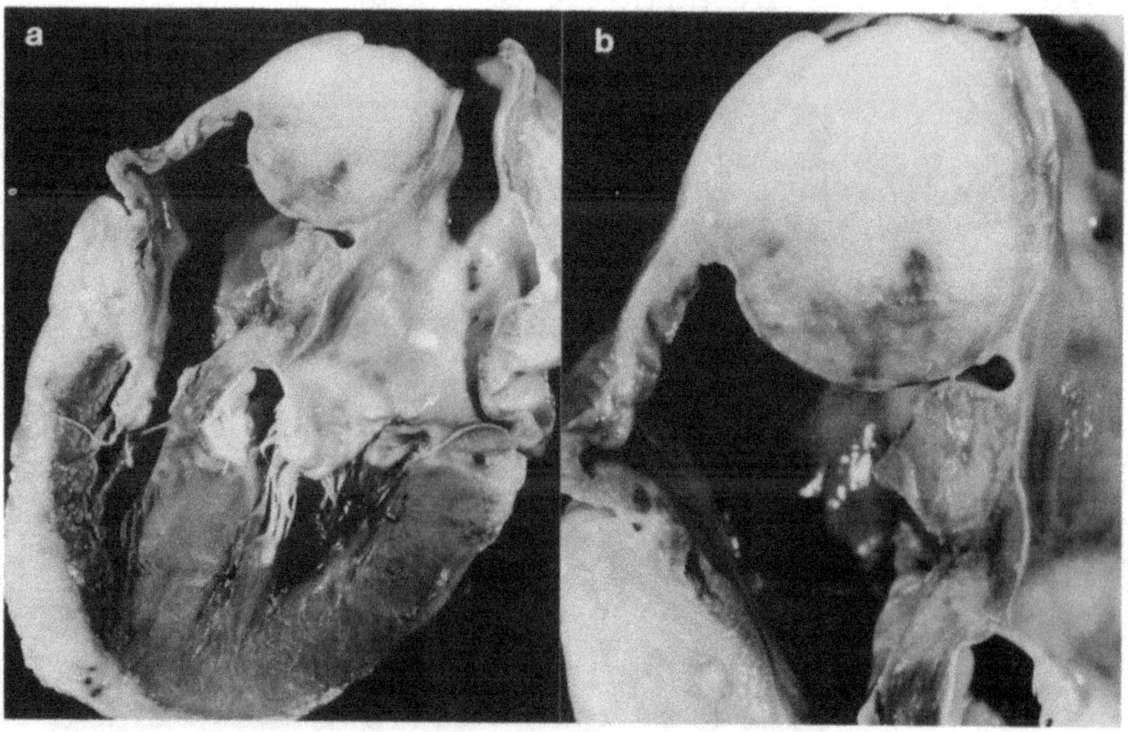

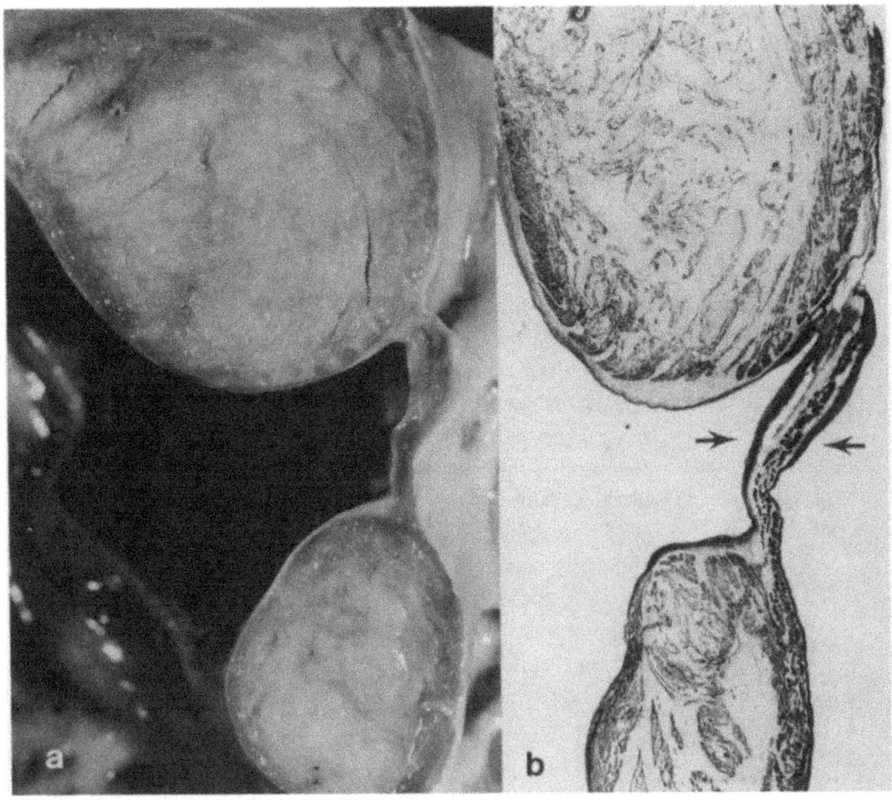

Figure 10. Gross (**a**) and histologic (**b**) section of the atrial septum of the heart of a 60-year old woman. Only minimal amounts of adipose tissue are present in the fossa ovalis (**arrows**). Movat stain ×25 (**b**).

12-lead QRS voltage measured by the method of Siegel and Roberts (22) ranged from 59 to 266 mm (mean 131 ± 51). Patients with an atrial septum ≥3 cm had a significantly higher frequency of atrial arrhythmias (75% vs. 18%) and larger total 12-lead QRS voltages (150 vs. 115 mm) than those of patients with an atrial septum <3 cm (Table 6).

Discussion

Measurement of atrial septal thickness. One difference in our study from those published previously on this subject is

Figure 11. Normal atrial septum (DCMEO 78-04-284) with a maximal thickness of 6 mm in its cephalad portion and no fatty deposit. The fossa ovalis membrane (**arrows**) measures <1 mm in thickness. LA = left atrium; RA = right atrium.

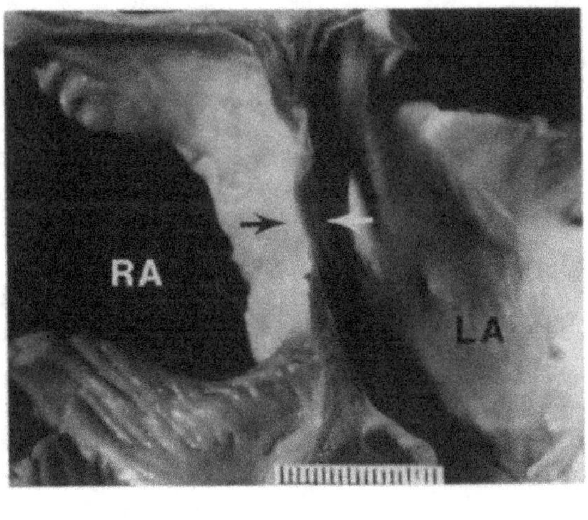

Table 3. Comparison of the Clinical and Morphologic Findings in Patients With Small (septal thickness <3 cm) and Large (septal thickness ≥3 cm) Fatty Deposits in the Atrial Septum

	Atrial Septal Thickness <3 cm (n = 59)		Atrial Septal Thickness ≥3 cm (n = 21)	
Age (yr), range (mean)	48–91 (68)		51–85 (71)	
Men	43 (73%)*		9 (43%)*	
Atrial arrhythmias	19/56 (34%)*		12/20 (60%)*	
Systemic hypertension	31/56 (55%)*		15/21 (71%)*	
Body weight (kg), range (mean)	55–95 (78)		55–125 (84)	
Heart weight (g), range (mean)	300–915 (520)*		335–880 (565)*	
Heart floats in water	37/53 (70%)*		15/16 (94%)*	
No. of coronary arteries with >75% ↓ in CSA by plaque				
4	2 (4%)	42 (71%)	1 (5%)	11 (52%)
3	10 (17%)		3 (14%)	
2	15 (25%)		3 (14%)	
1	15 (25%)		4 (19%)	
0	17 (29%)		10 (48%)	
LV fibrosis	17 (29%)		5 (24%)	
LV necrosis	12 (20%)		3 (14%)	
Thickness of atrial septum (cm) range (mean)				
Cephalad portion	2.0–2.9 (2.1)*		3.0–6.0 (3.6)*	
Caudal portion	0.3–1.3 (1.0)		0.6–2.4 (1.2)	
Thickness of fat in atrioventricular groove (cm), range (mean)	0.7–2.6 (1.7)		0.9–2.5 (1.9)	
Thickness of fat over the right ventricle (cm), range (mean)	0.2–1.3 (0.7)		0.4–1.5 (0.8)	

*$p < 0.05$. Abbreviations as in Table 1.

Table 4. Comparison of Patients With Massive Fatty Deposits in the Atrial Septum With and Without Atrial Arrhythmias

	Atrial Arrhythmia	
	Present (n = 31)	Absent (n = 46)
Age (yr), range (mean)	52–84 (72)	48–91 (67)
Male/female	18 (58)/13 (42%)	31 (67)/15 (33%)
Systemic hypertension	18 (58%)	28 (61%)
Angina pectoris	9 (29%)	10 (22%)
Congestive heart failure	13 (42%)*	8 (17%)*
Diabetes mellitus	9 (29%)	10 (22%)
Corticosteroid therapy	5 (16%)	5/44 (11%)
Cancer	14 (45%)	14 (30%)
≥1 CA with >75% ↓ in CSA by plaque	21 (68%)	31 (67%)
Heart weight (g), range (mean)		
Men	410–915 (605)	345–800 (585)
Women	315–880 (545)*	300–680 (470)*
Heart floats	17/25 (68%)	34/42 (81%)
Maximal thickness of the atrial septum (cm)	2.0–5.5 (2.9)*	2.0–6.0 (2.3)*
Mitral annular calcium	8 (26%)	12 (26%)
Myocardial infarction		
Healed	8 (26%) } 14 (45%)	9 (20%) } 18 (40%)
Acute	4 (13%)	6 (13%)
Both healed and acute	2 (6%)	3 (7%)

*$p < 0.05$. Abbreviations as in Table 1.

the method chosen to measure the thicknesses of the atrial septum. In the present study, the atrial septum was incised in a coronal fashion, with the incision extending through the midportion of the fossa ovalis, which contains minimal amounts, if any, of fat and therefore is only ≈1 cm thick. By incising the atrial septum using the fossa ovalis as the landmark, the thickness of the cephalad portion was always greater than the thickness of the caudal portion of the septum. With this method of measuring the thickness of the atrial septum, 6 cm was the thickest and 1.5 cm was the thinnest atrial septum. Previous publications (5) have described larger atrial septa, but the method of measurement was never described precisely. If we had determined the thickness of the atrial septum by measuring, for example, the longitudinal thickness either anterior or posterior to the fossa ovalis, measurements two or more times as large as our maximal measurements would have resulted. The use of the fossa ovalis as the landmark for measuring atrial septal thickness also allows comparison of the necropsy measurements with those recorded by echocardiography-computed tomography and nuclear magnetic resonance (NMR) imaging.

Normally the atrial septum both cephalad and caudal to the fossa ovalis is <1 cm thick. In the present study, we focused primarily on patients with a maximal atrial septal thickness ≥2 cm. Because previous reports have included cases with <2 cm atrial septal thickness, we also included cases with maximal septal thickness ranging from 1.5 to 1.9 cm, so that these cases could be compared with others previously reported (Table 1).

Adipose tissue in other portions of the heart. When the atrial septum is massively infiltrated by fatty deposits, the amount of adipose tissue is always increased in other portions of the heart, mainly the subepicardial adipose tissue, particularly over the right ventricular wall and in the AV sulci. The fatty deposits may be so extensive that every square centimeter of ventricular myocardium is covered by adipose tissue. The huge deposits of fat in all portions of the heart made the heart in many of our patients lighter than water, such that 75% (52 of 69) of the hearts floated in water. The actual weight of the fat, measured in five of our patients, constituted 32% to 52% (mean 41%) of the total weight of the heart. The maximal thickness of the atrial septum in our patients with septa ≥2 cm correlated with the thickness of the subepicardial adipose tissue over the right ventricular myocardial wall ($r = 0.61$) and that in the AV sulcus ($r = 0.79$). Among our 80 patients, the body weight was available in 40 and the maximal thickness of atrial septum in these patients correlated with body weight ($r = 0.84$).

The adipose tissue in the heart may be the last site to disappear with weight loss. Support for this view is gained by the presence of huge quantities of cardiac fat in the 22 patients with fatal cancer, a number of whom were cachectic at necropsy. The maximal thickness of the atrial septum in the 22 patients with cancer was similar to that in the 56 patients without known cancer (2.5 vs. 2.6 cm).

In addition to the constant association of the massive atrial septal fatty deposits with massive deposits of fat in other portions of the heart and usually in other portions of the body, there also was near universal increase in heart weight: 77 (96%) of the 80 patients had an increased heart weight (>350 g in women, >400 g in men). Systemic hypertension, as might be expected because of the high prevalence of obesity, was present in 46 (60%) of 77 patients (Table 2). Significant atherosclerotic coronary artery disease was also common. Of the 80 patients, 53 (66%) had >75% narrowing in cross-sectional area of one or more major epicardial coronary arteries by atherosclerotic plaque and 33 (62%) of the 53 patients died from consequences of coronary artery disease.

Presence of atrial arrhythmias. Whether the frequency of atrial arrhythmias is greater in patients with massive atrial septal fatty deposits than in patients of similar age and gender without these deposits has been controversial. Among 122 cases of atrial septal fatty deposits reported by others (1–20), atrial arrhythmias of some type, including atrial premature complexes, were present in 56 (45%). Among our 80 patients with septa ≥2 cm thick, 31 (40%) had supraventricular arrhythmias. (This number and percent excludes atrial premature complexes.) In our patients, the frequency of atrial arrhythmias increased with increasing thickness of the atrial septa, such that 60% of the patients with an atrial septum ≥3 cm had atrial arrhythmias com-

Table 5. Electrocardiographic Findings in 28 Men and Women With Lipomatous Hypertrophy of the Atrial Septum

Pt No.	Age at Death (yr)/Gender	Interval From ECG to Death (days)	Heart Rate (beats/min)	Heart Rhythm	Interval (ms) PR	Interval (ms) QRS	Interval (ms) QTc	Conduction Abnormality	QRS Voltage (mm) 12-Lead	QRS Voltage (mm) I,II,III,R,L,F	QRS Voltage (mm) V_1–V_6	APC	LAA	HW (g)	LV Fibrosis	LV Necrosis	Thickness of Atrial Septum (cm)	≥1 CA >75% ↓ in CSA by Plaque	Cause of Death
									Men										
1	48/M	94	56	S	14	8	42	0	97	34	63	0	0	490	0	0	2.5	+	CAD
2	51/M	7	85	S	18	8	36	0	170	59	111	0	+	630	0	+	2.0	+	CAD
3	57/M	57	110	S	16	8	37	0	155	54	101	+	0	685	0	0	3.0	0	Cancer
4	64/M	23	82	S	15	9	28	0	139	59	80	+	+	470	0	0	2.5	0	Suicide
5	65/M	10	80	AF	—	12	—	Left BBB	241	95	146	–	–	450	+	+	3.0	+	CAD
6	68/M	1	56	S	18	10	44	0	93	34	59	+	+	490	0	0	2.0	+	CAD
7	70/M	3	72	J	17	14	44	Right BBB	118	53	65	0	+	520	0	+	2.5	+	CAD
8	70/M	1	124	AF	—	10	30	0	147	60	87	–	–	795	0	0	5.0	0	Infection
9	72/M	11	170	AT	—	11	26	IVCD	134	49	85	–	–	710	+	0	2.0	+	CAD
10	73/M	41	95	S	18	15	37	Right BBB,LPFB	94	49	45	+	+	690	+	0	2.9	+	Cancer
11	73/M	89	84	EA	22	13	41	Left BBB	112	50	62	+	–	550	0	0	3.4	+	AAA
12	84/M	5	120	AT	—	8	—	0	157	43	114	–	–	410	0	0	3.5	+	Cancer
Subtotal	67 ± 10/12M	29 ± 9	95 ± 30	6S	18 ± 2	10 ± 2	37 ± 6	5	140 ± 43	54 ± 17	87 ± 29	5 (63%)	6/7	576 ± 129	3	3	2.9 ± 0.9	9 (75%)	
									Women										
13	59/F	6	136	S	16	8	36	0	90	49	41	+	+	410	+	0	2.0	+	Cancer
14	60/F	1	125	S	16	9	36	0	91	20	71	0	0	680	+	+	3.0	+	CAD
15	70/F	41	82	S	17	10	44	0	127	60	67	+	+	550	0	+	2.0	+	CAD
16	71/F	9	89	S	18	9	38	0	125	52	67	0	+	630	0	+	2.2	+	CAD
17	72/F	15	85	S	20	10	40	0	93	23	70	0	+	330	0	0	2.0	0	Cancer
18	73/F	3	80	AF	—	9	40	0	158	52	106	–	–	680	0	0	2.7	+	CAD*
19	74/F	130	78	AF	—	9	—	0	133	51	82	–	–	540	0	0	3.5	0	Cancer
20	76/F	11	120	AT	—	8	—	0	266	80	186	–	–	450	0	0	3.0	0	—
21	77/F	6	146	AF	—	8	27	0	75	20	55	–	–	530	+	0	3.0	+	Infection
22	77/F	16	105	S	19	8	28	0	138	40	98	+	+	440	0	0	2.0	0	Leukemia
23	78/F	13	117	S	20	7	—	0	121	41	80	0	+	410	0	0	2.5	0	COPD
24	78/F	2	155	AF	—	10	—	0	110	34	76	–	–	540	0	0	3.3	0	Cancer
25	79/F	11	92	S	21	9	42	LAFB	88	50	38	0	+	420	0	0	2.0	+	COPD
26	79/F	455	100	S	20	8	38	0	217	71	146	0	+	500	0	0	3.5	0	Stroke
27	80/F	3	120	S	20	7	32	0	59	27	32	+	0	350	0	0	2.0	+	Cancer
28	83/F	39	132	AF	—	7	27	0	89	26	63	–	–	575	0	0	4.0	+	COPD
Subtotal	74 ± 7/16F	21 ± 16	110 ± 27	10S	19 ± 2	9 ± 1	36 ± 6	1	124 ± 53	43 ± 18	81 ± 39	4 (40%)	8/10	502 ± 108	3	3	2.7 ± 0.7	9 (56%)	
Total	70 ± 9/28	24 ± 9	103 ± 28	16S	18 ± 2	9 ± 2	36 ± 6	6 (18%)	131 ± 51	83 ± 36	47 ± 18	9 (50%)	14/17	545 ± 125	6	6	2.8 ± 0.7	18 (64%)	

*Died after mitral valve replacement for mitral regurgitation secondary to papillary muscle dysfunction. Subtotal and total values are presented as mean value ± SD or number (%) of patients. AAA = abdominal aortic aneurysm; AF = atrial fibrillation; APC = atrial premature complex; AT = (multifocal) atrial tachycardia; B = black; BBB = bundle branch block; COPD = chronic obstructive pulmonary disease; EA = ectopic atrial; ECG = electrocardiogram; IVCD = intraventricular conduction delay; J = junctional; LAA = left atrial abnormality; LAFB = left anterior fascicular block; LPFB = left posterior fascicular block; S = sinus; other abbreviations as in Table 1.

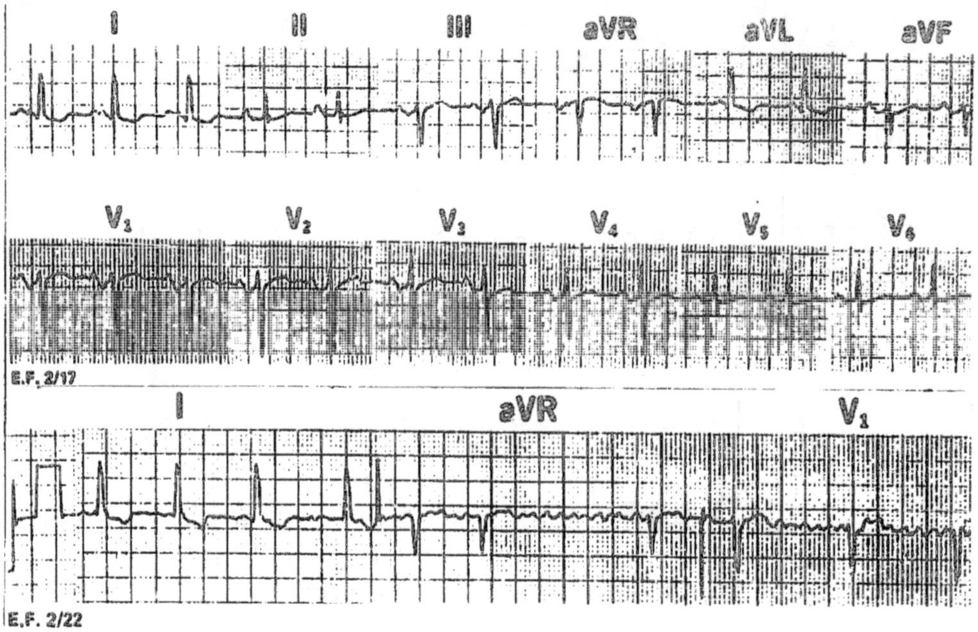

Figure 12. Electrocardiographic recordings obtained 5 days apart in a 74-year old white woman who died of lung cancer. At necropsy, the heart weighed 540 g, the atrial cavities were mildly enlarged and there were no scars in the left ventricular myocardium. The thickness of the atrial septum is 5.4 and 1.4 cm cephalad and caudal, respectively, to the fossa ovalis. **Upper two tracings,** Typical "dome and dip" P waves in sinus rhythm; **Lower tracing,** The rhythm is now atrial fibrillation.

pared with only 34% of the patients with an atrial septum 2 to 2.9 cm thick ($p < 0.01$). Furthermore, in the 31 patients with atrial arrhythmias the atrial septum was thicker than in patients without these arrhythmias (2.9 vs. 2.3 cm, $p < 0.01$) (Table 4). Finally, the similar frequency of significant coronary artery disease or myocardial infarction in the patients with and without atrial arrhythmias strongly supports the view that the atrial arrhythmias result in some way from the massive fatty deposits in the atrial septum.

Table 6. Comparison of the Clinical and Morphologic Findings in 28 Patients With Small (septal thickness <3 cm) and Large (septal thickness ≥3 cm) Fatty Deposits in the Atrial Septum in Whom a 12-Lead Electrocardiogram Was Available

	Atrial Septal Thickness <3 cm (n = 16)	Atrial Septal Thickness ≥3 cm (n = 12)
Age (yr) (mean)	(69)	(73)
Gender		
Men	7	5
Women	9	7
Systemic hypertension	10 (63%)	9 (75%)
Interval ECG to death (days)	19*	32*
Heart rhythm		
Sinus	13 (82%)*	3 (25%)*
Junctional	1 (6%)	0
Atrial tachycardia	1 (6%)	2 (17%)
Atrial fibrillation	1 (6%)	6 (50)%
Ectopic atrial rhythm	0	1 (8%)
Any atrial rhythm other than sinus	3 (18%)*	9 (75%)*
Conduction abnormality		
QRS voltage		
12-lead	115*	150*
Precordial leads	46	51
Limb leads	69*	99*
Heart weight (g)	515	520
LV fibrosis	3	3
LV necrosis	4	2
Thickness of atrial septum (cm)	2.2*	3.4*
≥1 CA with >75% ↓ in CSA by plaque	12 (75%)	6 (50%)

Kluge (2) was the first to mention a possible association between atrial arrhythmias and massive fatty deposits in the atrial septum. He described a 64-year old man with a 3-cm thick atrial septum and atrial tachycardia. The patient also had chronic obstructive pulmonary disease. Hutter and Page (4) described supraventricular arrhythmias in all 10 of their patients with an atrial septal thickness of 1 to 4 cm. Eight had premature atrial complexes that were often multifocal, three had wandering atrial pacemaker, three had multifocal atrial tachycardia and two had paroxysmal atrial tachycardia. One of the 10 patients had sick sinus syndrome and another 2 had atrial fibrillation. In five patients a peculiar P wave configuration (dome and dip P wave) was seen. We found similar P waves in 13 (67%) of our 16 patients in sinus rhythm (Fig. 12); 1 of our 13 patients had P waves suggestive of interatrial conduction block. At necropsy, the left atrium was dilated in only 1 (8%) of the 13 patients with sinus rhythm and an abnormal P wave configuration. Erhardt (15) speculated that the abnormal P waves in these patients result from normal downward activation of the right atrium from the sinus node, whereas the left atrium is electrically activated later in an upward fashion from the AV node. Four of the six patients reported on by Klein and Schaefer (17) with massive atrial septal fat diagnosed at necropsy had ECG abnormalities (intermittent sinoatrial block in two patients and atrial tachycardia and paroxysmal atrial fibrillation in one patient,

AV block in one). Only one patient had atherosclerotic coronary artery disease.

Other possible effects. Atrial arrhythmias appear to be the only functional consequence of massive fatty infiltrates in the atrial septum. Although other reports (6) have mentioned the possibility of obstruction to blood flow in the superior vena cava, coronary sinus, right pulmonary veins and right atrium, such obstruction has never been proved hemodynamically and none of our patients, even those with the thickest septa, had anatomic evidence of functional compression of adjacent vascular structures.

A potential danger of massive fatty infiltrates in the atrial septum is their confusion with neoplastic infiltration of the septum. Indeed, two patients have been reported (7,8) to have operative excision of the fatty mass in the atrial septum because cancer was suspected.

Diagnosis and nomenclature. In vivo diagnosis of massive fatty deposits in the atrial septum was reported first in 1982 with the use of computed tomography (13). Since then, a number of reports have described the diagnostic usefulness of echocardiography (8–12), computed tomography (11,12) and nuclear magnetic resonance imaging (8,10–12).

The best name for the massive fatty deposits in the atrial septum is still debated. We prefer the simple phrase "massive fatty deposits in the atrial septum" because it best describes the abnormality. The most common phrase is "lipomatous hypertrophy of the atrial septum," but the word "lipomatous" is incorrect because the fatty infiltrates are clearly not lipomas. In our view, the word "hypertrophy" should not be used to describe an infiltrate that should not be there in the first place. Thus, we suggest the simple descriptive phrase "massive fatty deposits in the atrial septum."

References

1. Prior JT. Lipomatous hypertrophy of cardiac interatrial septum: a lesion resembling hibernoma, lipoblastomatosis and infiltrating lipoma. Arch Pathol 1964;78:11–5.
2. Kluge WF. Lipomatous hypertrophy of the interatrial septum. Northwest Med 1969;68:25–30.
3. Page DL. Lipomatous hypertrophy of the cardiac interatrial septum: its development and probable clinical significance. Hum Pathol 1970;1:151–63.
4. Hutter AM, Page DL. Atrial arrhythmias and lipomatous hypertrophy of the cardiac interatrial septum. Am Heart J 1971;82:16–21.
5. McAllister HA, Fenoglio JJ. Tumors of the Cardiovascular System. Fascicle 15, Second Series. Atlas of Tumor Pathology. Armed Forces Institute of Pathology, Washington D.C. 1978:40–4.
6. McNamara RF, Taylor AE, Panner BJ. Superior vena caval obstruction by lipomatous hypertrophy of the right atrium. Clin Cardiol 1987;10:609–10.
7. Tschirkov A, Stegaru B. Lipomatous hypertrophy of interatrial septum presenting as recurring pericardial effusion and mistaken for constrictive pericarditis. Thorac Cardiovasc Surg 1979;27:400–3.
8. Fisher MS, Edmonds P. Lipomatous hypertrophy of the interatrial septum. Diagnosis by magnetic resonance imaging. J Comput Tomogr 1988;12:267–9.
9. Fyke FE III, Tajik AJ, Edwards WD, Seward JB. Diagnosis of lipomatous hypertrophy of the atrial septum by two-dimensional echocardiography. J Am Coll Cardiol 1983;1:1352–7.
10. Applegate PM, Tajik AJ, Ehman RL, Julsrud PR, Miller FA Jr. Two-dimensional echocardiographic and magnetic resonance imaging observations in massive lipomatous hypertrophy of the atrial septum. Am J Cardiol 1987;59:489–91.
11. Kindman LA, Wright A, Tye T, Seale W, Appleton C. Lipomatous hypertrophy of the interatrial septum: characterization by transesophageal and transthoracic echocardiography, magnetic resonance imaging, and computed tomography. J Am Soc Echocardiogr 1988;1:450–4.
12. Levine RA, Weyman AE, Dinsmore RE, et al. Noninvasive tissue characterization: diagnosis of lipomatous hypertrophy of the atrial septum by nuclear magnetic resonance imaging. J Am Coll Cardiol 1986;7:688–92.
13. Isner JM, Swan CS II, Mikus JP, Carter BL. Lipomatous hypertrophy of the interatrial septum: in vivo diagnosis. Circulation 1982;66:470–3.
14. Okel BB. The Wolff-Parkinson-White syndrome: report of a case with fatal arrhythmia and autopsy findings of myocarditis, interatrial lipomatous hypertrophy, and prominent right moderator band. Am Heart J 1968;75:673–8.
15. Erhardt LR. Abnormal atrial activity in lipomatous hypertrophy of the interatrial septum. Am Heart J 1974;87:571–6.
16. Reyes CV, Jablokow VR. Lipomatous hypertrophy of the cardiac interatrial septum: a report of 38 cases and review of the literature. Am J Clin Pathol 1970;72:785–8
17. Klein PJ, Schaefer HE. Das interatriale Lipom des Herzen. Z Krebsforsch 1973;79:11–8.
18. Crocker DW. Lipomatous infiltrates of the heart. Arch Pathol Lab Med 1978;102:69–72.
19. Kindblom LG, Svensson U. Multiple hibernomas of the heart: a case report. Acta Pathol Microbiol Scand 1977;85:122–6.
20. Inove T, Mohri N, Nagahara T, Takanashi R. A case report of "lipomatous hypertrophy of the cardiac interatrial septum," with a proposal for a new term "lipomatous hamartoma of the cardiac atrial septum." Acta Pathol Jpn 1988;38:1583–9.
21. Roberts WC, Roberts JD. The floating heart or the heart too fat to sink: analysis of 55 necropsy patients. Am J Cardiol 1983;52:1286–9.
22. Siegel RJ, Roberts WC. Electrocardiographic observations in severe aortic valve stenosis: correlative necropsy study to clinical hemodynamic and ECG variables demonstrating relation of 12-lead QRS amplitude to peak systolic transaortic pressure gradient. Am Heart J 1982;103:298–301.

Fatal Cor Pulmonale Caused by Extensive Tumor Emboli in the Small Pulmonary Arteries Without Emboli in the Major Pulmonary Arteries or Metastases in the Pulmonary Parenchyma

Michael J. Domanski, MD, Robert E. Cunnion, MD, Daniel J. Fernicola, MD, and William C. Roberts, MD

Microscopic-sized tumor emboli are an uncommon cause of cor pulmonale.[1–4] We report 2 patients who had precipitous terminal courses of respiratory insufficiency caused by extensive tumor emboli in the small pulmonary arteries.

Both patients were young (aged 38 and 27 years), both had recognized cancers (breast and pancreas) for short periods (12 and 9 months), and both had acute dyspnea for the first time beginning a short time before death (17 days and 1 day) with tachypnea and tachycardia. During the final acute dyspneic period, both had clear lung fields by chest radiographs and no neoplasm in the lung parenchyma at necropsy; both had elevated pulmonary arterial pressures (58/38 and 68/40 mm Hg), normal-sized cardiac silhouettes on chest radiograph and normal-sized hearts at necropsy (270 and 330 g); both had dilated right ventricular cavities (with normal-sized left ventricular cavities) and severe tricuspid regurgitation by echocardiogram; both had hypoxemia and respiratory alkalosis, and both had thrombocytopenia (40,000 and 44,000 cu mm) and anemia (hematocrits 33 and 27%). One patient (case 2) had schistocytes in peripheral blood. Pulmonary arteriogram (recorded only in patient 1) was normal (Figure 1); perfusion lung scan (recorded only in patient 2) was normal; cytology of pulmonary venous blood (analyzed only in patient 2) was positive for cancer cells. At necropsy, both had numerous small pulmonary arteries containing tumor emboli (Figure 2) without emboli in the major pulmonary arteries and without metastases in the pulmonary parenchyma, and both had widespread metastases in liver, lymph node and bone.

The 2 patients described in this study had rapidly progressive pulmonary and cardiovascular compromise resulting from extensive tumor emboli in the small pulmonary arteries. Diagnosis of this mechanism of dyspnea is rarely suspected antemortem.[2,3] Adenocarcinomas and trophoblastic neoplasms are the most frequently reported causes but other malignancies have been implicated.[3,5] Gastric carcinoma is the neoplasm giving rise most frequently to this syndrome.[5]

Patients generally present with dyspnea, tachypnea, tachycardia and hypoxemia with a normal chest radiograph and a nondiagnostic pulmonary arteriogram.[2,3,6] Progressive pulmonary hypertension is typical. Treatment is usually unsuccessful.[6] In our patient 1, a correct presumptive diagnosis was made based upon the clinical picture and the exclusion of large-artery thromboembolism by arteriography. Cytologic examination of pulmonary venous blood withdrawn through a wedged pulmonary artery catheter can be diagnostic,[7] as was the case in the second patient.

Small artery tumor emboli should be considered whenever a patient with a known malignancy presents

From the Clinical Trials and Cardiology and Pathology Branches, National Heart, Lung, and Blood Institute, and the Critical Care Medicine Department, National Institutes of Health, Bethesda, Maryland 20892. Manuscript received December 31, 1992, and accepted February 6, 1993.

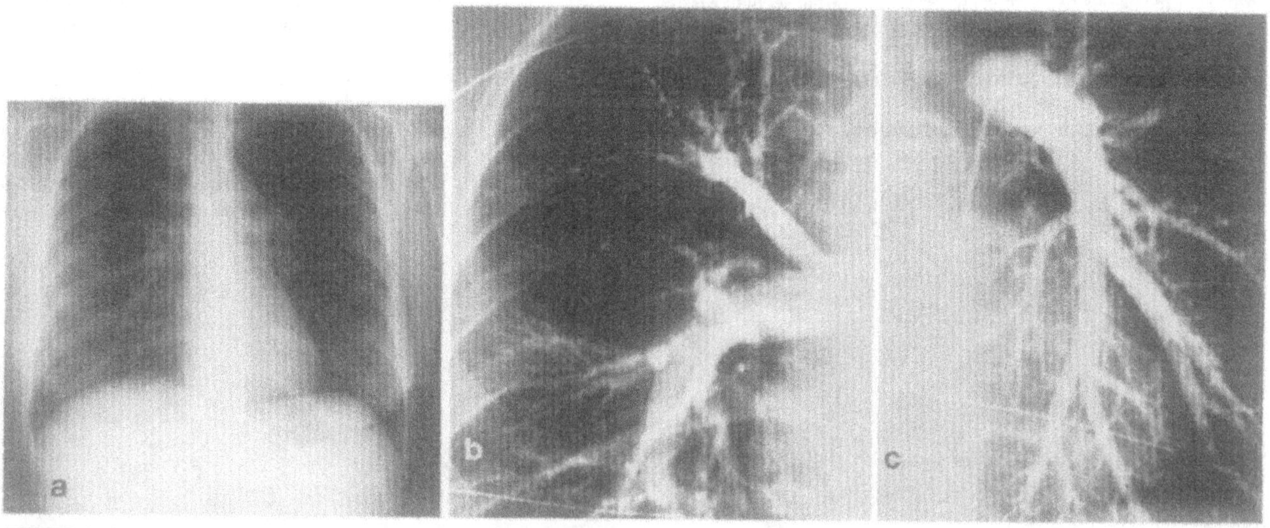

FIGURE 1. Case 1. Posteroanterior chest radiograph and pulmonary arteriograms. The chest radiograph *(a)*, obtained 2 days before death, is normal. No filling defects are seen on right *(b)* or left *(c)* pulmonary arteriograms obtained 1 day before death.

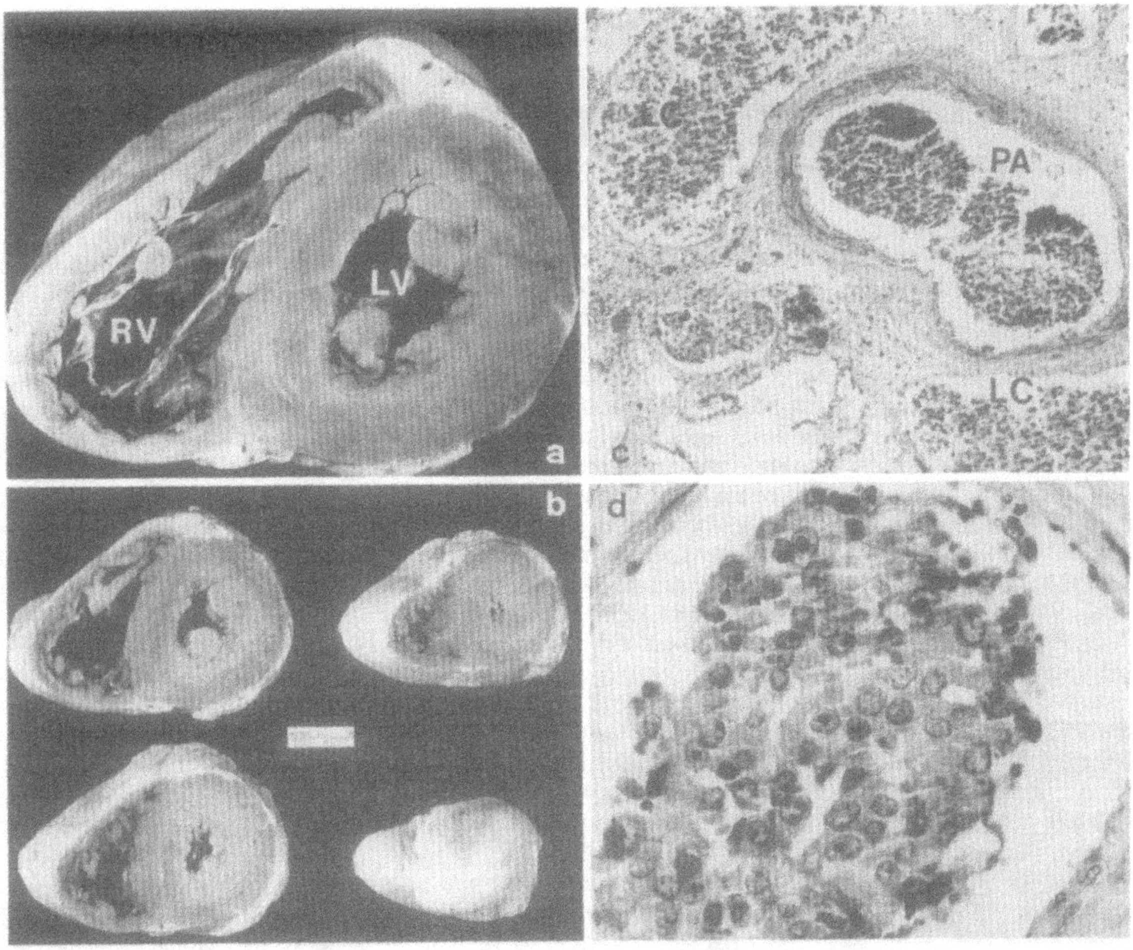

FIGURE 2. Case 1. Transverse cuts of the cardiac ventricles *(a and b)* showing a dilated right ventricle (RV) and a normal-sized left ventricle (LV). Microscopic sections of the lung show tumor emboli in *(c and d)* small pulmonary arteries (PA) and metastatic tumor in *(c)* lymphatic channels (LC). Hematoxylin-eosin stain × 100 *(c)*; Movat stain × 630 *(d)*; both reduced by 29%.

with progressive, unexplained dyspnea or pulmonary hypertension. Cytology of pulmonary venous blood may be diagnostic and antineoplastic therapy may be useful.

1. Kane RD, Hawkins HK, Miller JA, Noce PS. Microscopic pulmonary tumor emboli associated with dyspnea. *Cancer* 1975;36:1473–1482.
2. Marini JJ, Bilnoski W, Huseby JS. Acute cor pulmonale resulting from tumor microembolism. *West J Med* 1980;132:77–80.
3. Schriner RW, Ryu JH, Edwards WD. Microscopic pulmonary tumor embolism causing subacute cor pulmonale: a difficult antemortem diagnosis. *Mayo Clin Proc* 1991;66:143–148.
4. von Herbay A, Illes A, Waldherr R, Otto HF. Pulmonary tumor thrombotic microangiopathy with pulmonary hypertension. *Cancer* 1990;66:587–592.
5. Scully RE, ed. Case records of the Massachusetts General Hospital: case 30-1987. *N Engl J Med* 1987;317:225–235.
6. Altemus L, Lee R. Carcinomatosis of the lung with pulmonary hypertension: pathoradiologic spectrum. *Arch Intern Med* 1967;119:32–38.
7. Masson RG, Krikorian J, Lukl P, Evans GL, McGrath J. Pulmonary microvascular cytology in the diagnosis of lymphangitic carcinomatosis. *N Engl J Med* 1989; 321:71–76.

Are Autopsies Still Useful? Thank Goodness We Didn't Know. Not All Tumors Are Bad Tumors. Most of the Cavity Has to be Filled Before Trouble Occurs

An 80-year-old white woman fractured her hip and femur 5 days before a fatal pulmonary embolus. She was obese but never had symptoms of myocardial ischemia or cardiac dysfunction. Necropsy disclosed a myxoma attached to all of the fossa ovalis of the atrial septum and to a portion of the endocardium on the left atrial aspect of the septum both cephalad and caudal to the fossa ovalis (color figure below). The myxoma itself contained focal calcific deposits (radiograph in upper right of figure). Its caudal extension did not reach the level of the mitral annulus and therefore no "mitral" dysfunction resulted. The thickness of the atrial septum cephalad to the fossa measured just over 2.0 cm in maximal thickness due to heavy deposition of adipose tissue. The heart weighed 380 g. Large amounts of adipose tissue, primarily in the subepicardium, caused the heart to float in water. The coronary arteries were insignificantly narrowed and no lesions were present in the myocardial walls.

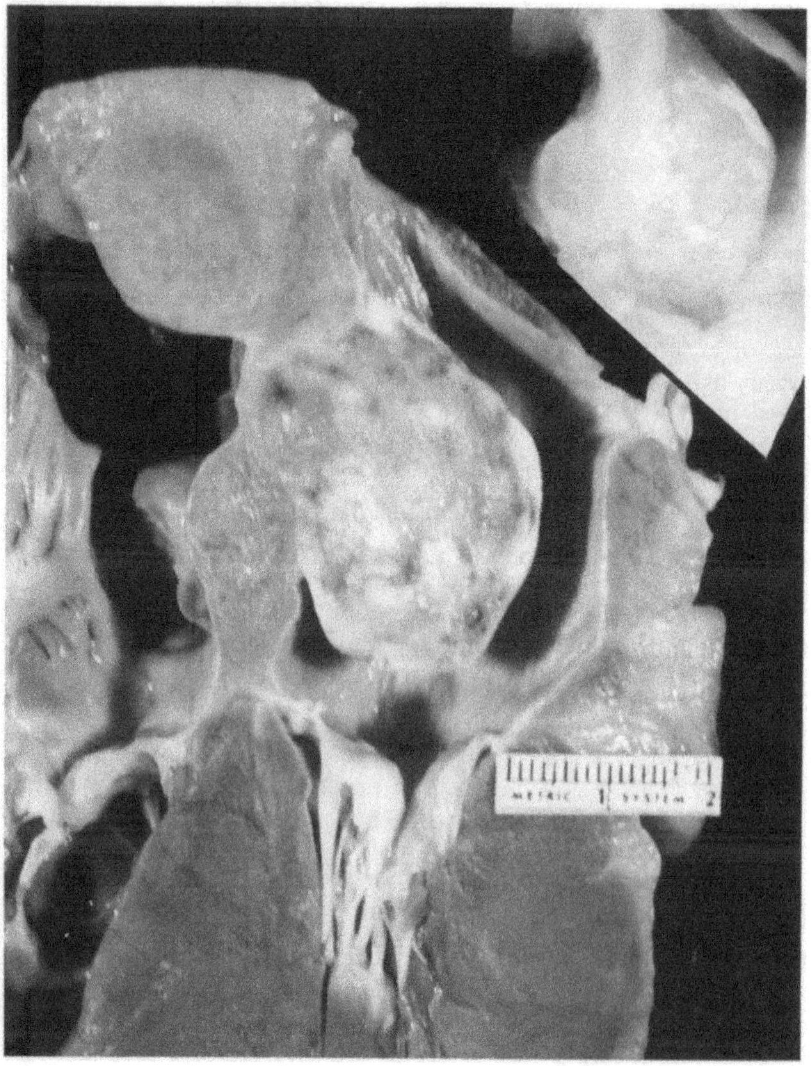

Conclusions: (1) Not all left atrial myxomas produce symptoms of cardiac dysfunction. (2) Not all myxomas are attached exclusively to the fossa ovale region of the atrial septum and therefore not all myxomas are attached to atrial septum by a small stalk. (3) The larger the site of attachment of the myxoma to the atrial septum, the shorter the extent of movement by the tumor during either phase of the cardiac cycle, and if the extent of the movement is short, mitral obstruction is infrequent. (4) The more extensive the calcific deposits within a myxoma, the older the tumor, but the amount of calcium correlates poorly with the size of the tumor. (5) Not all cardiac tumors require operative intervention. (6) Although most cardiac myxomas now are diagnosed by echocardiogram, a significant percent still are found for the first time only at necropsy.

Jamshid Shirani, MD
Richmond, Virginia
Jeffrey M. Isner, MD
Boston, Massachusetts
William C. Roberts, MD
Dallas, Texas
11 February 1993

Epicardial lipoma

Jamshid Shirani, MD,* and William C. Roberts, MD**
Bethesda, Md.

A 63-year-old man died of carcinoma of the pancreas. At necropsy the heart weighed 360 gm and was normal except for excessive subepicardial adipose tissue and a brownish 0.9 × 0.5 × 0.5 cm nodule weighing 0.5 gm attached by a stalk to the epicardial adipose tissue between the pulmonary trunk and the left atrial appendage (Fig. 1). The nodule consisted of mature fat cells surrounded by a fibrous tissue covering. Cardiac lipomas are rare. Approximately 25% arise from the epicardium.[1] All reported cardiac lipomas have been clinically silent. They, of course, need to be distinguished from other epicardial nodules such as aberrant thyroid glandular tissue.[2]

From the Pathology Branch, National Heart, Lung, and Blood Institute, National Institutes of Health, Bethesda.

*Present address: Division of Cardiology, Medical College of Virginia, Richmond.

**Present address: Baylor Cardiovascular Institute, 3500 Gaston Ave., Dallas, TX 75246.

AM HEART J 1993;126:1030.

0002-8703/93/$1.00 + .10 **4/4/48533**

REFERENCES

1. Harda K, Seki I, Kobayashi H, Okuni M, Sakurae I. Lipoma of the heart in a child. Clinical, echocardiographic, angiographic, and pathologic features. Jpn Heart J 1980;21:903-10.
2. Taylor MA, Bray M, Roberts WC. Aberrant thyroid gland attached to ascending aorta. Am J Cardiol 1986;57:708.

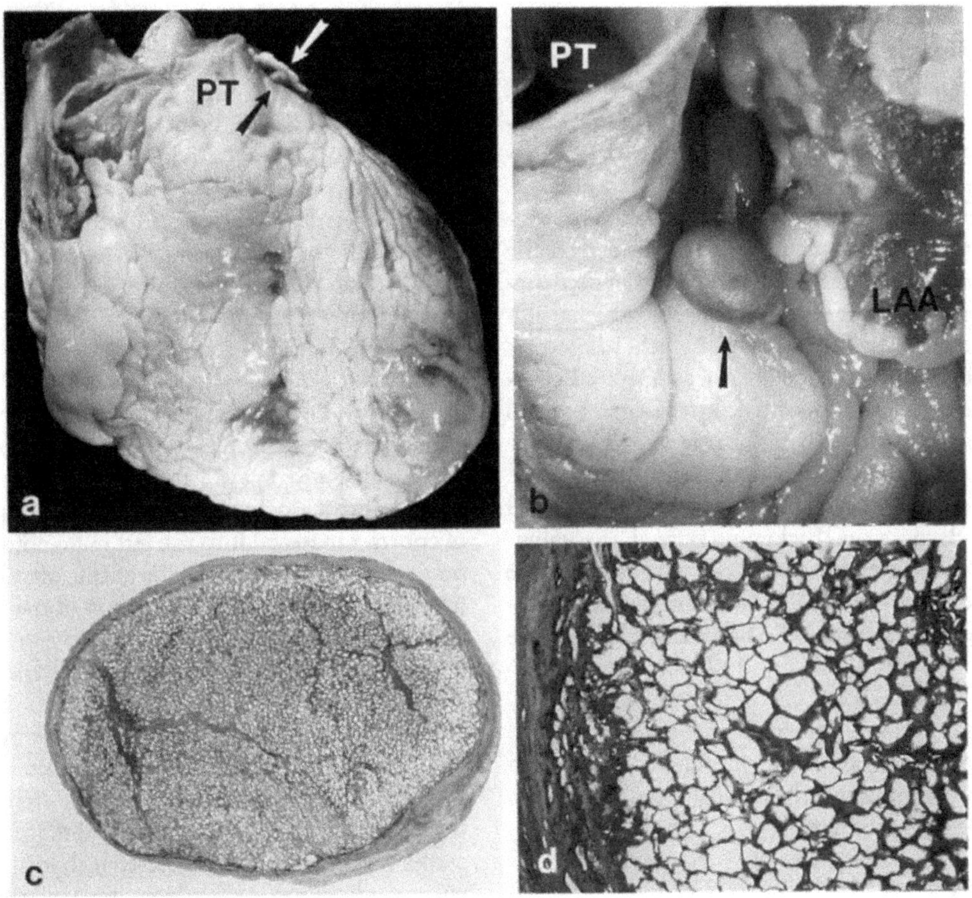

Fig. 1. Heart of 63-year-old man. **a,** View of anterior aspect of heart showing increased amounts of epicardial fat. *Arrows* point to lipoma. **b,** Close-up view of basal portion of anterior surface of heart showing lipoma *(arrow)* attached to epicardium by stalk between pulmonary trunk *(PT)* and left atrial appendage *(LAA)*. **c,** Histologic section of transected lipoma. Its outer portion consists of fibrous tissue. Interior consists of fat cells with some fibrous tissue strands. **d,** Higher power photomicrograph of lipoma with portion of its fibrous capsule. Movat stains, original magnification ×2.5 **(c)**, original magnification ×100 **(d)**.

Radiation-induced cardiovascular disease including stenosis of coronary ostium, coronary and carotid arteries, and aortic valve

Leigh Anne C. Harvey, MD, *Pathology Resident*; Samuel J. DeMaio, MD, *Cardiology Division*; and William C. Roberts, MD, *Baylor Cardiovascular Institute*

Clinical and necropsy findings are described in a 42-year-old man who received mediastinal irradiation (about 40 Gy) for Hodgkin's disease when he was 24 years old. He subsequently developed virtually every cardiovascular manifestation of radiation heart disease, including constrictive pericardial disease, complete occlusion of the ostium of a coronary artery, severe narrowing of the right coronary artery and of both carotid arteries, complete heart block (infranodal), hemodynamically confirmed aortic valve stenosis, and transmural right ventricular infarction.

Before the 1940s, the heart was considered a "radioresistant" organ. With the introduction of megavoltage radiotherapy for treatment of neoplasms, it became apparent that the heart could indeed be damaged by high-dose radiation, and numerous reports have documented such damage. The portion of the heart most frequently affected is the pericardium, the visceral and parietal aspects of which may eventually become thickened and adherent and cause myocardial constriction (1–4). The coronary arteries reside in the subepicardial adipose tissue; their lumens may be narrowed by atherosclerotic plaques, the development of which is greatly accelerated by irradiation. The myocardial wall frequently contains an increased amount of fibrous tissue, but usually no grossly visible myocardial lesions are seen in patients with radiation heart disease. Mural and valvular endocardium typically is focally thickened by fibrous tissue (4). Because the thickening is focal, the valvular involvement generally does not cause valvular dysfunction; if dysfunction does occur, it usually is pure regurgitation. Recently, we studied a man at necropsy who had received large-dose mediastinal irradiation 18 years earlier and 17 years later had hemodynamically demonstrated aortic valve stenosis, complete occlusion of a coronary ostium, coronary and carotid arterial stenosis, and other evidences of radiation-induced damage to vascular structures. A description of the extensive damage in this patient is the purpose of this report.

CASE DESCRIPTION

W.P., a 42-year-old white man who died on May 17, 1993, was well until age 24 years (1975) when he was found to have Hodgkin's disease, stage IA, with large supraclavicular and mediastinal lymph nodes. Following splenectomy he received approximately 40 Gy of irradiation to the upper mediastinum, lower neck, and axillary areas ("upper mantle"). At age 29 (1980), he developed clinical evidence of constrictive pericardial disease and underwent "total" pericardiectomy. The symptoms of cardiac dysfunction were relieved by this procedure.

He was then well until age 40 (April 1991, 25 months before death) when he developed respiratory symptoms, and pulmonary function tests disclosed evidence of both restrictive and obstructive pulmonary disease. During the next 2 years, he also had recurring acute pulmonary infections (cytomegalovirus, *Pseudomonas*) and pleural effusions. In April 1992, he had the first of several episodes of syncope. Examination in August 1992 disclosed a grade 3/6 harsh systolic murmur and a grade 2/6 blowing diastolic murmur over the precordium, loudest in the basal area. Echocardiogram disclosed thickening of the cusps of both mitral and aortic valves with poor mobility of the aortic valve cusps. Electrocardiogram showed sinus rhythm and complete right bundle branch block and later, complete heart block.

Cardiac catheterization on September 30, 1992, disclosed the following pressures in mm Hg: pulmonary artery, 19/10; right ventricle, 23/3; right atrium, mean 9; pulmonary arterial wedge, mean 6; left ventricle, 124/13; and aorta, 87/52, yielding on pullback of the catheter a peak systolic pressure gradient of 37 mm Hg between the left ventricle and aorta. The calculated aortic valve area was 1.2 cm^2 and the valve index, 0.59 cm^2/m^2. By left ventriculogram, the ejection fraction was 64%. Injection of contrast material into the left main coronary artery disclosed no narrowing of this artery or of the left anterior descending or left circumflex arteries The ostium of the right coronary artery could not be cannulated.

On October 1, 1992, an electrophysiologic study disclosed atrioventricular nodal block distal to the atrioventricular bundle. Wenckebach block occurred at atrial pacing with a cycle length of 490 milliseconds, and 2:1 block occurred at a cycle length of 470 milliseconds. Extra stimuli in the right ventricular outflow tract readily induced sustained monomorphic ventricular tachycardia that was easily terminated by burst pacing. An automatic pacer cardioverter-defibrillator was implanted.

The patient returned home and was treated daily with furosemide and enalapril. He remained in satisfactory condition until early May 1993, when a pacemaker lead was noted to have fractured. Following insertion of a new lead 7 days before death, he developed recurrent and progressive pulmonary insufficiency, his heart rate slowed, and he was found unresponsive in electromechanical dissociation.

Between September 28 and November 3, 1992, the serum total cholesterol was measured on at least 6 different occasions and ranged from 66 to 164 mg/dL (mean 121, median 129).

MORPHOLOGIC FINDINGS

At necropsy, the pleural spaces contained large, loculated effusions; the lungs were focally but extensively fibrotic; and histologic sections were compatible with chronic radiation pneumonitis. The epicardium was adherent by fibrous tissue to the surrounding structures. The heart weighed 420 g. Both atria were moderately dilated, and both ventricles were mildly dilated. The leaflets of all 4 cardiac valves were thickened by fibrous tissue, the mitral and aortic valves far more than the right-sided valves, and both left-sided valves also contained calcific deposits. The aortic valve cusps contained heavy calcific deposits on their aortic aspects; 1 cusp was made totally immobile by the deposits and was fixed in a ventricular diastolic position, and the mobility of the other 2 cusps also was limited (*Figure 1*). The adventitia of the sinus and proximal tubular portions of ascending aorta was severely thickened by dense, fibrous tissue, as was the adventitia about the arteries arising from the aortic arch (*Figure 2*). The

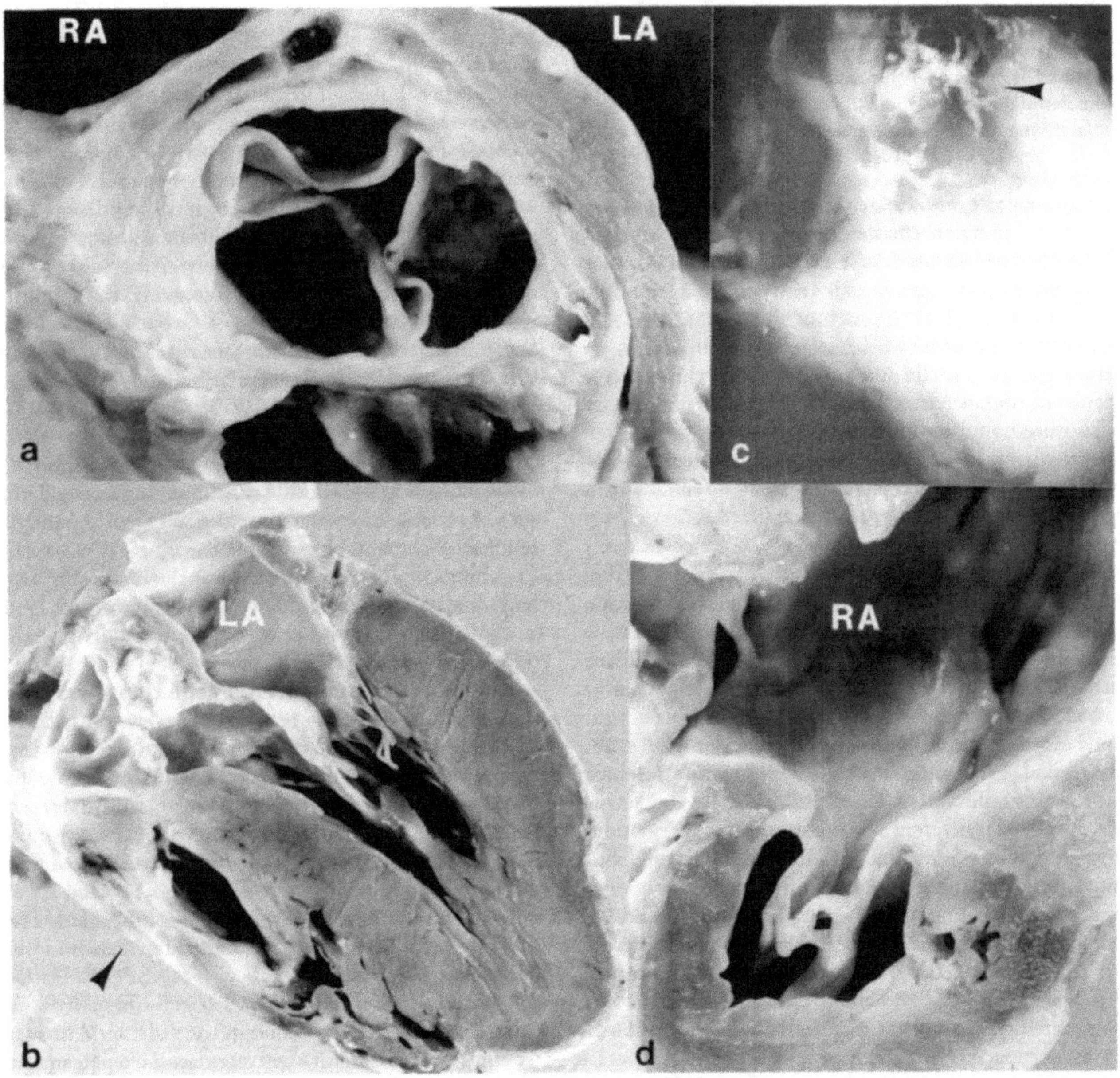

Figure 1. Photographs of the heart in the patient described. (**a**) Aortic valve from above. The cusps are thickened by fibrous tissue, and calcific deposits are present on the aortic aspects. LA = left atrial cavity, RA = right atrial cavity. (**b**) Long axis view showing the calcific deposits in the aortic valve. The arrow points to the right ventricular wall in the outflow tract, which is essentially replaced by fibrous tissue. (**c**) Radiograph of the heart showing heavy calcific deposits in the aortic valve cusps and also calcium at the posteromedial commissure area of the mitral valve. (**d**) Thickened tricuspid valve cusps and thickened mural endocardium of both right ventricle and right atrium.

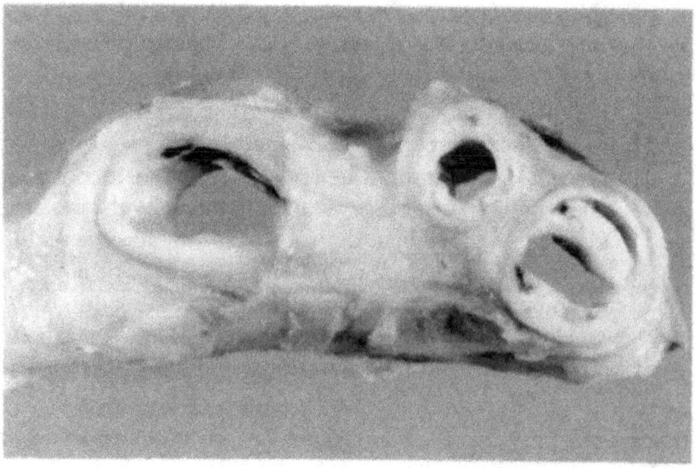

Figure 2. Great arteries arising from the aortic arch. The innominate artery is on the left and the left subclavian is on the right. All 3 contain atherosclerotic plaque. Doppler echocardiogram had shown considerable narrowing of both carotid arteries.

ostium of the right coronary artery was totally occluded by plaque. Small calcific deposits were present locally in all major epicardial coronary arteries. The lumen of the right coronary artery proximally was virtually totally occluded by plaque, and the left anterior descending coronary artery was narrowed up to 75% in cross-sectional area by plaque. Histologically, the adventitia of the major epicardial coronary arteries was thickened severely by dense fibrous tissue. No grossly visible foci of fibrosis or necrosis were noted in the left ventricular free wall or ventricular septum; in contrast, portions of the right ventricular wall, in its outflow tract, were completely replaced by fibrous tissue (*Figure 1*).

DISCUSSION

The heretofore described patient had evidence of radiation-induced heart disease. He had Hodgkin's disease at age 24 and received high doses of radiation to the mediastinum, including the heart. Five years later, he developed constrictive pericardial disease, and 17 years later, he developed a severe degree of heart block and hemodynamically confirmed aortic valve stenosis. At necropsy, he had typical morphologic features of radiation heart disease, including obliterative fibrous pericardial disease; fibrous replacement of the right ventricular wall (in its outflow tract) without grossly visible fibrosis of the left ventricular wall; obliteration of the aortic ostium of the right coronary artery; severe narrowing by plaque of the right coronary artery, with severe and extensive adventitial fibrosis (not a feature of atherosclerotic coronary artery disease) of all epicardial coronary arteries and thoracic aorta; focal fibrous thickening of the mural endocardium of the right atrium and right ventricle; and thickening of the valve cusps, particularly those of the aortic and mitral valves.

Hancock and associates (5) recently analyzed 2232 patients treated for Hodgkin's disease at Stanford University Medical Center, 2001 (90%) of whom had received mediastinal irradiation and 79% of whom had received doses of 40 Gy or more to the mediastinum. Of the 2232 patients, 88 (4%) died of heart disease: mode of death was acute myocardial infarction in 42 (48%), sudden coronary death (outside the hospital) in 13 (15%), ischemic cardiomyopathy in 11 (12%), radiation-induced pericardial disease in 14 (16%), valvular heart disease in 7 (8%), and doxorubicin-induced cardiomyopathy in 1 patient (1%). Of the 7 patients with valvular heart disease, 2 had infective endocarditis, 1 had a congenital valve abnormality, and 3 had aortic valve replacement. None of the 7 patients with valvular heart disease had a necropsy; or if so, the findings were not described, and therefore it is unclear if the valvular involvement was related to irradiation. The average interval between treatment for Hodgkin's disease and death from acute myocardial infarction or sudden unexpected cardiac arrest was 10.3 years (at an average age of 49 years), and from other types of cardiac disease, 11.3 years (at an average age of 51 years). The younger the patient at the time of radiation treatment, the greater was the risk of developing cardiac disease.

A number of case reports have described valvular abnormalities detected clinically many years after mediastinal irradiation, usually for Hodgkin's disease. In the 1991 publication by Carlson and associates (6), 35 previously reported cases (7–19) with valvular abnormalities were tabulated, and 3 additional patients were described (6). Subsequently, Suzuki and colleagues (20) reported an additional case. Of the total of 39 patients, 11 patients had echocardiographic evidence of thickening of the mitral (7 patients) or aortic valve (3 patients), or both (1 patient), without apparent valvular dysfunction; 6 patients had evidence of mitral regurgitation, 4 of aortic regurgitation, and 4 of both; 11 patients had evidence of aortic valve stenosis, including 5 with associated mitral regurgitation; 2 patients had pulmonic valve stenosis; and 1 had subpulmonic stenosis. None of the 39 patients had clinical evidence of mitral stenosis, and only 1 was reported to have associated tricuspid regurgitation. Seven of the 39 patients had attempted or actual replacement of the mitral (1 patient) or aortic (5 patients) valves, or both (1 patient), and 6 of these 7 patients had some degree of aortic valve stenosis (6, 11, 15, 17, 18).

Although narrowing of the major epicardial coronary arteries is a well-recognized complication of mediastinal irradiation, severe stenosis or total occlusion of a coronary ostium by this process, as occurred in our patient, is less recognized. Pilliere and colleagues (21) tabulated 11 reported patients with single coronary ostial stenosis following mediastinal radiotherapy, and at least 2 such patients with bilateral coronary ostial stenosis have been reported (22, 23). Orzan and associates (24) performed coronary angiography late after mediastinal irradiation in 15 patients, and 10 had evidence of coronary ostial stenosis, 9 of whom also had extensive involvement of other cardiac structures. Only 8 of the 15 patients had clinical evidence of myocardial ischemia.

Although myocardial lesions, usually interstitial myocardial fibrosis, are a recognized consequence of high-dose mediastinal irradiation, transmural right ventricular replacement fibrosis (right ventricular infarction), as occurred in our patient, has not been described previously as a consequence of this process.

High degrees of atrioventricular block, as occurred in our patient, are uncommon consequences of mediastinal irradiation. Orzan and associates (25) described 4 patients aged 31 to 46 years who developed complete heart block 13 to 20 years after therapeutic mediastinal irradiation for Hodgkin's disease. They also tabulated 18 previously reported patients with complete heart block from the same mechanism. Of these 18 patients, 11 were under 50 years of age when the complete heart block appeared, as occurred in our patient. The level of the atrioventricular block was infranodal in all but 2 patients with complete heart block. All patients with atrioventricular block of a high degree had other recognized consequences of radiation heart disease.

References

1. Cohn KE, Stewart JR, Fajardo LF, Hancock EW: Heart disease following radiation. *Medicine* 1967;46:281–298.
2. Fajardo LF, Stewart JR, Cohn KE: Morphology of radiation-induced heart disease. *Arch Pathol* 1968;86:512–519.
3. Ruckdeschel JC, Chang P, Martin RG, Byhardt RW, O'Connell MJ, Sutherland JC, Wiernik PH: Radiation-related pericardial effusions in patients with Hodgkin's disease. *Medicine* 1975;54:245–259.
4. Brosius FC III, Waller BF, Roberts WC: Radiation heart disease: analysis of 16 young (aged 15 to 33 years) necropsy patients who received over 3500 rads to the heart. *Am J Med* 1981;70:519–530.
5. Hancock SL, Tucker MA, Hoppe RT: Factors affecting late mortality from heart disease after treatment of Hodgkin's disease. *JAMA* 1993;270:1949–1955.
6. Carlson RG, Mayfield WR, Normann S, Alexander JA. Radiation-associated valvular disease. *Chest* 1991;99:538–545.
7. Stewart JR, Cohn KE, Fajardo LF, Hancock EW, Kaplan HS: Radiation-induced heart disease: a study of 25 patients. *Radiology* 1967;89:302–310.
8. Steinberg I: Effusive-constrictive radiation pericarditis: two cases illustrating value of angiocardiography in diagnosis. *Am J Cardiol* 1967;19:434–439.
9. Morton DL, Glancy DL, Joseph WL, Adkins PC: Management of patients with radiation-induced pericarditis with effusion: a note on the development of aortic regurgitation in two of them. *Chest* 1973;64:291–297.
10. Fouchard J, Joly J, Rousseau J, Herreman F: Pericardite constrictive et myocardite post-radiotherapique avec: insuffisance mitrale. *Semaine des Hopitaux* 1978;54:1283–1287.
11. Warda M, Khan A, Massumi A, Mathur V, Klima T, Hall RJ: Radiation-induced valvular dysfunction. *J Am Coll Cardiol* 1983;2:180–185.
12. Detrano RC, Yiannikas J, Salcedo EE: Two-dimensional echocardiographic assessment of radiation-induced valvular heart disease. *Am Heart J* 1984; 107:584–585.
13. Perrault DJ, Levy M, Herman JD, Burns BJ, Bar Schlomo BZ, Drunk MN, Wu WQ, McLaughlin PR, Gilbert BW: Echocardiographic abnormalities following cardiac radiation. *J Clin Oncol* 1985;3:546–551.
14. Pohjola-Sintonen S, Totterman K-J, Salmo M, Siltanen P: Late cardiac effects of mediastinal radiotherapy in patients with Hodgkin's disease. *Cancer* 1987;60:31–37.
15. Lederman GS, Sheldon TA, Chaffey JT, Herman TS, Gelman RS, Coleman CN: Cardiac disease after mediastinal irradiation for seminoma. *Cancer* 1987;60:772–776.
16. Moncure AC, Mark EJ: A 38-year-old woman with a history of radiation treatment for a malignant tumor in the right hemithorax and persistent chest pain and pleural abnormality. *N Engl J Med* 1987;316:1075–1083.
17. McEniery PT, Dorosti K, Schiavone WA, Pedrick TJ, Sheldon WC: Clinical and angiographic features of coronary artery disease after chest irradiation. *Am J Cardiol* 1987;60:1020–1024.
18. Hancock SL, Hoppe RT, Horning SJ, Rosenberg SA: Intercurrent death after Hodgkin disease therapy in radiotherapy and adjuvant MOPP trials. *Ann Intern Med* 1988;109:183–189.
19. Mauch P, Tarbell N, Weinstein H, Silver B, Goffman T, Osteen R, Zajac A, Coleman CN, Canellos G, Rosenthal D: Stage IA and IIA supradiaphragmatic Hodgkin's disease: prognostic factors in surgically staged patients treated with mantle and paraaortic irradiation. *J Clin Oncol* 1988; 6:1576–1583.
20. Suzuki M, Hamada M, Matsumoto Y, Hiwada K, Osuka Y. Aortic valvular disease and right coronary artery stenosis induced by mediastinal irradiation: report of a case. *Japanese Circ J* 1993;57:467–471.
21. Pillière R, Luquel L, Brun D, Jault F, Gandjbakhch I, Bourdarias JP: Ostial stenosis of the left main coronary artery after mediastinal radiotherapy: a case report. *Arch Mal Coeur Vaiss* 1991;84:869–872.
22. Deloche A, Bellin J, Hennetier J, Carpentier A: Post-irradiation coronary ostial stenosis treated by bilateral ostial endarterectomy. *Presse Med* 1987; 16:780–781.
23. Stegaru-Hellring B, Keller H, Bode G, Usadel KM, Wallwork J: Ostium stenosis of both coronary arteries and latent hypothyroidism as sequelae of radiotherapy in Hodgkin disease. *Z Kardiol* 1985;74:458–488.
24. Orzan F, Brusca A, Conte MR, Presbitero P, Figliomeni MC: Severe coronary artery disease after radiation therapy of the chest and mediastinum: clinical presentation and treatment. *Br Heart J* 1993;69:496–500.
25. Orzan F, Brusca A, Gaita F, Giustetto C, Figliomeni MC, Libero L: Associated cardiac lesions in patients with radiation-induced complete heart block. *Int J Cardiol* 1993;39:151–156.

A Unique Heart Disease Associated With a Unique Cancer: Carcinoid Heart Disease

LOCATION OF THE CARCINOID PRIMARY TUMOR

Carcinoid tumors are never primary in the heart and they infrequently metastasize to the heart. Nevertheless, patients with *ileal* carcinoid, the location of the primary tumor in nearly all patients who develop the carcinoid syndrome (flushing and diarrhea), when hepatic metastases are present, often develop distinctive lesions in the heart, always located in the right side of the heart, and occasionally also on the left side of the heart[1–3] (Figure 1). Patients with carcinoid tumor primary in the *ovary* associated with carcinoid heart disease are extremely rare, but in this circumstance typical carcinoid cardiac lesions may develop unassociated with hepatic carcinoid metastases, because the venous drainage from the ovaries is into the inferior vena cava.[4,5] When the primary carcinoid tumor arises in a pulmonary *bronchus*, the carcinoid lesions may be limited to the left-sided cardiac valves. In this circumstance, the liver may be devoid of carcinoid metastases. If hepatic carcinoid metastases are present and if carcinoid heart disease occurs, the distinctive fibrous lesions always involve the right side of the heart with or without involvement of one or both left-sided valves.

MORPHOLOGIC CHARACTERISTICS OF THE CARCINOID CARDIAC LESIONS

The distinctive carcinoid cardiac lesions consist of deposits of fibrous tissue *devoid of elastic fibers* on the ventricular aspect of the tricuspid valve leaflets and on the arterial aspect of the pulmonic valve cusps.[1–3,6] Occasionally, deposits also are seen on the ventricular aspects of the mitral leaflets and, very rarely and usually to a small extent, on the aortic aspects of the aortic valve cusps. Most patients with carcinoid heart disease have the distinctive fibrous lesions limited to the right side of the heart. Much less often, patients with right-sided lesions also have similar lesions on the left side of the heart, but in this circumstance the left-sided lesions are always smaller and of no functional significance. In the setting of bronchial carcinoid, the mitral valve lesions, however, may be so extensive that mitral stenosis has been a consequence, and right-sided carcinoid lesions may be absent.

COMPARISON OF CARCINOID SYNDROME PATIENTS WITH AND WITHOUT CARCINOID HEART DISEASE

Ross and Roberts[3] studied at necropsy 36 patients with the carcinoid syndrome, 21 (57%) of whom did and 15 (43%) of whom did not have carcinoid heart disease. The 2 groups were similar in mean age (54 vs 55 years), duration of clinical illness (4.7 vs 6.3 years), body weight (50 vs 52 kg), systemic blood pressure (117/77 vs 128/77 mm Hg), blood hematocrit (37% vs 36%), total serum protein (6.0 g/dl), and serum albumin (2.2 vs 2.6 g/dl). The 2 groups were significantly different in the frequency of the presence of precordial murmurs consistent with tricuspid regurgitation and/or pulmonic stenosis (95% vs 13%), cardiomegaly by chest radiography (38% vs 0), low voltage on electrocardiogram (47% vs 0), and location of the primary site of the carcinoid tumor. Total 12-lead electrocardiographic QRS voltage[3] was similar in each group (105 vs 132 mm) (10 mm = 1 mV). Of the patients with carcinoid heart disease, 43% died of cardiac causes; in contrast, none of those without carcinoid heart disease died of cardiac causes. Of the 21 subjects with carcinoid heart disease, 7 had left-sided cardiac involvement, but in none was it of functional significance. Thus, although carcinoid heart disease frequently is the cause of death in patients with the carcinoid syndrome, the development of carcinoid heart disease appears to be unrelated to the duration of symptoms of the carcinoid syndrome.

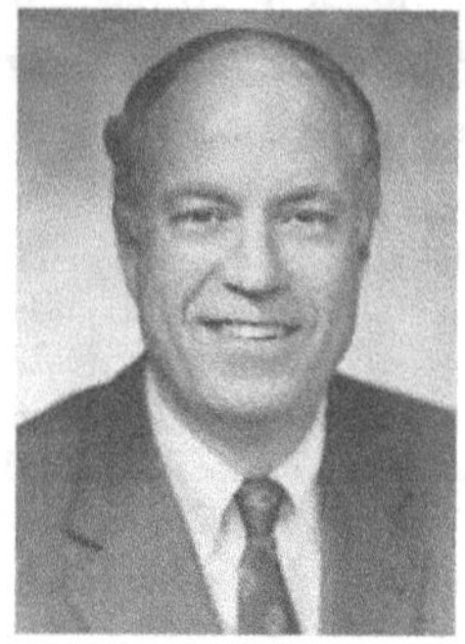

Clinical diagnosis of carcinoid heart disease can usually be established by noninvasive means. *Auscultation*, of course, is the first clue. In 20 (95%) of the 21 subjects studied by Ross and Roberts[3] with carcinoid heart disease and in 5 (33%) of the 15 subjects without carcinoid heart disease, 1 or more precordial murmurs were recorded. Of the 20 subjects with precordial murmurs and carcinoid heart disease, 8 had both systolic and diastolic murmurs and 12 had only systolic murmurs; of the 5 subjects with precordial murmurs but without carcinoid heart disease, the murmurs in all were systolic only. Thus, nearly all patients with carcinoid heart disease have precordial murmurs, and when the murmur has a diastolic component, diagnosis of carcinoid heart disease usually can be made with confidence.

The *systemic arterial blood pressure* is not helpful in either diagnosing carcinoid syndrome or distinguishing those with from those without carcinoid heart disease. Only 3 of the 36 subjects studied by Ross and Roberts[3] had indirect systolic systemic ar-

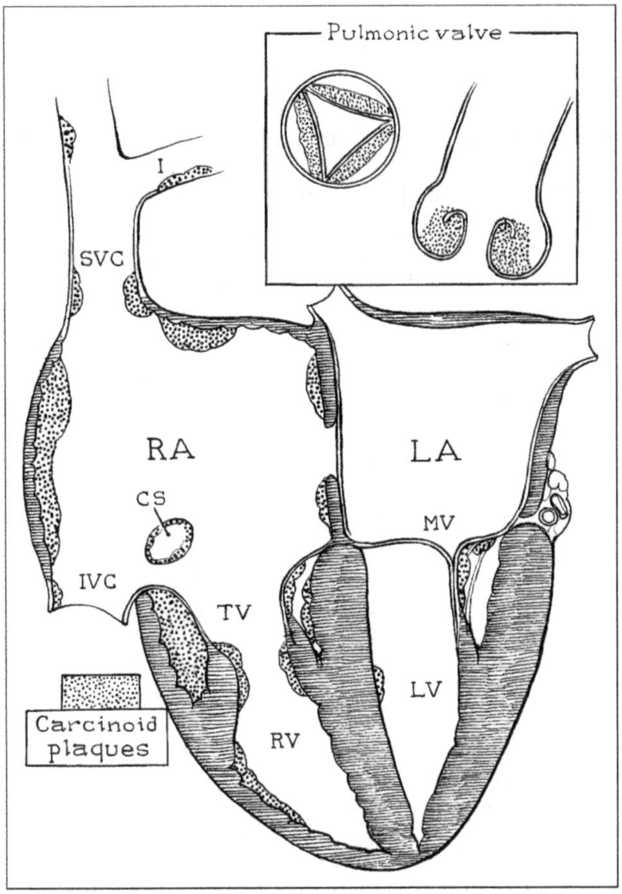

FIGURE 1. Diagram showing location of carcinoid fibrous plaques in *carcinoid heart disease.* CS = coronary sinus ostium; I = innominate vein; IVC = inferior vena cava; LA = left atrium; LV = left ventricle; MV = mitral valve; RA = right atrium; RV = right ventricle; SVC = superior vena cava; TV = tricuspid valve. Reproduced with permission from Ross EM and Roberts WC.[3]

terial pressures >140 mm Hg and/or diastolic arterial pressures >90 mm Hg: 1 of the 21 with and 2 of the 15 without carcinoid heart disease. The average peak systolic pressure was 117 mm Hg in the 21 subjects with and 128 mm Hg in the 15 subjects without carcinoid heart disease; the average diastolic pressure in both groups was 77 mm Hg.

Chest radiography is helpful in diagnosing carcinoid heart disease. The cardiothoracic ratio was >0.50 in 8 (38%) of the 21 subjects with carcinoid heart disease and in none of 15 subjects without carcinoid heart disease. Thus, the cardiothoracic ratio is not a very sensitive test for carcinoid heart disease, but it is specific.

The *resting electrocardiogram* is somewhat useful in distinguishing the subjects with from those without carcinoid heart disease. The sum of the QRS voltage in leads I, II, and III was ≤15 mm in 9 of the 21 subjects studied by Ross and Roberts[3] with and in none of the 15 subjects without carcinoid heart disease. The sum of the total 12-lead QRS voltage ranged from 58 to 227 mm (10 mm = 1 mV) in 34 subjects, and the mean values were not significantly different between the 2 groups (105 vs 132 mm) (normal >175 mm).[7] Evidence of right ventricular hypertrophy was rare. The R wave was greater than the S wave in either leads V_1 or V_2 in only 4 of the 19 subjects with and in none of the 15 subjects without carcinoid heart disease. Despite right atrial dilatation in the subjects with carcinoid heart disease, all 19 with and all 15 without carcinoid heart disease had sinus rhythm. The R-R interval was normal (≤0.20 seconds) in 18 of 19 subjects with and in 14 of 15 subjects without carcinoid heart disease. The width of the QRS complex was normal (≤0.12 second) in all subjects, irrespective of whether or not they had carcinoid heart disease. Thus, other than the higher frequency of low voltage in the subjects with carcinoid heart disease, the electrocardiogram was not helpful in distinguishing subjects with from those without carcinoid heart disease.

MORPHOLOGIC FEATURES OF CARCINOID HEART DISEASE

All of the 21 patients with carcinoid heart disease studied by Ross and Roberts[3] had involvement of both tricuspid and pulmonic valves by carcinoid plaques, and 19 of them also had carcinoid plaques on the mural endocardium of the right atrium and usually also on the mural endocardium of the right ventricle. The number of subjects with right-sided valvular dysfunction as a consequence of the carcinoid plaques on the valvular leaflets is less certain because of the relative difficulty in diagnosing by auscultation mild degrees of tricuspid and pulmonic valve dysfunction. In 2 of the 21 subjects with right-sided carcinoid heart disease, the degree of morphologic involvement of both valves was minimal and valvular function clearly was not affected. Of the remaining 19 subjects, 18 had precordial systolic and/or diastolic murmurs of grade 2/6 or greater intensity.

Although the composition and location of the carcinoid plaques on both right-sided cardiac valves are similar, the functional consequences of the carcinoid plaques are different. The deposits occur nearly entirely on the downstream side of the valvular leaflets, i.e., on the ventricular aspects of the septal and posterior tricuspid leaflets and on the pulmonary arterial side of the pulmonic valve cusps. On the anterior tricuspid valve leaflet, the deposits can be on both sides. The consequences of the "downstream" deposition is an adherence of the leaflet to the underlying mural endocardium (tricuspid septal and posterior leaflets) or to the underlying pulmonary arterial endothelium (pulmonic valve) via the carcinoid plaques. The fibrous tissue of the carcinoid plaque acts as a constricting substance such that the "ring" of both right-sided cardiac valves is made smaller than normal and at the same time leaflet mobility is diminished. The consequence is tricuspid regurgitation with or without some degree of stenosis. Nearly all patients with pure tricuspid regurgitation (no element of stenosis) have dilated valve rings, but patients with some degree of stenosis in addition to regurgitation do not have dilated annuli. Patients with carcinoid heart disease follow this principle.

Thus, patients with carcinoid heart disease have much more tricuspid regurgitation than stenosis, but usually there is some degree of stenosis, albeit small.

In contrast to the tricuspid valve, the dominant functional pulmonic valve lesion is stenosis, although all patients with stenosis have some degree of pulmonic regurgitation. The reason for the difference — compared with the tricuspid valve — is that the orifice of the normal pulmonic valve is much smaller initially than the orifice of the tricuspid valve. Thus, the constriction by deposition of carcinoid plaques within the pulmonic sinuses causes constriction of the pulmonic root with the production of pulmonic stenosis. Because the distal portions of the pulmonic cusps are inverted toward the sinuses and the mobility of the cusps is lost, some degree of regurgitation is inevitable in these patients who have any degree of pulmonic stenosis.

Although combined lesions of both mitral and aortic valves are fairly common as a consequence of either rheumatic heart disease or infective endocarditis, or both, combined lesions of both tricuspid and pulmonic valves are rare, and carcinoid is the only condition in which uniformly both — not just 1 — right-sided valves are involved. The 2 dominant functional consequences of right-sided carcinoid heart disease are pulmonic stenosis and tricuspid regurgitation. These 2 lesions in the same patient are particularly unfavorable because the pulmonic stenosis increases the degree of tricuspid regurgitation. A commonly employed method of producing chronic congestive heart failure in experimental animals is by banding the pulmonary trunk to create pulmonic stenosis, and excising or destroying 1 or more tricuspid valve cusps to make the valve purely regurgitant. Thus, right-sided carcinoid heart disease in essence creates this experimental model. If a patient with carcinoid heart disease had only dysfunction of the pulmonic or the tricuspid valve, probably the functional consequence would be insignificant. It is the combination of both right-sided valvular lesions — namely pulmonic stenosis and tricuspid regurgitation — that has the potential of being devastating.

ECHOCARDIOGRAPHIC FEATURES OF CARCINOID HEART DISEASE

Echocardiography, particularly cross-sectional, is helpful in diagnosing carcinoid heart disease. Callahan and associates[8] described retrospectively echocardiographic features in 20 patients with the carcinoid syndrome. By physical examination, 15 patients had a diagnosis of carcinoid heart disease and the other 5 did not. Both M-mode and cross-sectional echocardiographic examinations in the latter 5 patients disclosed no abnormal findings. Of the 15 patients with auscultatory evidence of carcinoid heart disease, 5 had normal M-mode and cross-sectional echocardiographic findings. The other 10, all of whom had tricuspid regurgitation by physical examination, had dilated right ventricular cavities, abnormal motion of the ventricular septum, and of the 9 in whom the tricuspid valve leaflets were visualized by cross-sectional echocardiography, strikingly abnormal tricuspid leaflets (thickened and retracted with fixed orifice). The pulmonic valve cusps were not visualized in any patient by M-mode echocardiography, but in the 4 in whom they were visualized by cross-sectional echocardiography, the pulmonic valve cusps were abnormal in each.

Howard and associates[9] prospectively examined by cross-sectional echocardiography 14 patients with the carcinoid syndrome, and 8 had definite abnormalities of 1 or both right-sided cardiac valves. Clinically, 7 had auscultatory evidence of tricuspid regurgitation including 1 with a diastolic rumble, and 5 of them had diffusely thickened and retracted tricuspid valve leaflets; the other 9 patients had normal tricuspid valves by echocardiography. Four patients by auscultation had evidence of pulmonic stenosis with or without pulmonic regurgitation. The pulmonic valve cusps were visualized by echocardiogram in 7 patients: 2 had retracted pulmonic cusps with decreased systolic motion (1 of whom had pulmonic stenosis by auscultation) and 5 had normal cusps (none of whom had auscultatory evidence of pulmonic stenosis).

Transesophageal echocardiography has proved to be more useful than transthoracic echocardiography for diagnosis of carcinoid heart disease. Lundin and associates[10] detected by the transesophageal approach tricuspid regurgitation in 22 (71%) of 31 patients with ileal carcinoid versus 18 (57%) by the transthoracic investigation. The transesophageal images allowed measurement of the thicknesses of the atrioventricular valve leaflets, and also the inner layer of the right atrial walls. The mean thicknesses of the anterior tricuspid leaflets were significantly greater than that of the anterior mitral leaflets, a difference not seen in controls. The patients with functional signs of severe carcinoid heart disease had significantly thicker mean right atrial inner layers than did those with less or no signs of right-sided cardiac disease.

Doppler echocardiography also has proved useful for diagnosis of carcinoid heart disease. Pellikka and colleagues[11] studied by echocardiogram 132 patients with the carcinoid syndrome and found that 74 (56%) had echocardiographic, including Doppler, features of carcinoid heart disease: 72 patients (97%) had shortened and thickened tricuspid valve leaflets; all 74 (100%) had Doppler evidence of tricuspid regurgitation (moderate or severe in 62 [90%]). Severe tricuspid regurgitation was characterized by a dagger-shaped Doppler spectral profile with an early peak pressure and rapid decline. The pressure half time was prolonged, a finding consistent with associated tricuspid valve stenosis. The pulmonic valve cusps were thickened, retracted, and immobile in 36 patients (59%) and the valve was so small that it could not be visualized in an additional 29 patients (39%). Of the 47 patients who had Doppler examination of the pulmonic valve, regurgitation was found in 38 (81%) and stenosis was present in 25

(53%). Left-sided valvular involvement was present in 5 patients (7%), 4 of whom had a patent foramen ovale or carcinoid metastases in the lung. Myocardial carcinoid tumor metastases were found in 3 (4%) of the 74 patients. Small pericardial effusions were present in 10 patients (14%). The patients with and without echocardiographic evidence of carcinoid heart disease did not differ with regard to sex, age, location of the primary tumor, duration of symptoms, or signs of the carcinoid syndrome (dermal flushing, diarrhea). Dyspnea was more frequent in those with than in those without carcinoid heart disease (54% vs 27%). Precordial murmurs were more frequent in those with than in those without carcinoid heart disease (92% vs 43%). Three-year survival of patients with compared to those without echocardiographic evidence of carcinoid heart disease was reduced (31% vs 68%).

MAGNETIC RESONANCE IMAGING AND COMPUTED TOMOGRAPHY IN CARCINOID HEART DISEASE

Magnetic resonance imaging and *computed tomography* also may be helpful in diagnosing carcinoid heart disease.[12] Although the findings usually simply corroborate those seen by echocardiography, supplemental information occasionally is supplied.

SERUM AND URINE TESTS IN CARCINOID HEART DISEASE

Measurement of circulating *serotonin* (5-hydroxytryptamine) or its principal metabolite, *5-hydroxyindole acetic acid* (5-HIAA), of course, is helpful in diagnosing the carcinoid syndrome, but it may not be helpful in differentiating the patients with and without carcinoid heart disease.[13] Roberts and Sjoerdsma[1] in their early (1964) study of 17 necropsy patients with the carcinoid syndrome, 9 with and 8 without carcinoid heart disease, found no significant difference in the urinary levels of 5-HIAA in those patients with and in those without carcinoid heart disease. More recently (1989), Himelman and Schiller[14] found higher peak levels of urinary 5-HIAA in their 17 patients with echocardiographic evidence of carcinoid heart disease and more severe hepatic dysfunction than in their 13 patients without carcinoid heart disease (331 ± 231 mg vs 58 ± 78 mg). Lundin and associates[15] studied 68 patients with proven mid-gut carcinoid tumors, 50 of whom had the carcinoid syndrome. Of the 68 patients, 61 (89%) had elevated urinary 5-HIAA levels. The 18 patients with advanced right-sided valve disease had significantly higher mean 5-HIAA urinary levels than did the patients without right-sided lesions or functionally insignficant ones (800 vs 210 μmol/day). Pellikka and associates[11] also observed higher levels of urinary 5-HIAA in their 74 patients with echocardiographic evidence of carcinoid heart disease than in their 58 patients without evidence of heart disease but with the carcinoid syndrome (270 vs 131 mg/day). The study by Robiolio et al,[16] utilizing the Duke Carcinoid Database of 604 patients with carcinoid tumors, found both plasma serotonin (1,130 vs 426 pmol/ml) and urinary 5-HIAA (219 vs 55 mg/day) strikingly higher in the 19 patients with proven carcinoid heart disease than in the 585 patients with carcinoid tumors (only some of whom had the carcinoid syndrome [flushing and diarrhea] but no carcinoid heart disease). Flushing and diarrhea was almost 3 times more common in patients with carcinoid heart disease than in those without the characteristic cardiac disease.

Other circulating substances have been found to be elevated in patients with carcinoid heart disease. Lundin and associates[15] found, for example, significantly higher plasma levels of *tachykinins neuropeptide K* and *substance P* in their patients with ileal carcinoid tumors with the most severe right-sided heart disease. Lundin and colleagues[17] found significantly higher plasma *atrial natriuretic peptide levels* in their patients with ileal carcinoid tumors with the most severe right-sided heart disease.

HEMODYNAMIC AND ANGIOGRAPHIC OBSERVATIONS IN CARCINOID HEART DISEASE

There are surprisingly few reported hemodynamic and angiographic observations in patients with carcinoid heart disease. Biörck and colleagues[18] in 1952 described a boy with "unusual cyanosis . . . with pulmonary stenosis and tricuspid insufficiency" who died shortly after injection of contrast material into the right ventricular cavity. Schwaber and Lukas[19] in 1962 described "hyperkinemia" associated with considerable cardiac failure in a patient with the carcinoid syndrome without associated carcinoid heart disease. Of the 17 necropsy patients with carcinoid heart disease described by Roberts and Sjoerdsma[1] in 1964, none had had cardiac catheterization performed, and of the 36 patients with carcinoid syndrome reported in 1986 by Ross and Roberts,[3] only 3 had had cardiac catheterization and 2 of them had been reported earlier by Roberts and colleagues.[2] In each of their 2 patients the right atrial pressures were quite high; the a-wave was 24 and the v-wave 34 mm Hg in 1 patient and 18 and 23 mm Hg, respectively, in the other patient. The latter patient had a right ventricular pressure of 45/13 mm Hg and a pulmonary arterial pressure of 20/8 mm Hg with a normal cardiac index (3.2 L/min/m^2). Each of the 2 patients had extensive right atrial carcinoid deposits. The authors suggested that the right atrial plaques make this chamber relatively inelastic and consequently not able to distend or to contract normally. This reduction in right atrial elasticity or distensibility significantly alters the hemodynamic findings in the right atrial pulse. Thus, in each of the 2 patients there was a greater elevation in right atrial pressures than would have been expected from the sizes of the tricuspid valve orifices observed at necropsy. These authors speculated that even mild tricuspid valve carcinoid disease might produce significant elevation of right atrial pressures because of associated right atrial carcinoid plaques, whereas an equal degree of rheumatic tricuspid disease might not cause right atrial hypertension.

More hemodynamic information was reported when valve replacement or valvuloplasty became a more common form of therapy in carcinoid heart disease. The degree of both tricuspid valve stenosis and pulmonic valve stenosis in patients with carcinoid heart disease appears to be rather small. The mean diastolic gradient between right atrium and right ventricle is usually <10 mm Hg, and the peak systolic pressure gradient between right ventricle and pulmonary trunk is nearly always <50 mm Hg, the latter, of course, being far less than that in the usual patient with congenital pulmonic valve stenosis. Because carcinoid involvement of both the tricuspid and pulmonic valves causes the cusps to retract toward their margins of attachment, the valvular orifices become fixed in an open position, which necessitates some degree of regurgitation of each valve. Because the tricuspid valve ring is initially much larger than the pulmonic valve "ring," similar degrees of deposition of carcinoid plaques on each of these 2 valve leaflets results in very different hemodynamic consequences. Stenosis is the major hemodynamic lesion involving the pulmonic valve, and regurgitation is the major hemodynamic lesion involving the tricuspid valve. The combination of pulmonic stenosis and tricuspid regurgitation is a very unfavorable hemodynamic combination because the former worsens the latter.

OPERATIVE TREATMENT OF CARCINOID HEART DISEASE

Cardiac valve replacement and/or *valvuloplasty* has been performed in some patients with carcinoid heart disease since 1963.[20] Most reports have been single case studies and these were reviewed by Ross and Roberts[3] up to 1985. In 1990 Lundin and associates[21] replaced both tricuspid and pulmonic valves with tissue valves in 4 patients: 1 died 5 days postoperatively and the other 3 were free of evidence of cardiac dysfunction 10, 12, and 38 months postoperatively. These authors also summarized outcomes in 25 previously reported patients having cardiac valve replacement for carcinoid heart disease. Knott-Craig and colleagues[22] reported results of mechanical valve replacement of the tricuspid valve in 10 patients combined with pulmonic valvectomy in 9 and pulmonic valve replacement (homograft) in 1: 4 patients died early and the remaining 6 were alive at 4, 4, 4, 7, 24, and 46 months postoperatively. These authors also reviewed 28 previously reported patients who had had tricuspid valve replacement for carcinoid heart disease. There was no significant difference in survival of patients with a bioprosthesis versus a mechanical prosthesis in the tricuspid valve position. For the entire group of 38 patients having tricuspid valve replacement for carcinoid heart disease, the 4-year survival was 48 ± 13%.

Connolly and colleagues[23] reported 26 patients having cardiac valve replacement for carcinoid heart disease and compared results with those in 40 patients with the carcinoid syndrome not having a cardiac operation. Nine patients (35%) died in the early postoperative period: of the 17 survivors, 8 were alive at a mean follow-up of 28 months and each of the 8 were symptomatically improved. The only predictor of operative mortality was low voltage (sum of QRS in I, II, and III ≤15 mm) on the preoperative electrocardiogram. Predictors of late survival included a lower preoperative urinary 5-HIAA level. And finally, Robiolio and associates[24] using the Duke Carcinoid Database, described results of bioprosthetic replacement of the tricuspid valve in 8 patients (2 also had open pulmonic valvuloplasty): 5 died within 30 days of the operation; 2 of the 3 survivors lived >10 years. Review of their 8 patients and 39 previously published valve replacement cases for carcinoid heart disease disclosed a 30-day mortality of 56% for patients >60 years of age and zero for those ≤60 years of age. Thus, although valve replacement may afford prolonged palliation for carcinoid heart disease, it is associated with a significant mortality risk.

A potential danger in using a bioprosthesis or any type of tissue valve for valve replacement in a patient with carcinoid heart disease is involvement of the bioprosthetic cusps by the same characteristic carcinoid fibrotic process that affected the native valves. Schoen and colleagues[25] described at necropsy typical carcinoid plaques on the cusps of the bioprosthesis in the tricuspid valve position, although bioprosthetic function at this time appeared to have been normal. Ridker and associates[26] described a patient who had replacement of the tricuspid valve with a porcine bioprosthesis and pulmonic valvulotomy, and when studied 11 years later had a stenotic (10 mm Hg mean diastolic gradient) bioprosthesis in the tricuspid valve position. The bioprosthesis was excised at reoperation and its cusps were thickened by both calcific deposits and typical carcinoid fibrous plaques. Ohri and colleagues[27] described typical carcinoid plaques that had developed on the cusps of a cryopreserved allograft which had been used to replace a native pulmonic valve only 3 months earlier because of carcinoid involvement. The patient continued to have pulmonary hypertension postoperatively and soon after operation developed pulmonic regurgitation which progressively worsened.

Balloon valvulotomy also has been performed in patients with carcinoid heart disease, and the results are mixed. Grant et al[28] reported 2 patients and each had balloon dilatation of stenotic pulmonic valves resulting from carcinoid heart disease. One patient had symptomatic benefit for 2 months and the other had no improvement. Onate and associates[29] performed balloon valvuloplasty of both tricuspid and pulmonic valves in 2 patients: 1 was not improved and the second became asymptomatic. Hargreaves and colleagues[30] described successful balloon dilatation of the pulmonic valve resulting from carcinoid heart disease.

William C. Roberts

William Clifford Roberts, MD
Editor in Chief
Baylor University Medical Center
Dallas, Texas 75246

1. Roberts WC, Sjoerdsma A. The cardiac disease associated with carcinoid syndrome (carcinoid heart disease). *Am J Med* 1964;36:5–34.
2. Roberts WC, Mason DT, Wright LD Jr. The non-distensible right atrium of carcinoid disease of the heart, *Am J Clin Pathol* 1965;44:627–631.
3. Ross EM, Roberts WC. The carcinoid syndrome: comparison of 21 necropsy subjects with carcinoid heart disease to 15 necropsy subjects without carcinoid heart disease. *Am J Med* 1986;79:339–354.
4. Oei SG, Kloosterman MD, Verhoeven ATHM. Primary ovarian carcinoid tumor in combination with carcinoid heart disease: a case report, *Eur J Obstet Gyn Reprod Biol* 1989;31:185–188.
5. Wilkowske MA, Hartmann LC, Mullany CJ, Behrenbeck T, Kvols LK. Progressive carcinoid heart disease after resection of primary ovarian carcinoid. *Cancer* 1994;73:1889–1991.
6. Ferrans VJ, Roberts WC. The carcinoid endocardial plaque. An ultrastructural study. *Human Pathol* 1976;7:387–409.
7. Odom H II, Davis JL, Dinh H, Baker BJ, Roberts WC, Murphy ML. QRS voltage measurements in autopsied men free of cardiopulmonary disease: a basis for evaluating total QRS voltage as an index of left ventricular hypertrophy. *Am J Cardiol* 1986;58:801–804.
8. Callahan JA, Wroblewski EM, Reeder GS, Edwards WD, Seward JB, Tajik AJ. Echocardiographic features of carcinoid heart disease. *Am J Cardiol* 1982;50:762–768.
9. Howard RJ, Drobac M, Rider WD, Keane TJ, Finlayson J, Silver MD, Wigle ED, Rakowski H. Carcinoid heart disease: diagnosis by two-dimensional echocardiography. *Circulation* 1982;66:1059–1065.
10. Lundin L, Landelius J, Andren B, Oberg K. Transesophageal echocardiography improves the diagnostic value of cardiac ultrasound in patients with carcinoid heart disease. *Br Heart J* 1990;64:190–194.
11. Pellikka PA, Tajik AJ, Khandheria BK, Seward JB, Callahan JA, Pitot HC, Kvols LK. Carcinoid heart disease. Clinical and echocardiographic spectrum in 74 patients. *Circulation* 1993;87:1188–1196.
12. Mirowitz SA, Gutierrez FR. MR and CT diagnosis of carcinoid heart disease. *Chest* 1993;103:630–631.
13. Oates JA. The carcinoid syndrome. *N Engl J Med* 1986;315:702–704.
14. Himelman RB, Schiller NB. Clinical and echocardiographic comparison of patients with the carcinoid syndrome with and without carcinoid heart disease. *Am J Cardiol* 1989;63:347–352.
15. Lundin L, Norheim I, Landelius J, Öberg K, Theodorsson-Norheim E. Carcinoid heart disease: relationship of circulating vasoactive substances to ultrasound-detectable cardiac abnormalities, *Circulation* 1988;77:264–269.
16. Ribiolio PA, Rigolin VH, Wilson JS, Harrison JK, Sanders LL, Bashore TM, Feldman JM. Carcinoid heart disease. Correlation of high serotonin levels with valvular abnormalities detected by cardiac catheterization and echocardiography. *Circulation* 1995;92:790–795.
17. Lundin L, Öberg K, Landelius J, Hansson HE, Wilander E, Theordorsson E. Plasma atrial natriuretic peptide in carcinoid heart disease, *Am J Cardiol* 1989;63:969–972.
18. Biörck G, Axen O, Thorson A. Unusual cyanosis in a boy with congenital pulmonary stenosis and tricuspid insufficiency. Fatal outcome after angiocardiography. *Am Heart J* 1952;44:143–148.
19. Schwaber JR, Lukas DS. Hyperkinemia and cardiac failure in the carcinoid syndrome, *Am J Med* 1962;32:846–853.
20. Wright PW, Mulder DG. Carcinoid heart disease. Report of a case treated by open heart surgery. *Am J Cardiol* 1963;12:864–868.
21. Lundin L, Hansson H-E, Landelius J, Öberg K. Surgical treatment of carcinoid heart disease. *J Thorac Cardiovasc Surg* 1990;100:552–561.
22. Knott-Craig CJ, Schaff HV, Mullany CJ, Kvols LK, Moertel CG, Edwards WD, Danielson GK. Carcinoid disease of the heart. Surgical management of ten patients. *J Thorac Cardiovasc Surg* 1992;104:475–481.
23. Connolly HM, Nishimura RA, Smith HC, Pellikka PA, Mullany CJ, Kvols LK. Outcome of cardiac surgery for carcinoid heart disease. *J Am Coll Cardiol* 1995;25:410–416.
24. Robiolio PA, Rigolin VH, Harrison JK, Lowe JE, Moore JO, Bashore TM, Feldman JM. Predictors of outcome of tricuspid valve replacement in carcinoid heart disease. *Am J Cardiol* 1995;75:485–488.
25. Schoen FJ, Hausner RJ, Howell JF, Beazley HL, Titus JL. Porcine heterograft valve replacement in carcinoid heart disease. *J Thorac Cardiovasc Surg* 1981;81:100–105.
26. Ridker PM, Chertow GM, Karlson EW, Neish AS, Schoen FJ. Bioprosthetic tricuspid valve stenosis associated with extensive plaque deposition in carcinoid heart disease. *Am Heart J* 1991;121:1835–1838.
27. Ohri SK, Schofield JB, Hodgson H, Oakley CM, Keogh BE. Carcinoid heart disease: early failure of an allograft valve replacement. *Ann Thorac Surg* 1994;58:1161–1163.
28. Grant SCD, Scarffe JH, Levy RD, Brooks NH. Failure of balloon dilatation of the pulmonary valve in carcinoid pulmonary stenosis. *Br Heart J* 1992;67:450–453.
29. Onate A, Alcibar J, Inguanzo R, Pena N, Gochi R. Balloon dilatation of tricuspid and pulmonary valves in carcinoid heart disease. *Texas Heart Inst J* 1993;20:115–119.
30. Hargreaves AD, Pringle SD, Boon NA. Successful balloon dilatation of the pulmonary valve in carcinoid heart disease. *Intern J Cardiol* 1994;45:150–151.

Primary and Secondary Neoplasms of the Heart

In the last 40 years cardiac neoplasms have progressed from clinical curiosities described primarily in numerous case reports with diagnosis mainly at autopsy to fairly rapid antemortem diagnosis and frequent curative operative therapy. Diagnosis has been greatly facilitated by 2-dimensional echocardiography and, in select cases, the use of magnetic resonance imaging or computed tomography.

CLASSIFICATION

There is no perfect classification for cardiac neoplasms. Like any organ or tissue, neoplasms involving the heart may be primary or secondary. The primary ones may be benign or malignant and the secondary or metastatic ones are, by definition, malignant. The metastatic neoplasms are far more frequent than are the primary neoplasms by at least a 30 to 1 ratio.[1,2] The various frequencies of the primary benign and primary malignant tumors vary from report to report, approximately 0.1% to 0.3% in most autopsy series. A recent list of primary benign neoplasms gathered by investigators at the Armed Forces of Pathology is listed in Table I, and those primary malignant tumors encountered are listed in Table II.[3] The frequencies of the metastatic neoplasms also vary from report to report, but nearly all studies have listed carcinoma of the lung as the most commonly encountered metastatic tumor at autopsy followed by cancer of the breast, lymphoma, and leukemia (Table III). The order of frequency of metastases is different, however, if the frequency of each different type of tumor with metastasis to the heart is determined. For example, Table IV lists the frequencies of metastases to the heart in each of 100 cases of each of 20 separate tumors: melanoma has the highest frequency of metastases to the heart followed by malignant germ cell tumor, leukemia, lymphoma, cancer of the lung, and then the various sarcomas.[3]

LOCATION OF CARDIAC NEOPLASMS

Cardiac neoplasms may involve only the endocardium, only the myocardium, only the epicardium, or various combinations (Figure 1). By far the most common location of metastatic cardiac neoplasm is epicardium.[4] Neoplasms limited to parietal pericardium without extension into epicardium are not considered cardiac neoplasms. The epicardial tumor deposits may be multifocal or single, or they may be extensive and essentially diffuse or nearly so. Likewise, the intramyocardial masses may be focal or multifocal. The most common location for intramyocardial masses is left ventricular free wall and ventricular septum, portions of the heart, of course, with the greatest myocardial mass. The endocardial neoplasms are the intracavitary ones. They may involve a single cardiac cavity or >1. They may be limited to either the right or left side of the heart or they may involve both. It is the intracavitary tumors that produce obstruction to inflow into the heart or into a ventricular cavity or outflow from a ventricular cavity. The intracavitary neoplasms are the ones that may partially dislodge and produce either pulmonary or systemic emboli, or both. The intracavitary deposits are the ones with the potential of producing the triad of obstruction, embolization, and constitutional symptoms.

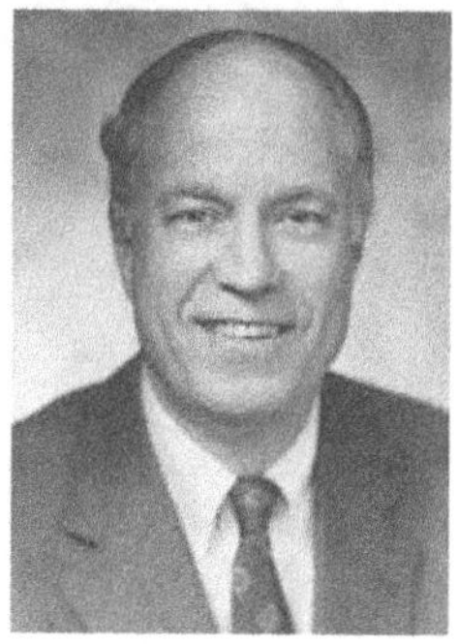

TABLE I Primary *Benign* Neoplasms of the Heart (1976–1993)*

Tumor†	Total	Surgical	Autopsy	Age ≤15 Years at Diagnosis
Myxoma	114	102	12	4
Rhabdomyoma	20	6	14	20
Fibroma	20	18	2	13
Hemangioma	17	10	7	2
Atrioventricular nodal	10	0	10	2
Granular-cell	4	0	4	0
Lipoma	2	2	0	0
Paraganglioma	2	2	0	0
Myocytic hamartoma	2	2	0	0
Histiocytoid cardiomyopathy	2	0	2	2
Inflammatory pseudotumor	2	2	0	1
Fibrous histiocytoma	1	0	1	0
Epitheloid hemangio-endothelioma	1	1	0	0
Bronchogenic cyst	1	1	0	0
Teratoma	1	0	1	1
Totals	199	146 (73%)	53 (27%)	45 (23%)

*Modified from: Burke A, Virmani R. Atlas of Tumor Pathology. Tumors of the Heart and Great Vessels. Washington, DC: Armed Forces Institute of Pathology 1996:231.

†Excludes papillary fibroelastoma and lipomatous hypertrophy of the atrial septum.

TABLE II Primary *Malignant* Tumors of the Heart (1976–1993)*

Tumor	Total	Surgical	Autopsy	Age ≤15 Years at Diagnosis
Sarcoma	137 (95%)	116	21	11 (8%)
Angio	33	22	11	1
Unclassified	33	30	3	3
Fibrous histiocytoma	16	16	0	1
Osteo	13	13	0	0
Leiomyo	12	11	1	1
Fibro	9	9	0	1
Myxo	8	8	0	1
Rhabdomyo	6	2	4	3
Synovial	4	4	0	0
Lipo	2	0	2	0
Schwannoma	1	1	0	0
Lymphoma	7 (5%)	1	6	0
Totals	144 (100%)	117 (81%)	27 (19%)	11 (8%)

*Modified from: Burke A, Virmani R. Atlas of Tumor Pathology. Tumors of the Heart and Great Vessels. Washington, DC: Armed Forces Institute of Pathology 1996:231.

TABLE III Metastatic Neoplasms in the Heart at Necropsy—Order of Frequency of Cancers Encountered*

Primary Tumor	Total Autopsies	Metastases to Heart
1. Lung	1,037	180 (17%)
2. Breast	685	70 (10%)
3. Lymphoma	392	67 (17%)
4. Leukemia	202	66 (33%)
5. Esophagus	294	37 (13%)
6. Uterus	451	36 (8%)
7. Melanoma	69	32 (46%)
8. Stomach	603	28 (5%)
9. Sarcoma	159	24 (15%)
10. Oral cavity & tongue	235	22 (9%)
11. Colon & rectum	440	22 (5%)
12. Kidney	114	12 (11%)
13. Thyroid gland	97	9 (9%)
14. Larynx	100	9 (9%)
15. Germ cell	21	8 (38%)
16. Urinary bladder	128	8 (6%)
17. Liver & biliary tract	325	7 (2%)
18. Prostate gland	171	6 (4%)
19. Pancreas	185	6 (3%)
20. Ovary	188	2 (1%)
21. Nose (interior)	32	1 (3%)
22. Pharynx	67	1 (1%)
23. Miscellaneous	245	0
	6,240	653 (10%)

*Modified from: Burke and Virmani (who combined studies of McAllister HA and Fenoglio JJ Jr). Tumors of the Cardiovascular System Atlas of Tumor Pathology. Washington, DC: Armed Forces Institute of Pathology 1978: 111–119; and Mukai K, Shinkai T, Tominaga K, Shomosato Y. The incidence of secondary tumors of the heart and pericardium: a 10-year study. *Jpn N Clin Oncol* 1988;18:195–201.

SPECIFIC BENIGN PRIMARY CARDIAC NEOPLASMS

Myxoma: Myxomas are by far the most common type of primary cardiac tumor and 75% of them are located in the left atrial cavity (Figure 2), about 23% in the right atrial cavity (Figure 3), and about 2% in a ventricular cavity.[4–16] On rare occasion, the tumor is present in more than 1 cavity.[17] Generally, the neoplasm when located in the left atrium produces symptoms when it reaches about 70 g in size. Those in the right atrium that produce symptoms are usually about twice as large and sometimes several-fold larger. The cell of origin of the myxoma is still unclear.[5] How fast atrial myxomas grow has never been clarified. An attempt to answer this question was provided by a

TABLE IV *Metastatic* Neoplasms in the Heart at Necropsy: Order of Frequency of Metastases of Each Different Primary Tumor

Primary Tumor	Number of Autopsies	Percentage With Metastases to Heart*
Melanoma	100	46%
Germ cell	100	38%
Leukemia	100	33%
Lymphoma	100	17%
Lung	100	17%
Sarcoma	100	15%
Esophagus	100	13%
Kidney	100	11%
Breast	100	10%
Mouth & tongue	100	9%
Thyroid gland	100	9%
Uterus	100	8%
Urinary bladder	100	6%
Stomach	100	5%
Colon & rectum	100	5%
Prostate gland	100	4%
Pancreas	100	3%
Nose (interior)	100	3%
Ovary	100	1%
Pharynx	100	1%
Miscellaneous	100	0

*These percentages were obtained by combining studies by McAllister and Fenoglio and by Mukai et al. (see Table III).

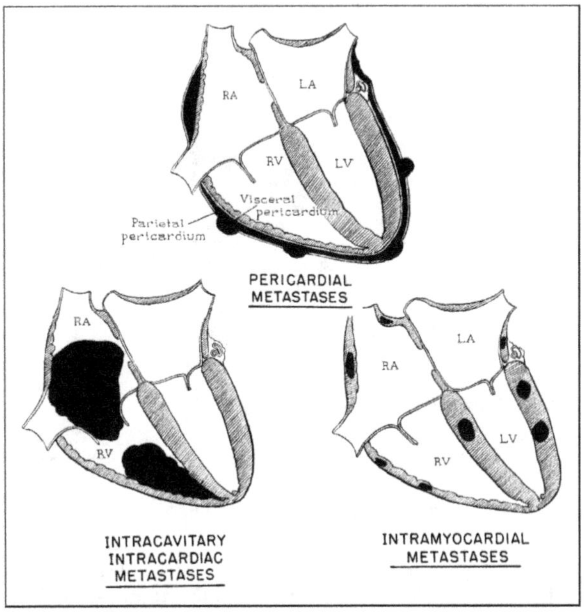

FIGURE 1. Diagram showing various locations of cardiac neoplasms involving the heart. LA = left atrium; LV = left ventricle; RA = right atrium; RV = right ventricle.

FIGURE 2. Clinically silent left atrial *myxoma* in a 60-year-old woman (A69-275) who died of metastatic carcinoid. The myxoma was not large enough to prolapse through the mitral orifice during ventricular diastole. *Left;* view from cephalad portion of the left atrium. *Center;* view of opened left atrium, mitral valve, and left ventricle. *Right;* longitudinal view showing attachment of the myxoma to the atrial septum by a relatively broad base. (Reproduced with permission from Ferrans VF and Roberts WC[5]).

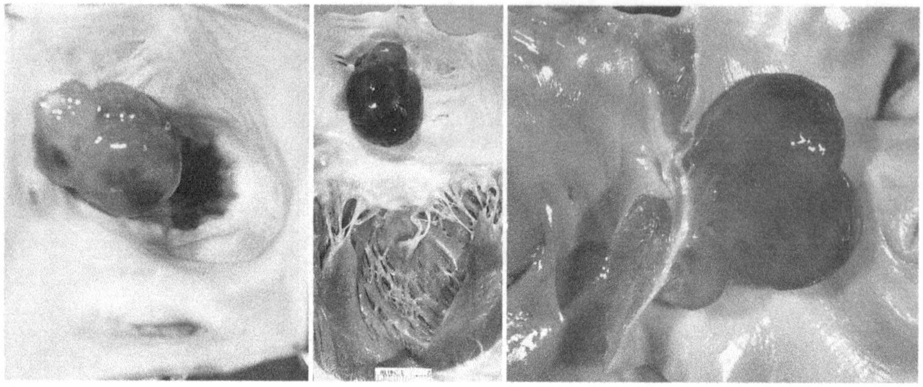

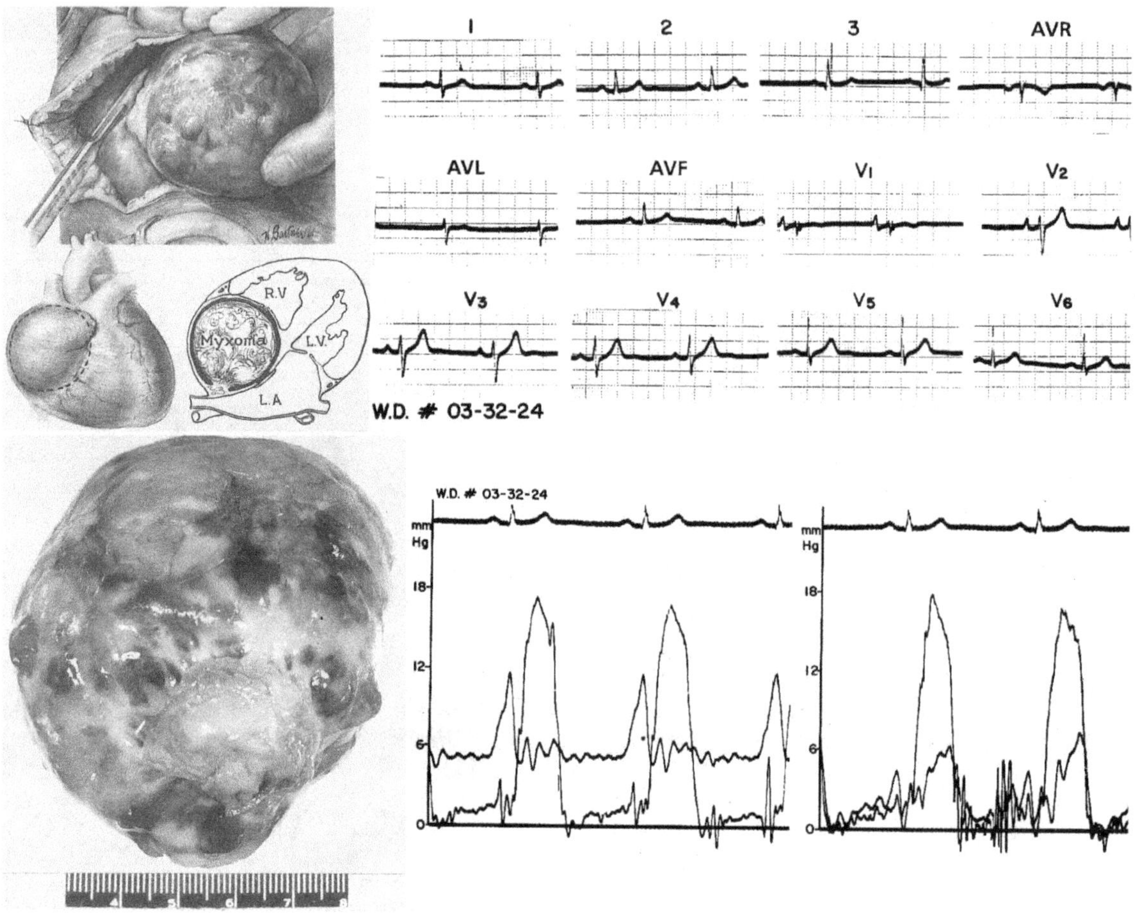

FIGURE 3. *Myxoma* excised from the right atrium from a 46-year-old man (S61-980) who had had evidence of cardiac dysfunction for 12 years. The tumor was attached to the atrial septum by a relatively small stalk (*lower left*). The myxoma weighed 142 g and its largest diameter was 8 cm. *Upper right;* electrocardiogram, Lower right; simultaneous right atrial and right ventricular pressure tracings before and after excision of the myxoma.

study that examined size of recurrent myxomas and divided that size in grams by the interval between the first operation and the second one.[18] It was estimated that recurrent left atrial myxomas grow on average of 0.15 cm/month or 1.8 cm/year, or an average of 1.2 g/month or 14 g/year. Whatever the exact growth rate may be, it appears that both recurrent and initial left atrial myxomas grow rather rapidly. Morphologic diagnosis of myxoma is readily made by gross inspection, and their appearance is clearly different from thrombi. The surface is smooth but irregular, shiney, and usually multicolored. Some contain calcific deposits, sometimes extensive ones, and those with calcific deposits appear to embolize very infrequently. The calcium may limit the growth potential of a myxoma. Attachment is nearly always to the atrial septum if the tumor is in the left atrium and the stalk is most commonly much smaller than the maximal diameter of the mass. On occasion, the site of attachment to the atrial septum is broad. The mean age of patients with sporadic myxoma is 56 years and 70% are women.

Familial cardiac myxomas constitute approxi-

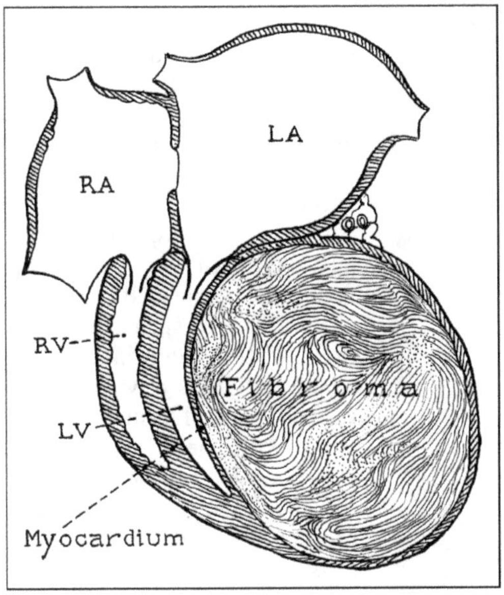

FIGURE 4. Diagram of an intramyocardial *fibroma* seen at necropsy in a 5-month-old boy (A-07-92) who was found dead in his crib. The neoplasm had been diagnosed by biopsy during the child's first few days of life. It was considered nonresectable.

mately 10% of all patients with myxomas and the transmission is an autosomal dominant one. The familial myxomas occur in younger patients (mean age 25) than the nonfamilial ones and they have less female gender predominance. The myxomas in the familial syndrome are much more liable (50% of the time) to be multiple and to have a ventricular cavity location (13% as compared with about 2% in the nonfamilial or sporadic patients with myxomas). These patients typically have exterior facial freckling; they have noncardiac myxomas (breast or skin) and also endocrine neoplasms. Both the NAME (nevi, atrial myxoma, neurofibromata, and ephelides) and the LAMB (lentigines, atrial myxoma, and balloon nevi) syndromes are associated with the familial variety of cardiac myxoma. Chromosomal abnormalities for atrial myxoma on chromosome 2 (Carney's) and chromosome 12 (Kiras-genes) have been described.

Myxomas probably present the most varied clinical picture of all primary cardiac neoplasms.[6,8,9] Several major syndromes have been observed including presentation with signs of emboli, obstruction to blood flow, and various constitutional syndromes. Fragments of tumor located in the right side of the heart may embolize to the lungs and those in the left side of the heart, of course, to various systemic organs. Diagnosis may be made on occasion by finding typical myxomatous endothelial-like cells which are elongated and spindle shaped with round or oval nuclei and prominent nucleoli in operatively removed emboli. Obstruction to blood flow may occur at the orifice of any valve, most commonly, of course, the mitral valve. Interference with flow through the mitral orifice may mimic signs of mitral stenosis, including signs of pulmonary congestion, diastolic apical rumble, opening snap, and accentuated first heart sounds. A murmur of mitral regurgitation may also be present as a result of chronic damage to the valve leaflets or to interference with proper closure of the valve by tumor. Differentiation between left atrial tumor and primary mitral stenosis is suggested by the influence of position on symptoms and on the intensity of the precordial murmurs and the opening snap.

The constitutional symptoms associated with atrial myxomas are protean and include fever, weight loss, Raynaud's phenomenon, digital clubbing, anemia, elevated erythrocyte sedimentation rate, elevated leuko-

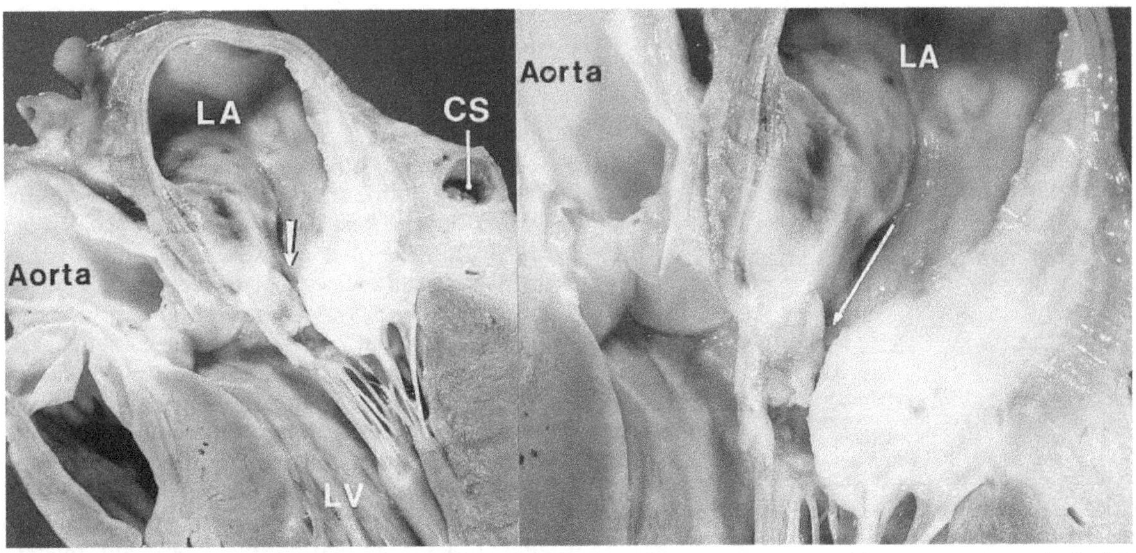

FIGURE 5. *Primary cardiac sarcoma,* undifferentiated type, causing mitral stenosis in a 46-year-old woman (A90-2) who had been well until 8 months before death. Cardiac catheterization disclosed a 20-mm Hg mean diastolic gradient between the pulmonary artery wedge position and left ventricle (LV). Right ventricular pressure was 105/18 mm Hg. The neoplasm is located in the walls of the left atrium (LA) and in both anterior and posterior mitral leaflets. The patient is described in detail elsewhere)[39] CS = coronary sinus. (Reproduced with permission from Domanski et al[39].)

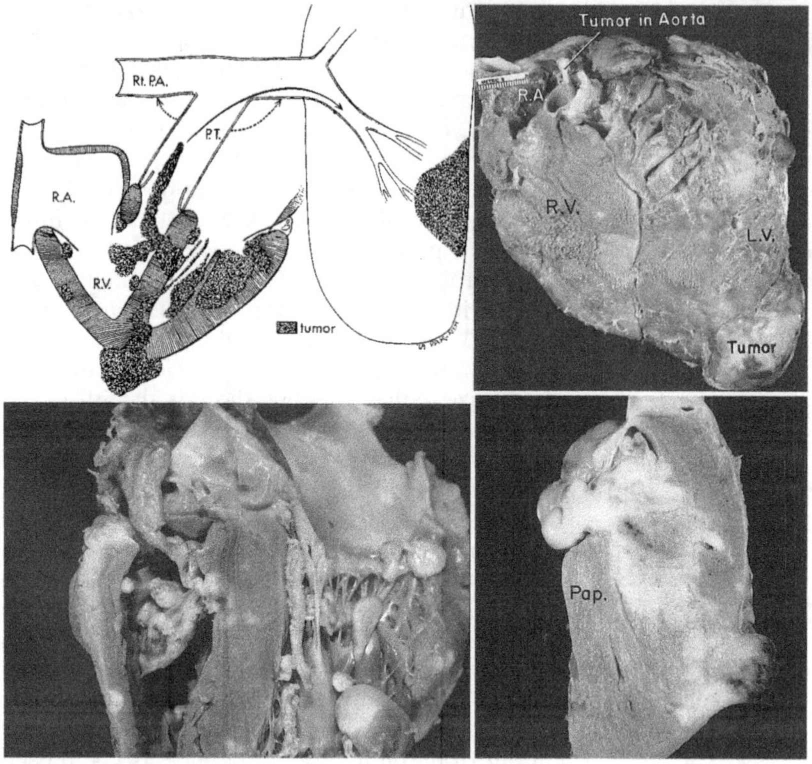

FIGURE 6. ***Primary cardiac sarcoma,*** **undifferentiated type, with neoplastic emboli to lungs and other organs in a 26-year-old man (A69-149) who had been well until 3 months before death.** ***Upper right;*** **exterior of heart containing blood, fibrin, and tumors.** ***Lower left;*** **opened right ventricle (R.V.), left ventricle (L.V.), left atrium, and aortic valve showing numerous tumor deposits.** ***Lower right;*** **section of left ventricular wall showing neoplasm extending through the entire wall and with extension beneath posterior mitral leaflet and through the epicardium. Pap. = papillary muscle; RA = right atrium; Rt. P.A. = right pulmonary artery.**

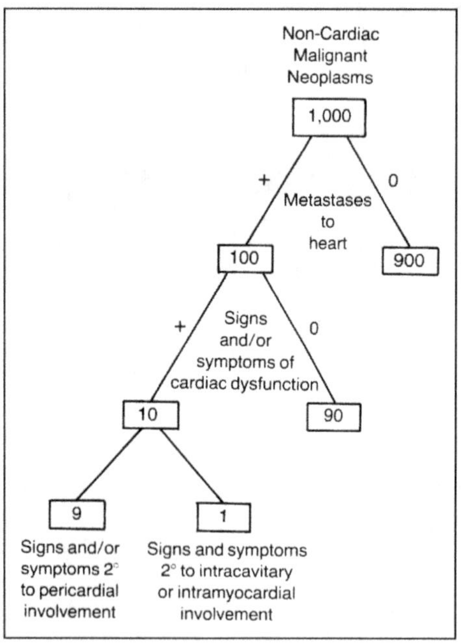

FIGURE 7. Diagram showing the relative frequency of cardiac metastases producing cardiac dysfunction.

cyte count, decreased platelet count, positive seroreactive protein, and abnormal serum proteins (usually increased gamma globulins). These constitutional symptoms may mimic infective endocarditis, collagen vascular disease, or occult malignancy.

Right atrial myxoma has occasionally migrated to the left atrial cavity via a patent foramen ovale with resultant systemic hypoxemia.[19,20]

The proper treatment of myxoma in any cavity of the heart is operative resection because there is no medicine known to shrink myxomas or to prevent their continued growth.[4,10] Some surgeons advise a biatrial approach for full visualization of both sides of the heart and then complete removal of a left or right atrial myxoma, excising the full thickness of the atrial septum if the neoplasm is attached to the region of the fossa ovalis. If a large portion of the atrial septum is removed, a cloth patch or parietal pericardium must be used to close the defect. Because fragmentation and embolization of the tumor is an ever present threat, vigorous palpation and other manipulations of the heart should be avoided until cardiopulmonary bypass is initiated. Most surgeons usually induce ventricular standstill with cardioplegia solution before manipulating the heartto reduce the possibility of fragmentation of portions of the tumor. Left atrial myxomas have been removed successfully during pregnancy. On occasion, an atrioventricular valve has been so traumatized by the tumor's prolapsing through it during ventricular diastole that valve excision and replacement is necessary. Fortunately, recurrences of atrial myxomas are rare, and if they do recur, it is usually within 4 years after the initial resection.

Rhabdomyoma: The most common cardiac neoplasm in infants and children is rhabdomyoma.[21] There is some question as to whether this particular tumor is a true neoplasm or actually resembles a hamartoma. These neoplasms are usually multiple, most often involve the ventricular myocardium, and project into the cavity or move freely as a pedunculated mass.[22–24] Associated *tuberous sclerosis* is present in about one third of the patients. The diagnosis is suggested by the presence of yellow-brown angiofibromas (''adenoma sebaceum'') on the face, sublingual fibromas around the fingernails, café au lait spots, and subcutaneous nodules. Presenting symptoms may be caused by obstruction to inflow into or outflow from the ventricles, arrhythmias, atrioventricular block, pericardial effusion, and even sudden death.[25] These neoplasms may mimic pulmonic valve stenosis and produce hypoxic spells, resembling those seen in tetralogy of Fallot. These neoplasms are usually readily diagnosed by echocardiography, angiog-

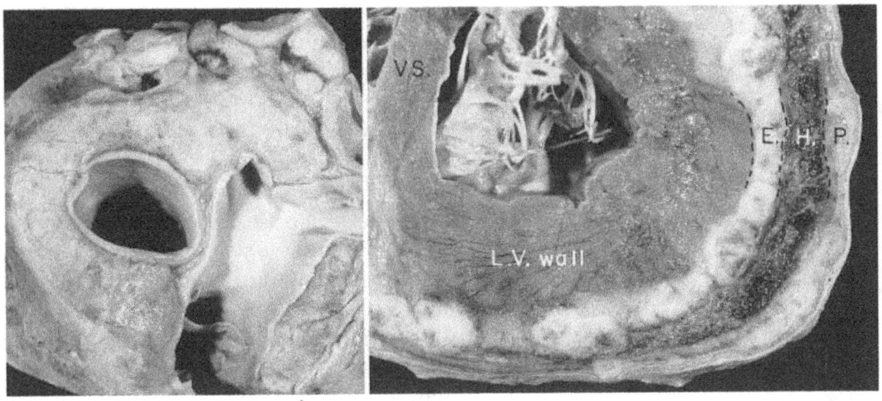

FIGURE 8. Metastatic *squamous-cell carcinoma of the lung* in a 61-year-old man (67A-531). Cardiac tamponade was the immediate cause of death. The entire heart and great vessels were encased in tumor. (Reproduced with permission from: Roberts WC, Spray TL. Pericardial heart disease. *Curr Prob Cardiol* 1977; (June);2(3):1–71.)

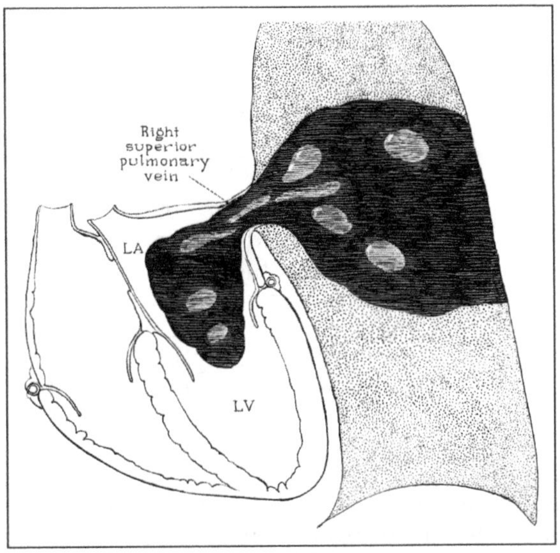

FIGURE 9. *Sarcoma,* undifferentiated type, in *lung* (primary uncertain) in a 29-year-old woman (A21-83) in whom echocardiogram disclosed tumor in the left atrium (LA) moving about "like a yo-yo." The left lung and its left atrial extension were operatively excised. LV = left ventricle.

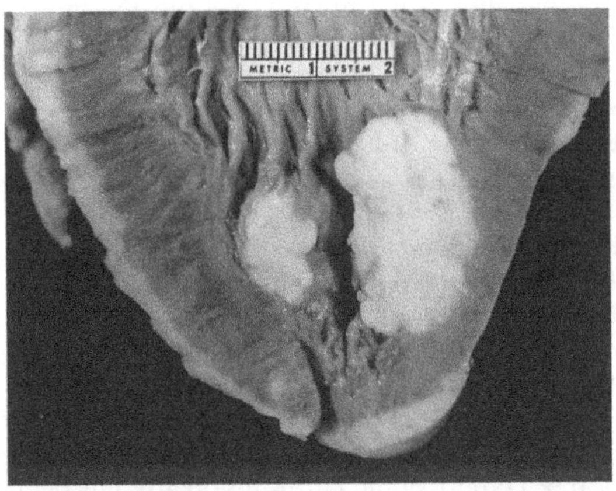

FIGURE 10. Opened left ventricle showing 2 asymptomatic apical neoplastic deposits from *adenocarcinoma in the lung* in a 59-year-old woman (A73-62). Another silent metastasis was in the right ventricular outflow tract but no metastasis was present in epicardium.

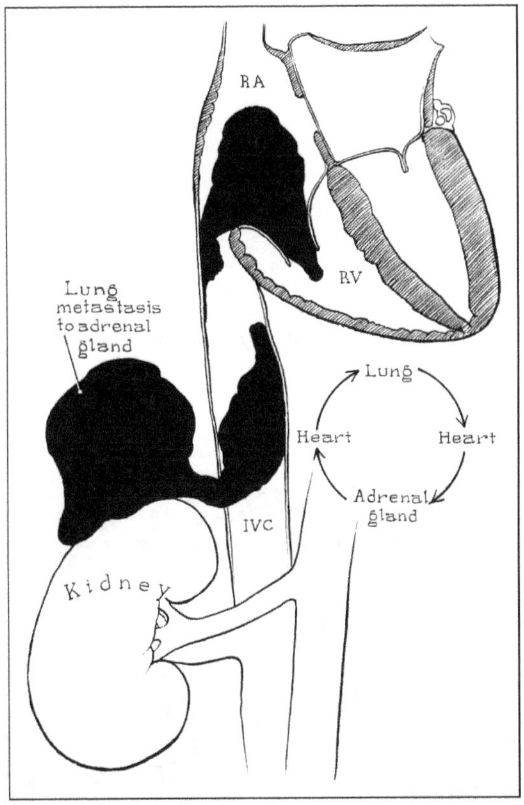

FIGURE 11. Diagram of metastatic *cancer of the lung* to the right adrenal gland with extension into the inferior vena cava (IVC) and then into the right atrium (RA) and right ventricle (RV) in a 57-year-old man (DCVAH #84A-121). Echocardiogram showed the right atrial mass which prolapsed through the tricuspid valve in atrial diastole.

raphy, or magnetic resonance imaging. Prenatal detection of intracardiac rhabdomyoma by intrauterine echocardiography has been reported with successful operative removal. The occurrence of more than 1 tumor does not prevent operative intervention. On rare occasion, these tumors have produced ventricular tachycardia in infants, and this arrhythmia has disappeared following successful operative removal.

Fibroma: Fibromas are usually intramural within a ventricular wall (Figure 4).[3,26] Most also occur in infants and children. Calcific deposits may be present within the neoplasm. Sudden death has occurred in about one third of the patients, presumably the result of a conduction defect or arrhythmia or obstruction to outflow from a ventricle. Left-axis deviation has been seen on electrocardiogram. Total or partial resection

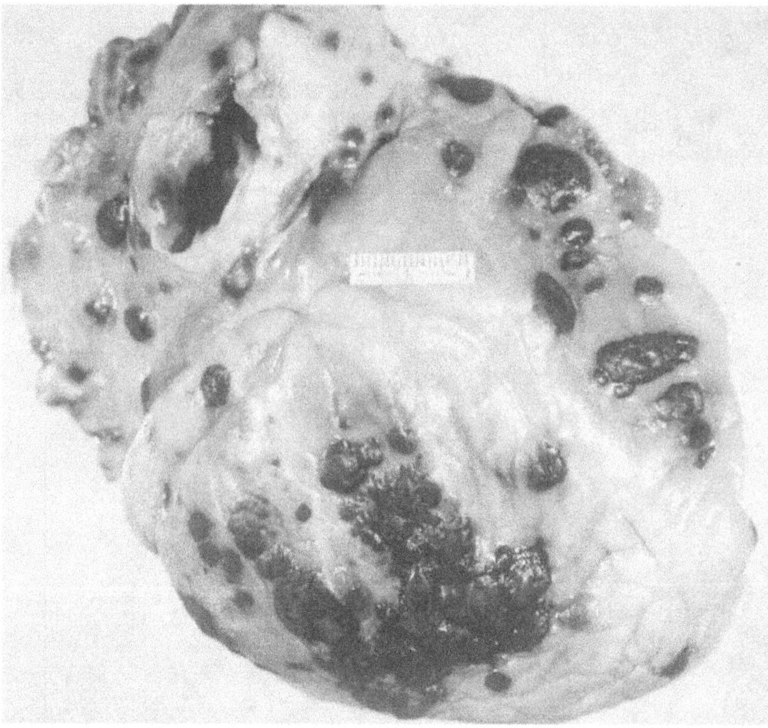

FIGURE 12. Exterior of posterior surface of the heart with clinically silent multiple metastases of *melanoma* in a 33-year-old man (A77-220).

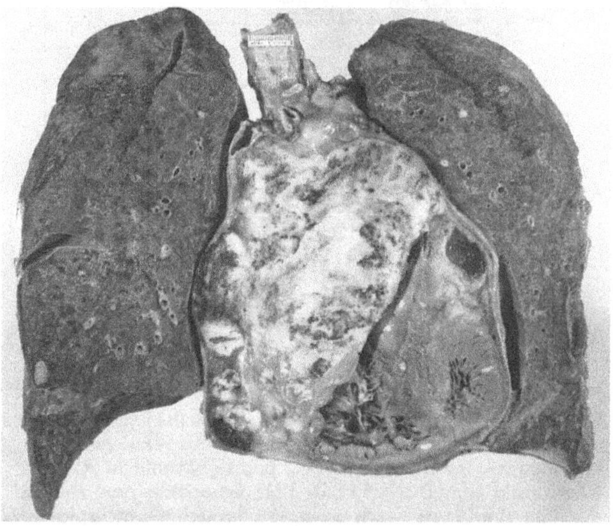

FIGURE 13. Metastatic *melanoma* to the heart in a 53-year-old man (A75-41). During life a pericardial friction rub was audible and the neck veins were quite distended. The parietal pericardium is everywhere adherent to epicardium. The superior vena cava, right atrium, right ventricle, and pulmonary trunk were severely compressed by the tumor. (Reproduced with permission from: Roberts WC, Spray TL. Pericardial heart disease. Curr Probl Cardiol 1977;(June);2(3)1–71.)

of the neoplasm may relieve obstruction with an excellent probability of long-term survival.

Lipoma: Lipomas involving the heart may be extremely small and represent incidental necropsy findings, or they may be massive.[27–30] The largest cardiac neoplasm ever reportedly apparently was an intrapericardial lipoma. They may be mistaken for pericardial cysts, they may cause pericardial effusion, or they may be asymptomatic and are suggested by a widened mediastinum on chest radiograph. Intramyocardial lipomas are encapsulated and usually small. Lipomas also have been located on cardiac valves and here they may simulate vegetations or myxomas.[29] Magnetic resonance imaging permits preoperative identification of these fatty tumors.

Hemangioma: These tumors are best diagnosed by coronary angiography which yields a characteristic "tumor blush." Spontaneous resolution without treatment has been reported. Total excision is usually not possible.

SPECIFIC MALIGNANT PRIMARY CARDIAC NEOPLASMS

Angiosarcoma: Nearly all primary malginant cardiac neoplasms are sarcomas, and the most frequent one is angiosarcoma.[31–35] It characteristically originates from the right atrium. The large quantity of vascular channels within these tumors and the subsequent large quantity of blood flowing through them may produce a continuous precordial murmur. About 25% of all angiosarcomas will, at least in part, be intracavitary, producing valvular obstruction, right-sided heart failure, and hemorrhagic pericardial tamponade. The course is rapid with widespread metastases and operative intervention is usually unsuccessful.

Rhabdomyosarcoma: Rhabdomyosarcoma is the second most frequent primary sarcoma of the heart, and, like angiosarcoma, it is most common in males.[36–38] In contrast, however, to angiosarcoma, no single cardiac chamber has a predilection for this neoplasm. Indeed, the neoplasm may be in all 4 cardiac chambers, or at least in more than 1, and obstruction may occur in 1 or more valve orifices. Again, prognosis is poor, survival is short, and operative intervention is usually futile.

Miscellaneous: Fibrosarcoma, liposarcoma, primary malignant lymphoma, and occasional sarcomas of other cell types constitute the remaining but infrequent primary malignant cardiac neoplasms (Figures 5 and 6). All of these neoplasms may obstruct valvular orifices or obliterate chambers and/or produce peripheral emboli.[39] Hypertrophic cardiomyopathy has been suggested by heavy tumorous infiltrations into the ventricular septum.[40]

METASTATIC NEOPLASMS TO THE HEART

Metastatic or secondary tumors of the heart with a primary in another body organ or tissue are far more frequent than are primary tumors of the heart.[41] The

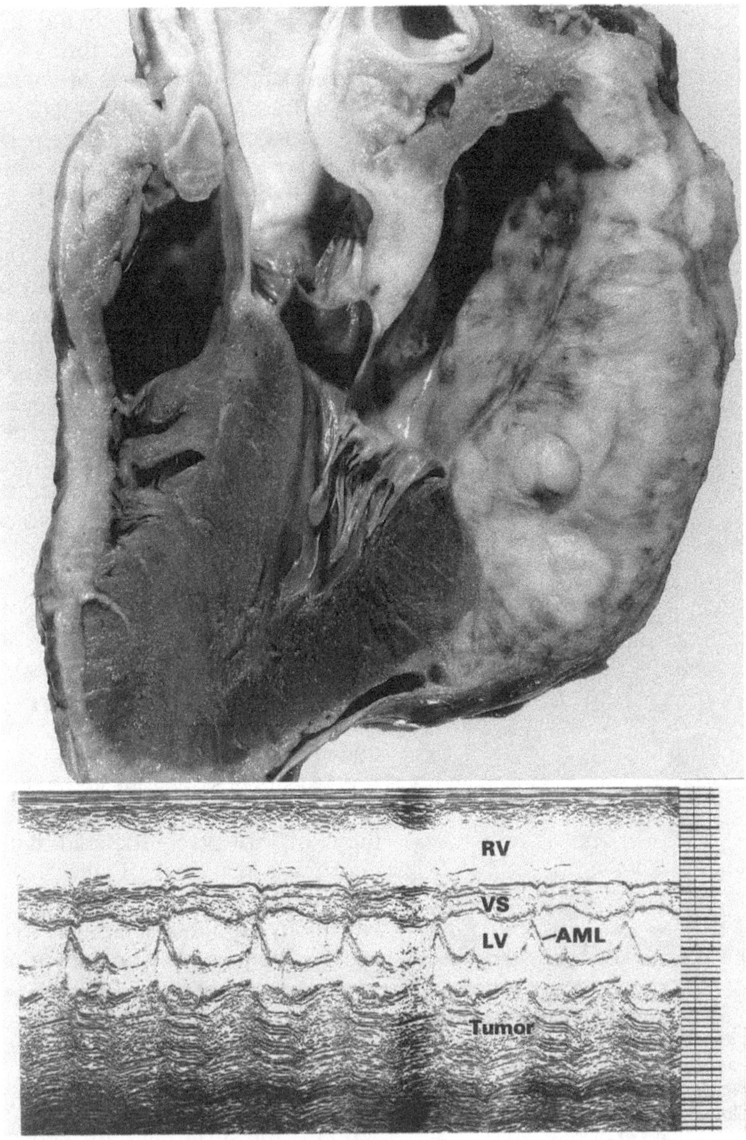

FIGURE 14. ***Cardiac histiocytic lymphoma*** **in a 64-year-old woman (A77-172) who had had evidence of congestive heart failure for 7 months. The cause of the heart failure was not apparent until necropsy. The patient is described in detail elsewhere.[57]** ***Upper;*** **longitudinal view of heart showing posterior wall of left atrium to be massively thickened by the neoplasm.** ***Lower;*** **echocardiogram showing the tumor behind the more basal portion of left ventricle (LV). AML = anterior mitral leaflet; RV = right ventricle; VS = ventricular septum. (Reproduced with permission from Roberts et al.[57])**

secondary tumors are far more commonly carcinomas than sarcomas simply because carcinomas are far more common than are sarcomas. Diagnosis can be suspected whenever cardiac manifestations occur in a patient diagnosed with a primary tumor in an organ or tissue other than the heart. The development of cardiac enlargement, tachycardia, arrhythmias, or heart failure in the presence of neoplasm elsewhere in the body is highly suggestive of cardiac metastases. Only rarely is metastatic tumor limited to the heart. Thus, the presence of metastatic tumor in the heart usually indicates widespread metastases in a number of body organs. On rare occasion, cardiac involvement may be the first or only expression of a noncardiac primary neoplasm. The most common sign is tamponade.[42] Direct invasion of the heart via the vena cava or pulmonary veins may lead to obstruction of an atrioventricular valve as well as to pulmonary or systemic emboli, or both.[43–45]

Only a minority of patients with metastases to the heart develop signs and/or symptoms of cardiac dysfunction as a result of the cardiac metastases. As shown in Figure 7, only about 10% of patients with cardiac metastases develop signs and/or symptoms of cardiac dysfunction, and of them 90% result from pericardial involvement and only about 10% from intracavitary or intramyocardial involvement.

Specific types of metastatic neoplasms to the heart: *Carcinoma of the lung* and *carcinoma of the breast* tend to invade parietal pericardium and then visceral pericardium leading to myocardial constriction and/or pericardial effusion (Figure 8). Another common presentation of cancer of the lung is to invade the pulmonary veins within the lung with spread of the cancer within the lumen of the pulmonary veins into the left atrium, which in turn can continue into the mitral orifice sometimes causing obstruction of that orifice (Figure 9).[46,47] Isolated or multiple left ventricular neoplastic deposits also are common (Figure 10). Metastatic cancer from the lung to the adrenal gland also may extend into the inferior vena cava and then into the right side of the heart (Figure 11), just as can primary adrenal gland or renal cancer.[48] Cancer of the lung or breast surrounding the main right or left pulmonary artery can lead to pulmonary arterial obstruction.[49]

Melanoma has the highest frequency of metastases to the heart per 100 cases of any neoplasm.[50,51] The metastases may be anywhere in the heart and usually melanotic metastases invade the walls of all 4 cardiac chambers and also epicardium and endocardium (Figures 12 and 13). The cancers in these patients are in so many body organs that the presence of the neoplasm in the heart is almost incidental.

Leukemia commonly invades the heart.[52] In the days before platelet transfusions, extensive hemorrhages into the myocardial walls and into endocardium and epicardium was commonly found in patients with fatal leukemia of various types. Histologically, leukemic infiltration between myocardial cells is quite common and sometimes gross deposits of leukemic cells are visible within the heart. A few patients with leukemia present with pericardial effusion, which is usually hemorrhagic. Large calcific deposits in the right side of the heart have been reported.[53]

Lymphoma also has a very high frequency of metastases to the heart.[54–59] Nearly 25% of patients with

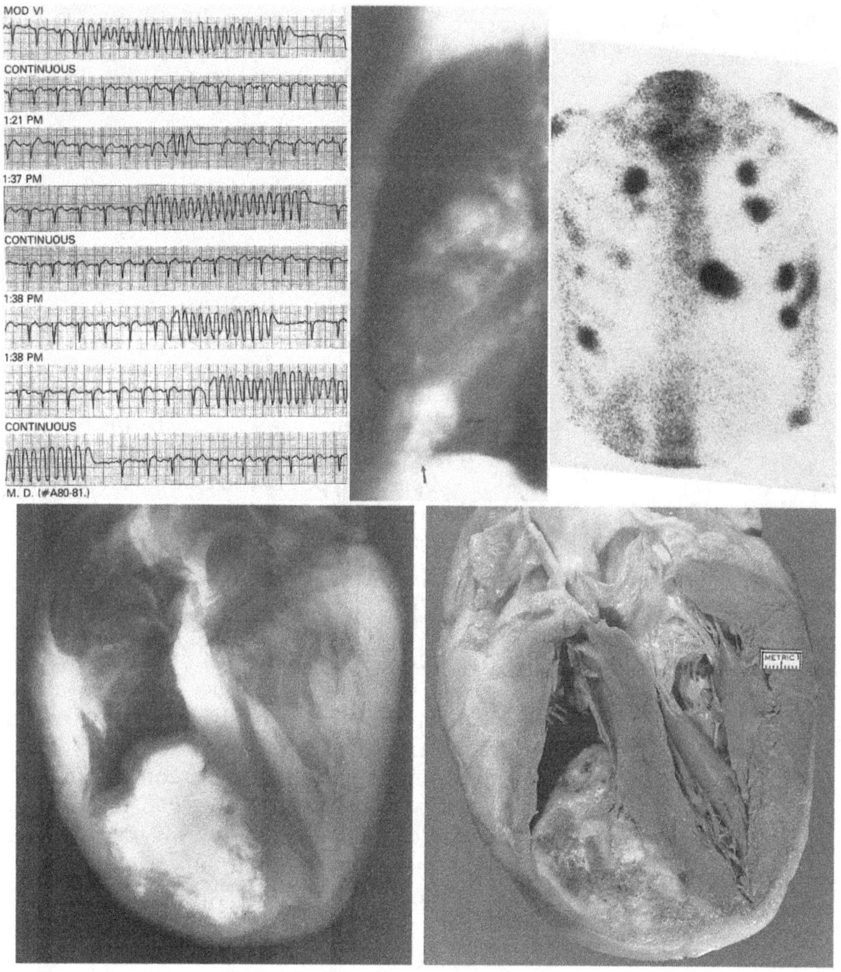

FIGURE 15. ***Osteogenic sarcoma*** **to the heart in a 39-year-old woman (A80-81) with a large calcified tumor in the right ventricle. This patient, who was ill for 20 months, had episodic ventricular tachycardia (*upper left*) during her last 20 months. *Upper middle;* lateral chest radiograph showing a calcified tumor (*arrows*) in the right ventricle (*lower left and lower right*). The computed tomogram (*upper right*) also shows the calcified right ventricular tumor as well as multiple metastases in the lungs and bones. The patient is described elsewhere.[60] (Reproduced with permission from Seibert et al.[60])**

lymphomas of various types have lymphoma involving epicardium, myocardium, or endocardium, or combinations (Figure 14). In contrast to leukemic involvement, the lymphomatous deposits are usually grossly discernible.

Some cancers, like *osteognic sarcoma,* may have calcium within them (Figure 15).[60,61]

NON-NEOPLASTIC CONDITIONS IN THE HEART OR PERICARDIUM FREQUENTLY MISTAKEN FOR CARDIAC NEOPLASM

Pericardial cyst: Pericardial or mesothelial cysts are the most frequent benign "tumors" of the pericardium. These cysts are generally asymptomatic and found on "routine" chest radiograph.[62] About a quarter of the patients, however, develop various symptoms including chest pain, dyspnea, cough, and tachycardia as a consequence of a pericardial cyst. The cysts are usually outside the pericardial cavity and, therefore, they really should not be considered "cardiac tumors."

Teratoma: Teratomas are actually extracardiac in at least 99% of the cases, but still within the pericardial cavity.[63–65] They arise and receive their blood supply from the ascending aorta or pulmonary trunk, presumably through the vasa vasorum. Most are found in infants and children and primarily in females. Recurrent serious pericardial effusion in children should suggest intrapericardial teratoma. Because these tumors may become quite large, they may cause compression of various cardiac chambers with subsequent symptoms therefrom.

Lipomatous hypertrophy of the atrial septum: Massive fatty infiltration of the atrial septum is an extremely common condition occurring almost exclusively in persons over 50 years of age, and usually over 65 years of age (Figure 16).[66] These lesions are essentially limited to obese people and they are always associated with enormous quantities of subepicardial adipose tissue, particularly enormous amounts of adipose tissue in the atrioventricular sulci. These hearts are almost always so fat that they float in water.[67] Normally the atrial septum is <1 cm in thickness. In patients with lipomatous hypertrophy of the atrial septum, the atrial septum cephalad to the fossa ovale may be as thick as 7 cm and the portion of atrial septum caudal to the fossa ovali may be as thick as 4 cm. Enormous infiltration of fat in the atrial septum may be associated with atrial arrhythmias. It is probably the only atrial arrhythmia that is treatable, possibly curable, by transient starvation. The importance of lipomatous hypertrophy of the atrial septum in the context of "cardiac tumors" is that these patients should not be operated on to remove fat from the atrial septum. The treatment is simply weight loss. These fatty deposits may be diagnosed by echocardiography or computed tomography or magnetic resonance imaging.[68,69] Fat in the subepicardial adipose tissue has been confused by echocardiogram with pericardial effusion.[70]

Papillary fibroelastomas: These small avascular growths with multiple papillary fronds are located mainly on cardiac valves. They are common in older individuals. These lesions will be discussed in a future from-the-editor column.

Thrombi: These masses when within an intracardiac cavity may be indistinguishable from neoplasm by

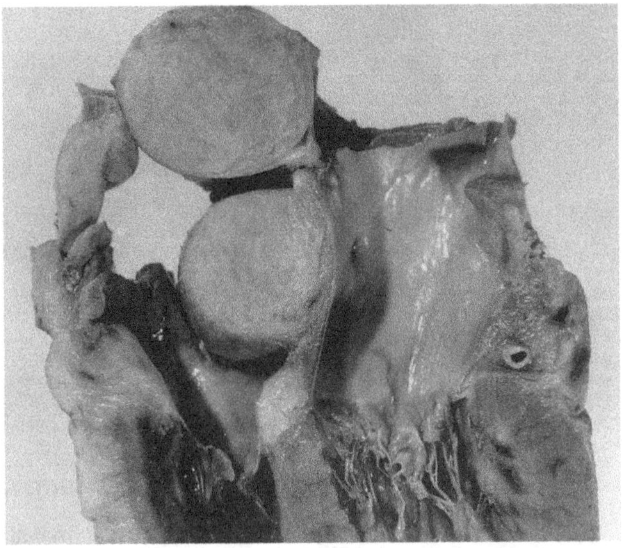

FIGURE 16. ***Lipomatous hypertrophy of the atrial septum*** **in a 74-year-old woman (GT #77A-42) with huge fatty deposits in the atrial septum (except for the fossa ovale area). (Reproduced with permission from: Shirani J, Roberts WC.[66])**

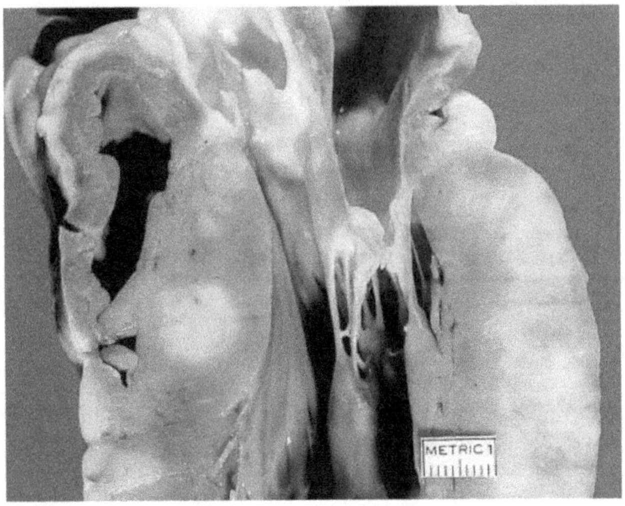

FIGURE 17. Longitudinal view of heart in a 27-year-old woman (DCMEO #83-10-670) with ***cardiac sarcoidosis*** **simulating cardiac neoplasms.**

echocardiogram or radiograph. Grossly, however, they are very different.

Sarcoid: When located in myocardium, sarcoid granuloma may grossly resemble neoplasm (Figure 17).[71–73]

CONSEQUENCES OF THERAPY FOR NEOPLASMS IN THE HEART OR MEDIASTINUM

Radiation heart disease: Radiation heart disease was first recognized after radiation therapy for Hodgkin's disease.[74–78] Some of the earlier patients with Hodgkin's disease received 8,000 rads, and that quantity of radiation caused consequences to pericardium, myocardium, and endocardium. The most common manifestation of radiation heart disease is pericardial effusion. The mechanism of the effusion is unclear. Fibrin deposits occur on both the visceral and parietal aspects of the pericardia. Because coronary arteries are located in subepicardial adipose tissue, they often receive the effects of radiation. Many patients have been reported to have coronary arterial narrowing at a very young age after radiation therapy, particularly patients with Hodgkin's disease. The intimal plaques resulting from radiation heart disease in actuality cannot be distinquished from plaques occurring from typical atherosclerosis. The distinquishing features of radiation heart disease involving the coronary arteries is extensive fibrous thickening of the adventitia, and also loss, focally or diffsely, of internal and external elastic membranes, particularly the latter. Narrowing of coronary ostia also are common in radiation heart disease. Radiation also can cause considerable scarring within the subepicardial adipose tissue. The second most common manifestation of radiation heart disease is mural endocardial thickening, most commonly of the right atrium and ventricle, but focally also in the left ventricle. The third most common manifestation of radiation heart disease is interstitial fibrosis and, depending on the portal of entry, it usually involves the anterior wall of the right ventricle more than any other portion of the heart.

Cardiac hemorrhages: Thrombocytopenia, particularly if persistent, often results in focal epicardial, myocardial, and mural endocardial hemorrhages. If the hemorrhages are located in conduction tissue, various degrees of heart block or arrhythmias may be the consequence.

Cardiac infection: The most common cardiac infections today in cancer patients are myocardial abscesses and mural endocardial and epicardial abscesses. These are particularly prevalent in patients with prolonged leukopenia.[79,80] Patients having unsuccessful bone-marrow transplantation are particularly prone to these infections, which usually are produced by fungi, not bacteria. Gas gangrene may involve the heart as well as most other body organs and tissues.[81]

Cardiac adiposity or the corticosteroid-treated heart: Patients with various types of cancers, particularly those with leukemia and lymphoma, and those developing cancer after transplantation of 1 or more body organs, usually receive corticosteroid therapy for prolonged periods. The consequence is excessive deposition of fat in the heart, mainly in the subepicardial areas.[82] These hearts may become so fatty that they float in water (buffalo hump of the heart), and this excessive subepicardial adipose tissue may simulate pericardial effusion.

Cardiac hemosiderosis: Normally the human body contains approximately 4 g of iron. If the deposits increase to about 25 g, iron deposits then are usually found within myocardial cells. Patients who receive 100 units of blood without associated bleeding diatheses can acquire approximately 25 g of iron within the body organs and tissues. In some patients with cancer, particularly leukemia, this situation may exist and the result is cardiac hemosiderosis.[83] These patients may be asymptomatic or they may develop features of dilated cardiomyopathy with heart failure. At times, ventricular arrhythmias may be a consequence. Myocardial restriction as a result of myocardial ironic deposits has occurred, but dilation is far more common.[84]

Anthracycline chemotherapy (doxorubicin and daunorubicin): Cardiac toxicity is a well-recognized complication of these agents and is frequently the dose-limiting factor in their administration.[85–87] Clinical toxicity is usually manifested by evidence of impaired left ventricular systolic function. Morphologic signs of toxicity may be present when clinical signs of toxicity are absent.

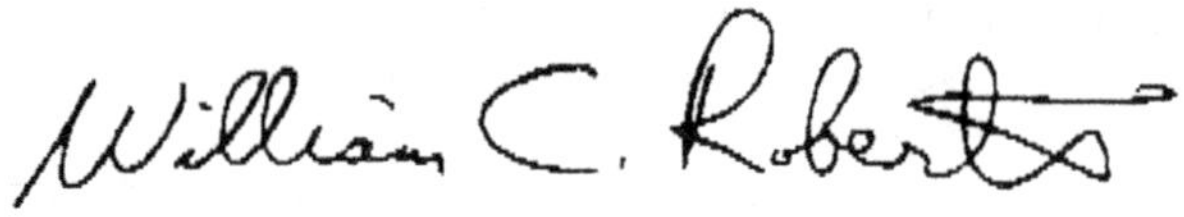

William Clifford Roberts, MD,
Editor in Chief
Baylor Cardiovascular Institute
Baylor University Medical Center
Dallas, Texas 75246

1. Lam KY, Dickens P, Chan ACL. Tumors of the heart. A 20-year experience with review of 12485 consecutive autopsies. *Arch Pathol Med* 1993;117:1027–1031.
2. Reynan K. Frequency of primary tumors of the heart. *Am J Cardiol* 1996;77:107.
3. Burke A, Virmani R. Atlas of Tumor Pathology. Third Series Fascicle 16. Tumors of the Heart and Great Vessels. Washington, DC: Armed Forces Institute of Pathology 1996:231.
4. Bahnson HT, Spencer FC, Andrus EC. Diagnosis and treatment of intracavitary myxomas of the heart. *Ann Surg* 1957;145:915–926.
5. Ferrans VJ, Roberts WC. Structural features of cardiac myxomas. Histology, histochemistry, and electron microscopy. *Human Pathol* 1973;4:111–146.
6. Peters MN, Hall RJ, Cooley DA, Leachman RD, Garcia E. The clinical syndrome of atrial myxoma. *JAMA* 1974;230:695–701.
7. Morgan DL, Palazola J, Reed W, Bell HH, Kindred LH, Beauchamp GD. Left heart myxomas. *Am J Cardiol* 1977;40:611–614.
8. St. John Sutton MG, Mercier L-A, Giuliani ER, Lie JT. Atrial myxomas. A review of clinical experience in 40 patients. *Mayo Clin Proc* 1980;55:371–376.
9. Markel ML, Waller BF, Armstrong WF. Cardiac myxoma. A review. *Medicine* 1987;66:114–125.
10. Murphy MC, Sweeney MS, Putnam JB Jr, Walker WE, Frazier OH, Ott DA, Cooley DA. Surgical treatment of cardiac tumors: a 25-year experience. *Ann Thorac Surg* 1990;49:612–618.
11. Tazelaar HD, Locke TJ, McGregor CGA. Pathology of surgically excised primary cardiac tumors. *Mayo Clin Proc* 1992;67:957–965.
12. Burke AP, Virmani R. Cardiac myxomas: a clinicopathologic study. *Am J Clin Pathol* 1994;100:671–680.
13. Morrow AG, Kahler RL, Reis RL. Primary myxoma of the right ventricle. Clinical, hemodynamic and angiographic findings before and following operative treatment. *Am J Med* 1966;40:954–960.
14. Hickie JB, Gibson H, Windsor HM. "The wrecking ball": right atrial myxoma. *Med J Aust* 1970;2:82–86.
15. Hada Y, Wolfe C, Murray GF, Craig E. Right ventricular myxoma. Case report and review of phonocardiographic and auscultatory manifestations. *Am Heart J* 1980;100:871–877.
16. Massumi R. Bedside diagnosis of right heart myxomas through detection of palpable tumor shocks and audible plops. *Am Heart J* 1983;105:303–310.
17. Leonhardt ET, Kullenberg KP. Bilateral atrial myxomas with multiple arterial aneurysms—a syndrome mimicking polyarteritis nodosa. *Am J Med* 1977;62:792–794.
18. Malekzadeh S, Roberts WC. Growth rate of left atrial myxoma. *Am J Cardiol* 1989;64:1075–1076.
19. Talley RC, Baldwin BJ, Symbas PN, Nutter DO. Right atrial myxoma. Unusual presentation with cyanosis and clubbing. *Am J Med* 1970;48:256–260.
20. Goldschlager A, Popper R, Goldschlager N, Gerbode F, Prozan G. Right atrial myxoma with right to left shunt and polycythemia presenting as congenital heart disease. *Am J Cardiol* 1972;30:82–86.
21. Chan HSL, Sonley MJ, Moës CAF, Daneman A, Smith CR, Martin DJ. Primary and secondary tumors of childhood involving the heart, pericardium, and great vessels. A report of 75 cases and review of the literature. *Cancer* 1985;56:825–836.
22. Fenoglio JJ Jr, McAllister HA, Ferrans VJ. Cardiac rhabdomyoma: a clinicopathologic and electron microscopic study. *Am J Cardiol* 1976;38:241–251.
23. Smythe JF, Dyck JD, Smallhorn JF, Freedom RM. Natural history of cardiac rhabdomyoma in infancy and childhood. *Am J Cardiol* 1990;66:1247–1249.
24. Burke AP, Virmani R. Cardiac rhabdomyoma, a clinicopathologic study. *Mod Pathol* 1991;4:70–74.
25. Biancaniello TM, Meyer RA, Gaum WE, Kaplan S. Primary benign intramural ventricular tumors in children: pre- and post-operative electrocardiographic, echocardiographic, and angiocardiographic evaluation. *Am Heart J* 1982;103:852–857.
26. Williams DB, Danielson GK, McGoon DC, Feldt RH, Edwards WD. Cardiac fibroma. Long-term survival after excision. *J Thorac Cardiovasc Surg* 1982;84:230–236.
27. Estevez JM, Thompson DS, Levinson JP. Lipoma of the heart. Review of the literature and report of 2 autopsied cases. *Arch Pathol* 1964;77:638–642.
28. Moulton AL, Jaretzki A III, Bowman FO Jr, Silverstien EF, Bregman D. Massive lipoma of the heart. *NY State J Med* 1976;76:1820–1825.
29. Dollar AL, Wallace RB, Kent KM, Burkhart MW, Roberts WC. Mitral valve replacement for mitral lipoma associated with severe obesity. *Am J Cardiol* 1989;64:1405–1407.
30. Shirani J, Roberts WC. Epicardial Lipoma. *Am Heart J* 1993;126:1030.
31. Bear PA, Moodie DS. Malignant primary cardiac tumors. The Cleveland Clinic Experience, 1956–1986. *Chest* 1987;92:860–862.
32. Putman JB Jr, Sweeney MS, Colon R, Lanza LA, Frazier OH, Cooley DA. Primary cardiac sarcomas. *Ann Thorac Surg* 1991;51:906–910.
33. Burke AP, Cowan D, Virmani R. Primary sarcomas of the heart. *Cancer* 1992;69:387–395.
34. Glancy DL, Morales JB, Roberts WC. Angiosarcoma of the heart. *Am J Cardiol* 1968;21:413–419.
35. Herrmann MA, Shankerman RA, Edwards WD, Shub C, Schaff HV. Primary cardiac angiosarcoma: a clinicopathologic study of six cases. *J Thorac Cardiovasc Surg* 1992;103:655–664.
36. Shrivastava S, Jacks JJ, White RS, Edwards JE. Diffuse rhabdomyomatosis of the heart. *Arch Pathol Lab Med* 1977;101:78–90.
37. Hajar R, Roberts WC, Folger GM Jr. Embryonal botryoid rhabdomyosarcoma of the mitral valve. *Am J Cardiol* 1986;57:376.
38. Hui KS, Green LK, Schmidt WA. Primary cardiac rhabdomyosarcoma: definition of a rare entity. *Am J Cardiovasc Pathol* 1988;2:19–29.
39. Domanski MJ, Delaney TF, Kleiner DE Jr, Goswitz M, Agatston A, Tucker E, Johnson M, Roberts WC. Primary sarcoma of the heart causing mitral stenosis. *Am J Cardiol* 1990;66:893–895.
40. Isner JM, Falcone MW, Virmani R, Roberts WC. Cardiac sarcoma causing "ASH" and simulating coronary heart disease. *Am J Med* 1979;66:1025–1030.
41. Abraham DP, Reddy V, Gattusa P. Neoplasms metastatic to the heart: review of 3314 consecutive autopsies. *Am J Cardiovasc Pathol* 1990;3:195–198.
42. Adenle AD, Edwards JE. Clinical and pathologic features of metastatic neoplasms of the pericardium. *Chest* 1982;81:166–169.
43. MacLowry JD, Roberts WC. Metastatic choriocarcinoma of the lung. Invasion of pulmonary veins with extension into the left atrium and mitral orifice. *Am J Cardiol* 1966;18:938–941.
44. Labib SB, Schick EC Jr, Isner JM. Obstruction of right ventricular outflow tract caused by intracavitary metastatic disease: analysis of 14 cases. *J Am Coll Cardiol* 1992;19:1664–1668.
45. Domanski MJ, Cunnion RE, Fernicola DJ, Roberts WC. Fatal cor pulmonale caused by extensive tumor emboli in the small pulmonary arteries without emboli in the major pulmonary arteries or metastases in the pulmonary parenchyma. *Am J Cardiol* 1993;72:233–234.
46. Onuigbo WI. Direct extension of cancer between pulmonary veins and the left atrium. *Chest* 1972;62:444–446.
47. Weg IL, Mehra S, Azueta V, Rosener F. Cardiac metastasis from adenocarcinoma of the lung. Echocardiographic-pathologic correlation. *Am J Med* 1986;80:108–112.
48. Kadir S, Coulam CM. Intracaval extension of renal cell carcinoma. *Cardiovasc Intervent Radiol* 1980;3:180–183.
49. Waller BF, Fletcher RD, Roberts WC. Carcinoma of the lung causing pulmonary arterial stenosis. *Chest* 1981;79:589–591.
50. Glancy DL, Roberts WC. The heart in malignant melanoma. A study of 70 autopsy cases. *Am J Cardiol* 1968;21:555–571.
51. Waller BV, Gottdiener JS, Virmani R, Roberts WC. The "charcoal heart". Melanoma to the cor. *Chest* 1980;77:671–676.
52. Roberts WC, Bodey GP, Wertlake PT. The heart in acute leukemia. A study of 420 autopsy cases. *Am J Cardiol* 1968;21:388–412.
53. Waller BF, Roberts WC. Systolic clicks caused by rocks in the right heart chambers. *Am Heart J* 1981;102:459–460.
54. Roberts WC, Glancy DL, DeVita VT Jr. Heart in malignant lymphoma

(Hodgkin's disease, lymphosarcoma, reticulum cell sarcoma and mycosis fungoides). A study of 196 autopsy cases. *Am J Cardiol* 1968;22:85–107.
55. Terry LN, Kligerman MM. Pericardial and myocardial involvement by lymphomas and leukemias. *Cancer* 1970;25:1003–1008.
56. McDonnell PJ, Mann RB, Bulkley BH. Involvement of the heart by malignant lymphoma: a clinicopathologic study. *Cancer* 1982;49:944–951.
57. Roberts CS, Gottdiener JS, Roberts WC. Clinically undetected cardiac lymphoma causing congestive heart failure. *Am Heart J* 1990;120:1239–1242.
58. Holladay AO, Siegel RJ, Schwartz EA. Cardiac malignant lymphoma in acquired immune deficiency syndrome. *Cancer* 1992;70:2203–2207.
59. Moore JA, DeRan BP, Minor R, Arthur J, Fraker TD. Transesophageal echocardiographic evaluation of intracardiac lymphoma. *Am Heart J* 1992;124: 514–516.
60. Seibert KA, Rettenmier CW, Waller BF, Battle WE, Levine AS, Roberts WC. Osteogenic sarcoma metastatic to the heart. *Am J Med* 1982;73:136–141.
61. Burke AP, Virmani R. Osteosarcomas of the heart. *Am J Surg Pathol* 1991;15:289–295.
62. Feigin DS, Fenoglio JJ, McAllister HA, Madewell JR. Pericardial cysts: a radiologic-pathologic correlation and review. *Radiology* 1977;125:15–20.
63. Reynolds JL, Donahue JK, Pearce CW. Intrapericardial teratoma: a cause of acute pericardial effusion in infancy. *Pediatrics* 1969;4:71–78.
64. DeGeeter B, Kretz JG, Nisand I, Eisenmann B, Kieny MT, Kieny R. Intra-pericardial teratoma in a newborn infant: Use of fetal echocardiography. *Ann Thorac Surg* 1983;35:664–666.
65. Brabham KR, Roberts WC. Cardiac-compressing intrapericardial teratoma at birth. *Am J Cardiol* 1989;63:386–387.
66. Shirani J, Roberts WC. Clinical, electrocardiographic and morphologic features of massive fatty deposits ("lipomatous hypertrophy") in the atrial septum. *J Am Coll Cardiol* 1993;22:226–238.
67. Roberts WC, Roberts JD. The floating heart or the heart too fat to sink: analysis of 55 necropsy patients. *Am J Cardiol* 1983;52:1286–1289.
68. Applegate PM, Taijk AJ, Ehman RL, Julsrud PR, Miller FA Jr. Two-dimensional echocardiographic and magnetic resonance imaging observations in massive lipomatous hypertrophy of atrial septum. *Am J Cardiol* 1987;59:489–491.
69. Kindman LA, Wright A, Tye T, Seale W, Appleton C. Lipomatous hypertrophy of the interatrial septum: characterization of transesophageal and transthoracic echocardiography, magnetic resonance imaging, and computed tomography. *J Am Soc Echocardiogr* 1988;1:450–454.
70. Isner JM, Carter BL, Roberts WC, Bankoff MS. Subepicardial adipose tissue producing echocardiographic appearance of pericardial effusion. Documentation by computed tomography and necropsy. *Am J Cardiol* 1983;51:565–569.
71. Roberts WC, McAllister HA Jr, Ferrans VJ. Sarcoidosis of the heart. A clinicopathologic study of 35 necropsy patients (group I) and review of 78 previously described necropsy patients (group II). *Am J Med* 1977;63:86–108.
72. Virmani R, Bures JC, Roberts WC. Cardiac sarcoidosis: a major cause of sudden death in young individuals. *Chest* 1980;77:423–428.
73. Shirani J, Roberts WC. Subepicardial myocardial lesions. *Am Heart J* 1993; 125:1346–1352.
74. Morton DL, Kagar AR, Roberts WC, O'Brien KP, Holmes EC, Adkins PC. Pericardiectomy for radiation-induced pericarditis with effusion. *Ann Thorac Surg* 1969;8:195–208.
75. Serpik A, Lowenbraum S, Sheinbrot S, Brace K, Belcher V, Roberts WC. Possible radiation pericarditis in Hodgkin's disease. *Cancer Chemo Report* 1970; 54:199–208.
76. McReynolds RA, Gold GL, Roberts WC. Coronary heart disease after mediastinal irradiation for Hodgkin's disease. *Am J Med* 1976;60:39–45.
77. Brosius FC III, Waller BF, Roberts WC. Radiation heart disease. Analysis of 16 young (aged 15 to 33 years) necropsy patients who received over 3,500 rads to the heart. *Am J Med* 1981;70:519–530.
78. Harvey LAC, DeMaio SJ, Roberts WC. Radiation-induced cardiovascular disease including stenosis of coronary ostium, coronary and carotid arteries, and aortic valve. *Baylor University Med Ctr Proc* 1994;7:33–36.
79. Ihde DC, Roberts WC, Marr KC, Brereton HD, McGuire WP, Levine AS, Young RC. Cardiac candidiasis in cancer patients. *Cancer* 1978;41:2364–2371.
80. Ross EM, Macher AM, Roberts WC. *Aspergillus Fumigatus* thrombi causing total occlusion of both coronary arterial ostia, all four major epicardial coronary arteries and coronary sinus and associated with purulent pericarditis. *Am J Cardiol* 1985;56:499–500.
81. Roberts WC, Berard CW. Gas gangrene of the heart in clostridial septicemia. *Am Heart J* 1967;74:482–488.
82. Bulkley BH, Roberts WC. The heart in systemic lupus erythematous and the changes induced in it by corticosteriod therapy. A study of 36 necropsy patients. *Am J Med* 1975;58:243–264.
83. Buja LM, Roberts WC. Iron in the heart. Etiology and clinical significance. *Am J Med* 1971;51:209–221.
84. Cutler DJ, Isner JM, Bracey AW, Hufnagel CA, Conrad PW, Roberts WC, Kerwin DM, Weintraub AM. Hemochromatosis heart disease: an unemphasized cause of potentially reversible restrictive cardiomyopathy. *Am J Med* 1980;69: 923–928.
85. Buja LM, Ferrans VJ, Mayer RJ, Roberts WC, Henderson ES. Cardiac ultrastructural changes induced by daunorubicin therapy. *Cancer* 1973;32:771–788.
86. Buja LM, Ferrans VJ, Roberts WC. Drug-induced cardiomyopathies. *Adv Cardiol* 1974;13:330–348.
87. Isner JM, Ferrans VJ, Cohen SR, Witkind BG, Virmani R, Gottdiener JS, Beck JR, Roberts WC. Clinical and morphologic cardiac findings after anthracycline chemotherapy. Analysis of 64 patients studied at necropsy. *Am J Cardiol* 1983;51:1167–1174.

Papillary Fibroelastomas of the Heart

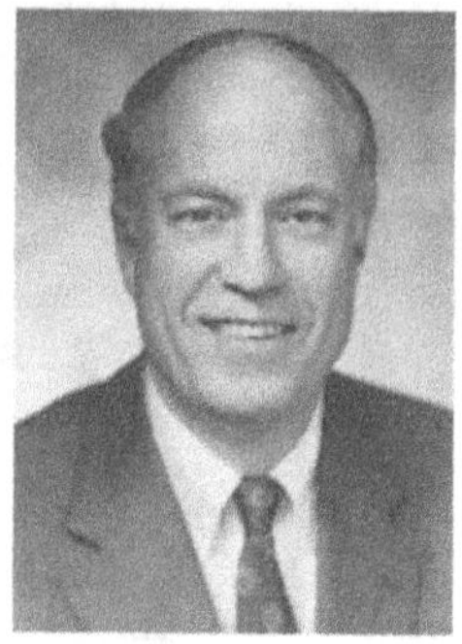

These are small avascular growths with multiple papillary fronds most commonly located on cardiac valves, mainly the aortic and mitral (Figure 1).[1–4] They are never present at birth, but are seen, at least on valves, primarily in older persons. They consist of fibrous tissue covered by an elastic membrane which in turn is covered by endocardium. Occasionally (about 15%), they also occur on left ventricular and/or ventricular septal mural endocardium,[15–14] particularly in patients with small or relatively small ventricular cavities, such as in patients with mitral stenosis (Figure 2)[9,12,13] or hypertrophic cardiomyopathy (Figures 3 and 4).[5,11] When located on the aortic valve, they usually are located on the ventricular aspects of the cusps in the more central portions but they also occur on the aortic aspects of these cusps usually near the margins.[15–20] When occurring on the mitral valve leaflets, they are usually on the atrial aspects near the margins.[21–28] In patients with mitral stenosis or hypertrophic cardiomyopathy, however, they involve the ventricular aspects of the anterior mitral leaflet and they sometimes are seen on chordae tendineae and mural endocardium, particularly over the papillary muscles. These lesions appear to result from contact of one valve leaflet with another or one mural endocardial surface with another.

A number of patients have been reported with papillary fibroelastomas and evidence of *stroke*[19–21,26,27,29–33] or loss of vision.[34] Whether the stroke was connected in any way with the cardiac fibroelastomas is debatable (in my view). Some patients have been in their 20s or 30s without other predisposing features or findings commonly associated with cerebral infarction, and the occurrence of stroke in the younger age group certainly is suggestive of a connection. In contrast to myxoma, where myxomatous material has been seen in systemic emboli, however, histologic findings of papillary fibroelastomas have not been observed in a cerebral artery in a patient with stroke and cardiac papillary fibroelastomas. Furthermore, the papillary fibroelastomas are firmly attached to valvular or mural endocardium and, therefore, dislodgement of a fibroelastoma would appear extremely unlikely. Thrombus, however, is occasionally superimposed on papillary fibroelastomas and it may be that the thrombus is the material that is dislodged and responsible for the stroke.

Additionally, *angina pectoris*,[33] *acute myocardial infarction*,[35–38] and *sudden death*[39] have been observed in patients with cardiac papillary fibroelastomas, mainly on the aortic valve. These papillary

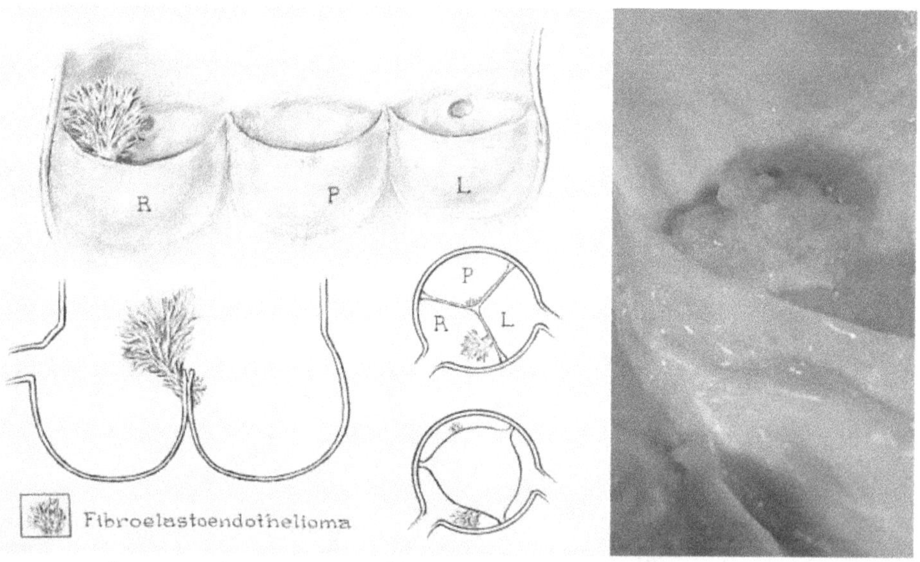

FIGURE 1. Fibroelastomas on the aortic valve in a 66-year-old man (FSH#85A-95) who had an *acute myocardial infarction* of the posterior left ventricular wall with subsequent fatal rupture of the posteromedial papillary muscle. The epicardial coronary arteries were severely narrowed by atherosclerotic plaque. *Left,* 1 fibroelastoma was located on the aortic aspect of the right (R) cusp, and during ventricular systole (*bottom right*), it was located close to the ostium of the right coronary artery. If the fibroelastoma had been located more centrally on the right cusp it theoretically could have contacted the ostium of the right coronary artery during ventricular systole. *Right,* photograph of the fibroelastoma on the right cusps. L = left cusp; P = posterior cusp.

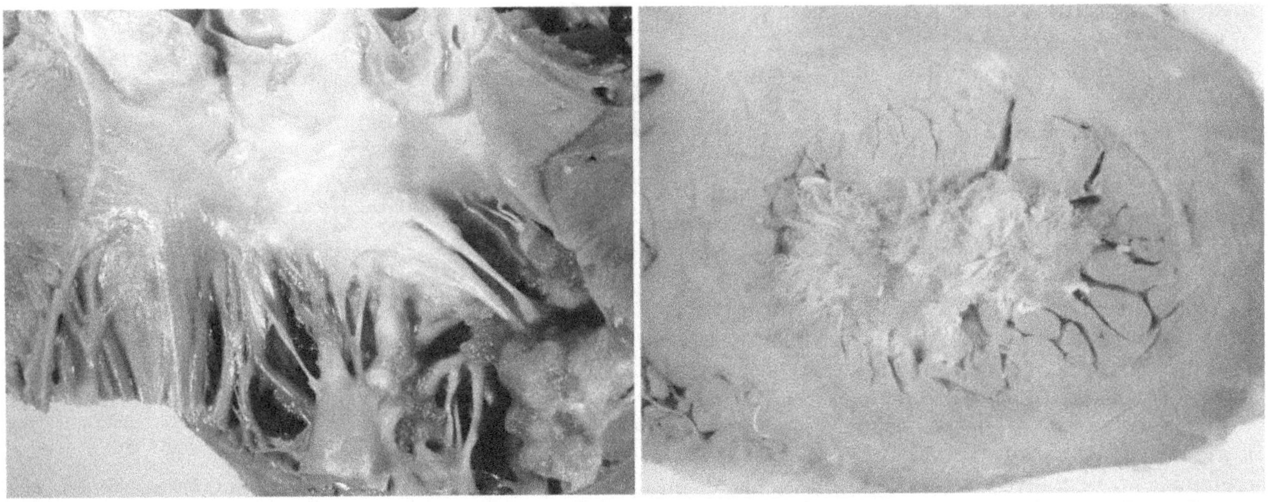

FIGURE 2. Multiple fibroelastomas in a 49-year-old woman (GT#83A-14) with *mitral stenosis. Left,* opened left ventricular outflow tract showing numerous elastofibromas attached to the ventricular aspect of the mitral leaflets and to their chordae tendineae and papillary muscles. One fibroelastoma is also located on the ventricular aspect of the posterior aortic valve cusp. *Right,* view of left ventricle showing papillary fibroelastomas filling the cavity.

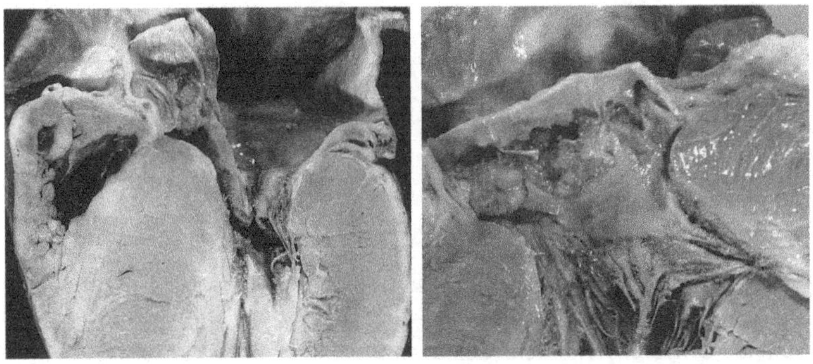

FIGURE 3. Multiple papillary fibroelastomas in a 36-year-old woman (A67-121) with *hypertrophic cardiomyopathy.* The left ventricular-aortic peak systolic pressure gradient was 75 mm Hg and the heart weighed 450 g. *Left,* longitudinal anterior to posterior cut exposing the left ventricular outflow tract, left atrium, and right ventricular outflow tracts. The fibroelastomas are located on the ventricular aspects of both anterior and posterior mitral leaflets and their chordae tendineae and papillary muscles and also on the aortic valve cusps. *Right,* opened aortic valve and left ventricular outflow tract demonstrating fibroelastomas on the ventricular aspects of all 3 aortic valve cusps, on the mural endocardium in apposition to anterior mitral leaflet, and also on the ventricular aspects of the anterior mitral leaflet.

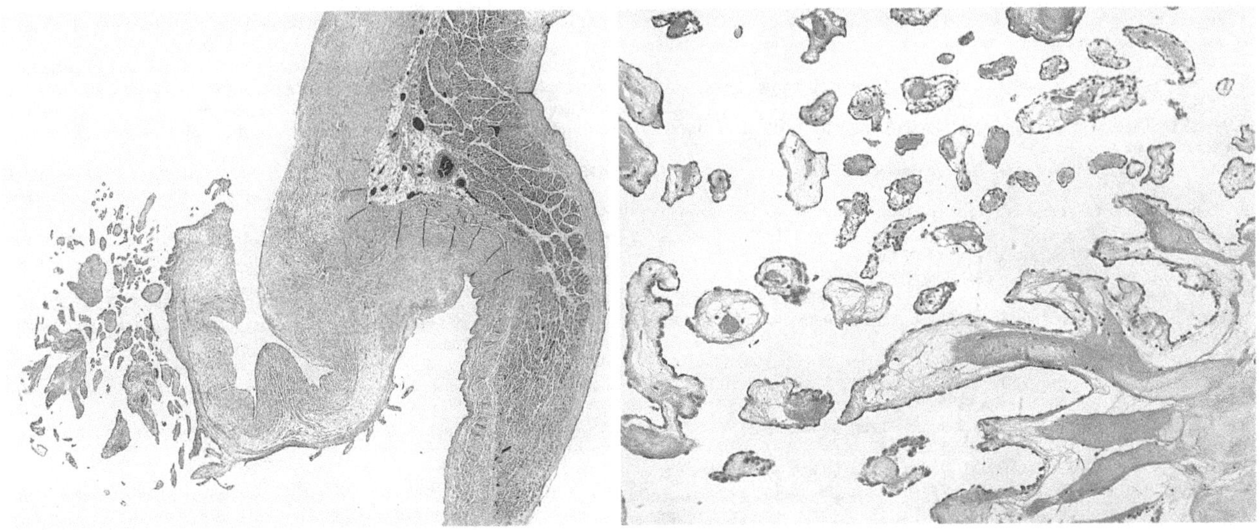

FIGURE 4. Photomicrographs of papillary fibroelastomas from the patient described in Figure 3. *Left,* view of aortic valve cusps with multiple fibroelastomas on the ventricular aspect of the cusps. *Right,* close-up view of the papillary fibroelastoma. Hematoxylin-eosin stains, left, ×15; right, ×84; reduced by 30%.

growths may also obstruct an aortic ostium of a coronary artery.[40,41]

On rare occasion, papillary fibroelastomas have been observed on the right side of the heart, mainly the tricuspid valve.[42–47]

Papillary fibroelastomas have been operatively excised from cardiac valves and/or mural endocardium in patients with evidence of stroke or other peripheral events and a few patients have had cardiac valve replacement.[9,11,13,14,19,20,22–24,29,30,34,37,41,45,47] When papillary fibroelastomas are detected by echocardiography in asymptomatic patients, operative excision rarely appears warranted. Whether operative excision or valve replacement is beneficial for papillary fibroelastomas in patients with cerebral or myocardial ischemic events is unsettled. I wonder if anticoagulation in these patients may be preferable to operative excision or valve replacement. There are no long-term follow-up studies available to answer these questions.

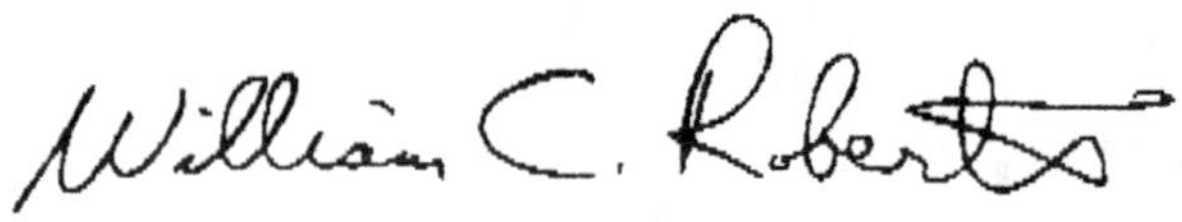

William Clifford Roberts, MD
Editor in Chief
Baylor Cardiovascular Institute
Baylor University Medical Center
Dallas, Texas 75246

1. Raeburn C. Papillary fibro-elastic hamartomas of the heart valves. *J Pathol Bacteriol* 1953;65:371–374.
2. Heath D, Best PV, Davis BT. Papilliferous tumors of the heart valves. *Br Heart J* 1961;23:20–24.
3. Nassar SGA, Parker JC Jr. Incidental papillary endocardial tumor. *Arch Pathol* 1971;92:370–376.
4. Fisbein MC, Ferrans VJ, Roberts WC. Endocardial papillary elastofibromas. Histologic, histochemical, and electron microscopical findings. *Arch Pathol* 1975;99:335–341.
5. Roberts WC. Valvular, subvalvular, and supravalvular aortic stenosis: morphologic features. *Cardiovasc Clin* 1973;5:97–126.
6. Heath D, Thompson IM. Papillary "tumors" of the left ventricle. *Br Heart J* 1965;29:950–954.
7. Burn CG, Bishop MB, Davies JNP. A stalked papillary tumor of the mural endocardium. *Am J Clin Pathol* 1969;51:344–346.
8. Flotte T, Pinar H, Feiner H. Papillary elastofibroma of the left ventricular septum. *Am J Surg Pathol* 1980;4:585–588.
9. Almagro UA, Perry LS, Choi H, Pintar K. Papillary fibroelastoma of the heart. Report of six cases. *Arch Pathol Lab Med* 1982;106:318–321.
10. Ong LS, Nanda NC, Barold SS. Two-dimensional echocardiographic detection and diagnostic features of left ventricular papillary fibroelastoma. *Am Heart J* 1982;103:917–918.
11. Topol EJ, Biern RO, Reitz BA. Cardiac papillary fibroelastoma and stroke. Echocardiographic diagnosis and guide to excision. *Am J Med* 1986;80:129–132.
12. Kalman JM, Lubicz S, Brennan JB, Vernon-Roberts E, Calafiore P. Multiple cardiac papillary fibroelastoma and rheumatic heart disease. *Aust N Z J Med* 1991;21:744–746.
13. Bedi HS, Sharma VK, Mishra M, Kasliwal RR, Trehan N. Papillary fibroelastoma of the mitral valve associated with rheumatic mitral stenosis. *Eur J Cardiothorac Surg* 1995;9:54–55.
14. Allen KB, Goldin M, Mitra R. Transaortic video-assisted excision of a left ventricular papillary fibroelastoma. *J Thorac Cardiovas Surg* 1996;112:199–201.
15. Campbell M, Carling W. Sudden death due to a fibrinous polyp of the aortic valve. *Guy's Hosp Rep* 1934;84:41–42.
16. Butterworth JS, Poindexter CA. Papilloma of cusp of the aortic valve: report of a patient with sudden death. *Circulation* 1973;48:213–215.
17. Cha SD, Incarvito J, Fernandez J, Chang KS, Maranhao V, Gooch AS. Giant Lambl's excrescences of papillary muscle and aortic valve: echocardiographic, angiographic, and pathologic findings. *Clin Cardiol* 1981;4:51–54.
18. Gopal A, Li Mandri G, King DL, Marboe C, Homma S. Aortic valve papillary fibroelastoma. A diagnosis by transthoracic echocardiography *Chest* 1994;105: 1885–1887.
19. Ragni T, Grande AM, Cappuccio G, Arbustini E, Grasso M, Tramarin R, Vigano M. Embolizing fibroelastoma of the aortic valve. *Cardiovasc Surg* 1994; 2:639–641.
20. Shahian DM, Labib SB, Chang G. Cardiac papillary fibroelastoma. *Ann Thorac Surg* 1995;59:538–541.
21. Fowles RE, Miller DC, Ebgert BM, Fitzgerald JW, Popp RL. Systemic embolization from a mitral valve papillary endocardial fibroma detected by two-dimensional echocardiography *Am Heart J* 1981;102:128–130.
22. Groton ME, Soltanzadeh H. Mitral valve fibroelastoma. *Ann Thorac Surg* 1989;47:605–607.
23. Gallo R, Kumar N, Prabhakar G, Awada A, Maalouf Y, Duran CM. Papillary fibroelastoma of mitral valve chorda. *Ann Thorac Surg* 1993;55:1576–1577.
24. Shapiro OM, Willimason WA, Dugan JM. Papillary fibroelastoma of the mitral valve. *Cardiovasc Surg* 1993;1:599–601.
25. Mann J, Parker DJ. Papillary fibroelastoma of the mitral valve. a rare cause of transient neurological deficits. *Br Heart J* 1994;71:6.
26. Pinelli G, Carteaux JP, Mertes PM, Civit T, Trinh A, Villemot JP. Mitral valve tumor revealed by stroke. *J Heart Valve Dis* 1995;4:199–201.
27. Zamora RL, Adelberg DA, Berger AS, Huettner P, Kaplan HJ. Branch retinal artery occlusion caused by a mitral valve papillary fibroelastoma *Am J Opthalmol* 1995;119:325–329.
28. Colucci V, Alberti A, Bonacina E, Gordini V. Papillary fibroelastoma of the mitral valve. A rare cause of embolic events. *Tex Heart Inst J* 1995;22:327–331.
29. McFadden PM, Lacy JR. Intracardiac papillary fibroelastoma: an occult cause of embolic neurologic deficit. *Ann Thorac Surg* 1987;43:667–669.
30. Brown RD Jr, Khandheria BK, Edwards WD. Cardiac papillary fibroelastoma: a treatable cause of transient ischemic attack and ischemic stroke detected by transesophageal echocardiography. *Mayo Clinic Proc* 1995;70:863–868.
31. Ighoghossian N, Trouillas P, Perinetti M, Barthelet M, Ninet J, Loire R. Lambl's excrescence: an uncommon cause of cerebral embolism. *Rev Neurol* 1995;151:583–585.
32. Kasarskis EJ, O'Connor W, Earle G. Embolic stroke from cardiac papillary fibroelastomas. *Stroke* 1988;19:1171–1173.
33. Zull DN, Diamond M, Beringer D. Angina and sudden death resulting from papillary fibroelastoma of the aortic valve. *Ann Emerg Med* 1985;14:470–473.
34. Shirani J, Bradlow JA, Metbeyeva P, Losada M, Factor SM, Strom JA, Sisto D. Transient loss of vision as the presenting symptom of papillary fibroelastoma of aortic valve. *Cardiovasc Pathol* 1997,6:237–240.
35. Richard J, Castello R, Dressler FA, Willman VL, Nashed A, Lewis B, Labovitz AJ. Diagnosis of papillary fibroelastoma of the mitral valve complicated by non-Q wave infarction with apical thrombus. trans-esophageal and transthoracic echocardiography study. *Am Heart J* 1993;126:710–712.
36. Etienne Y, Jobic Y, Houel JF, Barra JA, Boschat J, Meunier M, Penther P. Papillary fibroelastoma of the arotic valve with myocardial infarction: echocardiographic diagnosis and surgical excision. *Am Heart J* 1994;127:443–445.
37. Eckstein FS, Chafers HJ, Grote J, Mugge A, Borst HG. Papillary fibroelastoma of the aortic valve presenting with myocardial infarction. *Ann Thorac Surg* 1995;60:206–208.
38. Grote J, Mugge A, Schfers JH, Daniel WG, Lichtlen PR. Multiplane transesophageal echocardiography detection of a papillary fibroelastoma of the aortic valve causing myocardial infarction. *Eur Heart J* 1995;16:426–429.
39. Harris LS, Adelson L. Fatal coronary embolism from a myxomatous polyp of the aortic valve: an unusual cause of sudden death. *Am J Clin Pathol* 1965;43:61–64.
40. Boone S, Higginson LA, Walley VM. Endothelial papillary fibroelastoma arising in and around the aortic sinus, filling the ostium of the right coronary artery. *Arch Pathol Lab Med* 1992;116:135–137.
41. Mazzucco A, Bortolotti U, Thiene G, Dan M, Stritoni P, Scutari M, Stellin G. Left ventricular fibroelastoma with coronary embolization. *Eur J Cardiothorac Surg* 1989;3:471–473.
42. Anderson KR, Fiddler FI, Lie JR. Congenital papillary tumor of the tricuspid valve: an unusual cause of right ventricular outflow obstruction in a neonate with trisomy E. *Mayo Clin Proc* 1977;52:665–669.
43. Frumin H, O'Donnell L, Kerin NZ, Levine F, Nathan LE, Klein SP. Two-dimensional echocardiographic detection and diagnostic features of tricuspid papillary fibroelastoma. *J Am Coll Cardiol* 1983;2:1016–1018.
44. Mohan JC, Goel PK, Gambhir DS, Khanna SK, Arora R. Calcified mobile papillary fibroelastoma of the tricuspid valve a case report. *Indian Heart J* 1987;39:237–239.
45. Wolfe JT III, Finck SJ, Safford RE, Perselin ST. Tricuspid valve papillary fibroelastoma: echocardiographic characterization. *Ann Thorac Surg* 1991;51: 116–118.
46. Neerukonda SK, Jantz RD, Vijay NK, Narrod JA, Schoonmaker FW. Pulmonary embolization of papillary fibroelastoma arising from the tricuspid valve. *Tex Heart Inst J* 1991;18:132–135.
47. Ganjoo AK, Johnson WD, Gordon RT, Jain DP, Lang GE, Shankar VS. Tricuspid papillary fibroelastoma causing syncopal episodes. *J Thorac Cardiovasc Surg* 1996;112:551–553.

Cardiac Neoplasms

William C. Roberts

OVERVIEW

Primary cardiac tumors involving the heart may either be benign or malignant. Most of the benign tumors are myxomas, which are most commonly located in the left atrium. Primary malignant neoplasms usually involve the myocardium and the interior of the cardiac cavities, whereas metastatic neoplasms to the heart most commonly involve pericardium, and pericardial effusion and constriction are the most common consequences. Computed tomography and magnetic resonance imaging are becoming the most useful instruments of precision to diagnosis cardiac tumors. A number of nonneoplastic conditions in the heart or pericardium are frequently mistaken for cardiac neoplasms including pericardial cysts, teratoma, lipomatous hypertrophy of the atrial septum, papillary fibroelastoma, thrombi, and sarcoid. There are a number of cardiac consequences of malignancy including radiation heart disease, cardiac hemorrhages, cardiac infection, and cardiac adiposity or the corticosteroid treated heart, cardiac hemosiderosis, and anthracycline chemotherapy. Carcinoid heart disease is a unique type of heart disease associated with a unique type of cancer.

W. C. Roberts: Baylor Cardiovascular Institute, Baylor University Medical Center, Dallas, Texas 75246

HISTORICAL PERSPECTIVE

In the last 40 years, cardiac neoplasms have progressed from clinical curiosities described primarily in numerous case reports with diagnosis mainly at autopsy to fairly rapid antemortem diagnosis and frequent curative operative therapy. Diagnosis has been greatly facilitated by two-dimensional echocardiography and, in select cases, the use of magnetic resonance imaging or computed tomography.

CLASSIFICATION

There is no perfect classification for cardiac neoplasms. Like any organ or tissue, neoplasms involving the heart may be primary or secondary. The primary ones may be benign or malignant, and the secondary or metastatic ones are, by definition, malignant. The metastatic neoplasms are far more frequent than are the primary neoplasms by at least a 30 to 1 ratio (1,2). The various frequencies of the primary benign and primary malignant tumors vary from report to report, approximately 0.1% to 0.3% in most autopsy series. A recent list of primary benign neoplasms gathered by investigators at the Armed Forces Institute of Pathology is listed in Table 1, and those primary malignant tumors encountered are listed in Table 2 (3). The frequencies of the metastatic neoplasms also vary from

TABLE 1. *Primary benign neoplasms of the heart (1976–1993)*

Tumor*	Total	Surgical	Autopsy	Age ≤15 years at diagnosis
Myxoma	114	102	12	4
Rhabdomyoma	20	6	14	20
Fibroma	20	18	2	13
Hemangioma	17	10	7	2
Atrioventricular nodal	10	0	10	2
Granular-cell	4	0	4	0
Lipoma	2	2	0	0
Paraganglioma	2	2	0	0
Myocytic hamartoma	2	2	0	0
Histiocytoid cardiomyopathy	2	0	2	2
Inflammatory pseudotumor	2	2	0	1
Fibrous histiocytoma	1	0	1	0
Epitheloid hemangioendothelioma	1	1	0	0
Bronchogenic cyst	1	1	0	0
Teratoma	1	0	1	1
Totals	199	146 (73%)	53 (27%)	45 (23%)

Source: Modified from Burke A, Virmani R. *Atlas of Tumor Pathology. Tumors of the Heart and Great Vessels.* Washington, DC: Armed Forces Institute of Pathology, 1996:231.

* Excludes papillary fibroelastoma and lipomatous hypertrophy of the atrial septum.

report to report, but nearly all studies have listed carcinoma of the lung as the most commonly encountered metastatic tumor at autopsy, with cancer of the breast, followed by lymphoma and leukemia as the next leading causes (Table 3). The order of frequency of metastases is different, however, if the frequency of each different type of tumor with metastasis to the heart is determined. For example, Table 4 lists the frequencies of metastases to the heart in each of 100 cases of each of 20 separate tumors: melanoma has the highest frequency of metastases to the heart followed by malignant germ cell tumor, leukemia, lymphoma, cancer of the lung, and then the various sarcomas (3).

LOCATION OF CARDIAC NEOPLASMS

Cardiac neoplasms may involve only the endocardium, only the myocardium, only the epicardium, or various combinations (Fig. 1). By far the most common location of metastatic cardiac neoplasm is the epicardium. Neoplasms limited to parietal pericardium without extension into the epicardium are not considered cardiac neoplasms. The epicardial tumor deposits may be multifocal or single, or they may be extensive and essentially diffuse or nearly so. Likewise, the intramyocardial masses may be focal or multifocal. The most common location for intramyocardial masses is the left ventricular free wall and ventricular septum, the portions of the heart, of course, with the greatest myocardial mass. The endocardial neoplasms are the intracavitary ones. They may involve a single cardiac cavity or more than one. They may be limited to either the right or left side of the heart, or they may involve both. Intracavitary tumors produce obstruction to inflow into the heart or into a ventricular cavity or outflow from a ventricular cavity. The intracavitary neoplasms are the ones that may partially dislodge and produce either pulmonary or systemic emboli or both. The intracavitary deposits have the potential of producing the triad of obstruction, embolization, and constitutional symptoms.

TABLE 2. *Primary malignant tumors of the heart (1976–1993)*

Tumor	Total	Surgical	Autopsy	Age ≤15 years at diagnosis
Sarcoma	137 (95%)	116	21	11 (8%)
Angio	33	22	11	1
Unclassified	33	30	3	3
Fibrous histiocytoma	16	16	0	1
Osteo	13	13	0	0
Leiomyo	12	11	1	1
Fibro	9	9	0	1
Myxo	8	8	0	1
Rhabdomyo	6	2	4	3
Synovial	4	4	0	0
Lipo	2	0	2	0
Schwannoma	1	1	0	0
Lymphoma	7 (5%)	1	6	0
Totals	144 (100%)	117 (81%)	27 (19%)	11 (8%)

Source: Modified from Burke A, Virmani R. *Atlas of Tumor Pathology. Tumors of the Heart and Great Vessels.* Washington, DC: Armed Forces Institute of Pathology, 1996:231.

TABLE 3. *Metastatic neoplasms in the heart at necropsy in the order of frequency of cancers encountered*

Primary tumor	Total autopsies	Metastases to heart*
1. Lung	1037	180 (17)
2. Breast	685	70 (10)
3. Lymphoma	392	67 (17)
4. Leukemia	202	66 (33)
5. Esophagus	294	37 (13)
6. Uterus	451	36 (8)
7. Melanoma	69	32 (46)
8. Stomach	603	28 (5)
9. Sarcoma	159	24 (15)
10. Oral Cavity and tongue	235	22 (9)
11. Colon and rectum	440	22 (5)
12. Kidney	114	12 (11)
13. Thyroid gland	97	9 (9)
14. Larynx	100	9 (9)
15. Germ cell	21	8 (38)
16. Urinary bladder	128	8 (6)
17. Liver and biliary tract	325	7 (2)
18. Prostate gland	171	6 (4)
19. Pancreas	185	6 (3)
20. Ovary	188	2 (1)
21. Nose (interior)	32	1 (3)
22. Pharynx	67	1 (1)
23. Miscellaneous	245	0
Totals	6240	653 (10)

Source: Modified from Burke and Virmani who combined studies of McAllister HA and Fenoglio JJ Jr. *Tumors of the Cardiovascular System. Atlas of Tumor Pathology.* Washington, DC: Armed Forces Institute of Pathology, 1978:111–119, and Mukai K, Shinkai T, Tominaga K, Shomosato Y. The incidence of secondary tumors of the heart and pericardium: A 10-year study. *Jpn J Clin Oncol* 1988; 18: 195–201.

* Numbers in parentheses are percentages.

TABLE 4. *Metastatic neoplasms in the heart at necropsy: order of frequency of metastases of each different primary tumor*

Primary tumor	Number of autopsies	Percent with metastases to heart*
1. Melanoma	100	46
2. Germ cell	100	38
3. Leukemia	100	33
4. Lymphoma	100	17
5. Lung	100	17
6. Sarcoma	100	15
7. Esophagus	100	13
8. Kidney	100	11
9. Breast	100	10
10. Mouth and tongue	100	9
11. Thyroid gland	100	9
12. Uterus	100	8
13. Urinary bladder	100	6
14. Stomach	100	5
15. Colon and rectum	100	5
16. Prostate gland	100	4
17. Pancreas	100	3
18. Nose (Interior)	100	3
19. Ovary	100	1
20. Pharynx	100	1
21. Miscellaneous	100	0

* These percentages were obtained by combining studies by McAllister and Fenoglio and by Mukai et al. McAllister HA and Fenoglio JJ Jr. *Tumors of the Cardiovascular System. Atlas of Tumor Pathology.* Washington, DC: Armed Forces Institute of Pathology, 1978; 111–119. Mukai K, Shinkai T, Tominaga K, Shomosato Y. The incidence of secondary tumors of the heart and pericardium: A 10-year study. *Jpn J Clin Oncol* 1988; 18:195–201.

TECHNIQUES FOR DIAGNOSING CARDIAC NEOPLASMS

Symptoms and Physical Signs

The various signs and symptoms produced by the various cardiac neoplasms are determined primarily by the tumor's location in the heart. Physical examination is rarely diagnostic (4–6).

Pericardial (specifically epicardial) involvement is the most common type of involvement by metastatic neoplasms to the heart (7). Neoplastic pericardial disease is usually asymptomatic and detected only as an incidental finding at autopsy. Signs of cardiac tamponade may be the initial or later manifestation of neoplastic pericardial disease. In patients with epicardial constriction by neoplasm, dyspnea is most common followed by chest pain, cough, orthopnea, and hepatomegaly. Distal cardiac sounds and a pericardial friction rub are infrequent.

Intramyocardial neoplasms are usually clinically silent. Occasionally there are disturbances of conduction or rhythm, and both of these disturbances are determined primarily by the actual location of the tumor. The sudden development of complete heart block or high degrees of atrioventricular block or asystole are suggestive of myocardial involvement. A wide range of arrhythmias may be produced, including atrial fibrillation or flutter, paroxysmal atrial tachycardia with or without block, nodal rhythm, ventricular premature complexes, ventricular tachycardia, and ventricular fibrilla-

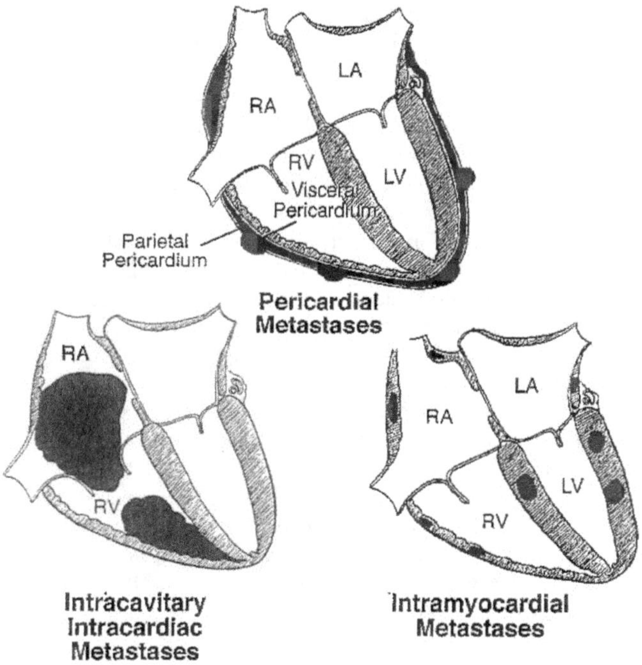

FIG. 1. Diagram showing various locations of cardiac neoplasms involving the heart. RA = right atrium; LA = left atrium; LV = left ventricle; RV = right ventricle.

tion. On occasion, intramyocardial tumors impair ventricular function resulting in confusion with restrictive cardiomyopathy or hypertrophic cardiomyopathy.

Left atrial cavitary neoplasms may produce signs and symptoms often mimicking those of mitral valve disease, especially mitral stenosis, including dyspnea, orthopnea, paroxysmal nocturnal dyspnea, pulmonary edema, cough, hemoptysis, chest pain, peripheral edema, and fatigue. Additionally, some patients, particularly those with left atrial myxoma, may lose weight, become pale, faint, and have cardiac arrest. Left atrial tumors may produce symptoms suddenly or intermittently, and sometimes they come and go depending on body position. Although most symptoms produced by left atrial tumors are nonspecific, the occurrence of paroxysmal symptoms that occur characteristically in a particular body position and are out of proportion to the clinical findings should raise suspicion of a left atrial myxoma.

Right atrial cavitary neoplasms, if large enough, produce signs and symptoms of right-sided heart failure, including peripheral edema, ascites, hepatomegaly, and prominent ''a'' waves in the jugular venous pulse. It may take years from the symptomatic presentation to the correct diagnosis. The development of right-sided heart failure may be rapidly progressive and is often associated with new systolic or diastolic precordial murmurs or both. The murmurs generally are the result of obstruction to the tricuspid valve orifice by the neoplasm, of tricuspid regurgitation caused by the tumor's interference with valve closure, or of direct destruction of the tricuspid valve leaflets by the tumor's movement in the tricuspid valve orifice. Signs of pulmonary embolism and pulmonary hypertension may occur. If the right atrial pressure rises to levels greater than that of the left atrium and if the foramen ovale is patent (15% of population), a right-to-left shunt may be the consequence, and systemic hypoxia, cyanosis, clubbing, and polycythemia may result. Evidence of superior or inferior vena caval obstruction, hepatomegaly, and ascites may occur. An early diastolic rumbling murmur alone or in combination with a holosystolic murmur, which increases with inspiration, usually indicates tricuspid regurgitation. A protodiastolic ''tumor plop'' also may occur with right atrial tumors. The jugular venous pressure may be elevated and the ''a'' wave within the venous system may be quite prominent.

Right ventricular cavitary neoplasms often present with right-sided heart failure as a result of an obstruction to right ventricular filling or outflow, and the consequences include peripheral edema, hepatomegaly, ascites, dyspnea, syncope, and cardiac arrest. A systolic ejection murmur at the left sternal border is usually present. Neoplastic emboli to peripheral pulmonary arteries may cause pulmonary hypertension. If the neoplasm extends into the pulmonary trunk, it may interfere with pulmonic valve closure, resulting in pulmonic regurgitation. The jugular veins are frequently distended with a prominent ''a'' wave and a Kussmaul's sign.

Left ventricular cavitary neoplasms are probably most frequently located at the apex of this chamber and, as a consequence, are usually clinically silent. Those in the left ventricular outflow tract may lead to obstruction to outflow, producing syncope or evidence of heart failure. Chest pain also may occur. A neoplasm in the left ventricular outflow tract may cause a precordial systolic murmur. The intensity of the murmur and the level of the blood pressure may vary with position.

Electrocardiogram

The electrocardiogram is usually nonspecific (8,9), but it could be far more useful than has been appreciated in the past. The problem has been that the electrocardiogram may be recorded when diagnosis is first considered, but subsequently electrocardiograms are not taken very frequently toward the end of the patient's life. One study (8) compared findings on electrocardiogram in patients with malignant lymphoma who had cardiac lymphoma to another group of patients with lymphoma who did not have cardiac involvement. The percentage with abnormal tracings (62%) was similar in each of the two groups. Fewer than half the patients had more than one electrocardiogram during the entire illness. Findings included sinus tachycardia; low voltage; ectopic tachycardia, including atrial fibrillation; atrial flutter; atrial tachycardia; atrial ventricular block, including prolonged PR interval; second- and third-degree block; premature ventricular complexes; right or left axis deviation; right bundle branch block; T-wave abnormalities, and ST-T wave changes of usually nonspecific nature. The suddent development of some of these electrocardiographic findings in a patient who previously lacked these changes is suggestive evidence of cardiac involvement.

Radiograph

The chest radiograph may be helpful, particularly when an epicardial neoplasm is present (10). Enlargement of the cardiac silhouette, mediastinal widening, a hilar mass, or an irregular contour of the cardiac silhouette may suggest pericardial involvement. Calcium within an intracardiac neoplasm can be seen on occasion by chest radiograph or fluoroscopy. The lung fields may have a paucity of pulmonary markings in patients with large right atrial or right ventricular neoplasms. Patients with neoplasms in the left atrium may have pulmonary changes similar to those in mitral stenosis. Likewise, left ventricular neoplasms causing obstruction to left ventricular inflow or outflow may produce similar pulmonary arterial vascular changes.

Echocardiogram

More cardiac tumors today are diagnosed by echocardiography (Table 5), at least initially, than by any other instrument of precision. Diagnosis of left atrial myxoma, the most common primary tumor of the heart, has been one of the principal uses of echocardiography since the introduction of the technique (11–15). The classic left atrial myxoma is a mobile echogenic mass that is in the body of the left atrium in ventricular systole and passes into the mitral orifice in ventricular diastole. Occasionally, an echocardiogram will detect a left atrial myxoma which is small or not close to the mitral orifice, and it is therefore clinically silent. M-mode echocardiography was the first technique used to detect intracardiac tumors and particularly left atrial myxomas. Two-dimensional echocardiography obviously improved the ability to detect tumors in chambers other than those in the left atrium. Although it is usually possible to detect intracardiac tumors with transthoracic echocardiography, the transesophageal examination produces, as a rule, spectacular images and makes diagnosis, particularly of atrial masses, relatively easy (16,17). The transesophageal examination not only offers a higher sensitivity for detecting left atrial tumors, for example, but also permits a clearer picture of the attachment or stalk of the tumor and more precise characterization of the size, shape, and location of the mass. A major advantage of echocardiography is its ability to provide serial studies. Thus, by this technique, one may see progressive increase in size of a neoplasm or detect

TABLE 5. *Imaging techniques for the diagnosis of cardiac tumors*

	Radiography	CT	Angiography	MRI	Echocardiography
Primary benign tumors					
Myxoma	+*	++	+++	++++	+++++
Pericardial cyst	++	+++	0	+++++	+
Lipoma	+	+++	+	+++++	+++
Fibroelastoma	0	0	0	+++	+++++
Rhabdomyoma	0	+	+	++++	+++++
Fibroma	0	+		++++	++++
Primary malignant tumors					
Sarcoma	+	++	++	+++++	+++
Mesothelioma	+	+++	+	+++++	++
Lymphoma	++	+++	+	+++++	++
Secondary tumors					
Direct extension	+	+++	++	+++++	+++
Venous extension	0	+	+++	++++	++++
Metastatic spread	+	++	+	++++	++

Source: From Salcedo EE, Cohen GI, White RD, Davison MB. Cardiac tumors: diagnosis and management. *Curr Prob Cardiol* 1992 (Feb); 17:75–137.

* 0 = of no use; + = of limited use; ++ = may be of use; +++ = useful; ++++ = very useful; +++++ = preferred diagnostic tool.

recurrence once the initial tumor is excised. The echocardiogram also has been useful in detecting intracardiac tumors other than myxomas, including rhabdomyomas and rhabdomyosarcomas, neoplasms that occur primarily in infants and are located usually in the ventricles. The echocardiogram is also helpful in detecting metastases to the heart. This is particularly true in neoplasms that migrate up the inferior vena cava into the right side of the heart, such as renal cell carcinoma or adrenal cell carcinoma. Echocardiography, particularly transesophageal, has been extremely helpful in detecting mediastinal or extracardiac masses, which may compress the cardiac structure.

Computed Tomogram

The computed tomogram is useful in diagnosing cardiac tumors (18,19); it may be especially useful in defining the degree of intramyocardial extension or the lack thereof and whether the tumor is present in adjacent extracardiac structures. Ultrafast computed tomography, a technique that uses electron-beam technology, has a short scanning acquisition time that eliminates the motion artifacts occurring with conventional computed tomography. This new approach appears to be particularly well suited for assessing intracardiac masses.

Magnetic Resonance Imaging

Compared with computed tomography, magnetic resonance imaging appears to be of greater value in delineating cardiac tumors (20). It may be able to depict the size, shape, and surface characteristics of the tumor more clearly than computed tomography. This technique also can provide information regarding tissue composition that can help to differentiate neoplasms from thrombi.

Angiogram

A cardiac catheterization and selective angiography are no longer necessary in all patients with cardiac neoplasms, because adequate preoperative information can usually be obtained by echocardiography, computed tomography, or magnetic resonance imaging. For cases in which the latter three techniques have not fully defined the location and attachment of the neoplasm, in which all four chambers of the heart have not been well delineated, or in which another type of cardiac condition is suspected (such as coronary arterial narrowing), then cardiac catheterization with angiography might be necessary. Angiography in patients with cardiac neoplasms is particularly useful in detecting compression or displacement of cardiac cavities or large masses, and the magnitude of the intracavitary filling defects. The most frequent angiographic findings are intracavitary filling defects, which may be either fixed or mobile, lobulated or smooth, and attached over a broad base or by a narrow stalk. Coronary angiography is sometimes helpful in visualizing the vascular supply of the neoplasm and the relation of the neoplasm to the coronary arteries. The vascular pattern is not helpful, however, in differentiating benign from malignant tumors. In contrast to the other diagnostic techniques, cardiac catheterization can be a bit risky in patients with intracardiac neoplasms because the catheter may dislodge a fragment of the tumor with resulting embolus. Thus, the noninvasive techniques are preferred before cardiac catheterization in a patient suspected of having an intracardiac mass. The transseptal approach to the left atrium is not advised if a left atrial tumor is suspected, because the stalk of the left atrial myxoma is usually attached to the fossa ovale membrane, where the transseptal catheter courses.

SPECIFIC BENIGN PRIMARY CARDIAC NEOPLASMS

Myxoma

Myxomas are by far the most common type of primary cardiac tumor and 75% of them are located in the left atrial cavity (Fig. 2), about 23% in the right atrial cavity (Fig. 3), and about 2% in a ventricular cavity (21–33). On rare occasion, the tumor is present in more than one cavity (34). Generally, when located

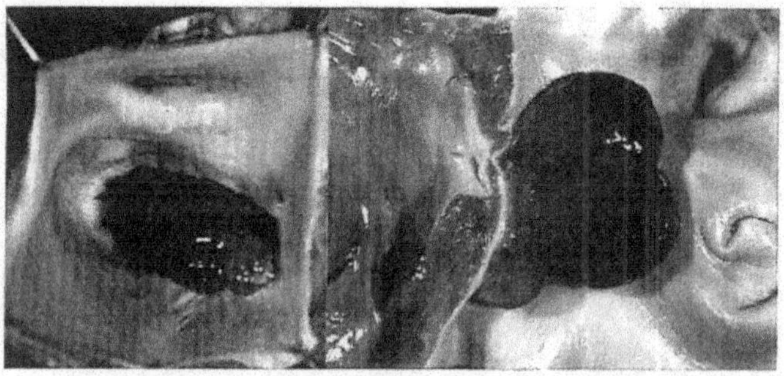

FIG. 2. Left atrial myxoma in a 60-year-old woman (A69-275) who died of metastatic carcinoid and never had clinical evidence of heart disease. The myxoma was not large enough to prolapse through the mitral orifice during ventricular diastole. *Left:* View of left atrium cephalad. *Right:* Longitudinal view showing attachment of the myxoma to the atrial septum by a relatively broad base.

in the left atrium, the neoplasm produces symptoms when it reaches about 70 in size. Those in the right atrium that produce symptoms are usually about twice as large and sometimes several-fold larger. The cell of origin of the myxoma is still unclear (22). How fast atrial myxomas grow has never been clarified. An attempt to answer this question was provided by a study that examined size of recurrent myxomas and divided that size in grams by the interval between the first operation and the second one (35). It was estimated that recurrent left atrial myxomas grow an average of 0.15 cm per month or 1.8 cm per year, or an average of 1.2 g per month or 14 g per year. Whatever the exact growth rate may be, both recurrent and initial left atrial myxomas appear to grow rather rapidly. Morphologic diagnosis of myxoma is readily made by gross inspection, and their appearance is clearly different from thrombi. The surface is smooth but irregular, shiny, and usually multicolored. Attachment is nearly always to the atrial septum if the tumor is in the left atrium, and the stalk is most commonly much smaller than the maximal diameter of the mass. On occasion, the site of attachment

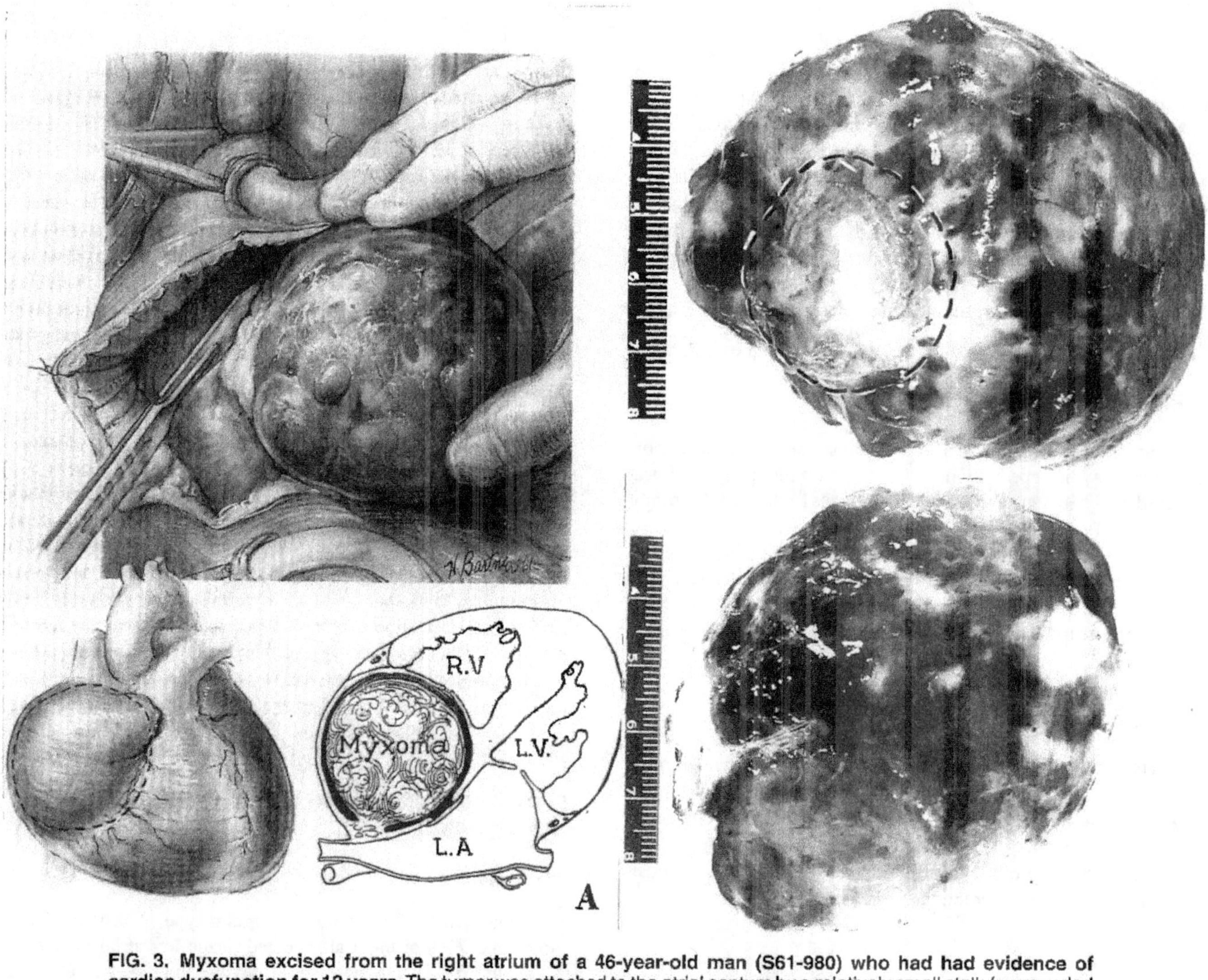

FIG. 3. Myxoma excised from the right atrium of a 46-year-old man (S61-980) who had had evidence of cardiac dysfunction for 12 years. The tumor was attached to the atrial septum by a relatively small stalk (surrounded by dashed circle [*upper right*]). The myxoma weighed 142 g and its largest diameter was 8 cm. A view of the cut section of the tumor is shown in the lower right.

to the atrial septum is broad. The mean age of patients with sporadic myxoma is 56 years, and 70% are women.

Familial cardiac myxomas constitute approximately 10% of all myxomas, and they appear to have an autosomal dominant transmission. These occur in younger patients (mean age 25) and have less female gender predominance. The myxomas in the familial syndrome are much more liable (50% of the time) to be multiple and to have a ventricular cavity location (13% as compared with <1% in the nonfamilial or sporadic patients with myxomas). These patients typically have exterior facial freckling; they have noncardiac myxomas (breast or skin) and also endocrine neoplasms. Both the NAME (nevi, atrial myxoma, neurofibromata, ephelides) and the LAMB (lentigines, atrial myxoma, and balloon nevi) syndromes are associated with the familial variety of cardiac myxoma. Chromosomal abnormalities for atrial myxoma on chromosome 2 (Carney's) and chromosome 12 (Ki-ras genes) have been described.

Myxomas probably present the most varied clinical picture of all primary cardiac neoplasms (4–6,23,25,26). Several major syndromes have been observed, including presentation with signs of emboli, obstruction to blood flow, and various constitutional syndromes. Fragments of tumor located in the right side of the heart may embolize to the lungs, and of those in the left side of the heart, of course, to various systemic organs. Diagnosis may be made, on occasion, by finding typical myxomatous endothelial-like cells—which are elongated and spindle shaped with round or oval nuclei and prominent nucleoli—in surgically removed emboli.

Obstruction to blood flow may occur at the orifice of any valve, most commonly, of course, the mitral valve. Interference with flow through the mitral orifice may mimic signs of mitral stenosis, including signs of pulmonary congestion, diastolic apical rumble, opening snap, and accentuated first heart sounds. A murmur of mitral regurgitation may also be present as a result of chronic damage to the valve leaflets or to interference with proper closure of the valve by tumor. Differentiation between left atrial tumor and primary mitral stenosis is suggested by the influence of position on symptoms and on the intensity of the precordial murmurs and the opening snap. Right atrial myxoma has occasionally migrated to the left atrial cavity via a patent foramen ovale with resulting systemic hypoxemia (36,37).

The constitutional symptoms associated with atrial myxomas are protean and include fever, weight loss, Raynaud's phenomenon, digital clubbing, anemia, elevated erythrocyte sedimentation rate, elevated leukocyte count, decreased platelet count, positive seroreactive protein, and abnormal serum proteins (usually increased gamma globulins). These constitutional symptoms may mimic infective endocarditis, collagen vascular disease, or occult malignancy.

The proper treatment of myxoma in any cavity of the heart is operative resection because no medicine is known to shrink myxomas or to prevent their continued growth (21,27). Some surgeons advise a biatrial approach for full visualization of both sides of the heart and then complete removal of a left or right atrial myxoma, excising the full thickness of the atrial septum if the neoplasm is attached to the region of the fossa ovalis. If a large portion of the atrial septum is removed, a patch must be used to close the defect. Because fragmentation and embolization of the tumor is an ever present threat, vigorous palpation and other manipulations of the heart should be avoided until cardiopulmonary bypass is initiated. Most surgeons usually induce ventricular standstill with cardioplegia solution before manipulating the heart in order to reduce the possibility of fragmentation of portions of the tumor. Left atrial myxomas have been removed successfully during pregnancy. On occasion, an atrioventricular valve has been so traumatized by the tumor's prolapsing through it during ventricular diastole that valve excision and replacement is necessary. Fortunately, recurrences of atrial myxomas are rare, and if they do recur, it is usually within a 4-year period.

Rhabdomyoma

The most common cardiac neoplasm in infants and children is rhabdomyoma (38). There is some question whether this particular tumor is a true neoplasm or actually resembles a hamartoma. These neoplasms are usually multiple, most often involve the ventricular myocardium, and project into the cavity or move freely as a pedunculated mass (39–41). Associated tuberous sclerosis is present in about one third of the patients. The diagnosis is suggested by the presence of yellow-brown angiofibromas ("adenoma sebaceum") on the face, sublingual fibromas around the fingernails, café au lait spots, and subcutaneous nodules. Presenting symptoms may be caused by obstruction to inflow to or outflow from the ventricles, arrhythmias, atrioventricular block, pericardial effusion, and even sudden death (42). These neoplasms may mimic pulmonic valve stenosis and produce hypoxic spells, resembling those seen in tetralogy of Fallot. These neoplasms are usually readily diagnosed by echocardiography, angiography, or magnetic resonance imaging. Prenatal detection of intracardiac rhabdomyoma by intrauterine echocardiography has been reported with successful operative removal. The occurrence of more than one tumor does not prevent operative intervention. On rare occasion, these tumors have produced ventricular tachycardia in infants, and this arrhythmia has disappeared following successful operative removal.

Fibroma

Fibromas are usually intramural within a ventricular wall (Fig. 4) (3,43). Most also occur in infants and children. Calcific deposits may be present within the neoplasm. Sudden death has occurred in about a third of the patients, presumably the result of a conduction defect, arrhythmia, or obstruction to outflow from a ventricle. Left axis deviation has been seen on electrocardiogram. Total or partial resection of the neoplasm may relieve obstruction with an excellent probability of long-term survival.

Lipoma

Lipomas involving the heart may be extremely small and represent incidental necropsy findings, or they may be massive (44–47). The largest cardiac neoplasm ever reportedly apparently was an intrapericardial lipoma. They may be mistaken for pericardial cysts, they may cause pericardial effusion, or they may be asymptomatic and suggested by a widened mediastinum on chest radiograph. Intramyocardial lipomas are encapsulated and usually small. Lipomas also have been located on cardiac valves, where they may simulate vegetations or myxomas (46). Magnetic resonance imaging permits preoperative identification of these fatty tumors.

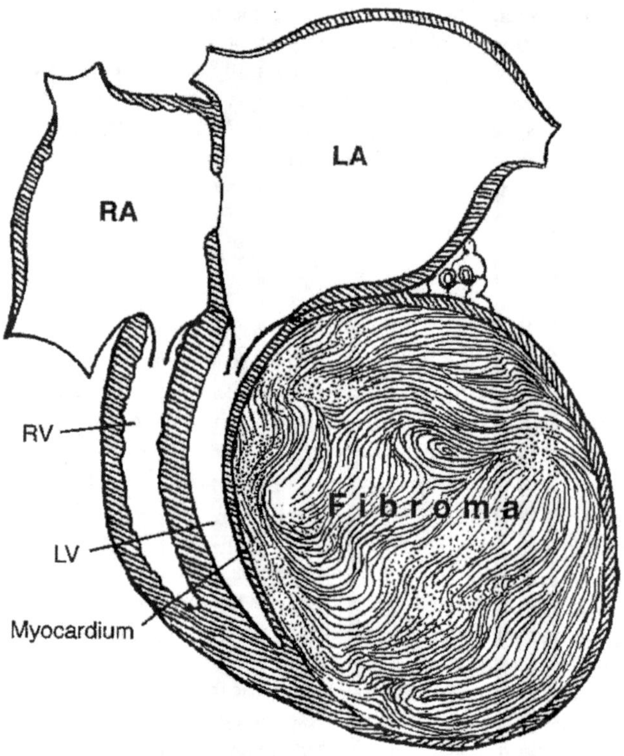

FIG. 4. Diagram of an intramyocardial fibroma seen at necropsy in a 5-month-old boy (A-07-92) who was found dead in his crib. The neoplasm had been diagnosed by biopsy during the child's first few days of life. It was considered nonresectable.

Hemangioma

Hemangiomas are best diagnosed by coronary angiography, which yields a characteristic "tumor blush." Spontaneous resolution without treatment has been reported. Total excision is usually not possible.

SPECIFIC MALIGNANT PRIMARY CARDIAC NEOPLASMS

Angiosarcoma

Nearly all primary malignant cardiac neoplasms are sarcomas, and the most frequent one is angiosarcoma (48–52), which characteristically originates from the right atrium or from the epicardium of the right atrium. The large quantity of vascular channels within these tumors and the subsequent large quantity of blood flowing through them may produce a continuous precordial murmur. About 25% of all angiosarcomas will, at least in part, be intracavitary with valvular obstruction and cause right-sided heart failure and pericardial tamponade with a hemorrhagic-type fluid. The course is rapid with widespread metastases and operative intervention is usually unsuccessful.

Rhabdomyosarcoma

Rhabdomyosarcoma is the second most frequent primary sarcoma of the heart, and, like angiosarcoma, it is most common in males (53–55). In contrast to angiosarcoma, however, no single cardiac chamber has a predilection for this neoplasm. Indeed, the neoplasm may be in all four cardiac chambers, or at least in more than one, and obstruction may occur in one or more valve orifices. Again, prognosis is poor, survival is short, and operative intervention is usually futile.

Miscellaneous

Fibrosarcoma, liposarcoma, primary malignant lymphoma, and occasional sarcomas of other cell types constitute the remaining but infrequent primary malignant coronary neoplasms (Figs. 5–7). All of these neoplasms may obstruct valvular orifices or obliterate chambers and/or produce peripheral emboli (56). Hypertrophic cardiomyopathy has been suggested by heavy tumorous infiltrations of the ventricular septum (57).

METASTATIC NEOPLASMS TO THE HEART

Metastatic or secondary tumors of the heart with a primary in another body organ or tissue are far more frequent than are

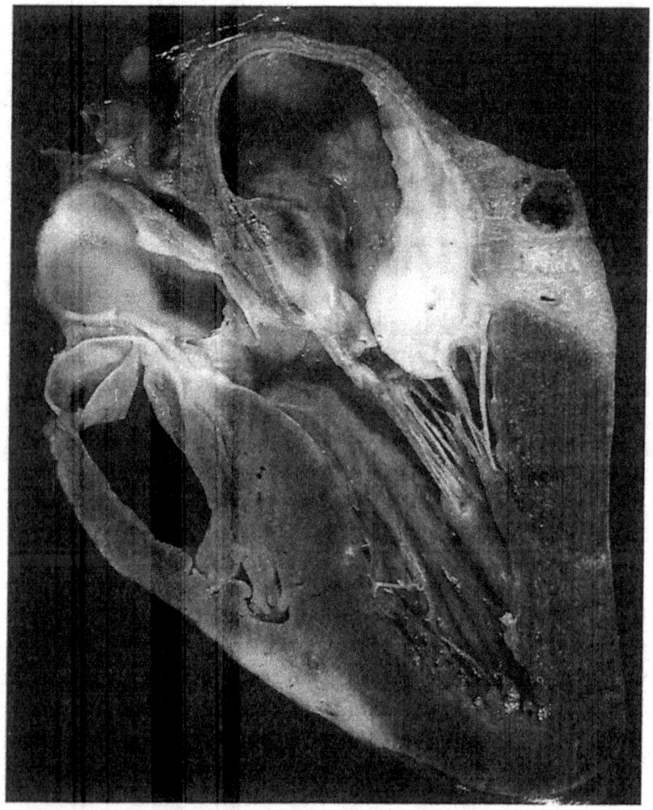

FIG. 5. Primary cardiac sarcoma, undifferentiated type, causing mitral stenosis in a 46-year-old woman (A90-2) who had been well until 8 months before death. Cardiac catheterization disclosed a 20-mm Hg mean diastolic gradient between the pulmonary artery wedge position and left ventricle. The right ventricular pressure was 105/18 mm Hg. The neoplasm is located in the walls of left atrium and in both arteries and posterior mitral leaflets. The patient is described in detail elsewhere (56). (From Domanski et al. Primary sarcoma of the heart causing mitral stenosis. *Am J Cardiol* 1990; 66:893–895, with permission.)

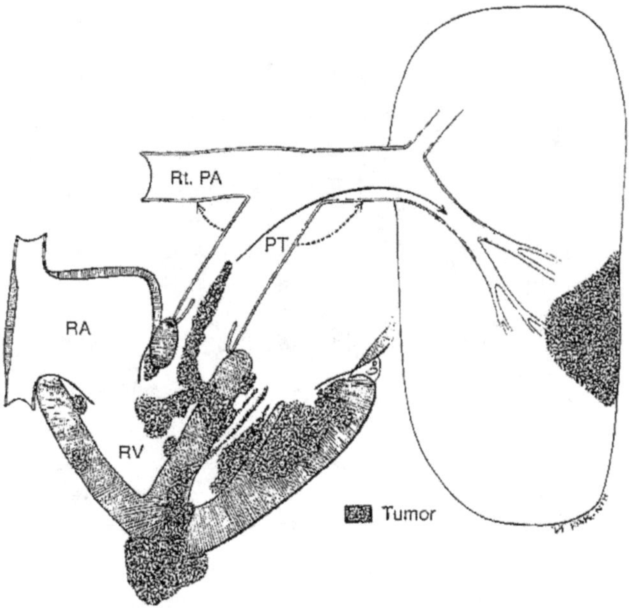

FIG. 6. Primary cardiac sarcoma, undifferentiated type, with neoplastic emboli to lung and other organs in a 26-year-old man (A69-149) who had been well until 3 months before death.

primary tumors of the heart (58). The secondary tumors are far more commonly carcinomas than sarcomas simply because carcinomas are far more common. Diagnosis can be suspected whenever cardiac manifestations occur in a patient diagnosed with a primary tumor in an organ or tissue other than the heart. The development of cardiac enlargement, tachycardia, arrhythmias, or heart failure in the presence of neoplasm elsewhere in the body is highly suggestive of cardiac metastases. Only rarely is metastatic tumor limited to the heart. Thus, the presence of metastatic tumor in the heart usually indicates widespread metastases in a number of body organs. On rare occasion, cardiac involvement may be the first or only expression of a noncardiac primary neoplasm. The most common sign is tamponade (59). Direct invasion of the heart via the vena cava or pulmonary veins may lead to obstruction of an atrioventricular valve, as well as to pulmonary or systemic emboli or both (60–62).

Carcinoma of the lung and carcinoma of the breast tend to invade the parietal pericardium and then the visceral pericardium, leading to myocardial constriction and/or pericardial effusion (Fig. 8). Another common presentation of cancer of the lung is invasion of the pulmonary veins within the lung, with spread of the cancer within the lumen of the pulmonary veins into the left atrium. From there, the cancer which in turn can continue into the mitral orifice, sometimes causing obstruction of that orifice (63,64) (Fig. 9). Metastatic cancer from the lung to the adrenal gland also may extend into the inferior vena cava and then into the right side of the heart (Fig. 10), just as can primary adrenal gland or renal cancer (65). Cancer of the lung or breast surrounding the main right or left pulmónary artery can lead to pulmonary arterial obstruction (66).

Melanoma has the highest frequency of metastases to the heart per 100 cases of any neoplasm (67,68). The metastases may be anywhere in the heart; usually melanotic metastases invade the walls of all four cardiac chambers and also the epicardium and endocardium (Fig. 11). The cancers in these patients are in so many body organs that the presence of the neoplasm in the heart is almost incidental.

Leukemia commonly invades the heart (69). In the days before platelet transfusions, extensive hemorrhages into the myocardial walls and into the endocardium and epicardium were commonly found in patients with fatal leukemia of various types. Histologically, leukemic infiltration between myocardial cells is quite common, and sometimes gross deposits of leukemic cells are visible within the heart. A few patients with leukemia present with pericardial effusion, which is usually hemorrhagic. Large calcific deposits in the right side of the heart have been reported (70).

Lymphoma also has a very high frequency of metastases to the heart (71–76). Nearly 25% of patients with lymphomas of various types have lymphoma involving the epicardium, myocardium, or endocardium, or combinations. In contrast to leukemic involvement, the lymphomatous deposits are usually grossly discernible.

Some cancers, like osteognic sarcoma, may have calcium within them (77,78) (Fig. 12).

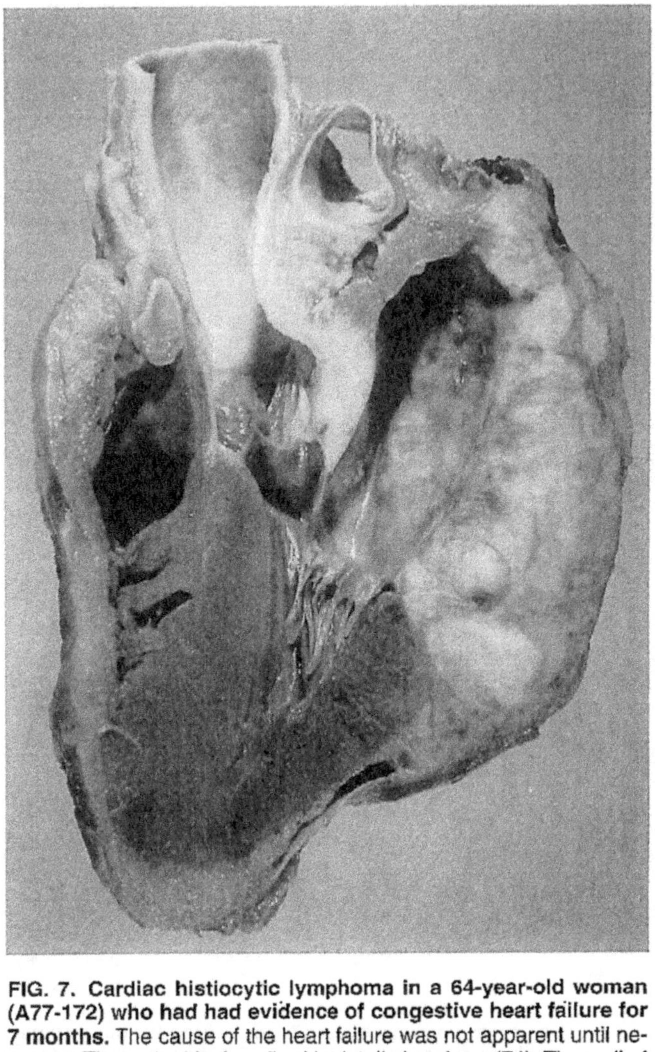

FIG. 7. Cardiac histiocytic lymphoma in a 64-year-old woman (A77-172) who had had evidence of congestive heart failure for 7 months. The cause of the heart failure was not apparent until necropsy. The patient is described in detail elsewhere (74). The wall of the left atrium is massively thickened by the neoplasm. (From Roberts CS, Gottdiener JS, Roberts WC. Clinically undetected cardiac lymphoma causing congestive heart failure. *Am Heart J* 1990; 120: 1239–1242, with permission.)

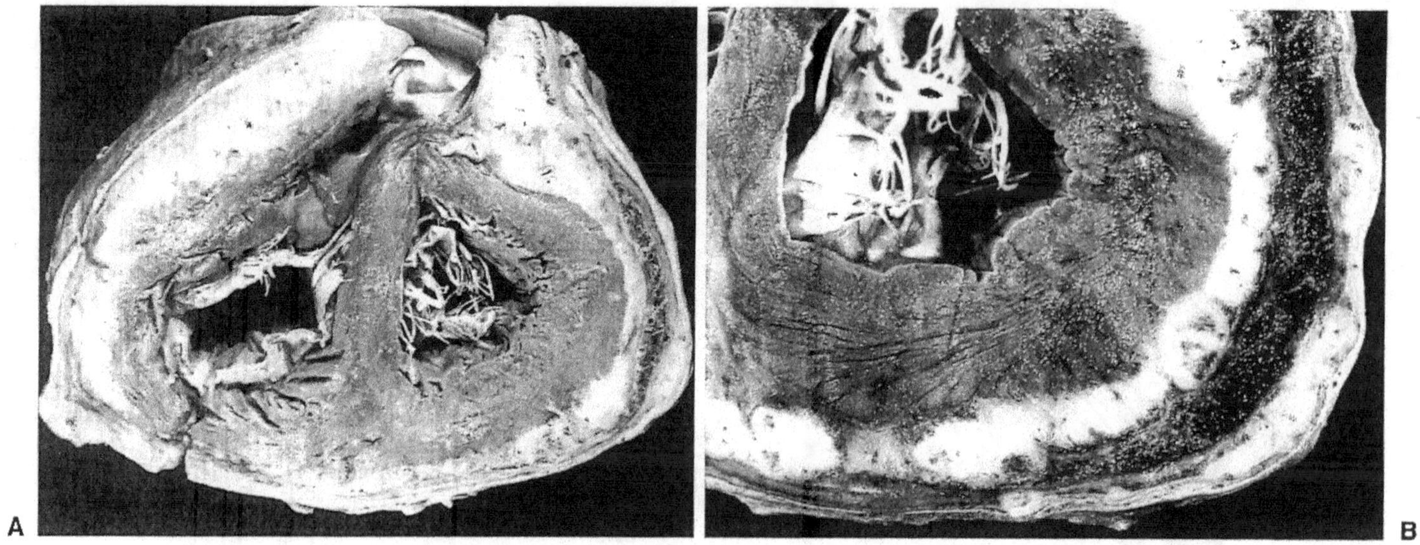

FIG. 8. Metastatic squamous-cell carcinoma of the lung in a 61-year-old man (67A-531). Cardiac tamponade was the immediate cause of death. The entire heart and great vessels were encased in tumor. (From Roberts WC and Spray TL. Pericardial heart disease. *Curr Prob Cardiol* 1977; 2(June):1–71, with permission.)

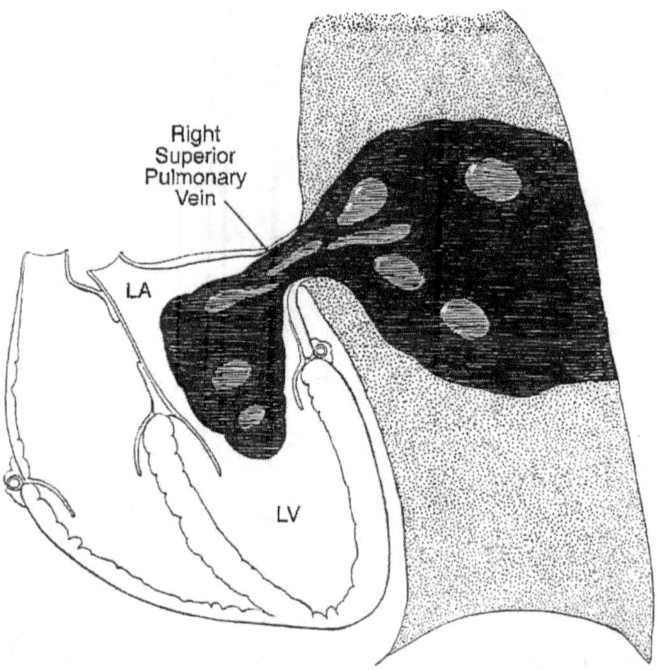

FIG. 9. Sarcoma, undifferentiated type, in lung (primary uncertain, possibly in pulmonary vein) in a 29-year-old woman (A21-83) in whom echocardiogram disclosed the tumor in the left atrium moving about "like a yo-yo." The left lung and its left atrial extension were operatively excised. IVC = inferior vena cava; RA = right atrium; RV = right ventricle.

NONNEOPLASTIC CONDITIONS IN THE HEART OR PERICARDIUM FREQUENTLY MISTAKEN FOR CARDIAC NEOPLASM

Pericardial Cyst

Pericardial or mesothelial cysts are the most frequent benign "tumors" of the pericardium. These cysts are generally asymptomatic and found on "routine" chest radiograph (79). About a quarter of the patients, however, develop various symptoms including chest pain, dyspnea, cough, tachycardia, as a consequence of a pericardial cyst. The cysts are usually outside the pericardial cavity and, therefore, they really should not be considered "cardiac tumors."

Teratoma

Teratoma are actually extracardiac in at least 99% of the cases, but still within the pericardial cavity (80–82) (Fig. 13). They arise and receive their blood supply from the ascending aorta or pulmonary trunk, presumably through the vasa vasorum. Most are found in infants and children and primarily in females. Recurrent serous pericardial effusion in children should suggest intrapericardial teratoma. Because these tumors may become quite large, they may cause compression of various cardiac chambers and resulting symptoms.

Lipomatous Hypertrophy of the Atrial Septum

Massive fatty infiltration of the atrial septum is an extremely common condition occurring almost exclusively in persons over 50 years of age and usually over 65 years of age (Fig. 14) (83). These lesions are essentially limited to obese people, and they are always associated with enormous quantities of subepicardial adipose tissue, particularly enormous amounts of adipose tissue in the atrioventricular sulci. These hearts are almost always so fat that they

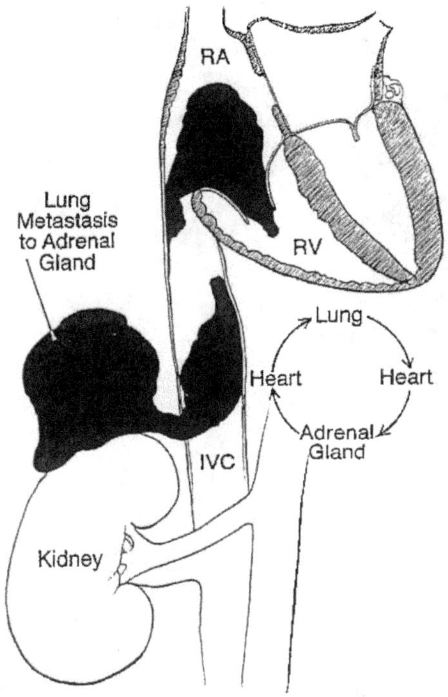

FIG. 10. Diagram of metastatic cancer of the lung to the right adrenal gland with extension into the inferior vena cava and then into the right side of the heart in a 57-year-old man (DCVAH #84A-121). Echocardiogram showed the right atrial mass, which prolapsed through the tricuspid valve in atrial systole.

float in water (84). Normally the atrial septum is less than 1 cm in thickness. In patients with lipomatous hypertrophy of the atrial septum, the atrial septum cephalad to the fossa ovale may be as thick as 7 cm, and the portion of atrial septum caudal to the fossa ovali may be as thick as 4 cm. Enormous infiltration of fat into the atrial septum may be associated with atrial arrhythmias. It is probably the only atrial arrhythmia that is treatable, possibly curable, by transient starvation. The importance of lipomatous hypertrophy of the atrial septum in the context of "cardiac tumors" is that these patients should not be operated on to remove fat from the atrial septum. The treatment is simply weight loss. These fatty deposits may be diagnosed by echocardiography, computed tomography, or magnetic resonance imaging (85,86). Fat in the subepicardial adipose tissue has been confused by echocardiogram with pericardial effusion (87).

Papillary Fibroelastomas

Papillary fibroelastomas are small avascular growths with multiple papillary fronds usually limited to cardiac valves, mainly the aortic and mitral, and they are common in older persons (88–91). They consist of fibrous tissue covered by an elastic membrane, which in turn is covered by endocardium. Occasionally (about 15%), they also occur on left ventricular or ventricular septal mural endocardium (92–101), particularly in patients with small or relatively small ventricular cavities, such as patients with hypertrophic cardiomyopathy (92,98) or mitral stenosis with or without aortic valve stenosis (96,99,100). When located on the aortic valve, papillary fibroelastomas are usually found on the ventricular aspects of the cusps in the more central portions. They also occur on the aortic

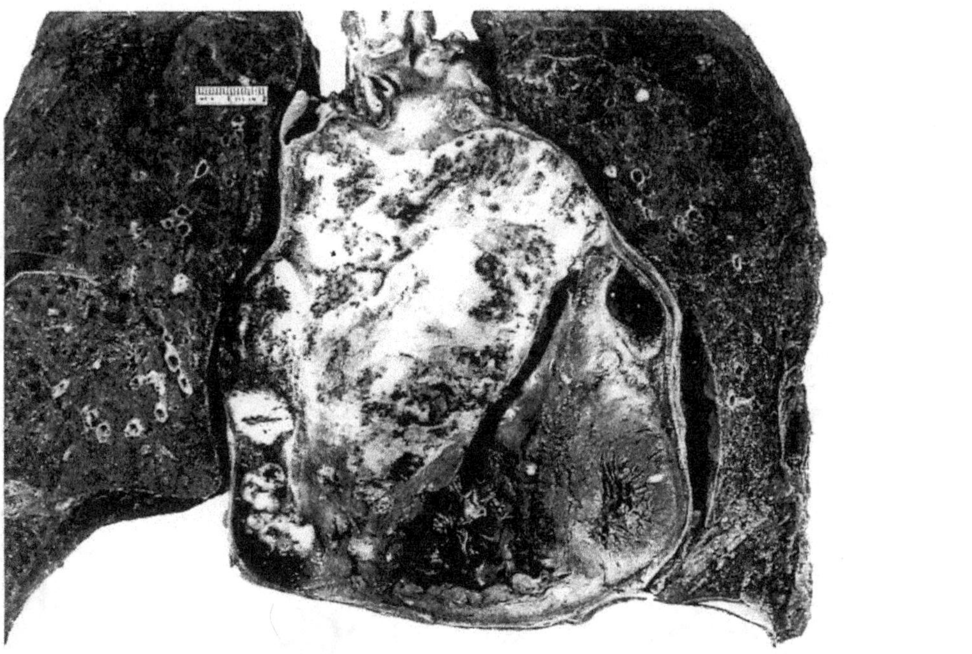

FIG. 11. Metastatic melanoma to the heart in a 53-year-old man (A75-41). During life, a pericardial friction rub was audible, and the neck veins were quite distended. The parietal pericardium is everywhere adherent to the epicardium. The superior vena cava, right atrium, right ventricle, and pulmonary trunk are severely compressed by the tumor. (From Roberts WC and Spray TL. Pericardial heart disease. *Curr Prob Cardiol* 1977; 2(June):1–71, with permission.)

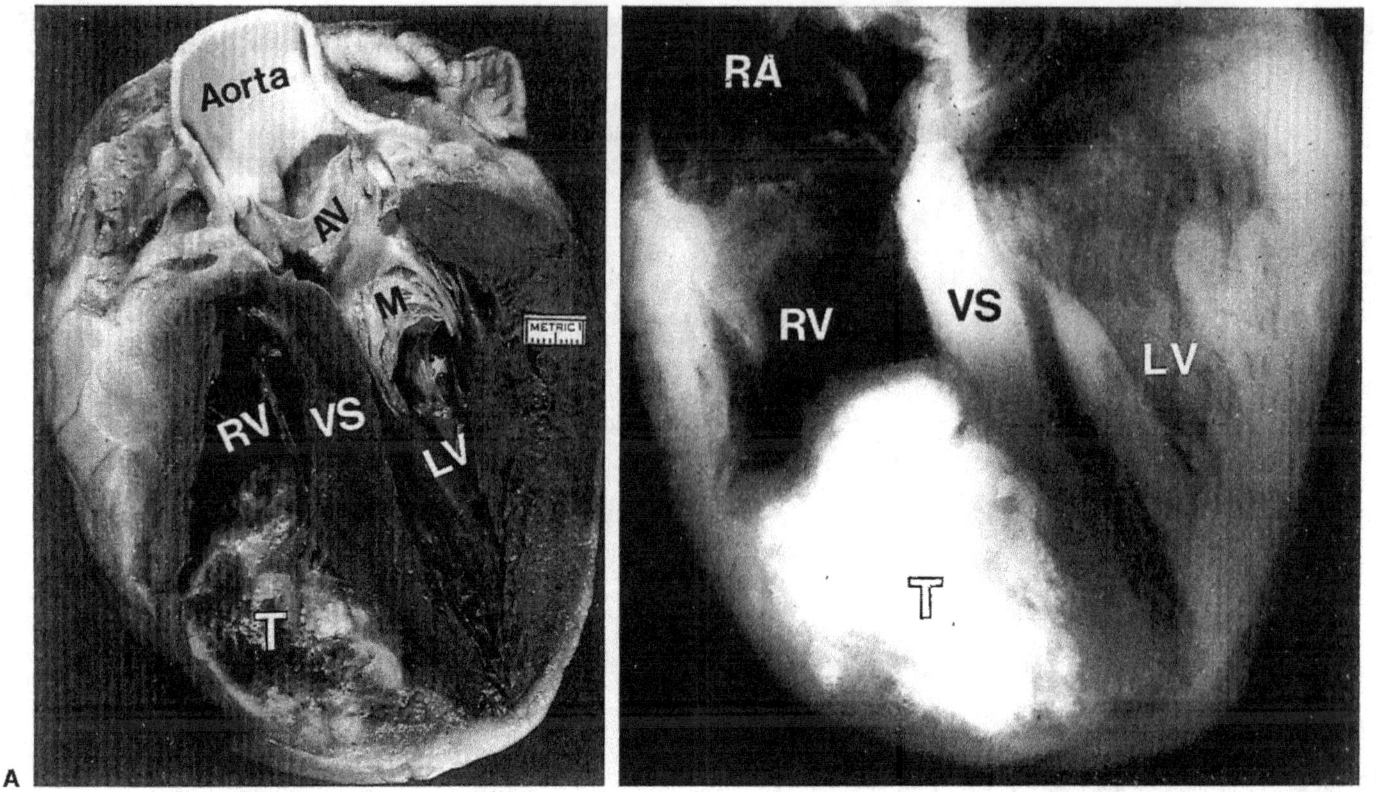

FIG. 12. Osteogenic sarcoma to the heart in a 39-year-old woman (A80-81) with a large calcified tumor (T) in the right ventricle (RV). This patient, who was ill for 20 months, had episodic ventricular tachycardia during her last 10 months. AV = aortic valve; M = mitral leaflet; LV = left ventricle; RA = right atrium; VS = ventricular septum. The patient is described elsewhere (77). (From Seibert KA, Rettenmier CW, Waller BF, et al. Osteogenic sarcoma metastatic to the heart. *Am J Med* 1982; 73:136–141, with permission.)

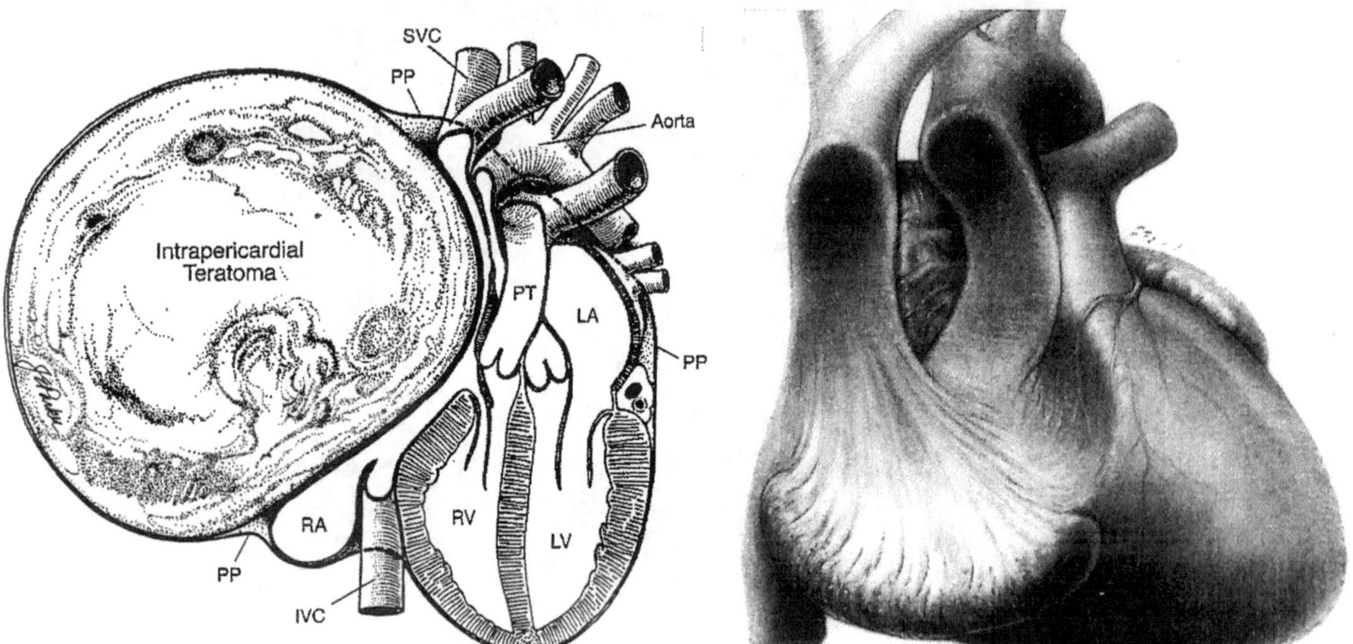

FIG. 13. Intrapericardial teratoma in a stillborn. The infant's heart weighed 8 g and the tumor, which greatly compressed the heart, 20 g. (From Brabham KR, Roberts WC. Cardiac-compressing intrapericardial teratoma at birth. *Am J Cardiol* 1989; 63:386–387, with permission.)

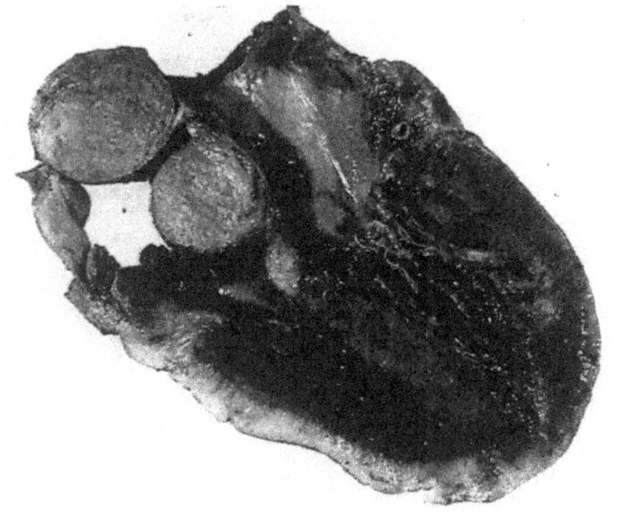

FIG. 14. Lipomatous hypertrophy of the atrial septum in a 74-year-old woman (GT #77A-42) with huge fatty deposits in the atrial septum (except for the fossa ovale area). (From Shirani J, Roberts WC. Clinical, electrocardiographic and morphologic features of massive fatty deposits ("lipomatous hypertrophy") in the atrial septum. *J Am Coll Cardiol* 1993; 22:226–238, with permission.)

aspects of these cusps, usually near the margins (102–107). On the mitral valve leaflets, they are usually on the atrial aspects near the margins (108–115). In patients with hypertrophic cardiomyopathy or mitral stenosis, they may be on the ventricular aspects of the anterior mitral leaflet and sometimes in mural endocardium, particularly over the papillary muscles. These lesions may be the result of contact of one valve leaflet with another or one mural endocardial surface with another.

A number of patients have been reported with papillary fibroelastomas and evidence of stroke (106–108, 113,114,116–120). Whether the stroke was truly connected in any way with the cardiac fibroelastomas is debatable. Some patients have been in their 20s or 30s without other predisposing features or findings commonly associated with cerebral infarction, and the occurrence of stroke in the younger age group is suggestive of a connection. In contrast to myxoma, where myxomatous material has been seen in systemic emboli, however, histologic findings of papillary fibroelastomas have not been observed in a cerebral artery in a patient with stroke and cardiac papillary fibroelastomas. Furthermore, the papillary fibroelastomas are firmly attached to valvular or mural endocardium, and dislodgement of a fibroelastoma therefore would appear unlikely. Thrombus, however, is occasionally superimposed on papillary fibroelastomas, and it may be that the thrombus is the material which is dislodged and responsible for the stroke.

Additionally, angina pectoris (120), acute myocardial infarction (121–125), and sudden death (121,126) have been observed in patients with cardiac papillary fibroelastomas, mainly on the aortic valve. These papillary growths may also obstruct an aortic ostium of a coronary artery (127,128). On rare occasion, papillary fibroelastomas have been observed on the right side of the heart, mainly the tricuspid valve (129–134).

Papillary fibroelastomas have been operatively excised from the cardiac valve and/or mural endocardium in patients with evidence of stroke or other peripheral events, and a few patients have had cardiac valve replacement (96,98,100,101,106,107,109–111, 116,117,124,128,132,134). When papillary fibroelastomas are detected by echocardiography in asymptomatic patients, operative excision rarely appears warranted.

Thrombi

Thrombi within an intracardiac cavity may be indistinguishable from neoplasm by echocardiogram or radiograph. Grossly, however, they are very different.

Sarcoid

When located in myocardium, sarcoid granuloma may grossly resemble neoplasm (135–137).

CONSEQUENCES OF THERAPY FOR NEOPLASMS IN THE HEART OR MEDIASTINUM

Radiation Heart Disease

Radiation heart disease was first recognized after radiation therapy for Hodgkin's disease (138–142). Some of the earlier patients with Hodgkin's disease received 8,000 rads, which adversely affected the pericardium, myocardium, and endocardium. The most common manifestation of radiation heart disease is pericardial effusion. The mechanism of the effusion is unclear. Fibrin deposits occur on both the visceral and parietal aspects of the pericardia. Because coronary arteries are located in subepicardial adipose tissue, they often receive the effects of radiation. Many patients have been reported to have coronary arterial narrowing at a very young age after radiation therapy, particularly patients with Hodgkin's disease. The intimal plaques resulting from radiation heart disease in actuality cannot be distinguished from plaques occurring from typical atherosclerosis. The distinguishing feature of radiation heart disease involving the coronary arteries is extensive fibrous thickening of the adventitia, and also loss, focally or diffusely, of internal and external elastic membranes, particularly the latter. Narrowing of coronary ostia is also common in radiation heart disease. In addition, radiation can cause considerable scarring within the subepicardial adipose tissue. The second most common manifestation of radiation heart disease is mural endocardial thickening, most commonly of the right atrium, and ventricle, but focally also in the left ventricle. The third most common manifestation of radiation heart disease is interstitial fibrosis, depending on the portal of entry, it usually involves the anterior wall of the right ventricle more than any other portion of the heart.

Cardiac Hemorrhages

Thrombocytopenia, particularly if persistent, often results in focal epicardial, myocardial, and mural endocardial hemorrhages. If the hemorrhages are located in conduction tissue, various degrees of heart block or arrhythmias may be the consequence.

Cardiac Infection

The most common cardiac infections today in cancer patients are myocardial abscesses and mural endocardial and epicardial abscesses. These are particularly prevalent in patients with prolonged leukopenia (143,144). Patients having unsuccessful bone-marrow transplantation are particularly prone to these infections, which usually are produced by fungi, not bacteria. Gas gangrene may involve the heart as well as most other body organs and tissues (145).

Cardiac Adiposity or the Corticosteroid-Treated Heart

Patients with various types of cancers, particularly those with leukemia and lymphoma, and those developing cancer after transplantation of one or more body organs, usually receive corticosteroid therapy for prolonged periods. The consequence is excessive deposition of fat in the heart, mainly in the subepicardial areas (146). These hearts may become so fatty that they float in water (buffalo hump of the heart), and this excessive subepicardial adipose tissue may simulate pericardial effusion.

Cardiac Hemosiderosis

Normally the human body contains approximately 4 g of iron. If the deposits increase to about 25 g, iron deposits are then usually found within myocardial cells. Patients who receive 100 units of blood without associated bleeding diatheses can acquire approximately 25 g of iron within the body organs and tissues. This situation may exist in some patients with cancer, particularly leukemia, and the result is cardiac hemosiderosis (147). These patients may be asymptomatic, or they may develop features of dilated cardiomyopathy with heart failure. At times, ventricular arrhythmias may be a consequence. Myocardial restriction as a result of myocardial ironic deposits has occurred, but dilation is far more common (148).

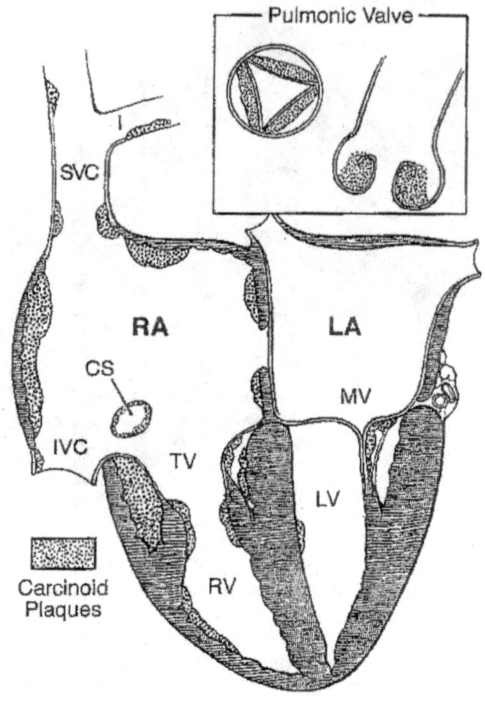

FIG. 15. Diagram showing location of carcinoid fibrous plaques in carcinoid heart disease. CS = coronary sinus ostium; I = innominate vein; IVC = inferior vena cava; LA = left atrium; LV = left ventricle; MV = mitral valve; RA = right atrium; RV = right ventricle; SVC = superior vena cava; TV = tricuspid valve. (From Ross EM, Roberts WC. The carcinoid syndrome: comparison of 21 necropsy subjects with carcinoid heart disease to 15 necropsy subjects without carcinoid heart disease. *Am J Med* 1986; 79:339–354, with permission.)

Anthracycline Chemotherapy (Doxorubicin and Daunorubicin)

Cardiac toxicity is a well-recognized complication of doxorubicin and daunorubicin and is frequently the dose-limiting factor in their administration (149–151). Clinical toxicity is usually manifested by evidence of impaired left ventricular systolic function. Morphologic signs of toxicity may be present when clinical signs of toxicity are absent.

A UNIQUE HEART DISEASE ASSOCIATED WITH A UNIQUE CANCER: CARCINOID HEART DISEASE

Carcinoid tumors are never primary in the heart, and they rarely metastasize to the heart. Nevertheless, patients with ileal, bronchial, or ovarian carcinoid, when hepatic metastases are present, often develop distinctive lesions in the heart, particularly in the right side (152–156) (Fig. 15). The distinctive lesions consist of deposits of fibrous tissue devoid of elastic fibers on the ventricular aspect of the tricuspid valve leaflets and on the arterial aspect of the pulmonic valve leaflets. Occasionally, deposits also are seen on the ventricular aspects of the mitral leaflets and, very rarely and usually to a small extent, on the aortic aspects of the aortic valve cusps. These lesions may result in tricuspid regurgitation and stenosis and pulmonic valve stenosis and regurgitation. Surprisingly, patients with carcinoid heart disease, compared to patients with metastatic carcinoid disease without carcinoid heart disease, have similar life spans after diagnosis of the carcinoid syndrome. The syndrome is diagnosed primarily by the presence of facial flushing and diarrhea.

Ross and Roberts (155) studied at necropsy 36 patients with metastatic carcinoid: 21 (57%) with and 15 (43%) without carcinoid heart disease. The two groups were similar in mean age (54 years vs. 55 years), duration of clinical illness (4.7 years vs. 6.3 years), body weight (50 kg vs. 52 kg), systemic blood pressure (117/77 mm Hg vs. 128/77 mm Hg), blood hematocrit levels (37% vs. 36%), total serum protein levels (6.0 g/dl), and serum albumin levels (2.2 g/dl vs. 2.6 g/dl). The two groups differed in the frequency of the presence of precordial murmurs consistent with tricuspid regurgitation and/or pulmonic stenosis (95% vs. 13%), cardiomegaly by chest radiography (38% vs. 0), low voltage on electrocardiography (47% vs. 0), and location of the primary site of the carcinoid tumor. Total electrocardiographic 12-lead QRS voltage was similar in each group (105 mm vs. 132 mm) (10 mm = 1 mV). Of the patients with carcinoid heart disease, 43% died of cardiac causes; none of those without carcinoid heart disease died of cardiac causes. Of the 21 subjects with carcinoid heart disease, 7 had left-sided cardiac involvement, but in none was it of functional significance. Thus, although carcinoid heart disease frequently is the cause of death in patients with the carcinoid syndrome, the development of carcinoid heart disease is not related to the duration of symptoms of the carcinoid syndrome.

All of the 21 patients with carcinoid heart disease studied by Ross and Roberts (155) had involvement of both tricuspid and pulmonic valves by carcinoid plaques, and 19 of them also had carcinoid plaques on the mural endocardium of the right atrium and usually also on the mural endocardium of the right ventricle. The number of subjects with right-sided valvular dysfunction as a consequence of the carcinoid plaques on the valvular leaflets is less certain because of the relative difficulty in diagnosing by auscultation mild degrees of tricuspid and pulmonic valve dysfunction. In 2 of the 21 subjects with right-sided carcinoid heart disease, the degree of morphologic involvement of both valves was minimal and valvular function clearly was not affected. Of the remaining 19 subjects, 18 had precordial systolic and/or diastolic murmurs of grade 2/6 or greater intensity.

Although the composition and location of the carcinoid plaques on both right-sided cardiac valves are similar, the functional consequences of the carcinoid plaques are different. The deposits occur nearly entirely on the downstream side of the valvular leaflets, that is, on the ventricular aspects of the septal and posterior tricuspid leaflets and on the pulmonary arterial side of the pulmonic valve cusps. On the anterior tricuspid valve leaflet, the deposits can be on both sides. The consequence of the "downstream" deposition is an adherence of the leaflet to the underlying mural endocardium (tricuspid septal and posterior leaflets) or to the underlying pulmonary arterial endothelium (pulmonic valve) via the carcinoid plaques. The fibrous tissue of the carcinoid plaque acts as a constricting substance such that the "ring" of both right-sided cardiac valves is made smaller than normal and, at the same time, leaflet mobility is diminished. The consequence is tricuspid regurgitation with or without some degree of stenosis. Nearly all patients with pure tricuspid regurgitation (no element of stenosis) have dilated valve rings, but patients with some degree of stenosis in addition to regurgitation do not have dilated annuli. Patients with carcinoid heart disease follow this principle. Thus, patients with carcinoid heart disease have much more tricuspid regurgitation than stenosis, but usually there is some degree of stenosis, albeit small.

In contrast to the tricuspid valve, the dominant functional pulmonic valve lesion is stenosis, although all patients with stenosis have some degree of pulmonic regurgitation. The reason for the difference from the tricuspid valve is that the orifice of the normal pulmonic valve is much smaller initially than the orifice of the tricuspid valve. Thus, the constriction by deposition of carcinoid plaques within the pulmonic sinuses causes constriction of the pulmonic root with the production of pulmonic stenosis. Because the distal portions of the pulmonic cusps are inverted toward the sinuses and the mobility of the cusps is lost, some degree of regurgitation is inevitable in patients who have any degree of pulmonic stenosis.

Although combined lesions of both mitral and aortic valves are fairly common as a consequence of rheumatic heart disease, infective endocarditis, or both, combined lesions of both tricuspid and pulmonic valves are rare, and carcinoid heart disease is the only condition in which uniformly both—not just one—right-sided valves are involved. The two dominant functional consequences of right-sided carcinoid heart disease are pulmonic stenosis and tricuspid regurgitation. These two lesions in the same patient are particularly unfavorable because pulmonic stenosis increases the degree of tricuspid regurgitation. A commonly employed method of producing chronic congestive heart failure in experimental animals is by banding the pulmonary trunk to create pulmonic stenosis, and excising or destroying one or more tricuspid valve cusps to make the valve purely regurgitant. Thus, right-sided carcinoid heart disease, in essence, creates this experimental model. If a patient with carcinoid heart disease had only dysfunction of the pulmonic or the tricuspid valve, the functional consequence probably would be insignificant. The combination of both right-sided valvular lesions—namely pulmonic stenosis and tricuspid regurgitation—has the potential of being devastating.

Clinical diagnosis of carcinoid heart disease can usually be established by noninvasive means. Auscultation, of course is the first clue. In Ross and Roberts' study (155), 20 (95%) of 21 subjects with carcinoid heart disease and 5 (33%) of 15 subjects without carcinoid heart disease had one or more precordial murmurs. Of the 20 subjects with precordial murmurs and carcinoid heart disease, 8 had both systolic and diastolic murmurs and 12 had only systolic murmurs; of the 5 subjects with precordial murmurs but without carcinoid heart disease, all the murmurs were systolic only. Thus, nearly all patients with carcinoid heart disease have precordial murmurs, and when the murmur has a diastolic component, diagnosis of carcinoid heart disease can be made with confidence.

The systemic arterial blood pressure is not helpful in either diagnosing carcinoid syndrome or distinguishing those with from those without carcinoid heart disease. Only 3 of the 36 subjects studied by Ross and Roberts (155) had indirect systolic systemic arterial pressures of more than 140 mm Hg and/or diastolic arterial pressures of more than 90 mm Hg: 1 of the 21 with carcinoid heart disease and 2 of the 15 without it. The average peak systolic pressure was 117 mm Hg in the 21 subjects with carcinoid heart disease and 128 mm Hg in the 15 subjects without it. The average diastolic pressure in both groups was 77 mm Hg.

Chest radiography is helpful in diagnosing carcinoid heart disease. The cardiothoracic ratio was more than 0.50 in 8 (38%) of the 21 subjects with carcinoid heart disease and in none of 15 subjects without it. Thus, the cardiothoracic ratio is not a very sensitive test for carcinoid heart disease, but it is specific.

The resting electrocardiogram is somewhat useful in distinguishing subjects with and without carcinoid heart disease. In Ross and Roberts' study (155), the sum of the QRS voltage in leads I, II, and III was 15 mm or less in 9 of the 21 subjects with carcinoid heart disease and in none of the 15 subjects without the disease. The sum of the total 12-lead QRS voltage ranged from 58 mm to 227 mm (10 mm = 1 mV) in 34 subjects, and the mean values did not differ significantly between the two groups (105 mm vs. 132 mm). Evidence of right ventricular hypertrophy was rare. The R wave was greater than the S wave in either lead V_1 or V_2 in only 4 of the 21 subjects with carcinoid heart disease and in none of the 15 subjects without it. Despite right atrial dilatation in most of the subjects with carcinoid heart disease, all 21 with and all 15 without carcinoid heart disease had sinus rhythm. The R-R interval was normal (0.20 sec or less) in 18 of 21 subjects with the disease and in 14 of 15 subjects without it. The width of the QRS complex was normal (0.12 sec or less) in all subjects, irrespective of whether they had carcinoid heart disease. Thus, other than the higher frequency of low voltage in the subjects with carcinoid heart disease, electrocardiography was not helpful in distinguishing between subjects with and without carcinoid heart disease.

Echocardiography, particularly cross-sectional, is helpful in diagnosing carcinoid heart disease. Callahan and associates (157) described retrospectively echocardiographic features in 20 patients with the carcinoid syndrome. By physical examination, 15 patients had a diagnosis of carcinoid heart disease and the other 5 did not. Both M-mode and cross-sectional examinations in the latter 5 patients disclosed no abnormal findings. Of the 15 patients with auscultatory evidence of carcinoid heart disease, 5 had normal M-mode and cross-sectional echocardiographic findings. The other

THE FUTURE

Improvement of chemotherapy will almost certainly improve outcome of primary and metastatic cancer involving the heart. ■

10, all of whom had tricuspid regurgitation by physical examination, had dilated right ventricular cavities, abnormal motion of the ventricular septum, and of the 9 in whom the tricuspid valve leaflets were visualized by cross-sectional echocardiography, strikingly abnormal tricuspid leaflets (thickened and retracted with fixed orifice). The pulmonic valve cusps were not visualized in any patient by M-mode echocardiography, but in the four in whom they were visualized by cross-sectional echocardiography, the pulmonic valve cusps were abnormal in each.

Howard and associates (158) prospectively examined by cross-sectional echocardiography 14 patients with the carcinoid syndrome, and 8 had definite abnormalities of one or both right-sided cardiac valves. Clinically, five had auscultatory evidence of tricuspid regurgitation, and all five had diffusely thickened and retracted tricuspid valve leaflets; the other nine patients had normal tricuspid valves by echocardiography. Four patients by auscultation had evidence of pulmonic stenosis with or without pulmonic regurgitation. The pulmonic valve cusps were visualized by echocardiography in seven patients: two had retracted pulmonic cusps with decreased systolic motion (one of whom had pulmonic stenosis by auscultation), and five had normal cusps (none of whom had auscultatory evidence of pulmonic stenosis).

Right-sided cardiac valve excision with or without valve replacement or valve commissurotomy or annuloplasty has been carried out in some patients with carcinoid heart disease. The interval from onset of symptoms and signs of congestive heart failure to cardiac valve operation in 15 patients collected from published reports by Ross and Roberts (160) ranged from 3 to 60 months (mean 14) and the interval from onset of symptoms of the carcinoid syndrome to cardiac valve operation ranged from 0.5 to 33 years (mean 10). Preoperatively, at least 12 of the 15 patients had hemodynamic evidence of tricuspid valve stenosis with mean diastolic pressure gradients between right atrium and right ventricle ranging from 4 to 24 mm Hg (mean 9). Of 15 patients, 14 had tricuspid regurgitation, which was graded as severe at angiography in at least 7 patients. Pullback pressures between pulmonary artery and right ventricle were recorded in 14 patients, 12 of whom had peak systolic pressure gradients ranging from 3 to 50 mm Hg (average 29). The presence or absence of pulmonic regurgitation as determined by pulmonary angiography was noted in 12 patients, and only 2 apparently had regurgitation into the right ventricle during ventricular diastole. Of the 15 patients, 14 had tricuspid valve procedures: replacement in 13 and annuloplasty in 1; 10 patients had pulmonic valve procedures: commissurotomy in 6, replacement in 3, and excision only in 1. Of the 15 patients, 8 had died at the time of the report: 4 within 2 months of operation, and 1 each 4, 8, 24, and 72 months after the operation. The other 7 patients were alive 4 to 132 months (median 23) after the operation.

CONTROVERSIES AND PERSONAL PERSPECTIVES

Benign cardiac tumors should constantly be kept in mind because so many of them are entirely curable by operative therapy. It is not bad to overlook metastatic cancer to the heart because virtually no cancers metastasize to the heart without metastasizing to other body organs and usually multiple other body organs. Cardiac tumors, whether primary or secondary, can simulate more common types of cardiac disease, and this fact should always be kept in mind.

REFERENCES

1. Lam KY, Dickens P, Chan ACL. Tumors of the heart. A 20-year experience with review of 12485 consecutive autopsies. *Arch Pathol Med* 1993; 117:1027–1031.
2. Reynan K. Frequency of primary tumors of the heart. *Am J Cardiol* 1996; 77: 107.
3. Burke A, Virmani R. *Atlas of Tumor Pathology.* Third Series Fascicle 16. *Tumors of the Heart and Great Vessels.* Washington, DC: Armed Forces Institute of Pathology, 1996:231.
4. Goodwin JF. The spectrum of cardiac tumors. *Am J Cardiol* 1968; 21:307–314.
5. Harvey WP. Clinical aspects of cardiac tumors. *Am J Cardiol* 1968; 21:328.
6. Salcedo EE, Cohen GI, White RD, Davison MB. Cardiac tumors: Diagnosis and management. *Curr Prob Cardiol* 1992 (Feb); 17:75–137.
7. Roberts WC, Spray TL. Pericardial heart disease. *Curr Prob Cardiol* 1977 (June); 2:1–71.
8. Roberts WC, Glancy DL, DeVita VT Jr. Heart in malignant lymphoma (Hodgkin's disease, lymphosarcoma, reticulum cell sarcoma and mycosis fungoides). A study of 196 autopsy cases. *Am J Cardiol* 1968; 22:85–107.
9. Lindsay J, Jr, Goldberg SD, Roberts WC. Electrocardiogram in neoplastic and hematologic disorders. In Rios JD, ed. *Clinical Electrocardiographic Correlations.* Philadelphia: FA Davis, 1977:225–242.
10. Steiner RE. Radiologic aspects of cardiac tumors. *Am J Cardiol* 1968; 21: 344–356.
11. Bass NM, Sharratt GJP. Left atrial myxoma diagnosed by echocardiography with observation on tumor movement. *Br Heart J* 1973; 35:1332.
12. Giuliani ER, Lemur F, Schattenberg T. Unusual echocardiographic findings in a patient with left atrial myxoma. *Mayo Clin Proc* 1978; 53:469.
13. Obeid AI, Marvasti M, Parker F, Rosenberg J. Comparison of transthoracic and transesophageal echocardiography in diagnosis of left atrial myxoma. *Am J Cardiol* 1989; 63:1006–1008.
14. Pernod J, Piwnica A, Duret JC. Right atrial myxoma: An echocardiographic study. *Br Heart J* 1978; 40–201.
15. Melier J, Teichholz LE, Pichard AD, et al. Left ventricular myxoma: Echocardiographic diagnosis and review of the literature. *Am J Med* 1977; 63:816–823.
16. Reeder GS, Khandheria BK, Seward JB, Taijk AJ. Transesophageal echocardiography and cardiac masses. *Mayo Clin Proc* 1991; 66:1101–1109.
17. Mugge A, Daniel WG, Haverich A, Lichtlen PR. Diagnosis of noninfective cardiac mass lesions by two-dimensional echocardiography: Comparison of the transthoracic and transesophageal approaches. *Circulation* 1991; 83:70–78.
18. Monocada R, Baker M, Salinas M, et al. Diagnostic role of computed tomography in pericardial heart disease: Congenital defects, thickening, neoplasms, and effusions. *Am Heart J* 1982; 103:263–282.
19. Bateman TM, Sethna DH, Whiting JS, et al. Comprehensive noninvasive evaluation of left atrial myxomas using cardiac cinecomputed tomography. *J Am Coll Cardiol* 1987; 9:1180–1183.
20. Boxer RA, LaCorte MA, Singh S, et al. Diagnosis of cardiac tumors in infants by magnetic resonance imaging. *Am J Cardiol* 1985; 56:831–832.
21. Bahnson HT, Spencer FC, Andrus EC. Diagnosis and treatment of intracavitary myxomas of the heart. *Ann Surg* 1957; 145:915–926.
22. Ferrans VJ, Roberts WC. Structural features of cardiac myxomas. Histology, histochemistry, and electron microscopy. *Hum Pathol* 1973; 4:111–146.
23. Peters MN, Hall RJ, Cooley DA, et al. The clinical syndrome of atrial myxoma. *JAMA* 1974; 230:695–701.
24. Morgan DL, Palazola J, Reed W, et al. Left heart myxomas. *Am J Cardiol* 1977; 40:611–614.
25. St. John Sutton MG, Mercier L-A, Giuliani ER, Lie JT. Atrial myxomas: A review of clinical experience in 40 patients. *Mayo Clin Proc* 1980; 55:371–376.
26. Markel ML, Waller BF, Armstrong WF. Cardiac myxoma: A review. *Medicine* 1987; 66:114–125.
27. Murphy MC, Sweeney MS, Putnam JB Jr, et al. Surgical treatment of cardiac tumors: A 25-year experience. *Ann Thorac Surg* 1990; 49:612–618.

28. Tazelaar HD, Locke TJ, McGregor CGA. Pathology of surgically excised primary cardiac tumors. *Mayo Clin Proc* 1992; 67:957–965.
29. Burke AP, Virmani R. Cardiac myxomas: A clinicopathologic study. *Am J Clin Pathol* 1994; 100:671–680.
30. Morrow AG, Kahler RL, Reis RL. Primary myxoma of the right ventricle. Clinical, hemodynamic and angiographic findings before and following operative treatment. *Am J Med* 1966; 40:954–960.
31. Hickie JB, Gibson H, Windsor HM. "The wrecking ball": Right atrial myxoma. *Med J Aust* 1970; 2:82–86.
32. Hada Y, Wolfe C, Murray GF, Craig E. Right ventricular myxoma. Case report and review of phonocardiographic and auscultatory manifestations. *Am Heart J* 1980; 100:871–877.
33. Massumi R. Bedside diagnosis of right heart myxomas through detection of palpable tumor shocks and audible plops. *Am Heart J* 1983; 105:303–310.
34. Leonhardt ET, Kullenberg KP. Bilateral atrial myxomas with multiple arterial aneurysms—A syndrome mimicking polyarteritis nodosa. *Am J Med* 1977; 62: 792–794.
35. Malekzadeh S, Roberts WC. Growth rate of left atrial myxoma. *Am J Cardiol* 1989; 64:1075–1076.
36. Talley RC, Baldwin BJ, Symbas PN, Nutter DO. Right atrial myxoma. Unusual presentation with cyanosis and clubbing. *Am J Med* 1970; 48:256–260.
37. Goldschlager A, Popper R, Goldschlager N, et al. Right atrial myxoma with right to left shunt and polycythemia presenting as congenital heart disease. *Am J Cardiol* 1972; 30:82–86.
38. Chan HSL, Sonley MJ, Moës CAF, et al. Primary and secondary tumors of childhood involving the heart, pericardium, and great vessels: A report of 75 cases and review of the literature. *Cancer* 1985; 56:825–836.
39. Fenoglio JJ Jr, McAllister HA, Ferrans VJ. Cardiac rhabdomyoma: A clinicopathologic and electron microscopic study. *Am J Cardiol* 1976; 38:241–251.
40. Smythe JF, Dyck JD, Smallhorn JF, Freedom RM. Natural history of cardiac rhabdomyoma in infancy and childhood. *Am J Cardiol* 1990; 66:1247–1249.
41. Burke AP, Virmani R. Cardiac rhabdomyoma: A clinicopathologic study. *Mod Pathol* 1991; 4:70–74.
42. Biancaniello TM, Meyer RA, Gaum WE, Kaplan S. Primary benign intramural ventricular tumors in children: Pre- and post-operative electrocardiographic, echocardiographic, and angiocardiographic evaluation. *Am Heart J* 1982; 103: 852–857.
43. Williams DB, Danielson GK, McGoon DC, et al. Cardiac fibroma: Long-term survival after excision. *J Thorac Cardiovasc Surg* 1982; 84:230–236.
44. Estevez JM, Thompson DS, Levinson JP. Lipoma of the heart. Review of the literature and report of 2 autopsied cases. *Arch Pathol* 1964; 77:638–642.
45. Moulton AL, Jaretzki A III, Bowman FO Jr, et al. Massive lipoma of the heart. *NY State J Med* 1976; 76:1820–1825.
46. Dollar AL, Wallace RB, Kent KM, et al. Mitral valve replacement for mitral lipoma associated with severe obesity. *Am J Cardiol* 1989; 64:1405–1407.
47. Shirani J, Roberts WC. Epicardial lipoma. *Am Heart J* 1993; 126:1030.
48. Bear PA, Moodie DS. Malignant primary cardiac tumors. The Cleveland Clinic Experience, 1956–1986. *Chest* 1987; 92:860–862.
49. Putman JB Jr, Sweeney MS, Colon R, et al. Primary cardiac sarcomas. *Ann Thorac Surg* 1991; 51:906–910.
50. Burke AP, Cowan D, Virmani R. Primary sarcomas of the heart. *Cancer* 1992; 69:387–395.
51. Glancy DL, Morales JB, Roberts WC. Angiosarcoma of the heart. *Am J Cardiol* 1968; 21:413–419.
52. Herrmann MA, Shankerman RA, Edwards WD, et al. Primary cardiac angiosarcoma: A clinicopathologic study of six cases. *J Thorac Cardiovasc Surg* 1992; 103:655–664.
53. Shrivastava S, Jacks JJ, White RS, Edwards JE. Diffuse rhabdomyomatosis of the heart. *Arch Pathol Lab Med* 1977; 101:78–90.
54. Hajar R, Roberts WC, Folger GM Jr. Embryonal botryoid rhabdomyosarcoma of the mitral valve. *Am J Cardiol* 1986; 57:376.
55. Hui KS, Green LK, Schmidt WA. Primary cardiac rhabdomyosarcoma: Definition of a rare entity. *Am J Cardiovasc Pathol* 1988; 2:19–29.
56. Domanski MJ, Delaney TF, Kleiner DE Jr, et al. Primary sarcoma of the heart causing mitral stenosis. *Am J Cardiol* 1990; 66:893–895.
57. Isner JM, Falcone MW, Virmani R, Roberts WC. Cardiac sarcoma causing "ASH" and simulating coronary heart disease. *Am J Med* 1979; 66:1025–1030.
58. Abraham DP, Reddy V, Gattusa P. Neoplasms metastatic to the heart: Review of 3314 consecutive autopsies. *Am J Cardiovasc Pathol* 1990; 3:195–198.
59. Adenle AD, Edwards JE. Clinical and pathologic features of metastatic neoplasms of the pericardium. *Chest* 1982; 81:166–169.
60. MacLowry JD, Roberts WC. Metastatic choriocarcinoma of the lung: Invasion of pulmonary veins with extension into the left atrium and mitral orifice. *Am J Cardiol* 1966; 18:938–941.
61. Labib SB, Schick EC Jr, Isner JM. Obstruction of right ventricular outflow tract caused by intracavitary metastatic disease: analysis of 14 cases. *J Am Coll Cardiol* 1992; 19:1664–1668.
62. Domanski MJ, Cunnion RE, Fernicola DJ, Roberts WC. Fatal cor pulmonale caused by extensive tumor emboli in the small pulmonary arteries without emboli in the major pulmonary arteries or metastases in the pulmonary parenchyma. *Am J Cardiol* 1993; 72:233–234.
63. Onuigbo WI. Direct extension of cancer between pulmonary veins and the left atrium. *Chest* 1972; 62:444–446.
64. Weg IL, Mehra S, Azueta V, Rosener F. Cardiac metastasis from adenocarcinoma of the lung. Echocardiographic-pathologic correlation. *Am J Med* 1986; 80:108–112.
65. Kadir S, Coulam CM. Intracaval extension of renal cell carcinoma. *Cardiovasc Intervent Radiol* 1980; 3:180–183.
66. Waller BF, Fletcher RD, Roberts WC. Carcinoma of the lung causing pulmonary arterial stenosis. *Chest* 1981; 79:589–591.
67. Glancy DL, Roberts WC. The heart in malignant melanoma: A study of 70 autopsy cases. *Am J Cardiol* 1968; 21:555–571.
68. Waller BV, Gottdiener JS, Virmani R, Roberts WC. The "charcoal heart": Melanoma to the cor. *Chest* 1980; 77:671–676.
69. Roberts WC, Bodey GP, Wertlake PT. The heart in acute leukemia: A study of 420 autopsy cases. *Am J Cardiol* 1968; 21:388–412.
70. Waller BF, Roberts WC. Systolic clicks caused by rocks in the right heart chambers. *Am Heart J* 1981; 102:459–460.
71. Roberts WC, Glancy DL, DeVita VT Jr. Heart in malignant lymphoma (Hodgkin's disease, lymphosarcoma, reticulum cell sarcoma and mycosis fungoides): A study of 196 autopsy cases. *Am J Cardiol* 1968; 22:85–107.
72. Terry LN, Kligerman MM. Pericardial and myocardial involvement by lymphomas and leukemias. *Cancer* 1970; 25:1003–1008.
73. McDonnell PJ, Mann RB, Bulkley BH. Involvement of the heart by malignant lymphoma: a clinicopathologic study. *Cancer* 1982; 49:944–951.
74. Roberts CS, Gottdiener JS, Roberts WC. Clinically undetected cardiac lymphoma causing congestive heart failure. *Am Heart J* 1990; 120:1239–1242.
75. Holladay AO, Siegel RJ, Schwartz EA. Cardiac malignant lymphoma in acquired immune deficiency syndrome. *Cancer* 1992; 70:2203–2207.
76. Moore JA, DeRan BP, Minor R, et al. Transesophageal echocardiographic evaluation of intracardiac lymphoma. *Am Heart J* 1992; 124:514–516.
77. Seibert KA, Rettenmier CW, Waller BF, et al. Osteogenic sarcoma metastatic to the heart. *Am J Med* 1982; 73:136–141.
78. Burke AP, Virmani R. Osteosarcomas of the heart. *Am J Surg Pathol* 1991; 15: 289–295.
79. Feigin DS, Fenoglio JJ, McAllister HA, Madewell JR. Pericardial cysts: A radiologic-pathologic correlation and review. *Radiology* 1977; 125:15–20.
80. Reynolds JL, Donahue JK, Pearce CW. Intrapericardial teratoma: A cause of acute pericardial effusion in infancy. *Pediatrics* 1969; 4:71–78.
81. DeGeeter B, Kretz JG, Nisand I, et al. Intrapericardial teratoma in a newborn infant: Use of fetal echocardiography. *Ann Thorac Surg* 1983; 35:664–666.
82. Brabham KR, Roberts WC. Cardiac-compressing intrapericardial teratoma at birth. *Am J Cardiol* 1989; 63:386–387.
83. Shirani J, Roberts WC. Clinical, electrocardiographic and morphologic features of massive fatty deposits ("lipomatous hypertrophy") in the atrial septum. *J Am Coll Cardiol* 1993; 22:226–238.
84. Roberts WC, Roberts JD. The floating heart of the heart too fat to sink: analysis of 55 necropsy patients. *Am J Cardiol* 1983; 52:1286–1289.
85. Applegate PM, Taijk AJ, Ehman RL, et al. Two-dimensional echocardiographic and magnetic resonance imaging observations in massive lipomatous hypertrophy of atrial septum. *Am J Cardiol* 1987; 59:489–491.
86. Kindman LA, Wright A, Tye T, et al. Lipomatous hypertrophy of the interatrial septum: Characterization of transesophageal and transthoracic echocardiography, magnetic resonance imaging, and computed tomography. *J Am Soc Echocardiogr* 1988; 1:450–454.
87. Isner JM, Carter BL, Roberts WC, Bankoff MS. Subepicardial adipose tissue producing echocardiographic appearance of pericardial effusion. Documentation by computed tomography and necropsy. *Am J Cardiol* 1983; 51:565–569.
88. Raeburn C. Papillary fibro-elastic hamartomas of the heart valves. *J Pathol Bacteriol* 1953; 65:371–374.
89. Heath D, Best PV, Davis BT. Papilliferous tumors of the heart valves. *Br Heart J* 1961; 23:20–24.
90. Nassar SGA, Parker JC Jr. Incidental papillary endocardial tumor. *Arch Pathol* 1971; 92:370–376.
91. Fisbein MC, Ferrans VJ, Roberts WC. Endocardial papillary elastofibromas. Histologic, histochemical, and electron microscopical findings. *Arch Pathol* 1975; 99:335–341.
92. Roberts WC. Valvular, subvalvular, and supravalvular aortic stenosis: morphologic features. *Cardiovasc Clin* 1973; 5:97–126.
93. Heath D, Thompson IM. Papillary "tumors" of the left ventricle. *Br Heart J* 1965; 29:950–954.
94. Burn CG, Bishop MB, Davies JNP. A stalked papillary tumor of the mural endocardium. *Am J Clin Pathol* 1969; 51:344–346.
95. Flotte T, Pinar H, Feiner H. Papillary elastofibroma of the left ventricular septum. *Am J Surg Pathol* 1980; 4:585–588.
96. Almagro UA, Perry LS, Choi H, Pintar K. Papillary fibroelastoma of the heart. Report of six cases. *Arch Pathol Lab Med* 1982; 106:318–321.
97. Ong LS, Nanda NC, Barold SS. Two-dimensional echocardiographic detection and diagnostic features of left ventricular papillary fibroelastoma. *Am Heart J* 1982; 103:917–918.
98. Topol EJ, Biern RO, Reitz BA. Cardiac papillary fibroelastoma and stroke. Echocardiographic diagnosis and guide to excision. *Am J Med* 1986; 80: 129–132.
99. Kalman JM, Lubicz S, Brennan JB, et al. Multiple cardiac papillary fibroelastoma and rheumatic heart disease. *Aust N Z J Med* 1991; 21:744–746.
100. Bedi HS, Sharma VK, Mishra M, et al. Papillary fibroelastoma of the mitral

valve associated with rheumatic mitral stenosis. *Eur J Cardiothorac Surg* 1995; 9:54–55.
101. Allen KB, Goldin M, Mitra R. Transaortic video-assisted excision of a left ventricular papillary fibroelastoma. *J Thorac Cardiovasc Surg* 1996; 112: 199–201.
102. Campbell M, Carling W. Sudden death due to a fibrinous polyp of the aortic valve. *Guy's Hosp Rep* 1934; 84:41–42.
103. Butterworth JS, Poindexter CA. Papilloma of cusp of the aortic valve: Report of a patient with sudden death. *Circulation* 1973; 48:213–215.
104. Cha SD, Incarvito J, Fernandez J, et al. Giant Lambl's excrescences of papillary muscle and aortic valve: Echocardiographic, angiographic, and pathologic findings. *Clin Cardiol* 1981; 4:51–54.
105. Gopal A, Li Mandri G, King DL, et al. Aortic valve papillary fibroelastoma: A diagnosis by transthoracic echocardiography. *Chest* 1994; 105:1885–1887.
106. Ragni T, Grande AM, Cappuccio G, et al. Embolizing fibroelastoma of the aortic valve. *Cardiovasc Surg* 1994; 2:639–641.
107. Shahian DM, Labib SB, Chang G. Cardiac papillary fibroelastoma. *Ann Thorac Surg* 1995; 59:538–541.
108. Fowles RE, Miller DC, Ebgert BM, et al. Systemic emoblization from a mitral valve papillary endocardial fibroma detected by two-dimensional echocardiography. *Am Heart J* 1981; 102:128–130.
109. Groton ME, Soltanzadeh H. Mitral valve fibroelastoma. *Ann Thorac Surg* 1989; 47:605–607.
110. Gallo R, Kumar N, Prabhakar G, et al. Papillary fibroelastoma of mitral valve chorda. *Ann Thorac Surg* 1993; 55:1576–1577.
111. Shapiro OM, Willimason WA, Dugan JM. Papillary fibroelastoma of the mitral valve. *Cardiovasc Surg* 1993; 1:599–601.
112. Mann J, Parker DJ. Papillary fibroelastoma of the mitral valve: A rare cause of transient neurological deficits. *Br Heart J* 1994; 71:6.
113. Pinelli G, Carteaux JP, Mertes PM, et al. Mitral valve tumor revealed by stroke. *J Heart Valve Dis* 1995; 4:199–201.
114. Zamora RL, Adelberg DA, Berger AS, et al. Branch retinal artery occlusion caused by a mitral valve papillary fibroelastoma. *Am J Opthalmol* 1995; 119: 325–329.
115. Colucci V, Alberti A, Bonacina E, Gordini V. Papillary fibroelastoma of the mitral valve: A rare cause of embolic events. *Tex Heart Inst J* 1995; 22:327–331.
116. McFadden PM, Lacy JR. Intracardiac papillary fibroelastoma: An occult cause of embolic neurologic deficit. *Ann Thorac Surg* 1987; 43:667–669.
117. Brown RD Jr, Khandheria BK, Edwards WD. Cardiac papillary fibroelastoma: A treatable cause of transient ischemic attack and ischemic stroke detected by transesophageal echocardiography. *Mayo Clinic Proc* 1995; 70:863–868.
118. Nighoghossian N, Trouillas P, Perinetti M, et al. Lambl's excrescence: An uncommon cause of cerebral embolism. *Rev Neurol* 1995; 151:583–585.
119. Kasarskis EJ, O'Connor W, Earle G. Embolic stroke from cardiac papillary fibroelastomas. *Stroke* 1988; 19:1171–1173.
120. Zull DN, Diamond M, Beringer D. Angina and sudden death resulting from papillary fibroelastoma of the aortic valve. *Ann Emerg Med* 1985; 14:470–473.
121. Marvasti MA, Obeid AT, Cohen PS, et al. Successful removal of papillary endocardial fibroma. *Thorac Cardiovasc Surg* 1983; 31:254–255.
122. Richard J, Castello R, Dressler FA, et al. Diagnosis of papillary fibroelastoma of the mitral valve complicated by non-Q wave infarction with apical thrombus: Transesophageal and transthoracic echocardiography study. *Am Heart J* 1993; 126:710–712.
123. Etienne Y, Jobic Y, Houel JF, et al. Papillary fibroelastoma of the arotic valve with myocardial infarction: Echocardiographic diagnosis and surgical excision. *Am Heart J* 1994; 127:443–445.
124. Eckstein FS, Chafers HJ, Grote J, et al. Papillary fibroelastoma of the aortic valve presenting with myocardial infarction. *Ann Thorac Surg* 1995; 60: 206–208.
125. Grote J, Mugge A, Schfers JH, et al. Multiplane transesophageal echocardiography detection of a papillary fibroelastoma of the aortic valve causing myocardial infarction. *Eur Heart J* 1995; 16:426–429.
126. Harris LS, Adelson L. Fatal coronary embolism from a myxomatous polyp of the aortic valve: An unusual cause of sudden death. *Am J Clin Pathol* 1965; 43: 61–64.
127. Boone S, Higginson LA, Walley VM. Endothelial papillary fibroelastoma arising in and around the aortic sinus, filling the ostium of the right coronary artery. *Arch Pathol Lab Med* 1992; 116:135–137.
128. Mazzucco A, Bortolotti U, Thiene G, et al. Left ventricular fibroelastoma with coronary embolization. *Eur J Cardiothorac Surg* 1989; 3:471–473.
129. Anderson KR, Fiddler FI, Lie JR. Congenital papillary tumor of the tricuspid valve: An unusual cause of right ventricular outflow obstruction in a neonate with trisomy E. *Mayo Clin Proc* 1977; 52:665–669.
130. Frumin H, O'Donnell L, Kerin NZ, et al. Two-dimensional echocardiographic detection and diagnostic features of tricuspid papillary fibroelastoma. *J Am Coll Cardiol* 1983; 2:1016–1018.
131. Mohan JC, Goel PK, Gambhir DS, et al. Calcified mobile papillary fibroelastoma of the tricuspid valve: A case report. *Indian Heart J* 1987; 39:237–239.
132. Wolfe JT III, Finck SJ, Safford RE, Perselin-ST. Tricuspid valve papillary fibroelastoma: Echocardiographic characterization. *Ann Thorac Surg* 1991; 51: 116–118.
133. Neerukonda SK, Jantz RD, Vijay NK, et al. Pulmonary embolization of papillary fibroelastoma arising from the tricuspid valve. *Tex Heart Inst J* 1991; 18: 132–135.
134. Ganjoo AK, Johnson WD, Gordon RT, et al. Tricuspid papillary fibroelastoma causing syncopal episodes. *J Thorac Cardiovasc Surg* 1996; 112:551–553.
135. Roberts WC, McAllister HA Jr, Ferrans VJ. Sarcoidosis of the heart: A clinicopathologic study of 35 necropsy patients (Group I) and review of 78 previously described necropsy patients (Group II). *Am J Med* 1977; 63:86–108.
136. Virmani R, Bures JC, Roberts WC. Cardiac sarcoidosis: A major cause of sudden death in young individuals. *Chest* 1980; 77:423–428.
137. Shirani J, Roberts WC. Subepicardial myocardial lesions. *Am Heart J* 1993; 125:1346–1352.
138. Morton DL, Kagar AR, Roberts WC, et al. Pericardiectomy for radiation-induced pericarditis with effusion. *Ann Thorac Surg* 1969; 8:195–208.
139. Serpik A, Lowenbraum S, Sheinbrot S, et al. Possible radiation pericarditis in Hodgkin's disease. *Cancer Chemo Rep* 1970; 54:199–208.
140. McReynolds RA, Gold GL, Roberts WC. Coronary heart disease after mediastinal irradiation for Hodgkin's disease. *Ann J Med* 1976; 60:39–45.
141. Brosius FC III, Waller BF, Roberts WC. Radiation heart disease: Analysis of 16 young (aged 15 to 33 years) necropsy patients who received over 3,500 rads to the heart. *Am J Med* 1981; 70:519–530.
142. Harvey LAC, DeMaio SJ, Roberts WC. Radiation-induced cardiovascular disease including stenosis of coronary ostium, coronary and carotid arteries, and aortic valve. *Baylor Univ Med Ctr Proc* 1994; 7:33–36.
143. Ihde DC, Roberts WC, Marr KC, et al. Cardiac candidiasis in cancer patients. *Cancer* 1978; 41:2364–2371.
144. Ross EM, Macher AM, Roberts WC. *Aspergillus fumigatus* thrombi causing total occlusion of both coronary arterial ostia, all four major epicardial coronary arteries and coronary sinus and associated with purulent pericarditis. *Am J Cardiol* 1985; 56:499–500.
145. Roberts WC, Berard CW. Gas gangrene of the heart in clostridial septicemia. *Am Heart J* 1967; 74:482–488.
146. Bulkley BH, Roberts WC. The heart in systemic lupus erythematous and the changes induced in it by corticosteroid therapy: A study of 36 necropsy patients. *Am J Med* 1975; 58:243–264.
147. Buja LM, Roberts WC. Iron in the heart: Etiology and clinical significance. *Am J Med* 1971; 51:209–221.
148. Cutler DJ, Isner JM, Bracey AW, et al. Hemochromatosis heart disease: An unemphasized cause of potentially reversible restrictive cardiomyopathy. *Am J Med* 1980; 69:923–928.
149. Buja LM, Ferrans VJ, Mayer RJ, et al. Cardiac ultrastructural changes induced by daunorubicin therapy. *Cancer* 1973; 32:771–788.
150. Buja LM, Ferrans VJ, Roberts WC. Drug-induced cardiomyopathies. *Adv Cardiol* 1974; 13:330–348.
151. Isner JM, Ferrans VJ, Cohen SR, et al. Clinical and morphologic cardiac findings after anthracycline chemotherapy: Analysis of 64 patients studied at necropsy. *Am J Cardiol* 1983; 51:1167–1174.
152. Roberts WC, Sjoerdsma A. The cardiac disease associated with carcinoid syndrome (carcinoid heart disease). *Am J Med* 1964; 36:5–34.
153. Roberts WC, Mason DT, Wright LD Jr. The non-distensible right atrium of carcinoid disease of the heart. *Am J Clin Pathol* 1965; 44:627–631.
154. Ferrans VJ, Roberts WC. The carcinoid endocardial plaque: An ultrastructural study. *Hum Pathol* 1976; 7:387–409.
155. Ross EM, Roberts WC. The carcinoid syndrome: Comparison of 21 necropsy subjects with carcinoid heart disease to 15 necropsy subjects without carcinoid heart disease. *Am J Med* 1986; 79:339–354.
156. Oates JA. The carcinoid syndrome. *N Engl J Med* 1986; 315:702–704.
157. Callahan JA, Wroblewski EM, Reeder GS, et al. Echocardiographic features of carcinoid heart disease. *Am J Cardiol* 1982; 50:762–768.
158. Howard RJ, Drobac M, Rider WD, et al. Carcinoid heart disease: Diagnosis by two-dimensional echocardiography. *Circulation* 1982; 66:1059–1065.

Neoplasms involving the heart, their simulators, and adverse consequences of their therapy

William Clifford Roberts, MD

Primary cardiac tumors involving the heart may be either benign or malignant. Most of the benign tumors are myxomas, which are most commonly located in the left atrium. Primary malignant neoplasms usually involve the myocardium and the interior of the cardiac cavities, whereas neoplasms metastatic to the heart most commonly involve pericardium, and pericardial effusion and constriction are the most common consequences. Computed tomography and magnetic resonance imaging are becoming the most useful instruments of precision for the diagnosis of cardiac tumors. Pericardial cysts, teratomas, lipomatous hypertrophy of the atrial septum, papillary fibroelastomas, thrombi, and sarcoid are frequently mistaken for cardiac neoplasms. There are a number of cardiac consequences of malignancy, including radiation heart disease, cardiac hemorrhages, cardiac infection, cardiac adiposity or the corticosteroid-treated heart, cardiac hemosiderosis, and toxicity due to anthracycline chemotherapy.

In the past 40 years, our recognition of cardiac neoplasms has progressed from clinical curiosities described primarily in numerous case reports with diagnosis mainly at autopsy to fairly rapid antemortem diagnosis and frequent curative operative therapy. Diagnosis has been greatly facilitated by 2-dimensional echocardiography and, in select cases, the use of magnetic resonance imaging (MRI) or computed tomography (CT). This article describes a classification of cardiac neoplasms, their location, techniques for diagnosis, and specific benign and malignant neoplasms. It also describes secondary tumors of the heart and conditions frequently mistaken for cardiac neoplasms. It closes with a section on adverse consequences of therapy.

CLASSIFICATION

There is no perfect classification for cardiac neoplasms. As in any organ or tissue, neoplasms involving the heart may be primary or secondary. The primary ones may be benign or malignant, and the secondary or metastatic ones are, by definition, malignant. Metastatic neoplasms are far more frequent than primary neoplasms by a ratio of at least 30 to 1 (1, 2).

The frequencies of the primary benign and primary malignant tumors vary from report to report, approximately 0.1% to 0.3% in most autopsy series. A list of primary benign neoplasms gathered by investigators at the Armed Forces Institute of Pathology is presented in *Table 1*, and primary malignant tumors encountered are listed in *Table 2* (3). The frequencies of the metastatic neoplasms also vary from report to report, but nearly all studies have listed carcinoma of the lung as the most frequently encountered secondary tumor at autopsy, with cancer of the breast, lymphoma, and leukemia as the next leading causes (*Table 3*). The order of frequency of secondary tumors is different, however, if the frequency of each different type of tumor that metastasizes to the heart is determined. For example, *Table 4* lists the frequencies of metastases to the heart in 100 cases of each of 20 separate tumors; melanoma has the highest frequency of metastases to the heart, followed by malignant germ cell tumor, leukemia, lymphoma, cancer of the lung, and then the various sarcomas (3).

Table 1. Primary benign neoplasms of the heart (1976–1993)*

Tumor†	Total	Surgical	Autopsy	Age <15 years at diagnosis
Myxoma	114	102	12	4
Rhabdomyoma	20	6	14	20
Fibroma	20	18	2	13
Hemangioma	17	10	7	2
Atrioventricular nodal	10	0	10	2
Granular cell	4	0	4	0
Lipoma	2	2	0	0
Paraganglioma	2	2	0	0
Myocytic hamartoma	2	2	0	0
Histiocytoid cardiomyopathy	2	0	2	2
Inflammatory pseudotumor	2	2	0	1
Fibrous histiocytoma	1	0	1	0
Epithelioid hemangioendothelioma	1	1	0	0
Bronchogenic cyst	1	1	0	0
Teratoma	1	0	1	1
Totals	199	146 (73%)	53 (27%)	45 (23%)

*Modified from Burke A, Virmani R. *Atlas of Tumor Pathology. Tumors of the Heart and Great Vessels.* Washington, DC: Armed Forces Institute of Pathology, 1996:231.
†Excludes papillary fibroelastoma and lipomatous hypertrophy of the atrial septum.

From the Baylor Heart and Vascular Center and the Division of Cardiology, Department of Internal Medicine, and Department of Pathology, Baylor University Medical Center, Dallas, Texas.

Corresponding author: William C. Roberts, MD, Baylor Heart and Vascular Center, Baylor University Medical Center, 3500 Gaston Avenue, Dallas, Texas 75246 (e-mail: wc.roberts@baylordallas.edu).

Table 2. Primary malignant tumors of the heart (1976–1993)*

Tumor	Total	Surgical	Autopsy	Age <15 years at diagnosis
Sarcoma	137 (95%)	116	21	11 (8%)
Angio	33	22	11	1
Unclassified	33	30	3	3
Fibrous histiocytoma	16	16	0	1
Osteo	13	13	0	0
Leimyo	12	11	1	1
Fibro	9	9	0	1
Myxo	8	8	0	1
Rhabdomyo	6	2	4	3
Synovial	4	4	0	0
Lipo	2	0	2	0
Schwannoma	1	1	0	0
Lymphoma	7 (5%)	1	6	0
Totals	144 (100%)	117 (81%)	27 (19%)	11 (8%)

*Modified from Burke A, Virmani R. *Atlas of Tumor Pathology. Tumors of the Heart and Great Vessels.* Washington, DC: Armed Forces Institute of Pathology, 1996:231.

Table 3. Metastatic neoplasms in the heart at necropsy: order of frequency of cancers encountered*

Primary tumor	Total autopsies	Metastases to heart
1. Lung	1037	180 (17%)
2. Breast	685	70 (10%)
3. Lymphoma	392	67 (17%)
4. Leukemia	202	66 (33%)
5. Esophagus	294	37 (13%)
6. Uterus	451	36 (8%)
7. Melanoma	69	32 (46%)
8. Stomach	603	28 (5%)
9. Sarcoma	159	24 (15%)
10. Oral cavity and tongue	235	22 (9%)
11. Colon and rectum	440	22 (5%)
12. Kidney	114	12 (11%)
13. Thyroid gland	97	9 (9%)
14. Larynx	100	9 (9%)
15. Germ cell	21	8 (38%)
16. Urinary bladder	128	8 (6%)
17. Liver and biliary tract	325	7 (2%)
18. Prostate gland	171	6 (4%)
19. Pancreas	185	6 (3%)
20. Ovary	188	2 (1%)
21. Nose (interior)	32	1 (3%)
22. Pharynx	67	1 1%)
23. Miscellaneous	245	0
	6240	653 (10%)

*Modified from Burke A, Virmani R. *Atlas of Tumor Pathology. Tumors of the Cardiovascular System.* Washington, DC: Armed Forces Institute of Pathology, 1978:111–119, and Mukai K, Shinkai T, Tominaga K, Shomosato Y. The incidence of secondary tumors of the heart and pericardium: a 10-year study. *Jpn N Clin Oncol* 1988;18:195–201. Burke and Virmani combined studies of McAllister HA and Fenoglio JJ Jr.

Table 4. Metastatic neoplasms in the heart at necropsy: order of frequency of metastases of each different primary tumor

Primary tumor	Number of autopsies	Percentage with metastases to the heart*
Melanoma	100	46
Germ cell	100	38
Leukemia	100	33
Lymphoma	100	17
Lung	100	17
Sarcoma	100	15
Esophagus	100	13
Kidney	100	11
Breast	100	10
Mouth and tongue	100	9
Thyroid gland	100	9
Uterus	100	8
Urinary bladder	100	6
Stomach	100	5
Colon and rectum	100	5
Prostate gland	100	4
Pancreas	100	3
Nose (interior)	100	3
Ovary	100	1
Pharynx	100	1
Miscellaneous	100	0

*Modified from Burke A, Virmani R. *Atlas of Tumor Pathology. Tumors of the Cardiovascular System.* Washington, DC: Armed Forces Institute of Pathology, 1978:111–119, and Mukai K, Shinkai T, Tominaga K, Shomosato Y. The incidence of secondary tumors of the heart and pericardium: a 10-year study. *Jpn N Clin Oncol* 1988;18:195–201. Burke and Virmani combined studies of McAllister HA and Fenoglio JJ Jr.

LOCATION OF CARDIAC NEOPLASMS

Cardiac neoplasms may involve only the endocardium, only the myocardium, only the epicardium, or any combination of these (*Figure 1*). By far the most common location of metastatic cardiac neoplasm is the epicardium. Neoplasms limited to parietal pericardium without extension into the epicardium are not considered cardiac neoplasms. The epicardial tumor deposits may be multifocal or single, or they may be extensive and essentially diffuse or nearly so. Likewise, the intramyocardial masses may be focal or multifocal. The most common locations for intramyocardial masses are the left ventricular free wall and the ventricular septum, which are, of course, the portions of the heart with the greatest myocardial mass. The endocardial neoplasms are the intracavitary ones. They may involve a single cardiac cavity or more than one. They may be limited to either the right or left side of the heart, or they may involve both. Intracavitary tumors produce obstruction to inflow into the heart or into a ventricular cavity or outflow from a ventricular cavity. The intracavitary neoplasms are the ones that may partially dislodge and produce either pulmonary or systemic emboli or both. They have the potential of producing the triad of obstruction, embolization, and constitutional symptoms.

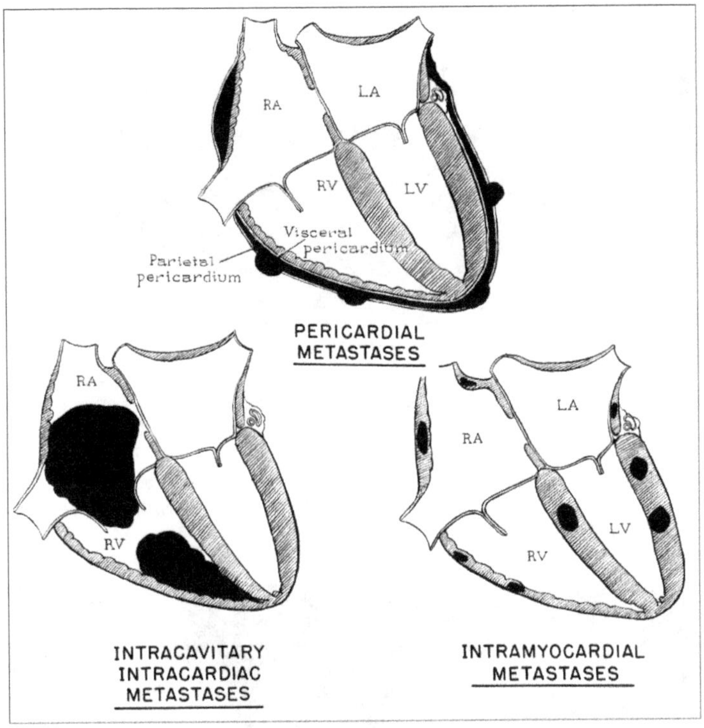

Figure 1. *Various locations of cardiac neoplasms.* RA indicates right atrium; LA, left atrium; LV, left ventricle; RV, right ventricle. Reprinted from Roberts WC. Primary and secondary neoplasms of the heart. *Am J Cardiol* 1977;80:671–682 with permission from Excerpta Medica Inc.

TECHNIQUES FOR DIAGNOSING CARDIAC NEOPLASMS

Symptoms and physical signs

The signs and symptoms produced by the various cardiac neoplasms are determined primarily by the tumor's location in the heart. Physical examination is rarely diagnostic (4–7).

Electrocardiogram

The electrocardiogram is usually nonspecific (8, 9), but it could be far more useful than has been appreciated in the past. The problem has been that the electrocardiogram may be recorded when diagnosis is first considered, but subsequently electrocardiograms are not taken very frequently as the disease progresses. One study compared electrocardiographic findings in patients with malignant lymphoma who had cardiac involvement with another group of patients with lymphoma who did not have cardiac involvement (8). The percentage with abnormal tracings (62%) was similar in the 2 groups. Fewer than half the patients had >1 electrocardiogram during the entire illness. Findings included sinus tachycardia; low voltage; ectopic tachycardia, including atrial fibrillation; atrial flutter; atrial tachycardia; atrial ventricular block, including prolonged PR interval; second- or third-degree block; premature ventricular complexes; right or left axis deviation; right bundle branch block; T-wave abnormalities; and ST-T wave changes, usually of nonspecific nature. The sudden development of some of these electrocardiographic findings in a patient who previously lacked these changes suggests cardiac involvement.

Radiograph

The chest radiograph may be helpful, particularly when an epicardial neoplasm is present (10). Enlargement or an irregular contour of the cardiac silhouette, mediastinal widening, or a hilar mass may suggest pericardial involvement. Calcium within an intracardiac neoplasm can be seen on occasion by chest radiograph or fluoroscopy. The lung fields may have a paucity of pulmonary markings in patients with large right atrial or right ventricular neoplasms. Patients with neoplasms in the left atrium may have pulmonary changes similar to those in mitral stenosis. Left ventricular neoplasms causing obstruction to left ventricular inflow or outflow may produce similar pulmonary arterial vascular changes.

Echocardiogram

More cardiac tumors today are diagnosed by echocardiography, at least initially, than by any other instrument of precision. Diagnosis of left atrial myxoma has been one of the principal uses of echocardiography since the introduction of the technique (11–15). The classic left atrial myxoma is a mobile echogenic mass that is in the body of the left atrium in ventricular systole and passes into the mitral orifice in ventricular diastole. Occasionally, an echocardiogram will detect a left atrial myxoma that is small or not close to the mitral orifice, and it is therefore clinically silent.

Although it is usually possible to detect intracardiac tumors with transthoracic echocardiography, the transesophageal examination produces spectacular images and makes diagnosis, particularly of atrial masses, relatively easy (16, 17). The transesophageal examination not only offers a higher sensitivity for detecting left atrial tumors, for example, but also permits a clearer picture of the attachment or stalk of the tumor and more precise characterization of the size, shape, and location of the mass. A major advantage of echocardiography is its ability to provide serial studies. Thus, this technique may be used to monitor progressive increase in size of a neoplasm or detect recurrence once the initial tumor is excised.

The echocardiogram has been useful in detecting intracardiac tumors other than myxomas, including rhabdomyomas and rhabdomyosarcomas, neoplasms that occur primarily in infants and are usually located in the ventricles. The echocardiogram is also helpful in detecting metastases to the heart. This is particularly true in neoplasms that migrate up the inferior vena cava into the right side of the heart, such as renal cell carcinoma or adrenal cell carcinoma. Echocardiography, particularly transesophageal, has been extremely helpful in detecting mediastinal or extracardiac masses, which may compress the cardiac structure.

Computed tomogram

CT is useful in diagnosing cardiac tumors (18, 19); it may be especially useful in defining the degree of intramyocardial extension or the lack thereof and determining whether the tumor is present in adjacent extracardiac structures. Ultrafast CT appears to be particularly well suited for assessing intracardiac masses.

Magnetic resonance imaging

MRI appears to be of greater value than CT in delineating cardiac tumors (20). It may be able to depict the size, shape, and surface characteristics of the tumor more clearly than CT. This technique also can provide information regarding tissue composition that can help to differentiate neoplasms from thrombi.

Angiogram

A cardiac catheterization and selective angiography are no longer necessary in all patients with cardiac neoplasms because adequate preoperative information can usually be obtained by echocardiography, CT, or MRI. For cases in which the latter 3 techniques have not fully defined the location and attachment of the neoplasm, in which all 4 chambers of the heart have not been well delineated, or in which another type of cardiac condition is suspected (such as coronary arterial narrowing), cardiac catheterization with angiography might be necessary.

Angiography in patients with cardiac neoplasms is particularly useful in detecting compression or displacement of cardiac cavities or large masses and determining the magnitude of the intracavitary filling defects. The most frequent angiographic findings are intracavitary filling defects, which may be fixed or mobile, lobulated or smooth, and attached over a broad base or by a narrow stalk. Coronary angiography is sometimes helpful in visualizing the vascular supply of the neoplasm and the relation of the neoplasm to the coronary arteries. The vascular pattern is not helpful, however, in differentiating benign from malignant tumors.

In contrast to the other diagnostic techniques, cardiac catheterization can be a bit risky in patients with intracardiac neoplasms, because the catheter may dislodge a fragment of the tumor with resulting embolus. Thus, the noninvasive techniques are preferred to cardiac catheterization in a patient suspected of having an intracardiac mass. The transseptal approach to the left atrium is not advised if a left atrial tumor is suspected, because the stalk of the left atrial myxoma is usually attached to the fossa ovale membrane, where the transseptal catheter courses.

SPECIFIC BENIGN PRIMARY CARDIAC NEOPLASMS

Myxoma

Myxomas are by far the most common type of primary cardiac tumor; 75% of them are located in the left atrial cavity (*Figures 2* and *3*), about 23% in the right atrial cavity (*Figure 4*), and about 2% in a ventricular cavity (21–33) (*Figure 5*). On rare occasions, the tumor is present in >1 cavity. Generally, when located in the left atrium, the neoplasm produces symptoms when it reaches about 7 cm in size. Neoplasms in the right atrium that produce symptoms are usually about twice as large and sometimes several times larger. The cell of origin of the myxoma is still unclear (22, 34–36).

How fast atrial myxomas grow has never been clarified. An attempt to answer this question was provided by a study that examined the size of recurrent myxomas and divided their mass in grams by the interval between the first and second operations (37). It was estimated that recurrent left atrial myxomas grow an average of 0.15 cm per month or 1.8 cm per year, or an average of 1.2 g per month or 14 g per year. Whatever the exact growth rate may be, both recurrent and initial left atrial myxomas appear to grow rather rapidly (38, 39).

Morphologic diagnosis of myxoma is readily made by gross inspection, and its appearance is clearly different from that of thrombi. The surface is smooth but irregular, shiny, and usually multicolored. Although there are exceptions (29–32, 40–43), the tumor is nearly always attached to the atrial septum if it is in the left atrium, and the stalk is most commonly much smaller than

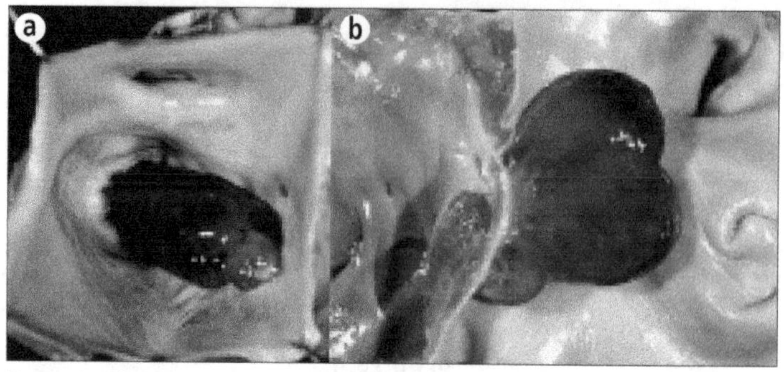

Figure 2. Clinically silent *left atrial myxoma* found at necropsy in a 60-year-old woman who died of metastatic carcinoid. The myxoma was not large enough to prolapse through the mitral orifice during ventricular diastole. **(a)** Cephalad view of the left atrium. **(b)** Longitudinal view showing attachment of the myxoma to the atrial septum by a relatively broad base. Reprinted with permission from Roberts WC, Perloff JK. Mitral valvular disease. A clinicopathologic survey of the conditions causing the mitral valve to function abnormally. *Ann Intern Med* 1972;77:939–975.

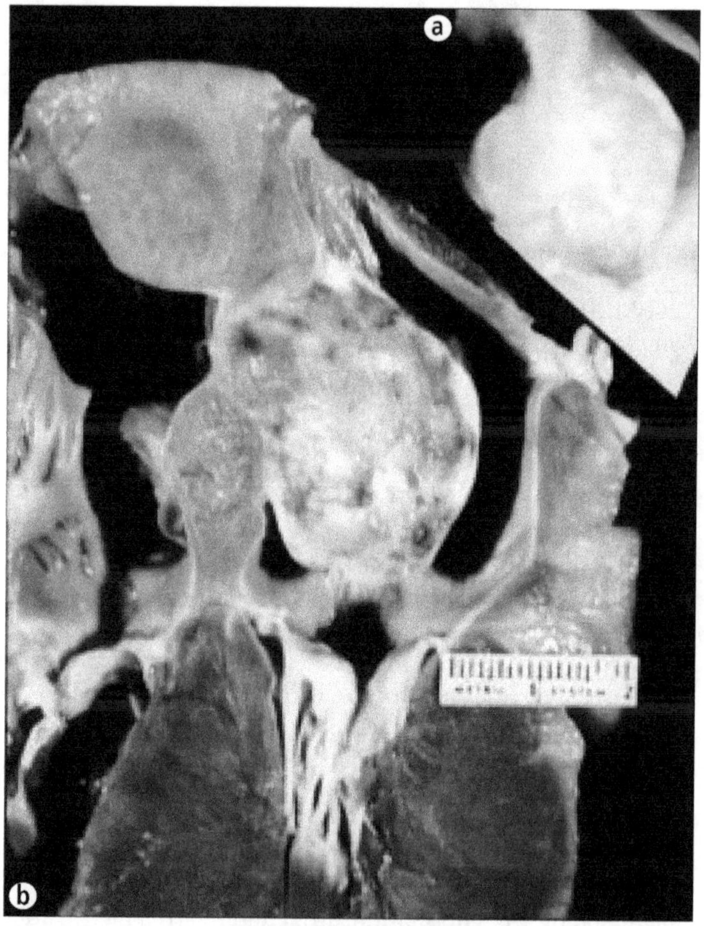

Figure 3. Clinically silent *left atrial myxoma* discovered at necropsy in an 80-year-old woman who fractured her hip and femur 5 days before a fatal pulmonary embolus. She had never had symptoms of cardiac dysfunction or myocardial ischemia. **(a)** A radiograph showing calcific deposits in the myxoma. **(b)** A longitudinal view of the myxoma arising from the fossa ovale area and from the atrial septum both cephalad and caudal to it. The cephalad portion of the atrial septum was thickened mainly by adipose tissue (lipomatous hypertrophy of the atrial septum). Reprinted from Shirani J, Isner JM, Roberts WC. Are autopsies still useful? Thank goodness we didn't know. Not all tumors are bad tumors. Most of the cavity has to be filled before trouble occurs. *Am J Cardiol* 1993;72:371–372 with permission from Excerpta Medica Inc.

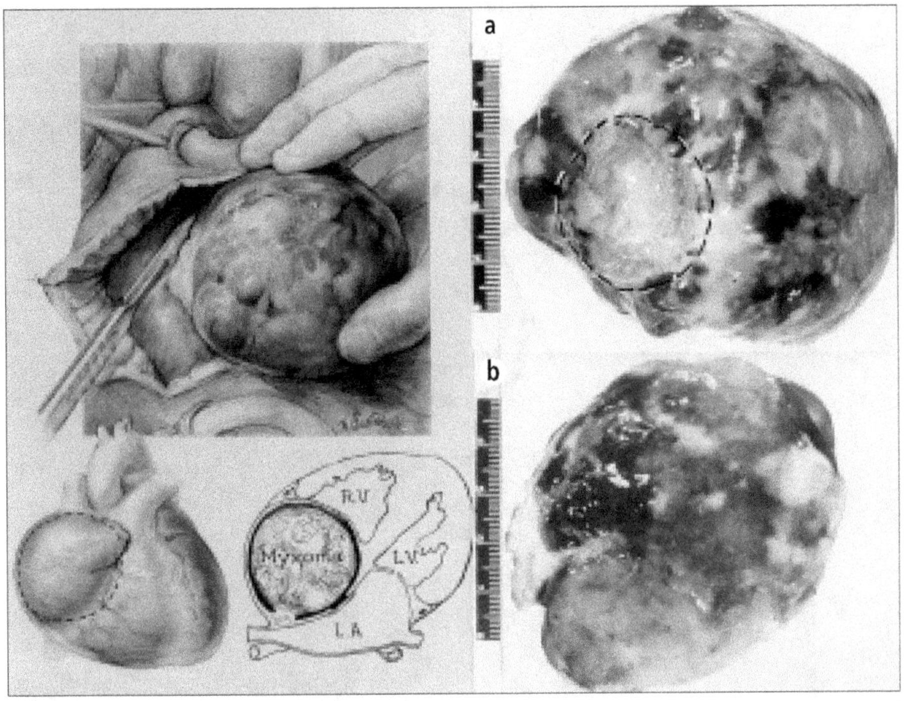

Figure 4. *Right atrial myxoma* operatively excised from the right atrium of a 46-year-old man who had had evidence of cardiac dysfunction for 12 years. **(a)** The tumor was attached to the atrial septum by a relatively small stalk (surrounded by dashed circle). The myxoma weighed 142 g, and its largest diameter was 8 cm. **(b)** A view of the cut section of the tumor. Reprinted from Roberts WC. Primary and secondary neoplasms of the heart. *Am J Cardiol* 1997;80:671–682 with permission from Excerpta Medica Inc.

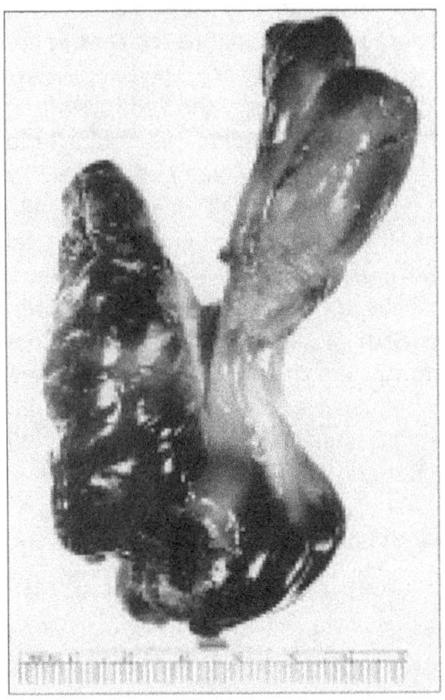

Figure 5. *Right ventricular myxoma* operatively excised in a 21-year-old man who was well until 10 months before excision of the cardiac tumor, when he had the first of 3 syncopal episodes during exertion. A precordial murmur was heard for the first time after the first syncopal spell. When he was examined shortly before the cardiac operation, a grade 4/6 holosystolic murmur was audible and was loudest along the left sternal border. Catheterization showed the right ventricular pressure to be 63/5 and the pulmonary arterial pressure to be 15/7, yielding a 45-mm Hg peak systolic pressure gradient. Angiography disclosed a large filling defect in the right ventricle. The right ventricular tumor weighed 82 g. During each ventricular systole, the tumor extended out the outflow tract to contact the bifurcation of the pulmonary trunk. Reprinted with permission from Lindsay J Jr, Goldberg SD, Roberts WC. Electrocardiogram in neoplastic and hematological disorders. *Cardiovasc Clin* 1977;8(3):225–242.

the maximal diameter of the mass. On occasion, the site of attachment to the atrial septum is broad. The mean age of patients with sporadic myxoma is 56 years, and at least 75% are women. During the past 10 years at Baylor University Medical Center, at least 15 left atrial myxomas have been excised; 14 were in women.

Familial cardiac myxomas constitute approximately 10% of all myxomas, and they appear to have an autosomal-dominant transmission (44). These occur in younger patients (mean age, 25 years) and have less female gender predominance. The myxomas in the familial syndrome are much more liable to be multiple (50% of the time) and to have a ventricular cavity location (13% compared with <1% in the nonfamilial or sporadic myxomas). Patients with familial myxoma typically have exterior facial freckling; they have noncardiac myxomas (breast or skin) and also endocrine neoplasms. Both the NAME (nevi, atrial myxoma, neurofibromas, ephelides) and the LAMB (lentigines, atrial myxoma, and balloon nevi) syndromes are associated with the familial variety of cardiac myxoma. Chromosomal abnormalities for atrial myxoma have been described on chromosome 2 (Carney's) and chromosome 12 (Ki-*ras* genes).

Myxomas probably present the most varied clinical picture of all primary cardiac neoplasms (4–6, 23, 25, 26, 45). Several major syndromes have been observed, including presentation with signs of emboli, obstruction of blood flow, and various constitutional syndromes. Fragments of tumor located in the right side of the heart may embolize to the lungs, and those in the left side of the heart, of course, to various systemic organs. Diagnosis may be made, on occasion, by finding typical myxomatous endothelial-like cells—which are elongated and spindle shaped with round or oval nuclei and prominent nucleoli—in surgically removed emboli.

Obstruction of blood flow may occur at the orifice of any valve, most commonly, of course, the mitral valve. Interference with flow through the mitral orifice may mimic signs of mitral stenosis, including signs of pulmonary congestion, diastolic apical rumble, opening snap, and accentuated first heart sounds. A murmur of mitral regurgitation may also be present as a result of chronic damage to the valve leaflets or of interference with proper closure of the valve by tumor. Differentiation between a left atrial tumor and primary mitral stenosis is suggested by the influence of position on symptoms and on the intensity of the precordial murmurs and the opening snap.

The constitutional symptoms associated with atrial myxomas include fever, weight loss, Raynaud's phenomenon, digital clubbing, anemia, elevated erythrocyte sedimentation rate, elevated leukocyte count, decreased platelet count, positive seroreactive protein, and abnormal serum proteins (usually increased gamma globulins). These constitutional symptoms may mimic infective endocarditis, collagen vascular disease, or occult malignancy. A myxoma also may become infected (46).

The proper treatment of myxoma in any cavity of the heart is operative resection, because no medicine is known to shrink myxomas or to prevent their continued growth (21, 27, 33). Some surgeons advise a biatrial approach for full visualization of both sides of the heart and then complete removal of a left or right atrial myxoma, excising the full thickness of the atrial septum if the neoplasm is attached to the region of the fossa ovalis. If a large portion of the atrial septum is removed, a patch must be used to close the defect. Because fragmentation and embolization of the tumor is an ever-present threat, vigorous palpa-

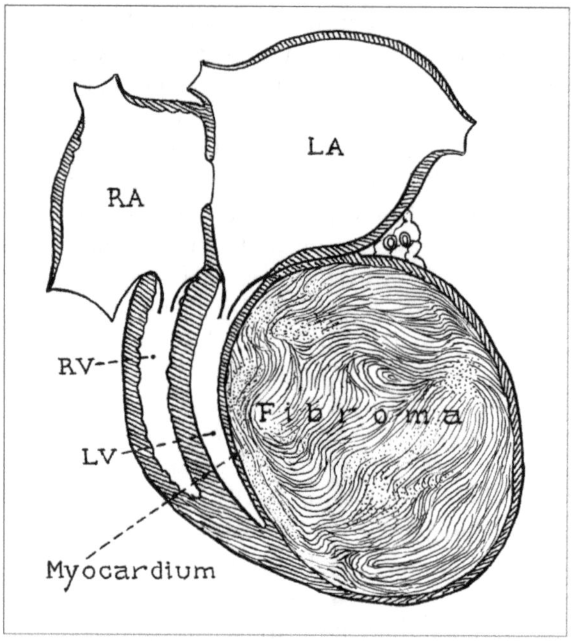

Figure 6. Diagram of an *intramyocardial fibroma* seen at necropsy in a 5-month-old boy who was found dead in his crib. The neoplasm had been diagnosed by biopsy during the child's first few days of life. It was considered nonresectable. Reprinted from Roberts WC. Primary and secondary neoplasms of the heart. *Am J Cardiol* 1997; 80:671–682 with permission from Excerpta Medica Inc.

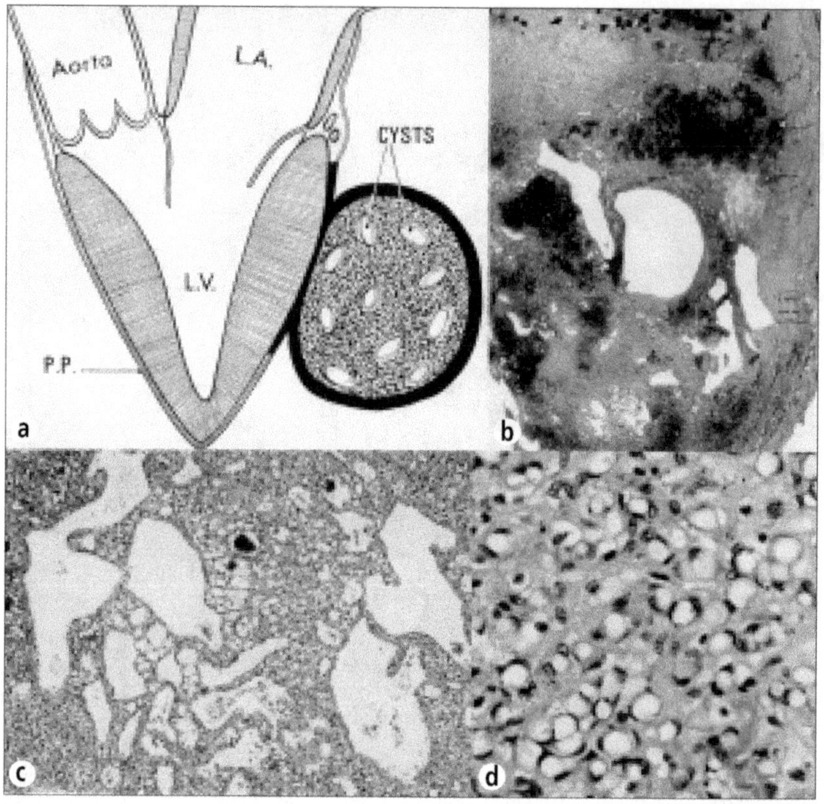

Figure 7. Benign *hemangioma of the epicardium.* This 36-year-old man suddenly developed transient but severe anterior chest pain a few hours after playing basketball. When he was examined after the pain had disappeared, there was a 3 × 3–cm area of precordial pulsation and a grade 2/6 short systolic murmur. Fluoroscopy disclosed a mass along the left cardiac border, which enlarged during ventricular systole. Left ventricular angiography, however, showed a smooth endocardial surface and no aneurysm. Coronary angiography showed the left circumflex artery to be dilated and tortuous and the left anterior descending and right arteries to be normal. The pressures (in mm Hg) were pulmonary artery, 28/14; right ventricle, 28/9; right atrial mean, 9; pulmonary artery wedge mean, 13; left ventricle, 118/19; and aorta, 118/80. **(a)** The electrocardiogram showed left axis deviation. At thoracotomy, a nonexpansile, solid, 7 × 3 × 2–cm mass was found on the posterolateral surface of the left ventricle. The tumor was covered by a capsule attached to the epicardium of the left ventricle, which was involved by the tumor. On sectioning, the tumor was cystic, hemorrhagic, and firm. **(b, c, d)** Histologically, the tumor consisted of numerous small and large vascular channels lined by either mesothelial or endothelial cells. Between the vascular channels was fibrous tissue containing hemosiderin deposits. The tumor was judged to be benign. Hematoxylin-eosin stains: (b) ×15, (c) ×63, and (d) ×400. Reprinted with permission from Roberts WC, Spray TL. Pericardial heart disease. *Curr Probl Cardiol* 1977;2(3):1–71.

tion and other manipulations of the heart should be avoided until cardiopulmonary bypass is initiated. Most surgeons induce ventricular standstill with cardioplegia solution before manipulating the heart to reduce the possibility of fragmentation of portions of the tumor. Left atrial myxomas have been removed successfully during pregnancy. On occasion, an atrioventricular valve has been so traumatized by the tumor's prolapsing through it during ventricular diastole that valve excision and replacement are necessary. Fortunately, recurrences of atrial myxomas are rare, and if they do recur, the recurrence usually occurs within 4 years of surgical resection of the initial tumor (38, 39).

Rhabdomyoma

The most common cardiac neoplasm in infants and children is rhabdomyoma (47). There is some question whether this particular tumor is a true neoplasm or a hamartoma. These neoplasms are usually multiple, most often involve the ventricular myocardium, and project into the cavity or move freely as a pedunculated mass (48–50). Associated tuberous sclerosis is present in about one third of the patients. The diagnosis is suggested by the presence of yellow-brown angiofibromas ("adenoma sebaceum") on the face, subungual fibromas around the fingernails, café au lait spots, and subcutaneous nodules. Presenting symptoms may be caused by obstruction to inflow to or outflow from the ventricles, arrhythmias, atrioventricular block, or pericardial effusion; at times the "presenting symptom" is sudden death (51). These neoplasms may mimic pulmonic valve stenosis and produce hypoxic spells resembling those seen in tetralogy of Fallot. They are usually readily diagnosed by echocardiography, angiography, or MRI. Prenatal detection of intracardiac rhabdomyoma by intrauterine echocardiography has been reported. The occurrence of >1 tumor does not prevent operative intervention. On rare occasions, these tumors have produced ventricular tachycardia in infants, and this arrhythmia has disappeared following successful operative removal.

Fibroma

Fibromas usually appear within a ventricular wall (i.e., intramural) (3, 52) (*Figure 6*). Most also occur in infants and children. Calcific deposits may be present within the neoplasm. Sudden death has occurred in about a third of the patients, presumably the result of a conduction defect, arrhythmia, or obstruction to outflow from a ventricle. Left axis deviation has been seen on electrocardiogram. Total or partial resection of the neoplasm may relieve obstruction with an excellent probability of long-term survival.

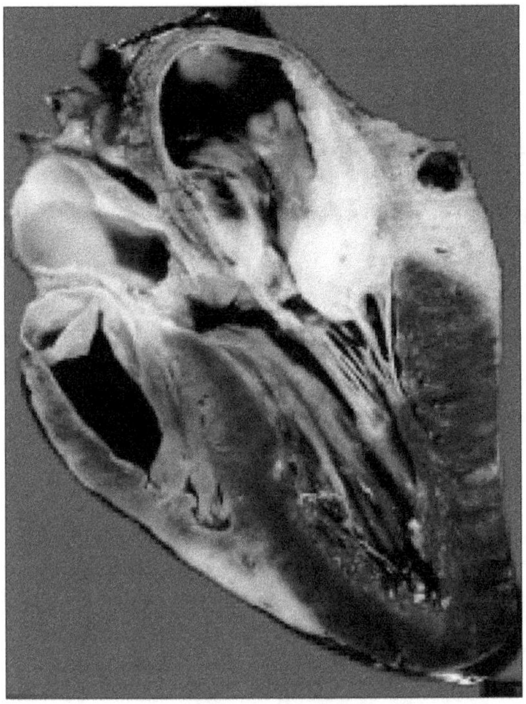

Figure 8. *Primary cardiac sarcoma,* undifferentiated type. This tumor caused mitral stenosis in a 46-year-old woman who had been well until 8 months before death. Cardiac catheterization disclosed a 20–mm Hg mean diastolic gradient between the pulmonary artery wedge position and left ventricle. The right ventricular pressure was 105/18 mm Hg. The neoplasm was located in the walls of the left atrium and in both anterior and posterior mitral leaflets. Reprinted from Domanski MJ, Delaney TF, Kleiner DE Jr, Goswitz M, Agatston A, Tucker E, Johnson M, Roberts WC. Primary sarcoma of the heart causing mitral stenosis. *Am J Cardiol* 1990;66:893–895 with permission from Excerpta Medica Inc.

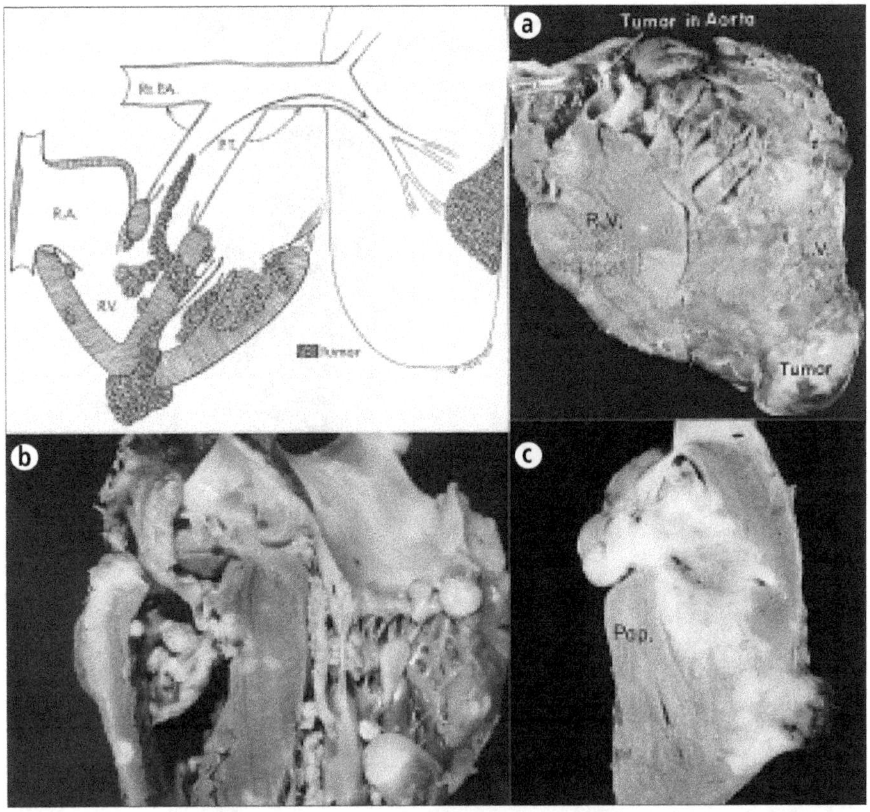

Figure 9. *Primary cardiac sarcoma,* undifferentiated type, with neoplastic emboli to the lung and other organs in a 26-year-old man who had been well until 3 months before death. **(a)** Exterior of the heart containing blood, fibrin, and tumor. **(b)** Opened right ventricle (RV), left ventricle (LV), left atrium, and aortic valve showing numerous tumor deposits. **(c)** Section of the left ventricular wall showing the neoplasm extending through the entire wall and with extension beneath the posterior mitral leaflet and through the epicardium. Pap indicates papillary muscle; RA, right atrium; Rt PA, right pulmonary artery. Reprinted from Roberts WC. Primary and secondary neoplasms of the heart. *Am J Cardiol* 1997;80:671–682 with permission from Excerpta Medica Inc.

Lipoma

Lipomas involving the heart may be extremely small and represent incidental necropsy findings, or they may be massive (53–56). The largest cardiac neoplasm ever reported apparently was an intrapericardial lipoma. They may be mistaken for pericardial cysts, cause pericardial effusion, or be asymptomatic and suggested by a widened mediastinum on chest radiograph. Intramyocardial lipomas are encapsulated and usually small. Lipomas also have been located on cardiac valves, where they may simulate vegetations or myxomas (55). MRI permits preoperative identification of these fatty tumors.

Hemangioma

Hemangiomas are best diagnosed by coronary angiography, which yields a characteristic "tumor blush." Spontaneous resolution without treatment has been reported. Total excision is possible only in some cases *(Figure 7)*.

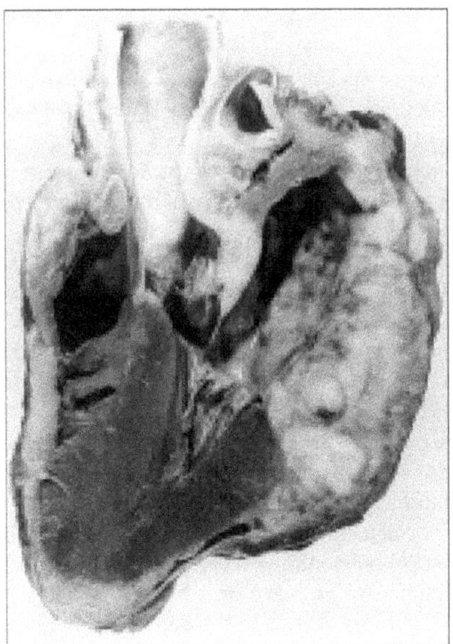

Figure 10. *Primary cardiac histiocytic lymphoma.* This 64-year-old woman had had evidence of congestive heart failure for 7 months. The cause of the heart failure was not apparent until necropsy. The wall of the left atrium was massively thickened by the neoplasm. Reprinted with permission from Roberts CS, Gottdiener JS, Roberts WC. Clinically undetected cardiac lymphoma causing congestive heart failure. *Am Heart J* 1990; 120:1239–1242.

SPECIFIC MALIGNANT PRIMARY CARDIAC NEOPLASMS

Angiosarcoma

Nearly all primary malignant cardiac neoplasms are sarcomas, and the most frequent one is angiosarcoma (57–62), which characteristically originates from the right atrium or from the epicardium of the right atrium. The large quantity of vascular channels within these tumors and the subsequent large quantity of blood flowing through them may produce a continuous precordial murmur. About 25% of all angiosarcomas are, at least in part, intracavitary with valvular obstruction and cause right-sided heart failure and pericardial tamponade with a hemorrhagic-type fluid. The course is rapid with widespread metastases, and operative intervention is usually unsuccessful.

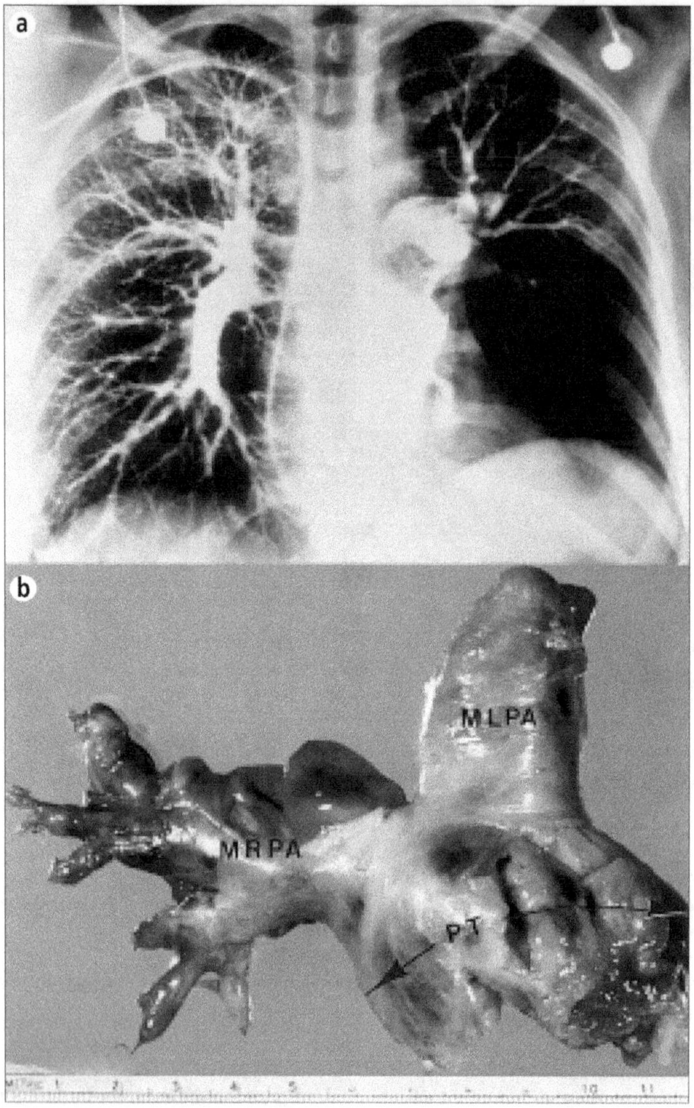

Figure 11. *Primary sarcoma of the pulmonary trunk.* This 34-year-old woman was well until 20 days before operative excision of the tumor, when she suddenly experienced severe substernal chest pain with radiation to both arms, associated with dyspnea and nausea, while climbing stairs. A minute or so later she fainted; she awoke about 15 minutes later lying on the floor in a pool of urine. Shortly thereafter she was hospitalized. She appeared healthy. A grade 3/6 systolic, ejection-type precordial murmur, loudest in the pulmonic area, was heard. The lungs were clear. The electrocardiogram was normal. Chest radiograph showed enlargement of the "pulmonary segment." The following pressures in mm Hg were recorded: intrapulmonary pulmonary artery, 20/10; pulmonary trunk, 60/25; right ventricle, 60/18; right atrial mean, 7; pulmonary arterial wedge mean, 11; and aorta, 100/60. **(a)** Angiography with injection into the right ventricular cavity disclosed large filling defects in the pulmonary trunk and in both right main and left main pulmonary arteries with total lack of filling of arteries to the lower half of the left lung and markedly diminished filling of those to the upper left lung. **(b)** At thoracotomy, the large tumor completely filled the pulmonary trunk (PT) and main right (MRPA) and left (MLPA) pulmonary arteries, and it was excised. The tumor was attached to the pulmonary trunk over a large base. Histologically, the tumor was an undifferentiated sarcoma. Although the early postoperative course was unremarkable and the pulmonary arterial and right ventricular pressures returned to normal, repeat right ventricular angiogram 7 months postoperatively disclosed a filling defect in the pulmonary trunk. She then underwent resection of the pulmonary trunk containing the sarcoma recurrence and replacement with a graft. Reprinted from Shmookler BM, Marsh HB, Roberts WC. Primary sarcoma of the pulmonary trunk and/or right or left main pulmonary artery—a rare cause of obstruction to right ventricular outflow. Report on two patients and analysis of 35 previously described patients. *Am J Med* 1977;63:263–272 with permission from Excerpta Medica Inc.

Rhabdomyosarcoma

Rhabdomyosarcoma is the second most frequent primary sarcoma of the heart, and, like angiosarcoma, it is most common in males (63–65). In contrast to angiosarcoma, however, this neoplasm has no predilection for a specific cardiac chamber. Indeed, the neoplasm may be in all 4 cardiac chambers, or at least in >1, and obstruction may occur in ≥1 valve orifice. Again, prognosis is poor, survival is short, and operative intervention is usually futile.

Miscellaneous

Fibrosarcoma, liposarcoma, primary malignant lymphoma, and occasional sarcomas of other cell types constitute the remaining but infrequent primary malignant coronary neoplasms (66–69) (*Figures 8–10*). All of these neoplasms may obstruct valvular orifices, obliterate chambers, obstruct arteries exiting the heart (*Figure 11*), and produce peripheral emboli (70). Hypertrophic cardiomyopathy has been suggested by heavy tumorous infiltrations of the ventricular septum (71).

METASTATIC NEOPLASMS TO THE HEART

Metastatic or secondary tumors of the heart with a primary tumor in another body organ or tissue are far more frequent than primary tumors of the heart (72) (*Figure 12*). The secondary tumors are far more commonly carcinomas than sarcomas simply because carcinomas are far more common. The diagnosis can be suspected whenever cardiac manifestations occur in a patient diagnosed as having a primary tumor in an organ or tissue other than the heart. The development of cardiac enlargement, tachycardia, arrhythmias, or heart failure in the presence of a neoplasm elsewhere in the body is highly suggestive of cardiac metastases. Only rarely are metastases limited to the heart. Thus, the presence of a metastatic tumor in the heart usually indicates widespread metastases in a number of body organs. On rare occasions, cardiac involvement may be the first or only expression of a noncardiac primary neoplasm. The most common sign is tamponade (73). Direct invasion of the heart via the vena cava or pulmonary veins may lead to obstruction of an atrioventricular valve; it may also lead to pulmonary or systemic emboli or both (74–76).

Carcinoma of the lung and *carcinoma of the breast* tend to invade the parietal pericardium and then the visceral pericardium, leading to myocardial constriction and/or pericardial effusion (*Figure 13*). Another presentation of lung cancer is invasion of the pulmonary veins within the lung, with spread of the cancer within the lumen of the pulmonary veins into the left atrium. From there, the cancer can continue into the mitral orifice, sometimes causing obstruction (77, 78) (*Figure 14*). Cancer in mediastinal lymph nodes also may obstruct pulmonary arteries (*Figure 15*). In addition, lung cancer metastases in the adrenal gland may extend into the inferior vena cava and then into the right side of the heart (*Figure 16*), just as primary adrenal gland or renal cancer may (79). Cancer of the lung or breast surrounding the main right or left pulmonary artery can lead to pulmonary arterial obstruction (80). Carcinoma of the lung may also invade the myocardium from the endocardial side only (*Figure 17*).

Of all neoplasms, *melanoma* has the highest frequency of metastases to the heart per 100 cases (81, 82). The metastases

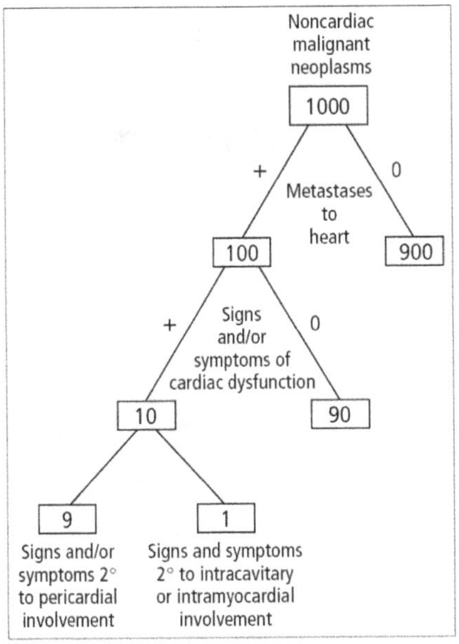

Figure 12. *Relative frequencies of cardiac metastases producing cardiac dysfunction.* Reprinted from Roberts WC. Primary and secondary neoplasms of the heart. *Am J Cardiol* 1997;80: 671–682 with permission from Excerpta Medica Inc.

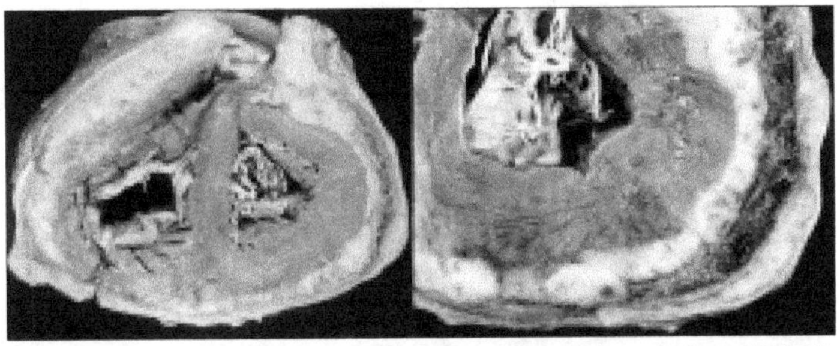

Figure 13. *Squamous cell carcinoma of the lung metastatic to the heart.* This 61-year-old man had fatal cardiac tamponade. The entire heart and great vessels were encased in tumor. Reprinted with permission from Roberts WC, Spray TL. Pericardial heart disease. *Curr Probl Cardiol* 1977;2(3):1–71.

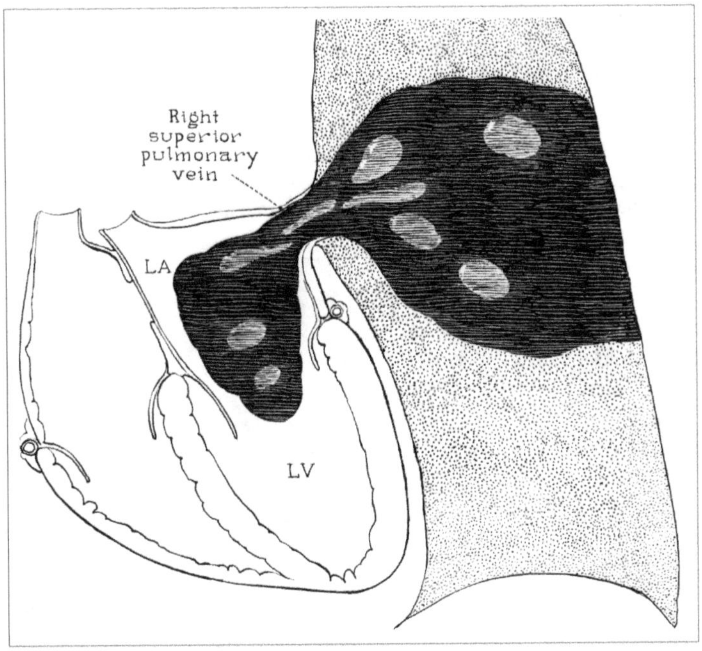

Figure 14. *Sarcoma, undifferentiated type, in the lung* (primary uncertain, possibly in the pulmonary vein). In this 29-year-old woman, an echocardiogram disclosed the tumor in the left atrium (LA) moving about "like a yo-yo." The left lung and its left atrial extension were operatively excised. LV indicates left ventricle. Reprinted from Roberts WC. Primary and secondary neoplasms of the heart. *Am J Cardiol* 1977;80:671–682 with permission from Excerpta Medica Inc.

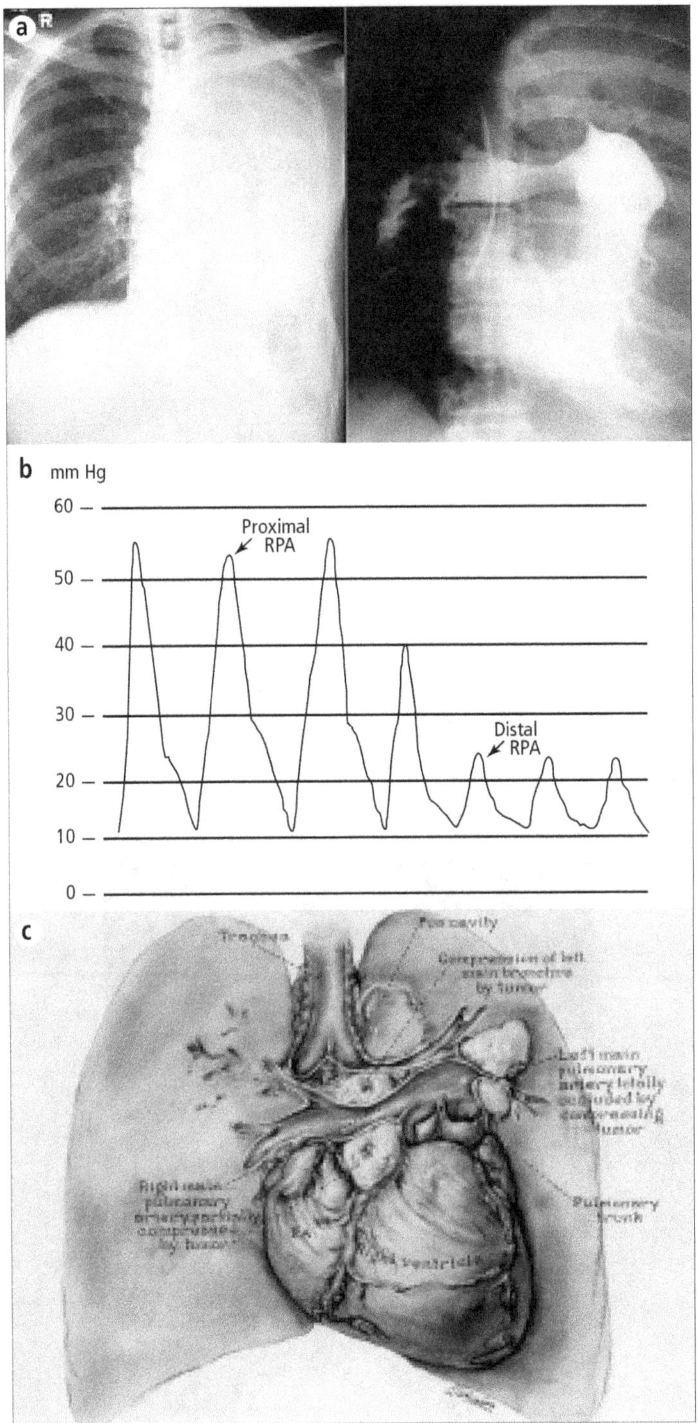

Figure 15. *Carcinoma of the lung causing pulmonary arterial stenosis.* This 55-year-old man had been well until 11 months before death, when left anterior chest pain and dyspnea first appeared and tissue from the left main bronchus disclosed small cell carcinoma. **(a)** Chest roentgenogram disclosed complete opacification of the left lung field. Precordial examination disclosed wide splitting of the second heart sound at the base, increased intensity of the pulmonic component of the second sound, and a grade 3/6 systolic murmur over the entire precordium, loudest at the upper left sternal border. **(b)** Cardiac catheterization disclosed the pressure (in mm Hg) in the distal right pulmonary artery to be 22/10; pulmonary trunk, 55/10; and right ventricle, 55/10. A right ventricular angiogram showed severe narrowing of the left main and moderate narrowing of the right main pulmonary arteries. **(c)** At necropsy, cancer was widespread in both lungs, and both the left main bronchus and left main pulmonary artery were severely compressed by tumor deposits. RA indicates right atrium. Reprinted with permission from Waller BF, Fletcher RD, Roberts WC. Carcinoma of the lung causing pulmonary arterial stenosis. *Chest* 1981;79:589–591.

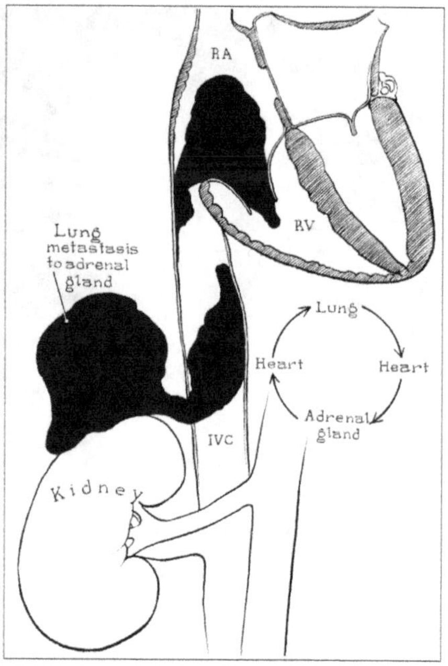

Figure 16. *Cancer of the lung metastatic to the right adrenal gland with extension into the inferior vena cava (IVC) and then into the right side of the heart.* An echocardiogram in this 57-year-old man showed the right atrial mass, which prolapsed through the tricuspid valve in atrial systole. RA indicates right atrium; RV, right ventricle. Reprinted from Roberts WC. Primary and secondary tumors of the heart. *Am J Cardiol* 1997;80:671–682 with permission from Excerpta Medica Inc.

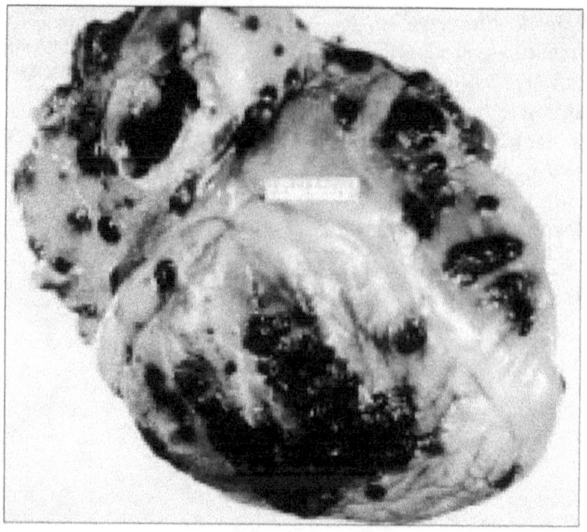

Figure 19. *Melanoma metastatic to the heart.* Shown here is the posterior surface of the heart with clinically silent multiple metastases in a 33-year-old man.

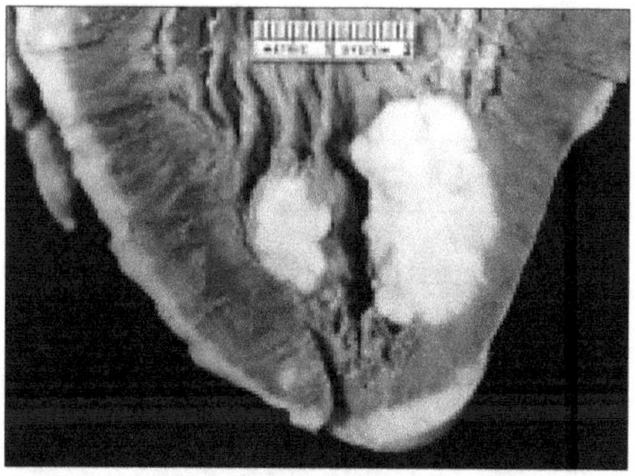

Figure 17. *Adenocarcinoma of the lung metastatic to the heart.* In this 59-year-old woman, silent metastases were present in the apex of the left ventricle and in the right ventricular outflow tract (not shown). Reprinted from Roberts WC. Primary and secondary neoplasms of the heart. *Am J Cardiol* 1997;80:671–682 with permission from Excerpta Medica Inc.

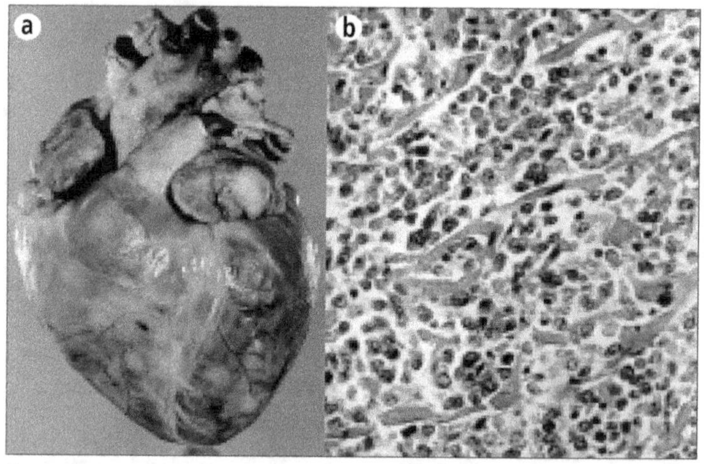

Figure 20. *Acute lymphocytic leukemia involving the heart.* This 18-month-old girl's illness lasted only 3 weeks. She died of massive intracerebral hemorrhage (platelet count, 5000/mm^3). **(a)** Necropsy disclosed nodular leukemic infiltrates in numerous organs, including the heart. Leukemic nodules were present in the walls of all 4 chambers. **(b)** The myocardial fibers in a tumor nodule were widely separated by leukemic cells. Hematoxylin-eosin stain, ×360. Reprinted from Roberts WC, Bodey GP, Wertlake PT. The heart in acute leukemia. A study of 420 autopsy cases. *Am J Med* 1968;21:388–412 with permission from Excerpta Medica Inc.

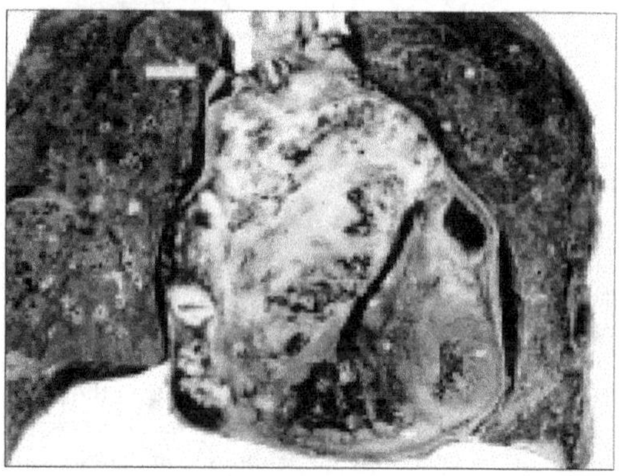

Figure 18. *Melanoma metastatic to the heart.* In this 53-year-old man, a pericardial friction rub was audible, and the neck veins were quite distended. The parietal pericardium at necropsy was everywhere adherent to the epicardium. The superior vena cava, right atrium, right ventricle, and pulmonary trunk were severely compressed by the tumor. Reprinted with permission from Roberts WC, Spray TL. Pericardial heart disease. *Curr Probl Cardiol* 1977;2(3):1–71.

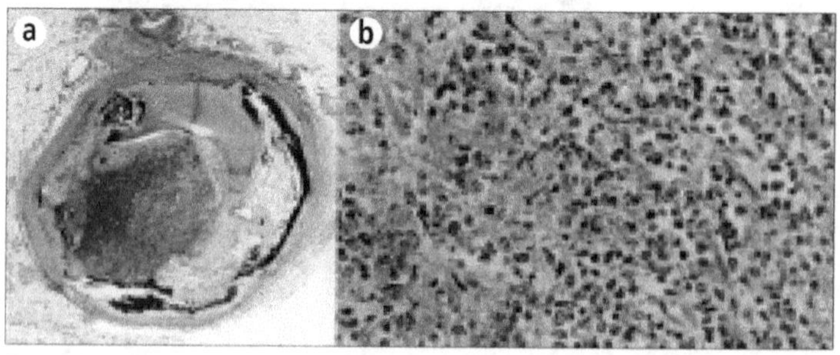

Figure 21. *Acute myelogenous leukemia in an epicardial coronary artery.* During the final day of his illness, this 41-year-old man developed hypotension, tachypnea, and diaphoresis without chest pain. An electrocardiogram was not recorded. Necropsy disclosed severe diffuse coronary arterial atherosclerosis, complete occlusion of the right coronary artery, and focal scars in the left ventricular wall. **(a)** The final occlusion of the coronary artery was produced by leukemic cells. **(b)** A photomicrograph of leukemic cells in the coronary artery (hematoxylin-eosin stain, ×315). Reprinted from Roberts WC, Bodey GP, Wertlake PT. The heart in acute leukemia. A study of 420 autopsy cases. *Am J Med* 1968;21:388–412 with permission from Excerpta Medica Inc.

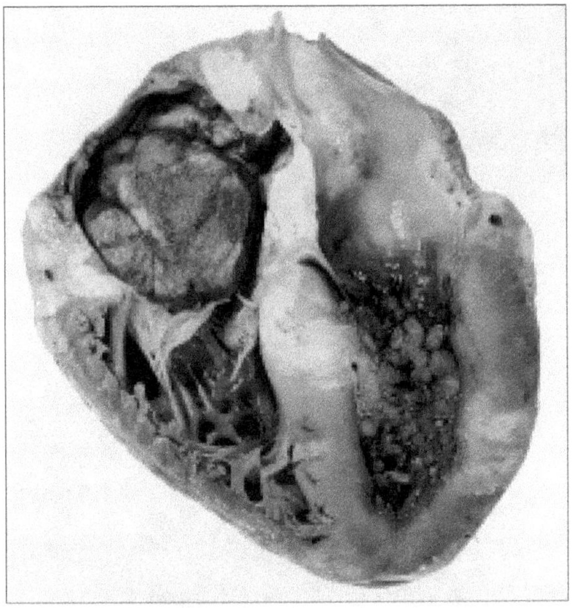

Figure 22. *Lymphoma of the heart.* This 38-year-old man with AIDS developed complete heart block and a large hemorrhagic pericardial effusion. A large tumor resided within the right atrial cavity, and multiple tumor deposits (white in color) were present in the right atrioventricular sulcus, atrial septum, ventricular septum (cephalad portion), and left ventricular free wall.

may be anywhere in the heart; usually melanotic metastases invade the walls of all 4 cardiac chambers and also the epicardium and endocardium (*Figures 18* and *19*). The cancers in these patients are in so many body organs that the presence of the neoplasm in the heart is almost incidental. Resection of an intracardiac melanoma has been accomplished (83).

Leukemia commonly invades the heart (84). In the days before platelet transfusions, extensive hemorrhages into the myocardial walls and into the endocardium and epicardium were commonly found in patients with fatal leukemia of various types. Histologically, leukemic infiltration between myocardial cells is quite common, and sometimes gross deposits of leukemic cells are visible within the heart (*Figure 20*). A few patients with leukemia present with pericardial effusion, which is usually hemorrhagic. Large calcific deposits in the right side of the heart have been reported (85). Leukemic cells have even caused obstruction of coronary arteries containing atherosclerotic plaques (*Figure 21*).

Lymphoma also has a very high frequency of metastases to the heart (8, 86–88). Nearly 25% of patients with lymphomas of various types have involvement of the epicardium, myocardium, endocardium, or some combination. In contrast to leukemic involvement, the lymphomatous deposits are usually grossly discernible (*Figure 22*).

Some cancers, like *osteogenic sarcoma*, may have calcium within them (89–91) (*Figure 23*). Others may not (*Figure 24*). Adenocarcinoma of the colon may also nearly obliterate the right ventricular cavity (*Figure 25*). Some sarcomas may involve the wall

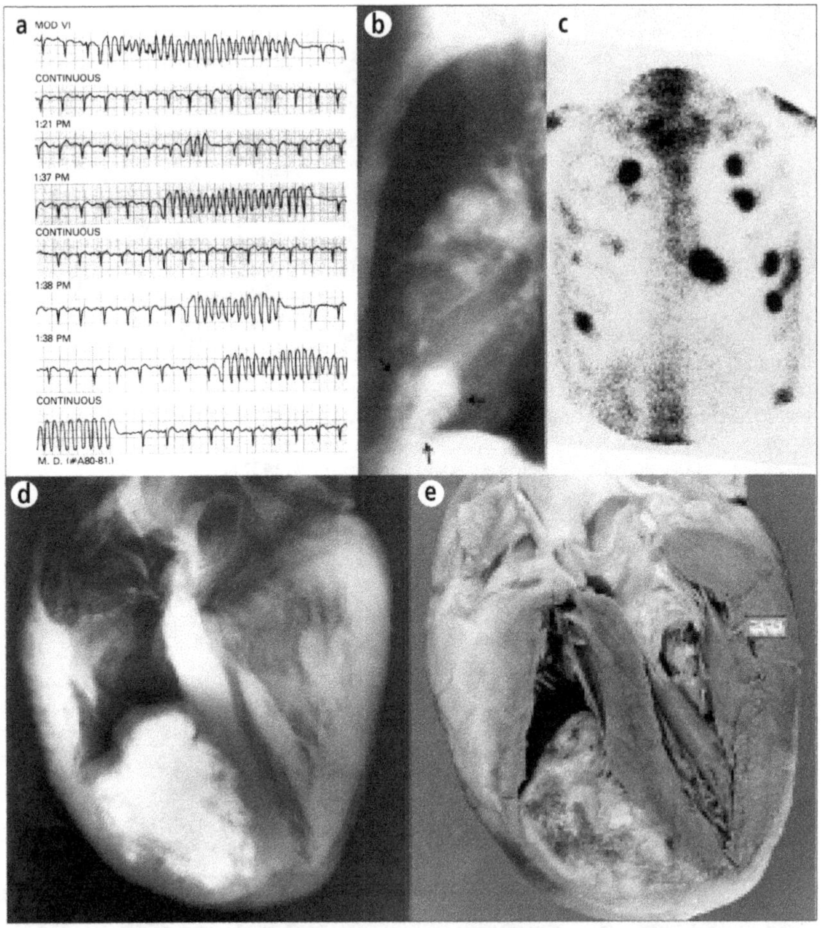

Figure 23. *Osteogenic sarcoma metastatic to the heart.* **(a)** This 39-year-old woman, who was ill for 20 months, had episodic ventricular tachycardia during her last 10 months. **(b)** The lateral chest radiograph shows a calcified tumor in the right ventricle (arrows). **(c)** The computed tomogram also shows the calcified tumor in the right ventricle as well as multiple metastases in the lungs and bone. **(d, e)** A large calcified tumor was present in the right ventricle. Reprinted from Seibert KA, Rettenmier CW, Waller BF, Battle WF, Levine AS, Roberts WC. Osteogenic sarcoma metastatic to the heart. *Am J Med* 1982;73:136–141 with permission from Excerpta Medica Inc.

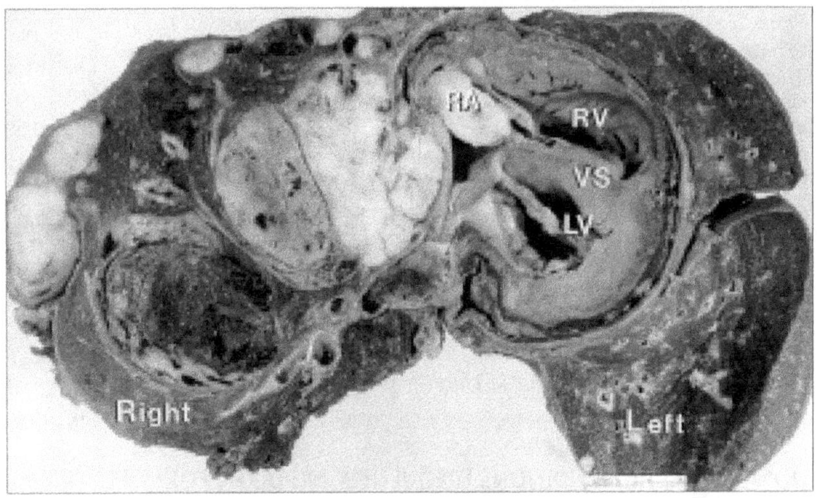

Figure 24. *Osteogenic sarcoma metastatic to the heart.* This 24-year-old man whose primary tumor was in the tibia had widespread pulmonary and cardiac (epicardium and right atrial [RA] cavity) metastases. Transverse cut of the lungs and heart showing multiple metastatic masses. RV indicates right ventricular cavity; VS, ventricular septum; LV, left ventricular cavity. Reprinted from Seibert KA, Rettenmier CW, Waller BF, Battle WE, Levine AS, Roberts WC. Osteogenic sarcoma metastatic to the heart. *Am J Med* 1982;73:136–141 with permission from Excerpta Medica Inc.

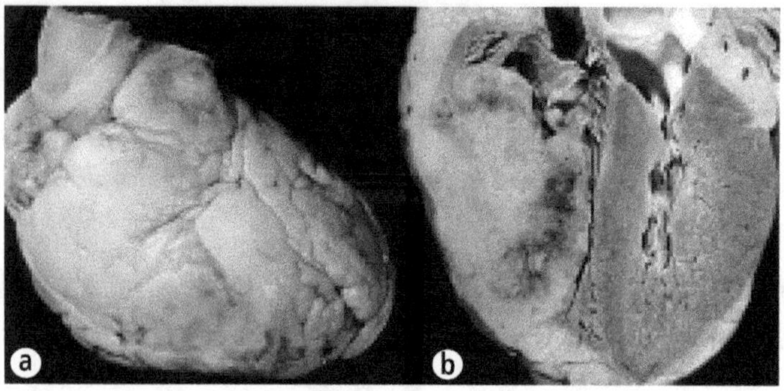

Figure 25. *Adenocarcinoma from the colon metastatic to the heart.* This 70-year-old woman had widespread metastases. **(a)** She had multiple deposits of tumor in the epicardium. **(b)** Much of the right ventricular cavity was filled with tumor. Reprinted with permission from Lindsay J Jr, Goldberg SD, Roberts WC. Electrocardiogram in neoplastic and hematological disorders. *Cardiovasc Clin* 1977;8(3):225–242.

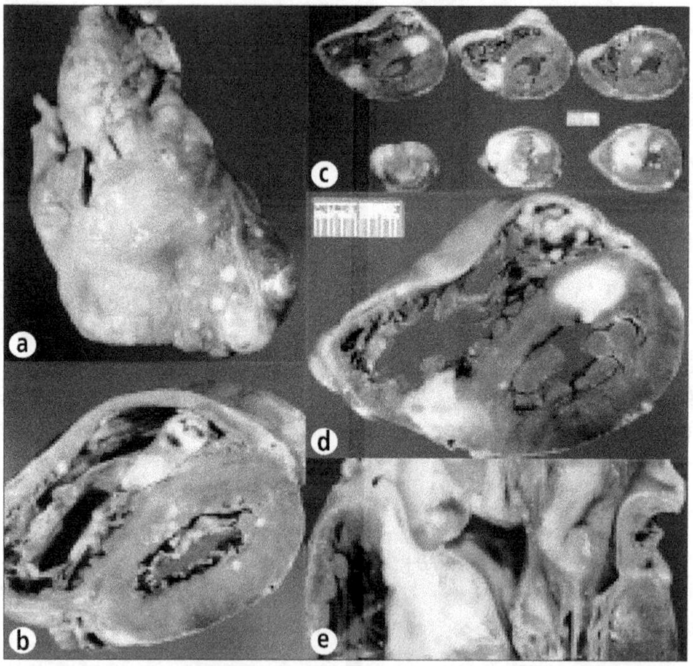

Figure 26. *Sarcoma metastatic to the heart.* This 30-year-old woman was found to have complete heart block and widespread metastatic cancer shortly before dying suddenly. The site of the primary tumor was never determined, but histologically the tumor was an undifferentiated sarcoma. **(a)** View of the heart showing numerous tumor deposits on the epicardial surface and over the aorta and pulmonary trunk. **(b)** Transverse section of the cardiac ventricles showing tumor deposits in the walls and a right ventricular intracavitary deposit. **(c)** Six "slices" of the ventricular walls showing multiple tumor deposits. **(d)** Close-up view of one "slice." **(e)** Longitudinal view of the most basal portion of the heart showing complete replacement of the most cephalad portion of the ventricular septum. This tumor deposition caused the complete heart block.

of all chambers as well as being located within 1 or more cavities and in the epicardium *(Figure 26)*. Others may obstruct a valve orifice *(Figure 27)*.

NONNEOPLASTIC CONDITIONS FREQUENTLY MISTAKEN FOR CARDIAC NEOPLASM

Pericardial cyst

Pericardial or mesothelial cysts are the most frequent benign "tumors" of the pericardium. These cysts are generally asymptomatic and found on "routine" chest radiograph (92) *(Figure 28)*. About a quarter of the patients, however, develop various symptoms, including chest pain, dyspnea, cough, and tachycardia, as a consequence of a pericardial cyst. The cysts are usually outside the pericardial cavity and, therefore, really should not be considered cardiac tumors.

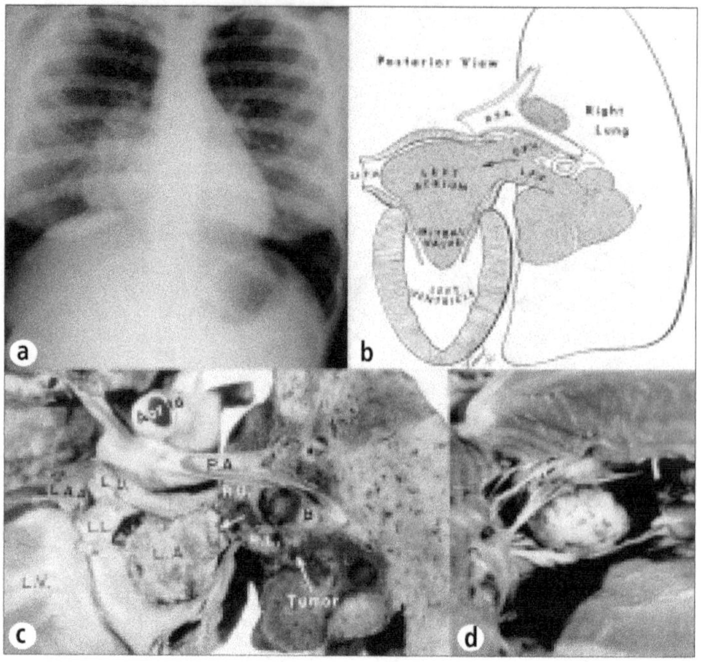

Figure 27. *Choriocarcinoma metastatic to the heart.* This 28-year-old woman died of disseminated choriocarcinoma 3 months after delivering a normal infant by cesarean section. The electrocardiogram, recorded 1 day before death, showed prominent P waves and large QRS complexes. **(a)** A chest roentgenogram 2 weeks before death showed a mass in the right lung and a normal-sized heart. **(b)** At necropsy, the mass in the right lung had invaded the major right pulmonary veins and via these veins extended into the left atrium and mitral valve orifice, obstructing the latter. **(c)** The left atrium (LA) containing the choriocarcinoma is shown from the back. **(d)** View of the mitral valve from the left ventricle containing the "tongue" of the choriocarcinoma. RU and RL indicate right upper and lower pulmonary vein; LU and LL, left upper and lower pulmonary vein; LAA, left atrial appendage; LA, left atrium containing the neoplasm; LV, left ventricle; B, bronchus; PA, pulmonary artery. Reprinted from MacLowery JD, Roberts WC. Metastatic choriocarcinoma of the lung. Invasion of pulmonary veins with extension into the left atrium and mitral orifice. *Am J Cardiol* 1966;18:938–941 with permission from Excerpta Medica Inc.

Teratoma

Teratomas are extracardiac in at least 99% of cases but are still within the pericardial cavity (93–95) *(Figure 29)*. They arise and receive their blood supply from the ascending aorta or pulmonary trunk, presumably through the vasa vasorum. Most are found in infants and children, primarily in females. Recurrent serous pericardial effusion in children should suggest intrapericardial teratoma. Because these tumors may become quite large, they may compress various cardiac chambers and therefore produce symptoms.

Lipomatous hypertrophy of the atrial septum

Massive fatty infiltration of the atrial septum is an extremely common condition occurring almost exclusively in persons >50 years of age and usually in individuals >65 years of age (96) *(Figure 30)*. These lesions are essentially limited to obese people, and they are always associated with enormous quantities of subepicardial adipose tissue, particularly in the atrioventricular sulci.

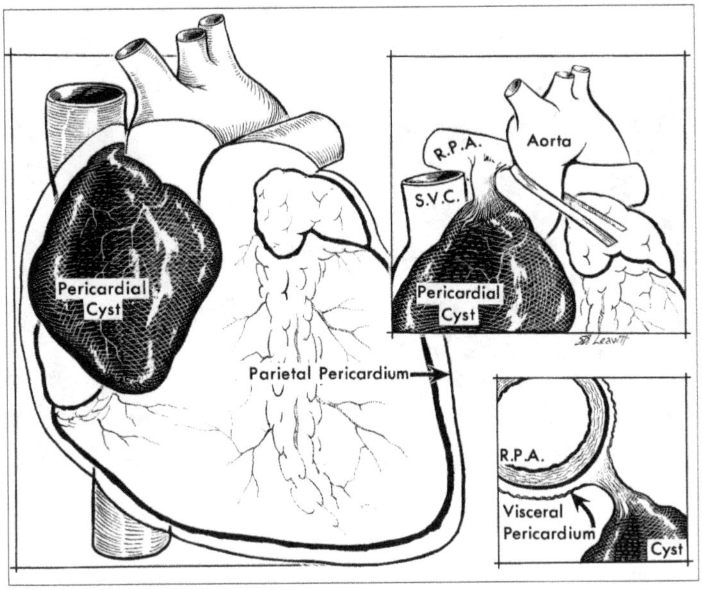

Figure 28. A *pericardial cyst* that was an incidental necropsy finding in a 75-year-old woman. The cyst, which contained serous fluid, overlay the right atrium and arose from a pedicle attached to the right main pulmonary artery (RPA). SVC indicates superior vena cava. Reprinted with permission from Roberts WC, Spray TL. Pericardial heart disease. *Curr Probl Cardiol* 1977;2(3):1–71.

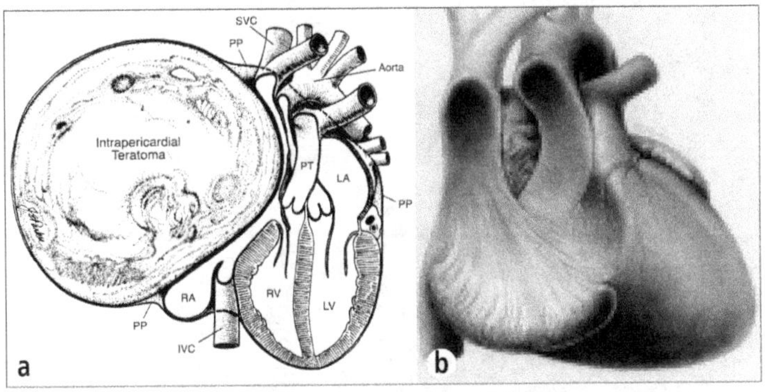

Figure 29. *Intrapericardial teratoma.* This stillborn child's heart weighed 8 g and the tumor, which weighed 20 g, greatly compressed the heart. Reprinted from Brabham KR, Roberts WC. Cardiac-compressing intrapericardial teratoma at birth. *Am J Cardiol* 1989;63:386–387 with permission from Excerpta Medica Inc.

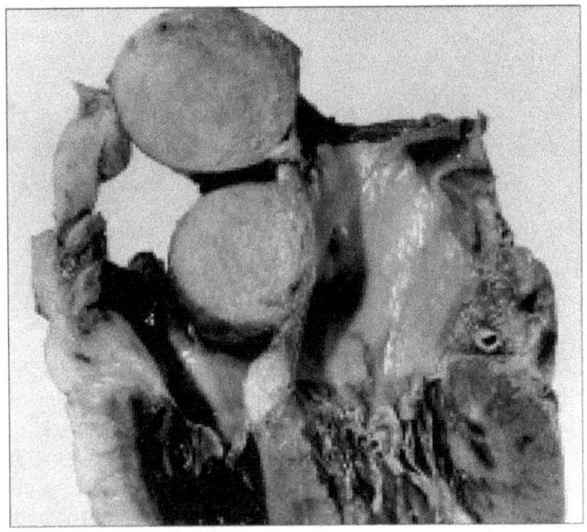

Figure 30. *Lipomatous hypertrophy of the atrial septum* in a 74-year-old woman with huge fatty deposits in the atrial septum (except for the fossa ovale area). Reprinted with permission from the American College of Cardiology (Shirani J, Roberts WC. Clinical, electrocardiographic and morphologic features of massive fatty deposits ("lipomatous hypertrophy") in the atrial septum. *J Am Coll Cardiol* 1993;22:226–238).

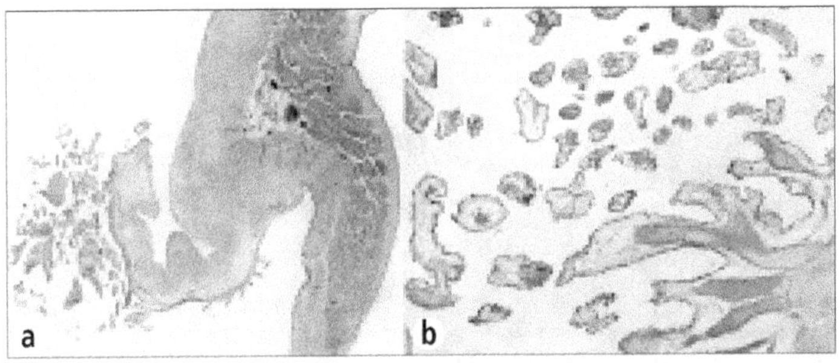

Figure 31. Photomicrographs of *papillary fibroelastoma* in a 36-year-old woman with hypertrophic cardiomyopathy and severe left ventricular outflow obstruction. These fibroelastomas were on the ventricular aspects of the aortic valve, on the atrial aspect of the mitral leaflets, and on the left ventricular mural endocardium. **(a)** View of an aortic valve cusp with multiple fibroelastomas on the cusp. **(b)** Close-up view of the fibroelastoma. Hematoxylin-eosin stains: (a) ×15, (b) ×84. Reprinted from Roberts WC. Papillary fibroelastomas of the heart. *Am J Cardiol* 1997;80:973–975 with permission from Excerpta Medica Inc.

These hearts are almost always so fat that they float in water (97). Normally, the atrial septum is <1 cm in thickness. In patients with lipomatous hypertrophy of the atrial septum, the atrial septum cephalad to the fossa ovale may be as thick as 7 cm, and the atrial septum caudal to the fossa ovale may be as thick as 4 cm. Extensive infiltration of fat into the atrial septum may be associated with atrial arrhythmias. These patients should not be operated on to remove fat from the atrial septum. The treatment is simply weight loss. The fatty deposits may be diagnosed by echocardiography, CT, or MRI (98, 99). Fat in the subepicardial adipose tissue has been confused with pericardial effusion on echocardiogram (100).

Papillary fibroelastomas

Papillary fibroelastomas are small avascular growths with multiple papillary fronds usually limited to cardiac valves, mainly the aortic and mitral; they are common in older persons (101) (*Figure 31*). They consist of fibrous tissue covered by an elastic membrane, which in turn is covered by endocardium. In about 15% of patients, they also occur on left ventricular or ventricular septal mural endocardium (102–111), particularly in patients with small or relatively small ventricular cavities, such as in patients with hypertrophic cardiomyopathy (102, 108) or mitral stenosis with or without aortic valve stenosis (106, 109, 110). When located on the aortic valve, papillary fibroelastomas are usually found on the ventricular aspects of the cusps in the more central portions. They also occur on the aortic aspects of these cusps, usually near the margins (112–115). On the mitral valve leaflets, they are usually on the atrial aspects near the margins (116–123). In patients with hypertrophic cardiomyopathy or mitral stenosis, they may be on the ventricular aspects of the anterior mitral leaflet and sometimes on mural endocardium, particularly over the papillary muscles. These lesions may be the result of contact of one valve leaflet with another or one mural endocardial surface with another.

A number of cases of papillary fibroelastomas and stroke have been reported (114–117, 121, 122, 124–128). Whether the stroke was truly connected with the cardiac fibroelastomas is

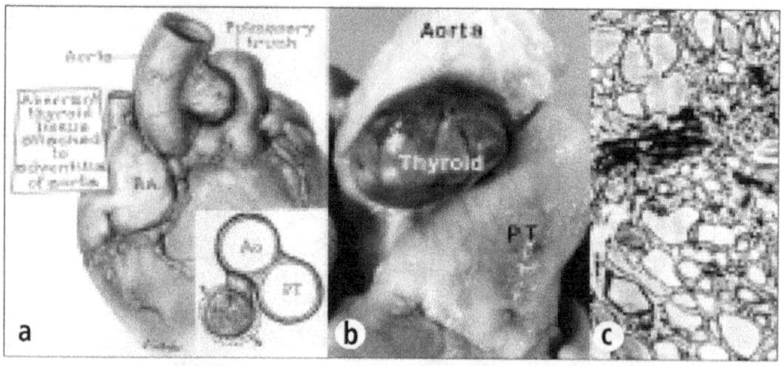

Figure 32. *Aberrant thyroid gland attached to the ascending aorta.* This 47-year-old man, who died of intracerebral hemorrhage soon after injecting heroin into a vein, at necropsy was found to have a brownish-red nodule weighing 15 g and measuring 3.0 × 2.3 × 1.5 cm attached to the adventitia of the ascending aorta. **(a)** A drawing of the location of the aberrant thyroid gland. **(b)** A photograph of the aberrant gland. **(c)** A photomicrograph of a portion of the nodule showing the thyroid gland (hematoxylin-eosin stain, ×80). Ao indicates aorta; PT, pulmonary trunk; RA, right atrium. Reprinted from Taylor MA, Bray M, Roberts WC. Aberrant thyroid gland attached to ascending aorta. *Am J Cardiol* 1986;57:708 with permission from Excerpta Medica Inc.

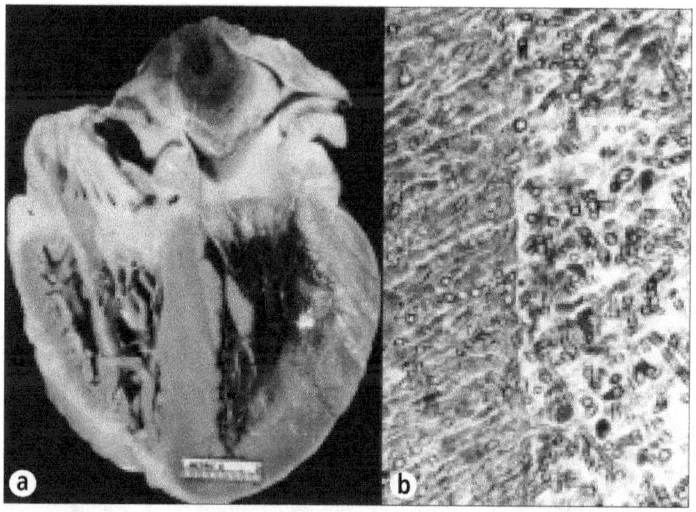

Figure 33. *Mucormycosis of the heart.* This 15-year-old boy had acute myelocytic leukemia for 6 months. One month before death, acute bilateral pneumonia developed. **(a)** Necropsy disclosed hemorrhagic necrotizing pneumonia and a fungus ball occluding the right pulmonary veins and invading the left atrial cavity. **(b)** A photomicrograph of mucor organisms in the left atrial mass (hematoxylin-eosin stain, ×400). Reprinted with permission from Buchbinder NA, Roberts WC. Active infective endocarditis confined to mural endocardium. A study of 6 necropsy patients. *Arch Pathol* 1972;93:435–440.

debatable. Some patients have been in their 20s or 30s without other predisposing features or findings commonly associated with cerebral infarction, and the occurrence of stroke in the younger age group is suggestive of a connection. In contrast to myxoma, tissue from which has been seen in systemic emboli, papillary fibroelastomas have not been observed by histologic studies in a cerebral artery of any patient with cardiac papillary fibroelastomas who had a stroke. Furthermore, the papillary fibroelastomas are firmly attached to valvular or mural endocardium, and dislodgment of a fibroelastoma therefore would appear unlikely. Thrombus, however, is occasionally superimposed on papillary fibroelastomas, and thrombus may be the material that is dislodged and is responsible for the stroke.

Angina pectoris (128), acute myocardial infarction (129–133), and sudden death (129, 134) have been observed in patients with cardiac papillary fibroelastomas, mainly on the aortic valve. These papillary growths may obstruct an aortic ostium of a coronary artery (135, 136). On rare occasions, papillary fibroelastomas have been observed on the right side of the heart, mainly on the tricuspid valve (137–140).

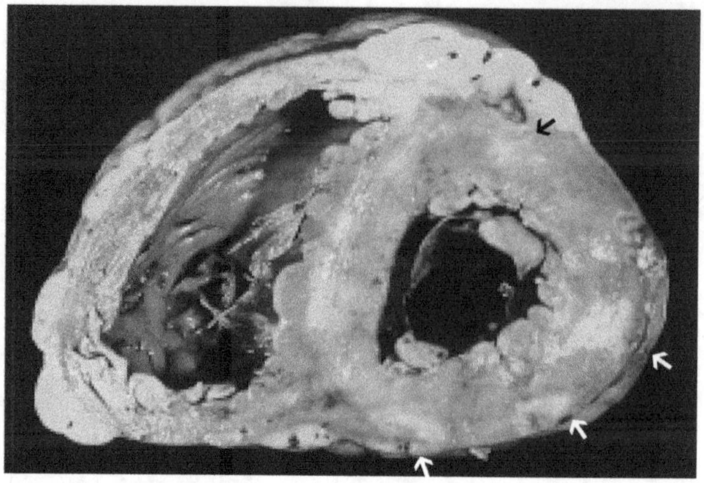

Figure 34. *Myocardial abscesses after bone marrow transplantation for chronic myelogenous leukemia.* This 31-year-old morbidly obese man had a bone marrow transplant 24 days before his death. Thereafter he had many complications, including aspergillosis septicemia and pneumonia. Necropsy disclosed numerous aspergillosis abscesses in the ventricular myocardial walls and also on the ventricular mural myocardium (arrows).

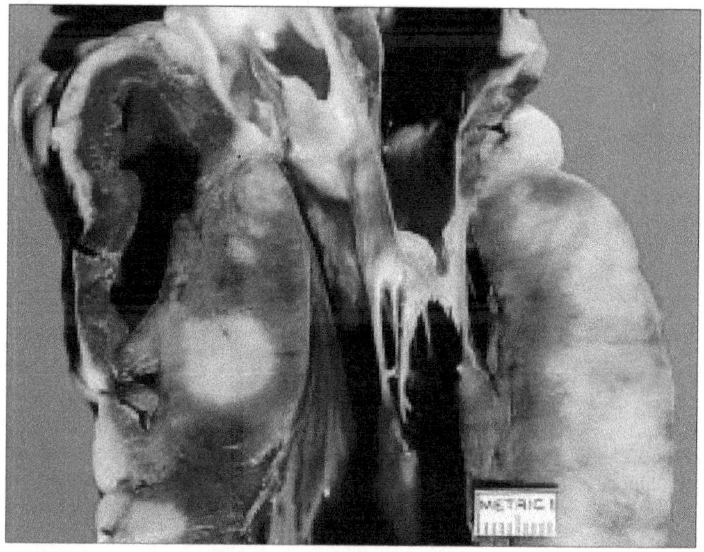

Figure 35. *Sarcoid heart disease.* Longitudinal view of the heart in a 27-year-old woman who died suddenly outside the hospital. Necropsy disclosed widespread sarcoid granulomas in many body organs, including the heart as shown here. The left ventricular sarcoid infiltrations were primarily subepicardial. Grossly, these sarcoid deposits were similar to neoplastic deposits. Reprinted with permission from Shirani J, Roberts WC. Subepicardial myocardial lesions. *Am Heart J* 1993;125:1346–1352.

Papillary fibroelastomas have been operatively excised from the cardiac valve and/or mural endocardium in patients with evidence of stroke or other peripheral events, and a few patients have had cardiac valve replacement (106, 108, 110, 111, 114, 115, 117–119, 124, 125, 132, 136, 138, 140). When papillary fibroelastomas are detected by echocardiography in asymptomatic patients, operative excision rarely appears warranted.

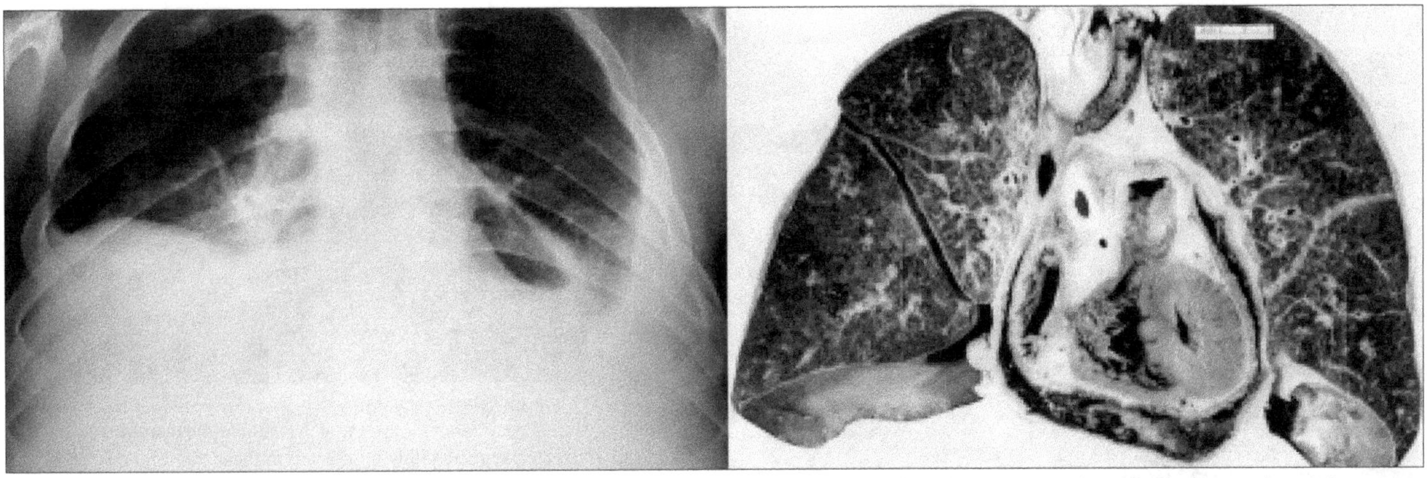

Figure 36. *Radiation heart disease for Hodgkin's disease.* This 26-year-old man was found to have Hodgkin's disease 27 months earlier by biopsy of a painless nodule in the neck. He received about 13,000 rads to the neck and mediastinum. He died from pericardial tamponade. Shown here is a radiograph with air in the pericardial sac. Both the parietal and visceral pericardia were thickened, and a large pericardial effusion was present. Reprinted from Roberts WC, Glancy DL, DeVita VT Jr. Heart in malignant lymphoma (Hodgkin's disease, lymphosarcoma, reticulum cell sarcoma and mycosis fungoides). A study of 196 autopsy cases. *Am J Cardiol* 1968;22:85–107 with permission from Excerpta Medica Inc.

Thrombi

Thrombi within an intracardiac cavity may be indistinguishable from neoplasm by echocardiogram or radiograph. Grossly, however, they are very different.

Thyroid gland

Aberrant thyroid tissue may be located with the pericardial sac (141) *(Figure 32)*.

Calcium

Calcium deposits may occur within any cardiac cavity, and some may be large (85, 142).

Abscess

Large abscesses, mainly of fungal origin, may replace portions of cardiac wall, protrude from the endocardial surfaces (mural endocarditis), and potentially obstruct inflow into or outflow from a cardiac chamber (143). *Figure 33* shows mucormycosis obstructing a pulmonary vein and occupying a portion of the left atrial cavity. These abscesses are especially common after unsuccessful bone marrow transplantation *(Figure 34)*.

Sarcoid

When located in myocardium, sarcoid granuloma may grossly resemble neoplasm (144–146) *(Figure 35)*.

CONSEQUENCES OF THERAPY FOR NEOPLASMS IN THE HEART

Radiation heart disease

Radiation heart disease was first recognized after radiation therapy for Hodgkin's disease (147–150). Some of the earlier patients with Hodgkin's disease received >8000 rads, which adversely affected the pericardium, myocardium, and endocardium. The most common manifestation of radiation heart disease is pericardial effusion *(Figure 36)*. Fibrin deposits occur on both the visceral and parietal aspects of the pericardia. Because coronary arteries are located in subepicardial adipose tissue, they often receive the effects of radiation. Many patients, particularly patients with Hodgkin's disease, have been reported to have coronary arterial narrowing at a very young age after radiation therapy. The intimal plaques resulting from radiation heart disease cannot be distinguished from plaques occurring from typical atherosclerosis. The distinguishing feature of radiation heart disease involving the coronary arteries is extensive fibrous thickening of the adventitia, as well as loss, focally or diffusely, of internal and external elastic membranes, particularly the latter *(Figure 37)*. Narrowing of coronary ostia also is common in radiation heart disease (150). In addition, radiation can cause considerable scarring within the subepicardial adipose tissue. The second most common manifestation of radiation heart disease is mural endocardial thickening, most commonly of the right atrium and ventricle, but focally also in the left ventricle. Its third most common manifestation is interstitial fibrosis; its location depends on the portal of entry, but it involves the anterior wall of the right ventricle more than any other portion of the heart *(Figure 37)*. Radiation in excess also can cause focal thickening of valves *(Figure 38)*.

Cardiac hemorrhages

Thrombocytopenia, particularly if persistent, often results in focal epicardial, myocardial, and mural endocardial hemorrhages. If the hemorrhages are located in conduction tissue, various degrees of heart block or arrhythmias may be the consequence.

Cardiac infection

The most common cardiac infections today in cancer patients are myocardial abscesses and mural endocardial and epicardial abscesses. These are particularly prevalent in patients with prolonged leukopenia (143, 151, 152). Patients having unsuccessful bone marrow transplants are particularly prone to these infections, which usually are produced by fungi, not bacteria. Gas gangrene may involve the heart as well as most other body organs and tissues (153).

Cardiac adiposity or the corticosteroid-treated heart

Patients with various types of cancers, particularly leukemia or lymphoma, and those developing cancer after organ transplan-

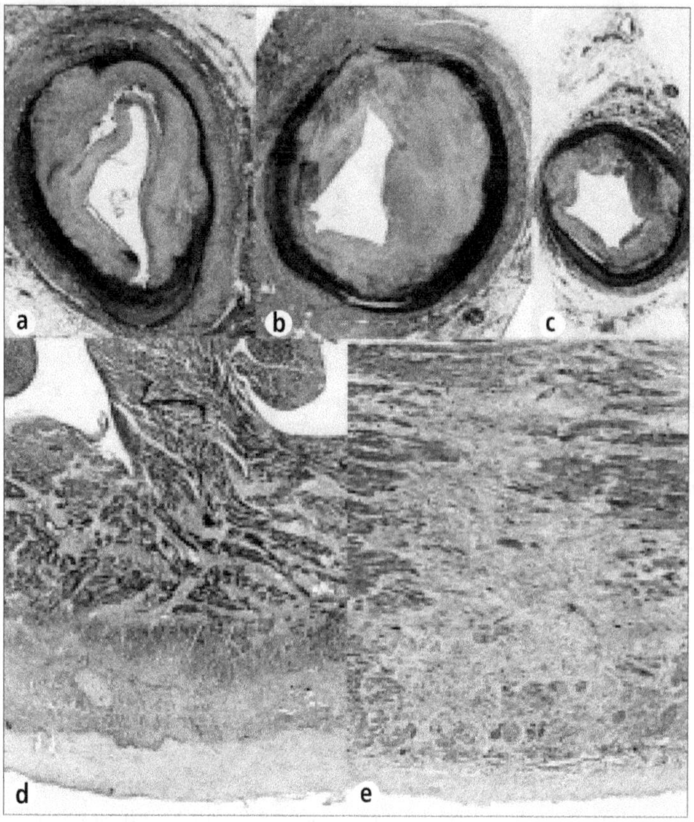

Figure 37. *Radiation heart disease.* On routine chest radiograph at age 24, this 33-year-old man was found to have bilateral hilar masses, and histologic examination of one of the hilar nodes disclosed Hodgkin's disease. He received approximately 8000 rads to his mediastinum, 5000 from an anterior portal. Thereafter, he was asymptomatic until 2½ hours before death when he developed severe substernal chest pain followed by hypotension and a malignant ventricular arrhythmia. Necropsy showed considerable luminal narrowing of the **(a)** right, **(b)** left anterior descending, and **(c)** left circumflex coronary arteries, mainly by fibrous tissue with focal medial atrophy and very impressive adventitial fibrosis. The epicardium over both the **(d)** right and **(e)** left ventricular walls was focally thickened by fibrous tissue, and the amount of interstitial and replacement fibrosis (subepicardial) was extensive in both ventricular walls. Movat stains (a, b, c), each ×16. Movat stain (d), ×34. Hematoxylin-eosin stain (e), ×54. Reprinted from McReynolds RA, Gold GL, Roberts WC. Coronary heart disease after mediastinal irradiation for Hodgkin's disease. *Am J Med* 1976;60:39–45 with permission from Excerpta Medica Inc.

tation usually receive corticosteroid therapy for prolonged periods. The consequence is excessive deposition of fat in the heart, mainly in the subepicardial areas (154). These hearts may become so fatty that they float in water (buffalo hump of the heart), and this excessive subepicardial adipose tissue may simulate pericardial effusion (97, 100).

Cardiac hemosiderosis

Normally the human body contains approximately 4 g of iron. If the iron level increases to about 25 g, iron deposits are usually found within myocardial cells. Patients who receive 100 units of blood without associated bleeding diatheses can acquire approximately 25 g of iron within the body organs and tissues. This situation may exist in some patients with cancer, particularly leukemia, and the result is cardiac hemosiderosis (155). These patients may be asymptomatic or may develop features of dilated cardiomyopathy with heart failure. At times, ventricular arrhythmias may be a consequence. Myocardial restriction as

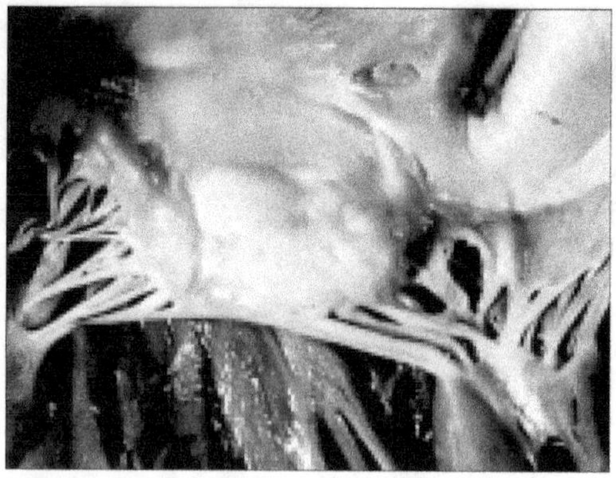

Figure 38. *Radiation heart disease.* Shown here is a focally thickened anterior mitral leaflet in a 30-year-old man who received approximately 11,000 rads to the mediastinum 5 years earlier for Hodgkin's disease. Although there was no valve dysfunction, the amount of focal leaflet scarring was abnormal for a 30-year-old man and suggested that this unusual leaflet scarring was a consequence of the earlier radiation. Reprinted from Brosius FC III, Waller BF, Roberts WC. Radiation heart disease. Analysis of 16 young (aged 15 to 33 years) necropsy patients who received over 3,500 rads to the heart. *Am J Med* 1981;70:519–530 with permission from Excerpta Medica Inc.

a result of myocardial iron deposits has occurred, but dilation is far more common (156).

Anthracycline chemotherapy (doxorubicin and daunorubicin)

Cardiac toxicity is a well-recognized complication of doxorubicin and daunorubicin and is frequently the dose-limiting factor in their administration (157–159). Clinical toxicity is usually manifested by evidence of impaired left ventricular systolic function. Morphologic signs of toxicity may be present when clinical signs of toxicity are absent.

1. Lam KY, Dickens P, Chan ACL. Tumors of the heart. A 20-year experience with a review of 12,485 consecutive autopsies. *Arch Pathol Lab Med* 1993;117:1027–1031.
2. Reynen K. Frequency of primary tumors of the heart. *Am J Cardiol* 1996; 77:107.
3. Burke A, Virmani R. *Atlas of Tumor Pathology. Tumors of the Heart and Great Vessels*. Washington, DC: Armed Forces Institute of Pathology, 1996:231.
4. Goodwin JF. The spectrum of cardiac tumors. *Am J Cardiol* 1968;21:307–314.
5. Harvey WP. Clinical aspects of cardiac tumors. *Am J Cardiol* 1968;21:328–343.
6. Salcedo EE, Cohen GI, White RD, Davison MB. Cardiac tumors: diagnosis and management. *Curr Probl Cardiol* 1992;17(2):73–137.
7. Roberts WC, Spray TL. Pericardial heart disease. *Curr Probl Cardiol* 1977; 2(3):1–71.
8. Roberts WC, Glancy DL, DeVita VT Jr. Heart in malignant lymphoma (Hodgkin's disease, lymphosarcoma, reticulum cell sarcoma and mycosis fungoides). A study of 196 autopsy cases. *Am J Cardiol* 1968;22:85–107.
9. Lindsay J Jr, Goldberg SD, Roberts WC. Electrocardiogram in neoplastic and hematologic disorders. In Rios JD, ed. *Clinical Electrocardiographic Correlations*. Philadelphia: FA Davis, 1977:225–242.
10. Steiner RE. Radiologic aspects of cardiac tumors. *Am J Cardiol* 1968;21:344–356.
11. Bass NM, Sharratt GP. Left atrial myxoma diagnosed by echocardiography, with observations on tumor movement. *Br Heart J* 1973;35:1332–1335.
12. Giuliani ER, Lemire F, Schattenberg TT. Unusual echocardiographic findings in a patient with left atrial myxoma. *Mayo Clin Proc* 1978;53:469–472.

13. Obeid AI, Marvasti M, Parker F, Rosenberg J. Comparison of transthoracic and transesophageal echocardiography in diagnosis of left atrial myxoma. *Am J Cardiol* 1989;63:1006–1008.
14. Pernod J, Piwnica A, Duret JC. Right atrial myxoma: an echocardiographic study. *Br Heart J* 1978;40:201–203.
15. Meller J, Teichholz LE, Pichard AD, Matta R, Litwak R, Herman MV, Massie KF. Left ventricular myxoma: echocardiographic diagnosis and review of the literature. *Am J Med* 1977;63:816–823.
16. Reeder GS, Khandheria BK, Seward JB, Tajik AJ. Transesophageal echocardiography and cardiac masses. *Mayo Clin Proc* 1991;66:1101–1109.
17. Mugge A, Daniel WG, Haverich A, Lichtlen PR. Diagnosis of noninfective cardiac mass lesions by two-dimensional echocardiography: comparison of the transthoracic and transesophageal approaches. *Circulation* 1991;83:70–78.
18. Moncada R, Baker M, Salinas M, Demos TC, Churchill R, Love L, Reynes C, Hale D, Cardoso M, Pifarre R, Gunnar RM. Diagnostic role of computed tomography in pericardial heart disease: congenital defects, thickening, neoplasms, and effusions. *Am Heart J* 1982;103:263–282.
19. Bateman TM, Sethna DH, Whiting JS, Chaux A, Berman DS, Forrester JS. Comprehensive noninvasive evaluation of left atrial myxomas using cardiac cine-computed tomography. *J Am Coll Cardiol* 1987;9:1180–1183.
20. Boxer RA, LaCorte MA, Singh S, Shapiro J, Schiller M, Goldman M, Stein HL. Diagnosis of cardiac tumors in infants by magnetic resonance imaging. *Am J Cardiol* 1985;56:831–832.
21. Bahnson HT, Spencer FC, Andrus EC. Diagnosis and treatment of intracavitary myxomas of the heart. *Ann Surg* 1957;145:915–926.
22. Ferrans VJ, Roberts WC. Structural features of cardiac myxomas. Histology, histochemistry, and electron microscopy. *Hum Pathol* 1973;4:111–146.
23. Peters MN, Hall RJ, Cooley DA, Leachman RD, Garcia E. The clinical syndrome of atrial myxoma. *JAMA* 1974;230:695–701.
24. Morgan DL, Palazola J, Reed W, Bell HH, Kindred LH, Beauchamp GD. Left heart myxomas. *Am J Cardiol* 1977;40:611–614.
25. St. John Sutton MG, Mercier L-A, Giuliani ER, Lie JT. Atrial myxomas: a review of clinical experience in 40 patients. *Mayo Clin Proc* 1980;55:371–376.
26. Markel ML, Waller BF, Armstrong WF. Cardiac myxoma: a review. *Medicine (Baltimore)* 1987;66:114–125.
27. Murphy MC, Sweeney MS, Putnam JB Jr, Walker WE, Frazier OH, Ott DA, Cooley DA. Surgical treatment of cardiac tumors: a 25-year experience. *Ann Thorac Surg* 1990;49:612–618.
28. Tazelaar HD, Locke TJ, McGregor CGA. Pathology of surgically excised primary cardiac tumors. *Mayo Clin Proc* 1992;67:957–965.
29. Burke AP, Virmani R. Cardiac myxomas. A clinicopathologic study. *Am J Clin Pathol* 1993;100:671–680.
30. Morrow AG, Kahler RL, Reis RL. Primary myxoma of the right ventricle. Clinical, hemodynamic and angiographic findings before and following operative treatment. *Am J Med* 1966;40:954–960.
31. Hickie JB, Gibson H, Windsor HM. "The wrecking ball": right atrial myxoma. *Med J Aust* 1970;2:82–86.
32. Hada Y, Wolfe C, Murray GF, Craige E. Right ventricular myxoma. Case report and review of phonocardiographic and auscultatory manifestations. *Am Heart J* 1980;100:871–877.
33. Schaff HV, Mullany CJ. Surgery for cardiac myxomas. *Semin Thorac Cardiovasc Surg* 2000;12:77–88.
34. Chopra P, Ray R, Airan B, Talwar KK, Venugopal P. Appraisal of histogenesis of cardiac myxoma: our experience of 78 cases and review of literature. *Indian Heart J* 1999;51:69–74.
35. Pucci A, Gagliardotto P, Zanini C, Pansini S, diSumma M, Mollo F. Histopathologic and clinical characterization of cardiac myxoma: review of 53 cases from a single institution. *Am Heart J* 2000;140:134–138.
36. Lindner V, Edah-Tally S, Chakfe N, Onody T, Eisenmann B, Walter P. Cardiac myxoma with glandular component: case report and review of the literature. *Pathol Res Pract* 1999;195:267–272.
37. Malekzadeh S, Roberts WC. Growth rate of left atrial myxoma. *Am J Cardiol* 1989;64:1075–1076.
38. Shinfeld A, Katsumata T, Westaby S. Recurrent cardiac myxoma: seeding or multifocal disease? *Ann Thorac Surg* 1998;66:285–288.
39. Bortolotti U, Scioti G, Guglielmi C, Milano A, Nardi C, Tartarini G. Recurrent myxoma of the left ventricle. Case report and review of the literature. *J Cardiovasc Surg (Torino)* 1999;40:233–235.
40. Das AK, Reddy KS, Suwanjindar P, Fulmer A, Siquiera C Jr, Floten HS, Starr A. Primary tumors of the aorta. *Ann Thorac Surg* 1996;62:1526–1528.
41. Chakfe N, Kretz JG, Valentin P, Geny B, Petit H, Popescu S, Edah-Tally S, Massard G. Clinical presentation and treatment options for mitral valve myxoma. *Ann Thorac Surg* 1997;64:872–877.
42. Murphy DP, Glazier DB, Krause TJ. Mitral valve myxoma. *Ann Thorac Surg* 1997;64:1169–1170.
43. Thongcharoen P, Laksanabunsong P, Thongtang V. Left ventricular outflow tract obstruction due to a left ventricular myxoma: a case report and review of the literature. *J Med Assoc Thai* 1997;80:799–806.
44. Singh SD, Lansing AM. Familial cardiac myxoma—a comprehensive review of reported cases. *J Ky Med Assoc* 1996;94:96–104.
45. Panos A, Kalangos A, Sztajzel J. Left atrial myxoma presenting with myocardial infarction. Case report and review of the literature. *Int J Cardiol* 1997;62:73–75.
46. Revankar SG, Clark RA. Infected cardiac myxoma. Case report and literature review. *Medicine (Baltimore)* 1998;77:337–344.
47. Chan HSL, Sonley MJ, Moes CAF, Daneman A, Smith CR, Martin DJ. Primary and secondary tumors of childhood involving the heart, pericardium, and great vessels: a report of 75 cases and review of the literature. *Cancer* 1985;56:825–836.
48. Fenoglio JJ Jr, McAllister HA Jr, Ferrans VJ. Cardiac rhabdomyoma: a clinicopathologic and electron microscopic study. *Am J Cardiol* 1976; 38:241–251.
49. Smythe JF, Dyck JD, Smallhorn JF, Freedom RM. Natural history of cardiac rhabdomyoma in infancy and childhood. *Am J Cardiol* 1990;66:1247–1249.
50. Burke AP, Virmani R. Cardiac rhabdomyoma: a clinicopathologic study. *Mod Pathol* 1991;4:70–74.
51. Biancaniello TM, Meyer RA, Gaum WE, Kaplan S. Primary benign intramural ventricular tumors in children: pre- and postoperative electrocardiographic, echocardiographic, and angiocardiographic evaluation. *Am Heart J* 1982;103:852–857.
52. Williams DB, Danielson GK, McGoon DC, Feldt RH, Edwards WD. Cardiac fibroma: long-term survival after excision. *J Thorac Cardiovasc Surg* 1982;84:230–236.
53. Estevez JM, Thompson DS, Levinson JP. Lipoma of the heart. Review of the literature and report of 2 autopsied cases. *Arch Pathol* 1964;77:638–642.
54. Moulton AL, Jaretzki A III, Bowman FO Jr, Silverstein EF, Bregman D. Massive lipoma of heart. *N Y State J Med* 1976;76:1820–1825.
55. Dollar AL, Wallace RB, Kent KM, Burkhart MW, Roberts WC. Mitral valve replacement for mitral lipoma associated with severe obesity. *Am J Cardiol* 1989;64:1405–1407.
56. Shirani J, Roberts WC. Epicardial lipoma. *Am Heart J* 1993;126:1030.
57. Bear PA, Moodie DS. Malignant primary cardiac tumors. The Cleveland Clinic experience, 1956 to 1986. *Chest* 1987;92:860–862.
58. Putnam JB Jr, Sweeney MS, Colon R, Lanza LA, Frazier OH, Cooley DA. Primary cardiac sarcomas. *Ann Thorac Surg* 1991;51:906–910.
59. Burke AP, Cowan D, Virmani R. Primary sarcomas of the heart. *Cancer* 1992;69:387–395.
60. Glancy DL, Morales JB Jr, Roberts WC. Angiosarcoma of the heart. *Am J Cardiol* 1968;21:413–419.
61. Herrmann MA, Shankerman RA, Edwards WD, Shub C, Schaff HV. Primary cardiac angiosarcoma: a clinicopathologic study of six cases. *J Thorac Cardiovasc Surg* 1992;103:655–664.
62. Butany J, Yu W. Cardiac angiosarcoma: two cases and a review of the literature. *Can J Cardiol* 2000;16:197–205.
63. Shrivastava S, Jacks JJ, White RS, Edwards JE. Diffuse rhabdomyomatosis of the heart. *Arch Pathol Lab Med* 1977;101:78–80.
64. Hajar R, Roberts WC, Folger GM Jr. Embryonal botryoid rhabdomyosarcoma of the mitral valve. *Am J Cardiol* 1986;57:376.
65. Hui KS, Green LK, Schmidt WA. Primary cardiac rhabdomyosarcoma: definition of a rare entity. *Am J Cardiovasc Pathol* 1988;2:19–29.
66. Pessotto R, Silvestre G, Luciani GB, Anselmi M, Pasini F, Santini F, Mazzucco A. Primary cardiac leiomyosarcoma: seven-year survival with combined surgical and adjuvant therapy. *Int J Cardiol* 1997;60:91–94.
67. Babatasi G, Massetti M, Galateau F, Khayat A. Leiomyosarcoma of the pulmonary veins extending into the left atrium or left atrial leiomyosar-

coma: multimodality therapy. *J Thorac Cardiovasc Surg* 1998;116:665–667.
68. Minardi G, Pulignano G, Sentinelli S, Narducci C, Giovannini M. Left atrial leiomyosarcoma: double occurrence and double recurrence—report of one case. *J Am Soc Echocardiogr* 1998;11:1171–1176.
69. Pins MR, Ferrell MA, Madsen JC, Piubello Q, Dickersin GR, Fletcher CD. Epithelioid and spindle-celled leiomyosarcoma of the heart. Report of 2 cases and review of the literature. *Arch Pathol Lab Med* 1999;123:782–788.
70. Domanski MJ, Delaney TF, Kleiner DE Jr, Goswitz M, Agatston A, Tucker E, Johnson M, Roberts WC. Primary sarcoma of the heart causing mitral stenosis. *Am J Cardiol* 1990;66:893–895.
71. Isner JM, Falcone MW, Virmani R, Roberts WC. Cardiac sarcoma causing "ASH" and simulating coronary heart disease. *Am J Med* 1979;66:1025–1030.
72. Abraham KP, Reddy V, Gattusa P. Neoplasms metastatic to the heart: review of 3314 consecutive autopsies. *Am J Cardiovasc Pathol* 1990;3:195–198.
73. Adenle AD, Edwards JE. Clinical and pathologic features of metastatic neoplasms of the pericardium. *Chest* 1982;81:166–169.
74. MacLowry JD, Roberts WC. Metastatic choriocarcinoma of the lung. Invasion of pulmonary veins with extension into the left atrium and mitral orifice. *Am J Cardiol* 1966;18:938–941.
75. Labib SB, Schick EC Jr, Isner JM. Obstruction of right ventricular outflow tract caused by intracavitary metastatic disease: analysis of 14 cases. *J Am Coll Cardiol* 1992;19:1664–1668.
76. Domanski MJ, Cunnion RE, Fernicola DJ, Roberts WC. Fatal cor pulmonale caused by extensive tumor emboli in the small pulmonary arteries without emboli in the major pulmonary arteries or metastases in the pulmonary parenchyma. *Am J Cardiol* 1993;72:233–234.
77. Onuigbo WI. Direct extension of cancer between pulmonary veins and the left atrium. *Chest* 1972;62:444–446.
78. Weg IL, Mehra S, Azueta V, Rosner F. Cardiac metastasis from adenocarcinoma of the lung. Echocardiographic-pathologic correlation. *Am J Med* 1986;80:108–112.
79. Kadir S, Coulam CM. Intracaval extension of renal cell carcinoma. *Cardiovasc Intervent Radiol* 1980;3:180–183.
80. Waller BF, Fletcher RD, Roberts WC. Carcinoma of the lung causing pulmonary arterial stenosis. *Chest* 1981;79:589–591.
81. Glancy DL, Roberts WC. The heart in malignant melanoma: a study of 70 autopsy cases. *Am J Cardiol* 1968;21:555–571.
82. Waller BF, Gottdiener JS, Virmani R, Roberts WC. The "charcoal heart": melanoma to the cor. *Chest* 1980;77:671–676.
83. Chen RH, Gaos CM, Frazier OH. Complete resection of a right atrial intracavitary metastatic melanoma. *Ann Thorac Surg* 1996;61:1255–1257.
84. Roberts WC, Bodey GP, Wertlake PT. The heart in acute leukemia: a study of 420 autopsy cases. *Am J Cardiol* 1968;21:388–412.
85. Waller BF, Roberts WC. Systolic clicks caused by rocks in the right heart chambers. *Am Heart J* 1981;102(3 Pt 1):459–460.
86. McDonnell PJ, Mann RB, Bulkley BH. Involvement of the heart by malignant lymphoma: a clinicopathologic study. *Cancer* 1982;49:944–951.
87. Roberts CS, Gottdiener JS, Roberts WC. Clinically undetected cardiac lymphoma causing congestive heart failure. *Am Heart J* 1990;120:1239–1242.
88. Moore JA, DeRan BP, Minor R, Arthur J, Fraker TD Jr. Transesophageal echocardiographic evaluation of intracardiac lymphoma. *Am Heart J* 1992; 124:514–516.
89. Seibert KA, Rettenmier CW, Waller BF, Battle WE, Levine AS, Roberts WC. Osteogenic sarcoma metastatic to the heart. *Am J Med* 1982;73:136–141.
90. Burke AP, Virmani R. Osteosarcomas of the heart. *Am J Surg Pathol* 1991;15:289–295.
91. Zanella M, Falconieri G, Bussani R, Sinagra G, Della Libera D. Polypoid osteosarcoma of the left atrium: report of a new case with autopsy confirmation and review of the literature. *Ann Diag Pathol* 1998;2:167–172.
92. Feigin DS, Fenoglio JJ, McAllister HA, Madewell JR. Pericardial cysts: a radiologic-pathologic correlation and review. *Radiology* 1977;125:15–20.
93. Reynolds JL, Donahue JK, Pearce CW. Intrapericardial teratoma: a cause of acute pericardial effusion in infancy. *Pediatrics* 1969;43:71–78.
94. DeGeeter B, Kretz JG, Nisand I, Eisenmann B, Kieny MT, Kieny R. Intrapericardial teratoma in a newborn infant: use of fetal echocardiography. *Ann Thorac Surg* 1983;35:664–666.
95. Brabham KR, Roberts WC. Cardiac-compressing intrapericardial teratoma at birth. *Am J Cardiol* 1989;63:386–387.
96. Shirani J, Roberts WC. Clinical, electrocardiographic and morphologic features of massive fatty deposits ("lipomatous hypertrophy") in the atrial septum. *J Am Coll Cardiol* 1993;22:226–238.
97. Roberts WC, Roberts JD. The floating heart or the heart too fat to sink: analysis of 55 necropsy patients. *Am J Cardiol* 1983;52:1286–1289.
98. Applegate PM, Taijk AJ, Ehman RL, Julsrud PR, Miller FA Jr. Two-dimensional echocardiographic and magnetic resonance imaging observations in massive lipomatous hypertrophy of the atrial septum. *Am J Cardiol* 1987;59:489–491.
99. Kindman LA, Wright A, Tye T, Seale W, Appleton C. Lipomatous hypertrophy of the interatrial septum: characterization by transesophageal and transthoracic echocardiography, magnetic resonance imaging, and computed tomography. *J Am Soc Echocardiogr* 1988;1:450–454.
100. Isner JM, Carter BL, Roberts WC, Bankoff MS. Subepicardial adipose tissue producing echocardiographic appearance of pericardial effusion. Documentation by computed tomography and necropsy. *Am J Cardiol* 1983;51: 565–569.
101. Fishbein MC, Ferrans VJ, Roberts WC. Endocardial papillary elastofibromas. Histologic, histochemical, and electron microscopical findings. *Arch Pathol* 1975;99:335–341.
102. Roberts WC. Valvular, subvalvular and supravalvular aortic stenosis: morphologic features. *Cardiovasc Clin* 1973;5:97–126.
103. Heath D, Thompson IM. Papillary "tumors" of the left ventricle. *Br Heart J* 1967;29:950–954.
104. Burn CG, Bishop MB, Davies JNP. A stalked papillary tumor of the mural endocardium. *Am J Clin Pathol* 1969;51:344–346.
105. Flotte T, Pinar H, Feiner H. Papillary elastofibroma of the left ventricular septum. *Am J Surg Pathol* 1980;4:585–588.
106. Almagro UA, Perry LS, Choi H, Pintar K. Papillary fibroelastoma of the heart. Report of six cases. *Arch Pathol Lab Med* 1982;106:318–321.
107. Ong LS, Nanda NC, Barold SS. Two-dimensional echocardiographic detection and diagnostic features of left ventricular papillary fibroelastoma. *Am Heart J* 1982;103:917–918.
108. Topol EJ, Biern RO, Reitz BA. Cardiac papillary fibroelastoma and stroke. Echocardiographic diagnosis and guide to excision. *Am J Med* 1986;80:129–132.
109. Kalman JM, Lubicz S, Brennan JB, Vernon-Roberts E, Calafiore P. Multiple cardiac papillary fibroelastomas and rheumatic heart disease. *Aust N Z J Med* 1991;21:744–746.
110. Bedi HS, Sharma VK, Mishra M, Kasliwal RR, Trehan N. Papillary fibroelastoma of the mitral valve associated with rheumatic mitral stenosis. *Eur J Cardiothorac Surg* 1995;9:54–55.
111. Allen KB, Goldin M, Mitra R. Transaortic video-assisted excision of a left ventricular papillary fibroelastoma. *J Thorac Cardiovasc Surg* 1996;112:199–201.
112. Campbell M, Carling W. Sudden death due to a fibrinous polyp of the aortic valve. *Guy's Hosp Rep* 1934;84:41–42.
113. Gopal A, Li Mandri G, King DL, Marboe C, Homma S. Aortic valve papillary fibroelastoma. A diagnosis by transthoracic echocardiography. *Chest* 1994;105:1885–1887.
114. Ragni T, Grande AM, Cappuccio G, Arbustini E, Grasso M, Tramarin R, Vigano M. Embolizing fibroelastoma of the aortic valve. *Cardiovasc Surg* 1994;2:639–641.
115. Shahian DM, Labib SB, Chang G. Cardiac papillary fibroelastoma. *Ann Thorac Surg* 1995;59:538–541.
116. Fowles RE, Miller DC, Egbert BM, Fitzgerald JW, Popp RL. Systemic embolization from a mitral valve papillary endocardial fibroma detected by two-dimensional echocardiography. *Am Heart J* 1981;102:128–130.
117. Gorton ME, Soltanzadeh H. Mitral valve fibroelastoma. *Ann Thorac Surg* 1989;47:605–607.
118. Gallo R, Kumar N, Prabhakar G, Awada A, Maalouf Y, Duran CM. Papillary fibroelastoma of mitral valve chorda. *Ann Thorac Surg* 1993;55:1576–1577.
119. Shapira OM, Williamson WA, Dugan JM. Papillary fibroelastoma of the mitral valve. *Cardiovasc Surg* 1993;1:599–601.
120. Mann J, Parker DJ. Papillary fibroelastoma of the mitral valve: a rare cause of transient neurological deficits. *Br Heart J* 1994;71:6.

121. Pinelli G, Carteaux JP, Mertes PM, Civit T, Trinh A, Villemot JP. Mitral valve tumor revealed by stroke. *J Heart Valve Dis* 1995;4:199–201.
122. Zamora RL, Adelberg DA, Berger AS, Huettner P, Kaplan HJ. Branch retinal artery occlusion caused by a mitral valve papillary fibroelastoma. *Am J Ophthalmol* 1995;119:325–329.
123. Colucci V, Alberti A, Bonacina E, Gordini V. Papillary fibroelastoma of the mitral valve. A rare cause of embolic events. *Tex Heart Inst J* 1995;22:327–331.
124. McFadden PM, Lacy JR. Intracardiac papillary fibroelastoma: an occult cause of embolic neurologic deficit. *Ann Thorac Surg* 1987;43:667–669.
125. Brown RD Jr, Khandheria BK, Edwards WD. Cardiac papillary fibroelastoma: a treatable cause of transient ischemic attack and ischemic stroke detected by transesophageal echocardiography. *Mayo Clin Proc* 1995;70:863–868.
126. Nighoghossian N, Trouillas P, Perinetti M, Barthelet M, Ninet J, Loire R. [Lambl's excrescence: an uncommon cause of cerebral embolism.] *Rev Neurol (Paris)* 1995;151:583–585.
127. Kasarskis EJ, O'Connor W, Earle G. Embolic stroke from cardiac papillary fibroelastomas. *Stroke* 1988;19:1171–1173.
128. Zull DN, Diamond M, Beringer D. Angina and sudden death resulting from papillary fibroelastoma of the aortic valve. *Ann Emerg Med* 1985;14:470–473.
129. Marvasti MA, Obeid AI, Cohen PS, Giambartolomei A, Parker FB. Successful removal of papillary endocardial fibroma. *Thorac Cardiovasc Surg* 1983;31:254–255.
130. Richard J, Castello R, Dressler FA, Willman VL, Nashed A, Lewis B, Labovitz AJ. Diagnosis of papillary fibroelastoma of the mitral valve complicated by non-Q-wave infarction with apical thrombus: transesophageal and transthoracic echocardiographic study. *Am Heart J* 1993;126(3 Pt 1):710–712.
131. Etienne Y, Jobic Y, Houel JF, Barra JA, Boschat J, Meunier M, Penther P. Papillary fibroelastoma of the aortic valve with myocardial infarction: echocardiographic diagnosis and surgical excision. *Am Heart J* 1994; 127:443–445.
132. Eckstein FS, Schafers HJ, Grote J, Mugge A, Borst HG. Papillary fibroelastoma of the aortic valve presenting with myocardial infarction. *Ann Thorac Surg* 1995;60:206–208.
133. Grote J, Mugge A, Schafers HJ, Daniel WG, Lichtlen PR. Multiplane transesophageal echocardiography detection of a papillary fibroelastoma of the aortic valve causing myocardial infarction. *Eur Heart J* 1995;16:426–429.
134. Harris LS, Adelson L. Fatal coronary embolism from a myxomatous polyp of the aortic valve: an unusual cause of sudden death. *Am J Clin Pathol* 1965;43:61–64.
135. Boone S, Higginson LA, Walley VM. Endothelial papillary fibroelastomas arising in and around the aortic sinus, filling the ostium of the right coronary artery. *Arch Pathol Lab Med* 1992;116:135–137.
136. Mazzucco A, Bortolotti U, Thiene G, Dan M, Stritoni P, Scutari M, Stellin G. Left ventricular papillary fibroelastoma with coronary embolization. *Eur J Cardiothorac Surg* 1989;3:471–473.
137. Anderson KR, Fiddler GI, Lie JR. Congenital papillary tumor of the tricuspid valve: an unusual cause of right ventricular outflow obstruction in a neonate with trisomy E. *Mayo Clin Proc* 1977;52:665–669.
138. Wolfe JT III, Finck SJ, Safford RE, Persellin ST. Tricuspid valve papillary fibroelastoma: echocardiographic characterization. *Ann Thorac Surg* 1991; 51:116–118.
139. Neerukonda SK, Jantz RD, Vijay NK, Narrod JA, Schoonmaker FW. Pulmonary embolization of papillary fibroelastoma arising from the tricuspid
140. Ganjoo AK, Johnson WD, Gordon RT, Jain DP, Lang GE, Shankar VS. Tricuspid papillary fibroelastoma causing syncopal episodes. *J Thorac Cardiovasc Surg* 1996;112:551–553.
141. Taylor MA, Bray M, Roberts WC. Aberrant thyroid gland attached to ascending aorta. *Am J Cardiol* 1986;57:708.
142. Dean DC, Pamukcoglu T, Roberts WC. Rocks in the right ventricle. A complication of congenital right ventricular infundibular obstruction associated with chronic pulmonary parenchymal disease. *Am J Cardiol* 1969; 23:744–747.
143. Buchbinder NA, Roberts WC. Active infective endocarditis confined to mural endocardium. A study of six necropsy patients. *Arch Pathol* 1972; 93:435–440.
144. Roberts WC, McAllister HA Jr, Ferrans VJ. Sarcoidosis of the heart: a clinicopathologic study of 35 necropsy patients (group I) and review of 78 previously described necropsy patients (group II). *Am J Med* 1977;63:86–108.
145. Virmani R, Bures JC, Roberts WC. Cardiac sarcoidosis: a major cause of sudden death in young individuals. *Chest* 1980;77:423–428.
146. Shirani J, Roberts WC. Subepicardial myocardial lesions. *Am Heart J* 1993;125(5 Pt 1):1346–1352.
147. Morton DL, Kagan AR, Roberts WC, O'Brien KP, Holmes EC, Adkins PC. Pericardiectomy for radiation-induced pericarditis with effusion. *Ann Thorac Surg* 1969;8:195–208.
148. McReynolds RA, Gold GL, Roberts WC. Coronary heart disease after mediastinal irradiation for Hodgkin's disease. *Am J Med* 1976;60:39–45.
149. Brosius FC III, Waller BF, Roberts WC. Radiation heart disease: analysis of 16 young (aged 15 to 33 years) necropsy patients who received over 3,500 rads to the heart. *Am J Med* 1981;70:519–530.
150. Harvey LAC, DeMaio SJ, Roberts WC. Radiation-induced cardiovascular disease including stenosis of coronary ostium, coronary and carotid arteries, and aortic valve. *BUMC Proceedings* 1994;7(3):33–36.
151. Ihde DC, Roberts WC, Marr KC, Brereton HD, McGuire WP, Levine AS, Young RC. Cardiac candidiasis in cancer patients. *Cancer* 1978;41:2364–2371.
152. Ross EM, Macher AM, Roberts WC. *Aspergillus fumigatus* thrombi causing total occlusion of both coronary arterial ostia, all four major epicardial coronary arteries and coronary sinus and associated with purulent pericarditis. *Am J Cardiol* 1985;56:499–500.
153. Roberts WC, Berard CW. Gas gangrene of the heart in clostridial septicemia. *Am Heart J* 1967;74:482–488.
154. Bulkley BH, Roberts WC. The heart in systemic lupus erythematosus and the changes induced in it by corticosteroid therapy. A study of 36 necropsy patients. *Am J Med* 1975;58:243–264.
155. Buja LM, Roberts WC. Iron in the heart. Etiology and clinical significance. *Am J Med* 1971;51:209–221.
156. Cutler DJ, Isner JM, Bracey AW, Hufnagel CA, Conrad PW, Roberts WC, Kerwin DM, Weintraub AM. Hemochromatosis heart disease: an unemphasized cause of potentially reversible restrictive cardiomyopathy. *Am J Med* 1980;69:923–928.
157. Buja LM, Ferrans VJ, Mayer RJ, Roberts WC, Henderson ES. Cardiac ultrastructural changes induced by daunorubicin therapy. *Cancer* 1973;32:771–788.
158. Buja LM, Ferrans VJ, Roberts WC. Drug-induced cardiomyopathies. *Adv Cardiol* 1974;13:330–348.
159. Isner JM, Ferrans VJ, Cohen SR, Witkind BG, Virmani R, Gottdiener JS, Beck JR, Roberts WC. Clinical and morphologic cardiac findings after anthracycline chemotherapy. Analysis of 64 patients studied at necropsy. *Am J Cardiol* 1983;51:1167–1174.

Sex Distribution in Cardiac Myxomas

Dong Hi Anthony Yoon, MD, and William Clifford Roberts, MD

During the last 15 years at Baylor University Medical Center, 15 patients have had operative excision of a cardiac myxoma. All tumors were located in the left atrium and 14 patients (93%) were female. This report summarizes some findings in these 15 patients and reviews some previously published reports concerning sex distribution of operatively excised cardiac myxomas.

• • •

Pertinent findings in the 15 patients are listed in Table 1. The histologic slides of the atrial tumors were reexamined by 1 of us (WCR) to confirm that each was a myxoma.

Of the 1,195 patients who had atrial myxomas operatively excised and reported by others,[1–25] 796 patients (67%) were female and 399 patients (33%) were male (Table 2). Their ages ranged from 2.5 to 97 years. Three additional studies[26–28] included intracardiac myxomas either operatively excised or found at autopsy (Table 3); of the 80 patients included in these 3 studies, 57 patients (71%) were female and 23 patients (29%) were male. The only report[29] we found describing more males than females with atrial myxomas was from the Armed Forces Institute of Pathology, and their cases are derived almost entirely from armed forces hospitals, which, of course, provide care mainly for males. Their 107 cases of cardiac myxomas included operatively excised myxomas and those found at necropsy: 50 cases (47%) were female and 57 cases (53%) were male.

• • •

Thus, cardiac myxomas, like rheumatic mitral stenosis, occur predominately in females.

From the Departments of Internal Medicine and Pathology and the Heart & Vascular Institute, Baylor University Medical Center, Dallas, Texas. Dr. Roberts' address is: Baylor Heart & Vascular Institute, Baylor University Medical Center, 621 N Hall St., Dallas, Texas 75246.
Manuscript received March 25, 2002; revised manuscript received and accepted May 1, 2002.

1. Ennker J, Daniel W, Doehring W, Oelert H. Surgical experience with left atrial myxomas. *Herz* 1983;8:227–233.
2. Shimizu T, Iyomasa Y, Nakashima N. Fourteen cases of left atrial myxoma with emphasis on related histology. *Jpn J Surg* 1983;13:1–5.
3. Semb BKH. Surgical considerations in the treatment of cardiac myxoma. *J Thorac Cardiovasc Surg* 1984;87:251–259.
4. Hanson EC, Gill CC, Razavi M, Loop FD. The surgical treatment of atrial myxomas. Clinical experience and late results in 33 patients. *J Thorac Cardiovasc Surg* 1985;89:298–303.
5. Guiloff AK, Flege JB, Callard GM, Dunn EJ, Wilson JM, Wright CB. Surgery of left atrial myxomas. Report of eleven cases and review of the literature. *J Cardiovasc Surg* 1986;27:194–200.
6. Dein JR, Frist WH, Stinson EB, Miller DC, Baldwin JC, Oyer PE, Jamieson S, Mitchell RS, Shumway NE. Primary cardiac neoplasm. Early and late results of surgical treatment in 42 patients. *J Thorac Cardiovasc Surg* 1987;93:502–511.
7. Burakovsky VI, Zuckerman GI, Kossatch GA, Golossovskaya MA, Javorskaya LA. Surgical treatment of cardiac myxomas. *J Thorac Cardiovasc Surg* 1988; 96:800–805.
8. Larsson S, Lepore V, Kennergren C. Atrial myxomas: results of 25 years' experience and review of the literature. *Surgery* 1989;105:695–698.
9. Nomeir A-M, Watts LE, Seagle R, Joyner CR, Corman C, Prichard RW. Intracardiac myxomas: twenty-year echocardiographic experience with review of the literature. *J Am Soc Echocardiogr* 1989;2:139–150.
10. Murphy MC, Sweeney MS, Putnam JB Jr, Walker WE, Frazier OH, Ott DA, Cooley DA. Surgical treatment of cardiac tumors: a 25-year experience. *Ann Thorac Surg* 1990;49:612–618.
11. Bortolotti U, Maraglino G, Rubino M, Santini F, Mazzuco A, Milano A, Fasoli G, Livi U, Thiene G, Gallucci V. Surgical excision of intracardiac myxomas: a 20-year follow-up. *Ann Thorac Surg* 1990;49:449–453.
12. Sellke FW, Lemmer JH Jr, Vandenberg BF, Ehrenhaft JL. Surgical treatment of cardiac myxomas: long-term results. *Ann Thorac Surg* 1990;50:557–561.
13. Blondeau P. Primary cardiac tumors—French studies of 533 cases. *Thorac Cardiovasc Surg* 1990;38:192–195.
14. Moggio RA, Pucillo AL, Schechter AG, Pooley RW, Sarabu MR, Reed GE. Primary cardiac tumors. Diagnosis and management in 14 cases. *N Y State J Med* 1992;92:49–52.
15. Tazelaar HD, Locke TJ, McGregor CGA. Pathology of surgically excised primary cardiac tumors. *Mayo Clin Proc* 1992;67:957–965.
16. Lijoi A, Scoti P, Faveto C, Canale C, Parodi E, Passerone GC, Dottori V, Venere G. Surgical management of intracardiac myxomas. A 16-year experience. *Tex Heart Inst J* 1993;20:231–234.
17. Actis Dato GM, De Benedictis M, Actis Data A Jr, Ricci A, Sommariva L, De Paulis R. Long term follow-up of cardiac myxomas (7-31 years). *J Cardiovasc Surg* 1993;34:141–143.
18. Meyns B, Vancleemput J, Flameng W, Daenen W. Surgery for cardiac myxoma. *Eur J Cardiothorac Surg* 1993;7:437–440.
19. MacGowan SW, Sidhu P, Aherne T, Luke D, Wood AE, Neligan MC, McGovern E. Atrial myxoma: national incidence, diagnosis and surgical management. *Irish J Med Sci* 1993;162:223–226.
20. Kabbani SS, Jokhadar M, Meada R, Jamil H, Abdun F, Sandouk A, Nabhani F. Atrial myxoma: report of 24 operations using the biatrial approach. *Ann Thorac Surg* 1994;58:483–488.
21. Shimono T, Makino S, Kanamori Y, Kinoshita T, Yada I. Left atrial myxomas. Using gross anatomic tumor types to determine clinical features and coronary angiographic findings. *Chest* 1995;107:674–679.
22. Jones DR, Warden HE, Murray GF, Hill RC, Graeber GM, Cruzzavala JL,

TABLE 1 Findings in 15 Patients With Myxomas Excised from Left Atrium at Baylor University Medical Center from 1985 to 2001

Systemic Embolus (H, B, S, K)	Age (yrs)/ Sex	Attached to FO	Largest Diameter (cm)	Wt (g)	CA	No. of Coronary Arteries Narrowed >50%	Pressures (mm Hg) PA (SD)	PAW (Mean)	LV (SD)	SA (SD)	PAW-LV (MDG)	EF (%)	Systemic Embolus (H, B, S, K)	Hct (%)	ESR (mm/hr)	Tumor Plop Sound	Symptoms D	CP
1	25F	+	5.0	—	O	–	24/10	13	117/10	115/74	3	66	0	38	—	O	+	+
2	43F	+	3.5	—	+	0	31/14	—	—	149/80	—	55	0	30	—	O	O	O
3	43F	0	5.0	—	+	1	—	—	91/15	91/52	—	50	+ (H,B)	41	81	O	O	O
4	47F	+	2.2	—	+	0	—	—	—	120/60*	—	50	0	21	—	O	+	O
5	49F	+	5.5	—	+	0	65/30	25	—	96/67	—	70	0	26	84	+	+	O
6	50F	+	6.3	—	O	–	—	—	—	110/60*	—	—	0	38	—	O	+	+
7	53F	+	7.6	—	+	0	—	—	—	140/90*	—	55	0	38	41	O	+	+
8	61F	+	5.5	—	+	0	25/9	7	147/6	149/59	1	75	+ (B)	40	50	O	O	O
9	66F	+	4.0	—	+	0	21/8	—	—	131/86*	—	—	0	46	—	O	O	O
10	70F	+	3.5	44	O	–	—	—	—	160/80*	—	—	0	33	—	O	+	O
11	70F	+	2.5	34	+	0	40/24	24	94/9	97/53	15	60	0	37	—	O	+	+
12	72M	+	5.5	—	+	3	35/6	6	—	126/49	—	35	+ (B)	42	—	O	+	O
13	72F	0	8.0	—	+	0	44/18	18	—	110/57	—	68	0	34	—	+	+	+
14	77F	+	6.5	31	+	0	68/32	30	—	138/78*	22	46	+ (B)	31	61	O	+	+
15	83F	+	6.0	36	O	–	—	—	—	140/10*		—	+ (B)	36	—	O	O	O

*Indirect measurement.

B = brain; CA = coronary angiogram; CP = chest pain; D = dyspnea; EF = ejection fraction; ESR = erythrocyte sedimentation rate; FO = fossa ovale; H = heart; Hct = hematocrit; K = kidney; V = left ventricle; mdg = mean diastolic gradient; PA = pulmonary artery; PAW = pulmonary artery wedge pressure; Pt = patient; S = spleen; SA = systemic artery; Wt = weight; + = positive or present; O = negative or absent.

TABLE 2 Ages and Gender of Previously Reported Operatively Excised Atrial Myxomas

First Author/ Reference Number (years)	Years Patients Studied	No. of Patients	Females	Males	Age Range (years) (mean)	Myxoma		Location of Solitary Myxoma			
						Solitary	Multiple	LA	RA	LV	RV
Ennker[1] (1983)	1974–1982	16	12 (75%)	4 (25%)	26–72 (50)	16	0	16	0	0	0
Shimizu[2] (1983)	1968–1981	14	8 (57%)	6 (43%)	16–71 (44)	14	0	14	0	0	0
Semb[3] (1984)	1968–	18	14 (78%)	4 (22%)	(52)	17	1	15	2	0	0
Hanson[4] (1985)	1957–1981	33	28 (85%)	5 (15%)	17–70 (48)	33	0	31	0	2	0
Guiloff[5] (1986)	1971–1982	11	8 (73%)	3 (27%)	16–69 (53)	10	1	10	0	0	0
Dein[6] (1987)	1961–1986	27	19 (70%)	8 (30%)	13–79 (50)	27	0	25	2	0	0
Burakovsky[7] (1988)	—	40	26 (65%)	14 (35%)	—	39	1	31	5	1	2
Larsson[8] (1989)	1961–1985	20	11 (55%)	9 (45%)	26–72 (52)	20	0	16	3	0	1
Nomeir[9] (1989)	1968–1988	35	23 (66%)	12 (34%)	19–75 (45)	—	—	—	—	—	—
Murphy[10] (1990)	1964–1989	63	39 (62%)	24 (38%)	21–81 (51)	63	0	57	6	0	0
Bortolotti[11] (1990)	1968–1988	54	35 (65%)	19 (35%)	7–68 (48)	54	0	46	6	0	2
Sellke[12] (1990)	1965–1988	22	16 (73%)	6 (27%)	16–76 (50)	21	1	17	3	0	1
Blondeau[13] (1990)	1961–1988	440	286 (65%)	154 (35%)	2.5–82	434	6	364	47	2	11
Moggio[14] (1992)	1979–1989	11	10 (91%)	1 (9%)	—	11	0	11	0	0	0
Tazelaar[15] (1992)	1957–1991	76	51 (67%)	25 (33%)	13–80 (53)	—	—	—	—	—	—
Lijoi[16] (1993)	1977–1992	26	14 (54%)	12 (46%)	33–81 (63)	26	0	22	2	1	1
Dato[17] (1993)	1961–1985	14	5 (36%)	9 (64%)	29–52 (42)	14	0	14	0	0	0
Meyns[18] (1993)	1971–1991	32	23 (72%)	9 (28%)	36–78 (57)	32	0	31	0	0	1
MacGowan[19] (1993)	1977–1991	26	18 (69%)	8 (31%)	14–75 (51)	24	2	24	0	0	0
Kabbani[20] (1994)	1978–1993	23	15 (65%)	8 (35%)	4–71 (36)	22	1	21	1	0	0
Shimono[21] (1995)	1981–1992	26	15 (58%)	11 (42%)	—	26	0	26	0	0	0
Jones[22] (1995)	1964–1994	20	13 (65%)	7 (35%)	18–76 (55)	20	0	17	3	0	0
Premaratne[23] (1995)	1974–1993	35	28 (80%)	7 (20%)	11–79 (48)	34	1	32	2	0	0
Lukács[24] (1997)	1974–1994	50	33 (66%)	17 (34%)	16–81 (55)	46	4	42	3	0	1
Bjessmo[25] (1997)	1954–1996	63	46 (73%)	17 (27%)	15–76 (51)	62	1	56	6	0	0
Totals		1,195	796 (67%)	399 (33%)		1,065	19	938	91	6	20

LA = left atrium; LV = left ventricle; RA = right atrium; RV = right ventricle.

TABLE 3 Ages and Gender of Previously Reported Atrial Myxomas Operatively Excised or Found at Autopsy

First Author	Year	Years Patients Studied	Total Patients	Females	Males	Age Range (years) Mean	Myxoma		Location of Solitary Myxoma			
							Solitary	Multiple	LA	RA	LV	RV
Bulkley[26]	1979	1928–1978	24	17 (71%)	7 (29%)	24–74	24	0	22	2	0	0
Sutton[27]	1980	1957–1977	40	27 (68%)	13 (32%)	17–73 (44.5)	39	1	32	7	0	0
Poole[28]	1984	1943–1981	16	13 (81%)	3 (19%)	33–97 (54)	16	0	14	1	1	0

Abbreviations as in Table 2.

Gustafson RA, Vasilakis A. Biatrial approach to cardiac myxomas: a 30-year clinical experience. *Ann Thorac Surg* 1995;59:851–856.

23. Premaratne S, Hasaniya NW, Arakaki HY, Mugiishi MM, Mamiya RT, McNamara JJ. Atrial myxomas: experiences with 35 patients in Hawaii. *Am J Surg* 1995;169:600–603.

24. Lukács L, Lengyel M, Szedö F, Haán A, Nagy L, Thomka I, Kassai I. Surgical treatment of cardiac myxomas: a 20-year follow-up. *Cardiovasc Surg* 1997;5:225–228.

25. Bjessmo S, Ivert T. Cardiac myxoma: 40 years' experience in 63 patients. *Ann Thorac Surg* 1997;63:697–700.

26. Bulkley BH, Hutchins GM. Atrial myxomas: a fifty year review. *Am Heart J* 1979;97:639–643.

27. St. John Sutton MG, Mercier L-A, Giuliani ER, Lie JT. Atrial myxomas. A review of clinical experience in 40 patients. *Mayo Clin Proc* 1980;55:371–376.

28. Poole GV Jr, Breyer RH, Holliday RH, Hudspeth AS, Johnston FR, Cordell AR, Mills SA. Tumors of the heart: surgical considerations. *J Cardiovasc Surg* 1984;25:5–11.

29. Burke AP, Virmani R. Cardiac myxoma. A clinicopathologic study. *Am J Clin Pathol* 1993;100:671–680.

Tumor Excision Versus Valve Replacement for Papillary Fibroelastoma Involving the Mitral Valve

Mohammad Zaim Nawaz, MD[†], Allison Richey Lander, MD[a], Jeffrey M. Schussler, MD[a], Paul Arthur Grayburn, MD[b], Baron Lloyd Hamman, MD[b], and William Clifford Roberts, MD*[c,d]

We recently encountered a young man who had 3 strokes and a mass found by echocardiography on his mitral valve, which as a consequence was replaced. The tumor both grossly and histologically was a classic papillary fibroelastoma (PF). The patient's condition stimulated a discussion regarding whether excision of the PF or replacement of the valve containing it might be the preferred procedure. In an attempt to answer the question posed, patients previously reported in an English publication since the first mitral valve operation for PF involving an otherwise normal valve were reviewed.

• • •

A 37-year-old previously healthy house painter noted right-sided weakness unassociated with headache shortly after arising at 7 A.M. It resolved within minutes, but at about 8:30 A.M. right hemiplegia appeared and it persisted. By 10:00 A.M. he had arrived at the emergency room and right-sided weakness in both arm and leg was still present. He was in no distress. He did not smoke, drink alcohol, or use drugs intravenously. His body mass index was 19 kg/m^2. His blood pressure was 145/90 mm Hg initially, but 3 hours later and thereafter was about 120/85 mm Hg. No precordial murmur was heard. Electrocardiogram disclosed no abnormalities. The heart rate was 75 beats/min, and he was in sinus rhythm. A computed tomogram disclosed a remote cerebral infarct but no acute cerebral lesions. Magnetic resonance imaging of the head disclosed an acute infarct involving the left internal capsule and total occlusion of the left middle cerebral artery about 1.5 cm from its origin. The carotid and vertebral arteries were normal. The serum total cholesterol was 253, low-density lipoprotein cholesterol 197, high-density lipoprotein cholesterol 30, and triglycerides 166 mg/dl. The platelet count, prothrombin time, partial thromboplastin time, antithrombin III, protein C, protein S, anti-cardiolipin antibody, antinuclear antibody, and homocystine levels were normal. Factor V Leiden, platelet nuclear antibody 20210, and rapid plasma reagin were negative. By 5 P.M., the right-sided weakness had disappeared.

Cerebral angiography performed within 24 hours disclosed a non-occlusive thrombus in the arterior division of the left middle cerebral artery. During recovery from the procedure, he again developed aphasia and right upper extremity weakness. A repeat angiogram showed that the thrombus (embolus) had migrated, totally obstructing flow. Intraarterial thrombolysis (tissue-plaminogen activator) was performed with restoration of flow to the anterior division of the middle cerebral artery and full recovery of voice and strength.

A transesophageal echocardiogram revealed a 0.9 × 0.7 cm mass on the atrial aspect of the anterior mitral leaflet with slight mitral regurgitation (Figure 1). Blood cultures were negative. Coronary angiography disclosed normal epicardial coronary arteries. At cardiotomy, the anterior mitral leaflet with the mass was resected and a St. Jude Medical (27 mm) prosthesis inserted. Early postoperatively, he developed transient complete heart block (ventricular rate 45 beats/min). On postoperative day 15 he was dyspneic and weak, and found to have cardiac tamponade. A pericardial "window" was created. When seen 3 months after operation, he was asymptomatic.

The operatively excised anterior mitral leaflet, its chordae, and the mass together weighed 0.88 g (Figure 2). The leaflet and chordae were normal. Histologic study of the mass on the anterior leaflet showed it to be a classic PF.

• • •

The described patient had a single PF on the atrial aspect of his anterior mitral leaflet, 3 transient strokes, an angiographically demonstrated embolus in a middle cerebral artery that was lysed by a thrombolytic agent, and operative excision of the anterior mitral leaflet followed by mitral valve replacement. It is presumed that the source of the cerebral embolus was a thrombus on the PF, which dislodged and migrated to a cerebral artery. At the mitral operation no thrombus was seen on the PF and gross and histologic examination of the PF disclosed no evidence of thrombus. Nevertheless, there is supporting evidence from previously reported cases that such a mechanism is the cause of the stroke in our patient as in others. Of the 45 previously published cases of PF involving the mitral valve,[1–42] at least 3 patients with an operatively excised PF on the mitral valve were shown by gross and histologic study to have a thrombus superimposed on the PF.[4,28,36] Additionally, a patient with an

[a]Department of Internal Medicine, Baylor University Medical Center; [b]Department of Internal Medicine (Division of Cardiology) and [c]Department of Cardiothoracic Surgery, and [d]Department of Pathology, Baylor Heart & Vascular Institute, Baylor University Medical Center, Dallas, Texas. Manuscript received September 21, 2005; revised manuscript received and accepted November 15, 2005.

*Corresponding author: Tel: 214-820-7911; Fax: 214-820-7533.

E-mail address: wcroberts@BaylorHealth.edu (W.C. Roberts).

[†]Cardiovascular Medicine Fellow, Scott & White Hospital, Texas A & M University, Temple, Texas.

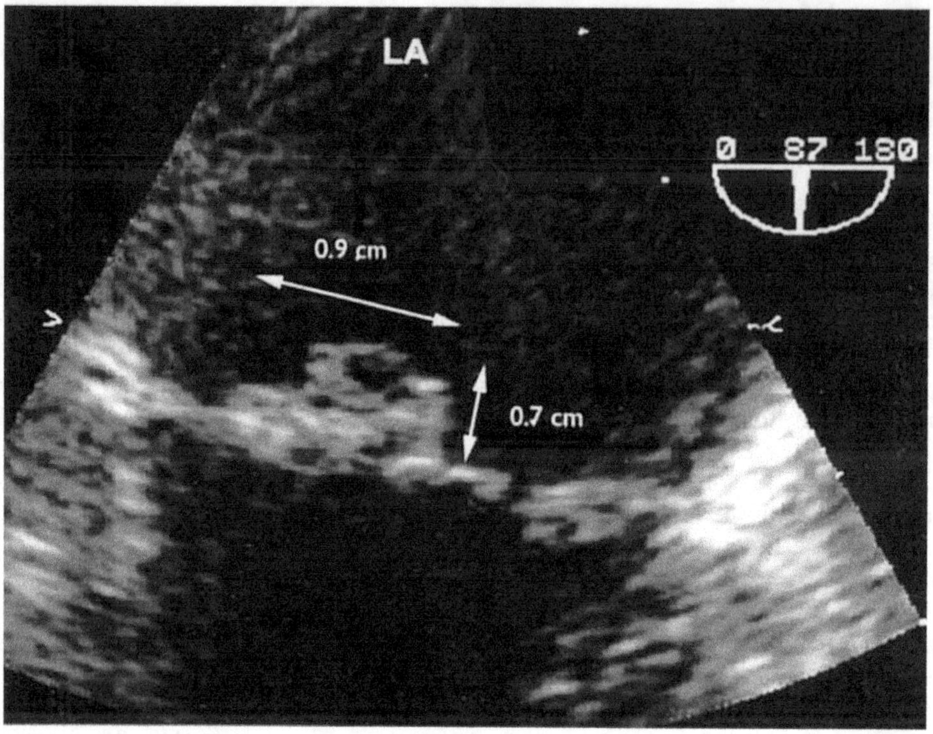

Figure 1. Transesophageal echocardiogram showing the elastofibroendothelioma on the atrial aspect of the anterior mitral leaflet. LA=left atrium.

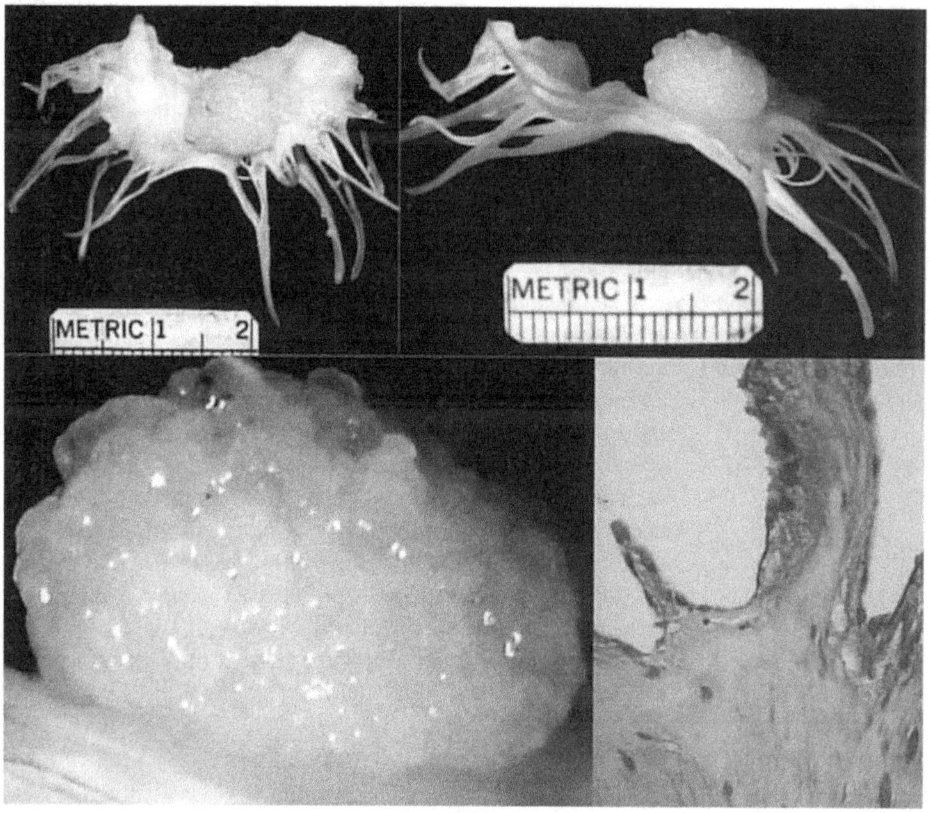

Figure 2. Photographs of the operatively excised anterior mitral leaflet containing the elastofibroendothelioma (EFE) on its atrial aspect *(left upper, right and lower left)* and photomicrograph of a portion of the elastofibroendothelioma. The *upper right photograph* shows the extent of the protrusion of the EFE into the mitral orifice. The *lower left* is a very close up of the EFE. The photomicrograph is stained by the Movat method, and shows the endothelial cells lining the frons and the underlying fibrous and myxoid tissue. The photographs were taken by Ms. Jong Mi Ko.

Table 1
Reported patients having papillary fibroelastoma on the mitral valve and operative excision with or without leaflet repair

Case	Year of Report	First Author	Age (years) at MV Operation	Gender	TIA or Stroke	Cardiac Arrest	AMI	Largest Diameter (cm) of PF	Length of Follow-up After MV Operation (months)	Mitral Leaflet Involved	Chordae Tendineae Involved
1	1981	Shub[1]	55	F	0	0	0	1.0	—	Anterior	+
2	1983	Marvasti[2]	24	M	+	0	0	1.0	16	Posterior	+
3	1986	Topol[3]	27	M	+	0	0	1.5	6	Anterior	0
4	1987	McFadden[4]	41	F	+	0	0	0.5	—	Anterior	0
5	1988	Kasarskis[5]	43	F	+	0	0	1.8	—	Anterior	0
6	1988	Kasarskis[5]	52	M	+	0	0	1.3	36	Posterior	0
7	1989	Akagawa[6]	39	M	0	0	0*	2.5	—	Neither	+
8	1991	Mazzucco[7]	25	M	0	0	+	1.0	—	Anterior	0
9	1992	Valente[8]	31	M	0	0	+	1.7	—	Neither	+
10	1993	Gallo[9]	21	M	+	0	0	0.8	—	Anterior	+
11	1993	Thomas[10]	70	F	0	0	0*	1.5	—	Anterior	0
12	1993	Richard[11]	62	M	0	0	+	1.5	—	Anterior	0
13	1993	Braile[12]	15	M	0	0	0	2.6	6	Anterior	0
14	1993	Shapira[13]	73	F	0	0	0*	1.5	—	Posterior	0
15	1994	Zamora[14]	37	F	+***	0	0	0.8	—	Posterior	0
16	1994	Meyer[15]	38	M	0	0	0**	1.2	—	Posterior	0
17	1995	Pinelli[16]	27	F	+	0	0	0.7	6	Anterior	0
18	1995	Brown[17]	40	F	+	0	0	0.6	—	Anterior	+
19	1996	Hicks[18]	36	M	0	0	0*	0.6	—	Anterior	+
20	1996	Muir[19]	46	M	+	0	0	0.6	—	Anterior	0
21	1996	Menezes[20]	3	M	+	0	0	—	6	Anterior	+
22	1996	Ni[21]	31	F	+	0	0	1.0	—	Anterior	0
23	1997	Tkebuchava[22]	50	M	0	0	0**	1.0	5	Neither	+
24	1998	Moraes[23]	39	M	0	+	+	0.7	6	Anterior	0
25	1998	Al-Mohammad[24]	64	F	+	0	0	1.0	44	Anterior	+
26	1998	Mayer[25]	44	F	0	+	0	—	—	Anterior	0
27	1998	Conte[26]	40	F	+	0	0	1.5	12	Posterior	0
28	1998	Pacini[27]	72	F	+	0	0	4.0	12	Neither	+
29	1999	Grinda[28]	33	M	+	0	0	1.0	36	Anterior	0
30	1999	Sankar[29]	33	F	+	0	0	0.5	—	Anterior	0
31	1999	Howard[30]	39	M	0	+	+	0.7	3	Anterior	0
32	1999	DiMattia[31]	40	M	0	0	0	1.0	3	Anterior	+
33	1999	DiMattia[31]	50	M	0	0	+	1.2	—	Anterior	+
34	2000	Sastre-Garriga[32]	39	M	+	0	0	0.9	—	Posterior	0
35	2000	Sastre-Garriga[32]	32	F	+	0	0	1.5	—	Posterior	0
36	2000	Gölbasi[33]	32	M	+	0	0	1.0	—	Anterior	0
37	2000	Karaeren[34]	21	M	+	0	0	1.5	—	Anterior	0
38	2000	Toda[35]	78	F	+	0	0	0.8	4	Posterior	0

* Chest pain; ** palpitations; ***retinal artery occlusion.
AMI = acute myocardial infarction; MV = mitral valve; PF = papillary fibroelastoma; TIA = transient ischemic attack.

Table 2
Reported patients having papillary fibroelastoma on mitral valve and mitral valve replacement

Case	Year of Report	First Author	Age (years) at MV Operation	Gender	TIA or Stroke	Cardiac Arrest	AMI	Largest Diameter (cm) of PF	Length of Follow-up After MV Operation (months)	Mitral Leaflet Involved	Chordae Tendineae Involved
1	1981	Fowles[36]	35	M	+	+	+	1.0	—	Posterior	0
2	1987	Dien[37]	25	M	+	+	0	—	81	Posterior	0
3	1989	Gorton[38]	77	F	+	0	0	2.0	9	Both	+
4	1994	Mann[39]	59	M	+	0	0	2.3	12	Neither	+
5	1995	Colucci[40]	66	F	+	0	0	1.5	12	Anterior	+
6	1998	Bailbé[41]	31	M	+	0	0	0.8	18	Unknown	+
7	2001	Shing[42]	34	M	+	0	0	1.0	6	Anterior	0

Abbreviation as in Table 2.

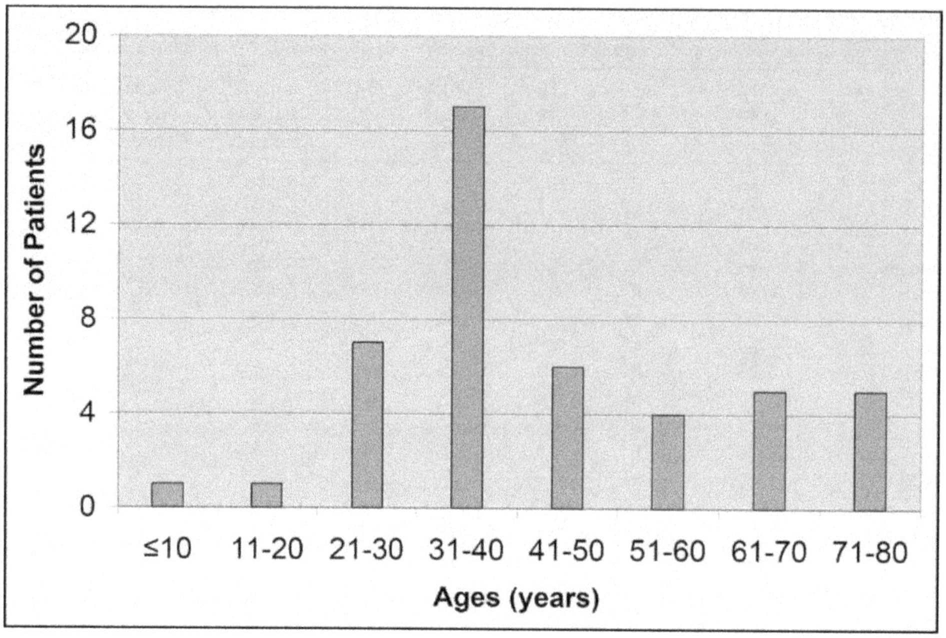

Figure 3. Ages (years) at time of mitral valve operations of 47 previously reported patients with papillary fibroelastoma involving the mitral valve.

PF involving a pulmonic valve also had superimposed thrombus on it.[43] In our patient and in the 45 previously reported patients with an PF on the mitral valve, no other source of embolism other than the PF could be demonstrated. Thus, it is reasonable to believe that mitral PF was the source of systemic embolism in our patient. It is not fragments of the PF which embolized, it is the thrombus superimposed on the PF.

Reports published in English of patients with PF involving an otherwise normal (except for aging changes) mitral valve with operative excision or mitral replacement produced 45 individual reports.[1–42] Those having operative excision of the mitral PF are listed in Table 1; those having mitral replacement are listed in Table 2, and the findings in both groups are summarized in Figure 3. All but 3 of 45 patients presented with either stroke and/or transient ischemic attack, and/or nonfatal cardiac arrest, and/or acute myocardial infarction. Although the patients ranged in age from 3 to 78 years, 28 (62%) were <40 years old (Figure 3). Men were seen slightly more frequently than women (62% vs 38%). A precordial murmur was usually absent. The PFs on 1 or both mitral leaflets, i.e., excluding the 5 cases in which the PF involved only the chordae tendineae, were usually small; of the 37 patients in whom the PF involved a mitral leaflet and the largest diameter was reported, the PF was ≤1.5 cm in 35 (95%), and the largest had a maximal diameter of 2.6 cm. In contrast, in 4 of the 5 patients in whom the PF spared a mitral leaflet and involved only its chordae tendineae, the maximal diameter of the PF was >1.7 cm (range 1.7 to 4.0). In only 1 of the 45 patients reported was the weight of the operatively excised PF recorded, and that was 0.29 g.

Of the 45 reported patients, 38 (84%) had PF excision and 7 (16%) had valve replacement. The argument for valve excision, of course, is that a mechanical prosthesis with its mandatory anticoagulation thereafter or a bioprosthesis with its inevitable degeneration is avoided. The argument for valve replacement is that worry of thrombus formation at the base of the excised PF and the potential regrowth of an PF on the valve are no longer possibilities. Recurrence, however, of an PF at the site of a previously excised PF has never been reported. Although all 45 previously reported cases presented as individual case reports (Tables 1 to 2; Figure 3) survived the operative period, follow-up information is scant at best. Of the 45 patients, follow-up information >1 month after the mitral operation was described in only 21 patients (47%) and ranged from 3 to 81 months (mean 16; median 9), and in 15 of the 21 patients (71%), the follow-up was ≤12 months. Thus, the preferred type of operative intervention remains unclear, but logic for most of these patients favors PF excision without valve replacement.

The data in the previously described cases came from individual case reports and included only cases where the PF was located on the mitral valve and was either excised or the mitral valve replaced. Two large collections[44,45] of cases of PF confirmed histologically after operative excision or at necropsy were not included in our analysis because both studies included all cases of cardiac PF irrespective of where the PF was located in the heart, and data on the cases involving only the mitral valve was limited.

Klarich and associates[44] included 4 cases of PF involving a mitral leafet among 12 cases of PF involving a cardiac valve having operative intervention: 3 had operative excision of the mitral PF and 1 had mitral replacement.

The latter patient had a flail anterior mitral leafet and that was the reason for the mitral replacement, not the presence of a PF on the mitral valve. Follow-up information on these 4 cases was not available.

Gowda and associates[45] reported on 725 cases of cardiac PF confirmed either at operation or autopsy, and 180 (25%) involved the mitral valve (223 cases involved the aortic valve, 65 cases the tricuspid valve, 43 the pulmonic valve, and the remainder presumably a non-valvular site). Surgical excision was performed in 325 patients and valve replacement in 42 patients. No recurrence of PF occurred in the patients having valve excision. It was not possible to separate data in the cases in whom the PF was located on the mitral valve from those involving other cardiac valves or only the mural endocardium.

1. Shub C, Tajik AJ, Seward JB, Edwards WD, Pruitt RD, Orszulak TA, Pluth JR. Cardiac papillary fibroelastoms. Two-dimensional echocardiographic recognition. *Mayo Clin Proc* 1981;56:629–633.
2. Marvasti MA, Obeid AI, Cohen PS, Giambartolomei A, Parker FB. Successful removal of papillary endocardial fibroma. *Thorac Cardiovasc Surg* 1983;31:254–255.
3. Topol EJ, Biern RO, Reitz BA. Cardiac papillary fibroelastoma and stroke. Echocardiographic diagnosis and guide to excision. *Am J Med* 1986;80:129–132.
4. McFadden PM, Lacy JR. Intracardiac papillary fibroelastoma: an occult cause of embolic neurologic deficit. *Ann Thorac Surg* 1987;43:667–669.
5. Kasarskis EJ, O'Connor W, Earle G. Embolic stroke from cardiac papillary fibroelastomas. *Stroke* 1988;19:1171–1173.
6. Akagawa H, Kawara T, Hirano A, Sugiwara S, Ogata M, Aoyagi S, Kosuga K, Ohishi K, Koga M. Excision of papillary endocardial tumor. *J Cardiovasc Surg* 1989;30:47–49.
7. Mazzucco A, Faggian G, Bortolotti U, Bonato R, Pittarello D, Centonze G, Thiene G. Embolizing papillary fibroelastoma of the mitral valve. *Tex Heart Inst J* 1991;18:62–66.
8. Valente M, Basso C, Thiene G, Bressan M, Stritoni P, Cocco P, Fasoli G. Fibroelastic papilloma: a not-so-benign cardiac tumor. *Cardiovasc Pathol* 1992;1:161–166.
9. Gallo R, Kumar N, Prabhakar G, Awada A, Maalouf Y, Duran CMG. Papillary fibroelastoma of mitral valve chorda. *Ann Thorac Surg* 1993;55:1576–1577.
10. Thomas MR, Jayakrishnan AG, Desai J, Monaghan MJ, Jewitt DE. Transesophageal echocardiography in the detection and surgical management of a papillary fibroelastoma of the mitral valve causing partial mitral valve obstruction. *J Am Soc Echocardiogr* 1993;6:83–86.
11. Richard J, Castello R, Dressler FA, Willman VL, Nashed A, Lewis B, Labovitz AJ. Diagnosis of papillary fibroelastoma of the mitral valve complicated by non-Q-wave infarction with apical thrombus: transesophageal and transthoracic echocardiographic study. *Am Heart J* 1993;126:710–712.
12. Braile DM, Rossi MA, Jacob JLB, Thevenard RS, Suzigan S, Ramos SG. Cystic fibroelastoma of the mitral valve:report of a case. *J Thorac Cardiovasc Surg* 1993;106:1228–1230.
13. Shapira OM, Williamson WA, Dugan JM. Papillary fibroelastoma of the mitral valve. *Cardiovasc Surg* 1993;1:599–601.
14. Zamora RL, Adelberg DA, Berger AS, Huettner P, Kaplan HJ. Branch retinal artery occlusion caused by a mitral valve papillary fibroelastoma. *Am J Ophthalmol* 1995;119: 325–329.
15. Meyer AH, Clements SD Jr., Sadel SM, Shanewise JS, Gravanis MB. Papillary fibroelastoma of the cardiac valves. *Heart Dis Stroke* 1994;3:318–319.
16. Pinelli G, Carteaux J-P, Mertes PM, Civit T, Trinh A, Villemot J-P. Mitral valve tumor revealed by stroke. *J Heart Valve Dis* 1995; 4:199–201.
17. Brown RD Jr., Khandheria BK, Edwards WD. Cardiac papillary fibroelastoma: a treatable cause of transient ischemic attack and ischemic stroke detected by transesophageal echocardiography. *Mayo Clin Proc* 1995;70: 863–868.
18. Hicks KA, Kovach JA, Frishberg DP, Wiley TM, Gurczak PB, Vernalis MN. Echocardiographic evaluation of papillary fibroelastoma: a case report and review of the literature. *J Am Soc Echocardiogr* 1996;9:353–360.
19. Muir KW, McNeish IBM, Grosset DG, Metcalfe M. Visualization of cardiac emboli from mitral valve papillary fibroelastoma. *Stroke* 1996;27:1133–1134.
20. de Menezes IC, Fragata J, Martins FM. Papillary fibroelastoma of the mitral valve in a 3-year-old child: case report. *Pediatr Cardiol* 1996;17:194–195.
21. Ni Y, von Segesser LK, Dirsch O, Schneider J, Jenni R, Turina M. Cardiac papillary fibroelastoma. *Thorac Cardiovasc Surg* 1996;44: 257–260.
22. Tkebuchava T, von Segesser LK, Gallino A, Dirsch O, Turina MI. Cardiac papillary fibroelastoma excision combined with reconstructive surgery. *Jpn Heart J* 1997;38:457–462.
23. Moraes D, Philippides GJ, Shapira OM. Papillary fibroelastoma of the mitral valve with systemic embolization. *Circulation* 1998;98: 1251–1252.
24. Al-Mohammed A, Pambakian H, Young C. Fibroelastoma: case report and review of literature. *Heart* 1998;79:301–304.
25. Mayer K, Niederhaeuser U, Jenni R. Cardiac papillary fibroelastoma with cerebral and coronary embolic events. *Heart* 1998;79:307.
26. Conte FJ, Katz AS. Fibroelastoma and embolic stroke. *Circulation* 1998;97:1648.
27. Pacini D, Farneti PA, Leone O, Galli R. Cardiac papillary fibroelastoma of the mitral valve chordae. *Euro J Cardiothorac Surg* 1998;13:322–324.
28. Grinda J-M, Couetil JP, Chauvaud S, D'Attellis N, Berrebi A, Fabiani J-N, Deloche A, Carpentier A. Cardiac valve papillary fibroelastoma: surgical excision for revealed or potential embolization. *J Thorac Cardiovasc Surg* 1999;117:106–110.
29. Sankar NM, Odayan MK, Morris M, Peterson H, Hanna WM. Cardiac valvular papillary fibroelastoma. A report of 2 cases. *Tex Heart Inst J* 1999;26:298–299.
30. Howard RA, Aldea GS, Shapira OM, Kasznica JM, Davidoff R. Papillary fibroelastoma: increasing recognition of a surgical disease. *Ann Thorac Surg* 1999;68:1881–1885.
31. Di Mattia DG, Assaghi A, Mangini A, Ravagnan S, Bonetto S, Fundaro P. Mitral valve repair for anterior leaflet papillary fibroelastoma: two case descriptions and a literature review. *Euro J Cardiothorac Surg* 1999;15:103–107.
32. Sastre-Garriga J, Molina C, Montaner J, Mauleon A, Pujadas F, Codina A, Álvarez-Sabin J. Mitral papillary fibroelastoma as a cause of cardiogenic embolic stroke: report of two cases and review of the literature. *Euro J Neurol* 2000;7:449–453.
33. Gölbasi Z, Çiçek D, Aydogdu S, Can C. Papillary fibroelastoma of mitral valve. A rare cause of transient ischemic attack in the young. *Jpn Heart J* 2000;41:525–526.
34. Karaeren H, Ilgenli TF, Celik T, Deveci S, Kuralay E, Barcin C, Uzun M, Genc C, Demirtas E. Papillary fibroelastoma of the mitral valve with systemic embolization. *Echocardiography* 2000;17:165–167.
35. Toda R, Iguro Y, Moriyama Y, Matsumoto H, Taira A. Papillary fibroelastoma on the mitral valve. *Jpn J Thorac Cardiovasc Surg* 2000;48:132–134.
36. Fowles RE, Miller DC, Egbert BM, Fitzgerald JW, Popp RL. Systemic embolization from a mitral valve papillary endocardial fibroma detected by two-dimensional echocardiography. *Am Heart J* 1981;102:128–130.
37. Dein JR, Frist WH, Stinson EB, Miller DC, Baldwin JC, Oyer PE, Jamieson S, Mitchell RS, Shumway NE. Primary cardiac neoplasms. Early and late results of surgical treatment in 42 patients. *J Thorac Cardiovasc Surg* 1987;93:502–511.
38. Gorton ME, Soltanzadeh H. Mitral valve fibroelastoma. *Ann Thorac Surg* 1989;47:605–607.
39. Mann J, Parker DJ. Papillary fibroelastoma of the mitral valve: a rare cause of transient neurological deficits. *Br Heart J* 1994;71:6.
40. Colucci V, Alberti A, Bonacina E, Gordini V. Papillary fibroelastoma of the mitral valve. A rare cause of events. *Tex Heart Inst J* 1995;22: 327–331.
41. Bailbé M, Coisne D, Babin P, Corbi P, Menu P, Rosier MP, Couderq C, Pouget Abadie JF,

Gil R, Neau JP. Fibroélastome papillaire. Une étiologie rare des accidents vasculaires cérébraux du sujet jeune. *Rev Méd Interne* 1998;19:119–122.

42. Shing M, Rubenson DS. Embolic stroke and cardiac papillary fibroelastoma. *Clin Cardiol* 2001;24:346–347.

43. Fekete PS, Nassar VH, Talley JD, Boedecker EA. Cardiac papilloma. A case report with evidence of thrombotic origin. *Arch Pathol Lab Med* 1983;107:246–248.

44. Klarich KW, Enriquez-Sarano M, Gura GM, Edwards WD, Tajik AJ, Seward JB. Papillary fibroelastoma: echocardiographic characteristics for diagnosis and pathologic correlation. *J Am Coll Cardiol* 1997;30:784–790.

45. Gowda RM, Khan IA, Nair CK. Mehta NJ, Vasavada BC, Sacchi TJ. Cardiac papillary fibroelastoma: a comprehensive analysis of 725 cases. *Am Heart J* 2003;146:404–410.

Preoperative exclusion of significant coronary artery disease by 64-slice CT coronary angiography in a patient with a left atrial myxoma

Rafic F. Berbarie, MD, Mohammed K. Aslam, MD, Johannes J. Kuiper, MD, Gregory J. Matter, MD, Alan W. Martin, MD, William C. Roberts, MD, and Jeffrey M. Schussler, MD

A 49-year-old man without any significant past medical history presented to the emergency department with complaints of diplopia, paresthesias in both arms, vertigo, tinnitus in the right ear, and dysarthria. Physical examination was unremarkable. A computed tomographic (CT) scan of the head was normal. These symptoms resolved within several hours, consistent with a transient ischemic attack. Magnetic resonance imaging of the brain revealed acute infarcts in the left cerebellar hemisphere and in the right occipital lobe, suggesting a thromboembolic source.

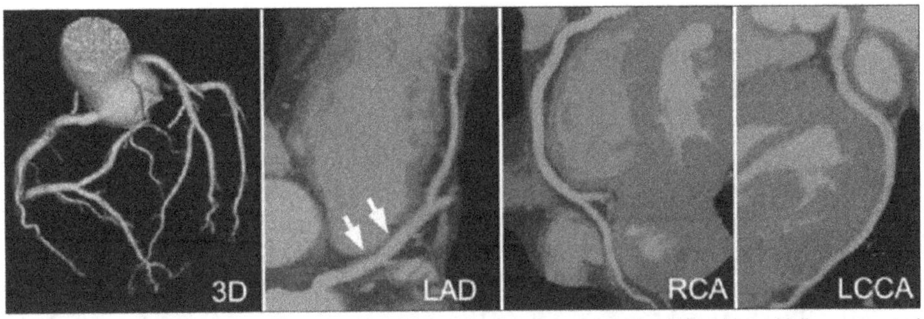

Figure 1. Three-dimensional reconstruction of the patient's coronary arteries (3D) with multislice computed tomography. Curved reformat images of the left anterior descending (LAD) coronary artery, right coronary artery (RCA), and left circumflex coronary artery (LCCA) reveal only minimal plaque in the proximal LAD (arrows).

Transesophageal echocardiography disclosed a 2 × 2-cm mass attached to the left atrial aspect of the atrial septum, and surgical excision was planned. As the patient was considered to have a very low risk for the presence of significant arterial narrowing, he underwent a 64-slice cardiac CT scan rather than invasive coronary angiography. The scan demonstrated minimal plaque in the coronary arteries *(Figure 1)*. The left atrial mass was also well visualized on both the axial slices and also with three-dimensional imaging *(Figure 2a–c)*. Subsequently, the patient's left atrial mass was excised without complication, and the mass was a typical myxoma *(Figure 2d, e)*.

This case demonstrates how, in the future, routine invasive coronary angiography may not be necessary as part of the workup for noncoronary cardiac surgery. In this instance, significant concomitant coronary artery disease was effectively excluded with multislice CT rather than an invasive procedure, thus allowing the surgery to proceed without a cardiac catheterization. In addition, CT imaging assisted with long-term prognostic information, as it suggested the need for the patient to be on cholesterol reduction therapy by demonstrating the early presence of coronary atherosclerosis.

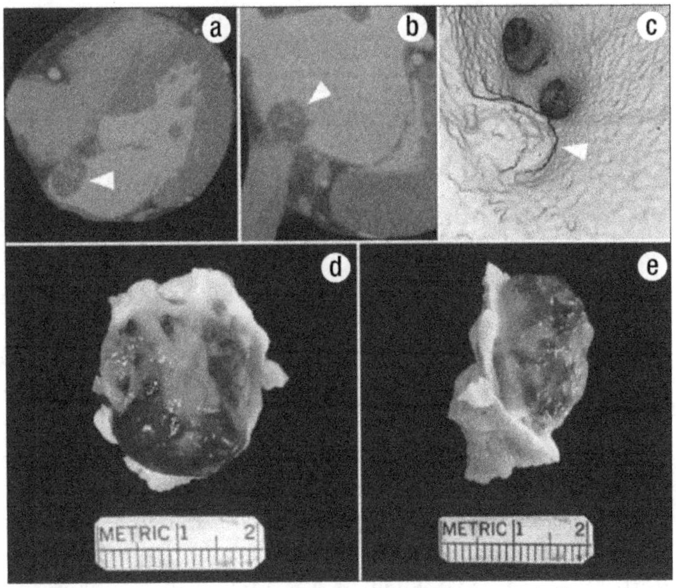

Figure 2. (a, b) Axial slices from the patient's multislice computed tomographic scan demonstrating the myxoma attached to the left atrial aspect of the atrial septum (arrowheads). **(c)** The myxoma (arrowhead) shown via a "navigator" view inside the left atrium. The orifices of the right pulmonary veins can also be appreciated. **(d, e)** The excised 2 × 2-cm myxoma.

Heart failure resulting from chemotherapy for testicular neoplasm: a follow-up on a patient reported 20 years earlier

David Dmitry Boltan, MD, Shelley Anne Hall, MD, and William Clifford Roberts, MD

In 1986 Doll and associates (1) from Phoenix and Nashville reported on 4 patients who developed acute vascular ischemic events after cisplatin-based combination chemotherapy for germ-cell tumor of the testis. Case 1 in their study is the patient described here 20 years later.

• • •

A 47-year-old man, who was born in July 1959, had been well until August 1982, when at age 23 he noted a left-upper-quadrant mass and bilateral testicular enlargement. A computed tomography examination a year later disclosed a retroperitoneal mass. The patient's serum alpha-fetoprotein level was 4058 mg/mL. Bilateral orchiectomy showed yolk sac carcinoma. The patient was treated at 3-week intervals with 4 cycles of cisplatin 20 mg/m^2 body surface area intravenously on days 1 through 5; vinblastine, 0.15 mg/kg body weight intravenously on days 1 and 2; and bleomycin, 30 units intravenously weekly for 12 weeks.

A complete remission was obtained, but over the next year the patient developed Raynaud's phenomenon affecting the digits in his fingers. In June 1985, 18 months after completion of chemotherapy, he developed substernal chest pain, and a series of electrocardiograms and cardiac enzyme tests were consistent with anterior wall acute myocardial infarction. In September 1985, 3 months later, coronary angiography showed no abnormalities. Administration of ergonovine maleate precipitated chest discomfort accompanied by diffuse right coronary spasm exceeding 40% diameter reduction. Anginal symptoms and coronary spasm were promptly relieved by nitroglycerin. A left ventriculogram showed anterolateral and apical hypokinesis and a mildly decreased ejection fraction.

In December 1985, the patient was hospitalized for overt heart failure. He continued to work without rehospitalization until 1992 (age 33), when he was advised to stop working because of heart failure. Atrial fibrillation appeared shortly thereafter, and it was paroxysmal. Cardiac catheterization in November 2002 disclosed normal right-sided cardiac pressures, normal pulmonary arterial wedge pressure (11 mm Hg), normal coronary arteries by angiogram, and a slightly decreased cardiac index (2.3 L/min/m^2).

In 1995 a stent was placed in an artery in the patient's leg for reasons that are unclear, and shortly thereafter he had 2 transient ischemic attacks. A thrombus was found in the left side of his heart, and warfarin was instituted. His left ventricular ejection fraction at that time was 24%, and the left ventricular cavity had a maximal diameter of 9.3 cm.

In April 1997, his serum total cholesterol was 249; low-density lipoprotein cholesterol, 184; high-density lipoprotein cholesterol, 34; and triglycerides, 156 mg/dL. He was placed on simvastatin 10 mg daily in 2000.

In April 2005 when he was 45, an echocardiogram continued to show the maximal left ventricular cavity diameter to be 9.3 cm, and there was generalized left ventricular hypokinesia with apical akinesia and an ejection fraction of about 10%. The serum total cholesterol now was 170; low-density lipoprotein cholesterol, 122; high-density lipoprotein cholesterol, 34; and triglycerides, 112 mg/dL. Repeat cardiac catheterization in July 2005 disclosed the following pressures in mm Hg: pulmonary artery wedge mean, 29, a 34, v 41; pulmonary artery, 51/26; and right atrial mean 6, a 10, v 9. The cardiac index was 1.9 L/min/m^2.

Cardiac transplantation was performed on September 18, 2005. Conversation with the patient on February 20, 2006, disclosed that he was asymptomatic and feeling well. The operatively excised native heart weighed 820 g. The amount of subepicardial adipose tissue was considerably increased such that the basal portion of the heart floated in formaldehyde. Both ventricular cavities but particularly the left one were greatly dilated *(Figure)*. Two transmural scars were present: one in the anterior wall and one in the posterior wall. The scarring extended from the apex to base. About half of the apical wall was scarred. In contrast, only a small portion of the anteroseptal wall was scarred in its most basal portion. The right coronary artery was narrowed about 50% in cross-sectional area at one site. The lumens of the left main, left anterior descending, and left circumflex coronary arteries were widely patent. Histologic sections of the ventricular walls confirmed the scarring. No foci or myofiber necrosis or inflammation were present.

From the Department of Internal Medicine (Boltan, Hall, Roberts) and the Department of Pathology (Roberts), Baylor Heart and Vascular Institute and Baylor University Medical Center, Dallas, Texas.

Corresponding author: William C. Roberts, MD, Baylor Heart and Vascular Institute, 621 North Hall Street, Dallas, Texas 75226 (e-mail: wc.roberts@BaylorHealth.edu).

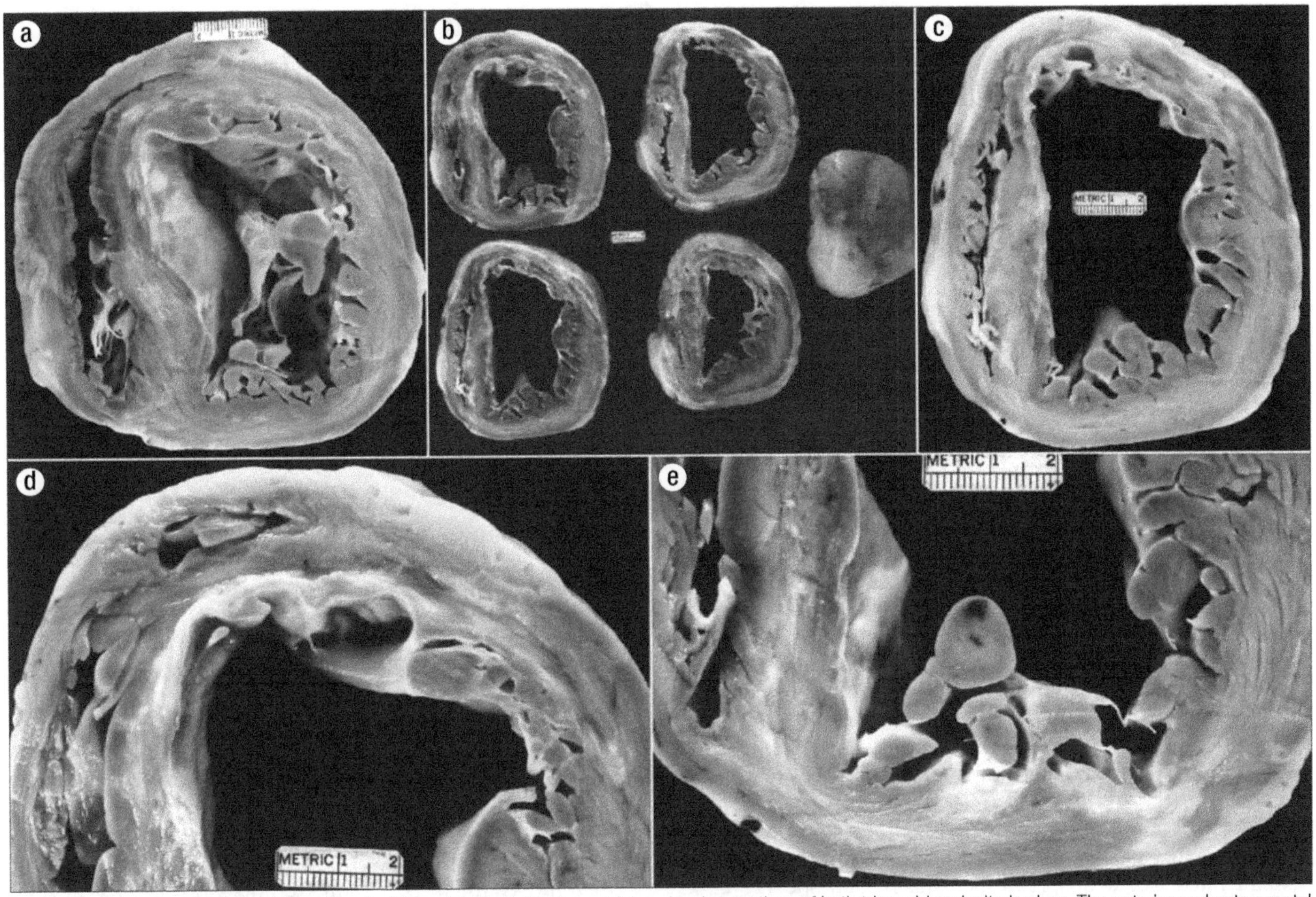

Figure. The native heart after cardiac transplantation. **(a)** View of both ventricles showing portions of both tricuspid and mitral valves. The anterior and anteroseptal walls are scarred. **(b)** View of 1-cm thick slices of the ventricles going from base (upper left) to apex (right). **(c)** Close-up view showing the transmural scar on the anterior wall. **(d)** Very close-up view of the anterior wall scar. **(e)** Very close-up view of the posterior wall scar. (Photographs by Jong Mi Ko.)

• • •

The patient described here had chemotherapy for a malignant testicular neoplasm. Although it eliminated the neoplasm, the chemotherapy produced vasospasm as confirmed by Raynaud's phenomenon; the precipitation of chest pain on administration of ergonovine maleate; and narrowing (up to 40% in diameter) of the right coronary artery. Eighteen months after completion of the chemotherapy, the patient, when only 25 years of age, had documented acute myocardial infarction. Three months later, an angiogram confirmed the presence of normal coronary arteries.

Examination of the operatively excised heart after cardiac transplantation disclosed 2 separate left ventricular scars, one anteriorly and one posteriorly, and a hugely dilated left ventricular cavity and essentially normal coronary arteries.

It is fairly well established that individuals who have an acute myocardial infarction and later appear to have normal coronary arteries have a good prognosis and indeed are generally free of clinical evidence of myocardial ischemia or heart failure (2). The patient described herein had 2 separate myocardial infarcts, and the extensiveness of the myocardial damage probably explains the degree of left ventricular dilatation and heart failure.

It is important to realize that the patient did not have coronary angiography *at the time of* the acute infarct but 3 months later. Therefore, we cannot be certain of the status of the coronary arteries at the time of the myocardial infarct. A thrombus or embolus in a coronary artery could have been present at the time of the infarct and could have retracted, organized, and recanalized subsequently such that it was angiographically "normal" later (3). Myocardial infarction as a consequence of coronary spasm has rarely if ever been confirmed.

In conclusion, chemotherapy destroyed the malignant cancer but also damaged the heart; the resulting heart failure would have been fatal had not cardiac transplantation intervened. The chemotherapy killed the cancer but at the same time destroyed the previously normal heart.

1. Doll DC, List AF, Greco FA, Hainsworth JD, Hande KR, Johnson DH. Acute vascular ischemic events after cisplatin-based combination chemotherapy for germ-cell tumors of the testis. *Ann Intern Med* 1986;105(1): 48–51.
2. Golzio PG, Orzan F, Ferrero P, Bobbio M, Bergerone S, Di Leo M, Trevi GP. Myocardial infarction with normal coronary arteries: ten-year follow-up. *Ital Heart J* 2004;5(10):732–738.
3. Arnett EN, Roberts WC. Acute myocardial infarction and angiographically normal coronary arteries. An unproven combination. *Circulation* 1976;53(3):395–400.

Carcinoid Heart Disease Without the Carcinoid Syndrome but With Quadrivalvular Regurgitation and Unsuccessful Operative Intervention

William Clifford Roberts, MD[a,b,d,*], Cyril Abie Varughese, DO[e], Jong Mi Ko, BA[d], Paul A. Grayburn, MD[b,d], Robert Frederick Hebeler, Jr., MD[c], and Elizabeth C. Burton, MD[a]

A 53-year-old woman is described who underwent mitral and aortic valve replacement and tricuspid valve annuloplasty for pure regurgitation at all 3 valve sites for unrecognized carcinoid heart disease without the carcinoid syndrome 22 days before death. Metastatic carcinoid was not recognized until necropsy, which disclosed a probable ovarian primary but with large hepatic metastases and left-sided cardiac involvement either greater than or equal to the right-sided involvement. Pulmonary hypertension, very unusual in carcinoid heart disease, persisted postoperatively and probably played a role in the patient's early death. Hepatic metastasis with ovarian primary is most unusual in this circumstance. **(Am J Cardiol 2011;107:788–792)**

It was in 1930, 80 years ago, when the first patient with a metastasizing carcinoid neoplasm associated with fibrous lesions on the right side of the heart was described.[1] In 1931, the first patient with metastasizing carcinoid syndrome (head and upper chest flushes and diarrhea) associated with fibrous lesions not only on the tricuspid and pulmonic valves but also on the anterior mitral leaflet and left ventricular mural endocardium was described.[2] Subsequently, of course, numerous reports have appeared describing clinical and morphologic features of the carcinoid syndrome and carcinoid heart disease.[2,3] Most patients have the primary carcinoid in the small intestine, widespread metastases, and specific carcinoid plaques limited to the right side of the heart.[2,3] The present report was prompted by study of a patient with severe mitral and aortic regurgitation leading to double valve replacement but without symptoms of the carcinoid syndrome but with metastasizing carcinoid.

Case Description

A 53-year-old mother of 6, who was born May 5, 1955, and died February 18, 2009, had been well until November 2008, when she noted exertional dyspnea, subcutaneous peripheral edema, and recurring palpitations, which proved to be runs of atrial fibrillation. The symptoms gradually worsened, with episodes of rapid heart rate, each lasting several minutes. On January 26, 2009, cardiac catheterization disclosed the following pressures in mm Hg: pulmonary arterial wedge mean 22, a wave 30, v wave 28; pulmonary trunk 56/10; right ventricle 56/18; right atrial mean 9, a wave 15, v wave 10; left ventricle 130/26; and aorta 127/58. Left ventriculography disclosed a normal-sized left ventricular cavity, with an ejection fraction of 60% and 4+/4+ mitral regurgitation. Aortography disclosed 4+/4+ aortic regurgitation. The coronary arteries were angiographically normal. Echocardiography showed thickened mitral and aortic valve cusps and a normal-sized left ventricle (Figure 1).

On January 27, 2009, the mitral and aortic valves were replaced with mechanical prostheses (#20 ATS Medical [Minneapolis, Minnesota] in the aortic position and #29 St. Jude Medical [St. Paul, Minnesota] in the mitral position). A Maze procedure was also performed as well as tricuspid valve annuloplasty. The operatively excised valves are shown in Figures 2 and 3. The 6-day postoperative hospital course was characterized by a weight gain of 6.6 kg (from 76.7 to 83.3 kg), sinus rhythm, and gradual ambulation.

On February 13, 2009, the patient was rehospitalized because of increasing weakness and dyspnea, evidence of gastrointestinal bleeding (on warfarin with an international normalized ratio of 4.7), and large pleural and pericardial effusions. The blood hemoglobin level was 11.1 g/dl, and the hematocrit was 35%. The serum bilirubin level was 1.4 mg/dl; alkaline phosphatase, 295 U/L; aspartate aminotransferase, 210 U/L; and alanine aminotransferase, 147 U/L. The blood urea nitrogen level was 17 mg/dl and glucose 96 mg/dl. The brain natriuretic peptide level was 430 pg/ml (normal range <100). Echocardiography now showed a normal-sized, normally functioning left ventricle, a very dilated and dysfunctional right ventricle, and large pericardial and right pleural effusions (Figure 4). Approximately 1,800 ml of serous fluid was drained from the right pleural space. Shortly thereafter, the patient had a cardiac arrest and died.

At necropsy, classic carcinoid neoplasms were present in the right ovary (2.3 × 2.1 × 1.9 cm), the liver (2 hemorrhagic and necrotic carcinoid masses, 10 × 9 × 9 and 3 × 3 × 3 cm;

[a]Departments of Pathology, [b]Internal Medicine (Cardiology), and [c]Cardiothoracic Surgery; [d]Baylor Heart and Vascular Institute, Baylor University Medical Center; and [e]Department of Internal Medicine, Methodist Dallas Medical Center, Dallas, Texas, USA. Manuscript received September 1, 2010; revised manuscript received and accepted October 11, 2010.

*Corresponding author: Tel: 214-820-7911; fax: 214-820-7533.

E-mail address: wc.roberts@baylorhealth.edu (W.C. Roberts).

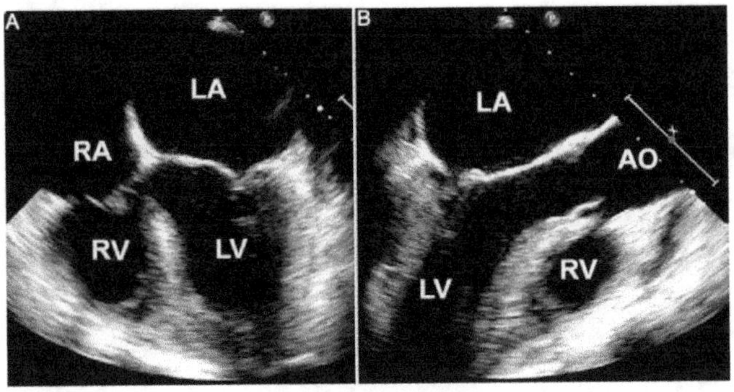

Figure 1. Preoperative (1 day) echocardiograms in the patient are described. *(A)* Four-chamber view showing the thickened mitral and tricuspid leaflets and the normal-sized right ventricular and left ventricular cavities. *(B)* Long-axis view again showing the thickened mitral leaflets and also a thickened aortic valve cusp. AO = aorta; LA = left atrium; LV = left ventricle; RA = right atrium; RV = right ventricle.

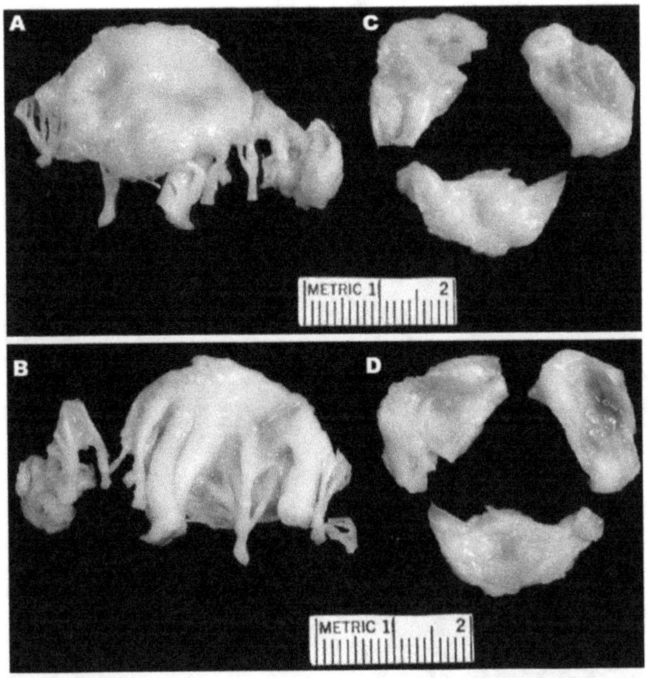

Figure 2. Photographs of the operatively excised mitral *(A,B)* and aortic *(C,D)* valves. *(A)* View of the atrial aspect of the anterior mitral leaflet. *(B)* View of the ventricular aspect of the anterior mitral leaflet with marked fibrous thickening of the chordae tendineae. A fragment of posterior leaflet with attached papillary muscle is also visible. *(C)* Focally thickened ventricular aspect of the tricuspid aortic valve. *(D)* Aortic aspect.

liver weight 2,100 g); the serosa of the bowel (1 nodule) and uterus (1 nodule); the adrenal glands (multiple small nodules); the pancreas (1 nodule, 0.3 cm); and the heart (multiple microscopic-sized nodules). Sections of the tumors in the liver, ovary, and adrenal glands were positive for neuron-specific enolase.

The heart (Figures 5 to 8) weighed 370 g. The coronary arteries were free of atherosclerotic plaque. The left ventricular cavity was small, and the right ventricular cavity was very dilated. No myocardial foci of fibrosis or necrosis were present, except in the posteromedial left ventricular papillary muscle, which was fibrotic. Both atria were dilated, the right more than the left. The pulmonic valve cusps were thickened, and the anterior cusp was rigid and immobile. The foramen ovale was closed.

Comments

Our patient underwent mitral and aortic valve replacement and tricuspid valve annuloplasty for pure mitral, aortic, and tricuspid valve regurgitation. Examination of the operatively excised valves suggested an appearance similar to that described in patients having taken fenfluramine-phentermine for weight reduction. The patient, however, denied having ever taken that medication. Postoperatively, the patient's condition worsened, and she died 22 days after the operation. Necropsy disclosed carcinoid tumors in 1 ovary, both adrenal glands, the liver, the pancreas, the serosal surfaces of the uterus and bowel, and the heart (intramyocardial). There was never evidence of the carcinoid syndrome (flushing, diarrhea), and the presence of the carcinoid neoplasm was not diagnosed until necropsy, which also disclosed evidence of carcinoid heart disease involving both right-sided cardiac valves as well as both left-sided valves.

The primary in the patient described was not certain, but the ovary appeared to be the most logical site. Only 1 of the 2 ovaries was involved, and the cancerous nodule was >2 cm in diameter. Hepatic metastasis of carcinoid with ovarian primary, however, is quite unusual.[4,5] Chatterjee and Heather[6] found hepatic carcinoid metastases in only 1 of 35 reported cases with primary carcinoid in the ovary. Although our patient had only 2 carcinoid metastases in the liver, both were large.

In our patient, carcinoid heart disease involved all 4 cardiac valves: the pulmonic valve to a worse extent than the aortic valve, but the mitral valve to a worse extent than the tricuspid valve. Although the pulmonic valve was heavily involved by the carcinoid process, there was no pressure gradient across the valve, although the end-diastolic pressures in both the pulmonary trunk and the right ventricle were similar, indicating pure pulmonic regurgitation.

Is the electrocardiogram helpful in patients with malignant carcinoid in diagnosing carcinoid heart disease? No. Ross and Roberts[3] examined electrocardiograms in 34 patients with the carcinoid syndrome: the total 12-lead QRS voltages[7] in the 19 patients with carcinoid heart disease ranged from 58 to 227 mm (mean 105; standardization 10 mm) and in the 15 patients without carcinoid heart disease from 89 to 192 mm (mean 132). Twelve-lead QRS voltages in 16 men aged 44 to 74 years (mean 55) without cardiovascular disease ranged from 84 to 159 mm (mean 124) and heart weight from 288 to 392 g (mean 351).[8] Thus, in groups of patients with the carcinoid syndrome, those with carcinoid heart disease have lower total 12-lead QRS voltages, but much overlap occurred between the 2 groups. Our patient had a total 12-lead QRS voltage of 127 mm. The duration of the P-R, QRS, and Q-T intervals and heart rates at rest were similar in the 2 groups with and without carcinoid heart disease.

The presence of pulmonary hypertension in our patient is most unusual in carcinoid heart disease and reasonably

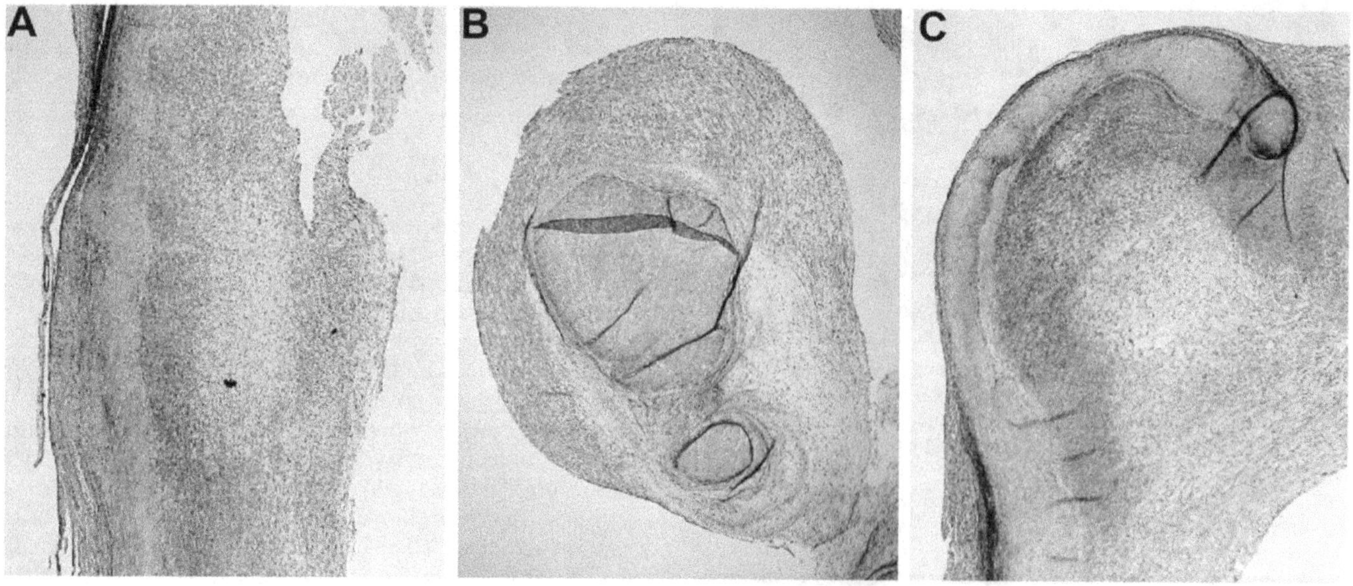

Figure 3. Photomicrograph of anterior mitral leaflet *(A)*, chordae tendineae *(B)*, and aortic valve cusp *(C)*. The underlying leaflet and chordae are normal, but both are quite thickened by superimposed cellular fibrous tissue devoid of elastic fibrils. The sinus portion of the aortic valve is filled with cellular fibrous tissue devoid of elastic fibers *(C)*. Elastic van Gieson's stains (100×).

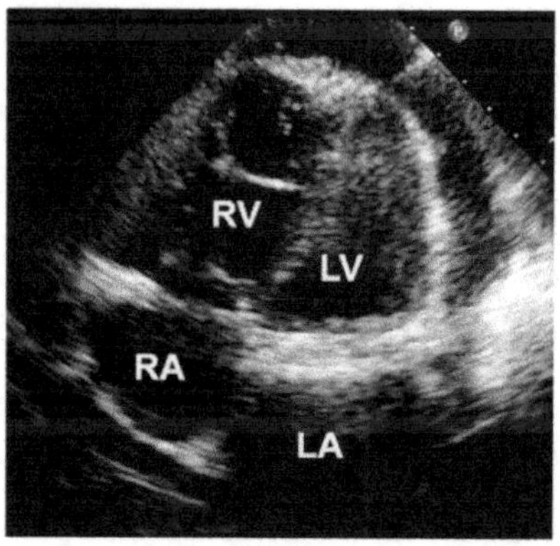

Figure 4. Four-chamber echocardiogram shortly before death in the patient described. The right ventricular cavity is severely dilated, whereas the left ventricle (LV) is not dilated. LA = left atrium; RA = right atrium; RV = right ventricle.

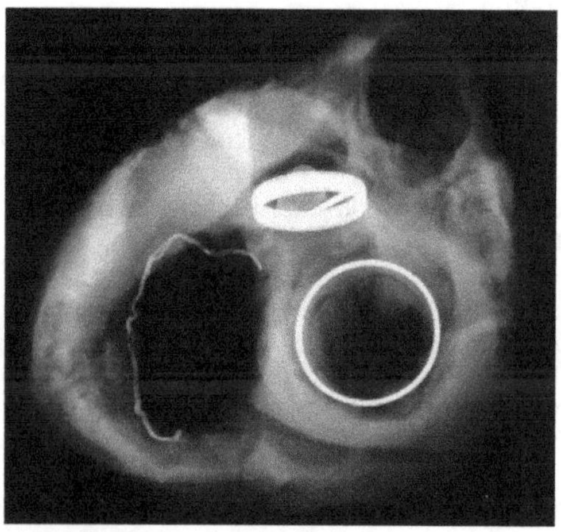

Figure 5. X-ray of the heart at necropsy. Prostheses are present in the mitral and aortic valve positions, and a ring is in the tricuspid valve annular position. The left ventricular cavity is not dilated, whereas the right ventricular cavity is considerably dilated.

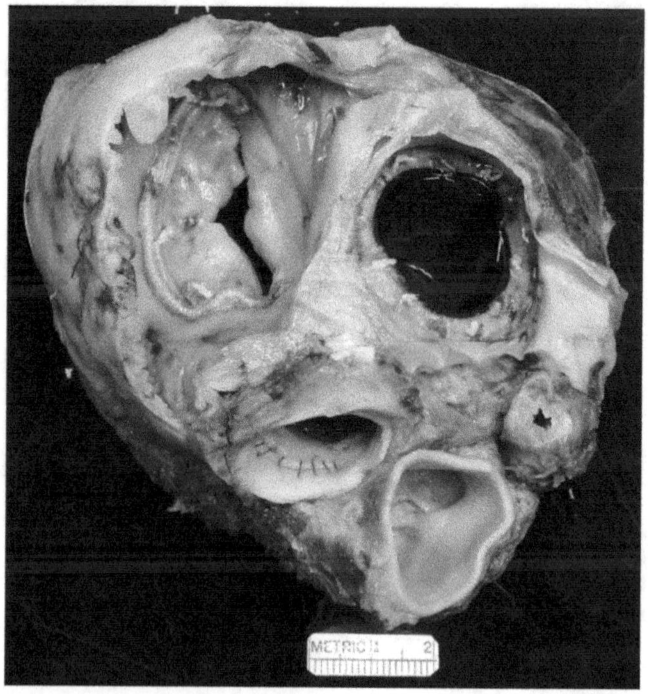

Figure 6. View of heart after removing the atrial walls and most of the ascending aorta and pulmonary trunk. The prosthesis in the mitral position fills the entire "floor" of the left atrium. The cloth-covered ring is visible in the tricuspid valve annulus.

can be attributed to the left-sided mitral disease.[9] The reason for its persistence postoperatively is unclear. The patient's symptoms worsened considerably postoperatively. The discs of the prostheses in both mitral and aortic positions moved without interference.

Cardiac valve replacement and/or "repair" for carcinoid heart disease is becoming more accepted, but nevertheless, outcomes are not always favorable.[9] In an early

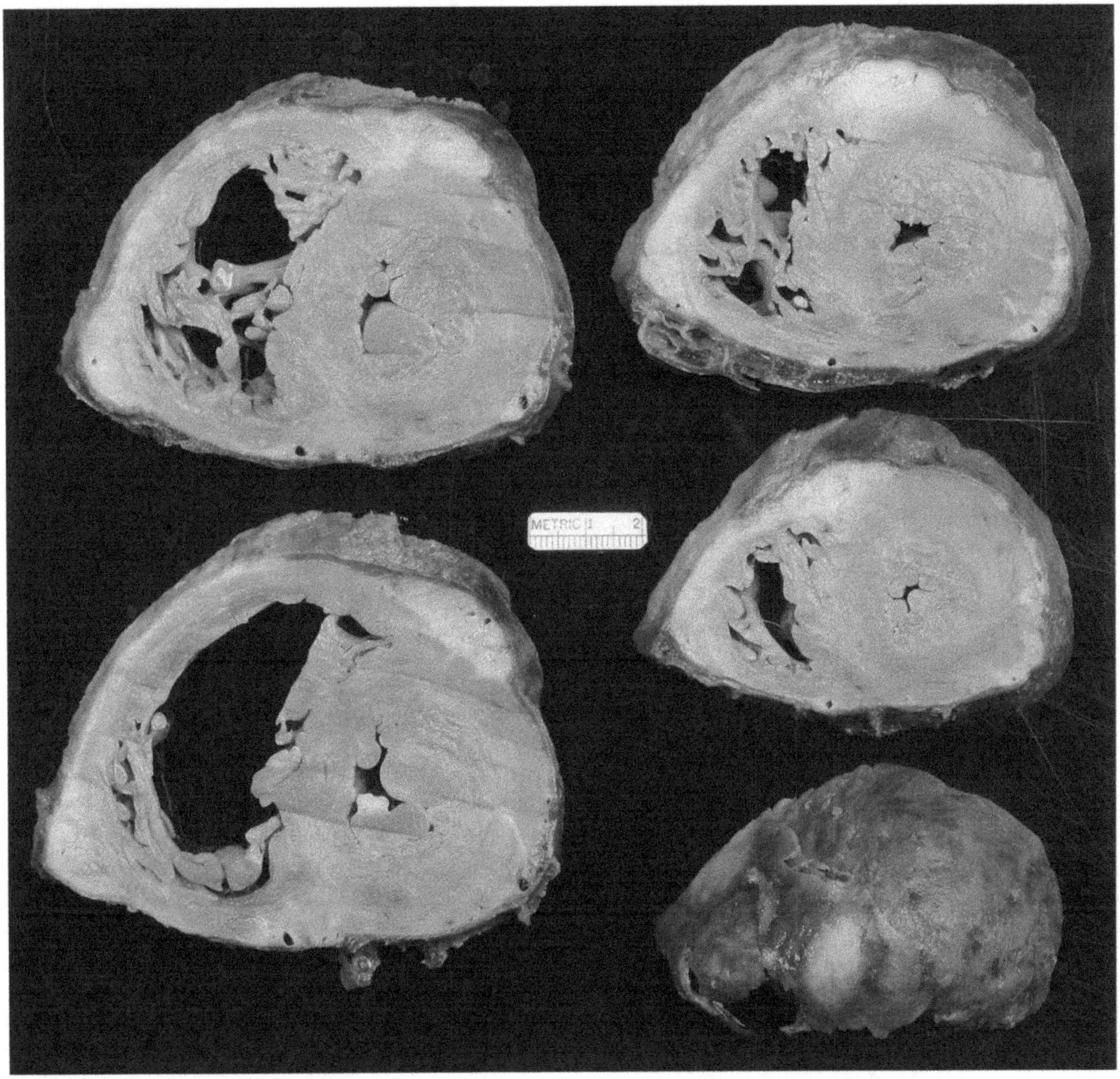

Figure 7. View of various "slices" of the cardiac ventricles showing the very small left ventricular cavity and the very dilated right ventricular cavity.

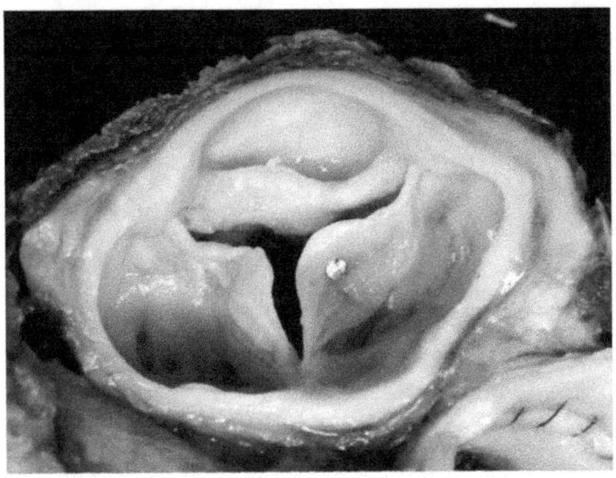

Figure 8. View of the pulmonic valve from above. The anterior cusp is very thick and immobile. The other 2 cusps are only mildly thickened by fibrous tissue.

report from the Mayo Clinic, 9 of 26 patients died in the early perioperative period and 9 others a mean of 19 months postoperatively. Only 4 of their 26 patients had mitral or aortic valve replacement, and none had both valves replaced, as did our patient. Although the mortality was higher, late operative survival (8 of 26 patients) resulted in considerable decrease (2 patients) or elimination (6 patients) of symptoms.[9] A later report from the same institution summarized results in 11 patients with carcinoid heart disease who underwent operation for left- and right-sided valve disease[10]: the tricuspid valve was replaced in all 11, the pulmonic in 3 (valvectomy in 7), the mitral valve in 6 (repair in 1), and the aortic valve in 4 (repair in 2). There were 2 perioperative deaths and 4 additional deaths in a mean follow-up period of 41 months. All but 1 operative survivor improved by ≥1 functional class. In retrospect, had the presence of carcinoid been recognized preoperatively or at operation in our patient, both tricuspid and pulmonic valves probably also would have been replaced (quadruple valve replacement).[11]

Acknowledgment: We thank Brad J. Roberts, BS, RCS, RDCS, for his help in preparing the echocardiogram.

1. Cassidy MA. Abdominal carcinomatosis with probable adrenal involvement. *Proc Roy Soc Med* 1930;24:139–141.
2. Roberts WC, Sjoerdsma A. The cardiac disease associated with the carcinoid syndrome (carcinoid heart disease). *Am J Med* 1964;36: 5–34.
3. Ross EM, Roberts WC. The carcinoid syndrome: comparison of 21 necropsy subjects with carcinoid heart disease to 15 necropsy subjects without carcinoid heart disease. *Am J Med* 1985;79:339–353.
4. Chaoqalit N, Connolly HM, Schaff HV, Webb MJ, Pellikka PA. Carcinoid heart disease associated with primary ovarian carcinoid tumor. *Am J Cardiol* 2004;93:1314–1315.
5. Rabban JT, Lerwill MF, McCluggage WG, Grenert JP, Zaloudek CJ. Primary ovarian carcinoid tumors may express CDX-2: a potential pitfall in distinction from metastatic intestinal carcinoid tumors involving the ovary. *Int J Gynecol Pathol* 2009;28:41–48.
6. Chatterjee K, Heather JC. Carcinoid heart disease from primary ovarian carcinoid tumors. *Am J Med* 1968;45:643–648.
7. Siegel RJ, Roberts WC. Electrocardiographic observations in severe aortic valve stenosis: correlative necropsy study to clinical, hemodynamic, and ECG variables demonstrating relation of 12-lead QRS amplitude to peak systolic transaortic pressure gradient. *Am Heart J* 1982;103:210–221.
8. Odom H II, Davis L, Dinh HA, Baker BJ, Roberts WC, Murphy ML. QRS voltage measurements in autopsied men free of cardiopulmonary disease: a basis for evaluating total QRS voltage as an index of left ventricular hypertrophy. *Am J Cardiol* 1986;58:801–804.
9. Connolly HM, Nishimura RA, Smith HC, Pellikka PA, Mullany CJ, Kvols LK. Outcome of cardiac surgery for carcinoid heart disease. *J Am Coll Cardiol* 1995;25:410–416.
10. Connolly HM, Schaff HV, Mullany CJ, Rubin J, Abel MD, Pellikka PA. Surgical management of left-sided carcinoid heart disease. *Circulation* 2001;104:I36–I40.
11. Arghami A, Connolly HM, Abel MD, Schaff HV. Quadruple valve replacement in patients with carcinoid heart disease. *J Thorac Cardiovasc Surg* 2010;140:1432–1434.

Cardiac Transplantation in Adults With Aortic Valve Disease With Focus on the Bicuspid Aortic Valve

William Clifford Roberts, MD[a,b,d,*], Carey Camille Roberts[d,e], Jong Mi Ko, BA[d], Shelley Anne Hall, MD[a,d], and John Edward Capehart, MD[c]

The frequency of congenitally bicuspid aortic valves in patients having cardiac transplantation (CT) is unknown. We reviewed 243 explanted hearts in patients having CT at Baylor University Medical Center, Dallas from June 1997 through November 2011 to determine the frequency of a bicuspid aortic valve in this population. Of the 243 explanted hearts, 7 (2.9%) were found to have a congenitally bicuspid aortic valve: 3 had severe aortic valve stenosis and before CT had had the aortic valve replaced; the other 4 had normally functioning bicuspid valves and underwent CT for cardiomyopathy (ischemic in 1, idiopathic in 2, and hypertrophic in 1). Review of previously published reports of CT and aortic valve disease disclosed that 4 patients had had aortic valve replacement (AVR) from 2 to 8 years before CT, 3 had AVR or aortic valve repair of the donor heart at the time of CT, and 4 had AVR or transcatheter aortic valve implantation from 1 to 14 years after CT. Some of these aortic valve replacements, before, at the time of, or after CT were in patients with congenitally bicuspid aortic valves. In conclusion, congenitally bicuspid aortic valves were found in 7 of 243 explanted hearts in patients having CT at a single medical center in a 14-year period: 4 had functioned normally and 3 were severely stenotic. Previous reports of patients having AVR or repair before, during, and after CT were reviewed. **(Am J Cardiol 2012;109:1212–1214)**

Cardiac transplantation (CT) is performed mainly in patients with ischemic or idiopathic dilated cardiomyopathy and infrequently in patients with valvular heart disease. This report describes the frequency of finding a bicuspid aortic valve in patients undergoing CT at a single medical center in a 14-year period and reviews previously published reports of patients having aortic valve replacement (AVR) or repair before, at the time of, and after CT.

Methods

From June 1997 through November 2011, CT was performed at Baylor University Medical Center, Dallas in 243 patients and in each the recipient heart was submitted to the cardiovascular division of the surgical pathology department. Each heart was examined and described by 1 of the authors (W.C.R.) and photographed. Among the 243 hearts studied, 9 had structural (primary) cardiac valve disease: 1 had had mitral valve replacement 2 times, originally for rheumatic mitral stenosis; 1 had replacement of both mitral and aortic valves for pure regurgitation secondary to radiation therapy for Hodgkin's disease many years previously; and the remaining 7 patients had congenitally bicuspid aortic valves, 3 stenotic valves had been replaced and the other 4 were functionally normal (Table 1).

This study was approved by the institutional review board at Baylor University Medical Center and informed consent was waived.

Results

Pertinent data in each of the 7 patients—all men—are presented in Table 1. Four of the 7 patients (cases 1 to 4) had normally functioning congenitally bicuspid aortic valves discovered during examination of the recipient heart: 2 of these patients had idiopathic dilated cardiomyopathy,[1] 1 had hypertrophic cardiomyopathy, and 1 had ischemic cardiomyopathy.

The remaining 3 patients (cases 5 to 7) had had AVR for aortic valve stenosis and all 3 had congenitally bicuspid aortic valves (Figure 1). Case 7 also had coronary artery bypass grafting at the time of AVR. The interval from AVR to CT in these 3 patients was 8, 4.7, and 5.2 years, respectively. During the interval from AVR to CT, heart failure persisted and eventually progressed in each to New York Heart Association class IV without evidence of significant dysfunction of the mechanical prosthesis or the bioprosthesis in the aortic valve position. Case 6 had a left ventricular assist device inserted 5 months before CT. All 3 patients had left ventricular ejection fractions during the months before CT of ≤20%. All 3 patients are alive as of October 28, 2011. The hearts in each of the 3 patients who had CT after AVR had very dilated left ventricular cavities (maximum internal diameter 5.5, 6.0, and 7.5 cm, respectively), hearts of increased weight (650, 730, and 615 g, respectively, not including the portion of the atrial walls to which the donor heart was connected), and 2 had transmural left ventricular

Departments of [a]Internal Medicine (Division of Cardiology), [b]Pathology, [c]Cardiothoracic Surgery, and [d]Baylor Heart and Vascular Institute, Baylor University Medical Center, Dallas, Texas; [e]Junior, The University of Georgia, Athens, Georgia. Manuscript received November 29, 2011; revised manuscript received and accepted December 1, 2011.

The study was funded by the Baylor Health Care System Foundation, Dallas, Texas.

*Corresponding author: Tel: 214-820-7911; fax: 214-820-7533.

E-mail address: wc.roberts@baylorhealth.edu (W.C. Roberts).

Table 1
Pertinent data in seven men having cardiac transplantation and congenitally bicuspid aortic valves with or without aortic valve replacement

Patient Number	Age at CT (years)	Diagnosis	AVR	Year of AVR	Interval (years) AVR → CT	LVAD	BMI (kg/m²)	LVEF (%)	Date of CT	HW (g)	LV Diameter (cm)	RV Diameter (cm)	CABG	CABG Date	LV Scar
1	35	HC	0	—	—	+	28.2	5	10/13/2011	435	6.0	1.0	0	—	0
2	46	IDC	0	—	—	+	29.9	15	12/23/2001	565	5.0	2.5	0	—	0
3	47*	IDC	0	—	—	+	30.3	10	4/25/2001	705	5.0	3.0	0	—	0
4	60	IC	0	—	—	0	27.5	7	7/1/2011	635	8.0	5.0	+	2005	+
5	30	AS	+ (SJM)	1991	8	0	25.0	10	10/14/1999	650	5.5	2.8	0	—	+
6	56	AS	+ (Bio)	2002	4.7	+	28.3	5	7/1/2007	730	6.0	4.0	0	—	0
7	65	AS	+ (SJM)	1997	5.2	0	18.4	20	1/16/2003	615	7.5	3.0	+	1997	+

— = not applicable; AS = aortic stenosis; AVR = aortic valve replacement; Bio = bioprosthesis; BMI = body mass index; CABG = coronary artery bypass grafting; CT = cardiac transplantation; HC = hypertrophic cardiomyopathy; HW = heart weight; IC = ischemic cardiomyopathy; IDC = idiopathic dilated cardiomyopathy; LV = left ventricular; LVAD = left ventricular assist device; LVEF = left ventricular ejection fraction; RV = right ventricular; SJM = St. Jude Medical mechanical prosthesis.
* Died March 22, 2011, or 10 years after cardiac transplantation.

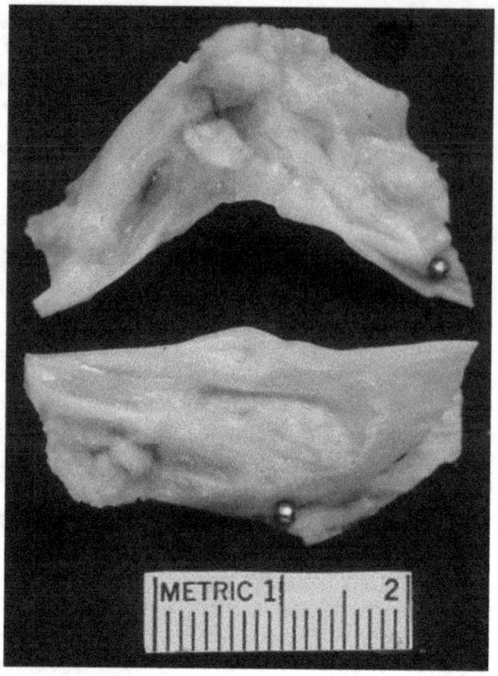

Figure 1. Case 6 (Table 1). Operatively excised severely stenotic congenitally bicuspid aortic valve.

scars, only 1 (case 7) of whom had narrowed coronary arteries. Case 6 had focally thickened left ventricular mural endocardium (possibly the consequence of the left ventricular assist device inserted 5 months previously).

Discussion

A common denominator in each of the heretofore described men was the presence of a congenitally malformed bicuspid aortic valve. In 4, the malformed valve functioned normally and was unrecognized during life. CT was performed in 2 of them because of idiopathic dilated cardiomyopathy, in 1 for ischemic cardiomyopathy, and in 1 for hypertrophic cardiomyopathy.

The remaining 3 patients had AVR for aortic stenosis superimposed on their malformed valve and of them 1 had concomitant coronary bypass grafting. The decision to do CT in these 3 patients rather than repeat AVR was based on the presence of progressively worsening heart failure without evidence of dysfunction of the mechanical prosthesis or bioprosthesis in the aortic valve position, extremely dilated left ventricular cavities (≥5 cm) in ventricular systole, and extremely low left ventricular ejection fractions (≤20%). These 3 patients may have had underlying dilated cardiomyopathy in addition to aortic stenosis.

The frequency of congenitally malformed aortic valves is unclear but probably is about 1% of the population, an involvement of about 3 million Americans.[2] In the present study, 7 congenitally malformed valves were found in 243 patients undergoing CT.

The present report is not the first to describe aortic valve disease and CT (Figure 2). Park et al[3] described a 33-year-old man who underwent orthotopic CT after 2 previous valve replacements for active infective endocarditis involving the native mitral and aortic valves followed by infection

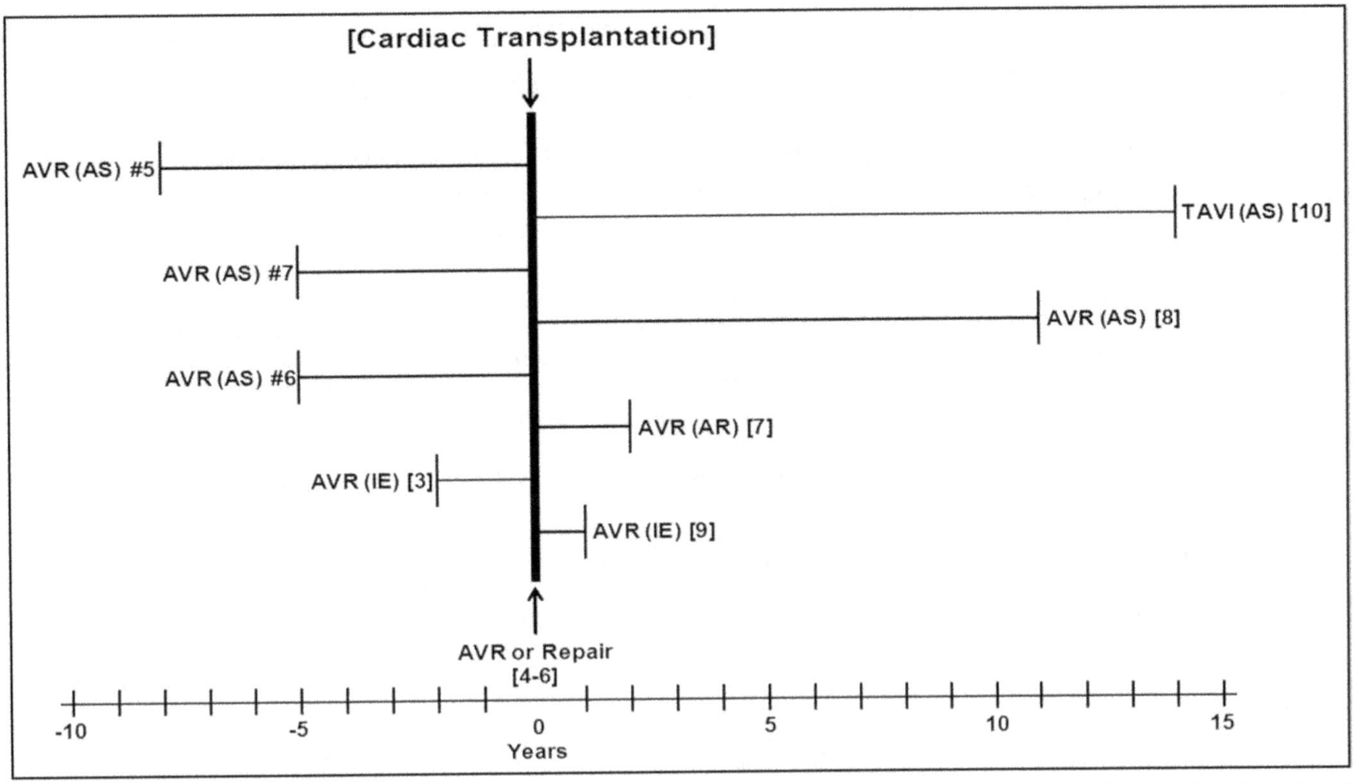

Figure 2. This diagram shows the present cases (5 to 7) and the previously reported patients *(reference in brackets)* having cardiac transplantation and aortic valve replacement or repair, before, at the time of, or after cardiac transplantation. Time in years *(horizontal axis)* is presented before (minus), at the time of, and after cardiac transplantation for aortic stenosis (AS) and/or regurgitation (AR). Several patients clearly had malfunctioning congenitally bicuspid aortic valves. IE = infective endocarditis; TAVI = transcatheter aortic valve implantation (without replacement).

involving the prosthetic aortic valve. Navia et al[4] repaired a purely regurgitant aortic valve in the donor heart before using it for CT. Rao et al[5] and Larobina et al[6] found a donor's heart to have a very stenotic aortic valve and replaced it before CT. Goenen et al[7] found a donor heart to have a mildly regurgitant congenitally bicuspid aortic valve, used the heart for CT, but 2 years after CT did AVR in the donor heart because of development of severe aortic regurgitation. Joyce et al[8] described severe aortic stenosis involving a congenitally bicuspid aortic valve in a donor heart 11 years after CT with successful AVR. Sayeed et al[9] performed AVR for infective endocarditis in a donor heart a year after CT. And finally, Seiffert et al[10] performed successfully transcatheter aortic valve implantation (without replacement) in a 67-year-old heart transplant recipient for severe symptomatic aortic stenosis 14 years after CT.

1. Roberts WC, Siegel RJ, McManus BM. Idiopathic dilated cardiomyopathy: analysis of 152 necropsy patients. *Am J Cardiol* 1987;60:1340–1355.
2. Roberts WC. The congenitally bicuspid aortic valve. A study of 85 autopsy cases. *Am J Cardiol* 1970;26:72–83.
3. Park SJ, Sullivan HJ, Lonchyna V, Hinkamp TJ, Pifarre R. Heart transplantation for complicated and recurrent early prosthetic valve endocarditis. *J Heart Lung Transplant* 1993;12:802–803.
4. Navia JL, Atik FA, Marullo A, Starling RC, Garcia M, Vega PR, Smedira NG, McCarthy PM. Bench repair of donor aortic valve with minimal access orthotopic heart transplantation. *Ann Thorac Surg* 2005;80:313–315.
5. Rao JN, Prendergast B, Dark JH. Orthotopic heart transplantation with concurrent aortic valve replacement and coronary artery bypass grafting. *J Heart Lung Transplant* 2000;19:897–899.
6. Larobina ME, Mariani JA, Rowland MA. Aortic valve replacement for aortic stenosis during orthotopic cardiac transplant. *Ann Thorac Surg* 2008;86:1979–1982.
7. Goenen MJ, Jacquet L, De Kock M, Van Dyck M, Schoevardts JC, Chalant CH. Aortic valve replacement thirty-one months after orthotopic heart transplantation. *J Heart Lung Transplant* 1991;10:604–607.
8. Joyce DL, Russell SD, Conte JV, Cattaneo SM. Aortic valve replacement in a diseased bicuspid valve eleven years after transplantation. *Interact Cardiovasc Thorac Surg* 2009;8:594–595.
9. Sayeed R, Drain AJ, Sivasothy PS, Large SR, Wallwork J. Aortic valve replacement for late infective endocarditis after heart-lung transplantation. *Trans Proc* 2005;37:4537–4539.
10. Seiffert M, Meyer S, Franzen O, Conradi L, Baldus S, Schirmer J, Deuse T, Costard-Jaeckle A, Reichenspurner H, Treede H. Transcatheter aortic valve implantation in a heart transplant recipient: a case report. *Trans Proc* 2010;42:4661–4663.

Clues to Diagnosing Carcinoid Heart Disease as the Cause of Isolated Right-Sided Heart Failure

Carey Camille Roberts, BS[a,b], Rohit J. Parmar, MD[b,c], Paul A. Grayburn, MD[b,c], Gautam R. Patankar, MD[b,c], Jong Mi Ko, BA[b], Baron L. Hamman, MD[d], and William Clifford Roberts, MD[b,c,e,*]

Described herein is a 67-year-old woman who underwent replacement of both tricuspid and pulmonic valves because of severe isolated right-sided systolic heart failure. The cause of the heart failure preoperatively was believed to be the result of left breast radiation a year earlier. At operation, however, the pulmonic valve was excised and a biopsy of the stiff-walled right atrium was performed, and histologic examination of each was classic of carcinoid heart disease. She never awoke postoperatively. Postoperatively, computed tomography disclosed numerous masses in the liver. Retrospectively, clues to the presence of carcinoid heart disease include thickening of both the tricuspid and pulmonic valve leaflets by echocardiogram, a pressure gradient, albeit small, across the pulmonic valve, the plastering of the septal tricuspid-valve leaflet to the ventricular septum, the total absence of left-sided heart disease, and the presence of extremely low 12-lead QRS electrocardiographic voltage. **(Am J Cardiol 2014;114:1623–1626)**

The most common cause of right-sided heart failure is left-sided heart failure. Isolated right-sided heart failure is far less common than that associated with left-sided heart failure, and usually results from pulmonary disease (parenchymal, vascular and/or bellows-system abnormalities), all of which produce pulmonary hypertension. Constrictive pericardial diseases and isolated congenital pulmonic-valve stenosis are far less common causes. Carcinoid heart disease as a cause of right-sided heart failure is rare, but distinctive clues to its presence are usually discernible[1–6] (Figure 1). This report describes a patient with undiagnosed carcinoid heart disease and discusses certain clinical clues which may have established the proper diagnosis and prevented the unsuccessful right-sided double-valve replacement.

Case Description

This 67-year-old white woman apparently had been in her usual state of health until age 57 when she had a knee replacement (December 2001) because of osteoarthritis. An electrocardiogram at the time showed total 12-lead QRS voltage to be 158 mm (measured with normal [10 mm] standardization [10 mm = 1 mV]) (Figure 2). At age 66 (2012), she underwent left breast lumpectomy for confirmed cancer and received radiation to that breast and to the left

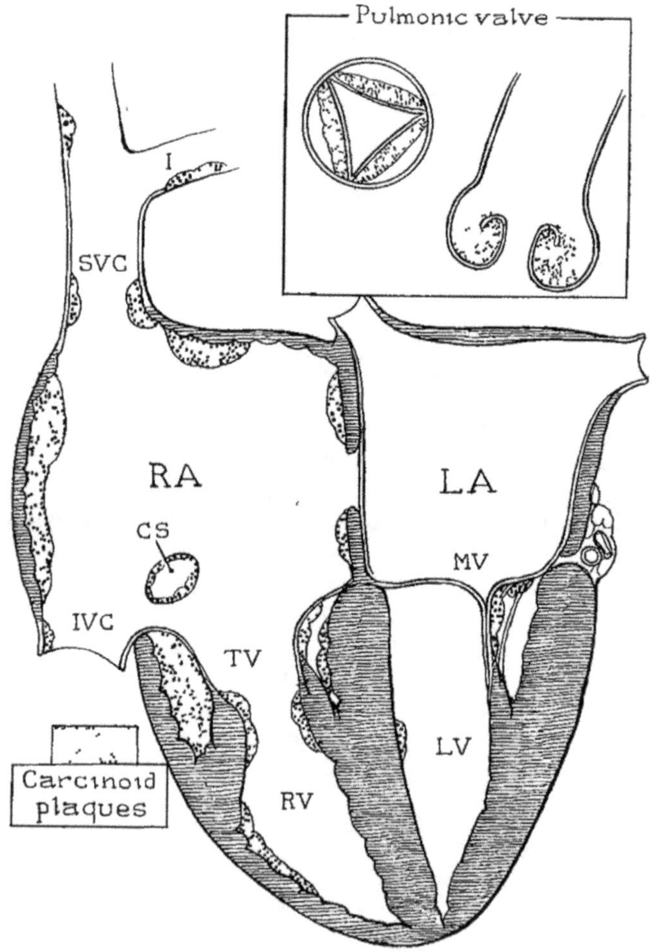

Figure 1. Diagram showing the usual location of carcinoid plaques in patients with carcinoid heart disease. CS = coronary sinus ostium; I = innominate vein; IVC = inferior vena cava; LA = left atrium; LV = left ventricle; MV = mitral valve; RA = right atrium; RV = right ventricle; SVC = superior vena cava; TV = tricuspid valve. Reproduced with permission from the authors (Ross EM and Roberts WC) and the publisher (Elsevier).[4]

[a]Second Year, Georgetown University School of Medicine, Washington, DC and [b]The Baylor Heart and Vascular Institute, Departments of [c]Internal Medicine (Division of Cardiology), [d]Cardiothoracic Surgery, and [e]Pathology, Baylor University Medical Center, Dallas, Texas. Manuscript received July 23, 2014; revised manuscript received and accepted August 15, 2014.

Support for this investigation was provided by the Baylor Health Care System Foundation through the Cardiovascular Research Review Committee in cooperation with the Baylor Heart and Vascular Institute.

See page 1626 for disclosure information.

*Corresponding author: Tel: (214) 820-7911; fax: (214) 820-7533.

E-mail address: wc.roberts@baylorhealth.edu (W.C. Roberts).

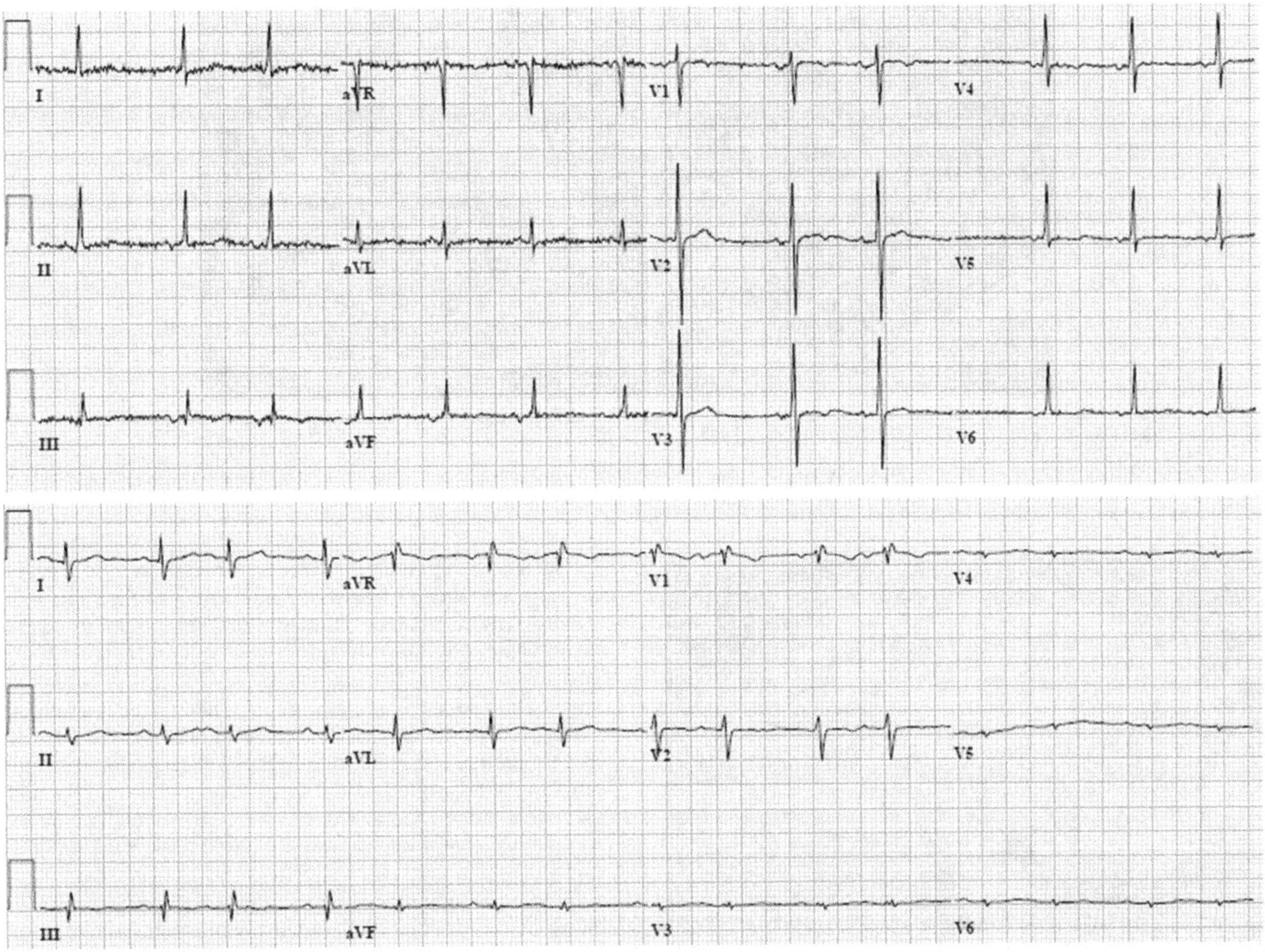

Figure 2. Electrocardiograms of the described patient at age 57 (December 2001) (*upper*) showing total 12-lead QRS voltage to be 158 mm (measured with normal [10 mm] standardization [10 mm = 1 mV]). Electrocardiogram from same patient 11 years later at age 66 (2012) (*lower*) with right-sided heart failure showing total 12-lead QRS voltage to be 51 mm, the presence of incomplete right bundle branch block, and atrial premature complexes.

axillary region. At age 67, peripheral edema, abdominal swelling, and weight gain appeared and each progressively worsened over a 6-month period during which time she gained 40 pounds. Examination in August 2013 confirmed the presence of anasarca. Facial flushing, diarrhea or labile blood pressure, if present, was not recorded. A precordial murmur was described as absent. An electrocardiogram now showed total 12-lead QRS of 51 mm; incomplete right bundle branch block and atrial premature complexes (Figure 2). Echocardiogram disclosed both pulmonic and tricuspid valve regurgitation, thickening of both valvular leaflets, immobility of the tricuspid valve leaflets, severe dilatation of both right sided chambers, and no dilatation of the left-sided chambers (Figure 3). Cardiac catheterization disclosed the following pressures in mm Hg: pulmonary artery, 30/10; right ventricle, 43/18; right atrial mean 18 with V wave 25 and pulmonary arterial wedge mean 8. The cardiac index was 1.4 L/min/m^2. The left ventricular ejection fraction was approximately 60%. Coronary angiography disclosed insignificant narrowing (<30% diameter reduction).

In September 2013, the pulmonic valve was replaced with a homograft and the tricuspid valve, with a bioprosthesis (Edwards, Magna Ease). The tricuspid valve leaflets and chordae were sclerotic. Early postoperatively, excessive bleeding necessitated reexploration. Computed tomographic examination of the heart during the post-operative period disclosed an enlarged liver (23 cm in greatest dimension) containing innumerable masses (Figure 4) and "… focal thickening of the cecum and terminal ileum." During the entire 10-day post-operative period, the patient never awoke and had fatal multi-organ "failure".

Examination of the operatively-excised thickened pulmonic valve and of a portion of the thickened right atrial wall disclosed classic changes of carcinoid heart disease (Figure 5). Necropsy was not performed.

Discussion

The patient described had some clinical features suggesting the presence of carcinoid heart disease. These

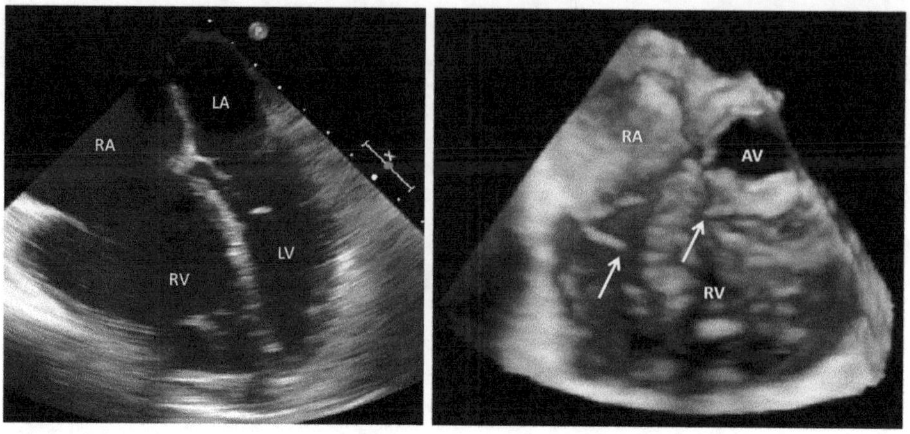

Figure 3. Transesophageal echocardiographic 4-chamber view showing right ventricular volume overload pattern with dilated right ventricle (RV) and right atrium (RA) and paradoxical ventricular septal motion. Left ventricle (LV) and left atrium (LA) are of normal size and there was no atrial septal defect (*left*). Three-dimensional short-axis view of the right atrium (RA), right ventricle (RV) and aortic valve (AV). The tricuspid leaflets (*arrows*) are shortened, thickened and immobile, consistent with carcinoid heart disease (*right*).

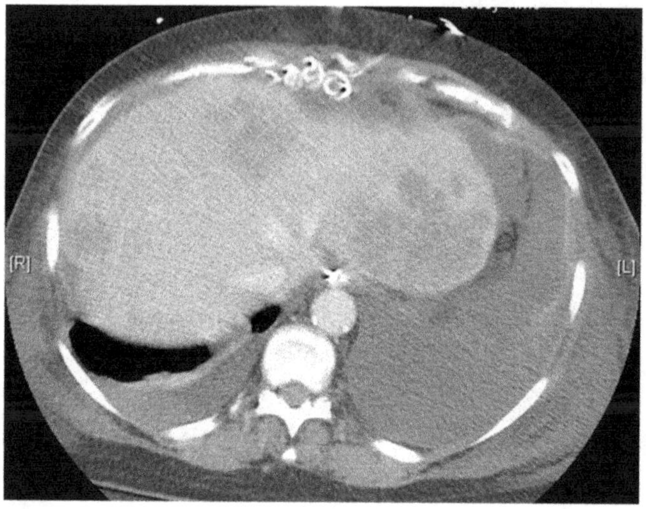

Figure 4. Computed tomographic image of the abdomen showing enlarged liver with innumerable masses.

features included severe isolated right-sided heart failure (anasarca), thickened pulmonic and tricuspid valve leaflets with severe regurgitation of both valves and some stenosis of the pulmonic valve, the absence of left-sided heart disease, the absence of pulmonary disease including the absence of pulmonary hypertension, the presence of extremely low total 12-lead QRS voltage on electrocardiogram, and, the clincher, the presence of classic superimposed fibromuscular tissue on the operatively excised pulmonic valve cusps and on the mural endocardium of the right atrium (which was biopsied).[1–6]

A major clue to diagnosis was the echocardiogram which showed severe right-sided dilatation unassociated with any left-sided dilatation or atrial septal defect. Additionally, both tricuspid and pulmonic valve leaflets were thickened and the tricuspid leaflets immobile, something not seen in patients with cor pulmonale. The echocardiogram also suggested the absence of pulmonary hypertension, a requirement for the presence of cor pulmonale. And, most important, there was no evidence of any pulmonary disease.

Because the patient had received radiation a year earlier for cancer of the left breast, the thickening of the right-sided valves was attributed clinically to the radiation-induced heart valve disease. An earlier study, however, had suggested that significant cardiac valve thickening secondary to radiation takes years as a rule to occur after completion of the radiation therapy.[7] The interval between the 2 events in our patient was no more than 1 year. Moreover, the radiation was limited to the left breast and axilla, yet only the right-sided heart valves were involved, a pattern more consistent with carcinoid heart disease than radiation injury.

Hemodynamic clues that carcinoid heart disease was the cause of the isolated right-sided heart failure was the pressure gradient—albeit small (13 mm Hg)—across the pulmonic valve. Such gradients across this valve do not occur in patients with cor pulmonale. The normal pulmonary arterial wedge pressure and the normal left ventricular end-diastolic pressures in the presence of the very elevated right atrial mean and right ventricular end-diastolic pressures rule out constrictive pericarditis as the cause of the isolated right-sided heart failure.

The extremely low QRS voltage on electrocardiogram fits the picture of carcinoid heart disease. Roberts and colleagues[8] studied total 12-lead QRS voltage in 11 different cardiac conditions (aortic stenosis, pure aortic regurgitation, pure mitral regurgitation, hypertrophic cardiomyopathy, idiopathic dilated cardiomyopathy, amyloid heart disease, cardiac adiposity and the carcinoid syndrome among others) and found that the 19 patients with carcinoid heart disease had the lowest 12-lead QRS voltage (mean 105) except for the 30 patients with cardiac amyloidosis who had a total 12-lead mean QRS voltage of 104 mm (measured with normal [10 mm] standardization [10 mm = 1 mV]). Our patient near the end of life preoperatively had a total 12-lead QRS voltage of 51 mm!

And finally, the finding by computed tomography of multiple masses in the liver occurs in nearly 100% of patients with the carcinoid syndrome with or without carcinoid heart disease.[4] In contrast, metastasis to the liver of a patient with carcinoma of the breast occurs in only about 20%.[9–13]

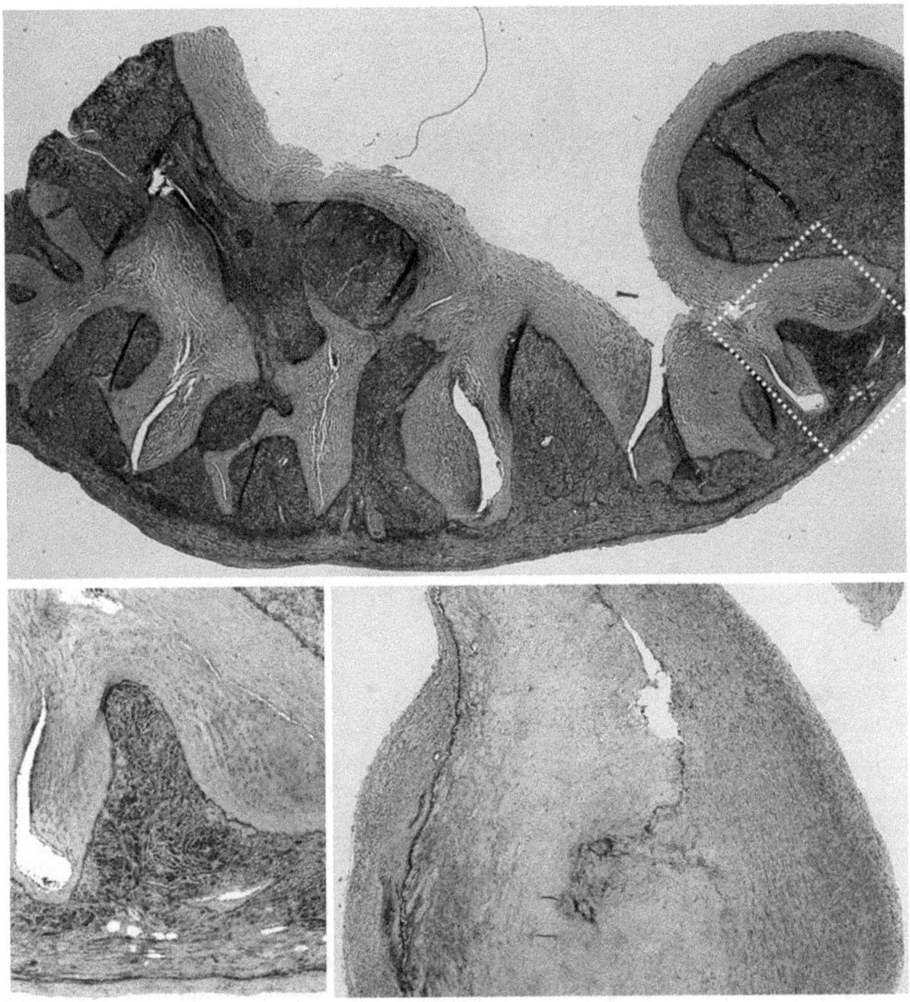

Figure 5. Histologic section of wall of right atrium (*top, lower left*) and pulmonic valve cusp (*lower right*). Carcinoid plaque (*stained green*) is superimposed on the mural endocardium of the right atrium and on the cusp and endocardium of the pulmonic valve. Movat stains: x20 (*upper*); x100 (*lower left*); x40 (*lower right*).

The superimposed fibromuscular tissue devoid of elastic fibers on the mural endocardium of right atrium and similar tissue superimposed on the pulmonic valve cusps is diagnostic of carcinoid heart disease.[1–6]

Disclosures

There are no conflicts of interest for any author.

1. Roberts WC, Sjoerdsma A. The cardiac disease associated with the carcinoid syndrome (carcinoid heart disease). *Am J Med* 1964;36:5–34.
2. Roberts WC, Mason DT, Wright LD Jr. The non-distensible right atrium of carcinoid disease of the heart. *Am J Clin Pathol* 1965;44:627–631.
3. Ferrans VJ, Roberts WC. The carcinoid endocardial plaque. An ultrastructural study. *Hum Pathol* 1976;7:387–409.
4. Ross EM, Roberts WC. The carcinoid syndrome: comparison of 21 necropsy subjects with carcinoid heart disease to 15 necropsy subjects without carcinoid heart disease. *Am J Med* 1985;79:339–354.
5. Roberts WC. A unique heart disease associated with a unique cancer: carcinoid heart disease. *Am J Cardiol* 1997;80:251–256.
6. Roberts WC, Varughese CA, Ko JM, Grayburn PA, Hebeler RF Jr, Burton EC. Carcinoid heart disease without the carcinoid syndrome but with quadrivalvular regurgitation and unsuccessful operative intervention. *Am J Cardiol* 2011;107:788–792.
7. Brosius FC 3rd, Waller BF, Roberts WC. Radiation heart disease. Analysis of 16 young (aged 15 to 33 years) necropsy patients who received over 3,500 rads to the heart. *Am J Med* 1981;70:519–530.
8. Roberts WC, Filardo G, Ko JM, Siegel RJ, Dollar AL, Ross EM, Shirani J. Comparison of total 12-lead QRS voltage in a variety of cardiac conditions and its usefulness in predicting increased cardiac mass. *Am J Cardiol* 2013;112:904–909.
9. Van Walsum GAM, de Ridder JAM, Verhoef C, Bosscha K, van Gulik TM, Hesselink EJ, Ruers TJM, van den Tol MP, Nagtegaal ID, Brouwers M, van Hillegersberg R, Porte RJ, Rijken AM, Strobbe LJA, de Wilt JHW. Resection of liver metastases in patients with breast cancer: survival and prognostic factors. *EJSO* 2012;38:910–917.
10. Mariani P, Servois V, Rycke YD, Bennett SP, Feron JG, Alumbarak MM, Reyal F, Baranger B, Pierga JY, Salmon RJ. Liver metastases from breast cancer: surgical resection or not? A case-matched control study in highly selected patients. *EJSO* 2013;39:1377–1383.
11. Kim JY, Park JS, Lee SA, Kim JK, Jeong J, Yoon DS, Lee HD. Does liver resection provide long-term survival benefits for breast cancer patients with liver metastasis? A single hospital experience. *Yonsei Med J* 2014;55:558–562.
12. Cummings MC, Simpson PT, Reid LE, Jayanthan J, Skerman J, Song S, McCart Reed AE, Kutasovic JR, Morey AL, Marquart L, O'Rourke P, Lakhani SR. Metastatic progression of breast cancer: insights from 50 years of autopsies. *J Pathol* 2014;232:23–31.
13. Elsberger B, Roxburgh CS, Horgan PG. Is there a role for surgical resections of hepatic breast cancer metastases? *Hepatogastroenterology* 2014;61:181–186.

Case report: whole exome sequencing of primary cardiac angiosarcoma highlights potential for targeted therapies

Leah Zhrebker[1,2*], Irene Cherni[3], Lara M. Gross[2], Margaret M. Hinshelwood[1], Merrick Reese[1,4], Jessica Aldrich[3], Joseph M. Guileyardo[5], William C. Roberts[2,5], David Craig[3], Daniel D. Von Hoff[6], Robert G. Mennel[1,4,7] and John D. Carpten[3]

Abstract

Background: Primary cardiac angiosarcomas are rare, but they are the most aggressive type of primary cardiac neoplasms. When patients do present, it is with advanced pulmonary and/or cardiac symptoms. Therefore, many times the correct diagnosis is not made at the time of initial presentation. These patients have metastatic disease and the vast majority of these patients die within a few months after diagnosis. Currently the treatment choices are limited and there are no targeted therapies available.

Case presentation: A 56-year-old male presented with shortness of breath, night sweats, and productive cough for a month. Workup revealed pericardial effusion and multiple bilateral pulmonary nodules suspicious for metastatic disease. Transthoracic echocardiogram showed a large pericardial effusion and a large mass in the base of the right atrium. Results of biopsy of bilateral lung nodules established a diagnosis of primary cardiac angiosarcoma. Aggressive pulmonary disease caused rapid deterioration; the patient went on hospice and subsequently died. Whole exome sequencing of the patient's postmortem tumor revealed a novel *KDR* (G681R) mutation, and focal high-level amplification at chromosome 1q encompassing *MDM4*, a negative regulator of TP53.

Conclusion: Mutations in *KDR* have been reported previously in angiosarcomas. Previous studies also demonstrated that *KDR* mutants with constitutive KDR activation could be inhibited with specific KDR inhibitors in vitro. Thus, patients harboring activating *KDR* mutations could be candidates for treatment with KDR-specific inhibitors.

Keywords: Cardiac angiosarcoma, Whole exome sequencing, Activating gene mutation, Targeted therapies

Background

Primary cardiac tumors are very rare; the reported incidence in most autopsy and surgery series varies from 0.001 to 0.3% [1–3]. Of tumors that arise in the heart, most are benign and approximately 25% are malignant. About 95% of the malignant tumors are sarcomas, and they comprise 10 to 15% of the total primary cardiac tumors. Sarcomas can develop in any site in the heart, but angiosarcomas, which account for a third of all sarcomas, normally originate in the right atrium near the atrioventricular groove [4, 5].

Initially, there are no noticeable symptoms for patients with cardiac angiosarcoma. When patients do present they tend to have locally advanced or metastatic disease. Most symptoms are related to intracardiac flow obstruction, pericardial effusion and tamponade, tumor embolism, and systemic or constitutional symptoms due to metastatic disease [6–8]. Lung metastases are common at presentation [4, 9]. Additionally, metastases have been reported in liver, lymph nodes, bone, adrenal glands, and to a lesser extent the central nervous system (CNS) and spleen [4, 9]. Due to the late stage at presentation, prognosis for patients with primary angiosarcoma of the heart is poor; median overall survival varies from 6 months or less for

* Correspondence: Leah.Zhrebker@BSWHealth.org
[1]Baylor Charles A. Sammons Cancer Center at Dallas, Baylor University Medical Center at Dallas, 3410 Worth Street, Dallas, TX 75246, USA
[2]Department of Internal Medicine, Baylor University Medical Center at Dallas, 3500 Gaston Ave, Dallas, TX 75246, USA
Full list of author information is available at the end of the article

untreated patients to 12 months for patients with incomplete tumor resection [6, 10–12]. Tumor often invades into the adjacent tissues, making complete resection challenging, if not impossible. In some cases, cardiac transplantation for patients with primary cardiac angiosarcoma has been reported, albeit with poor outcomes, with most patients dying from recurrence within 1 year of surgery. Cardiac transplantation is not currently recommended even for patients without evidence of metastatic disease due to lack of survival benefit to patients with transplantation [13–15].

Existing treatment strategies include resection for non-metastatic disease, chemotherapy, and radiation. There are limited data showing chemotherapy treatment algorithms for cardiac angiosarcoma. Currently used chemotherapies include traditional agents such as paclitaxel, docetaxel, and doxorubicin. Angiogenesis inhibitors, drugs that target the growth of endothelial cells, such as bevacizumab, sunitinib, and sorafenib, have been used as well. Although some therapies may extend the lifespan of patients when combined with other modalities [16], none of the traditional chemotherapies or newer agents have been shown to eradicate microscopic disease [17–20]. Lack of efficacy in existing treatment options highlights the need for targeted cancer therapies for patients with cardiac angiosarcoma.

To date, various studies investigated specific genes and pathways altered in angiosarcoma. V-Myc Avian Myelocytomatosis Viral Oncogene Homolog (*MYC*) amplified tumors are common in radiation-induced and lymphedema-associated angiosarcomas [21]. Moreover, Fms Related Tyrosine Kinase 4 (*FLT4*) and *MYC* co-amplification was observed in 25% of secondary angiosarcomas [22]. Point mutations in V-Ki-ras2 Kirsten rat sarcoma viral oncogene homolog (*KRAS*) oncogene were found in liver angiosarcoma [23]. In other reports, a primary skin angiosarcoma and liver angiosarcoma lacked expression of p16, the product of the Cyclin Dependent Kinase Inhibitor 2A (*CDKN2A*) gene [24–26]. A number of studies found high expression of mutated Tumor protein P53 (*TP53*) gene in the tumor cells of angiosarcoma from various tissues of origin [26–29]. Microarray expression studies revealed upregulation of a number of vascular-specific receptor tyrosine kinases, including Tyrosine Kinase with Immunoglobulin like and EGF Like Domains 1 (*TIE1*), Kinase Insert Domain Receptor (*KDR*), SNF Related Kinase (*SNRK*), TEK Receptor Tyrosine Kinase (*TEK*), and Fms Related Tyrosine Kinase 1 (*FLT1*) in angiosarcomas [30]. Further examination of these five genes by full-sequencing identified 10% of angiosarcoma patients harbored mutations in the *KDR* gene [30]. More recently, whole exome sequencing of primary and secondary angiosarcoma demonstrated mutations in the endothelial phosphatase, Protein tyrosine phosphatase, receptor type, B (*PTPRB*) and Phospholipase C, gamma 1 (*PLCG1*), a signal transducer of tyrosine kinase activators [31]. In the current study, we used custom-designed expanded exome capture to interrogate the genome of an aggressive primary cardiac angiosarcoma case using a genome-wide sequencing approach that included analysis of the annotated coding exome along with additional probes that allowed for genome-wide copy number analysis and the structural analysis of specific regions of the genome to capture translocations and inversions. This analysis allowed for a comprehensive assessment of the genomic landscape of this aggressive angiosarcoma.

Herein we describe the results of whole exome sequencing a primary, cardiac angiosarcoma. We found a novel *KDR* (G681R) mutation which is a putative ligand-independent activating mutation. Additionally, we discovered a focal high-level amplification at chromosome 1q encompassing MDM4 p53 binding protein homolog (*MDM4*), a negative regulator of TP53. We discuss potential therapeutic therapies which may be effective in treating patients with tumors containing these mutations/amplifications.

Case presentation

This case was presented previously [32]. Briefly, a 56-year-old Caucasian male was transferred to our hospital for possible pericardial window by cardiothoracic surgery after a transthoracic echocardiogram revealed a large pericardial effusion. A computed tomography scan of the chest revealed numerous pulmonary nodules surrounded by ground glass densities, along with small pleural effusions, and moderate to large pericardial effusion. Approximately 1250 ml of fluid was removed by pericardiocentesis, and the fluid was negative for the presence of infection or malignancy. Whole body positron emission tomography scan revealed a large, irregularly shaped, strikingly hypermetabolic cardiac lesion of probable right atrium origin (Fig. 1a). Moreover, there were extensive hypermetabolic pulmonary nodules in a background of ground glass infiltrates (Fig. 1b). A provisional diagnosis of cardiac sarcoma was made, and the patient underwent a left video-assisted thoracotomy, pericardial window and biopsy, and left lower lobe resection. Tumor cells in the lung nodules were both epitheliod and spindle-shaped in appearance. They were immunoreactive for Cluster of Differentiation (CD)31, CD34, and Factor VIII-related antigen, findings that were consistent with an angiosarcoma (Fig. 2). Given the aggressive nature of this cancer, the patient declined treatment and proceeded with in-hospital hospice where he expired on hospital day 19. Postmortem examination showed a large tumor was present in the right atrium attached just cephalad to the tricuspid valve annulus, anteriorly and laterally (Fig. 3). The tumor extended into

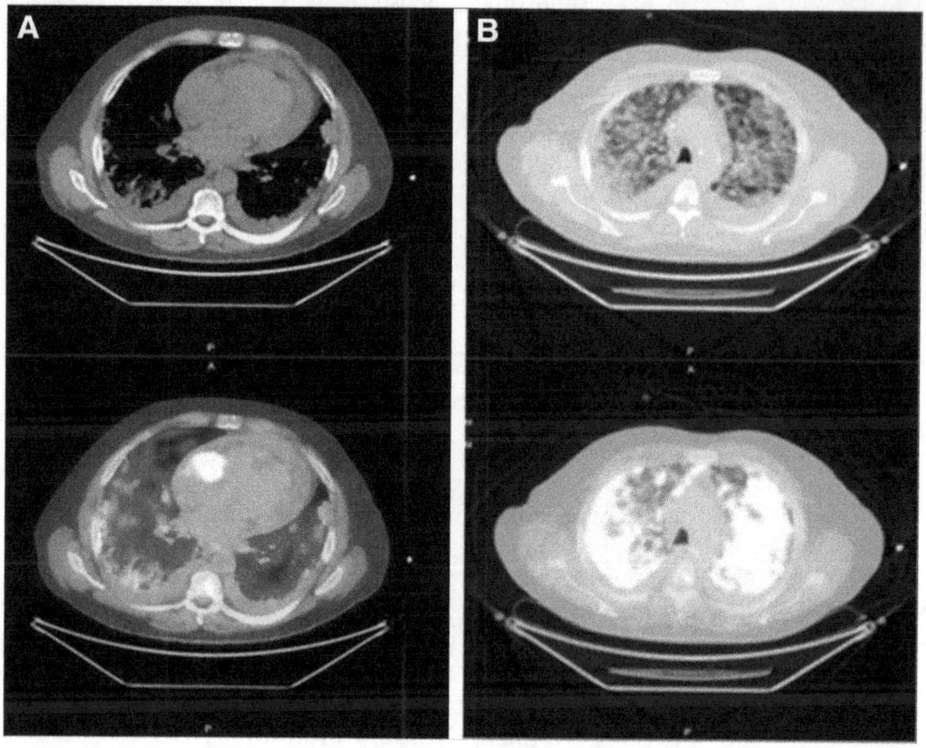

Fig. 1 Chest PET/CT Scan. **a** Chest PET/CT scan of the chest revealed abnormal uptake in the right atrium with an SUV of 14.9. **b** Chest PET/CT scan showed ground glass appearance and uptake indicative of nodules and pleural effusions in lungs; maximal SUVs of lung nodules were 9.0

the right atrioventricular sulcus. The right coronary artery was compressed by the tumor in the right atrioventricular sulcus. The neoplasm extended just slightly into the right ventricular wall but was not present in the ventricular septum, left ventricular free wall, or in the left atrial wall.

Methods

Immunohistochemistry

Immunohistochemical staining was performed on tissue sections of formalin-fixed, paraffin-embedded (FFPE) tumor samples using the BenchMarch System (Ventana Medical Systems, Inc., Tucson, AZ). The following primary antibodies were used: An anti-CD31 mouse monoclonal antibody from Dako North America, Inc. (Carpinteria, CA; M0823; lot # 00079267; 1:100 dilution), an anti-CD34 mouse monoclonal antibody from Ventana Medical Systems, Inc (790-2927; lot # 1327304B; 1:1 dilution), and a Factor VIII-related antigen rabbit polyclonal antibody from Cell Marque Corp. (Rocklin, CA; 250A; lot # 1113210A; 1:100 dilution).

Custom probe design for target enrichment

For this project, we used a set of custom baits (Agilent Technologies, Inc.; Cat# G9496C). Briefly, components of the expanded exome included the following probe groups: original baits from SureSelect Human All Exon V5, (Agilent Technologies, Inc.; Cat # 5190-6209), custom baits for select break point regions which can result in oncogenic fusions (as defined by the COSMIC database v67), and common tumor suppressor transcribed regions (Additional file 1: Table S1). Additionally, to aid in copy number alteration analysis, Agilent 44 k human comparative genomic hybridization (aCGH) probes (Agilent Technologies, Inc.) were supplemented in the regions where there was no strategic bait coverage (Additional file 2: Table S2). Expanded exome resulted in a custom 55.2 Mbp targeted design.

DNA isolation

Genomic DNA was isolated from frozen blood using the Qiagen QiaAmp DNA Blood Maxi Kit (Qiagen, Inc., Valencia, CA). Specifically, frozen blood (8 ml) was allowed to equilibrate to room temperature and supplemented with 2 ml of PBS. The mixture was then treated with Qiagen protease. Lysis buffer was added to the mixture and DNA isolation was conducted as written per the manufacturer's the protocol. DNA was eluted in 1000 μl of Buffer AE. The purified DNA was quantified using the Qubit 2.0 Fluorometer (Life Technologies, Grand Island, NY). Absorbance ratios (260/280 and 260/230) were obtained using Nanodrop spectrophotometer (Thermo Fisher Scientific, Inc. Waltham, MA). Tumor DNA was isolated from FFPE tissue using Qiagen

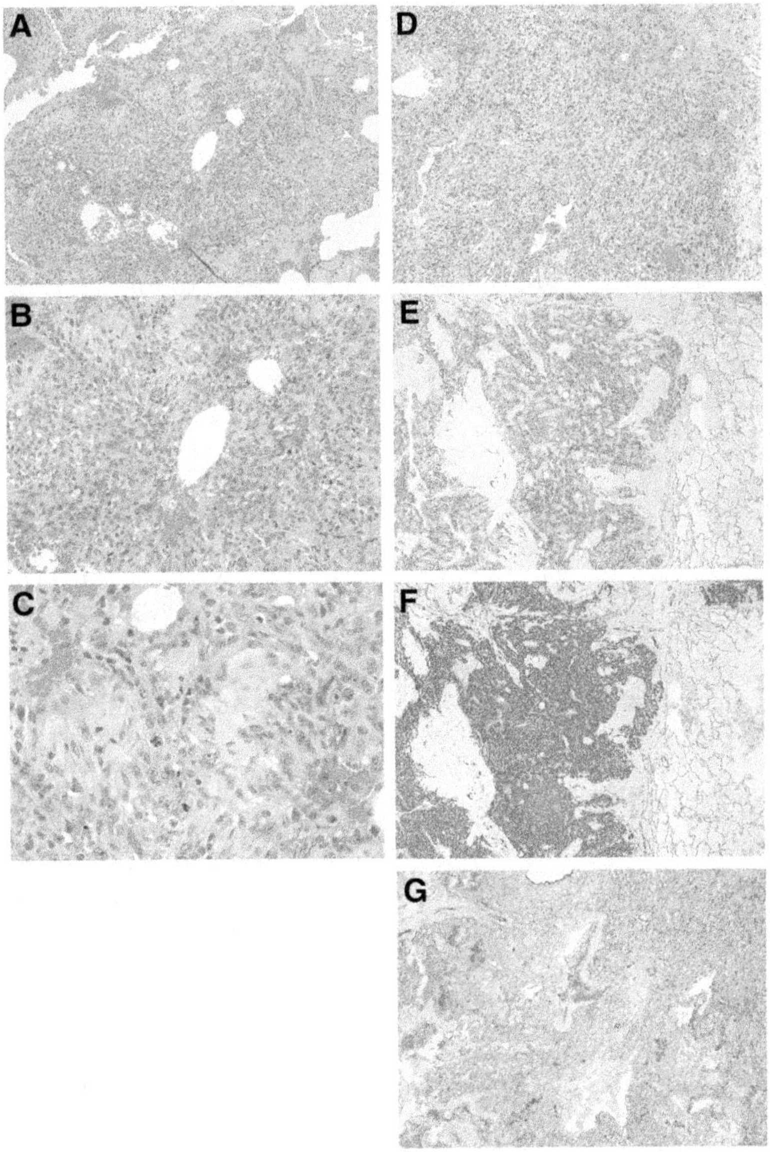

Fig. 2 Images of the tumor from the lung. **a-d** Hematoxyalin and eosin-stained tumor sections from lung nodules. **a** Low power magnification (40X) of tumor demonstrated nodules of tumor cells can be seen in a background of abundant, fresh blood cells. **b** Medium power magnification (100X) showed the tumor cells are both epitheliod and spindle-shaped in appearance. The epitheliod morphology predominates in this area of the tumor. **c** High power magnification (400X) illustrated the tumor cells have prominent nucleoli. A mitotic figure can be seen in the center of the image confirming the tumor is mitotically active. **d** Another view of the tumor showing both epitheliod and spindle-shaped tumor cells, but in this section the spindle-shaped cells predominant (40X). **e** Tumor cells stained positive for CD34, a vascular marker (40X). **f** Tumor cells showed intense signal for CD31, another vascular marker (40X). **g** Factor VIII-related antigen, another endothelial marker commonly used to identify vascular tumors, demonstrated positivity in the tumor cells (40X)

AllPrep DNA/RNA FFPE Kit (Qiagen). Briefly, slides with 5–10 μM thick FFPE sections were scraped into microcentrifuge tubes (two total) and treated with 640 μl of Qiagen Deparaffinization Solution. The resulting pellets were dried for 10 min at 37 °C and resuspended in 150 μl of Buffer PKD containing 10 μl proteinase K. After 15 min incubation at 56 °C, samples were cooled on ice for 3 min and then centrifuged at 20,000 x *g* for 15 min. Genomic DNA was isolated from the pellets according to manufacturer's instructions that included the optional RNAse treatment. Genomic DNA was eluted with 200 μl of buffer ATE and quantified using the Qubit 2.0 Fluorometer (Life Technologies) and Nanodrop spectrophotometer (Thermo Fisher Scientific, Inc.).

Whole exome library construction and target enrichment

Genomic DNA (500 ng) was sheared in 50 μl of TE low EDTA buffer employing the Covaris E210 system

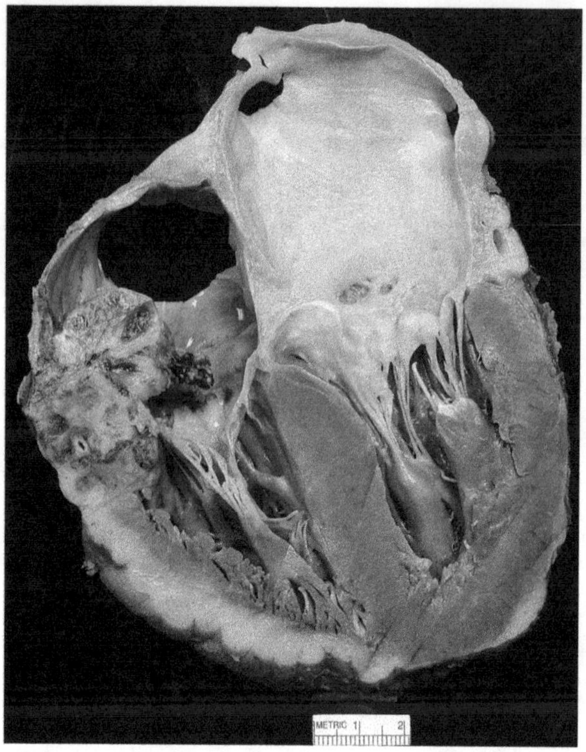

Fig. 3 Cardiac angiosarcoma the right atrium. The tumor was approximately 4 cm in diameter and attached just above the tricuspid valve annulus, extending anteriorly and laterally. The tumor extended into the right atrioventricular sulcus and was present throughout the atrioventricular sulcus shortly after the origin of the right coronary artery and extending posteriorly. For more gross images see Podduturi and Guileyardo [32]

(Covaris, Inc., Woburn, MA) to target fragment sizes of 150–200 bp. Fragmented DNA was then converted to an adapter-ligated whole genome library using the Kapa On-bead Library Prep kit (Kapa Biosciences, Inc., Wilmington, MA; Cat# KK8232) according to the manufacturer's protocol. SureSelect XT Adaptor Oligo Mix was utilized in the ligation step (Agilent Technologies, Inc.; Cat# 5190-3619). Pre-capture libraries were amplified using SureSelect XT primers (Cat# 5190-3620 and Cat# 5972-3694) for nine cycles. Amplified products were quantified and quality tested using Qubit® dsDNA BR Assay Kit (Life Technologies) and the Bioanalyzer DNA 1000 chip (Agilent Technologies, Inc.). Libraries were then hybridized to a custom Agilent SureSelect bait library (custom content regions are provided in Additional file 1: Table S1). Hybridization reactions were set up with 750 ng of the adapted library according to the SureSelect XT protocol with 24 h incubation at 65 °C followed by post-hybridization washes. SureSelect XT indexes were added to the individual libraries during the eight-cycle post-capture amplification step. Final captures were quantified and quality tested using Qubit® dsDNA HS Assay Kit (Life Technologies) and Bioanalyzer DNA HS chip (Agilent Technologies, Inc).

Whole exome sequencing and analysis

The sequencing pool was created by evenly combining four uniquely indexed captures into one pool which was sequenced across three lanes on Illumina HiSeq 2500 high output mode at 14 pM clustering density using paired-end reads (Illumina, Inc.). All sequencing reads were converted to industry standard FASTQ files using the Bcl Conversion and Demultiplexing tool (Illumina, Inc). Sequencing reads were aligned to the GRCh37 reference genome using the MEM module of Burrows-Wheeler Aligner (BWA) v0.7.8 [33] and SAMTOOLS v0.1.19 [33] to produce BAM files. After alignment, the base quality scores were recalibrated and joint small insertions and deletions (INDEL) realignment was performed on the BAM files using GATK v3.1-1 [34]. Duplicate read pairs were marked using PICARD v1.111 [35]. Final BAM files were then used to identify germline and somatic events. Germline SNP and INDELS were identified using GATK haplotype caller in the constitutional sample.

Somatic single nucleotide variations (SNVs) and INDELs were identified using SEURAT somatic variant caller [36]. Somatic copy number detection was based on a log2 comparison of normalized physical coverage (or clonal coverage) across tumor and normal whole exome sequencing data, where physical coverage was calculated by considering the entire region a paired-end fragment span. Normal and tumor physical coverage was then normalized, smoothed and filtered for highly repetitive regions prior to calculating the log2 comparison. Loss of Heterozygosity (LOH) is also deduced by calculating alternate allele frequencies for SNPs. Briefly, B-allele frequencies (BAF) are allele fraction of non-reference reads in the tumor at heterzogote common polymorphic SNPs (minor allele frequency >5%) from 1000 genomes [37] in the patient's germline. Only heterozygous SNPs are plotted determined from that patient's germline calls. We use the calculation alt/(ref + alt) where alt is B. This should be 50/50 unless loss of heterozygosity (LOH) or allele imbalance has occurred at that site. The BAF can then be plotted against map position to identify regions of LOH. Copy number analysis was also performed using the circular binary segmentation algorithm DNA copy within the BioConductor package [38]. Translocation detection was based on discordant read evidence in the tumor exome sequencing data compared to its corresponding normal data. In order for the structural variant to be called there needs to be greater than 7 read pairs mapping to both sides of the breakpoint [37]. Somatic structural rearrangements were identified through discordant read pairs using a previously published algorithm [39].

Annotation of somatic data

Somatic events are annotated using SNPeff (http://snpeff.sourceforge.net/), providing basic map position information as well as additional annotation fields for mutations and copy number events. For mutations, we use several functional prediction tools to help prioritize variants that might confer detrimental functional consequences. We use Mutation Assessor [40], Mutation Taster2 [41], and PolyPhen-2 [42]. Mutation Assessor uses a multiple sequence alignment (MSA), partitioned to reflect functional specificity, and generates conservation scores for each column to represent the functional impact of a missense variant [40]. A conservation score is combined with a specificity score to determine a functional impact score. Variants classed as 'neutral' or 'low' are predicted to not impact protein function, whereas variants classed as 'medium' or 'high' are predicted to result in altered function. Mutation Taster2 uses Bayesian classification and evolutionary conservation models to determine if a variant is likely neutral or deleterious [41]. PolyPhen-2 uses high-quality multiple protein sequence alignment and machine-learning classification to predict the impact of sequence variants (Benign, Probable Deleterious, or Deleterious) on the stability and function of a protein using structural and comparative evolutionary considerations [42].

Results

Somatic alterations in primary cardiac angiosarcoma

We performed next generation sequencing on tumor and germline DNA from a 56-year old male patient with diagnosed primary cardiac angiosarcoma using a 55.2 Mbp custom whole exome capture kit. Sequencing statistics are provided in Additional file 1: Table S1. On-target coverages of 282X for the tumor and 394X for the germline were achieved. Importantly, the tumor sample was FFPE and the blood was fresh. However quality sequencing data was generated from both samples evident by sequencing statistics. Importantly, we generated more sequencing reads from the tumor sample, but fewer of these sequencing reads aligned to the exome target regions as there were likely more low quality reads generated from this FFPE sample (Additional file 1: Table S1). Variant detection algorithms take into account read and base quality to help ensure accuracy in allele determination. This can also have effects on copy number analysis as well. A measure of the noise in log2(tumor/normal) copy number comparison or essentially log2(FFPE/Fresh) is the derivative log2ratio spread or DLR Spread (DLRS). The DLRS statistic describes the absolute value of the log2 ratio variance from each probe to the next, averaged over the entire genome [43]. It is a common measure of noise for CGH arrays [43]. We can also calculate DLRS for copy number from Next Generation Sequencing data using the same algorithm using coverage ratios rather than microarray probe intensities. We can use a similar DLRS threshold as CGH arrays for data of quality enough to make accurate copy number calls, where a DLRS of <0.3 represents low enough noise to make accurate gain and deletion calls. In our hands, copy number from fresh blood normal DNA and fresh *t*umor DNA typically averages DLRS <0.15, indicative of high quality data. The fresh blood sample and FFPE sample used in our study has a DLRS of 0.168 using the copy number tool, supporting high quality copy number analysis for our samples.

An overview of the tumor genome is provided in the form of a Circos plot (Fig. 4). Using SEURAT variant caller, we identified 57 somatic coding SNVs in this patient's tumor DNA (Additional file 1: Table S1). Recurrent *PTPRB* and *PLCG1* mutations have been previously reported in this tumor type [31]; however, no somatic coding mutations affecting either gene were found in our data set. Annotations of mutations were provided through SNPeff using several functional prediction algorithms including Mutation Assessor [40], Mutation Taster2 [41], and PolyPhen-2 [42]. Somatic mutations classified as medium or high by Mutation Assessor, Deleterious by MutationTaster2 and Polyphen2 were prioritized (Additional file 1: Table S1). Of note was the presence of a *KDR* mutation at position G681R mapping to the Immunoglobulin (Su(var)3–9, Enhancer-of-zeste, Trithorax (I-SET) protein domain (Fig. 4; Additional file 2: Table S2). Mutations in *KDR* that result in constitutive activation of the Vascular Endothelial Growth Factor Receptor 2 (VEGFR2) receptor leading to induction of angiogenesis signaling have been reported previously for other angiosarcoma tumors [30]. This KDR G681R mutation in the *KDR* gene to be damaging by all prediction algorithms, however the true functional consequences of this mutation are unknown. Another mutation predicted to be damaging by all three prediction algorithms was Cullin 3 (*CUL3*) R247Q (Additional file 1: Table S1). *CUL3* encodes cullin 3, a core component of the multiple cullin-RING-based BCR (BTB- CUL3-RBX1) E3 ubiquitin-protein ligase complexes which mediate the ubiquitination and subsequent proteasomal degradation of target proteins [44]. It is involved in Aurora Kinase and cell cycle control of G1/S checkpoint [45].

Custom probe tiling in our targeted assay allowed for even genome-wide copy number analysis. We detected whole chromosome gains of chromosomes 2, 4, 8 and 11 (Fig. 4). This tumor also displayed a low level broad gain that spanned chromosome (chr)17q12-qter. More focal events were detected at 1q, 8p and Xq (Fig. 4; Additional file 3: Figure S1). A focal gain was observed at chrXq28 that included a number of cancer testis antigens including Melanoma Antigen Family members (*MAGE*) *-A1, -A2, -A3, -A4, -A6, -A10, -A12, -2B, CTAG1A* and *CTAG2*. The chr1 event was characterized by an allele shift and several

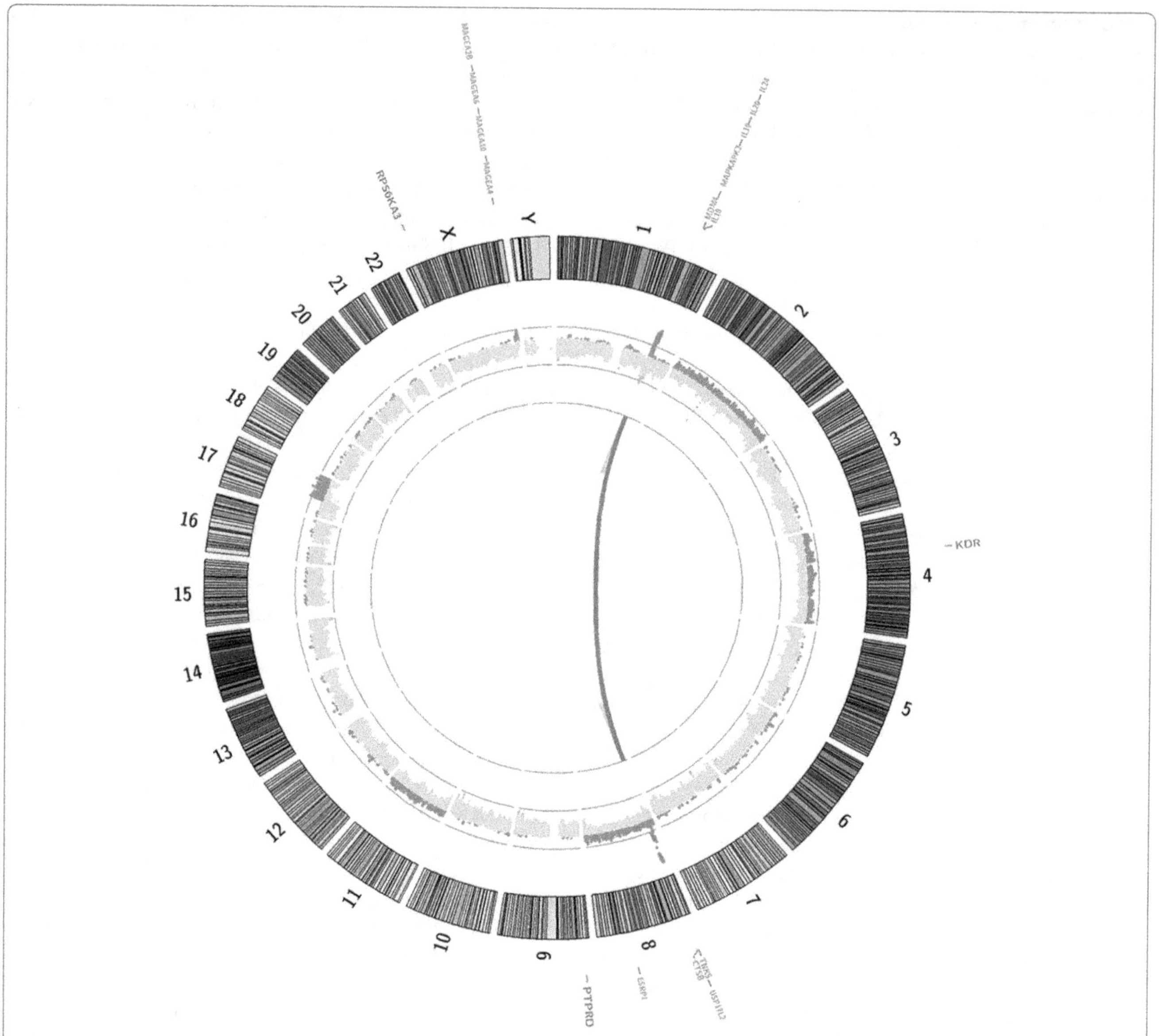

Fig. 4 Circos plot with whole exome sequencing summary. Copy number alterations (inside track, *red* = amplifications, *green* = deletions), Select somatic SNVs (outside track, *blue*) and structural events (*purple lines*)

focal regions of amplification spanning an approximate 7 Mb region at 1q32 (Additional file 2: Table S2 and Additional file 4: Figure S2). Regions of amplification at this locus encompassed a number of cancer-related genes including *MDM4,* Mitogen-Activated Protein Kinase-Activated Protein Kinase 2 (*MAPKAPK2*), and Phosphatidylinositol-4-Phosphate 3-Kinase Catalytic Subunit Type 2 Beta (*PIK3C2B*) and several interleukin genes including *IL10, IL19, IL20,* and *IL24* (Additional file 2: Table S2). The event at chr8p was also characterized by an allele shift and several focal regions of amplification and spanned an approximate 5 M region at 8p23 (Additional file 2: Table S2 and Additional file 5: Figure S3). This region encompassed tankyrase 1 gene, *TNKS,* which acts is an activator of the Wingless-Int (Wnt) signaling pathway [46]. It also contains the GATA Binding Protein 4 (*GATA4*) gene, which has highest expression in heart tissue and promotes cardiac myocyte enlargement [47]. Other significantly amplified genes found at the 8p23 locus included Ubiquitin Specific Peptidase 17-Like Family Member 2 (*USP17L2*), Cathepsin B (*CTSB*), and Epithelial Splicing Regulatory Protein 1 (*ESPR1*) (Additional file 2: Table S2).

Conclusions

In this report we characterized the genomic landscape of a rare primary cardiac angiosarcoma tumor taken postmortem from a 56 year old male patient. We have identified a number of somatic copy number events, mostly marked by amplifications, and SNV alterations in this patient's tumor. Our approach did not uncover any translocations that could result in oncogenic fusions previously reported in primary angiosarcomas [48, 49]. Copy number coupled with the translocation analysis suggested a presence of a circular chromosome harboring the *MDM4* gene. We were able to confirm our hypothesis by *in silico* reconstructing the discordant read pairs mapping to multiple regions on chr1 and chr8. Double minute chromosomes and homogeneously stained regions have been identified in several tumor types and are biologically complex extrachromosomal entities frequently harboring known oncogenes (i.e *MYC*) and/or oncogenic fusions [50]. Their origin in the nucleus is quite intriguing and is thought to arise as a result of several mechanisms including chromothripsis, a multi-step product of complex duplications and recombinations through non-homologous end joining. To our knowledge, there are no previous reports describing circular extrachromosomal DNA in primary angiosarcomas or angiosarcomas of the heart carrying *MDM4* gene. Future studies investigating frequency of this occurrence in primary cardiac angiosarcomas could add clinical value.

Another amplified region in this tumor genome mapped to chrXq28. This locus encompasses the *MAGE* gene cluster. Genes belonging to this cluster, cancer testis antigens (CTAs), often exhibit tumor-specific expression and are currently explored as immunotherapeutic targets in sarcomas [51], other solid tumors and hematologic malignancies [52]. Several ongoing preclinical and phase I trials are investigating vaccination-induced immunotherapeutic response in sarcoma patients with advanced disease (NCT02054104, NCT01313429, and NCT013441496).

Interestingly, a recent report describes an association between MAGE-A and MDM2 oncogene, E3 ubiquitin protein ligase (MDM2)/MDM4 complex in vitro in a human cell line model [53]. Specifically, MAGE-A was shown to compete with MDM4 for binding to MDM2 leading to elevated levels of free MDM4. Additionally, the group showed a positive correlation between MAGE-A and MDM4 by immunohistochemistry in primary breast cancer. Although we cannot comment on expression or protein levels of either MDM4 or MAGE in this patient's tumor, the co-amplification significance of multiple MAGE genes and MDM4 may merit further exploration in this tumor type.

Recently, another patient presented to our clinic with a cardiac angiosarcoma and a Foundation One genetic profile was performed on his tumor. A mutation of unknown significance in *KDR* was observed (N704del) in a region where other mutations, deletions, and insertions have been reported [54], including the patient described in the present study. Additionally, amplification of *MDM4* was found as was seen in our initial patient. Thus, from a potential therapeutic viewpoint one could one take away several points from these whole exome sequencing results (fully realizing this is from only two patients). Firstly, the *KDR*-G681R mutation, which occurs within the second I-SET domain of this protein, is novel. The G681 amino acid is highly conserved throughout evolution suggesting that it is a functionally relevant residue and based on prediction algorithms is potentially functionally relevant, however this would need to be validated through in vitro and/or in vivo cell-based mechanistic approaches. Although the true functional relevance of the mutation is currently unknown, this mutation would confer the strongest therapeutic targeting potential. One could consider a vascular endothelial growth factor receptor directed therapy such as bevacizumab, pazopanib, cabozantinib, vandetanib, ziv-aflibercept, or ramucirumab. Of note is that sorafenib and sunitnib inihibited KDR activity in vitro as previously noted by Antonescu and colleagues [30]. Secondly, there was high level focal amplification at 1q32, which contains the *MDM4* gene. Although there are multiple anticancer agents under clinical development which inhibit the structurally similar p53 binding protein MDM2 (e.g., the Nutlins etc.) there have not been any under development which inhibits MDM4 or MDMX (any MDM protein). But that has changed with the ongoing development of the agent ALRN-6924 an MDM2/MDMX dual inhibitor (which reactivates p53) [55]. That agent would be a potential match against the amplified MDM4 target. Although we have provided a relatively high resolution view of the genomic landscape of this tumor, further studies are needed to determine the effect of candidate cancer genes hypothesized from our analysis, and clinical validation of the frequency of these events in cardiac angiosarcomas.

Additional files

Additional file 1: Table S1. List of coordinates and genomic regions submitted to Sure Design software for custom bait selection. (DOCX 18 kb)

Additional file 2: Table S2. Basic Next Generation Sequencing Whole Exome Alignment Statistics. (DOCX 13 kb)

Additional file 3: Figure S1. Genome-wide chromosomal copy number plot outputs from 1A) copy number analysis, 1B) LOH and allelic imbalance analysis, 1C) segmentation algorithm copy number analysis, and 1D) ExomeCNV copy number analysis. 1A) chromosomal plots contain chromosomal map position in megabases on the X-axis, and the log2 fold change ratio information on the Y-axis. Regions of copy neutrality (ratios between log2FC -0.75 and +0.75) are black, regions of copy number gain (ratio > log2FC 0.75) are red, and regions of copy number loss (ratios < log2FC -0.75) are green. 1B) chromosomal plots contain chromosomal map position in megabases on the X-axis, and the B-allele frequency (BAF) on the Y-axis revealing chromosomal allelic imbalances. 1C) the copy number log2 fold change ratios (Y-axis) for each chromosome are colored alternately in green and black across the entirety of the genome map positions along the X-axis. 1D) chromosomal plots contain chromosomal map position in megabases on the X-axis, and the log2 fold change ratio information on the Y-axis derived from ExomeCNV. (ZIP 7726 kb)

Additional file 4: Figure S2. Chromosome 1 copy number plot outputs illustrating 1q32 amplification. Plots represent outputs from (2A upper panel) LOH and allelic imbalance analysis, and (2A lower panel) copy number analysis. 2A upper panel, chromosome 1 plot with map position in megabases on the X-axis, and the B-allele frequency (BAF) on the Y-axis revealing chromosomal allelic imbalances. 2A lower panel, chromosome 1 plot with map position in megabases on the X-axis, and the log2 fold change ratio information on the Y-axis. 2B shows 10 megabase zoomed region of chromosome 1 (1q32) amplicon. 2B upper panel, chromosome 1 zoomed in plot with map position in megabases on the X-axis, and the B-allele frequency (BAF) on the Y-axis revealing chromosomal allelic imbalance at this region. 2B lower panel, chromosome 1 zoomed in plot with map position in megabases on the X-axis, and the log2 fold change ratio information on the Y-axis. The map postion related to the *MDM4* gene locus is depicted as a purple line on each plot. (ZIP 1288 kb)

Additional file 5: Figure S3. Chromosome 8 copy number plot outputs illustrating 8p allelic imbalance and 8p23 amplification. Plots represent outputs from (upper panel) custom algorithm providing information on allelic imbalances, and (lower panel) copy number analysis. Upper panel, chromosome 8 plot with map position in megabases on the X-axis, and the B-allele frequency (BAF) on the Y-axis revealing chromosomal allelic imbalances. Lower panel, chromosome 8 plot with map position in megabases on the X-axis, and the log2 fold change ratio information on the Y-axis. (JPG 1099 kb)

Abbreviations

aCGH: array Comparative Genomic Hybridization; BAF: B-allele frequencies; BWA: Burrows-Wheeler Aligner; CD: Cluster of differentiation; CDKN2A: Cyclin Dependent Kinase Inhibitor 2A; chr: chromosome; CNS: Central nervous system; CTAG1A: Cancer/Testis Antigen 1A; CTAG2: Cancer/Testis Antigen 2; CTAs: Cancer testis antigens; CTSB: Cathepsin B; CUL3: Cullin 3; DLRS: Derivative log2ratio spread; ESPR1: Epithelial Splicing Regulatory Protein 1; FFPE: Formalin-Fixed, Paraffin-Embedded; FLT1: Fms Related Tyrosine Kinase 1; FLT4: Fms Related Tyrosine Kinase 4; GATA4: GATA Binding Protein 4; IL: Interleukin; INDELs: Insertions and deletions; I-SET domain: Immunoglobulin (Su(var)3-9, Enhancer-of-zeste, Trithorax); KDR: Kinase Insert Domain Receptor; KRAS: V-Ki-ras2 Kirsten rat sarcoma viral oncogene homolog; LOH: Loss of heterozygosity; MAGE-A1 – 2B: Melanoma Antigen Family Member A1 – 2B; MAPKAPK2: Mitogen-Activated Protein Kinase-Activated Protein Kinase 2; MDM2: MDM2 oncogene, E3 ubiquitin protein ligase; MDM4: MDM4 p53 binding protein homolog; MDMX: Any MDM protein; MSA: Multiple sequence alignment; MYC: V-Myc Avian Myelocytomatosis Viral Oncogene Homolog; PIK3C2B: Phosphatidylinositol-4-Phosphate 3-Kinase Catalytic Subunit Type 2 Beta; PLCG1: Phospholipase C, gamma 1; PTPRB: Protein tyrosine phosphatase, receptor type, B; SNRK: SNF Related Kinase; SNVs: Single nucleotide variations; TEK: TEK Receptor Tyrosine Kinase; TIE1: Tyrosine Kinase with Immunoglobulin like and EGF Like Domains 1; TNKS: Tankyrase 1; TP53: tumor protein P53; USP17L2: Ubiquitin Specific Peptidase 17-Like Family Member 2; VEGFR2: Vascular endothelial growth factor receptor 2; Wnt: Wingless-Int

Acknowledgements

We thank Robert Stoler, MD from the Baylor Cardiology Department for providing assistance in establishing the correct diagnosis of the patient and contributing to the patient's care. We thank Heather Webb, MD and Landis Griffeth, MD from the Baylor Radiology Department for the patient's images and interpretation of the images.

Funding

This study supported by the Department of Graduate Medical Education at the Baylor University Medical Center at Dallas.

Availability of data and materials

The datasets during and/or analyzed during the current study are available from JD Carpten on reasonable request.

Authors' contributions

LZ, JC, DVH, and MR conceived the concept of the case report and coordinated the design and data collection among all authors. LZ, JC, and DVH drafted the manuscript with significant contributions from MH, and IC. MH formatted the figures for publication. LZ, LG, MR, and RM were involved in all aspects of patient care and in providing clinical information for the case presentation. WR and JG were involved in all pathologic analysis including histopathological characterization of the primary and metastatic tumors and in generating the pathology figure. IC was responsible for tumor DNA isolation, somatic mutation profiling, and generation of Fig. 3. JA and DC were responsible for bioinformatics design and execution for primary and secondary data analysis. IC, DVH, and JC were responsible for the interpretation of the mutations/amplifications. All authors have read and approved the manuscript.

Competing interests

The authors declare that they have no competing interests.

Consent for publication

All authors gave their consent to publish this manuscript. Written informed consent was obtained from the family of the patient for publication of this case report and any accompanying images. A copy of the written consent is available for review by the Editor of this journal.

Ethics approval and consent to participate

This report adhered to the tenets of the Declaration of Helsinki and was approved exempt by the Baylor University Institutional Review Board (IRB #013-182). Consent to participate in this study was obtained from a direct relative of the patient in writing. The patient was deceased at the time of this study.

Author details

[1]Baylor Charles A. Sammons Cancer Center at Dallas, Baylor University Medical Center at Dallas, 3410 Worth Street, Dallas, TX 75246, USA. [2]Department of Internal Medicine, Baylor University Medical Center at Dallas, 3500 Gaston Ave, Dallas, TX 75246, USA. [3]Integrative Cancer Genomics, Translational Genomics Research Institute, 445N 5th Street, Phoenix, AZ 85004, USA. [4]Texas Oncology/US Oncology, 3410 Worth Street, Dallas, TX 75246, USA. [5]Anatomic Pathology and Clinical Pathology, Baylor University Medical Center at Dallas, 3600 Gaston Ave, Dallas, TX 75246, USA. [6]Clinical Translational Research Division Translational Genomics Research Institute, 445N 5th Street, Phoenix, AZ 85004, USA. [7]College of Medicine, Texas A&M Health Sciences Center, 3410 Worth Street, Dallas, TX 75246, USA.

Received: 19 January 2016 Accepted: 14 December 2016
Published online: 05 January 2017

References

1. Lam KY, Dickens P, Chan AC. Tumors of the heart. A 20-year experience with a review of 12,485 consecutive autopsies. Arch Pathol Lab Med. 1993; 117(10):1027–31.
2. Reynen K. Frequency of primary tumors of the heart. Am J Cardiol. 1996; 77(1):107.
3. Burke A, Virmani R. More on cardiac myxomas. N Engl J Med. 1996;335(19): 1462–3. author reply 63-4.
4. Janigan DT, Husain A, Robinson NA. Cardiac angiosarcomas. A review and a case report. Cancer. 1986;57(4):852–9.
5. Gal AA, Koss MN, McCarthy WF, Hochholzer L. Prognostic factors in pulmonary fibrohistiocytic lesions. Cancer. 1994;73(7):1817–24.
6. Burke AP, Tazelaar H, Butany JW, El-Demellawy D, Loire R, Geva T, Galvin JR, Veinot JP, Virmani R, Kamiya H, et al. Cardiac Sarcomas. In: William TD, Brambilla E, Muller-Hermelink HK, Harris CC, editors. Pathology and genetics tumours of the lung, pleura, thymus and heart. Lyon: IARC Press; 2004. p. 273–81.
7. Majano-Lainez RA. Cardiac tumors: a current clinical and pathological perspective. Crit Rev Oncog. 1997;8(4):293–303.
8. Meng Q, Lai H, Lima J, Tong W, Qian Y, Lai S. Echocardiographic and pathologic characteristics of primary cardiac tumors: a study of 149 cases. Int J Cardiol. 2002;84(1):69–75.
9. Glancy DL, Morales Jr JB, Roberts WC. Angiosarcoma of the heart. Am J Cardiol. 1968;21(3):413–9.
10. Roberts WC. Neoplasms involving the heart, their simulators, and adverse consequences of their therapy. Proc (Bayl Univ Med Cent). 2001;14(4):358–76.
11. Fernandes F, Soufen HN, Ianni BM, Arteaga E, Ramires FJ, Mady C. Primary neoplasms of the heart. Clinical and histological presentation of 50 cases. Arq Bras Cardiol. 2001;76(3):231–7.

12. Jimenez Mazuecos JM, Fuentes Manso R, Segovia Cubero J, Toquero Ramos J, Oteo Dominguez JF, Alonso-Pulpon Rivera L. Is heart transplantation for primary cardiac sarcoma a useful therapeutic option? Rev Esp Cardiol. 2003;56(4):408–11.
13. Crespo MG, Pulpon LA, Pradas G, Serrano S, Segovia J, Vegazo I, Salas C, Espana P, Silva L, Burgos R, et al. Heart transplantation for cardiac angiosarcoma: should its indication be questioned? J Heart Lung Transplant. 1993;12(3):527–30.
14. Talbot SM, Taub RN, Keohan ML, Edwards N, Galantowicz ME, Schulman LL. Combined heart and lung transplantation for unresectable primary cardiac sarcoma. J Thorac Cardiovasc Surg. 2002;124(6):1145–8.
15. Orlandi A, Ferlosio A, Roselli M, Chiariello L, Spagnoli LG. Cardiac sarcomas: an update. J Thorac Oncol. 2010;5(9):1483–9.
16. Ge Y, Ro JY, Kim D, Kim CH, Reardon MJ, Blackmon S, Zhai J, Coffey D, Benjamin RS, Ayala AG. Clinicopathologic and immunohistochemical characteristics of adult primary cardiac angiosarcomas: analysis of 10 cases. Ann Diagn Pathol. 2011;15(4):262–7.
17. Penel N, Marreaud S, Robin YM, Hohenberger P. Angiosarcoma: state of the art and perspectives. Crit Rev Oncol Hematol. 2011;80(2):257–63.
18. Maki RG, D'Adamo DR, Keohan ML, Saulle M, Schuetze SM, Undevia SD, Livingston MB, Cooney MM, Hensley ML, Mita MM, et al. Phase II study of sorafenib in patients with metastatic or recurrent sarcomas. J Clin Oncol. 2009;27(19):3133–40.
19. Chugh R, Wathen JK, Maki RG, Benjamin RS, Patel SR, Meyers PA, Priebat DA, Reinke DK, Thomas DG, Keohan ML, et al. Phase II multicenter trial of imatinib in 10 histologic subtypes of sarcoma using a bayesian hierarchical statistical model. J Clin Oncol. 2009;27(19):3148–53.
20. Agulnik M, Yarber JL, Okuno SH, von Mehren M, Jovanovic BD, Brockstein BE, Evens AM, Benjamin RS. An open-label, multicenter, phase II study of bevacizumab for the treatment of angiosarcoma and epithelioid hemangioendotheliomas. Ann Oncol. 2013;24(1):257–63.
21. Manner J, Radlwimmer B, Hohenberger P, Mossinger K, Kuffer S, Sauer C, Belharazem D, Zettl A, Coindre JM, Hallermann C, et al. MYC high level gene amplification is a distinctive feature of angiosarcomas after irradiation or chronic lymphedema. Am J Pathol. 2010;176(1):34–9.
22. Guo T, Zhang L, Chang NE, Singer S, Maki RG, Antonescu CR. Consistent MYC and FLT4 gene amplification in radiation-induced angiosarcoma but not in other radiation-associated atypical vascular lesions. Genes Chromosomes Cancer. 2011;50(1):25–33.
23. Przygodzki RM, Finkelstein SD, Keohavong P, Zhu D, Bakker A, Swalsky PA, Soini Y, Ishak KG, Bennett WP. Sporadic and Thorotrast-induced angiosarcomas of the liver manifest frequent and multiple point mutations in K-ras-2. Lab Invest. 1997;76(1):153–9.
24. Chang T-G, Wang J, Chen L-W, Chang H-W, Chen J-S, Cho C-L. Loss of expression of the p16 gene is frequent in malignant skin tumors. Biochem Biophys Res Commun. 1997;230(1):85–8.
25. Tannapfel A, Weihrauch M, Benicke M, Uhlmann D, Hauss J, Wrbitzky R, Wittekind C. p16INK4A-alterations in primary angiosarcoma of the liver. J Hepatol. 2001;35(1):62–7.
26. Weihrauch M, Markwarth A, Lehnert G, Wittekind C, Wrbitzky R, Tannapfel A. Abnormalities of the ARF-p53 pathway in primary angiosarcomas of the liver. Hum Pathol. 2002;33(9):884–92.
27. Naka N, Tomita Y, Nakanishi H, Araki N, Hongyo T, Ochi T, Aozasa K. Mutations of p53 tumor-suppressor gene in angiosarcoma. Int J Cancer. 1997;71(6):952–5.
28. Zu Y, Perle MA, Yan Z, Liu J, Kumar A, Waisman J. Chromosomal abnormalities and p53 gene mutation in a cardiac angiosarcoma. Appl Immunohistochem Mol Morphol. 2001;9(1):24–8.
29. Hayashi T, Koike K, Kumasaka T, Saito T, Mitani K, Terao Y, Ogishima D, Yao T, Takeda S, Takahashi K, et al. Uterine angiosarcoma associated with lymphangioleiomyomatosis in a patient with tuberous sclerosis complex: an autopsy case report with immunohistochemical and genetic analysis. Hum Pathol. 2012;43(10):1777–84.
30. Antonescu CR, Yoshida A, Guo T, Chang NE, Zhang L, Agaram NP, Qin LX, Brennan MF, Singer S, Maki RG. KDR activating mutations in human angiosarcomas are sensitive to specific kinase inhibitors. Cancer Res. 2009; 69(18):7175–9.
31. Behjati S, Tarpey PS, Sheldon H, Martincorena I, Van Loo P, Gundem G, Wedge DC, Ramakrishna M, Cooke SL, Pillay N, et al. Recurrent PTPRB and PLCG1 mutations in angiosarcoma. Nat Genet. 2014;46(4):376–9.
32. Podduturi V, Guileyardo JM. Primary cardiac angiosarcoma. Acad Forensic Pathol. 2014;4(1):123–6.
33. Li H, Handsaker B, Wysoker A, Fennell T, Ruan J, Homer N, Marth G, Abecasis G, Durbin R, Genome Project Data Processing S. The Sequence Alignment/Map format and SAMtools. Bioinformatics. 2009;25(16):2078–9.
34. McKenna A, Hanna M, Banks E, Sivachenko A, Cibulskis K, Kernytsky A, Garimella K, Altshuler D, Gabriel S, Daly M, et al. The Genome Analysis Toolkit: a MapReduce framework for analyzing next-generation DNA sequencing data. Genome Res. 2010;20(9):1297–303.
35. PICARD v1.111. http://broadinstitute.github.io/picard/.
36. Christoforides A, Carpten JD, Weiss GJ, Demeure MJ, Von Hoff DD, Craig DW. Identification of somatic mutations in cancer through Bayesian-based analysis of sequenced genome pairs. BMC Genomics. 2013;14:302.
37. Genomes Project C, Auton A, Brooks LD, Durbin RM, Garrison EP, Kang HM, Korbel JO, Marchini JL, McCarthy S, McVean GA, et al. A global reference for human genetic variation. Nature. 2015;526(7571):68–74.
38. Seshan VE, Olshen AR. DNAcopy: DNA copy number data analysis. 2016. In: R package version 1.44.0.
39. Liang WS, Aldrich J, Tembe W, Kurdoglu A, Cherni I, Phillips L, Reiman R, Baker A, Weiss GJ, Carpten JD, et al. Long insert whole genome sequencing for copy number variant and translocation detection. Nucleic Acids Res. 2014;42(2), e8.
40. Reva B, Antipin Y, Sander C. Predicting the functional impact of protein mutations: application to cancer genomics. Nucleic Acids Res. 2011;39(17), e118.
41. Schwarz JM, Rodelsperger C, Schuelke M, Seelow D. MutationTaster evaluates disease-causing potential of sequence alterations. Nat Methods. 2010;7(8):575–6.
42. Adzhubei I, Jordan DM, Sunyaev SR. Predicting functional effect of human missense mutations using PolyPhen-2. Curr Protoc Hum Genet. 2013; Chapter 7(Unit7):20.
43. Pinto D, Darvishi K, Shi X, Rajan D, Rigler D, Fitzgerald T, Lionel AC, Thiruvahindrapuram B, Macdonald JR, Mills R, et al. Comprehensive assessment of array-based platforms and calling algorithms for detection of copy number variants. Nat Biotechnol. 2011;29(6):512–20.
44. Zhang HF, Tomida A, Koshimizu R, Ogiso Y, Lei S, Tsuruo T. Cullin 3 promotes proteasomal degradation of the topoisomerase I-DNA covalent complex. Cancer Res. 2004;64(3):1114–21.
45. Sumara I, Peter M. A Cul3-based E3 ligase regulates mitosis and is required to maintain the spindle assembly checkpoint in human cells. Cell Cycle. 2007;6(24):3004–10.
46. Seimiya H, Smith S. The telomeric poly(ADP-ribose) polymerase, tankyrase 1, contains multiple binding sites for telomeric repeat binding factor 1 (TRF1) and a novel acceptor, 182-kDa tankyrase-binding protein (TAB182). J Biol Chem. 2002;277(16):14116–26.
47. Liang Q, De Windt LJ, Witt SA, Kimball TR, Markham BE, Molkentin JD. The transcription factors GATA4 and GATA6 regulate cardiomyocyte hypertrophy in vitro and in vivo. J Biol Chem. 2001;276(32):30245–53.
48. Dunlap JB, Magenis RE, Davis C, Himoe E, Mansoor A. Cytogenetic analysis of a primary bone angiosarcoma. Cancer Genet Cytogenet. 2009;194(1):1–3.
49. Gru AA, Becker N, Pfeifer JD. Angiosarcoma of the parotid gland with a t(12; 22) translocation creating a EWSR1-ATF1 fusion: a diagnostic dilemma. J Clin Pathol. 2013;66(5):452–4.
50. L'Abbate A, Macchia G, D'Addabbo P, Lonoce A, Tolomeo D, Trombetta D, Kok K, Bartenhagen C, Whelan CW, Palumbo O, et al. Genomic organization and evolution of double minutes/homogeneously staining regions with MYC amplification in human cancer. Nucleic Acids Res. 2014;42(14):9131–45.
51. Wilky BA, Goldberg JM. Immunotherapy in sarcoma: a new frontier. Discov Med. 2014;17(94):201–6.
52. Bodey B. Cancer-testis antigens: promising targets for antigen directed antineoplastic immunotherapy. Expert Opin Biol Ther. 2002;2(6):577–84.
53. Marcar L, Ihrig B, Hourihan J, Bray SE, Quinlan PR, Jordan LB, Thompson AM, Hupp TR, Meek DW. MAGE-A Cancer/Testis Antigens Inhibit MDM2 Ubiquitylation Function and Promote Increased Levels of MDM4. PLoS One. 2015;10(5):e0127713.
54. Forbes SA, Beare D, Gunasekaran P, Leung K, Bindal N, Boutselakis H, Ding M, Bamford S, Cole C, Ward S, et al. COSMIC: exploring the world's knowledge of somatic mutations in human cancer. Nucleic Acids Res. 2015;43(Database issue):D805–11.
55. Chang YS, Graves B, Guerlavais V, Tovar C, Packman K, To KH, Olson KA, Kesavan K, Gangurde P, Mukherjee A, et al. Stapled alpha-helical peptide drug development: a potent dual inhibitor of MDM2 and MDMX for p53-dependent cancer therapy. Proc Natl Acad Sci U S A. 2013;110(36):E3445–54.

Lipoma of the Mitral Valve

William C. Roberts, MD[a,b,c,d,*], Paul A. Grayburn, MD[a,b,c,d], and Baron L. Hamman, MD[a,b,c,d]

Described herein is a 67-year-old morbidly obese man who had a lipoma excised from his posterior mitral leaflet after it was found by echocardiogram. Findings in 6 other previously reported cases are reviewed. **(Am J Cardiol 2017;119:1121−1123)**

Every human heart contains some adipose tissue. It is most commonly located in the subepicardial regions, right ventricular free wall, and atrial septum. These fatty infiltrates are not localized or encapsulated but simply invade the subepicardial spaces or the spaces between the myocardial cells. On rare occasion, the adipose tissue cells are encapsulated forming distinct masses and then they can be called lipomas. They have been reported to occur in the atrial and ventricular cavities and walls [1−12] and in the atrioventricular valves.[13−18] Risk factors for these cardiac lipomas have not been delineated. This report was prompted by finding a mass on the mitral valve by echocardiogram, and that led to its operative excision and morphologic examination.

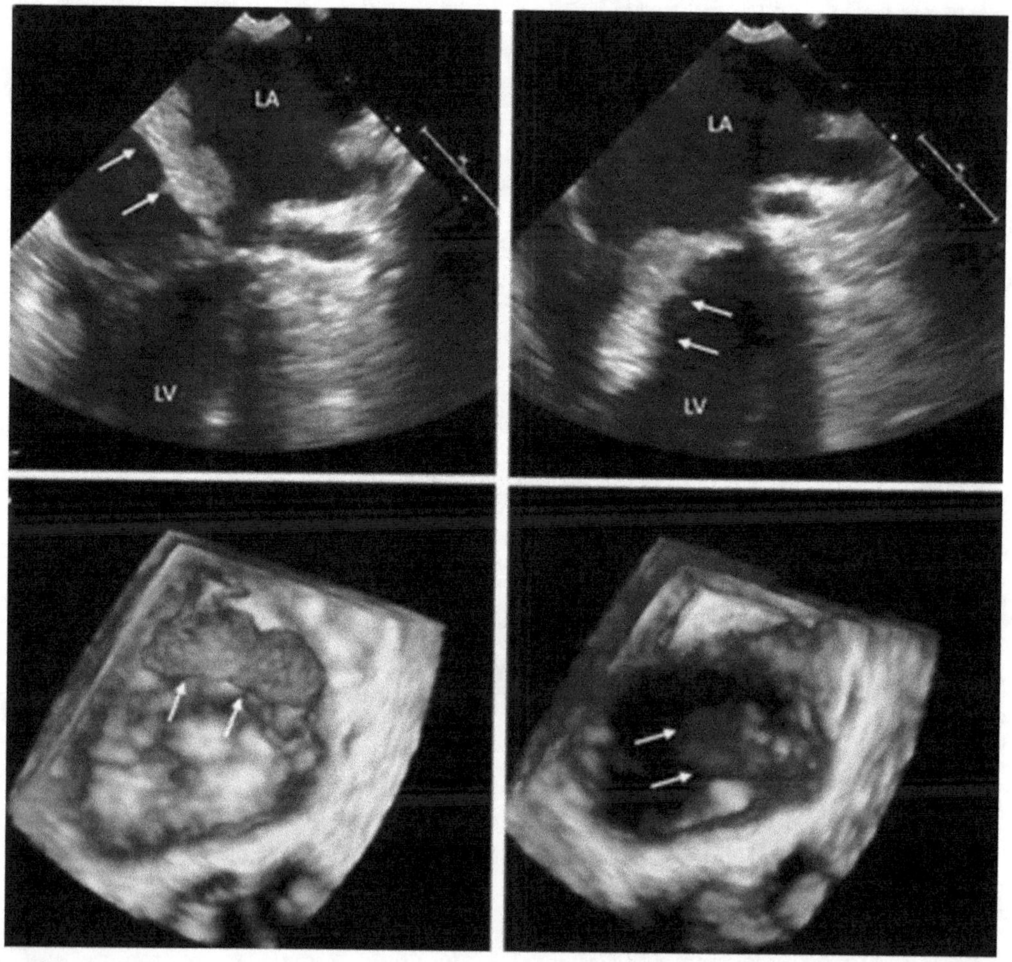

Figure 1. Transesophageal images of a large echo-dense mass attached to the medial scallop *(arrows)* of the posterior mitral leaflet. *Upper left*: End-systolic frame showing the mass extending cephalad into the left atrium (LA). *Upper right*: End-diastolic frame showing the mass extending into the left ventricle (LV). *Bottom left*: End-systolic 3-dimensional "surgeon's view" showing the mass from the left atrial aspect. *Bottom right*: End-diastolic 3-dimenional "surgeon's view" showing the mass in the LV.

[a]Baylor Heart and Vascular Institute, [b]Division of Cardiology, Department of Internal Medicine, [c]Department of Pathology, and [d]Department of Cardiothoracic Surgery, Baylor University Medical Center, Dallas, Texas. Manuscript received November 24, 2016; revised manuscript received and accepted November 29, 2016.

See page 1123 for disclosure information.

*Corresponding author: Tel: (214) 820-7911; fax: (214) 820-7533.

E-mail address: william.roberts1@BSWHealth.org (W.C. Roberts).

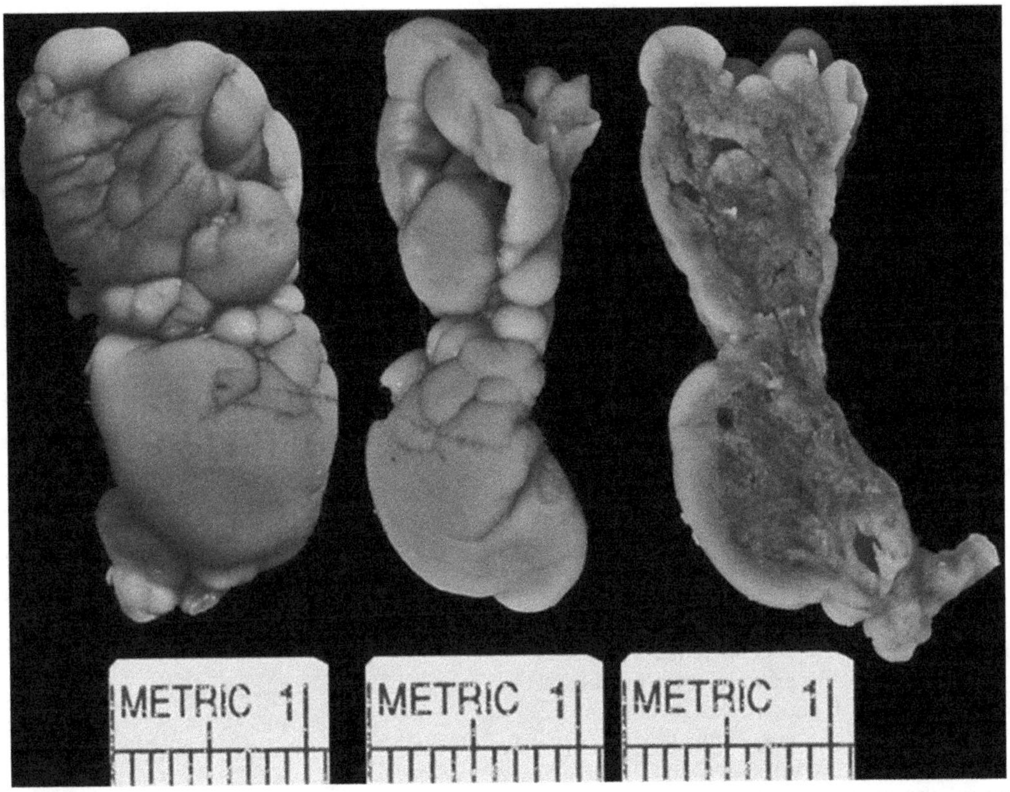

Figure 2. Photograph of the lipoma excised at operation. The *left* and *center* photos are exterior views showing the lumpy fatty deposits. The *right view* shows the necrotic interior of the lipoma.

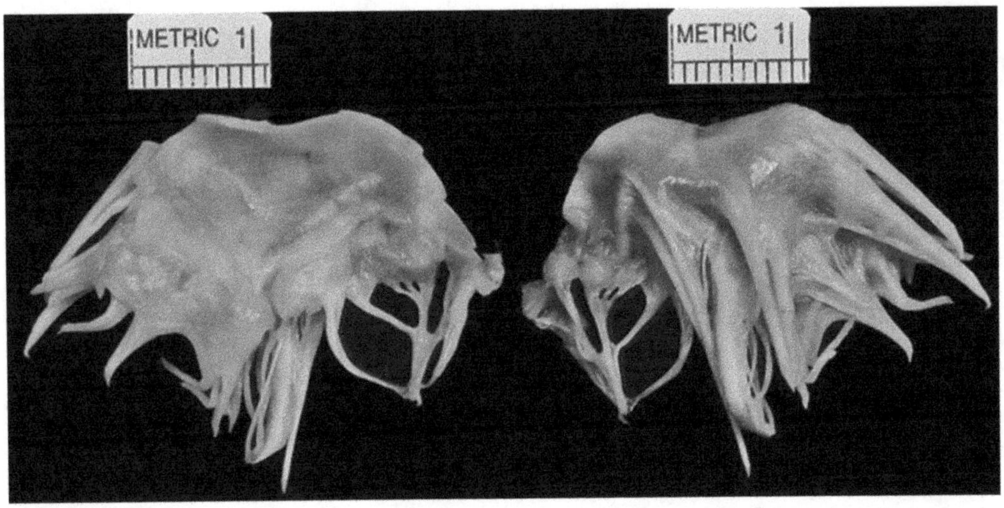

Figure 3. Operatively excised mitral valve. The *left photograph* shows the atrial aspect and the *right photograph*, the ventricular aspect.

Case Description

A 67-year-old man was hospitalized because of generalized weakness and exertional dyspnea for 3 weeks. In times past he had had periodic atrial fibrillation and had received a pacemaker. In the hospital, he was found to have pre-existing pneumonia and was treated accordingly. Because his symptoms could also have resulted from cardiac disease, an echocardiogram was performed and a mobile mass attached to the posterior mitral leaflet was found (Figure 1). The patient weighed 320 pounds and stood 74 inches in height (body mass index 41 kg/m^2). A precordial murmur was not present. At operation, the mass was attached by a single stalk to the posterior mitral leaflet. It was excised intact by incising the stalk and then the mitral valve was replaced by a metallic (ON-X 31/33) mechanical prosthesis. The mass weighed 2.30 g and histologically was a lipoma (Figure 2). Most of the interior of the mass consisted of necrotic adipose tissue cells. His postoperative course was uneventful. The excised anterior mitral leaflet is shown in Figure 3.

Table 1
Previously reported cases of lipomas involving the mitral valve

First Author (Year) [Reference]	Age (Yrs) at Excision	Sex	Leaflet Location on MV	Weight (g) of Lipoma	Operatively Excised	Symptoms Before Excision	Method of Diagnosis	MVR	MV Leaflet	Reason for Echo	MR	BMI (Kg/m^2)
1. Barberger-Gateau (1978) [13]	12	M	Posterior	4	+	0	Echo	+	Normal	Murmur	+	
2. Behnam (1983) [14]	16	F	Posterior	—	+	0	Echo	+	Normal	Murmur	+	
3. Anderson (1988) [15]	54	M	Posterior	—	+/−	+	Echo	+	Normal	Dizziness	+	
4. Dollar (1989) [16]	66	F	Posterior	2	+	+	Echo	+	Normal	Dyspnea	+	33
5. Vadmal (1998) [17]	5	M	Anterior	—	+	0	Echo	0	Normal	Murmur*	+	
6. Harth (2003) [18]	56	F	Anterior	3	+	0	Echo	0	Normal	"Thud"	+	
7. Present Case	67	M	Posterior	2.3	+	+	Echo	+	Normal	Dyspnea	+	41

BMI = body mass index; Echo = echocardiography; F = female; M = male; MR = mitral regurgitation; MV = mitral valve; MVR = mitral valve replacement.

— = no information available.

* This patient was known to have a perimembraneous ventricular septal defect.

Discussion

At least 6 reports have appeared (Table 1), each describing a single patient with a lipoma involving the mitral valve and in each the lipoma was operatively excised. In each of the 6 patients either the presence of a precordial murmur or abnormal sound (4 patients) or symptoms (2 patients) suggesting cardiac disease prompted the performance of an echocardiogram which provided the diagnosis. The lipoma involved the posterior mitral leaflet only in 4 patients and the anterior leaflet in 2. In 4 patients, the lipoma was firmly attached to the mitral leaflet with or without entangling the chordae tendineae and the valve was replaced; in 2 patients, the lipoma was attached to the anterior leaflet by a stalk, as in our patient, or by a small attachment and in both of these patients the valve was preserved. The fact that the interior of the lipoma in our patient was necrotic suggests that the lipoma had been in place for years. In only 1 previously reported patient was body weight or height or body mass index mentioned and that patient was obese. The presently described patient was morbidly obese (body mass index 41 kg/m^2). Both anterior and posterior leaflets in all 6 patients, as in the present patient, appeared to be normal in areas where the lipoma was not attached. In only 3 of the 6 patients was the operatively excised lipoma weighed (2 to 4 g). In the present patient it weighed 2.3 g. All patients survived the operative procedure without complications.

Disclosures

The authors have no conflicts of interest to disclose.

1. Crockett JE, Decker D, Reed W, Dunn M, Leger L. Lipoma of the heart. *Am J Cardiol* 1964;14:394–398.
2. Bradford JH, Nomeir AM, Watts LE. Left ventricular lipoma: echocardiographic and angiographic features. *South Med J* 1980;73:663–665.
3. Harada K, Seki I, Kobayashi H, Okuni M, Sakurai I. Lipoma of the heart in a child: clinical, echocardiographic, angiographic, and pathological features. *Jpn Heart J* 1980;21:903–910.
4. Zingas AP, Carrera JD, Murray CA III, Kling GA. Lipoma of the myocardium. *J Comput Assist Tomogr* 1983;7:1098–1100.
5. Hananouchi GI, Goff WB II. Cardiac lipoma: six-year follow-up with MRI characteristics, and a review of the literature. *Magn Reson Imaging* 1990;8:825–828.
6. Steger CM. Intrapericardial giant lipoma displacing the heart. *ISRN Cardiol* 2011:2011:243637.
7. Zhu SB, Zhu J, Liu Y, Wang RP. Surgical treatment of a giant symptomatic cardiac lipoma. *J Thorac Oncol* 2013;8:1341–1342.
8. Patris V, Argirious M, Lama N, Sakellaridis T, Charitos C. Trans-aortic excision of intraventricular lipoma with the assistance of arthroscopic camera. *J Thorac Dis* 2013;5:E140–E143.
9. Ismail I, Al-Khafaji K, Mutyala M, Aggarwal S, Cotter W, Hakim H, Khosia S, Arora R. Cardiac lipoma. *J Community Hosp Intern Med Perspect* 2015;5:28449.
10. Barbuto L, Ponsiglione A, Del Vecchio W, Altiero M, Rossi G, De Rosa D, Pisani A, Imbriaco M. Humongous right atrial lipoma: a correlative CT and MR case report. *Quant Imaging Med Surg* 2015;5:774–777.
11. Saikia MK, Kalita JP, Kapoor M, Phukon P, Malviya A, Padmanabhan A. Surgical resection of giant lipoma of interventricular septum presenting as RVOTO: a case report. *J Cardiovasc Dis Res* 2015;6:152–155.
12. Zhang HW, Zhong MH, Meng W, Zhang EY, Gu J, Hu J. Image section: intramuscular lipoma as an unusual cause of right ventricular outflow tract obstruction. *Echocardiography* 2016;33:328–329.
13. Barberger-Gateau P, Paquet M, Desaulniers D, Chenard J. Fibrolipoma of the mitral valve in a child: clinical and echocardiographic features. *Circulation* 1978;58:955–958.
14. Behnam R, Williams G, Gerlis L, Walker D, Scott O. Lipoma of the mitral valve and papillary muscle. *Am J Cardiol* 1983;51:1459–1460.
15. Anderson DR, Gray MR. Mitral incompetence associated with lipoma infiltrating the mitral valve. *Br Heart J* 1988;60:169–171.
16. Dollar AL, Wallace RB, Kent KM, Burkhart MW, Roberts WC. Mitral valve replacement for mitral lipoma associated with severe obesity. *Am J Cardiol* 1989;64:1405–1407.
17. Vadmal MS, Hajdu SI. Lipoma of the mitral valve in a child. *Ann Clin Lab Sci* 1998;28:242–245.
18. Harth M, Ruemmele P, Knuechel-Clarke R, Elsner D, Riegger G. Sclerosed lipoma of the mitral valve. *J Heart Valve Dis* 2003;12(6):722–725.

Papillary fibroelastoma in the left atrium

Charles S. Roberts, MD[a], Melissa M. Carry, MD[b], James W. Choi, MD[b], Paul A. Grayburn, MD[b,c], and William C. Roberts, MD[b,c]

[a]Department of Cardiac Surgery, Baylor University Medical Center, Dallas, Texas; [b]Division of Cardiology, Department of Internal Medicine, Baylor University Medical Center, Dallas, Texas; [c]Baylor Scott & White Heart and Vascular Institute, Baylor University Medical Center, Dallas, Texas

ABSTRACT
Described herein is a 71-year-old woman with previous angina pectoris who suddenly developed slurred speech and right-arm weakness. She was found to have significant coronary narrowing, a small mass in the left atrium attached to the endocardium near the orifice of the appendage, and multifocal punctate cerebral lesions in the distribution of the left middle cerebral artery. The left atrial mass was excised and confirmed to be a papillary fibroelastoma. Coronary bypass was also performed. It is believed that fibrin thrombus developed within the fronds of the fibroelastoma and embolized to the brain. Such lesions in the left atrium are exceedingly uncommon. She had no further emboli events.

KEYWORDS Angina pectoris; papillary fibroelastoma

Papillary fibroelastomas are commonly seen in the heart.[1] Most often they involve one or both left-sided cardiac valves, occasionally the tricuspid valve, and less frequently the mural endocardium of the left ventricle. Their occurrence on the left atrial mural endocardium is exceedingly rare. Such was the case, however, in the patient described herein.

CASE DESCRIPTION

A 71-year-old white woman, who was born in February 1947, was healthy until age 66 (February 2014) when she suddenly developed substernal chest pain that radiated to her left arm and prompted cardiac catheterization that disclosed narrowing (diameter reduction) of the coronary arteries as follows: left main 10%; left anterior descending 40%; left circumflex 10%; and right (proximally) 99%. A drug-eluting stent was inserted into the right coronary artery with relief of the stenosis. At the time, the left ventricular function was normal, and the four cardiac chambers were of normal size. Her total cholesterol was 130 mg/dL and low-density lipoprotein cholesterol was 47 mg/dL (on rosuvastatin).

Thereafter, she was well until age 71 (March 2018) when at home she suddenly developed slurred speech and right-arm weakness. By the time she arrived at the hospital within an hour, both speech and weakness had improved. Magnetic resonance imaging disclosed multifocal punctate acute infarcts in the cerebrum in the distribution of the left middle cerebral artery with a pattern suggestive of embolism. The electrocardiogram and troponin I level were normal. Her body mass index was 32 kg/m^2. Echocardiogram disclosed a small mass attached to the mural endocardium near the ostium of the left atrial appendage *(Figure 1)*. Erythrocyte sedimentation rate was 78 mm/h, hematocrit 38%, and C-reactive protein 14.3 mg/dL. Repeat coronary angiogram showed the following degrees of narrowing (diameter reduction): left main 10%; left anterior descending 70%; left circumflex 10%; left obtuse marginal 80%; and right 10%. The left ventricular size and wall motion were normal. The ejection fraction was 60%.

In June 2018, the left atrial mass (1.2×0.7 cm) was excised *(Figure 2)*, along with the underlying endocardium to which it was attached. A left internal mammary artery was anastomosed to the left anterior descending, and a saphenous venous conduit was anastomosed to the first obtuse marginal

Corresponding author: Charles S. Roberts, MD, Department of Cardiac and Thoracic Surgery, Baylor University Medical Center, 3900 Junius, Suite 415, Dallas, TX 75246 (e-mail: Charles.Roberts@BSWHealth.org)
Color versions of one or more of the figures in the article can be found online at www.tandfonline.com/ubmc.
Received November 15, 2018; Accepted November 19, 2018.

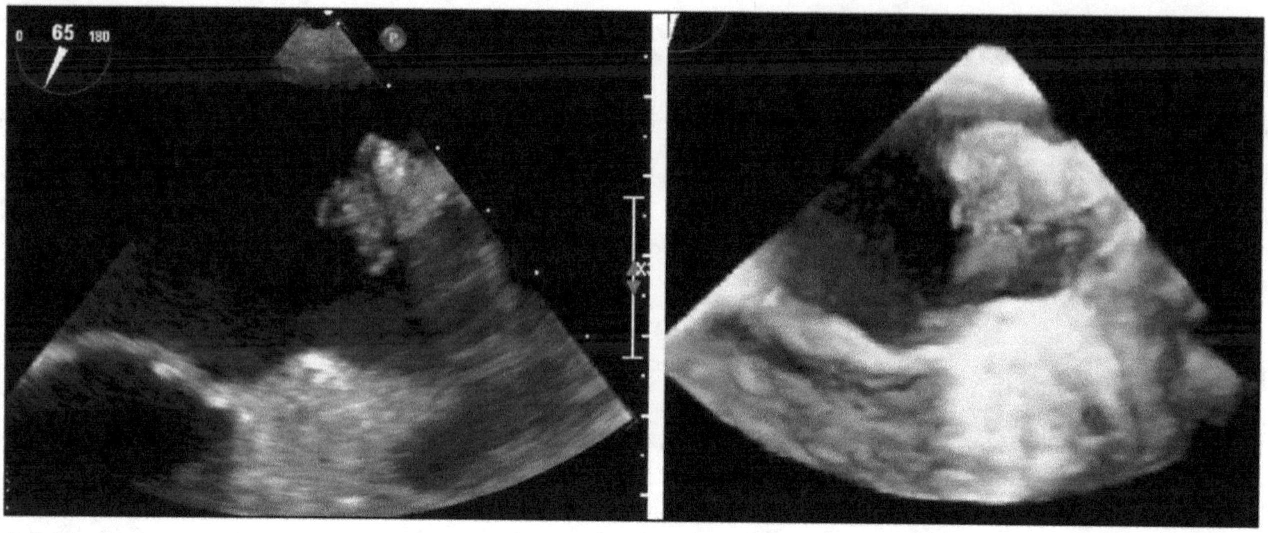

Figure 1. Echocardiogram.

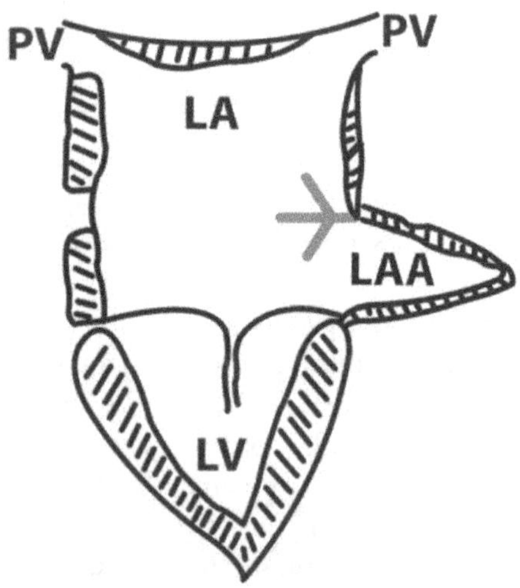

Figure 2. Diagram showing the location of the left atrial fibroelastoma.

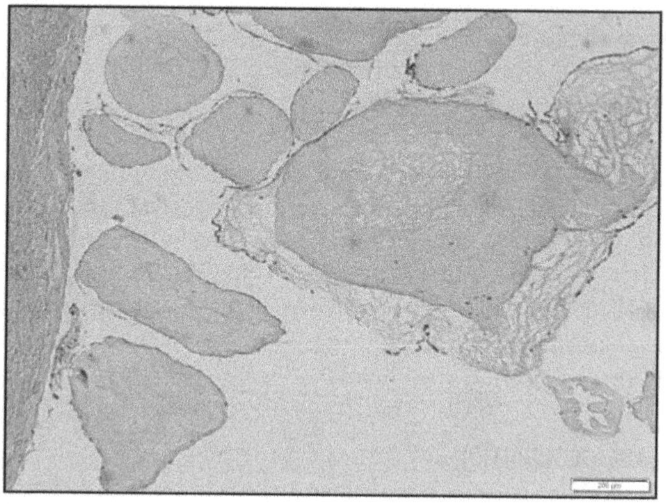

Figure 3. Photomicrograph of the left atrial mass showing the typical fronds. Hematoxylin/eosin stain, ×100.

coronary artery. The left atrial mass was a typical papillary fibroelastoma *(Figure 3)*. In October 2018 (4 months post-operative), the patient was asymptomatic.

DISCUSSION

Papillary fibroelastoma in the left atrium is rare. Gowda et al[2] reviewed 611 previously reported cases of papillary fibroelastoma in which the location of the tumor was described: 84% were located on one or more valvular cusps and 16% had a nonvalvular location. Of the latter, 12 (2%) overall were in the left atrial wall. Anastacio et al[3] described 23 patients with cardiac papillary fibroma. None occurred in the left atrium. The most common clinical consequence of a left-sided papillary fibroelastoma is transient ischemic attack or stroke, as occurred in the patient described who also had concomitant coronary bypass.

1. Roberts WC. Papillary fibroelastomas of the heart. *Am J Cardiol.* 1997;80(7):973–975.
2. Gowda RM, Khan I, Nair CK, Mehta NJ, Vasavada BC, Sacchi TJ. Cardiac papillary fibroelastoma: a comprehensive analysis of 725 cases. *Am Heart J.* 2003;146(3):404–410. doi:10.1016/S0002-8703(03)00249-7.
3. Anastacio MM, Moon MR, Damiano RJ Jr, Pasque MK, Maniar HS, Lawton JS. Surgical experience with cardiac papillary fibroelastoma over a 15-year period. *Ann Thorac Surg.* 2012;94(2):537–541. doi: 10.1016/j.athoracsur.2012.04.006.

www.ingramcontent.com/pod-product-compliance
Lightning Source LLC
LaVergne TN
LVHW062138200926
848484LV00007B/1829
9798888621547